MENTAL HEALTH–PSYCHIATRIC NURSING

A Holistic Life-Cycle Approach

MENTAL HEALTH–
PSYCHIATRIC NURSING

A Holistic Life-Cycle Approach

Second Edition

Cornelia Kelly Beck, R.N., Ph.D.

Professor, College of Nursing
Assistant Professor, Department of Psychiatry and Behavioral Sciences
College of Medicine
University of Arkansas for Medical Sciences
Little Rock, Arkansas

Ruth Parmelee Rawlins, R.N., M.S.E., C.S.

Doctoral Student
University of Alabama at Birmingham
Birmingham, Alabama
Assistant Professor, College of Nursing
University of Arkansas for Medical Sciences
Little Rock, Arkansas

Sophronia R. Williams, R.N., M.S.N.

Associate Professor, College of Nursing
University of Arkansas for Medical Sciences
Little Rock, Arkansas

Illustrated

THE C. V. MOSBY COMPANY

ST. LOUIS • WASHINGTON, D.C. • TORONTO • 1988

A TRADITION OF PUBLISHING EXCELLENCE

Editor　Linda L. Duncan
Assistant editor　Joanna May
Project manager　Suzanne Seeley
Design　John R. Rokusek
Production/editing　Teresa Breckwoldt, Kathy Burmann,
　　　　　　　　　Jeanne Genz, Sheila Jones, April Nauman,
　　　　　　　　　Timothy O'Brien, Jan Shelly

Second Edition

The C. V. Mosby Company
11830 Westline Industrial Drive, St. Louis, Missouri 63146

Library of Congress Cataloging-in-Publication Data

Mental health-psychiatric nursing.

　　Bibliography: p.
　　Includes index.
　　1. Psychiatric nursing.　I. Beck, Cornelia Kelly.
II.　Rawlins, Ruth Parmelee.　III. Williams, Sophronia R.
RC440.M355　1988　　　610.73'68　　　87-24815
ISBN 0-8016-0558-X

C/C/VH　9　8　7　6　5　4　3　2　1　01/A/086

To my husband, Barry, for his constant caring
To my children, Jason and Monica, for their understanding
To my parents, family, and friends
for their inspiration and support

Cornelia Kelly Beck

To my parents, from whom I learned perseverance
To my husband and daughters, for their patience and support
To all who love the challenges
of mental health–psychiatric nursing

Ruth Parmelee Rawlins

To my mother, my constant support
To the memory of my father

Sophronia R. Williams

CONTRIBUTORS

Ann Adams, R.N., M.N.Sc.
Veteran's Administration Hospital
Little Rock, Arkansas

Donna C. Aguilera, Ph.D., F.A.A.N.
Private Practice
Beverly Hills, California

Ellen A. Andruzzi, R.N., M.S.N.E., F.A.A.N.
Private Practice
Camp Springs, Maryland;
Member, Board of Directors
National Mental Health Association

Rose Therese Bahr, R.N., Ph.D., F.A.A.N.
Professor of Nursing and Associate Director
Gerontological Center
The Catholic University of America
Washington, D.C.

Bertram Bandman, Ph.D.
Professor of Philosophy
Brooklyn Center of Long Island University
Brooklyn, New York

Elsie L. Bandman, R.N., Ed.D., F.A.A.N.
Professor, Hunter-Bellevue School of Nursing
Hunter College of the City University of New York
New York, New York

Margaret T. Beard, R.N., Ph.D.
Professor, Texas Woman's University
Denton, Texas

Cornelia Kelly Beck, R.N., Ph.D.
Professor, College of Nursing
Assistant Professor
Department of Psychiatry and Behavioral Sciences
College of Medicine
University of Arkansas for Medical Sciences
Little Rock, Arkansas

Virginia Trotter Betts, M.S.N., J.D., R.N.
Professor, Department of Mental Health and
Organizational Behavior
Vanderbilt University School of Nursing
Nashville, Tennessee

E. Hope Bevis, R.N., M.S.N.
Private Practice
Denver, Colorado

Gloria Birkholz, R.N., J.D.
Private Practice
Assistant Professor, University of New Mexico
Albuquerque, New Mexico

Louise Truex Bradford, R.N., Ed.D.
Associate Professor, Harding University
Searcy, Arkansas

Charlene Uthoff Bradham, R.N., M.N.Sc.
Associate Professor
University of Arkansas at Little Rock
Little Rock, Arkansas

Lynne Brooks, Ph.D., R.N., C.N.A.
Chairperson and Associate Professor, Community Mental
Health
College of Nursing, University of South Alabama, Mobile,
Alabama;
Clinical Specialist in Psychiatry, Doctor's Hospital Affiliate
of Hospital Corporation of America
Mobile, Alabama

Elizabeth B. Brophy, R.N., Ph.D.
Assistant Professor, College of Nursing
Loyola University of Chicago
Chicago, Illinois

Mary Flo Bruce, R.N., Ph.D.
Day Treatment Center
Veterans' Administration Medical Center
Salt Lake City, Utah

Marilyn M. Bunt, R.N., Ph.D.
Dean and Professor, College of Nursing
Lewis University
Romeoville, Illinois

Sharon Elizabeth Byers, R.N., M.S.N., C.S.
Clinical Nurse Specialist
Hennepin County Mental Health Center
Minneapolis, Minnesota

Margery Chisholm, R.N., M.S., Ed.D.
Associate Professor and Associate Dean for Graduate
  Affairs
Boston University School of Nursing
Boston, Massachusetts;
Diplomate, American Board of Family Psychology;
Fellow, Orthopsychiatric Association

Bonnie Clayton, R.N., Ph.D.
Associate Professor, Graduate Program
College of Nursing, University of Utah
Salt Lake City, Utah

Patricia Ann Clunn, Ed.D., A.R.N.P., C.S.
Professor, University of Miami School of Nursing
Miami, Florida

Virginia Koch Drake, D.N.Sc., R.N., C.S.
Senior Clinician, Affiliate Medical Staff
San Antonio Children's Center;
Consultant, HCA Psychiatric Hospital;
Co-owner, Victim Assistance Network;
Private Practitioner
San Antonio, Texas

Janice Dyehouse, R.N., M.S.N.
Assistant Professor
College of Nursing and Health
University of Cincinnati
Cincinnati, Ohio

Nancy Kowal Ellis, M.S., R.N.
Practitioner/Teacher
Department of Psychiatric Nursing
Rush University and Rush-Presbyterian-St. Luke's Medical
  Center
Chicago, Illinois

Rauda Salkauskas Gelazis, R.N., M.N.Ed.
Assistant Professor, Ursuline College
Pepper Pike, Ohio;
Doctoral Student
Wayne State University
Detroit, Michigan

Carol R. Hartman, R.N., D.N.Sc., C.S.
Coordinator, Graduate Psychiatric–Mental Health Nursing
  Program
Boston College School of Nursing
Chestnut Hill, Massachusetts

Nancy Hedlund, R.N., Ph.D.
Coordinator of Nursing Research and Quality Assurance
The Queens Medical Center
Honolulu, Hawaii

Diane M. Helder, R.N., M.S.
Mental Health Clinical Specialist
Supervisor, Mercy Hospital and Medical Center
Chicago, Illinois

Sharon Holmberg, R.N., M.S.N.
Assistant Professor, Yale University
Clinical Nurse Specialist, Connecticut Mental Health
  Center
New Haven, Connecticut

Ann Hutton, R.N., M.S.
Assistant Professor, Psychosocial Nursing
College of Nursing, University of Utah
Salt Lake City, Utah

Finis Breckenridge Jeffrey
Honolulu, Hawaii

Margie N. Johnson, R.N., Ph.D.
Professor, Psychiatric–Mental Health Graduate Program
Texas Woman's University
Denton, Texas

Virginia Burke Karb, R.N., M.S.N.
Assistant Professor
University of North Carolina at Greensboro
Greensboro, North Carolina

Alice Kempe, R.N., M.Ed., M.S.N.
Assistant Professor, Ursuline College
Pepper Pike, Ohio

Sydney D. Krampitz, R.N., Ph.D.
Professor, Department of Psychiatric-Mental Nursing
Associate Dean and Director of Graduate Programs
School of Nursing, University of Kansas
Kansas City, Kansas

Becky Lancaster, R.N., M.S.N.
Instructor, University of Central Arkansas
Conway, Arkansas

Jeanette Lancaster, R.N., Ph.D., F.A.A.N.
Dean and Professor
Wright State University–Miami Valley
School of Nursing
Dayton, Ohio

Peggy A. Landrum, Ph.D., R.N.
Nurse Counselor
Texas Woman's University
Denton, Texas;
Private Practice, Mental Health Consultant
Houston, Texas

Judith R. Lentz, R.N., M.S.N.
Director of Clinical Services
Westheimer Day Hospital
Houston, Texas

Joyce S. Levy, R.N., M.S., C.S.
Psychiatric Liaison Nurse
The Cambridge Hospital, Cambridge, Massachusetts;
Lecturer on Psychiatry, Harvard Medical School
Boston, Massachusetts

Anita Lewis, R.N., M.S., C.S.
Psychiatric Liaison Nurse, Department of Nursing
Associate Director, Psychiatric Consultation/Liaison
   Service
Department of Psychiatry
New England Medical Center Hospitals, Inc.
Boston, Massachusetts

Eva Hester Lin, R.N., M.S.
Nurse Therapist
Montgomery County Health Department
Rockville, Maryland

Sonja H. Lively, R.N., M.S.
Assistant Professor
College of Nursing, University of Iowa
Iowa City, Iowa

Elizabeth Maloney, R.N., Ed.D
Associate Professor
Department of Nursing Education
Teachers College
Columbia University
New York, New York

Elizabeth Jane Martin, Ph.D., C.R.N.P., C.N.S.
Professor and Associate Dean
Graduate Academic Affairs and Director
Doctoral Program, University of Pittsburgh
Pittsburgh, Pennsylvania;
Board of Directors, American Holistic Nurses Association;
Editor, Journal of Holistic Nursing

Jackie Coombe Moore, R.N., M.N.Sc.
Assistant Professor
College of Nursing
University of Arkansas for Medical Sciences
Little Rock, Arkansas

Malinda Garner Pappas, R.N., M.N.Sc.
Clinical Nurse Specialist
John L. McClellan Memorial Veterans Hospital
Little Rock, Arkansas

Ruth P. Rawlins, R.N., M.S.E., C.S.
Doctoral Student, University of Alabama at Birmingham
Birmingham, Alabama;
Assistant Professor, College of Nursing
University of Arkansas for Medical Sciences
Little Rock, Arkansas

Martha Rhea, R.N., M.S.N.
Doctoral Student
School of Nursing
University of Utah
Salt Lake City, Utah

Linda Hannawalt Rickel, R.N., M.N.Sc.
Assistant Professor, College of Nursing
University of Arkansas at Pine Bluff
Pine Bluff, Arkansas

Michael Roark, Pharm. D.
Associate Director of Pharmacy Services
The Owen Company;
Maryland General Hospital
Baltimore, Maryland

Ethel Rosenfeld, R.N., M.S.E., C.S.
Associate Professor
University of Central Arkansas
Conway, Arkansas

Mary Patricia Ryan, R.N., Ph.D.
Associate Professor
Loyola University of Chicago
Chicago, Illinois

Judith A. Saifnia, R.N., M.N.Sc.
Psychiatric Clinical Nurse Specialist
Biofeedback Coordinator
St. Vincent's Infirmary
Little Rock, Arkansas

Rae Sedgwick, R.N., Ph.D., C.S.
Clinical Psychologist
Private Practice, Bonner Springs, Kansas;
Clinical and Consulting Staff, Bethany Medical Center
Kansas City, Kansas;
St. John Hospital and Cushing Memorial Hospital
Leavenworth, Kansas

Judith Eberle Seidenschnur, R.N., M.S.N. C.S.
Hospital Systems Review Coordinator
John L. McClellan Memorial Veterans Hospital
Little Rock, Arkansas

Carolyn Shannon, R.N., M.N.Sc.
Private Practice, Psychiatric–Mental Health
Little Rock, Arkansas;
Executive Director
Arkansas State Nurses' Association
Little Rock, Arkansas

Anne H. Shealy, R.N., M.S., C.S.
Assistant Professor, School of Nursing
University of Alabama
Birmingham, Alabama

Cathleen Shultz, R.N., Ed.D.
Dean, School of Nursing, Harding University
Searcy, Arkansas

Richard E. Stull, Ph.D.
Associate Professor of Pharmacology
College of Pharmacy
University of Arkansas for Medical Sciences
Little Rock, Arkansas

Sharon L. Thomas, R.N., M.A.
Marriage and Family Counselor
Englewood, Colorado

Toni Tripp-Reimer, R.N., Ph.D.
Professor, Director, Office of Research
College of Nursing, University of Iowa
Iowa City, Iowa

Patricia Wahl, R.N., Ph.D.
Assistant Dean, Graduate Program
College of Nursing and Health
University of Cincinnati
Cincinatti, Ohio

Barbara G. Williams, R.N., Ph.D.
Associate Professor, University of Central Arkansas
Conway, Arkansas

Sophronia R. Williams, R.N., M.S.N.
Associate Professor, College of Nursing
University of Arkansas for Medical Sciences
Little Rock, Arkansas

FOREWORD

Textbooks for nurses ought to enable students and practitioners to enlarge their current knowledge and to enrich their practice. At their best, such books present content that intermeshes contemporary and emerging perspectives related to nursing practice. The authors of this work have taken these responsibilities seriously.

This book describes accepted contemporary practices in mental health–psychiatric nursing, including various forms of psychotherapy, milieu therapy, crisis intervention, and others. Prevailing practices for such categories of dysfunction as impaired cognition and eating disorders are also included. Phenomena such as anxiety, loneliness, guilt, and other selected nursing diagnoses are discussed theoretically and in terms of relevant nursing interventions. The authors have considered important components of the current scope of mental health–psychiatric nursing practice, which has been greatly expanded over the past half century.

The book also takes into account several new perspectives that have recently emerged and seem to be gaining currency in nursing. For example, the subtitle of the book, *A Holistic Life Cycle Approach,* constitutes the authors' philosophical position from which principles of practice were derived and are set forth. In this view, nurses should eschew fragmentation of nursing practice. Instead, nurses should seek to provide comprehensive nursing services, within an "existential-humanistic" orientation. This approach considers the wholeness and integrity of persons and their capabilities for self-care. Therefore age, culture, family, community, and other content related to the holistic perspective are presented.

Another emerging direction is the effort within the profession to evolve a nursing model that is distinctly different from the medical model of practice. The significant difference lies in the phenomena to which the practices of each profession are addressed in this nursing textbook, psychiatric-medical diagnostic categories of the diseases called mental illness are *not* used. Instead, a broad range of psychosocial phenomena and human dysfunctions as observed by nurses in nursing situations are presented. Psychiatry, on the other hand, seems to be moving toward more biologically oriented practices, more in keeping with the traditional focus of physicians on pathophysiology. There is, of course, an area in which the practices of nurses intersect those of physicians, in psychiatric services. This textbook has taken this matter into account by discussions of somatic and pharmaceutical prescriptions and by description of the biological orientation of psychiatry.

A fairly recent development is the matter of accountability of professionals for the consequences of their services to people. This book considers accountability in several ways. First, nursing practice requires that nurses have adequate data about clients—their situation, the resources available to them, and so forth. Nurses obtain this vital information by using observation, the nursing process, various forms of assessment, and theory application. These topics are presented in separate chapters and in assessment sections in other parts of the book. Second, accountability is also considered in terms of quality assurance, ethics, legal matters, and the like.

This work is quite comprehensive, reflecting the expanded scope of mental health–psychiatric nursing today. The wide range of subject matter also reflects the authors' intent to present a blend of time-tested practices and new directions in the field of nursing. This text is another step forward in the effort to elucidate the nature of nursing. It has the particular merit of being in tune with several powerful contemporary trends in the field of mental health–psychiatric services for the people.

Hildegard E. Peplau, Ed.D., F.A.A.N
Professor Emerita, Rutgers

PREFACE

The intent of *Mental Health–Psychiatric Nursing: A Holistic Life-Cycle Approach* is to to provide a basic, comprehensive nursing text for the beginning student in mental health–psychiatric nursing. Since the basic concepts are defined behaviorally, this text is appropriate for use in either an integrated or a nonintegrated curriculum. The textbook will be most meaningful for students who have a general knowledge base in anatomy, physiology, psychology, sociology, and chemistry. In addition, an understanding of the nursing process and the relationship of a philosophy and conceptual framework to nursing practice will enhance the reader's use of the text. Chapters about issues, current treatment modalities, and mental health–psychiatric nursing across the life cycle may be of special interest to graduate students in nursing and to practicing mental health–psychiatric nurses.

In the first edition of *Mental Health–Psychiatric Nursing* our intent was to integrate content essential to the practice of mental health–psychiatric nursing into a holistic approach that addressed the five dimensions of the person as an organizing framework for the nursing process. For example, in the discussion of the person's physical dimension, the biological basis of behavior and the physiological manifestations of psychological processes were examined. In the discussion of the social dimension, the ethnic diversity of clients is addressed and the individual, family, and community were considered from an ecological perspective. The individual's self-responsibility in maintaining and promoting his health as well as participating in the restoration of his mental health was also a highlight of the text.

The second edition of our text is based on this same philosophy about nursing and the individual. The holistic philosophy is strengthened by emphasizing the discussion of holism and addressing the major ideas related to this concept. Nursing process continues to be the organizing framework for practice with strengthening of the implementation phase to make it more useful for the student and practitioner.

CONTENT

In the second edition we have attempted to reflect the latest research and trends in psychiatry and psychiatric nursing. Eight new chapters have been included:
Pain
Loneliness
Boredom
Manipulation
Community Mental Health Nursing
Family Therapy
Therapy with Clients with Psychophysiological Illness
Therapy with Clients with Eating Disorders
The most recent NANDA diagnoses that are pertinent to mental health–psychiatric nursing and DSM-III-R classifications are integrated throughout the text. Content on transactional analysis and the eclectic approach are added to the theoretical positions. The biological model is expanded in keeping with the current emphasis on the biological basis for psychiatric problems.

ORGANIZATION

Mental Health–Psychiatric Nursing continues to be divided into five parts. Part I is concerned with the foundations for the practice of mental health–psychiatric nursing. Included in this focus is an examination of a conceptual base for practice and selected philosophical positions about the nature of the person and the relationship of these positions to an understanding of mental health and illness. Theoretical approaches that contribute to the development of frameworks for mental health–psychiatric nursing are explored, including the work of nursing theorists. The organizing theme of Part I is a holistic approach to the individual within the five dimensions.

Part I also views the nursing process in mental health–psychiatric nursing as focusing on (1) basic communication, (2) the establishment of a therapeutic relationship, (3) the process of psychotherapy, and (4) cultural diversity in therapy. Skills and attitudes basic to this process are interwoven throughout the discussion. The five dimensions of the person are viewed as a basis for the effective use of self in developing a therapeutic relationship characterized by self-responsibility and advocacy. A detailed discussion of communication is included.

Part II focuses on the concepts that are basic to human functioning in health and illness throughout the life cycle. The concepts presented are anxiety, anger, guilt, hope-despair, flexibility-rigidity, dependence-independence, trust-mistrust, pain, loneliness, boredom, and manipulation. Each chapter begins with a discussion of the dynamics of these behaviors and the manifestations of these behaviors within the five dimensions of the individual. This second edition places more emphasis on the biological basis of these behaviors. Based on an organizing framework of the five dimensions, the steps in the nursing process are discussed with specific nursing interventions strengthened in the second edition. Each chapter includes a therapeutic interaction that exemplifies the concept and a summary of the nursing process is included in each chapter. Current research related to each concept and instruments for measuring related behaviors are included.

Presented in Part III is a description of specific treatment modalities designed for health promotion, maintenance, and restoration. Milieu, group, family, marital, and sex therapy as well as therapy with chronically distressed clients, dying clients, clients with psychophysiological illnesses, clients with eating disorders, victims of abuse, and clients with organic mental disorders are discussed. Crisis intervention and short-term psychotherapy are presented as modalities characterized by length of treatment. Psychotropic drugs, somatic therapies, and community mental health nursing are also presented. In addition, alternative forms of therapy, such as Feldenkrais and transcendental meditation, are included.

In Part IV, concepts and principles of mental health–psychiatric nursing are applied to the care of clients across the life cycle. The various periods of life discussed are infancy, childhood, adolescence, and young, middle, and aged adult years. For each life period, content essential to using the nursing process is presented. In addition, specific nursing interventions for mental health–psychiatric nursing are discussed for each stage of life. An assessment tool has been added to each life cycle chapter in the second edition.

An exploration of issues that are basic to the practice of mental health-psychiatric nursing in today's society is the focus of Part V. Value clarification and ethical principles are provided as bases for making decisions about professional practice issues. The chapter on legal issues includes a discussion of laws that have relevance for mental health–psychiatric nursing, the role of the nurse as a client advocate, and the responsibility of the nurse in effecting mental health care legislation. Issues and suggestions regarding research and various aspects of quality assurance, including credentialing, are also presented. The book concludes with a chapter on consultation-liaison nursing.

FEATURES

The manner in which content is structured is perceived as a study aid to reinforce the student's orientation to a holistic, conceptual approach to mental health–psychiatric nursing.

As in the first edition, we have begun each chapter with a list of student learning objectives. Within each chapter we have continued to highlight important concepts and information in tabular, boxed, or illustrative form, such as nursing diagnoses, DSM-III-R classifications, and psychopharmacological considerations. Many new Case Examples and Research Highlights have been included to facilitate understanding of clinical application. Sample nursing care plans for common problems are also featured.

The text is also extensively cross-referenced for easy location of selected topics. The table of contents contains a separate listing of where specific nursing diagnoses, DSM-III-R diagnoses, and discussions of personality disorders can be found in text. We have retained the glossary to familiarize students with key terms; these terms are italicized in text.

Because a thorough understanding of mental health–psychiatric nursing in its current state is facilitated by viewing its substance and issues within a historical perspective, each chapter contains a historical overview. For many chapters, we have included summaries of nursing process, presented within the holistic framework.

TERMINOLOGY AND LANGUAGE

The term *client* instead of *patient,* the traditional term in medicine, is used in this text in keeping with the current thinking that health care consumers have rights, responsibilities, and a participatory role in their care. "Patient" denotes a subservient or dependent position in relation to the caregiver and may imply that the consumer is passive, without responsibility, and subordinate to the caregiver. Use of the term client suggests a reciprocal relationship between consumer and caregiver.

We have attempted to delete evidence of sexism in the language of this textbook. However, this has not always been possible. Therefore, for clarity the client is referred to as "he" and the nurse is referred to as "she." No slight is intended to the growing numbers of men in nursing.

ACKNOWLEDGMENT

We greatly appreciate the expertise of the authors contributing chapters to this text. Without their continued efforts, a project of this magnitude would have been many years in the making. We also wish to thank the instructors, students, and clinicians who reviewed the second edition or who offered valuable comments and suggestions for the revision. Supportive friends and colleagues are too many to mention by name.

Linda Duncan, Editor, The C.V. Mosby Company, and Suzanne Seeley, Project Manager, are also gratefully acknowledged for their encouragement and support.

Cornelia Kelly Beck
Ruth Parmelee Rawlins
Sophronia R. Williams

CONTENTS

DETAILED CONTENTS

PART IV
Life-Cycle Phases

NANDA Classification of Nursing Diagnoses

DSM-III-R Classifications

Personality Disorders

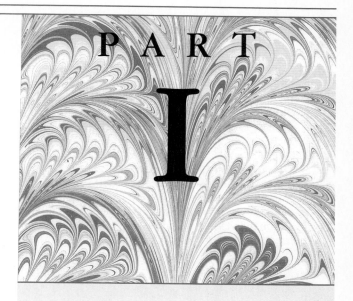

PART

I

Foundations for Practice

An important initial element in understanding the contemporary practice of mental health–psychiatric nursing is an awareness of the historical roots from which psychiatric nursing has emerged. Thus the text begins with an overview of the history of mental health–psychiatric nursing in Chapter 1. Both societal trends and changes in health care delivery are viewed as having an impact on the development of mental health–psychiatric nursing.

Just as contemporary practice has a basis in societal beliefs about mental health and illness, each nurse's beliefs direct her enactment of this practice. Major philosophical positions are discussed in Chapter 2, and holism is presented as the philosophical base for the ideas and approaches developed in this text.

Arising from various philosophical positions are the many theoretical approaches that form the basis for practice. Chapter 3 is an exposition of a variety of approaches from which nurses may choose.

Chapter 4, "Nursing Theorists' Approaches," describes the attempts of theorists in nursing to explain the phenomenon of nursing practice. The concepts and relationships that have emerged from these attempts are applied to the holistic approach to mental health–psychiatric nursing practice.

The next four chapters focus on the processes, attitudes, and skills that are basic to the practice of mental health–psychiatric nursing. Chapter 5 presents an examination of basic communication with emphasis on factors that facilitate or impede the development of therapeutic communication. Issues in therapeutic communication and methods for effecting behavior change through communication are also discussed. Chapter 6 addresses the development of a therapeutic relationship with clients. Application of the nursing process within the therapeutic relationship is presented as the process of psychotherapy in Chapter 7. Application of the nursing process to mental health psychiatric nursing is discussed in Chapter 8.

The next two chapters in Part I form an important core for this text because they provide the mental health–psychiatric nurse with a philosophical and behavioral approach to the individual. Chapter 9 represents the foundation for the holistic approach to the client, which is developed throughout the text. The way in which the process of psychotherapy differs among various cultures is the focus of Chapter 10.

With a sense of the past and a set of beliefs about the individual and mental health and mental illness, nurses are prepared to select theories from other disciplines as well as nursing theories to guide their practice with individuals, families, and communities.

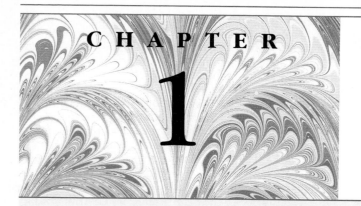

CHAPTER 1

HISTORICAL DEVELOPMENT

Nancy Hedlund   Finis Breckenridge Jeffery

After studying this chapter the learner will be able to:

Describe major trends in the development of treatment methods for mental illness.

Define and discuss the processes by which mental health–psychiatric nursing developed in the United States.

State the specific importance of the National Mental Health Act of 1946 and the Community Mental Health Centers Act of 1963 in moving mental health–psychiatric nursing into the community.

Describe the present and future challenges for mental health–psychiatric nursing.

Society has long had to deal with the actions of those considered deviant or crazy. Throughout most of history, relatives or friends cared for the mentally ill. Those without such support survived as best they could or were removed forcibly from society through banishment or execution. The treatment of unproductive members has been an unaffordable luxury for most societies. Some societies, such as certain American Indian tribes, have held the insane in high regard and have treated them as prophets or oracles. Other societies that could afford to be tolerant have permitted the insane the freedom to move about with little restraint. Only in recent decades have methods of treatment been developed that could be applied to a significantly large segment of the population.

The concept of people caring for the sick is an old one, but the specific role of nurses and nursing is relatively recent. As an organized profession, nursing originated in the middle-nineteenth century with the work of Florence Nightingale; however, nursing of the sick and wounded developed apart from care of the mentally ill, and practitioners of psychiatric nursing considered themselves distinct in training from their general hospital counterparts until well into the twentieth century. This distinction was removed when the nursing profession agreed that its members should receive one standard education, which occurred some years ahead of the development of advanced specialties.

Mental health–psychiatric nursing is a relatively recent development in the care of the mentally ill and exists primarily in the United States. Practitioners in this field are the beneficiaries of events in the separate disciplines of philosophy, psychology, psychiatry, and nursing, as well as the interdisciplinary interactions that have taken place over time. The practice of psychiatric nursing did not grow in a vacuum; concepts of philosophy and psychiatry were combined with the concepts of caring in nursing to produce the field as it is understood today. Originally, psychiatric nursing care consisted of little more than physical restraint. Only as more sophisticated approaches developed and the public demanded better treatment did nurses develop therapeutic systems of care. The complexity of the various kinds of treatment encouraged nurses to continue their education. The result is the relatively high percentage of psychiatric nurses who have advanced degrees and the substantial share of such degrees among the nursing profession in general. Although they have constituted only a relatively small percentage of all nurses, during the 1970s psychiatric nurses accounted for 30% of the doctorate degrees held among nurses as a whole.

Psychiatric nursing in the United States is unique in comparison to the field in other countries. Outside of Europe, psychiatry as a profession is little known; thus the low number of psychiatric nurses is not surprising. Even in Europe nurses play little role in treatment. In Western

Europe they still act in subordinate positions relative to that of the physician. One can only speculate about the activities they may be permitted to perform in the Soviet Union, given its use of psychiatric hospitals to control political dissidents.[6]

ORIGINS OF PSYCHIATRY
From Primitive Times to 500 AD

Psychology is defined as the study of the mind. As people began to contemplate what made them think, they realized that they could suffer from diseases of the mind as well as of the body, and psychiatry became the branch of medicine that specialized in such diseases. *Philosophy* is the term used to describe the search for understanding, by logical reasoning, about the basic truths and principles of the universe, of life, of morals, and of human perception; for example, Who are we? Where do we come from?

Restricting this philosophical search to the subject of mental illness, one can identify three trends[1]:

1. The organic approach, explaining diseases of the mind in physical terms
2. Cerebral explanations for mental disturbances
3. Use of magic to deal with inexplicable events

Early humans and their primitive descendants reacted to mental illness according to five different beliefs[12]:

1. The individual's soul had somehow fled the body; cure consisted of convincing the wandering soul to return.
2. A foreign body with magical powers had entered the body; cure required that it be extracted and neutralized.
3. Evil spirits had entered the body; these had to be exorcised before the victim could have relief.
4. An individual had somehow infringed on a taboo; this demanded ritualistic purification.
5. The individual had sinned, as in the Hebraic tradition and that of others attributing the affliction to sin; in which case the sin might or might not be expiated.

Early people confronted irrational behavior with fantastic or unreasonable responses; that is, whether the disease was physical or mental, and whether or not some form of actual treatment was involved, the effectiveness of healing was attributed to magic. This form of primitive medicine or primitive psychiatry was thought to effect a cure if the patient accepted and believed in the treatment. Ellenberger[12] identifies five key elements in the success of this kind of healing:

1. The healer occupied a central role in society.
2. Confidence was in the healer, not the medication.
3. Healers were invariably skilled and learned people, as defined by the particular culture.
4. Psychological methods of healing were most important.
5. The healing was almost always a public affair.

Jaynes[22] provides a fascinating explanation for this early approach to healing. He says that people originally were under the influence of the right or nonverbal side of the brain. They responded to what he calls the "inner voices" from the brain that in time came to be attributed to gods or superhuman forces; Jaynes argues, however, that many centuries ago the left side of the brain became dominant, and the perceived healing potential of these inner voices lost prominence as a method of care.

The correctness of Jaynes's ideas is still open to debate. For example, evidence also supports the theory that 2,500 years ago certain imaginative individuals developed concepts that laid the foundation for modern thought. These concepts included the idea that physical and mental afflictions can rationally be explained through cause and effect. Individual effort was also believed to play a role in cure. This "psychology without demons" developed over a long period and is one of the many significant contributions by the Greeks to Western culture.[1]

A study of the constructive development of ideas and culture of classical Europe offers an interesting contrast to a background of seemingly destructive and ruthless conquest. The Greek aristocracy, whether viewed as democratic or dictatorial, lacked concern for the fate of lower classes. Treatment and care of the mentally ill followed a similar line: afflicted members of the upper classes were cared for, but the less fortunate received little or no care.

Descriptions of the kinds of care practiced by the Greeks do not give credit to the philosophical concepts they developed. They believed humans were not subject to impersonal forces or demons that must be placated by symbolic offerings or rituals. Instead, people possessed within themselves the knowledge of their ills and the appropriate cure for them. Disputes would center on ways people could understand the universe, not on solving supernatural mysteries.

The Roman Empire followed a similar pattern, producing a remarkable legacy of ideas and culture. Its success can be traced to an emphasis on the virtues that produced victory in war and tight control of citizens in peace. Contemporary concern about the abundant human suffering this produced must be balanced with an appreciation of its obvious contributions to human achievement. The emphasis on military virtues was reflected in ideas about dealing with mentally ill people. The majority of the mentally ill were probably eliminated in some way as an unnecessary disturbance to the public order. Individuals who came from wealthy families were probably confined and treated in a kindly manner. Persons whose illness appeared "magical" were seen either as oracles or healers; they were often honored for their special view of reality.

Different approaches to the care of the mentally ill appear throughout the Middle East and Asia. The records are scant, but the majority of the mentally ill were probably removed as economic liabilities or hidden by their families. In some of these societies, such people were considered empowered with special gifts and protected as sources of power; they occupied important positions in society for religious and political purposes.

The Middle Ages

After the fall of the Roman Empire in 476 AD, concern for the less fortunate members of society tended to become the responsibility of the religious orders of the Roman Catholic church; it was not unusual, however, for lay workers to provide care in places where the church did not.

Saint Benedict of Nursia (480-543 AD) laid the foundations of monastic medicine.[1] Small centers staffed by members of religious orders offered sanctuary and care to the sick. The Greek tradition of rational medicine declined during the Middle Ages but was preserved to some extent in monastic libraries and even more so by the Arabs. These monastic orders accepted as their communal responsibility the task of ministering to the ill. They provided what physical comfort they could and put their trust in simple medicine and divine intervention to effect a cure.

At the beginning of the Middle Ages the mentally ill were treated not as outcasts but as persons to be helped. A few places, such as Gheel in Belgium, became famous for their care of psychotic individuals. This tolerance seems to have lasted until the fourteenth century, when a wave of general unrest swept through Europe. The insane were persecuted as witches. They would not again receive humane care on a consistent basis until the nineteenth century.[1]

Saint Augustine was one of the great figures of the early Middle Ages. Although not directly involved with care, he developed through his *Confessions* ideas about introspection and self-awareness that would provide a model for later developments in psychotherapy. As a Christian he believed that God acted directly in human affairs but that persons were responsible for their own actions. God was a necessary participant in the struggle with evil but was not viewed as acting alone.[1]

In the East the Byzantine Empire, until it fell in 1453, ruled half of the original Roman Empire. Perhaps its most important contribution was the preservation of Greek culture and medicine until the Renaissance.

Beginning in the seventh century the Byzantines faced the growing power of the Arab world, unified under the banner of Islam. The Arabs considered their mentally ill to be somehow divinely inspired and treated them with great kindness. A number of their philosophers also continued the Greek tradition of rational investigation, some of it dealing with irrational or disturbed actions.[24]

Throughout the Middle Ages, the insane received care ranging from good to poor. Despite a harsh environment, concern for their well-being persisted in their communities and families. This response would, in time, be replaced by the conviction that unacceptable behavior could be cured through the powers of the intellect. This belief in reason became the foundation of modern theories of mental health and treatment.

The Renaissance in Europe

In fifteenth-century Europe a spirit arose that would lead to increasing secularization and a weakening of the influence of religion on intellectual life and moral conduct. This spirit has been described as the Renaissance and included both the rediscovery of Greek and Roman culture and a frank and questioning attitude toward life. The religious Reformation accompanied the Renaissance and represented a powerful demand for fundamental change in the religious and political activities of the Roman Catholic church. As a result, the rational approach to the study of people and their place in the universe was resurrected, emphasizing the presence of internal and logical forces acting on the person in an orderly and predictable manner. This view forced individuals to consider themselves responsible for their own actions, not victims of dark and demonic forces. A consequence of this view was the idea that nonrational individuals are affected by factors that can be alleviated or cured by rational methods. Rather than appealing for divine intervention, the healer could use human methods.[16]

The transition to a more rational view of mental illness was not an instantaneous one. For the most part the mentally ill were still considered to be afflicted by evil spirits. They were often neglected and were even confined, beaten, and starved. Therefore the new spirit of rational treatment was paradoxically accompanied by a violent reaction by some people against the insane.[1] The decline in the authority of the Church was accompanied by attributions of increased power to the devil in the form of witches and sorcerers. Fear of those not viewed as normal resulted in such methods of control as burning at the stake for those accused of witchcraft, driving the insane outside the city walls, or paying sailors to carry them away on the "Ship of Fools," an image that remains in our collective consciousness.

Views of traditional European care for the mentally ill have probably been negatively influenced by highly publicized scenes of London's Hospital of Saint Mary of Bethlehem, which was popularly named "bedlam." Although these descriptions paint a dark picture, they actually occurred well after the significant reforms of the nineteenth century. In general, European society probably dealt with its sick much more humanely than these popular images suggest.

The American Experience

As an extension of the European experience, responses to the mentally ill in the United States reflected many of the same attitudes and treatments. The New World demanded a great deal of its inhabitants, and few resources remained for what might be considered humane care for the mentally ill. During the Colonial period the insane were left in the care of their families, who were judged the ones most responsible and most able to perform this task. Local government demonstrated no social obligation to erect special buildings to meet an unperceived need. The few eighteenth century institutions for the mentally ill were clearly places of last resort, designed for the custody of those with no family or friends.

Yet the picture is again replete with contrasts and so is probably not as grim as suggested. Even the famous example of American barbarity, the Salem witchcraft trials involving some mentally ill defendants, has been shown to be an aberration. With this one exception, the execution

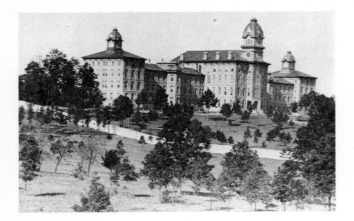

FIGURE 1-1 This photograph of the Arkansas Lunatic Asylum was taken in 1883 by L.W. Banks. (Courtesy of the Heiskell Library Collection at the Arkansas *Gazette*.)

of witches was a rare occurrence in American history.[10]

In the Jacksonian era (after 1820), Americans began to erect asylums for the insane at an increased rate.[35] (See Figure 1-1.) Although some might argue that this reflected a growing awareness of the problem and a more humane approach to its solution, it was more likely an attempt to promote the stability of a society at a time when the traditional ideas and practices of the new republic appeared outmoded, constricted, and ineffective. Before 1820 the insane had been judged an expected part of life and an unfortunate problem to be taken care of within the family. The new society of the Jacksonian era saw this deviant behavior as a reflection of the faulty organization of the community that required correction by the introduction of organized methods of care and treatment. The most effective solution lay in bringing healers and patients together at a centrally located site, an institution incorporating the latest ideas in architecture and treatment. In such a setting the chances for significant cure or improvement were enhanced.

The philosophy of the new asylums was to treat individuals who exhibited recent onset or milder symptoms of mental distress. Through the application of rational and humane methods of treatment, the patient could quickly be helped and returned to society. Such treatment included clean, well-ventilated surroundings and periods of discussion and reading when the patient's condition permitted. A strict schedule that included appropriate levels of work and reading therapy was followed from 5 AM until 9:30 PM. The reformers, as administrators considered themselves, were adamant that these institutions not become dumping grounds for the chronically ill but rather be short-term hospitals for persons with a good chance of being cured.

This optimistic concept broke down soon after the new asylums were occupied. Reformers such as Dorothea Dix had been tireless in their efforts to promote humane care and treatment for the mentally ill, but these efforts were hampered by the reality of increasing numbers of admissions for long-term care and the deterioration of facilities resulting from inadequate funds.[38] By the end of the Civil War the facilities had become custodial rather than therapeutic. The promise of reform built the asylums, but the functionalism of custody perpetuated them. By 1870 custody was definitely the norm, with increased use of *mechanical restraints* and harsh punishments. The asylum lost its place as a symbol of hope and instead became a forbidding place of last resort, the home of the incurable. Society, in turn, replaced its vision of cure and recovery with one of isolation from a disease that was now considered contagious. The America of the late nineteenth century grew fearful of mental illness and demanded protection from those who would spread the "contagion."[35]

The late nineteenth century can correctly be described as providing the context for the beginning of psychiatric nursing as it is understood today. Until this time, care of the insane was in the hands of the family or of poorly paid attendants whose sole function was custody and restraint. The nursing profession had begun in the 1850s with the work of Florence Nightingale, but her efforts were confined to nursing in general hospitals and treatment of physical illnesses. Nurses who advanced from this tradition would not claim kinship with nurses who worked with the insane until well into the twentieth century. Although this division seems strange today, it made perfectly good sense in the nineteenth century.

DEVELOPMENT OF PSYCHIATRIC NURSING
The Roots of Modern Psychiatric Nursing

Psychiatric nursing and nursing in general developed from the need for hospitals to provide socially acceptable levels of care for patients. Whereas many nurses found employment in various forms of private duty, the major impetus for the establishment of nursing as an organized profession can be traced to the demands of nineteenth century reformers for social services, such as hospital treatment of both physical and mental diseases. Hospitals differed in types of care and recruited suitably trained people to staff them.

General and mental hospitals differed little in the way they attracted nurses. As they sought to take care of patients, hospital administrators turned to women whose traditional function in society had been to provide care. Prompted by the ideas of Florence Nightingale, hospitals recruited women to provide the continuous service known as nursing. Although ideas of care have existed for as long as there have been people, the specifics of nursing were new. Thus hospitals created nursing education as they began to train nurses to meet the unique standards for general and psychiatric care.

The first mental hospital in the United States was built in 1773 in Williamsburg, Virginia; but the first training school for mental health nurses started at McLean Hospital, Waverly, Massachusetts in 1882. This school and those that followed ostensibly trained nurses for later employment. However, student nurses performed basically the same tasks as graduate nurses at far less cost. As a result, hospital training schools typically furnished the majority of nursing personnel providing nursing care in the insti-

TABLE 1-1 Peplau's history of psychiatric nursing

Date	Event
1773-1882	Psychiatric nursing did not exist as such. Psychiatric care was generally custodial and harsh.
1882-1914	Mental health nurses were trained and introduced into mental health facilities. New methods of treatment were applied that avoided the use of restraints. The mental hygiene movement began and emphasized prevention and more humane treatment. Nurses played a subordinate and custodial role as managers of the ward and keepers of the keys; their primary function was to implement treatment programs devised by others. Psychiatric nurse's training did not include much psychology or psychiatry.
1915-1935	The number of undergraduate programs, including courses in psychiatric nursing, increased to half of the existing programs by 1935. The first psychiatric nursing textbook was published. Some training at the postgraduate level for psychiatric nurses was given in psychiatric hospitals.
1936-1945	Three universities offered courses in postgraduate psychiatric nursing education. The establishment of the Mental Health and Psychiatric Nursing Project within the National League for Nursing Education brought psychiatric nursing into the mainstream of nursing.
1946-1959	Postgraduate education in psychiatric nursing was firmly established. The National League for Nursing assumed responsibility for the accreditation of psychiatric nursing curricula.

tution, but replaced them as they graduated with new enrollees. Whether in general or mental hospitals, the young profession had to face the fact that graduates of educational programs could not readily find jobs.[3]

Hildegard Peplau[32] wrote a concise history of psychiatric nursing that was completed shortly before the passage of the Community Mental Health Centers Act of 1963. She defined psychiatric nursing as both (1) a vital skill of general nursing practice to be acquired and used by all nurses, and (2) an area of clinical specialization to be practiced by those with a graduate education. Graduate education referred to a course of study leading to a certificate, diploma, or degree; increasingly it meant a baccalaureate degree. Today the term has come to refer to nurses with postbaccalaureate training.

Peplau divided her history into five periods. The events that occurred in each of these periods are summarized in Table 1-1.

The directive role played by the American Psychiatric Association (APA) during the early twentieth century partially illustrates the social status and image of nursing. For example, in 1906 the APA began a program to standardize the training of nurses in mental hospitals. Not until the mid-1930s did organized nursing actively initiate the definition of psychiatric nurses as a separate group with unique educational requirements.[34]

Esther Lucile Brown's influential study, *Nursing for the Future*,[7] was also of great importance to the nursing profession. She recommended that nursing increase its emphasis on mental health nursing, stressing the importance of integrating mental health nursing into a general curriculum and ending single-focus training schools in mental hospitals.

Peplau[32] concluded her optimistic view of the future of psychiatric nursing by raising some important questions and suggesting possible answers. She believed that the historic division of psychiatric and general nursing had been resolved, psychiatric nursing being recognized as an aspect of all nursing and a specialized field of advanced nursing practice. She advocated that the basic education of all nurses be unified and that those choosing to work in psychiatric hospitals receive an introduction to psychiatric concepts in the general curriculum, followed by a period of basic experience with psychiatric patients. The question of who would provide the basic psychiatric nursing experience—the psychiatric hospital or the school of nursing—was still unresolved.

Peplau[32] argued that a philosophy of psychiatric nursing had not yet been explicitly stated and was critical of the fact that organized symposia and papers by nurses about actual nursing practice were not available. She concluded in a hopeful statement about the exciting field of mental health nursing that much remained to be achieved with regard to improving standards and increasing the impact of nurses on the patient care environment.

Sills[36] discussed the history of psychiatric nursing, drawing largely from an unpublished paper by Peplau.[33] She took the story past 1959 into the period following the Community Mental Health Centers Act of 1963. She pointed out that two issues confronting the field in 1882 still remained: (1) dominance of untrained or poorly educated service personnel, and (2) uncertainty about where nurses should receive training for the care of emotionally troubled people.

The first issue has yet to be resolved. In a time of reduced public spending in health care and demands by nurses for better salaries, the attraction of low-cost and custodial personnel is high. The second concern, as Peplau noted, has been resolved in favor of the general nursing school over the single-focus school.

Sills explained that undergraduate programs were required to incorporate psychiatric nursing into their curricula after 1955. However, an appreciation of the impact of the 1963 Community Mental Health Centers Act was based on an analysis of what happened in the 1930s and after. During this transition nurses began to consider the presence of mental factors in all diseases, and basic nursing education included knowledge of psychiatric concepts.

In the aftermath of World War II the growing need for more psychiatric nurses and a consequent growth in postgraduate programs to prepare such specialists was made compellingly clear. War casualties included more than persons with physical wounds; the term *battle fatigue* described an equally disabling condition. Public awareness of the problems faced by soldiers and civilians was translated into a demand for legislation. A concrete plan for progress came with the National Mental Health Act of 1946. This legislation changed nursing practice to include more direct involvement of the nurse in communication and other therapies. In addition, it influenced nursing education to incorporate mental health content, improved the quality of care given to patients, and promoted research in patient care.

Changes such as these do not come about without the efforts of many dedicated individuals. Sills's classic analysis[36] singles out Theresa Muller and Hildegard Peplau as providing the field with a comprehensive framework for understanding psychiatric nursing. Muller[30] studied coping mechanisms for dealing with stress in everyday life. Peplau[31] defined the therapeutic roles that nurses have in the mental health setting.

Peplau, Gwen Tudor Will,[37] June Mellow,[27] and other nurse clinicians soon contributed the results of clinical studies to the literature, which helped create a substantial body of psychiatric nursing knowledge. This knowledge has helped to develop a professional climate in which the nurse is a coordinator of care, assembling a variety of treatment methods and helping determine those which are most effective. Opportunities for direct involvement in patient treatment have simultaneously increased.

Significantly more progressive attitudes and practices characterized care of the mentally ill as the twentieth century advanced. At the same time nursing knowledge in this arena was taking shape, ideas about teamwork in treating patients were defining treatment environments that were more therapeutic. The Community Mental Health Centers Act of 1963 had the dramatic effect of transferring much of the effort of the psychiatric nurse out of the institution and into the community. The thrust of this program was concern for mental health and the prevention of serious mental illness by means of early intervention and outpatient therapy.

The 1963 act was truly a visionary approach to widespread mental health problems that had long been ignored and neglected. As with any such movement, however, it produced its own problems as nurses and other health professionals worked to establish their own limits. Significant questions for nursing became the focus of debate: How should nurses prepare for this new role—in traditional hospitals or in the community? Should their preparation be united with that of social workers and other mental health workers, or should it be independent? Finally, once prepared, how should psychiatric nurses deal

with public health nurses within their own profession and social workers, psychiatrists, and psychologists from without? To understand the factors that led to the community mental health movement and subsequent controversy, one needs to consider the development of more progressive psychiatric treatment.

The two world wars provided at least two lessons significant to mental health–psychiatric nursing: (1) more effective short-term treatment for stress-related syndromes needed to be developed, and (2) more nurses with better training were needed to meet the demand for professional staff.

Important clinical understandings about short-term treatment were achieved as a result of treating soldiers experiencing posttraumatic stress syndromes or battle fatigue. A widespread belief up to that time suggested that war neuroses represented the continuation of preexisting neuroses. An alternative view, supported by empirical evidence, explained war neuroses as syndromes precipitated only by the combat experience, without preexisting emotional difficulty. Treatment in the stressful environment relatively near the front lines minimized the soldier's sense of guilt and shame and prevented him from identifying himself as a failure at the task. Withdrawal was not allowed, and the soldier seemed to fare better in overcoming his stress-related symptoms than if he were shipped "to the rear" or back to the States. Classic descriptions of this work are provided by Ferenczi and others,[15] Kardiner,[25,26] and Grinker and Spiegel.[18,19]

Psychiatric Nursing Today

Contemporary psychiatric nursing began with the inception of comprehensive community mental health centers and continues to the present. These years have been characterized by innovation, study, and consolidation of skills as nurses have moved into new roles emerging from the community mental health movement. Developments significantly shaping psychiatric nursing during this period can be classified as (1) developments in the organized profession, (2) developments in clinical practice, (3) developments in psychiatric nursing theory, (4) the holistic health movement, and (5) developments in the women's movement.

Developments in the profession. The 1946 National Mental Health Act stimulated development of graduate training programs and psychiatric nursing content in baccalaureate nursing programs. These strong graduate programs now permit specialization in education, administration, and clinical practice. Support for doctoral study by psychiatric nurses has made it possible for nurses to earn doctoral degrees in education, behavioral and physical sciences, and nursing.

Major events affecting contemporary psychiatric nursing include (1) delineation of levels of nursing through standards defined by the ANA, (2) formation of specialty subgroups with the ANA, and (3) *certification* of advanced practitioners in psychiatric nursing. The overall effect of these events is definition and assurance of quality in practice.

		Nursing practice method		
		Individual	Family	Group
Setting	Inpatient			
	Day treatment			
	Outpatient			

FIGURE 1-2 Two-way matrix. Nursing practice opportunities are created by variations in practice method and setting.

The ANA standards establish two levels of mental health–psychiatric nursing practice. The first level requires at least baccalaureate-level preparation in nursing; the second requires graduate education, supervised clinical experience, and skill and knowledge in practice. An example of a specialty subgroup within the ANA is the Division on Psychiatric and Mental Health Nursing; the formation of this subgroup has enabled practitioners to work together on issues and programs of common interest. Certification through the ANA has provided a mechanism for recognizing excellence in practice through examination, evidence of clinical competence, and achievement of appropriate education credentials. These ANA procedures and achievements are discussed in detail in Chapter 48.

Developments in clinical practice. Great diversity exists in contemporary mental health–psychiatric nursing practice with respect to methods and settings for practice. The diversity can be illustrated by a two-way matrix in which a large number of method-setting combinations are possible. Figure 1-2 shows a simple three-by-three matrix illustrating three practice methods (individual, family, and group therapeutic relationships) and three practice settings (inpatient, day treatment, and outpatient). The illustration reveals how different practice situations can occur. In reality, all the possible method-setting combinations shown in a full two-way matrix probably do not occur. Rather, the matrix is a way of thinking about how method and setting combine in different forms to create different clinical practice experiences. In the following discussion a number of typical settings for mental health–psychiatric nursing practice will briefly be reviewed to show both the diversity of these settings and the nature of some of the improvements in psychiatric nursing care.

Inpatient facilities vary in the length of time the client typically stays in the hospital and the type of institution providing the care. Inpatient stay can vary from a few days to a few years. Most comprehensive community mental health centers have short-stay inpatient units; those that do not have such units have arrangements with a nearby institution to provide this care. State mental hospitals also provide inpatient care. Finally, inpatient units can be found in general hospitals and private psychiatric institutions.

Although one kind of unit cannot be definitely established as better than another, comparisons are typically made because people naturally try to decide whether or when one option of care is a better choice than another. Accordingly, the following factors can be used to describe variations that can influence the quality of inpatient units. First, the ratio of nurses to clients varies greatly. Some units are staffed by a nurse for every three or four clients, whereas others have one nurse on duty to supervise care on three or four wards. The stereotypical picture of an old state hospital "back ward" is one in which psychiatric aides or technicians staff the unit and a nurse supervises an entire building containing several wards.

In the past most inpatient wards were locked and nurses carried keys. Many psychiatric nursing leaders today speak about this type of ward as outmoded. However, across the United States many back ward units still exist, nurses in certain settings are still very much the keepers of the keys, and some psychiatric inpatients still see very little of a psychiatric nurse. On the other hand, many inpatient unit nurses are active members of the treatment team, clients are responsible for remaining in the unit, and the ratio of well-trained staff to clients is excellent.

A second factor interacts with the first: the underlying philosophy of the institution determines the treatment offered. For example, some inpatient treatment settings strongly emphasize the therapeutic potential of the client's social milieu.[17] Nurses in these settings work with other members of the team to develop therapeutic relationships with clients and environmental situations that help clients to develop skills in coping with daily events.

In other settings, a strong medical model prevails in which intensive psychotherapy between client and psychiatrist (often a resident) is the main focus of care. In such settings it is not unusual for the nurse's role to be that of a social chairperson; the client's nursing care is limited to social conversation, card games, and recreational outings. The ability of the nurse to establish therapeutic communication with the client has little value in these settings, and may even be discouraged or prohibited.

In some settings strongly influenced by the medical model the client is under the care of a private psychiatrist who makes brief rounds each day and leaves the remainder of the client's care to the hospital staff. In these settings it is not unusual to find clients who are being treated with large doses of medication or electroconvulsive therapy. The treatment modalities are typically justified by defining them as methods of increasing the client's accessibility to therapeutic interaction; however, others believe these treatments reduce the client's accessibility because of the side effects of drowsiness, confusion, and memory loss. Nurses in these settings typically monitor patients' vital signs, orientation, and safety in performing activities of daily living. The care is supportive in nature, often with only limited attention to the development of social or therapeutic relationships.

A third factor is the family's attitude toward the client. Family reactions vary, influenced by variables such as social class and culture. What matters is whether family members support the client or withdraw, whether they offer understanding or condemnation, and whether the client will return to a supportive family system or hostility and rejection.

When evaluating the quality of care in a given psychiatric nursing setting, the wisest approach is to refrain from making a judgment without firsthand experience or valid data. Several of the most progressive psychiatric nursing environments currently exist in public facilities where nurses are responsible for the majority of the client's daily care and interaction. From a psychiatric nursing standpoint, some of the least progressive treatment settings can be found in prestigious and highly regarded institutions. This means that a poor client may receive the most progressive care and a well-to-do client may receive the least; however, this is not necessarily a pattern. Quality of care cannot be predicted by knowing the name of the institution, whether it is a state or private facility, or whether it is in a nice neighborhood.

Outpatient facilities are characterized by even greater diversity and are usually influenced by far fewer traditions. That is, the development of outpatient care has largely occurred in the last 20 to 30 years, primarily influenced by the community mental health movement. Outpatient services can be found in mental health clinics, schools, churches, prisons, storefronts, and hospital emergency departments. Every type of care except inpatient care is available in these settings; sometimes even a short stay of a few hours or a day is the treatment of choice.

Community practice settings include private practice activities, consultation, and community organizations as well as employment in schools, industries, and child care facilities. Activities are typically conducted out of an office if the person is in private practice; otherwise, they are part of an organized system of mental health services. Nurses are now commonly found to be practicing in these independent roles (private practice, consultation, and community organizations).

A major difficulty for nurses in establishing a private practice is the problem of being paid for services. In many instances nurses are not reimbursed through *third-party payment*—even nurses with certification—for psychiatric nursing services. The alternative, undesirable to many nurses, is to restrict their practice to well-to-do people who can afford to pay full or sliding-scale fees. Charges by psychiatric nurses in private practice are said to range from no fee or a few dollars per therapy hour for the indigent client up to $40 to $60 for the full-fee client. Nurses practicing in consultative roles may charge anywhere from a $100 to $500 per day or more. The considerable variance in earnings in private practice is probably caused by problems associated with third-party reimbursement as well as the reluctance of nurses to share facts about their fees. This is certainly different from the pattern observed among psychoanalysts who charge approximately the same fee in almost any community.

Employment in schools, industry, and child care facilities is characterized by a wide variation in work roles. These systems increasingly have recognized the applications of mental health–psychiatric nursing in such areas as counseling, teaching, group discussions, and home visits. The high degree of effectiveness achieved by mental health nurses in prevention-related activities has made possible both specialized and generic nursing roles in these settings.

An interesting trend in the community arena is the increasing evidence of concern and involvement on the part of psychiatric nurses in studying and attempting to treat social problems that have mental health implications. For example, many psychiatric nurses now work with problems such as child abuse and other forms of family violence, abortion and family planning, single parenting, poverty, and crisis hot lines. This trend can be explained by the influence of the community mental health movement in which prevention is a central component. Additional impetus derives from the fact that nursing is substantially a profession of women, and women are often the beneficiaries of the programs designed to alleviate many of these social problems. Today professional women have become especially sensitive to the social problems that severely harm women.

Developments in psychiatric nursing theory. Study of this text will reveal a great deal about current thought in psychiatric nursing and in other mental health professions. These ideas will not be reviewed here, since they are thoroughly discussed elsewhere in this book; however, the development of psychiatric nursing thought over the past 20 to 30 years should be contemplated as this book is studied. Some psychiatric nurses are troubled by the fact that no dramatically new ideas or thinkers seem to have emerged—at least not in significant numbers—since the outstanding contributions of Peplau, Mellow, Orlando, and others in the 1950s and early 1960s. Are we falling behind or failing to progress? An alternative explanation is that the full impact of the community mental health movement, especially the role of the nurse as therapist, is still unfolding. The latter explanation places our progress at a satisfactory point in the evolution of psychiatric nursing thought.

The holistic health movement. The philosophy of holistic health will be discussed at length in Chapter 2. Its importance for psychiatric nursing lies in the reawakening of concern about the relationship of mind to body. The holistic health movement functions in large part as an analog to the consumer movement in which individuals now seek and demand the right and responsibility for decisions concerning their own health. Self-help groups form to aid individuals in confronting everything from a minor disorder to terminal cancer. Public interest in learning how to expand the powers of the mind has grown as rapidly as interest in physical fitness. In addition, an individual can work to increase his score on intellectual tests by applying physical and mental techniques that maximize the brain's logical processes.

The obvious problem with applying these concepts to the field of mental health is variability in the personal commitment of the client. Self-improvement requires desire, energy, and resources; often the mentally ill individual displays symptoms of the opposite nature. To compound the problem, families often provide little support or even contribute significantly to the problem.

The challenge of the holistic health movement in mental health is to deal with these considerable barriers in such a way as to help the individual while simultaneously developing a sense of caring in the community. Society still collectively applauds the efforts of the physically ill or handicapped to carve our meaningful lives but retreats to suspicion and a desire for retribution in response to the plight of the depressed, homeless, or mentally ill. As difficult as it is to treat the problems of the mentally ill, the major problem is still the responses of individual citizens and the community.

Although challenges to effective treatment of the mentally ill exist, recognition of these obstacles implies the existence of a cure or at least a commitment to finding one. As successful methods of applying holistic principles are developed, treatment of borderline cases as well as the chronically ill will be improved. As frontiers in space and energy are approached, it is important to remember that the greatest and most complex frontier of all remains within the individual.

Developments in the women's movement. Nursing is primarily a profession of women. Rich detail about the parallels between the women's movement and the nursing profession is provided by contemporary authors who have sought to overcome obstacles to economic security and social status encountered by the profession.[3,29]

At the turn of the century, nurses advancing the cause of nursing and women advancing the right of women to vote were in many instances the same individuals, actively seeking to change their society. However, today's transitions in nursing and in the women's movement have resulted in a substantial degree of separation between the two. No leading feminist theorist and few feminist activists are nurses, even though many nurses actively promote the concerns of women through feminist groups and political activities. Some contemporary nurse leaders express concern that the social changes now promoted by feminist thought only "trickle down" through the society to nursing rather than originating in nursing as they did in the past. Others indicate optimism over nursing's reemergence in the social fabric of today's women's movement, as evidenced by increased involvement in women's health and heightened concern about current sociopolitical issues affecting women.

Major issues of the contemporary women's movement have become critical issues for nursing as well, significantly affecting professional, political, and personal arenas. For example, professional issues involving collaboration and autonomy in the workplace have emerged as central to nursing's definition of its place in health care and in society. Increased competition has brought status concerns and economic goals to the forefront as nurses have sought higher and more powerful organizational positions and greater economic rewards for their services. A few nurses have found their way into public office, in addition to those who have sought political influence through professional roles within nursing. Nurses have also confronted the same personal issues about career and family life as other women, as they have sought to integrate parenthood and career roles in a society that still rewards the more "male" career role model of full-time work with no disruptions for childbirth and child care. Recent court rulings may influence society to loosen its rigid stance regarding pregnancy and child care by making it easier, if not more acceptable, for men and women to take parental leave following childbirth.

Psychiatric Nursing in the Future

A look into future decades and beyond raises interesting questions. How will psychiatric nursing evolve? How will our society respond to the distressed and socially deviant? What changes will occur in the mental health disciplines, and how will key professionals work together? These questions cannot be answered with ease. Rather, more questions can be posed and possible trends described.

Government support of services, training, and research will probably continue to decline, a problem with which nursing has struggled for some time. Continued expectations of more resources as a solution to problems is neither realistic nor justifiable. The population of the United States continues to increase in size and diversity. For some time, unemployment has been high and this trend will apparently continue; growing numbers of persons are untrained, illiterate, and poor to marginal in economic status. In response, our country would probably do well to operate on the assumption that widespread public resources will not be applied to problems of social deviance, disorder, and distress.

The decline of government support poses a dilemma, however, only if social problems continue to rise in seriousness and frequency. An alternative prediction is that reduced resources will spark increased capacities for self-reliance in individuals, families, communities, and states. The tension between government as provider and government as controller has produced a society much more willing to accept what government offers but less willing to accept the way the government's controls seem to infringe on individual liberties. A more hopeful view of the future is that growing numbers of people will take responsibility for their own needs and extend this concern in a realistic way to their families and communities.

How, then, will mental health–psychiatric nursing change? Already responsiveness in the profession can be seen in increased involvement in social problems. Practice, research, and education all reveal this shift in emphasis. Nevertheless, as a group of professionals, mental health–psychiatric nurses are at risk for becoming spread too thin. That is, limited expansions in public services indicate that "more is better" solutions cannot be applied. Rather, new activities within the private and public sectors need to be sought so that creative responses to social problems can evolve. For example, emphasis on self-care is now established in the thinking of many health care professionals and many lay persons in the community. Self-help groups and activities related to problems in living are also appearing, suggesting that the instinct to support others during difficult times is alive and well. These activities will play an increasingly critical role with people experiencing distress, as is evidenced in contemporary self-help groups for cancer patients and their families and for people with long-term psychiatric problems. Nurses play instrumental roles in these groups, as consultants in health education and community organization matters and as facilitators of a renewed demonstration of family and community involvement.

Science will present a significant challenge to the content and even the existence of the psychiatric nursing role. Many mental health professionals believe we have moved into an era in which biological and physiological factors and consequences of mental illness are to be the leading topics of research and critical thought. After successful achievement of "answers" to interpersonal questions, but failure to show that mental illness can be effectively prevented or eliminated by interpersonally oriented treatment methods, other solutions need to be sought. Simultaneously, dramatic scientific inroads have been made with respect to depression, schizophrenia, borderline syndrome, violence, and other important mental health problems. Accordingly, psychiatric nursing will be faced with certain painful realities.

First, psychiatric nurses have not generally been researchers into the origins or processes of disorders, especially with respect to biological and physiological factors. Second, the interpersonal techniques at which nurses have worked so hard to become proficient will not be given as much credence in the years to come if biological treatment of these conditions becomes the norm. If psychiatric disorders become manageable, as with administration of lithium or antiseizure medication (even if the exact pharmacological mechanism is not known), extensive interpersonal care may not be required. Much literature and research supports the fact that removal of symptoms can effect a return of the client to a satisfactory life without a recurrence of the same or a substitute symptom and without extensive psychotherapy or counseling to relieve the so-called underlying psychodynamic condition.

Mental health–psychiatric nursing needs to successfully confront two challenges in the coming decades: (1) nurses will need to actively participate in establishing the conditions under which interpersonal treatment methods are effective in preventing or relieving mental disorders, and (2) nurses will need to actively participate in establishing the conditions under which mental health–psychiatric nursing practice interacts with new treatment methods emerging from psychobiological research in preventing or relieving mental disorders. Accomplishment of these goals requires becoming more knowledgeable about research methods and data analysis and the physiological processes that will be studied by other scientists interested in mental health problems. Coinvestigative roles will be significant research avenues for the involvement of nurses, since it is likely that a relatively small number of psychiatric nurses in the immediate future will have the biological or physiological research expertise to be forerunners in this field. Better research and more complete answers will emerge as a result of this willingness and ability to collaborate; however, this collaboration can be undertaken only from a base of expertise in the field.

In the political arena the possibilities are limitless. Major issues to be confronted include the following: first, advocacy of public support for treatment, training, and research relating to the mental health requirements of the United States. Broader definitions need to be created that include serious social problems relating to violence against children and older adults. Funding for treatment, training, and research will need to be made available to all mental health disciplines, not just medicine, which receives the majority of funding at the present time. Second, as an internal goal, nursing will need to establish and maintain clearer standards for producing scholarly work and for integrating that work into the mainstream of knowledge used by mental health professionals. Third, nurses must remain active advocates of the interests of women and the women's movement. Tenuous links between the women's movement and nursing need to be strengthened. The women's movement seeks to improve society's regard for women and their contributions in the home and in the workplace. As society changes, nurses can more effectively participate in efforts to improve the health care of the nation and the status of nursing within this framework.

In conclusion, mental health–psychiatric nursing faces a period of necessary consideration of important political, economic, scientific, and social realities in its analysis of how to proceed. Strongly conservative political forces now oppose the liberal ideas that shaped the evolution of the community mental health movement of the late fifties and early sixties. Major cutbacks in public spending for social services accompanied by increased defense spending have characterized recent attempts to create economic stability. Some observers note that social responses reveal greater unrest and disorder in certain sectors; others point out the significance of the theory of relative deprivation to analyses of perceived despair because improvements in social conditions that heighten expectations have also resulted in disappointment and increased dissatisfaction.

More opportunity than risk characterizes the immediate future. Choices range from embarking on independent practice roles to undertaking the academic study necessary to become clinical researchers. Psychiatric nurses can work and develop collectively with other nurses and collaborate with other health professionals; becoming advocates in the community and devoting their energies to creating institutional forms of care that respond to the human condition are current opportunities. Efforts to promote better third-party reimbursement of mental health nursing services and working to achieve better compensation for nurses in institutional roles mean clients will have more opportunity to experience the holistic form of care that characterizes modern-day mental health–psychiatric nursing.

BRIEF REVIEW

The psychiatric nurse's treatment of mental health problems is a relatively recent response to an age-old human dilemma: What is the best way to care for an individual who is mentally ill? Through the ages this care has been the product of two different traditions, one stressing a need to appease magical or supernatural forces, the other attempting to understand, through rational methods, the causes and cure of the disease.

The development of mental hospitals in the United States during the nineteenth century created the need for trained nurses to manage wards and "keep the keys." As psychiatric treatments have improved, the role of the psychiatric nurse has expanded to a therapeutic role. Appropriate standards of education have developed to match the needs of the profession.

Training of psychiatric nurses has changed from experience acquired solely in mental hospitals to enrollment in general schools of nursing. Concepts of psychiatric care have been added to the curriculum that all nursing students complete. Nurses specialize today by means of postgraduate training, and psychiatric nurses have been supported in this by extensive federal aid, primarily as a result of the National Mental Health Act of 1946.

The Community Mental Health Centers Act of 1963 has been a powerful impetus in moving care out of the hospital into the community. This was a natural development in a field in which prevention has become an important concept. Some of the consequences of this expansion of services have brought nurses into conflict with other mental health professionals. The resolution of this conflict promises to be an important factor in determining the future course of psychiatric nursing.

The holistic health movement represents the desire to treat the client as the sum total of all his parts. It incorporates many attributes of consumerism by stressing the need for the individual to be responsible for and knowledgeable about the creation and maintenance of a healthy state of existence.

The psychiatric nurse today confronts opportunity and risk in the present and in the future. Practicing in a variety of settings, the psychiatric nurse integrates conflicting values of tradition and progress. The future challenges psychiatric nursing to find creative responses to decreasing public support, increasing emphasis on biological theories of mental disorder, and the perception that mental problems and social disorder are on the rise. The importance of nursing care in treatment of the mentally ill and the socially deviant will be confirmed through continued commitment to progress in research, practice, and education. In each instance opportunity is abundant.

REFERENCES AND SUGGESTED READINGS

1. Alexander, F., and Selesnick, S.: The history of psychiatry, New York, 1966, Harper & Row, Publishers, Inc.
2. American Nurses Association Council on Psychiatric and Mental Health Nursing: Guidelines for private practice, Pacesetter, p. 3, Spring 1985.
3. Ashley, J.: Hospitals, paternalism and the role of the nurse, New York, 1976, Teachers College Press.
4. Bailey, H.: Nursing mental diseases, New York, 1920, The Macmillan Co.
5. Beers, C.: A mind that found itself, ed. 7, Garden City, N.Y., 1948, Doubleday & Co., Inc.
6. Block, S., and Reddaway, P.: Psychiatric terror: how Soviet psychiatry is used to suppress dissent, New York, 1977, Basic Books, Inc., Publishers.
7. Brown, E.L: Nursing for the future, New York, 1948, Russell Sage Foundation.
8. Chamberlain, J.: The role of the federal government in development of psychiatric nursing, Journal of Psychosocial Nursing and Mental Health Services **21**(4):11, 1983.
9. Church, O.M.: Emergence of training programs for asylum nursing at the turn of the century, Advances in Nursing Science **7**(2):35, 1985.
10. Davidson, J., and Lytle, M.: After the fact: the art of historical detection, vol. 1, New York, 1982, Alfred A. Knopf, Inc.
11. Davis, E.D., and Pattison, E.M.: The psychiatric nurse's role identity, American Journal of Nursing **79**:298, 1979.
11a. Donahue, M.P.: Nursing: the finest art—an illustrated history, St. Louis, 1985, The C.V. Mosby Co.
12. Ellenberger, F.: The discovery of the unconscious, New York, 1970, Basic Books, Inc., Publishers.
13. Fagin, C.M.: Psychiatric nursing at the crossroads: quo vadis, Perspectives in Psychiatric Care **19**(3-4):99, 1981.
14. Fagin, C.M.: Concepts for the future: competition and substitution, Journal of Psychosocial Nursing and Mental Health Services **21**(3):36, 1983.
15. Ferenczi, S., and others: Psychoanalysis and the war neuroses, New York, 1921, International Psychoanalytic Press.
16. Foucalt, M.: Madness and civilization, New York, 1965, Pantheon Books, Inc.
17. Greenblatt, M., York, R., and Brown, E.L.: From custodial to therapeutic patient care in mental hospitals, New York, 1955, Russell Sage Foundation.
18. Grinker, R., and Spiegel, J.: War neurosis in North Africa, New York, 1943, Josiah Macy, Jr. Foundation.
19. Grinker, R., and Spiegel, J.: Men under stress, New York, 1945, Blakiston.

20. Hardin, S., and Durham, J.: First rate: structure, process and effectiveness of nurse psychotherapy, Journal of Psychosocial Nursing and Mental Health Services 23(5):8, 1985.

21. Hume, T.B.: General principles of community psychiatry. In Arieti, S., editor: American handbook of psychiatry, vol. 3, New York, 1966, Basic Books, Inc., Publishers.

22. Jaynes, J.: The origin of consciousness in the breakdown of the bicameral mind, Boston, 1977, Houghton Mifflin Co.

23. Joint Commission on Mental Illness and Health: Action for mental health, New York, 1961, Basic Books, Inc., Publishers.

24. Kaplan, H.I., Freedman, A.M., and Sadock, B.J.: Comprehensive textbook of psychiatry/III, ed. 3, Baltimore, 1980, The Williams & Wilkins Co.

25. Kardiner, A.: Traumatic neuroses of war, New York, 1941, Paul B. Hoeber, Inc.

26. Kardiner, A.: Traumatic neuroses of war. In Arieti, S., editor: American handbook of psychiatry, New York, 1959, Basic Books, Inc., Publishers.

26a. Krauss, J.B.: Nursing, madness and mental health, Archives of Psychiatric Nursing 1:1, 1987.

27. Mellow, J.: The evolution of nursing therapy and its implications for education, doctoral dissertation, Boston, 1964, Boston University.

28. Mitsunaga, B.K.: Designing psychiatric/mental health nursing for the future: problems and prospects, Journal of Psychosocial Nursing and Mental Health Services 20(12):15, 1982.

29. Muff, J., editor: Socialization, sexism, and stereotyping: women's issues in nursing, St. Louis, 1982, The C.V. Mosby Co.

30. Muller, T.: Fundamentals of psychiatric nursing, Totowa, N.J., 1962, Littlefield, Adams & Co.

31. Peplau, H.: Interpersonal relations in nursing, New York, 1952, G.P. Putman's Sons.

32. Peplau, H.: Principles of psychiatric nursing. In Arieti, S., editor: American handbook of psychiatry, vol. 2, New York, 1959, Basic Books, Inc., Publishers.

33. Peplau, H.: Historical development of psychiatric nursing: a preliminary statement of some facts and trends, Paper presented at working conference on graduate education in psychiatric nursing, Williamsburg, Va., November, 1956. Reprinted in Smoyak, S.A., and Rouslin, S., editors: A collection of classics in psychiatric nursing literature, Thorofare, N.J., 1982, Charles B. Slack, Inc.

34. Roberts, M.: American nursing: history and interpretation, New York, 1954, The Macmillan Co., Publishers.

35. Rothman, D.: The discovery of the asylum, Boston, 1971, Little, Brown, & Co.

36. Sills, G.: Historical developments and issues in psychiatric mental health nursing. In Leininger, M., editor: Contemporary issues in mental health nursing, Boston, 1973, Little, Brown & Co.

37. Tudor, G.: Sociopsychiatric nursing approach to intervention in a problem of mutual withdrawal on a mental hospital ward, Psychiatry 15:193, 1952.

38. Wilson, D.: Stranger and traveler: the story of Dorothea Dix, American reformer, Boston, 1975, Little, Brown & Co.

ANNOTATED BIBLIOGRAPHY

Ashley, J.: Hospitals, paternalism and the role of the nurse, New York, 1976, Teachers College Press.

This important study traces the development of nursing in hospitals, exploring questions about why nurses have had so little influence on hospital management and health care delivery. Ashley argues that the problem is rooted in sexism and the exploitation of nurses over the years by hospital administrators and physicians. By illuminating the historical basis for contemporary problems, the author convincingly argues that nurses need to become more politically active in both health care and general social policy arenas.

Peplau, H.E.: Principles of psychiatric nursing. In Arieti, S., editor: American handbook of psychiatry, vol. 2, New York, 1959, Basic Books, Inc., Publishers.

A brief history of the development of psychiatric nursing until 1959 and a discussion of the role of the psychiatric nurse. This work was written shortly before the passage of the Community Mental Health Centers Act of 1963. The psychiatric nurse is depicted as working exclusively within a hospital setting. Evidently Peplau, a giant in this field, anticipated little more than anyone else the substantial changes that would shortly take place.

Roberts, M.M.: American nursing: history and interpretation, New York, 1954, The Macmillan Co., Publishers.

This is the "grand" book of nursing history, a work that, regrettably, provides a standard rarely equaled in later works. Roberts writes in a sympathetic yet unsparing style that clearly identifies the issue surrounding the development of nursing in the United States. Her work is meticulously documented and even today, 30 years later, is the best discussion of American nursing up to 1950. Unfortunately, throughout most of the period covered she does not deal with psychiatric nursing as it relates to nursing in general.

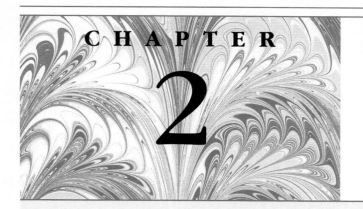

CHAPTER 2

PHILOSOPHICAL POSITIONS

Peggy A. Landrum

After studying this chapter the learner will be able to:

Discuss ways in which philosophy has influenced human life.

Examine contributions of philosophy to the Western health care system.

Describe the impact of philosophy on mental health–psychiatric nursing.

Identify components of various philosophical positions that have affected the nature of mental health–psychiatric nursing practice.

Identify the general view of human nature within the philosophical framework of holism.

Discuss the principles of holistic health care.

Philosophy plays an important role in all aspects of human life. Any conceptual base for mental health–psychiatric nursing has a foundation in philosophy. Personal and professional philosophies influence the nature and quality of mental health–psychiatric nursing care and thus affect both practitioner and client. The purposes of this chapter are (1) to introduce the concept of philosophy as a primary influence in human life, health care, and mental health–psychiatric nursing, (2) to briefly discuss several philosophical positions that are relevant to the understanding of health care in general and mental health–psychiatric nursing in particular, (3) to discuss the philosophical position of holism, and (4) to introduce basic principles of holistic health practice that may be used as guidelines in any setting to enhance the quality of the nurse-client relationship.

SIGNIFICANCE OF PHILOSOPHY
Philosophy and Human Nature

Philosophy has influenced every aspect of human life throughout recorded history. Philosophical thought probably occurred as soon as people began to question the nature of their own lives and their surroundings. Beliefs, expectations about life, and the meaning of human existence have been affected in profound ways by philosophical thinking. People have fought wars, explored new geographical areas, and developed technology based on their philosophical positions. Cultural attitudes and beliefs have made it possible for various political systems to evolve—from those flourishing on freedom of human thought and behavior to those thriving on practices such as slavery and human persecution. The meanings that people ascribe to life have also precipitated major changes in the course of history; those things that people value determine the direction of human development. Religions have been influenced by philosophy, as have ideals, goals, and standards of behavior. Throughout history, solutions to human problems and the acquisition of new knowledge have been interrelated with philosophy.

Individuals have a personal philosophy that consciously or unconsciously has an impact on their lives; this philosophy and its concomitant behaviors are partially determined by the culture in which they live. Personal philosophy determines how people view themselves, others, and the world in which they live. For instance, if one views the nature of people as essentially good, one is likely to approach people with positive expectations; if one believes that basic human nature is evil, one probably will have negative expectations. If one's personal philosophy asserts that people can exert some degree of control over their destiny, one is more likely to assume responsibility for oneself than if the belief is that outside or random forces control destiny. Personal philosophy regarding the environment will determine each individual's interaction with his physical surroundings; the result may be respectful or destructive.

One's philosophy is reflected in values, attitudes, beliefs, goals, and activities that are uniquely developed within each individual. Unique life circumstances—including familial, social, cultural, and environmental factors—contribute to the development of personal values. Many values and attitudes are learned from parents and families, from educational and religious institutions, and from personal and professional peer groups. Some are adopted through exposure to the media or literature. Each person needs to assume an active role in the development of a personal philosophy; otherwise, one's directions and goals may be determined more by others than by oneself.

Philosophy is not a static phenomenon; it constantly evolves and may be influenced by any aspect of one's life situation. As children, people incorporate certain values into their lives without question. This is necessary for socialization and survival. However, throughout life values are reevaluated to determine which are still relevant and which are no longer conducive to one's growth and development. Frequently, the shoulds and should nots that are learned as children need to be modified to serve people more appropriately as adults. For instance, in a child of an abusive family, an attitude of strong skepticism may be necessary; in an adult, this attitude may be maladaptive. As individuals move among different peer groups throughout their lives, they adopt some of the values and attitudes of each group. Personal philosophy influences receptiveness to new knowledge and beliefs; conversely, the acquisition of new knowledge and beliefs may affect overall personal philosophy.

Philosophy is a complementary partner of science; both are necessary and contribute to the quality of life. Science and technology provide necessary problem-solving tools; philosophy guides people in their use of these tools. Science analyzes the process and examines the facts, whereas philosophy seeks the meaning and value of the process and attempts to interpret the facts. Science reduces the whole into parts, and philosophy aims to reconstruct the parts in new ways that are more meaningful.

Philosophy and Health Care

The general philosophy of a society affects the nature of health care in that society. For example, in a society that views people as primarily in charge of their own destiny, health care is likely to encourage personal responsibility for disease prevention and for health promotion. If people believe that everything in the universe is interrelated, health care is likely to be approached with consideration of the many factors in a person's life contributing to health and illness. However, when cultural beliefs are such that mind and matter are two separate entities, physical and emotional problems are probably approached as separate, unrelated disturbances.

In health care, as in other areas of life, philosophy and science fulfill complementary roles. Both are necessary for the health care system to operate at its highest potential level. Science provides health care professionals with knowledge and technology that profoundly affect the quality of life and that often can make the difference between life and death; however, scientific expertise is used most effectively in a discriminate manner and within guidelines. Philosophy attempts to create a framework in which the health care system can apply its knowledge and technology in ways both meaningful and ethical to the client.

Any particular health care system develops its own philosophy, which is reflected in the values, attitudes, beliefs, goals, and activities of its health care practitioners and of the system as a whole. The philosophy of a health care system determines the general framework for the application of knowledge and technology, thus greatly affecting the nature and quality of health care delivery. Consideration of many facets is necessary when exploring the philosophy of a particular health care system. Because health care affects the quality and even the existence of individual human lives, the basic assumptions of the system about the value of human life are primary. The focus of the system is an important factor; it may be on the person or the disease, aimed toward prevention or cure, or health oriented or illness oriented. The system's view of the practitioner-client relationship and inherent beliefs about responsibility for health status influence the nature of health care. The practitioner-client relationship can range from authoritarian to coparticipatory and may or may not be considered a relevant aspect of the healing process; clients may be encouraged to assume a great deal of responsibility or discouraged from assuming any. In general the philosophy of a health care system determines how practitioners define and approach health and illness.

Philosophy and Mental Health–Psychiatric Nursing

The concept of mental health and illness has been recognized throughout history. Beliefs have changed as human culture and philosophy have changed. Different cultures have held different beliefs about mental illness. The definition of mental health or mental illness is based on the current philosophy and value systems of the society and culture. Individuals hold certain standards at any given time in the development of society; deviance from these standards has often been labeled as mental illness.

The philosophy of mental health–psychiatric nursing that this text embraces embodies the belief that people are multidimensional and in constant interaction with their environments. Nursing action focuses on people as they adapt to their environments, cope with illness, and pursue health.

Each nurse approaches mental health–psychiatric nursing in an individual way. To a large extent this approach is determined by the nurse's personal philosophy of life and concept of human nature. Each nurse has a philosophy that provides a framework for relationships with clients. One's values, attitudes, and beliefs about people and about mental health and illness dictate many aspects

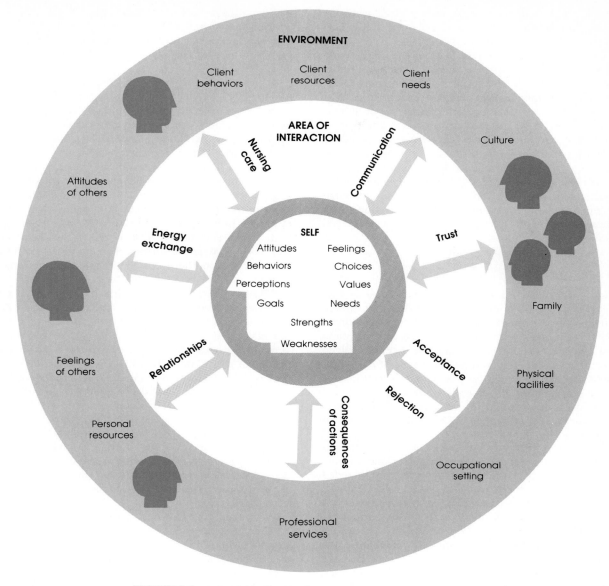

FIGURE 2-1 Awareness of self, of environment, and of interaction.

of nursing care. For example, nurses may value clients for who they are or concern themselves primarily with the illness or disease entity. Client perspectives may or may not be considered in the development of nursing care plans; primary emphasis may be on client needs or nurse-physician-institution needs. In addition, one's philosophy determines whether authoritarian or coparticipatory relationships are formed with clients and whether mental health and physical health are viewed as separate or inter-related entities. Tendencies to label or judge clients and to fear mental illness also affect nursing care. In general, personal philosophy affects how individuals fulfill the nursing role, which in turn affects the well-being of their clients.

Because personal philosophies have a great impact on the practice of mental health–psychiatric nursing, nurses

need to identify, and develop their own philosophical positions. To do so provides useful information about how nurses and clients may influence each other. This process begins with awareness of self, of environment, and of the interaction of the two. *Awareness of self* is developed as nurses clarify their values and beliefs, acknowledge their attitudes and opinions, and become consciously aware of the many choices and decisions that they constantly make. *Awareness of environment* includes recognition of client needs, belief systems, and behaviors; identification of the factors that contribute to health and illness in the client; and assessment of resources available to the client. *Awareness of interactions with the environment*—specifically with clients—is enhanced when nurses identify their specific feelings and thoughts about clients (including feelings of acceptance or rejection), evaluate the consequences of their actions toward clients, and learn to effectively differentiate between their own needs and client needs (Figure 2-1).

Awareness of self and others helps nurses effectively promote self-awareness in their clients. Nurses who possess this awareness are better able to authentically interact with clients rather than to recite stereotyped instructions or standard notions about how things are or should be. Those who have learned to evaluate their own strengths and weaknesses and to determine personal needs and goals are in a much stronger position to facilitate the same processes in clients. Awareness is the foundation of change; the more clients understand about themselves and their situations, the more likely they are to accurately identify their needs and to choose healthier ways of meeting them.

OVERVIEW OF PHILOSOPHIES
Preliterate Ideologies

In the earliest days of human existence most energy was necessarily devoted to survival. The reflective nature of human consciousness allowed an awareness of human mortality and a consequent concern for an uncertain and unknown future. Religious and magical concepts evolved to help cope with the uncertainty. Over tens of thousands of years humans adapted to environmental conditions as well by inventing tools, developing art forms, and creating social groups. They learned to cultivate food rather than simply gather it. Value and belief systems emerged that added order to human existence.

The practice of complicated magic and the use of symbolic rituals were intended to ensure safety and to help preliterate groups of people to obtain what they needed and wanted. Various forms of visions, such as dreams and sensing the invisible, were considered legitimate ways to acquire information and formed the basis for certain decisions. Misfortune was believed to be sent by evil spirits; good fortune, such as successful hunts or good crops, was often attributed to good spirits. In most of these cultures people felt a sense of continuity with other people and with the environment.

In preliterate cultures, the practice of magic and certain symbolic rituals was used to ensure the prevention of disease and injury. Outcomes of disease and injury were predicted by persons endowed with extrasensory powers and from dream interpretations. What is considered mental illness today was viewed as having various causes; among these were violation of taboos, refusal to participate in necessary rituals, loss of the soul from the body, possession by evil spirits, and witchcraft. In some cultures trephination, or surgical opening of the skull, was performed to release evil spirits or to allow the entrance of good spirits.

Shamanism evolved as a common practice in many preliterate cultures and is currently practiced in some parts of the world. A *shaman* is a person who has a special relationship to the spirit world that results in unique healing powers. Healing most often occurs when the shaman is in an altered state of consciousness. Public confessions by the afflicted individual and family, chants, symbolic rituals, and medicinal herbs are among the healing techniques of the shaman.

Chinese Perspective

Although human destiny initially depended on the gods, the value of human life and human virtue was recognized early in Chinese culture. As their civilization evolved, the Chinese considered destiny as primarily dependent on human actions and individual merit. Because human nature is considered essentially good, a strong sense of optimism exists in Chinese culture, and development of moral character is extremely important. Mencius (Chinese philosopher, c. 372-c. 289 BC) asserted four basic qualities of humans—love, righteousness, propriety, and wisdom. When nourished through moral training and social education, these develop; when neglected, they are lost.

Chinese doctrine also supports the concept of universal order; individuals, societies, and the physical universe are composed of the same elements and therefore reflect universal principles. Love of both people and things is very important, and harmony with nature is a primary goal of human life. Within the social order, the individual and society are equally significant and interdependent.[9]

Additionally, the natural cycles of the universe and of human life are intricately interrelated and respected. In Chinese philosophy *ch'i* is fundamental life energy that flows in orderly ways through the body along meridians. *Yin* and *yang* are polarized aspects of ch'i; yin is passive or negative energy, and yang is active or positive energy. An individual is healthy when the yin and yang energies are in balance; illness is viewed as a disturbance in this energy flow.

A primary focus of health care in Chinese culture is teaching people to prevent illness and to maintain and promote their own health. Responsibility for oneself is emphasized. When an individual's health problems are dealt with, attention is given to the whole person. This includes assessment of the flow of life energy, physical and emotional states, natural cycles, environmental influences, behavior, dreams, and current life situation. Any change from health to illness or illness to health develops gradually and includes many contributing factors rather than single causes and effects. Balance within the person and harmony with the environment are critical for health.[7] Because of the relatedness of everything in the universe, mind and body are not considered separate entities; mental functions are not specific to or located in any single part of an individual.

Chinese history acknowledges mental illness; ancient writings refer to insanity, dementia, violent behavior, and convulsions. Acute psychosis is sometimes attributed to loss of face or failure to fulfill family and social obligations; these conditions can lead to suicide. An aspect of Chinese life that may have a positive influence on mental health is that people are encouraged to make primary emotional and social attachments to groups as a whole rather than to specific individuals. This arrangement offers a broader support system than many other societies; an individual may be less likely to feel isolated and alone.

Eastern Indian Views

The most pervasive notion in Indian thought is the value of the subjective nature of humans. The highest value is to know one's true self, or *atman.* The atman is the most inward reality and the highest controlling power of a person. Because humans are the link between the supreme inward reality of spirit and the outward reality of matter, they are viewed as the center of the universe. A successful life is directly related to the degree of inwardness that a person deliberately pursues and attains, accounting for the Indian ideals of peace and quietism. This focus on the subjective nature of humans is not to be confused with a general retreat from the external world or with a passive approach to life. The universe is in constant motion in meaningful ways that provide order; one must act if one wants life.[26]

The natural and moral laws of the universe govern life conditions that complicate human efforts to pursue the inward search. The laws have to do with action, work, destiny, product, and effect, according to Buddhist tradition; adhering to these laws allows individuals to satisfy their duty. To not work through them is to work against universal energy and create further suffering and additional limitations in one's life.[12]

Yoga, a system designed to facilitate physical, mental, and spiritual development, is the primary method for enhancing the pursuit of inward consciousness. The purpose of yoga is to hasten the individual's movement through the distressful conditions of life and to reach *samadhi,* a state of total enlightenment in which the body, mind, and spirit function as a harmonious whole.[11]

In Indian thought the *prana* is the life energy that unites the physical body into a whole and organizes the life process. Pranic energy currents give vitality to the physical body and convey the psyche's activities throughout the body; they occur in relationship to the natural cycles of the universe and to the state of the individual. *Chakras* are centers of swirling pranic energy that act as centers of consciousness. The practice of yoga activates these chakras so that human energies are more balanced.

Ancient Indian writings indicated that health depended on one's cooperation with nature's laws. People who developed disease were believed to have violated moral laws or to be out of balance. The patient and the disease process were evaluated as a whole unit. Primary concerns, in addition to curing illness, were health promotion and longevity. Healers in ancient India had profound understanding of herbs and roots, an accurate knowledge of anatomy and physiology, and an awareness of the principles of some contagious diseases.[19]

In the *Atharuveda,* dated 700 BC, magic formulas were mentioned that counteracted demons and their human representatives. Early in their history the Indians differentiated the brain from the mind; they considered the heart the center of sensation and consciousness. Insanity was viewed as an imbalance within the person. At least four treatments for mental diseases were recognized: psychotherapy in the form of chanting, sacrifices, fasting, and purification rituals; drugs derived from plants or animals; divine agents such as sun, air, and water; and occasional physical or mental shocks.[14]

Ancient Greek Perspective

In the earliest days of Greek history the primary philosophical interest was in the order of nature as a whole; people were not viewed as objects of specific concern. Rather than having personal motivations, individuals were viewed as receiving feelings and ideas from external sources. In the fifth century BC, the Sophists believed that the true nature of the universe was mutable. Community action was emphasized because of the perceived inability of the individual alone to effect change.

Socrates (469-399 BC), following the Sophists, believed that nature was an ordered array of interactions rather than accidental chaos and that humans were a product of this ordered array. The soul allowed understanding and conscious direction of one's life, and diseases of the soul, such as ignorance and vice, were considered much worse than physical diseases. Socrates viewed the person as a physical body united with a nonphysical soul. The belief that mind and body are two separate, though interrelated, entities has occurred in many Western philosophies since the time of Socrates.

Plato (c. 429-347 BC), a student of Socrates, believed that mental health and justice were related. He contended that reason, spirit, and appetite are separate components of the psyche. Each part performs its unique task in a special way that enhances the person's ability to function in useful and healthy ways. Plato referred to such functioning as justice.

Plato viewed reason as the dominant and logical part of the psyche, in charge of coordinating information and feedback, making decisions and plans, and instructing the other parts to carry out their own tasks. For reason to function at its peak level, its primary requirement is truth. The spiritual element of the psyche is responsive to human and social matters. It provides energy both to fulfill the conclusions of reason and to assist in controlling the energy of appetite. Appetite is the part of the psyche that is the source of one's desires and cravings, and in excess is a liability. It is necessary to have manageable degrees of desire for things that are really important. The primary need of spirit is courage. The primary need of appetite is temperance. So for Plato truth, courage, and temperance—within the general context of justice—were needed to qualify a person as mentally healthy. Plato explained irrational events in behavior as an unavoidable aspect of human life; he expected people to deal with these events through reason.

Aristotle (384-322 BC), Plato's student for 20 years, believed that the mind is clearly distinguished, but is not

separate, from the body. Aristotle believed that regular catharsis was important to purge passion and to avoid violence. He viewed music, wine, and aphrodisiacs as therapeutic because of their tendency to arouse passion and
help the individual release repressed emotions.

Hippocrates (469-379 BC) believed that mental disease
is not supernatural or sacred but that it has certain characteristics and specific causes.[14] He believed that health
depended on interaction of the basic qualities in nature
and the body humors. If ill health occurred, an individual's
habits and any kind of irregularity that preceded illness
were noted. Therapeutic interventions were also based on
natural cycles. Dreams were used to gather information
and to heal physical ills. A particular treatment was to induce states of consciousness in which the unconscious
mind was instructed to heal body ills; this is evidence of
an early belief in Western culture that mind and body influence each other.[19]

The popular concept in the early Greek days was that
mental illness was caused by supernatural forces and possession by evil spirits that were sent by angry gods. Aimless wandering and violent behavior indicated mental disease. The personality functioned best when the appropriate interaction of internal and external forces had been
achieved.

Asceticism

The philosophy of *asceticism* (Greek *asketos,* one who
practices virtue) is basically a discipline of self-denial, renunciation, and detachment. The primary premise is that
human purpose is to know, love, and be united with a
spiritual force; this purpose takes precedence over the
love of humans and earthly things. Enlightened spiritual
states and salvation can only be attained through self-discipline and self-denial.

Asceticism was practiced in some Eastern religions and
also by proponents of some schools of Greek philosophy,
particularly by the Stoics and the Cynics. In the Roman
Empire ascetic practices were characteristic of certain
Gnostic sects who based their practices on the doctrine
that matter is evil and only spirit is good. Judeo-Christian
tradition asserts that humans are created in God's image;
when asceticism is practiced, the purpose is to achieve
peace with God through discipline of the body. Characteristics of early Christian asceticism were detachment from
the world, practice of celibacy, renunciation of personal
property, and martyrdom.

The highest value of asceticism is the dedication of
oneself to a mission, goal, purpose, or service that is divinely assigned. In the early history of nursing, society—
and nurses—viewed nursing as a mission that required
self-denial, dedication to duty, self-discipline, and the refusal of rewards. During this era asceticism was a primary
component of the philosophy of nursing and was particularly characteristic of nursing practice from the midnine-
teenth century through 1920. It did not disappear at this
time but became less dominant.

The ascetic influence affected both clients and nurses.
Redemption of the client's soul was the primary goal of
nursing care during the ascetic phase; this duty took priority over any other aspect of nursing care. It was not relevant that clients might have their own personal views of
the world and their particular situations, and the concept
of the client as a whole person with many kinds of needs
was not considered.

During this period, institutions for mental patients provided primarily custodial care. Because of large patient
populations and the severity of psychotic behavior, nursing care also was custodial; nurses did not deal with interpersonal or psychodynamic issues.[10] Early psychiatric
nursing texts written by both psychiatric nurses and psychiatrists,[3,29] advocated personal qualities such as patience, self-sacrifice, cheerfulness, courageousness, and
strong will for the psychiatric nurse to contend successfully with mental patients. As in other areas, nurses in
mental institutions worked long hours, functioned in poor
conditions, and collected low wages; service to clients
and physicians took precedence over the nurse's own
needs.

Romanticism

In the late eighteenth and early nineteenth centuries a
popular attitude of revolt against society and social institutions developed. This revolt included protest against established rules governing language, artistic form, and subjective matter. *Romanticism* was a social and esthetic
movement, characterized in art, literature, and music by
freedom of form, spontaneity of feeling, and a strong emphasis on imagination. The individual was glorified in accordance with personal merit rather than status; emotions,
imagination, and creative powers determined personal
merit. Self-fulfillment, emotionalism, freedom, and pursuit
of the ideal were valued and often found expression in
ways that were removed from reality and practicality. A
disposition to delight in the mysterious, the adventurous,
and the sentimental was evident; goals and aims were high
but often impractical.

Romanticism exerted a strong influence on nursing
from the early 1920s through the early 1940s, perhaps as
a reaction against the rigidity of the earlier ascetic nature
of nursing. During this time personal glory, emotionalism,
and adventure characterized the common view of nursing.
Service and loyalty to others often were ideal in nature;
nurses allowed physicians and hospitals to set the standards by which they practiced. Romanticism tended to encourage and idealize the dependence and subservience of
women; the parallel in nursing was dependence on physicians and hospitals. To a large degree nursing care was not
based on a rational foundation or on practical consequences for clients or nurses. Instead, the framework for
nursing practice followed the needs of the medical model
and of the hospital. Results of ascetic and romantic influences on nursing were similar in that autonomy, assertiveness, and independent thinking were not valued or rewarded. In return for their subservience, nurses did not
have to accept responsibility for themselves; physicians
and hospitals were willing to accept responsibility for
them.

Pragmatism

Pragmatism is a philosophy that focuses on practical consequences; ideas are valuable only in terms of their consequences. Intellectual concepts and theories are not significant if they make no practical difference; they must be applied in some way to everyday human existence and problem solving. Pragmatists are active rather than thoughtful and deal with facts rather than abstractions; they examine issues primarily to determine whether or not they serve a specific purpose.

Pragmatism was a useful philosophy for nursing to adopt during and following World War II, primarily to cope with the nurse shortage that ensued. Many problems of nursing care arose that demanded practical and expedient solution. Lack of sufficient nursing personnel and increases in patient populations of psychiatric hospitals created the necessity for delegation of many duties to ancillary personnel; thus nurses became to a large degree teachers and supervisors. Nursing care was primarily directed toward the specific problem or disease alone; other needs of the client often were not considered.

Response to the needs of physicians and institutions remained a priority of nursing during the early part of this era. Institutions providing health care became specialized according to diseases and to stages of illness. Psychiatric treatment units became more dynamic rather than custodial, and psychiatric nurses became more aware of interpersonal influences on behavior. The importance of therapeutic social interaction was recognized. The emergence of community psychiatry also created changes in the nursing role; mental illness was viewed as more than an isolated internal psychological problem.[10]

As psychiatric nurses were influenced by the pragmatic emphasis on applicability of ideas, they began to realize that nursing care could make a difference in client welfare. With this realization psychiatric nurses began to explore new ways to view clients that would be more effective. Focus on the client's perspective encouraged responsiveness to client needs. Consequently, there developed less emphasis on physician and hospital needs, and loyalties toward clients arose. When clients became the focus of nursing actions, nurses developed a sense of accountability to clients. Nurses could no longer allow physicians to assume responsibility for nursing care.[4]

Humanism

The basic tenets of *humanism* stress the importance of human abilities, aspirations, and achievements in the earthly life. Human nature is viewed as distinct from, though related to, the concrete physical universe and the metaphysical abstractions beyond it. Humanism received classical expression in the philosophy, literature, and art of ancient Greece and Rome but was submerged during the Middle Ages. It was revived when ancient culture was rediscovered during the Renaissance.

Renaissance humanism protested against the dogma of otherworldliness and the church. Humanists of the eighteenth century attacked political oppression, and those of the nineteenth century resisted attempts to interpret human nature through the categories and methods of the natural sciences.

Humanism today is a philosophical movement in which people and their interests, development, fulfillment, and creativity are made central and dominant. It is an ethical doctrine that particularly supports the right to human freedom. A universal tendency of humanists is to emphasize self-understanding, self-determination, and human responsibility. Humanists advocate that people develop individual goals based on their personal life experience.

Within nursing, humanism emphasizes the value and importance of being human and creates a sense of caring for the dignity and welfare of people. When the philosophical view of humanism guides mental health–psychiatric nursing practice, nurses are aware both of themselves and of clients in nursing interactions and are willing to assume responsibility for nursing care decisions. Within this approach, the person is the focus of nursing care, and the well-being of the client is the foundation of all nursing activities. The whole person, rather than only the specific disease or problem, receives attention. An accepting and nonjudgmental approach toward the client is valued, and clients are recognized as having the basic ability to make their own decisions concerning health care. The concern of nursing is to deal with the quality of life of each client and to help people as they strive toward their human potential.

Existentialism

The word *existentialism* was coined after World War I to designate the philosophical thinking of Karl Jaspers and Martin Heidegger. Both were indebted to the philosophy of Sören Kierkegaard (1813-1855), a nineteenth-century Danish theologian and philosopher. The writings of Jean-Paul Sartre brought existentialism to the attention of the English-speaking world after World War II. Existential philosophy is concerned with the essence of human existence rather than logic or science and developed out of a conviction that most academic philosophy is too remote from human life and death. Existentialists are especially concerned with the most extreme human experiences, such as anguish, despair, and confrontation with death, because they enable a person to realize the true nature of existence.

At least three main concerns are central to existentialism.[30] These concerns are as follows:

1. For individual existence rather than theories regarding general human nature because these theories often neglect the quality of uniqueness.
2. With the meaning and purpose of human lives on earth; inner experience is more important than objective truth.
3. With individual freedom, viewed as the most important and distinctively human property. People are free to choose their own attitudes, purposes, values, and way of life, and they must accept personal responsibility for these choices.

The most radical division of existential thought is between the religious and the atheistic. Kierkegaard rejected abstract theoretical philosophies and advocated the supreme importance of the individual and the individual's choices. He described three main ways of life (esthetic, ethical, and religious) and believed that each person must choose among them. He personally believed the religious way—Christianity in particular—to be the most desirable, but it could be reached only after struggling through the other two ways.

The views of Friedrich Nietzsche (1844-1900), the other main source of existential thought in the nineteenth century, were atheistic. He asserted that because religion and God are illusions people must rethink the nature of their lives, finding meaning and purpose in human terms alone. Nietzsche proposed that morality is individual and must come from within each person; if there were in fact an absolute morality and all people had knowledge of it, they would be stranded in a static and frozen position. To seek an absolute morality is to avoid the kind of consciousness that actually characterizes human existence itself, one consisting of change, process, and decision making.

Consciousness is the focus of twentieth-century existentialism, which asserts that individuals must each make their own choices with the full awareness that they are responsible for them and consequently responsible for the direction of their lives. This realization can be a lonely and frightening process; however, it is also a gratifying experience of change and growth and of fully appreciating one's potentials.

Existentialism in conjunction with humanism has influenced mental health–psychiatric nursing since the early 1960s. The implication derived from the conjunction is that nurses can neither understand clients through science or metaphysical systems alone, nor adequately relate to clients in terms of only their disease or problem. An isolated aspect of a client can neither explain how that client functions as a whole person nor indicate what the client needs. Only authentic, honest relationships with clients can help mental health–psychiatric nurses respond to the client as a whole person. This is not to say that scientific principles and attempts to predict human responses are excluded from nursing practice. However, an existentialist viewpoint makes it imperative that nurses accept the client's right to make choices about health care in particular and life-style in general.

Existentialism also supports the concept of accountability in nursing; nurses are free to make choices regarding nursing care and are responsible for personal and professional choices.

This is particularly true for mental health–psychiatric nurses who have established themselves as self-directed peers of other mental health practitioners and have exerted a major influence on nursing as a profession. Before nurses can assume responsibility for their choices, they must recognize the possibilities and alternatives. This necessitates that nurses become more aware of their own experience and that they be authentic and honest with themselves. The nurse-client relationship is viewed as an opportunity for both nurse and client to increase awareness, to experience freedom and growth, and to learn to make responsible choices.

HOLISTIC PHILOSOPHY AND HEALTH CARE

The philosophical position of holism is a useful construct in which to examine human nature and health care philosophy. Holism and holistic health have been described and definitions attempted from several perspectives. A basic premise inherent in all definitions is that living and nonliving entities are viewed in terms of "wholeness, relationships, processes, interactions, freedom and creativity."[6] The patterns of interrelationship within and among entities determine reality; thus it is inaccurate to consider individuals, societies, or things in isolation.

A holistic philosophy of health care simultaneously grows out of and integrates all of these concepts of human nature. It incorporates ideas and principles from several philosophical positions, such as the Eastern beliefs of China and India, humanism, and existentialism. Holistic health philosophy accepts the Chinese concept of universal order; everything in the universe is composed of the same elements. Therefore human nature is an intricate part of universal order, and harmony with nature is a primary value. A person's body is composed of active and passive energy forces; health exists when these energies are balanced, and illness occurs when they are disturbed. As in Chinese belief, holistic health care emphasizes prevention, personal responsibility, and mind-body unity.

A primary concept in holistic health, as in Indian philosophy, is the subjective nature of a person. To understand outward reality, individuals must seek to know and understand themselves. Health is viewed within the context of the importance of inward reality and of the natural laws of the universe; the two must be balanced. Person and disease are evaluated as one unit, and health promotion and longevity are valued.[19]

Humanism has contributed to holistic health care philosophy an emphasis on the value and importance of being human. In health care, the influence of humanism has directed attention toward the whole person rather than only the specific problem and has encouraged recognition of the basic ability and right of clients to choose a personal life path.

Existentialism has influenced holistic health care philosophy in several ways: (1) the concern for individual existence rather than theories regarding human nature, (2) the premise that inner experience provides people with meaning and purpose, and (3) the view that individuals make choices throughout life for which they are personally responsible. Existentialism implies that only through authentic, honest relationships with clients can health care providers understand how they function as whole persons; a crucial obligation is to encourage freedom, growth, and personal responsibility in relationships with clients.

A holistic orientation to health care, then, recognizes all aspects of a person as significant and considers how these interact to affect the whole person. Each individual is viewed as a whole person with physical, emotional, intellectual, social, and spiritual dimensions and as one who is in constant interaction with others and with the environment. What happens in each human dimension influences the others and consequently the whole person. All factors contribute to health and illness. The balance of all

TABLE 2-1 Summary of influence of philosophical positions on views of human nature, health care, and nursing

Position	View of Human Nature	View of Health Care	View of Nursing
Preliterate ideologies	Ruled by nonhuman forces Health and illness caused by good and evil spirits	Use of magic to appease spirits Trephination; transfer of disease to animals	
Chinese perspective	Importance of morality and harmony with nature Interdependence of person and society	Emphasis on prevention Health based on balanced flow of life energy; illness caused by disruption	
Eastern Indian views	Inward reality most important In constant process with universe	Health based on cooperation with natural and moral laws of universe Concern for health promotion and longevity	
Ancient Greek perspective	Nature as ordered rather than accidental Mind and body separate but interrelated	Importance of natural cycles Use of mind to heal physical ills	
Asceticism	Primary purpose to serve spiritual force Insignificance of physical needs Self-denial and self-discipline	Focus on redemption of client's soul	Primarily service and duty Tolerance of poor working conditions Dedication to a mission
Romanticism	Glorification of the individual Encouraged subservience of women Personal merit determined by superiority, not status Value of mystery, adventure, and sentiment	Idealization of service and loyalty to others	Lack of rational foundation or consideration of practical consequences Dependence on physicians and hospitals
Pragmatism	Focus on practical consequences Value of facts, not abstractions	Specialization according to disease and stage of illness	Focus on client perspectives Realization of impact of nursing care on client welfare
Humanism	Value of human abilities and aspirations; rejection of supernatural Resistance to methods of science	Emphasis on individual freedom in health choices	Attention to whole person rather than only disease process Acceptance of responsibility for nursing actions
Existentialism	Concern for essence of human existence, especially extreme experience Value of individual freedom and personal responsibility	Importance of accountability and responsibility by both clients and practitioners	Focus on authentic, honest relationships Importance of learning to make responsible choices
Holism	Reality in terms of relationships and processes Multidimensionality	Focus on context of health and illness Illness as opportunity for growth	Active partnership of client and nurse Emphasis on stress management and health promotion

dimensions of a person is valued. Thus no one human dimension, either within the person or as seen in that person's interactions with others, can be considered in isolation. Any attempt to consider only the social aspect or only the physical aspect, for instance, leaves one with an incomplete view of the whole person. If people are viewed in a fragmented way, the tendency is to interact with them in a fragmented manner.

Each individual actively participates in the development of conditions which either enhance health or encourage illness; thus personal responsibility is valued as a crucial component of a holistic orientation to health care. See Table 2-1 for a summary of philosophical positions.

HOLISTIC HEALTH PRINCIPLES OF PRACTICE

Holistic health principles of practice constitute a framework that can be used in any nursing care setting and that will enhance the quality of the nurse-client relationship. They are intended as guidelines to stimulate self-exploration and to improve the effectiveness of nursing care.

Human Uniqueness

Within a holistic health framework, each individual is considered unique. Complex factors, including human dimensions, comprise a person's view of himself, the world, health, and illness; an individual in a given situation cannot be equated with any other person. For any person, the interaction of different dimensions and the interaction of the person with the environment are unique.

This quality of uniqueness demands that people be viewed as requiring individualized approaches to health and illness. What is healthy for one person may be detrimental to another; what contributes to illness in one individual does not affect another. People meet their needs in each dimension in different ways. For example, one person may consider jogging an excellent form of exercise, and another may prefer aerobic dancing with a group of people. Group therapy may help one person who is depressed, whereas a form of individual therapy may help another. One person may effectively cope with social isolation through group participation, another through individual friendships, and still another through school or work involvement. Some individuals need many details to process, incorporate, and make decisions regarding new information; others are comfortable with very few details. One person may develop and express spirituality through meditation, another through organized religion.

In addition, individuals have different needs with respect to the achievement of balance within themselves and in their particular life situations. Recognition of these needs facilitates the attainment of health. For instance, the person who is physically fit but is unaware of feelings needs help in developing the emotional dimension. One who is able to express feelings well but is not able to solve problems in life situations may need to attend to the intellectual dimension. Another person who has well-developed problem-solving skills but cannot maintain a support system may need help in the development of the social dimension. Someone who has a well-developed social support system but experiences a loss of purpose in life may need to consider what is lacking in the spiritual dimension. The person who is attuned spiritually but neglectful of exercise or nutrition may need to direct some attention toward the physical dimension.

When an individual's uniqueness is not respected, health care may be approached in a way that has been effective with other clients but is not with this one. This is particularly likely if health care professionals consider only the disease process, the symptoms, or a label. When nurses limit a client to a category, they also limit their ability to perceive individual needs and innovative solutions. Labels encourage the use of identical interventions for similar sets of conditions in different individuals. This approach is sometimes useful and at other times is not. Sole reliance on labels makes it difficult to view the needs of the individual as a priority; instead, the application of standard interventions and the expectation of standard results become the priorities.

Context of Health and Illness

The philosophy of holistic health care asserts that health and illness must be considered within the context of the individual's life situation. People, including their states of health and illness, do not exist in isolation. They function within many settings, such as familial, occupa-

tional, communal, social, and cultural. The values, beliefs, and behaviors that develop from these settings influence health and illness. A holistic perspective acknowledges the significance of these factors. Families may offer a safe setting for the expression of feelings, or they may interact only on superficial levels. A person's work place may serve as a source of creative challenge or of chronic unrelieved stress. A community may provide areas for physical exercise and activities that encourage social interaction; a different community may appear physically unsafe and socially hostile. One individual may have a social network that is supportive of self-development and growth, and another may have friends who are unreliable and unresponsive to the individual's needs. Some cultures value verbal and nonverbal expressions of affection, whereas others view displays of affection with distaste.

When nurses are willing to view health and illness within the context of the individual's life, they are better able to understand the person's experience of health and illness. They are better able to understand that people with similar symptoms react in different ways, that individuals with similar disease processes do not necessarily respond to identical interventions, and that people differ in their perceptions of health and illness.

A person's life context to a large extent determines the options that are available at a given time. In any particular situation, people have access to various resources and not to others. The availability of financial, social, familial, and community resources will all influence the course of health and illness. A holistic perspective facilitates the identification and development of individual options and resources rather than assuming that what worked in one case will work in another.

Illness as Opportunity

Just as stressors are not inherently positive or negative, illness is not intrinsically good or bad. The primary factors that determine the impact of illness are one's attitudes toward it, what one is able to learn from it, and what growth one engages in as a result of the illness. Some people may view illness as a catastrophe that simply "happened" to them and over which they had no control. They see themselves as victims being persecuted by the illness (and often by other factors in their life situation). They view themselves as helpless and are tempted to give up. In contrast, other people are able to view illness as an opportunity to evaluate their current life situation, including the role of stressors. They view themselves as maintaining control of their lives and seek to discover the ways in which they may have contributed to the illness. They acknowledge that pertinent information is available in the illness, and they use this information to set new goals and move in new directions. This approach is consistent with holistic health philosophy, which asserts that there is personal meaning, or a message, in any illness. Discovering this message provides an opportunity for growth.

Illness may often be related to needs that a person has but is not meeting. People ideally strive to meet needs in the best available ways, such as asking for what they want, taking the time and space they need, or, in general, creating life to be what they want. However, when they are not conscious of or ignore certain needs, they may develop an illness or particular symptoms to meet their needs. This is usually an unconscious process and occurs when people do not have better coping mechanisms available to them.

The use of illness to meet one's needs may at first be a difficult issue to explore in one's own life. An initial and automatic response often is "but I don't want to be sick!" and this is certainly true. However, in a particular situation the person may not perceive any alternative. Possibly an individual is not even consciously aware of the need. A look at how one's situation changes as a result of illness, or what one gains from being ill or injured, will offer clues regarding needs that are not being met otherwise. These needs may be as simple as more time alone, less responsibility, or a few days' rest or as major as restructuring a relationship, changing jobs, or setting new priorities. If a person is forced to rest for a few days or to be dependent when the person normally is independent, dependence may be a need that the person is attempting to meet through illness. If illness or injury allows an individual to say "no" to certain demands without feeling guilty or provides permission to slow one's pace, perhaps one can learn to meet these needs in healthy ways.

At the very least, illness signals people to examine the stressors in their lives, the meaning that they ascribe to them, and their ways of coping with them. Their personal belief system and the meanings that they associate with various events and circumstances determine their range of possible responses. Illness and injury indicate that people need to reconsider these meanings and the ways in which they respond to life events. When individuals label an event as disastrous, they are likely to respond in harmful ways (such as by feeling helpless, hopeless, anxious, or panic-stricken); when they relabel the event as an opportunity for growth, they are able to respond in constructive ways (such as by feeling powerful, assertive, calm, and in charge of their lives). Illness is opportunity to the extent that one is willing to create different meanings that are more healthy and thus able to broaden the scope of one's responses.

Client-Nurse Partnership

Within a holistic health framework, the relationship between client and nurse is an active partnership, and responsibility in healing and growth is shared. Because an energy exchange occurs between the two, the relationship itself has a healing effect. Teaching and learning operate in both directions; thus the practitioner and the client both experience growth and change.

The nurse in a holistic health care setting attempts to create conditions that are conducive to healing and optimal health. The client's current belief system is the beginning framework, and from this point the nurse provides support and assists the client in finding healthy ways to meet individual needs. This process will include, but not be limited to, expansion of self-awareness, evaluation of life-style factors, identification of stressors and coping mechanisms, exploration of meanings of illness, exposure to alternative beliefs and response patterns, and implementation of healing modalities that are acceptable and appropriate for the client. Nurses are willing and able to share information and experience with clients rather than using their expertise to appear more powerful or more "professional." Actually nurses consider clients as the ultimate experts regarding their health and illness and respect the client's subjective experience as being highly relevant in the healing process.

Clients in a holistic setting are coparticipants in healing and health promotion, working closely with the nurse to determine necessary and appropriate interventions. To the greatest extent possible, clients maintain active roles in any treatment or decision-making process and actively seek relevant information. They do not consider themselves passive recipients of health care but learn to consider themselves the experts regarding their own needs and health status. In this way they are able to retain their sense of personal power rather than conceding it to the health care system, thus assuming the role of helpless victim. Clients learn to recognize that health and illness or injury are multidimensional, with many contributing factors and possible outcomes. They view themselves as whole persons with unique, valid needs and realize that many alternatives are available for meeting these needs. Rather than assuming that the nurse is able to decide for them, clients examine alternatives and choose from among them.

As a practitioner, the nurse's most powerful healing capacity comes from who she is and how she relates to others. Holistic nurses who pursue their own personal growth and strive toward optimal health for themselves are better able to facilitate healing and optimal health in others. Incorporating such qualities as self-awareness, personal responsibility, and balance into their own lives is a first step in enhancing these qualities in clients. The nurse's own willingness to examine stressors and choose healthier response patterns demonstrates what clients can do for themselves.

The client-nurse relationship will have some effect on both individuals. To a large extent, the nurse assumes the responsibility of making this a positive effect. Practitioners have the opportunity to influence clients so that they are better able to strive toward optimal health and get what they want out of life; at the same time practitioners have the opportunity to learn from each client and allow their own boundaries and experience of life to expand.

Self-Care

As implied in preceding sections, holistic health philosophy supports self-care as a valid and necessary component of the larger health care system. The formal health care system cannot provide all services associated with health and illness; it has no control over the choices that people make which contribute to health or illness, their responses to stressors, or their life-styles. Self-care proponents encourage individuals, families, and communities to assume more responsibility for health status improvement. Because people are, or can be, experts regarding themselves and their health, they can learn how to safely depend less on health professionals and more on themselves.

Self-care is based on the premise of personal responsibility and may range from health promotion behaviors to treatment of some illnesses, injuries, and chronic health conditions. A large portion of health care actually is self-care. Examples are stress management techniques, use of vitamins and over-the-counter medications, increased fluid intake, applications of heat or cold, use of Ace bandages, rest, and management of chronic conditions such as diabetes or asthma. Many common health problems can be prevented, alleviated, or eased by consumers, in many cases more efficiently and effectively than by the health care system.

Many factors, including cultural influence, familial patterns, personal value systems, and prior learning affect the individual's capacity for self-care. Appropriate self-care implies knowledge; thus a crucial element of self-care is health education. Because people engage in some form of self-care with or without adequate knowledge, health care practitioners have a responsibility to create every possible opportunity to disseminate accurate information concerning self-care concepts and skills. Such information may be made available through schools, churches, clinical settings, community centers, study groups, and formal classes. Self-care education that is based on the needs and current level of knowledge of the individual or community is likely to be the most acceptable and useful. A variety of approaches can be used to reach such diverse groups as children, adolescents, the elderly population, and minority groups.

Self-care is not an exclusive alternative to treatment by the health care system. However, with adequate knowledge about self-care, individuals are likely both to assume responsibility for their health and to recognize the importance of relationships with the health care system. The system operates in a consultant role, assisting and supplementing consumer skills. People who pursue self-care learn to coordinate their health services: how and when to best use professional assistance.

Health

Holistic health philosophy includes a primary focus on health promotion, or health as a positive process, rather than limiting itself to the elimination of illness. Health is more than the absence of disease; it is a dynamic, active process of continually striving to reach one's own balance and highest potentials. Health involves working toward optimal functioning in all areas. This process varies among people and even within individuals as they move from one situation or stage of life to another and is contingent on personal needs, imbalances, and individual perceptions of reality.

Health is a life-style that is conducive to optimal functioning, and therefore can be pursued only by the person, family, or community. Individuals create their own lifestyles through life choices. Because everything in one's life has an impact on health, each choice one makes leads toward or away from health. The goal is to improve one's ability and willingness to assess the impact on one's

choices on health and to make healthy choices. A major assumption of a healthy life-style is that individuals are each responsible for participating in the creation of their life situation so it promotes health.

In addition to personal responsibility, a positive adaptation to stress is an important aspect of health. People must learn to recognize stressors in all dimensions of life, eliminate those that are harmful, and choose healthy responses for those that they keep. This includes recognition of needs, strengths and weaknesses, and internal and external factors that affect all dimensions: physical, emotional, intellectual, social, and spiritual. Each person needs to determine whether activities, feelings, attitudes, beliefs, expectations, and interactions with others contribute to or detract from the quality of health status. One's ability to deal effectively with change and maintain a sense of control over life even while responding to change greatly contributes to health.

Illness or injury also stimulates the pursuit of health by providing information that the individual needs to restore balance and optimal functioning. It is often through such circumstances that he becomes aware of the changes that are necessary to obtain more of what he wants out of life. Individual and family health remains a goal and is possible even in acute or chronic illness or injury. Even when chronically ill or disabled, a person has an optimal functioning level. The focus is on maintaining optimal energy levels and striving toward one's health potential.

The meaning of health and genuinely healthy life-styles vary among individuals and are determined by both objective and subjective factors. Some objective components, such as nutrition, exercise, meditation, psychotherapy, visualization, development of healthy relationships, and positive belief patterns, are generally agreed upon as conductive to positive states of health. The relevance and usefulness of these objective factors, when applied to any particular individual, are determined by subjective factors such as cultural and familial belief systems, work and home environments, individual attitudes and values, the nature of the social network, past experiences, expectations for the future, and genetic predisposition. Holistic health practitioners consider objective and subjective factors while facilitating health in themselves and others.

BRIEF REVIEW

Philosophy has been a crucial factor in the evolution of human life, determining how people view themselves, others, and the universe in which they live. Individuals each have unique philosophies that are reflected in their values, attitudes, beliefs, goals, and activities; these influence their everyday lives through the choices that they make and the behaviors in which they engage. The relationship between philosophy and science is complementary; both contribute to the human quest for knowledge and understanding.

The health care system of any society is affected by the philosophy of that society. Both philosophy and the technology of science are necessary for health care to reach its highest potential. The philosophies of the health care system, the individual practitioner, and the client influence the quality of health care services.

Specifically philosophy is an integral part of mental health–psychiatric nursing. The personal and professional philosophies of nurses affect the nature of nursing care that they provide and the quality of relationships that they form with clients. For this reason nurses need to recognize and develop their own philosophical positions; the foundation of this process is awareness of self and others.

There have been numerous philosophies throughout the history of human existence, including asceticism, romanticism, pragmatism, humanism, existentialism, and holism; these have affected the quality of life, nature of health care, and, more specifically, approaches to mental health and mental illness. Nursing has evolved through various philosophical positions, all of which have influenced the nature of nursing practice. Several principles that evolve from these philosophical concepts may be used as guidelines for improving the quality of mental health-psychiatric nursing care.

The development of holistic health philosophy has been influenced by Chinese and Indian thought and by the more recent philosophical positions of humanism and existentialism. The person is viewed as a complex whole affected by many factors at any given time. Even though these variables each exert a particular influence, every factor alters the person's relationships with other influential forces. Thus it is most meaningful to view people in terms of their relationships rather than to analyze their various aspects in isolation.

REFERENCES AND SUGGESTED READINGS

1. Ackermann, R.J.: Beliefs and knowledge, New York, 1972, Anchor Books.
2. Ashley, J.A.: Hospitals, paternalism, and the role of the nurse, New York, 1976, Teachers College Press.
3. Bailey, H.: Nursing mental diseases, New York, 1920, Macmillan Publishing Company.
4. Bevis, E.O.: Framework for nursing practice. In Bower, F.L., and Bevis, E.O. co-editors: Fundamentals of nursing practice: concepts, roles, and functions, St. Louis, 1979, The C.V. Mosby Co.
5. Black, K.M.: An existential model for psychiatric nursing, Perspectives in Psychiatric Care **6:**178, 1968.
6. Blattner, B.: Holistic nursing, Englewood Cliffs, N.J., 1981, Prentice-Hall, Inc.
7. Bresler, D.E.: Chinese medicine and holistic health. In Hastings, A.C., Fadiman, J., and Gordon, J.S., editors: Health for the whole person, Boulder Co, 1980, Westview Press, Inc.
8. Cadwallader, E.H.: The main features of values experience, Journal of Value Inquiry **14:**229, 1980.
9. Chan, W.T.: The concept of man in Chinese thought. In Radhakrishnan, S., and Raju, P.T. editors: The concept of man, London, 1966, Allen & Unwin, Inc.
10. Critchley, D.L.: Evolution of the role. In Critchley, D.L., and Maurin, J.T. editors: The psychiatric mental health clinical specialist: theory, research and practice, New York, 1985, John Wiley & Sons, Inc.
11. Devi, I.: Renew your life through yoga: the Indra Devi method for relaxation through rhythmic breathing, Englewood Cliffs, N.J., 1963, Prentice-Hall, Inc.
12. Eliade, M.: Yoga: immortality and freedom, Princeton, N.J., 1969, Princeton University Press.
13. Farrell, F.: Western versus Chinese philosophy: cultural roots, Journal of Chinese Philosophy **8:**59, 1981.
14. Freedman, A.M., Kaplan, H.I., and Sadock, B.J.: Modern synopsis of comprehensive textbook of psychiatry/II, ed. 2, Baltimore, 1976, Williams & Wilkins.
15. Fuller, S.S.: Holistic man and the science and practice of nursing, Nurs. Outlook **26:**700, 1978.
16. Fumerton, R.: Reasons and value adjustments, J. Value Inquiry **8:**259, 1979.
17. Keyes, C.D.: Four types of value destruction, Washington, D.C., 1978, University Press of America, Inc.
18. Kollemorten, I., and others: Ethical aspects of clinical decision making, Journal of Medical Ethics **7:**67, 1981.
19. Krieger, D.: Foundations for holistic health nursing practices; the Renaissance nurse, Philadelphia, 1981, J.B. Lippincott Co.
20. Kurtz, P., editor: The humanist alternative: some definitions of humanism, Buffalo, 1973, Prometheus Books.
21. Laszlo, E., and Wilbur, J.B.: Value theory in philosophy and social science, New York, 1973, Gordon & Breach, Science Publishers, Inc.
22. Macklin, R.: Mental health and mental illness: some problems of definition and concept formation, Philosophy of Science **39:**341, 1979.
23. Moore, M.: Some myths about mental illness, Inquiry **18:**233, 1975.
24. Paterson, J.G., and Zderad, L.T.: Humanistic nursing, New York, 1976. John Wiley & Sons, Inc.
25. Price, J.I., Drake, R.E., and Hine, L.N.: Value assumptions in humanistic psychiatric nursing education, Perspectives in Psychiatric Care **12:**64, 1974.
26. Raju, P.T.: The concept of man in Indian thought. In Radhakrishnan, S., and Raju, P.T.: The concept of man, London, 1966, Allen & Unwin, Inc.
27. Riccardo, E.P.: Introduction to humanistic philosophy, Dubuque, Iowa, 1979, Kendall/Hunt Publishing Co.
28. Riehl, J.P., and Roy, C., editors: Conceptual models for nursing practice, New York, 1974, Appleton-Century-Crofts.
29. Sadler, W.S.: Psychiatric nursing, St. Louis, 1937, The C.V. Mosby Co.
30. Stevenson, L.: Seven theories of human nature, Oxford, England, 1974, Clarendon Press.
31. von Bertalanffy, L.: General system theory: foundations, development, applications, New York, 1968, George Braziller, Inc.

ANNOTATED BIBLIOGRAPHY

Bevis, E.O.: Framework for nursing practice. In Bower, F.L., and Bevis, E.O.: Fundamentals of nursing practice: concepts, roles, and functions, St. Louis, 1979, The C.V. Mosby Co.

Bevis discusses the influence of the following philosophical positions on the evolution of the nursing role: asceticism, romanticism, humanism, and existentialism. Examples of each of the philosophies' contribution to nurses' view of themselves and their clients throughout the history of professional nursing are given.

Critchley, D.L.: Evolution of the role. In Critchley, D.L., and Maurin, J.T. editors: The psychiatric mental health specialist: theory, research and practice, New York, 1985, John Wiley & Sons Inc.

Critchley offers a historical overview of the development of psychiatric nursing and the major forces in society, nursing, and medicine that have contributed to the development. Previous trends as well as current issues are discussed and related to the role of psychiatric mental health clinical specialist.

CHAPTER 3

THEORETICAL APPROACHES

Ann Adams   Elizabeth Maloney

After studying this chapter the learner will be able to:

Discuss the historical development of major theoretical approaches.

Identify key concepts associated with each selected theory.

Identify basic assumptions of each theoretical approach.

Discuss the application of selected theories to the therapeutic process.

---

common theme in nursing is the importance of theory-based practice. The use of theory as a basis for practice is one of the characteristics of a profession; it distinguishes professional from technical nursing practice. The nurse practices in highly complex settings, and few theories deal with all of the multiple, complex variables that affect a clinical problem. Undertaking the provision of care based on a holistic approach greatly compounds the challenge.

The theories presented in this chapter are used primarily for their explanatory value and bring significant understanding to clinical practice by providing frameworks for organizing and labeling perceptions of behavior. These theories also explain what that behavior means with respect to the individual in a specifically defined context.

The mental health–psychiatric nurse's basic beliefs about human nature and the meaning of mental health and illness provide the groundwork for the selection of theoretical approaches to psychiatric nursing. Other considerations in selecting a theoretical approach or combination of approaches to mental health–psychiatric nursing include the client's behavior, belief system, and resources; the treatment setting; and societal and political influences. The extent to which the thinking of mental health–psychiatric nurses has been influenced by theoretical approaches is evident in their *eclectic approach* as a basis for the nursing care they provide.

PSYCHOANALYTIC THEORY

A basic premise of psychoanalytic theory is that a person's overt behavior cannot be understood except by knowledge of his thoughts, feelings, and motives. Although some psychoanalytic theorists (such as Freud, Jung, and Erikson) emphasized intrapsychic functioning, others (such as Sullivan) focus on interpersonal experiences. The psychoanalytic approach emphasizes the unconscious and the *psychodynamics* of behavior. Two basic theoretical assumptions of psychodynamics are that present behavior is influenced by past experiences and that mental forces influence development and motivate behavior.

Intrapsychic

Sigmund Freud[19,20] developed the ideas that formed the foundation for psychoanalytic theory. He was the first theorist to develop a comprehensive theory of personality. One of his basic assumptions was that all behavior is meaningful. Even behavior that seems insignificant, such as slips of the tongue and forgetfulness, reveals significant information. Related to this assumption is the important role of the unconscious in influencing behavior. Anxiety (Chapter 11) is viewed as a motivator for behavior.

The personality consists of three major systems: the *id,* the *ego,* and the *superego.* Each system has specific characteristics and functions and interacts with the others

Historical Overview

DATE	EVENT
Pre-1800s	Approaches to the study of human behavior were nonscientific and almost exclusively in the domain of philosophy and theology. Scholars emphasized the biological foundation of behavior and believed the mind and body functioned independently. Philosophers and theologians focused on the conscious actions of the individual's free will, reason, and memory. These scholars studied the soul and attended to supernatural forces they believed governed behavior.
1800s	There was a transition from philosophy and theology to psychology and a scientific approach to the study of behavior. Experimental psychologists believed the field of psychology was the study of consciousness (mind) and that states of consciousness can be analyzed in terms of sensations, images, and feelings. A lasting contribution made by experimental psychologists is a framework for the measurement and study of individual differences. Psychologists associated with the functionalism school of thought also studied the conscious processes that affect behavior but were mainly interested in consciousness in relation to people's adaptation to the environment.
Early 1900s	Kraepelin and colleagues, proponents of the biological views of psychiatry, influenced research related to the biologic bases of behavior.
Mid-1900s	Psychoanalytic and behavioral schools of thought were dominant in the study of human behavior. Psychoanalytic theory emphasized unconscious mental processes. Psychoanalytic theorists also agreed that the early years of development are important. The behaviorists focused on mechanistic thinking and emphasized conscious control of behavior. The behaviorists used physiological concepts such as receptors, effectors, and conditioning as a basis for studying behavior and conducted experiments under controlled laboratory conditions. The learning theorists focused on learning in response to stimulus and reinforcement (reward) as the major basis for explaining behavior. The humanists were a dominant force that influenced the study of behavior. A goal of this group was to develop a multidisciplinary approach to the study of behavior that was broader than the behavioral and psychoanalytic approaches. The humanists emphasized the ability of individuals to assume responsibility for their behavior, basing their theory on the premise that the whole represents more than the sum of its parts.
1960s	American psychiatry shifted the focus of attention to the biological bases of behavior. General systems theory made its appearance and has since been continuously expanded. Symbolic interactionism became important to psychiatrists.
1970s	Flexibility of theoretical approaches was more apparent.
1980s	Increased interest in the biological explanation of mental health and mental illness.

causing behavior. When the functioning of the three systems is harmonious, individuals manifest relative stability. Discordant interaction among the three systems can lead to maladjusted behavior.

The id is the basic system of the personality structure and consists of all basic psychological processes that are present at birth. The id functions on a primitive level and is characterized by a lack of sense of time, irrationality, and a lack of logic. The id is amoral; that is, lacking moral sensibility. It is in contact with body processes, experiences the world subjectively and houses instinctual drives and *psychic energy (libido).*

The primary aim of the id is to experience pleasure and avoid pain. This tendency is referred to as the *pleasure principle.* When persons function according to the pleasure principle, they seek immediate gratification of needs, impulses, and wishes. Avoiding pain and seeking pleasure involves *primary process thinking.* Primary process thinking enables the individual to discharge tension by forming an image of the object that will remove the tension; for example, the infant has a hallucinatory experience involving a symbol for milk. This experience is referred to as *wish fulfillment.*

With maturation and the growing recognition that mental images do not satisfy needs, reality intervenes and the ego becomes differentiated from the id. Along with maturation, interactions with the environment and heredity influence the development of the ego. The ego is composed of processes and functions that mediate between the individual and the real "objective" world. The ego is the aspect of the personality that is in contact with reality.

The primary function of the ego is to mediate between the instinctual impulses and the environment to facilitate efficient satisfaction of the needs. In keeping with this function, the ego is the executive of the personality, maintaining harmony between the id, the superego, and the external world. The ego is the aspect of the personality that experiences anxiety and uses defense mechanisms to control the level of anxiety. The psychological functions of perception, memory, thinking, and action are also functions of the ego.

The *reality principle* and *secondary process thinking* govern the functions of the ego. The aim of the reality principle is to postpone immediate gratification until an appropriate object for satisfaction of the needs is available. This principle, then, functions in accord with the demands of reality. Secondary process thinking is logical, involving organized thought processes characterized by a causal relationship between events. This type of thinking is based on reality testing and consists of developing a plan of action as a result of problem solving.

The superego evolves from the ego in response to rewards and punishments from significant others. The superego begins its functions when the person has the capacity to identify with and internalize the prohibitions and demands of parental figures. This system is made up of two subsystems: the *conscience* and the *ego ideal.* The conscience is the prohibiting aspect of the superego and corresponds to the individual's conception of what parents consider morally wrong. The ego ideal is based on what parents consider morally good, and the individual strives to adhere to these ideals. The child learns what the parents perceive as morally good and bad through rewards and punishments. In addition to moral behavior are the ideals of beauty, strength, and success. To the extent that individuals are able to live up to the ideal standards of the superego, they experience inner satisfaction and increased self-esteem. When failure to fulfill one's ego ideals occurs, the person feels shame and a lowering of self-esteem. Failure to live up to moral standards leads to feelings of guilt. The superego may be in conflict with the id and ego as it fulfills its functions of (1) inhibiting the expression of id impulses, (2) persuading the ego to substitute moralistic goals for realistic ones, and (3) striving for perfection.

The id, ego, and superego need energy to fulfill their functions. Psychic energy (libido) is the form of energy used for the interaction of the id, ego, and superego. Psychic energy is body energy that is employed for psychological tasks such as thinking, perceiving, and remembering. Freud believed that each person has a specified amount of energy. The psychic energy used by the ego and superego is obtained from the id during the process of psychological development.

The psychic energy used by the three systems to perform their tasks is obtained from *instincts.* An instinct is an inborn psychological representation of a need. Body

TABLE 3-1 Freud's stages of psychosexual growth and development

Stage of Development	Critical Experiences	Developmental Task	Major Characteristics	Emergent Defense Mechanisms
Oral (birth to 18 months)	Weaning	Establishment of trusting dependence	Autoeroticism, narcissism, omnipotence, pleasure principle, frustration, dependence	Denial, introjection, projection
Anal (18 months to 3 years)	Toilet training	Development of sphincter control, self-control, feeling of autonomy	Reality principle, fear of loss of object love, approval and disapproval, beginning superego development	Sublimation, displacement
Phallic (3 to 5 years)	Oedipal conflict, castration anxiety	Establishment of sexual identity, beginning socialization	Differentiation between the sexes, superego more internalized	Identification, sublimation, reaction formation, undoing
Latency* (6 to 12 years)	Peer group experience, intellectual growth	Group identification	Superego influence in erotic interests, immense intellectual development	No new defense mechanisms; major operating defense mechanism, partial sublimations and reaction formation
Prepuberty and adolescence* (12 to 15 years)	Establishing heterosexual relationships	Development of social control over instincts	Identity, turmoil, needs of others	Intellectualization and asceticism
Genital (15 years to adult)	Sexual maturity	Resolution of dependence-independence conflict	Heterosexual relations	Use of all preceding defense mechanisms

*The latency and prepuberty and adolescence stages of psychosexual development were not included in Freud's original description of development. Anna Freud (1946) extended Freud's works when she described developments in these periods of life.

needs are the *source* of instincts. The *aim* of the instinct is to remove a body need. For example, the aim of the instinct of a hungry person is to remove the need of hunger. The *object* of the instinct is the means by which the aim is achieved. The *impetus,* or force, of the instinct is determined by the amount of energy used to achieve the aim. Freud believed that the source and aim of instincts remain constant throughout life unless the source is changed or eliminated by physical maturation. As new body needs emerge during development, new instincts may appear. The object various throughout life.

There are two categories of instincts: *life* instincts and *death* instincts. The aim of the life instinct is survival and propagation of the species. Hunger, sex, and thirst are examples of life instincts. Death instincts are also referred to as destructive and aggressive instincts.

Freud described three levels of consciousness that are closely related to structure of the personality. The levels of consciousness, referred to as the topographical theory of the mind, are *unconscious, preconscious,* and *conscious.* The unconscious level is the largest and consists of repressed memories, thoughts, and feelings. Instinctual impulses are in the unconscious and actively seek expression. Preconscious perception and memories are outside conscious awareness, but they are immediately available to consciousness when the need arises. These experiences require only recall to be brought into full awareness. Conscious experiences are those within conscious awareness at the moment. When attention is directed away from the experiences, they become preconscious.

Freud believed that the individual passes through a series of dynamically related predetermined stages of development, during which time sexual instincts undergo development and psychic energy becomes concentrated at specified *erogenous zones* of the body: the mouth, the anus, and the genitals. Tension becomes concentrated in these zones and can be relieved by manipulation of the region. The relief of tension is experienced as pleasure.

Freud referred to the first 5 years of development as pregenital; the individual's life is characterized by infantile

sexuality. He believed that the basic personality is formed by the end of the fifth year of life and that subsequent development builds on this basic structure. The stages of psychosexual development are summarized in Table 3-1. Failure to successfully achieve the tasks of each stage may lead to maladaptive traits (Table 3-2).

Carl Jung's analytic theory[33] is classified as psychoanalytic because of the emphasis placed on the role of the unconscious as a determinant of behavior. Jung described the structure of the personality, or *psyche,* as a composite of partial personalities that interact as a system. He believed that the psyche is the only thing people experience directly and know immediately. The *collective unconscious* is the most influential system of the personality. It is the inherited, racial foundation of the personality structure. The collective unconscious aspect of the psyche is a residue of the person's evolutionary development, an accumulation of experiences passed down from ancestors. Jung believed that this racial origin of the personality gives direction to the individual's behavior and determines, in part, what will become conscious and how the person will respond to experiences. That is, people are predisposed to certain experiences, and these predispositions are universal. Jung viewed fear of the dark and snakes and easily formed ideas about a supreme being as examples of predispositions.

The *ego,* which is the conscious mind, develops from the collective unconscious. The ego is the aspect of the personality that relates to the individual's feelings of identity and continuity. Perceptions, thoughts, memories, and feelings comprise the ego. In close contact with the ego is the individual's *personal unconscious,* which consists of experiences that were once conscious but that have been transformed by repression, suppression, or other mechanisms.

Archetypes are symbols derived from the collective experiences of the race. As structural components of the collective unconscious, archetypes relate to ideas, and modes of thought and provide clues to the hidden potentials and qualities of the person. The aim of the archetypical sym-

TABLE 3-2 Manifestations of failure to achieve developmental tasks

Stage of Development	Behavioral Manifestations
Oral	Behaviors centered around oral experiences, for example, smoking, obesity, substance (drug and alcohol) abuse; difficulty with trust; disturbed physiological (particularly gastrointestinal) reactions; pessimism; and excessive dependence, envy, and jealousy
Anal	Defiant behavior, bowel and bladder disorders; rage, diarrhea, constipation; obsessive-compulsive personality; perfectionism, stubbornness; and inability to control impulses and emotions
Phallic	Faulty sexual identity; problems with authority; sexual deviations; erotic attachment of male child to mother and of female child to father; phobic reactions; and conversion reactions
Latency	Lack of self-motivation in job; school problems, including lack of self-motivation; inability to accept proper social role; problems with relationships with persons of own sex; and behavior disorders such as stealing, lying, and sociopathic behaviors
Genital	Sexual acting out; excessively hostile attitudes toward authority; excessive dependence; unsatisfactory relationships with the opposite sex; serial marriages, and difficulty with sexual functioning such as frigidity and impotence

bols is the fulfillment of the individual personality as a whole. Jung believed that the archetypes are the source of the person's strength of will and inner resources that motivate him to discover his own personality.

Other systems of the personality, the persona, the anima and animus, and the shadow, develop from archetypes. Jung's conception of the *persona* is basically the same as other theorists' views of social role. The persona is a mask that a person wears in social situations. This mask is determined by the role assigned to the individual by society. The persona becomes a problem when the ego either identifies too closely with it or becomes too distant from it. Related to this problem is difficulty in differentiating between one's public self (persona) and one's private self.

The concepts of *anima* and *animus* relate to the essentially bisexual nature of people. The anima is the feminine archetype in the man, and the animus is the masculine archetype in the woman. The anima and animus develop from the racial unconscious experiences of man with woman and woman with man. These elements of the personality also evolve from the person's experiences with the parent of the opposite sex. Jung believed that people of each sex need to accept their bisexual archetype as reality, try to understand it, and integrate the archetype into the personality. The archetype will then serve a creative and constructive purpose.

The *shadow* archetype represents some of the unacceptable aspects and components of behavior. The shadow may operate within and outside consciousness; that is, the shadow archetype may account for an individual's lack of awareness of certain personal faults. To the extent that a person can accept the tendencies of the shadow as a part of himself, he is able to work toward wholeness of personality. Jung believed the shadow becomes more positive in the later half of life.

Jung's investigations led to theories about personality in middle and later years. Some of these views are presented in Chapters 42 and 43.

Erik Erikson[15] used Freud's psychoanalytic theory as a framework for his theory of personality. Erikson's primary goal was to build a bridge between psychosexual and psychosocial development. Thus he emphasized the importance of social and environmental factors within the home and community that influence development of the personality. He also extended Freud's theory by focusing on human development throughout the life cycle. The basis for some of his theoretical ideas is maladaptive behavior. However, unlike Freud, he derived the major portion of his theory from studies of the play activities of normal children and the functioning of young adolescents.

Erikson accepted many of Freud's ideas regarding the structure of the personality. Erikson used the terms *id, ego,* and *superego* and emphasized psychosocial development of the ego. He viewed the id and superego as horizontal polarities. The goal of the id is to meet its excessive and undisciplined wishes, whereas the superego strives to adhere to the internalized wishes of the parents and society. Erikson believed the superego is as barbaric as the id. The ego is the executive of the personality, assuming such functions as organizing external experiences, testing perceptual experiences, and governing action. These ego functions are considered positive and lead to control of the id's and superego's strivings and to a sense of oneself in a state of well-being.

Erikson accepted Freud's theory that instincts and psychic energy (libido) motivate behavior. Erikson believed that the libido is characterized by two dynamically op-

TABLE 3-3 Erikson's stages of psychosocial development

Stage of Development	Developmental Task	Major Characteristics
Oral-sensory (birth to 12 months)	Basic sense of trust versus mistrust	Mothering person viewed as significant
Anal-muscular (1 to 3 years)	Basic sense of autonomy versus shame and doubt	Ego skills; parallel play, negativism; ambivalence; self-control and will power; initial development of superego
Genital-locomotor (3 to 6 years)	Basic sense of initiative versus guilt	Cooperative play; fantasy; imitation of adults; development of conscience; directed and purposeful activities
Latency (6 to 12 years)	Basic sense of industry versus inferiority	Intellectual curiosity; government of behavior by rules and regulations; acculturation
Puberty and adolescence (12 to 18 years)	Basic sense of identity versus identity diffusion	Heterosexual relationships; establishment of identity
Young adult (18 to 25 years)	Basic sense of intimacy and solidarity versus isolation	Close personal relationships with adults of both sexes
Adulthood (25 to 45 years)	Basic sense of generativity versus stagnation	Creativity and productivity; parental sense; adjustment to life; lasting relationships
Maturity (older than 45 years)	Basic sense of ego integrity versus despair	Adjustment to changes; acceptance of culture; sense of continuity of past, present, and future; acceptance of death

posed strivings: a drive to live and an opposing drive to return to the earlier state before infancy. These drives are similar to Freud's life and death instincts and create a polarity. Erikson believed that the drives stimulate growth through the developmental stages.

Erikson's theory includes the three levels of awareness described by Freud: the *conscious,* the *preconscious,* and the *unconscious.* Erikson views the last two as most influential in the motivation of behavior.

Erikson described eight stages of development that are based on biological, psychological, and social events. The first five stages roughly parallel Freud's psychosexual developmental stages. The last three stages occur within adulthood. Each stage is characterized by a positive and a negative experience and an emotional crisis. Development involves a struggle between two poles, with experiences of the two essential for healthy growth. For example, the task of developing a sense of basic trust versus mistrust necessitates that the infant experience trust as well as mistrust to learn to differentiate between the two. Ultimately the infant needs to have more experiences with trust than with mistrust to grow psychologically. Erikson was optimistic in his views about continuous development throughout the life cycle and the possible opportunity for new solutions to problems at each stage. The eight stages and their related tasks are summarized in Table 3-3 and are discussed in Part IV of this text in relation to each phase of the life cycle.

Interpersonal

Harry Stack Sullivan,[67] credited with developing the most comprehensive theory of interpersonal relations, believed that the essence of being human is the capacity to live effectively in relationships with others. The influence of Freud's theory is evident in Sullivan's works. Social psychologists and anthropologists also greatly influenced his thinking about development. Sullivan believed the individual is a social being and that personality development is determined within the context of interactions with other humans. He recognized the influence of the person's biological system on development to the extent that the body is necessary for life. However, he believed society influences the individual's biological functions.

A central theme of Sullivan's theory is *anxiety* and its relationship to the formation of personality. He viewed anxiety as (1) a prime motivator of behavior, (2) a builder of self-esteem, and (3) the great educator in life. His ideas about anxiety are discussed in Chapter 10.

In keeping with his basic beliefs about the individual, Sullivan viewed the organization of personality as consisting of interpersonal experiences rather than intrapsychic ones. The *self-system* is a significant aspect of the personality that develops in response to anxiety. Disapproving and forbidding gestures during interactions with significant others contribute to the development of the self-system. In response to these gestures, *security operations* become a part of the self-system to help the individual avoid or minimize anxiety. The security operations include *sublimation, selective inattention,* and *dissociation.* Subli-

mation is an unconscious process of substituting a socially more acceptable activity pattern that partially satisfies a need for an activity that would give rise to anxiety. Selective inattention is an unconscious substitutive process by which many meaningful details of one's living that are associated with anxiety are not noticed. Sullivan believed selective inattention is a classic means by which individuals fail to profit from experiences related to problem areas. Dissociation is a system of processes for minimizing or avoiding anxiety by which parts of the individual's experiences called "not me" are kept out of consciousness. The self-system becomes unable to evaluate objectively the individual's behavior, and, because of this, Sullivan believed that the self-system is "the principal stumbling block to favorable changes in personality."[67]

Sullivan believed that at an early age individuals develop *personifications* that influence their perceptions of people throughout life. A personification is an image that individuals have of themselves and other people resulting from experiences with anxiety and satisfaction of needs. The basis for the development of personifications of self and others is the infant's early need-satisfaction experiences with the mothering one. Depending on the infant's experience, the mother is personified as a good mother or a bad mother. For example, because the infant experiences discomfort in his interaction with her, an anxious mother is personified as a bad mother. During development, the either-or personifications become fused and complex. When this fusion is not achieved, the individual goes through life with a polarized view of himself, other people, and situations. Everything is viewed in dichotomous terms such as black or white and good or bad.

Sullivan believed that during infancy (through sensations of the body and the caregiving of significant others in response to body needs) three personifications of "me" gradually evolve: *"good me," "bad me,"* and *"not me."* The "good me" results from experiences of approval and tenderness and leads to good feelings about onself. Experiences related to increasing anxiety states result in the "bad me." The "not me" evolves in response to overwhelming anxiety and results from experiences that are poorly grasped and that retain an uncanny quality like horror, dread, and awe. These personifications belong to the self-system.

Sullivan described the cognitive processes in terms of modes of experiences: *prototaxic, parataxic,* and *syntaxic.* The prototaxic mode of experience is the initial type and is characterized by sensations, feelings, and fragmented images of short duration. These experiences occur at random, are not connected logically, and leave memory traces as a basis for the next level of experience. This primitive type of experience is found during the early months of infancy and may be observed in deep psychotic states.

With the parataxic mode of experience, events that occur at the same time but are still not logically connected are viewed as being causally related. A child stated that every time he saw a police car there was an accident so he thought police cars caused accidents. This type of thinking is characteristic of development and is normally manifested throughout childhood. However, Sullivan believed that much of the individual's experience may not progress beyond this level. The parataxic mode of experience is frequently the foundation for adult prejudices and superstitious beliefs. The term *parataxic distortion* is used to label adult experiences in the parataxic mode.

The highest level of experience, which begins in the juvenile era, occurs in the syntaxic mode. Experiences that occur in this mode are logically interrelated and contribute to logical thinking. The syntaxic mode is characterized by consensually validated symbols: symbols accepted by enough people that they have a universal meaning. Sullivan believed that an individual can have meaningful relationships with others only when he has learned the syntaxic mode of experience.

Sullivan described six stages of personality development from birth to maturity that he divides according to the capacity for communication and integration of new interpersonal experiences. Experiences during each stage are influenced by those of the previous one. The personality achieves some degree of stability at the end of the juvenile era, but the personality continues to develop beyond this time and has the potential for corrective experiences. Sullivan believed that the juvenile and preadolescent eras contain the greatest opportunity for corrective experiences. The stages of personality development are summarized in Table 3-4.

Transactional

Eric Berne, the founder of transactional analysis, was trained in classic psychoanalysis. He departed from orthodox psychoanalysis when he developed his theory of transactional development; however, the influence of his psychoanalytic thinking is such that his theory can be grouped with the psychoanalytic theories of personality development.

Berne[5] assumed that the structure of the personality consists of *ego states.* An ego state is a coherent system of feelings and its related set of behavior patterns. The ego states are psychological realities in that they represent real people. Each person has three ego states: the Parent, the Adult, and the Child.

The Parent ego state is a collection of recordings of external events the person experienced during the first 5 years of life. Everything he saw the parental figures do and heard them say is recorded in the Parent. This ego state includes all of the rules and parental admonitions (the "shoulds" and "should nots") as well as some pleasant experiences. There are two forms of the Parent: the direct and the indirect. When the Parent is directly active, the message is "do as I do." Indirect influence of the Parent is evident when the individual adapts to the parents' requirement of the way they wanted him to respond. The message in this situation is "Don't do as I do, do as I *say* to do."

TABLE 3-4 Sullivan's stages of interpersonal growth and development

Stage of Development	Developmental Tools*	Developmental Task	Interpersonal Needs	Cognitive Mode of Experience
Infancy (birth to 1½ years)	Cry, mouth, satisfaction response, empathic communication, emergency reactions, autistic invention	Learning to count on others to meet needs	Need for contact	Prototaxic
Childhood (18 months to 6 years)	Language, anus, self, identification, anxiety, autistic invention, emergency reaction; anger, shame, guilt, and doubt	Learning to accept, in relative comfort, interferences with wishes	Need for adult participation in activities	Largely parataxic
Juvenile (6 to 9 years)	Competition, compromise, cooperation	Learning to form satisfactory relationships with compeers	Need for compeers Need for acceptance	Mostly syntaxic
Preadolescence (9 to 12 years)	Capacity to love, collaboration, consensual validation	Learning to relate to chum of same sex	Need for chum, friend, or loved one	Syntaxic
Early adolescence (12 to 14 years)	Lust, anxiety	Learning to become independent; learning to establish satisfactory relationships with members of the opposite sex	Need for intimacy	Syntaxic
Late adolescence (14 to 21 years)	Genital organs	Learning to become interdependent; learning to form durable sexual relationship with selected member of opposite sex	Need for heterosexual relationship	Fully syntaxic

*Experimentation, exploration, and manipulation are tools used during each stage of development.

The Child ego state represents archaic fears and expectations. It is characterized by autistic thinking comparable to what Freud designated as primary process thinking. The Child state records the child's response to internal events that he sees, hears, feels, and understands. Most of the information stored relates to feelings, because at the time the person made the recordings, he had no words with which to give meaning to his experiences. The Child ego state consists of negative and positive information. The negative information is a by-product of the demands of the socialization process. For example, toilet training placed demands on the child and caused frustration of his desires. On the basis of these negative experiences early in life the individual concludes "I'm not OK." Some positive aspects are curiosity, creativity, and a desire to explore and have fun. Because of these positive attributes, Berne believed the Child ego state was the most valuable part of the personality, because it allows access to pleasures experienced in childhood.

The Adult is characterized by reality testing and rational thinking, comparable to Freud's secondary process thinking. This ego state processes incoming information in accord with reality. The Adult state examines and regulates the activities of the Parent and Child. This ego state also makes decisions about what the individual will and will not do. These functions are essential for dealing with the outside world.

The ego states shift from one state of mind or one behavior pattern to another. Each ego state has its place and function and contributes to a healthy balance of the personality. When one or the other disturbs the balance, psychopathology may result.

Berne[6a] identified four life positions that underlie people's behavior:

1. "I'm not OK, you're OK"—the depressive, despair position
2. "I'm not OK, you're not OK"—the futility, giving-up position
3. "I'm OK, you're not OK"—the destructive, arrogant position
4. "I'm OK, you're OK"—the healthy, mature position

The first three positions are based on feelings. The fourth is based on thought. An individual can make a decision to move to a new position. These four positions are universal and learned during early development as the child has transactions with the parental figure. The positions are complex and contradictions may exist; however, each person usually has one basic position that governs his life and from which he plays out his games and scripts.

Berne[6] defined a psychological *game* as a type of human behavior that is predictable, stereotyped, usually destructive, and directed by hidden motives. During childhood, the individual is taught what games to play and how to play them. He then plays these games throughout his life, changing only such external events as place, person, and time. People tend to have a small collection of games that they use as a basis for their social relationships, and they find people with whom they can share these games. The games determine the use each individual will make of

opportunities in life. Games also determine the person's ultimate destiny, such as the "payoffs" in his marriage and career, and circumstances surrounding his death.

A *script* is the individual's unconscious life plan.[5] During development the individual makes decisions as to how he will live his life. The script is written unconsciously by the Child. Scripts as a complex set of transactions may or may not recur. A script is maintained by basic life positions, by games, and through strokes.

Strokes are the basic motivators of behavior.[5] Initially the infant needs strokes for survival. As he grows older symbolic expressions such as words and glances are meaningful strokes. Ideally strokes are positive and given in a kind, loving manner. However, negative strokes may be exchanged in some families. Negative strokes may be perceived as better than none at all and can also be important for survival. Stroking begins during the infant's earliest transactions with the mother.

A *transaction* is a unit of social intercourse. It is a stimulus from an ego state of one person and the corresponding response from the ego state of another person.[6a] The transactions that begin at birth continue throughout development. When any two or more people are in close proximity, sooner or later a transaction will take place. The simplest transactions are those in which both stimulus and response arise from the Adult state of each person. The Child-Parent are the next simplest transactions. Transactions may be:

1. Complimentary—when the response is what is appropriate and expected
2. Crossed—when communication is broken off
3. Ulterior—those transactions involving the activity of more than two ego states
4. Angular—those transactions involving all three ego states

The first transaction in the baby's life centers on getting his nourishment during the nursing situation. The rudiments of games are formed during these earliest transactions with the mother. As the child comprehends that he is separate from the mother and has some degree of independent existence, there is the beginning of Adult functioning. The infant begins to learn that he has some control of himself in that he is able to find the nipple and release it at will.

A new set of transactions develops as the child realizes he has to control his body in a way that is acceptable to people around him. Bowel training involves a long, complicated series of transactions that have the potential for development of maneuvers and games by the child and the mother.

The child next discovers that he has to share his mother with other people who are more powerful than he, such as the father, or a person the mother seems to prefer, such as a newborn sibling. The child, who is now 2 or 3 years old, develops games in his attempt to deal with the rivalries. At 4 to 7 years of age the child begins to make decisions, to take positions that justify the decisions, and to ward off influences that threaten his positions. The actions he takes determine his script (life plan) and affect his social relationships in later life.

As the child has transactions with other children and teachers at school, he tries out the games he learned at home. He sharpens some, tones down others, abandons some, and picks up new ones. He also tests decisions and positions. The influence of his family experiences is still evident in his transactions.

Adolescence is the first time the individual makes autonomous choices; however, these are still influenced by decisions made in early life. He reevaluates his basic decisions and positions in light of new experiences with peers. He fluctuates between using the actions learned early in life and trying out new ones. By his early twenties, the individual makes a decision to adhere to positions acquired earlier or modify his decisions. These decisions remain relatively constant until he reaches his forties, when he again struggles with new experiences that require reevaluating his basic positions. The remainder of life follows a similar pattern.

BEHAVIORAL THEORY

Behavioral theory is based on the premise that all behavior, adaptive and maladaptive, is a product of *learning.* Learning is a change in behavior that results from reinforcement. A related assumption is that, since behavior is learned, it can be unlearned and adaptive behavior can be substituted.

Conditioning is a type of learning. The classic work of **Pavlov**—the evoking of salivation in dogs with the ringing of a bell—is an example of a conditioned reflex and response. With training, the dogs associated the bell (stimulus) with food (reinforcement).

Neurotic symptoms are viewed as learned habits or responses that have been repeatedly reinforced. This view of the nature of the human condition has been considered both deterministic and reductionistic in that an individual's behavior is perceived to be under the control of past learned experiences and current environmental circumstances. This original view of behavior reduces human interaction to a set of mechanistic principles that preclude the concepts of freedom of choice, individual autonomy, and responsibility for one's destiny.

Behavioral therapists and theorists such as Albert Bandura[2] have emphasized the reciprocal interactive relationship between individuals and their environments; that is, individuals are seen as being active in influencing the environment, which in turn influences their behavior. In this newer approach, called social learning theory, clients are encouraged to be active participants in their therapy by defining problems, selecting objectives, and evaluating outcomes.

B.F. Skinner[65] is a behaviorist who avoided focusing on inner mental functioning such as repression and emphasized observable data when analyzing human behavior. He was interested in learning why the specific behavior started and what is happening in the current situation that makes it rewarding for the person to continue the behavior. His theory is based on *operant conditioning* techniques. Operant responses are emitted by the person rather than elicited by a stimulus. In operant conditioning, the subject actively manipulates the environment. This characteristic distinguishes Skinner's approach from the more passive Pavlovian conditioning.

One of the key concepts in Skinner's theory of operant conditioning is *reinforcement:* "any event, contingent upon the response of the organism, that alters the future likelihood of that response."[64] *Positive reinforcement* is a reward for selected behavior, and *negative reinforcement* brings anxiety-producing sanctions against whatever behavior is in progress. Thus continued rewards tend strongly to perpetuate desired behavior, whereas negative reinforcement is likely to extinguish undesirable behaviors.

Another concept of significance is *response frequency,* which refers to the frequency with which a response is expressed. In a treatment situation, the client's task is to adapt his repertoire of activities to behaviors approved by society and to abandon behaviors that are negatively sanctioned. This guidance of the individual in achieving the desired behavioral response is referred to as *shaping,* and the overall approach is called operant conditioning.

Joseph Wolpe[75] based many of his ideas on the concept that all behavior is learned; that is, individuals are conditioned to respond to a stimulus. Behavior, then, is a series of habitual responses to a familiar series of stimuli. Wolpe described neurosis as the use of maladaptive ways of responding in anxiety-producing situations.

Wolpe began developing his conditioning theory by producing experimental neurosis in animals in the mid-1940s. Based on this initial work, he developed a theory that considers anxiety as a generator of behavior. The individual with neurosis crystalizes the behavior as a way of coping. Wolpe hypothesized the *principle of reciprocal inhibition;* that is, if a pleasant or anxiety-reducing state is experienced at the same time the anxiety-provoking stimuli is introduced, this new experience diminishes the anxiety response to the stimuli.

A related concept basic to Wolpe's theory is *anxiety hierarchy.* Hierarchical relationships are established among anxiety-producing stimuli. With this approach, a more acceptable behavior is substituted for the symptom by learning another way of coping with the underlying anxiety. One such way developed by Wolpe is *systematic desensitization,* which is a counterconditioning technique for extinguishing maladaptive responses and replacing them with more acceptable (adaptive) responses. The details of this and related techniques are discussed later in this chapter.

John Dollard and **Neal Miller's** *stimulus-response theory*[13] emphasizes reinforcement or reward as the essential ingredient for the formation of a new stimulus response. They explored the determination of the conditions under which habits are formed and broken. A *habit* is a link of association between a stimulus and a response. Four concepts related to the learning process are basic to Dollard and Miller's theory: drive, cue, response, and reinforcement (reward).

A *drive* is a stimulus that has sufficient strength to impel the person into activity. *Primary drives,* which may be essential for survival, are innate and in close contact

TABLE 3-5 Piaget's stages of cognitive development

Stage of Development	Critical Experience	Major Characteristics
Sensorimotor (birth to 2 years)	Learning to recognize the permanence of objects	Goal-directed behavior; imitation in terms of make believe
Preoperational		
Preconceptual (2 to 4 years)	Symbolic mental activity; learning to think in terms of past, present, and future	Egocentrism; use of languae as major tool
Intuitive (4 to 7 years)	Learning to integrate concepts based on relationship	Comprehension of basic rules; increased exactness in imitation of reality
Stage of concrete operations (7 to 11 years)	Learning to use logic and objectivity in concrete thoughts	Classification of events; reversibility
Stage of formal operations (11 to 15 years)	Learning to think abstractly and logically	Use of scientific approach to problem solving

with physiological processes such as hunger, pain, and sex. These drives are important determinants of behavior to the extent that means for reduction of the drive stimuli are available to the person. The hunger drive of a person without the availability of sufficient food is strong and an important determinant of the person's behavior. *Secondary drives* evolve during the process of growth and incite and direct behavior. The stimuli of these drives generally replace those of the primary drives. The person learns to respond to secondary drive stimulation with appropriate adaptive activity, such as eating before primary drive stimuli (hunger pangs) are experienced.

A *cue* is a stimulus that determines the nature of the person's *response.* The time, place, and type of response are related to the cue. The response is learned in relationship to a given cue in the environment; during the process of growth, individuals learn a hierarchy of responses. *Reinforcements (rewards)* strengthen the connection between a given response and a particular cue and lead to a recurrence of repetition of the response. When the response is not reinforced, *extinction* of the behavior occurs.

Dollard and Miller believed that in the process of growth a person experiences *conflict,* which is opposition between two drives that are experienced simultaneously in response to the same situation. This concept is discussed in Chapter 11. The frustration-aggression hypothesis, which is basic to their theory of human behavior, is discussed in Chapter 12.

COGNITIVE THEORY

Jean Piaget's theory of cognition[56] is based on the assumption that human personality evolves from a composite of interrelated intellectual and affective functions. He believed that consciousness, judgment, and reasoning depend primarily on the evolving intellectual capacity of individuals to organize their experiences. Related to this assumption is his view that the total experiences of individuals shape their interests and the specific experiences they tend to pursue.

Piaget's theory of personality development describes the developing child as passing through four main, discrete states: the sensorimotor stage, the preoperational stage, the stage of concrete operations, and the stage of formal operations (Table 3-5). Each stage reflects a range of organizational patterns that occur in a definite sequence and within an approximate age span in the continuum of development.

Development is influenced by biological maturation, social experiences, and experiences with the physical environment. During the process of cognitive development, the individual strives to find equilibrium between himself and his environment. This striving, referred to as *adaptation,* depends on the interrelated processes of *assimilation* and *accommodation.* Assimilation is the process by which the child develops the ability to handle new situations and problems with his existing mechanisms. The process of change that enables the individual to manage situations that were previously beyond his abilities is accommodation. *Schema,* another concept related to the child's development, is an innate knowledge structure that allows the child to organize, in his mind, ways to behave in his environment. Interaction between the child and his environment is directed by changes in the cognitive processes that allow the child to adapt, accommodate, and assimilate so that he can adjust to his environment.

Albert Ellis's rational emotive theory (RET) of personality[14] was developed as a therapeutic approach and consists of four basic premises:

1. Essentially all people start with a basic set of values and assumptions that govern much of their lives. Once these assumptions are made, subsequent rational and irrational thinking and behaving can be accurately specified, understood, and worked with.
2. All humans want to survive and be relatively happy while surviving. He defines happy as satisfied and free from unnecessary pain.
3. Usually individuals want to live in and get along with members of a social group or community.
4. Individuals want to relate intimately (satisfactorily) with a few selected members of this group.

He believed that behaviors which support these basic values are rational and those which interfere with the attainment of the values are irrational.

Ellis considered the ABC theory of personality in health and illness central to RET theory: *A* is the *a*ctivating event, *B* is the person's *b*elief system about A, and *C* is the emotional *c*onsequence. A person's appropriate or inappropriate emotional response to an experience is determined by the person's belief system about the experience and not by the experience itself. For example, if a person feels depressed (point C) after being rejected for a job (point A), the rejection does not cause the feelings of depression. Rather, it is the person's beliefs (point B) about the rejection. Rational beliefs and appropriate feelings related to the experience motivate the person to work harder to achieve the goal. A person who has irrational beliefs and inappropriate feelings tends to become resigned to defeat.

Aron T. Beck[3] focused on cognitive distortions characteristically seen in depression. Much depression, according to Beck, is the result of irrational, distorted thinking. The cognitive distortions are of several types: *arbitrary inference,* in which a negative conclusion is drawn from insufficient evidence ("My boss didn't smile at me this morning; therefore I have done something terrible"); *overgeneralization,* in which what is true for one event is assumed to be true for all others ("I botched dinner last night; I am a stupid wife, a failure as a mother, and a rotten person"); *selective abstraction,* in which focus on one aspect of an event negates all other aspects ("My marriage is failing because of my self-centered demands"); and *magnification and minimization,* in which marked distortions occur in evaluating oneself ("My anger at my friend for being late has destroyed our friendship").

This process of distorted thinking develops from a set of rules one holds about oneself, others, and the world. These rules are called *underlying assumptions,* and the individual regards them as unquestionably true; they are so basic to one's belief system that they are rarely critically examined, except in therapy. In cognitive theory the underlying assumptions are the basis of conflict because they rigidly limit one's alternatives for solving ambiguous or new life situations. Some of these rules are assumptions of *entitlement* ("The world owes me a living"; "Things always work out for the best"; "I deserve better than this"), *perfection* ("Unless I do everything 100%, I'm useless"; "Unless I am perfect, no one will love me"; "A mistake is shameful"), and *expectations* ("A good mother never gets angry at her children"; "If he loves me, he'd understand me"; "I'm nothing without love"). Underlying assumptions generally divide the world into black-and-white alternatives. Therefore, each time an ambiguous situation is encountered, an underlying assumption triggers the distorted thinking pattern, producing *automatic thoughts,* a kind of habitual shorthand conclusion about the situation that is not subjected to crtical evaluation; for example, the boss passes by the secretory without smiling, and she *automatically* thinks, "He's going to fire me because I'm a terrible secretary," These thoughts arouse feelings of anger, helplessness, depression, or worthlessness, the hallmarks of a depressive episode.

SOCIOCULTURAL THEORIES

Sociocultural theories introduce a change in emphasis from the intrapsychic, individualistic approach to an action-oriented, community-based theory that links a sociocultural system to mental health.[43] This approach emphasizes social processes and their roles in mental illness.

George Mead's formulations[51] on *symbolic interactionism* are influenced by sociocultural theory. The major tenet of this theory is the concept of self that develops through interaction between the child and his significant others. The self comes into being through trying out or testing behaviors, retaining those which result in social approval and rejecting those which are not acceptable. This approach is an extremely complex action-interaction network that falls under the term *socialization.* The significant others teach the child the *rules* by which to live. These rules acknowledge sometimes explicit, other times implicit, norms defined by a particular culture. Deviation from these rules to any significant degree creates social or interpersonal pressures. In tandem with the rules is a set of *roles.* Deviation from the norms also may coincide with role rejection. As an example, failure to be a mother in the commonly accepted sense of the word depends on definitions of the mothering role in a given group or social setting. However, the heart of each definition has a recognizable core. To violate the core definition, to transgress the outer limits of the social definition may well lead to a *label.* The label may encompass a legal term (child abuse, for example) or a social definition ("poor mother").

Labels arise from norm deviations; these labels have a powerful force in deciding the fate of people who are tagged with terms such as "eccentric," "drunk," and "gambler." The label "crazy" is a familiar one; the consequences of acquiring a psychiatric label may be a lifelong liability. In every society and every cultural group within each society, there are acceptable behaviors, unacceptable behaviors, and behaviors that receive a temporary label because of some unusual circumstances perceived in the specific situation. Most of our everyday transactions are well within the "acceptable range"; those which exceed the usual expectations have been labeled deviant.

Thus social meaning, the consensus within a particular group, is at the heart of symbolic interactionism. Social meaning depends on *consensual validation;* that is, a sometimes almost imperceptible but constant checking on what a given situation means to one's reference group. The term *consensus* describes the device people use to establish social meaning.

Thomas Szasz,[68] a sociocultural theorist, also studied the effects of sociocultural variables on labeling behavior not conforming to social norms as deviant behavior. He recognized certain dangers in labeling others' behavior and believed that getting rid of the label is almost impossible despite social pressures to do so. He made an impact with his characterization of mental illness as a "myth." Szasz viewed mental illness as a label assigned to a group of persons who are unable or unwilling to conform to societal norms. These individuals are institutionalized in mental hospitals. This action is society's way of controlling disruptions of social life. His views served as a catalyst for reexamination of many legal, moral, and ethical factors in the confinement and treatment of clients with psychiatric problems.

Erving Goffman made lasting contributions to the study of behavior in the culture at large. His work, *Asylums,*[23] has been used extensively in the psychiatric world in assesment of the social factors that have an impact on patient residence in large public hospitals. Also derived from *Asylums* is the concept, *total institution.* A total institution is "a place of residence and work where a large number of like-situated individuals, cut off from the wider society for an appreciable period of time, together lead an enclosed, formally administered round of life."[23] The traditional state hospital is an example of a total institution. For one thing, it is possible for both "inmates" and staff members to remain at the hospital for long periods without leaving the grounds: food and other goods can be purchased in on-site stores, walks can be taken on the extensive grounds, gymnasiums are often available, movies are shown and other forms of recreation are available. There is a barrier to social interaction with the outside world. The institution, not the person's illness, is the most important factor in forming a mental hospital patient.

The concept of *stigma*[30] is also important in the care of the mentally ill. Goffman uses the term stigma to describe any attribute that makes one different or is discrediting in the categorization scheme employed by all societies, both large and small. The mentally ill, as well as many others who do not meet selected norms of a social group, are prominent in the discredited group.

Another movement pioneered by **Maxwell Jones**[29] is the concept of the therapeutic community. The term *therapeutic community* originated with **T.F. Main**[48] in 1946 when he was working with a group of demobilized, psychoneurotic former soldiers. The institution (hospital) was visualized as a community aimed at enhancing full participation in its daily life, resocialization and return to society. The means to achieve the goal is full participation in the microcosm that the ward or hospital represents. The concept of therapeutic community encompasses the use of the community's resources in a system of open and democratic communication.

GENERAL SYSTEMS THEORY

General systems theory is a science of "wholeness" characterized by dynamic interaction among the components of the system and between the system and the environment. A basic premise of systems theory is that a phenomenon cannot be understood independently of the system of which it is a part. General systems theory is also based on the assumption that an impact made on one component of a system affects the functioning of the total system. Instead of looking at parts of a person, for example, dealing only with the mind, general systems theory deals with both mind and body as they exist in a given environment. Systems can be persons, families, wards or care units in hospitals, educational centers, or shopping centers.

Ludwig von Bertalanffy[69] viewed a person as an active system in a larger system—the world. He considered the world a complex but well organized system. **Kurt Lewin**[47] suggested that each person or object exists in a particular field or environment. Within this person-field unit are two opposing forces: One set of forces producees change, and the other tends to halt change, thus upsetting the state of equilibrium. Lewin calls the direction that these forces take a *vector.* The psychobiological forces are made up of mind, body, and societal factors.

A *system* is a set of parts meshing with each other within a *boundary.* There are inputs, outputs, and throughputs across the boundary. Thus boundary lines delineating the shape of a system are an integral part of the systems concept.

Equilibrium, another important concept in the systems theory, refers to a balance among the parts of the system. The various parts inside the boundary have two possibilities: they can reach an even level, much as a scale can be balanced, or they can reach a steady state, in which they move dynamically through a process of exchange and rearrangements, maintaining a balanced relationship among all components. All systems tend to maintain a steady state, or a balance among the subsystems.

Feedback is another key feature of the systems theory, since systems maintain function and balance through communication. Feedback is necessary to communication. Since transmission of a message requires a sender and a receiver, the reply to the sender is described as feedback: literally "to feed back." The nature or kind of message sent determines how the return message will be structured or how long the interchange will last. A pleasant message usually will be received in a pleasant manner, whereas a curt, negative message can end the feedback loop at that point. Chapter 5 includes a more complete description of this process.

Certain concepts are related to the major terms just described. The first one, suggests that all living systems are open, with contacts across boundaries with input, output, and a functioning feedback system. A person is an open system in a state of constant exchange with other people (other psychological systems) as well as the environmental system, or physical world of components such as water, air, and food. According to the strict definition, no systems are truly closed, but a given system may have minimal inputs and outputs for a while.

EXISTENTIAL THEORY

Psychologists and psychiatrists in different areas of Europe in the 1940s and 1950s developed the initial existential orientation in psychiatry. Existentialism emphasized the totality of an individual's existence. The individual has responsibility for his own existence. Within this school of thought, recognition is given to the individual's values, his mode of being in the world and his religious qualities. Individuals are in a state of "becoming" which they control.

Each individual in living is forced to confront the ultimate existential dilemmas of death, isolation, and meaninglessness.[76] In this struggle the individual experiences anxiety, despair and dread. Suffering results. The individual uses maladaptive defenses to deny the inevitability of death, fails to accept freedom and therefore responsibility, fails to come to terms with individual isolation, and unsuccessfully struggles to develop individual meaning in life.

Erich Fromm,[21] generally allied with the interpersonal group, focused on the social and cultural aspects of human behavior, but primarily he was an existentialist in terms of theory. Fromm identified both positive and negative needs that must be met in a helpful, constructive way and, as with many existentialist theorists, saw as the ideal the individual who is free to live at the maximum of his particular capacities. Fromm clearly stated that this is the ideal but that often, as a result of family and cultural pressures, other patterns emerge.

Fromm is credited with developing the idea that *sadomasochism* is one "mechanism" that people use to escape from situations which interfere with expansion of their true selves. Sadistic and masochistic traits coexist in the person; they are opposite sides of the same coin and necessary for each other. A *sadist,* one who gains a feeling of power by inflicting pain on others, needs someone who is willing to incur the pain: the *masochist.* Both of these behaviors meet basic needs to relieve anxiety and to escape loneliness and powerlessness. In short, the behaviors are mechanisms of escape from what might be otherwise intolerable situations.

Fromm[23] developed several character types or prototypical constructions of general, observable kinds of personalities that are molded in the family and in the culture. A culture is influential in developing a set of characteristics common to most people in that group or society. Fromm has called this a *social character.* On top of this is built a unique pattern that interacts with the social character. Among the types developed are the *marketing character,* the *receptive character,* the *exploitative character,* the *hoarding character,* and the *productive character.*

HUMANISTIC THEORY

Because humanistic theory draws so heavily from existential theory, many refer to humanistic theory as existential-humanism.

Humanistic psychology is defined by a conception of the person as the most reliable source of knowledge about his own capabilities, resources, and characteristics. This psychology values all dimensions of the human condition from a holistic perspective: the physical, emotional, intellectual, social, and spiritual (see Chapter 9).

The humanists are similar to the ego psychologists in their emphasis on more conscious aspects of personality. According to the humanists, each person is an understanding, conscious, experiencing individual whose subjective impressions are at least as valid as the "hard data" of science. Personal growth or self-actualization is a response of the total person and, from the humanistic perspective, is among the most highly valued of goals. The current popularity of humanistic psychology is undoubtedly related to changing modern values such as personal freedom, individual responsibility, equality of opportunity, and protection of the land because it is the natural human environment. The humanists hold an optimistic view of human potentialities.

Among the diverse groups of theorists whose orientations are essentially consistent with the humanistic point of view are Frederick (Fritz) Perls, Abraham Maslow, Sidney Jourard, and R.D. Laing.

Perls[54,55] founded the gestalt theory. The major focus of this theory is the here and now; it encourages people to become aware of both psychological and physical functioning, since one affects and interacts with the other. Together they form a whole picture, or *gestalt.* Perls saw the individual as embedded or grounded in a situation with which he deals in terms of an open or a closed gestalt. The open gestalt is unformed, incomplete, or contains parts of a situation that remain as "unfinished business." When needs in the situation are met, the person can go on to another situation with a renewal of energy. Once this occurs, the gestalt is closed. The individual is encouraged to become aware of open gestalts, that is, to be himself in all facets of a situation and to devote his energies to moving toward closure of open gestalts. The open gestalts are anxiety-producing psychological states standing in the way of productive living and must be removed so that an objective and a subjective view of current reality are possible.

Maslow[49] viewed the personality as self-actualizing; that is, the ideal individual is one who is at the peak capacity of fulfilling his human potential. However, before peak fulfillment of an individual's capacity can occur, more basic needs, such as hunger, thirst, security, and physical safety, must be met. Thus Maslow devised a hierarchy of needs in the order of urgency of necessity for fulfillment. Once needs in the lower part of the hierarchy are fulfilled, those of a higher order can be met, such as the need to belong to a group, to be loved, to be looked on with esteem, and to have the respect of others. As the lower group of needs are met, the self is freed, or actualized, to create in whatever mode is suited to that person. An individual can then proceed to express himself in a personally creative way—in music, art, or as Maslow points out, by baking a superlative cake.

Jourard[30,31] discussed some of the self-actualizing, creative components of personality in his book *The Transparent Self.* The basic premise of his theory is that people who work with others in need must be in touch with their inner selves to the extent that they are genuinely relating as one person to another. This means that there is honesty in the relationship, not manipulative control or irrational use of interpersonal power. Jourard belived that the ability to disclose oneself to others is a sign of health and a distinct advantage in attempting to help others. A person who perceives himself as capable and who has adequate self-esteem will act in ways that indicate interpersonal capacity. Those who see themselves as nonfunctional, weak, and unable to relate to others will have too much anxiety to experience freedom in self-disclosure.

Laing,[37-39] a British psychiatrist, is perhaps best known for two things; his work with clients with schizophrenia and the publication of a book entitled *Knots* that expresses a series of communicative snarls in verse. Laing relates schizophrenia to lack of a core self; that is, the person so affected tries to assume roles that others have imposed from the outside, usually through family rules and metarules. *Metarules* are rules about rules, often unspoken. The environment, the individual's perception of the environment, and the family who pass along what their ancestors handed down to them all affect the individual. The individual then superimposes his unique perceptions or imaginings on the total picture. Laing called the process of handing down a set of patterns from one generation to another *mapping*. Each new generation has what was projected on and induced in it by the preceding generation. Of course, the preceding generation goes through the same process, and each generation develops its own response to all of the foregoing. Laing believed that at least three generations could be mapped.

STRESS THEORY

The development of the stress concept has contributed significantly to an understanding of the nature and causes of disease. Basic assumptions about stress have been applied to biological, psychological, and social behavior. Walter Cannon, Harold Wolff, Hans Selye, and R.S. Lazarus are among theorists who have made significant contributions to the development of the concept of stress.

Cannon[9,10] was the first physician to mention stress as a causative factor of disease. In developing his ideas about homeostasis, he described the strains and stresses resulting from pressure placed on specific mechanisms of the body that are necessary to maintain a steady state. He defines *homeostasis* as the maintenance of a normal steady state in the body. Fluid and electrolyte balance, body temperature control, nervous system control, and immune system response are homeostatic mechanisms that help maintain equilibrium.

Cannon applied the fight-light alert of the body to stress. He viewed disease as a fight to maintain the homeostatic balance of the body's tissues.

Wolff and Selye were the first to apply the term *stress* scientifically to medicine. **Wolff**[74] described stress as a dynamic state within the organism rather than an aspect of the external environment. He defined stress as an internal force produced by external forces or loads, and therefore viewed stress as the interaction between the external environment and the individual. Past experiences are a major factor in determining the response to stress.

Wolff[73,74] used a "protective reaction pattern" as a principal concept for the development of his ideas about stress. According to this pattern, threats to the physical integrity of the body cause a complex reaction to rid the body of the threat. Symbolic as well as physical threats initiate similar reactions. The reaction pattern involves alterations in feeling, body processes, and behavior.

Selye[63] developed a biochemical model of stress that focuses on an analysis of stress at the physiological and biochemical levels of functioning.[74] Selye defined stress as "a state manifested by a specific syndrome which consists of all the nonspecifically included changes within a biologic system." He viewed stress as the nonspecific response of the body to any demand made on it. The response is considered nonspecific in that no selectivity occurs and all or most parts of the body's systems must try to adjust to any specific agent of stress. Selye related stress to homeostasis when he described the body's adaptive response to cold by shivering. The goal of shivering is to return the body to its previous steady state.

A *stressor* produces stress. Any demand on the body, including those necessary to maintain life, are stressors. The body responds to both positive and negative stressors. Individuals experience multiple and constant stressors; these constitute the wear and tear on the body.

Selye believed that stressors to which people must adapt occur throughout life. Hereditary factors determine in part how an individual adapts to stress. However, the process by which all people adapt to stress is described by Selye as the *general adaptation syndrome* (GAS). GAS is the process by which the body's nonspecific responses to stress or noxious agents evolve through three stages of adaptation: (1) the *alarm reaction* (AR), (2) the *stage of resistance* (SR), and (3) the *stage of exhaustion* (SE).

The alarm reaction, the initial response to stress, is characterized by a generalized expression of the body's defense system. Selye found that no person can be maintained in the alarm reaction stage for an extended period without death ensuing. This recognition led him to identify and describe the stage of resistance; resistance to changes in the body organs lead to homeostasis and survival. The stage of exhaustion results from prolonged experiences with stress. The wear and tear on the body that accompanies this stage leads to premature aging. Selye believed that with most short-lived stressors, such as mental or physical exertion, only the first (AR) and second (SR) stages of GAS are manifested. People learn to adapt to the demands of their environment through repeated experiences with stages 1 and 2. Because SE is initiated by severe stress that may lead to death, it is not experienced as often as the other stages.

Selye believed that a person's adaptability is probably the most unique characteristic of life. The ability to adapt allows for the complexities of life, homeostasis, and resistance to stress.

Lazarus[41] proposed that the degree of reaction produced by a stressor is related to the subjective appraisal each individual makes of the event as threatening or nonthreatening. The Lazarus cognitive model of stress involves three phases: (1) *appraisal*, (2) *coping*, and (3) *outcome*.

Given a stressor, primary appraisal occurs as the person evaluates the stressor and the degree to which he is in danger. Secondary appraisal involves assessing the availability of adequate coping devices. Coping mechanisms can be palliative or involve direct action. The person meets or avoids the approaching threat when he takes direct action. Palliative mechanisms alter the distress the individual experiences in response to the event. The affectiveness of these actions leads to the overall outcome the event has on the person.

BIOLOGICAL THEORY

The biological explanation of mental illness is based on the assumption that the individual's biological development is influenced by genetics and organic factors that predispose a given individual to develop a psychiatric illness. Genetic factors include inherited diseases transmitted through defective genes from parents to children. Organic factors include chemical and physiological components of the person, which are influenced by the genetic factors. It is further assumed by some biological theorists that genetically or organically determined disorders are manifested as a result of certain kinds of environmental stresses.

Family, twin, and adoption studies have shown the important role of genetic factors in major psychiatric disorders. There is evidence that the incidence of schizophrenic disorders is much higher in the offspring of persons with schizophrenia than in the general population. Research also confirms a higher rate of bipolar disorder among children of parents with bipolar depression.

The studies of twins conducted by **Kallman**,[34] one of the first theorists to link genetics to mental illness, indicated that when one twin has schizophrenia the other has an 86% chance of having schizophrenia, especially when the twins are identical. Twins share an even higher occurrence (96%) of bipolar disorders.

In studies of biological and adoptive parents of matched groups of clients with schizophrenia, **Wender**[72] and his group found a significantly higher prevalence of schizophrenia and related disorders in the biological relatives of the adopted clients with schizophrenia than in the biological relatives of nonschizophrenic adoptees. These findings were apparent even when both groups of children were not raised by their biological parents but in adoptive homes that were comparative to those of the biological parents.

The earliest explanation of the biochemical causes of behavior was put forth in 1884 by Thudichum, who believed that mental illnesses were the external manifestations of poisons generated within the body. Presently, assumptions that biochemical factors underlie mental illness are based on two observations[17]: (1) the major psychoses, schizophrenia and affective disorders, have a strong familial tendency (genetic transmission), and (2) a large number of poisons, drugs, and somatic therapies are apparently capable of causing various forms of mental illness. Studies related to the chemical basis of mental illness have primarily focused on the role of the neurotransmitters. Many mental disorders may result from problems in the regulation of specific neurotransmitter systems including the production of dopamine, norepinephrine, and serotonin. There is neuron dysfunction with several major psychiatric disorders including schizophrenia and affective disorders.

Within the biological model, an interrelationship exists among mental functioning, the central nervous system, and the endocrine system. Cholinergic neuron malfunction has been hypothesized as contributing to some of the memory loss, emotional lability, and confusion in persons with Alzheimer's disease. Chronic brain disorders such as Huntington's chorea and Cushing's syndrome are thought to result from a combination of factors, including genes, hormones, and emotions. Vitamin deficiency syndromes may also result from an endocrine imbalance. For example, nutritional imbalances are suspected of contributing to the psychiatric instability of some women experiencing premenstrual syndrome and menopause.

The new science of *chromopsycophysiology* is based on the observation that almost every physiological process has a 24-hour cycle. This inner biological clock is responsible for homeostatic physiological functioning. In addition to the major 24-hour day-night cycle, other biological rhythms range from the microseconds of biochemical reactions, to the seconds of the heart cycle, to the 90-minute rapid eye movement (REM) cycle of dreaming, to the monthly menstrual cycle. The irregularity of these various cycles becomes apparent when there is a disruption because of disease, stress, or erratic synchronization, as seen in jet fatigue. Investigations are only beginning to determine relationships between abnormalities in biological rhythms and psychopathological conditions.

Extensive work dealing with an immunological abnormality in the blood of clients with schizophrenia has isolated a substance, taraxein, that researchers claim produces abnormal EEG activity and schizophrenic-like behavior. These studies conclude that schizophrenia may be an immunological disease.

Similarities between the catecholamines and the hallucinogen mescaline have been established. Studies have raised the question that an abnormal metabolite of the catecholamines may produce symptoms of schizophrenia.

Relationships between affective disorders and biogenic amines have been observed. Drugs that cause depletion of norepinephrine may produce depression. Elation or manic phases are associated with an increase in norepinephrine levels.

What has been referred to as a *medical model* of psychiatric care is encompassed within the biological theories. This model views mental illness as a diseased state of the mind, and is concerned with diagnosis, treatment, and prevention. Kraepelin's classification of psychoses influences the current classification of mental disorders into diagnostic categories. The DSM-III-R provides the specific criteria for making an accurate diagnosis. A group of psychiatrists called somatotherapists adhere strictly to the medical model, using electroconvulsive therapy (ECT) and a wide range of psychotropic medications.[27]

The theoretical approaches are summarized in Table 3-6 on pp. 43-44.

ECLECTIC APPROACH

An eclectic approach as a therapeutic modality encompasses the selection of the most appropriate theories and approaches from various orientations. If diverse theories are viewed as complementary perspectives of the truth of human beings rather than competing or exclusive, one can readily acknowledge the usefulness of all of these theories in a variety of nurse-client situations.

TABLE 3-6 Summary of theoretical approaches

Theory	Theorist	Emphases	Key Concepts
Psychoanalytic	Freud	The study of unconscious mental processes and the psychodynamics of behavior	Personality structure: id, ego, super-ego; libido, pleasure principle, reality principle, instincts; stages of psychosexual development
	Jung	The role of the unconscious as a determinant of behavior; the inherited racial foundation of personality structure	Collective unconscious, archetypes, persona, anima and animus, shadow
	Erikson	Psychosocial factors that influence development throughout the life cycle	Id, ego, superego; Conscious, pre-conscious, unconscious, developmental tasks; eight stages of biopsychosocial development
	Berne	Transactional development of the individual	Ego states, transactions; games, strokes, scripts
	Sullivan	Interpersonal experiences that influence development	Self-system, anxiety, security operations, personifications, modes of experience; stages of interpersonal growth and development
Behavioral	Pavlov	Mechanistic principles: individual's behavior is under the control of past learned experiences and current environmental circumstances	Conditioning; stimulus, reinforcement
	Skinner	Analysis of human behavior observed in the current situation	Operant conditioning; positive and negative reinforcement, response frequency, shaping
	Wolpe	Behavior is a series of habitual responses to a familiar series of stimuli	Principle of reciprocal inhibition, anxiety hierarchy, systematic desensitization
	Dollard and Miller	Reinforcement or reward as the essential ingredient for the formation of a new stimulus response	Drive: primary and secondary; habit, cue, response, reinforcement (rewards), extinction, conflict, frustration-aggression hypothesis
Cognitive	Piaget	The interrelationship of intellectual and affective functions in human development	Four discrete states in the stages of cognitive development; adaptation, assimilation, accommodation, schema
	Ellis	The values and assumptions that govern much of people's lives	ABC theory of rational emotive theory
	Beck	Cognitive distortions	Arbitrary inference, overgeneralization, selective abstraction, magnification and minimization, underlying assumptions, entitlement, perfection, automatic thoughts
Sociocultural	Mead	The development of self through the child's interaction with his significant others	Socialization, rules, roles, labels, consensual validation
	Szasz	The effects of sociocultural variables on labeling behavior that does not conform to social norms as deviant	Labels; mental illness as a "myth"
	Goffman	Social factors that have an impact on patient residence in large public hospitals	Total institution, stigma
	Jones	The hospital as a microcosm of the larger community	Therapeutic community
General Systems	Lewin	The interaction of the person-field as two opposing forces	System, boundary, equilibrium, feedback, vector
Existential	Fromm	Achievement of essence	Sadomasochism, social character
Humanism	Perls	The individual's awareness of his physical and psychological functioning	Gestalt
	Maslow	Fulfilling human potential	Hierarchy of needs, self actualization

Continued.

TABLE 3-6 Summary of theoretical approaches—cont'd

Theory	Theorist	Emphases	Key Concepts
Humanism—cont'd			
	Jourard	Self actualizing creative components of personality	Self-disclosure
	Laing	Schizophrenia and lack of a core self	Family rules, metarules, mapping
Stress	Cannon	The effect of strains and stresses of life on mechanisms of the body	Homeostasis, fight-flight, protective reaction pattern
	Wolff	Stress as a dynamic state within the organism	Protective reaction pattern
	Selye	Analysis of stress at the physiological and biochemical levels of functioning	Stressor, general adaptation syndrome: alarm reaction, stage of resistance, stage of exhaustion
	Lazarus	Cognitive model of stress	Appraisal, coping, outcome
Biological	Kallman	The influence of genetics and organic factors on the person's development of a psychiatric illness	Defective genes, environmental stresses
	Wender and others		

Nurse-client interaction is affected by many variables such as respective philosophies of life, values, motivations, time restrictions, and emotional and intellectual capabilities. Having a broad spectrum of theoretical approaches from which to select, the nurse is able to tailor interventions to the individual's needs or capabilities of the moment.

The following Case Example exemplifies an eclectic approach employed by a psychiatric nurse working with an adult woman who had survived severe long-term incestuous abuse as a child. Only those approaches that seemed most useful at different stages were applied.

Case Example

Laura is a 30-year-old woman who initially responded to a flier advertising a support-group for women who were sexually abused as children. The nurse of a local community mental health center facilitated this group. After a preliminary interview and assessment, Laura and the nurse decided that individual sessions would be initiated, the group experience to be an adjunct at a mutually agreed upon point. Laura and the nurse contracted to enter this process together. Weekly sessions lasted 1½ years.

After several sessions the nurse and Laura determined that similar to other survivors of long-term incestuous abuse, Laura was experiencing difficulties with the life issues of trust and self-worth. Specifically, Laura's long-term response to the sexual abuse was severely affecting her ability to establish and maintain intimate interpersonal relationships and to develop her potentials. Laura also exhibited an immobilizing reaction to rain storms.

Approaches

Psychoanalytic. Because long-term traumas existed during Laura's ego-formative years, the nurse selected an approach that used principles of psychoanalytic theory. This modified approach provided Laura an opportunity to examine the abuse within the context of life review, while developing insights into the psychogenic origins of her current problems. Interpretation and explanations were used as insight developed. During the course of the process the nurse became a surrogate nonabusing parent, and through support and acceptance, the therapeutic relationship provided opportunity for some degree of ego-restructuring and affirmation. Transferences, positive and negative, were discussed at appropriate times. For example, during one session the nurse reached up to scratch her head and Laura exhibited fear by wincing as if she were about to be struck. Laura acknowledged a fear that the nurse was going to strike her, as her father had. This transference was discussed, providing an opportunity for Laura to relate to the nurse in the here and now. Laura was able to move past the assumption that she had to be hurt in order to be cared about.

Behavioral. Several episodes of Laura's abuse occurred during thunderstorms. Laura developed a phobic response to adverse weather conditions. A desensitization tape was constructed that introduced sound recordings of water splashing, light rain, heavy rain, and finally thunderstorms with rain. These were gradually introduced following the relaxation exercise in the session. These relaxation exercises and eventually storm recordings were also practiced at home between sessions. Toward the end of the desensitization process, Laura and the nurse shared the experience of going into actual rain together. Laura slowly became reconditioned to the rain through relaxing and pleasurable events.

Cognitive. After approximately 6 months of sessions, the nurse suggested that Laura read a book, *Feeling Good,*[10] a self-help work that employs the techniques of cognitive therapy in identifying and modifying irrational thought assumptions and patterns. Laura did the suggested homework readings. Together in session, she and the nurse analyzed these readings. Laura was able to identify and diminish many of her automatic negative thought patterns and significantly reduce her tendency toward a depressive low self-esteem state.

Existential. Using gestalt "chair work" techniques, Laura emotionally expressed her long-withheld anger at the perpetrator father as well as grief and frustration about her unknowing, nonprotective mother. These exercises provided her with an experiential healing expression of her feelings. In addition, she was able to do this within a safe and supportive environment.

Once during a very difficult session in which Laura was evasive, noncooperative, and seemingly antagonistic, the nurse, after several traditional attempts at exploration and interpretation, stopped the process, admitting that she was confused and not quite certain what was happening. She then asked Laura if she was comfortable or satisfied with the way the session was going, or would she like to work with the nurse to begin again on a more authentic level. Laura responded that she was also confused. She immediately proceeded to deal with what was distressing her.

This demonstrates the existential use of the nurse as an authentic person, eliciting authenticity of behavior in the client. This new behavior in turn changes the nature of existence of the client—in this case from a shame-filled, secretive, and angry woman to one beginning to communicate more openly and responsibly.

Sociocultural. Understanding the nature of incestuous experiences and the tendency of the victim to maintain a sense of shame and secrecy, the nurse, after several individual sessions, encouraged Laura's participation in the support group for women survivors of childhood sexual abuse.

This group provided social support in which there was deep empathy among group members who had had similar experiences as children. Consensual-validation was shared as emotions and reactions were expressed. In addition, the group provided an excellent opportunity for the development of trust, intimacy, and communication skills.

During the course of the group, sociocultural conditions were examined that currently contribute to the abuse of children. Several group members, including Laura, became involved in sexual abuse prevention programs. These empowering activities greatly enhanced self-esteem.

This Case Example is representative of a nurse's use of a variety of client-appropriate paths to healing. Use of an eclectic method allows variability and expression of the nurses' and the clients' creative potentials. This process operates within the light of different theoretical orientations that examine the truth of human beings and how they live their lives and relate interpersonally as they share existence.

BRIEF REVIEW

Interest in the study of human behavior has existed for centuries; theology and philosophy provided the earliest focus on behavior. Experimental psychologists introduced a scientific approach to the study of behavior. They continued to focus on conscious aspects of the mind.

The psychoanalytic school of thought pioneered by Freud initiated a change in the focus of the motivators of behavior from conscious to unconscious processes. Therapists strive to develop insights, uncover basic conflicts, and restructure the personality.

Sullivan emphasized interpersonal relations in his theory of personality. Anxiety in human relations is central to his theory. In interpersonal therapy, both therapist and client actively participate in the process. Emphasis is on current issues and problems.

According to the behaviorists, the basis for behavior is learning in response to a stimulus response and reinforcement. Skinner, Wolpe, and Dollard and Miller focused on behavioral change. Therapeutic techniques are used to promote relearning experiences that in turn change behavior. Piaget, Ellis, and Beck focused on cognitive development and processes. Alteration in patterns of thinking is the goal of therapy.

Sociocultural theorists addressed the effects of social processes, conditions, and attitudes on individuals. Therapy involves the manipulation of these conditions, such as in a therapeutic community or groups. The focus is on developing harmony in human relations.

General systems theory emphasized wholeness. An impact made on one component of the system affects the functioning of the total system.

The existentialists gave consideration to personal responsibility and the here and now. Humanism emphasized health and human potential. The therapist participates in intense dialogue with the client, who assumes responsibility for establishing and achieving goals.

Cannon, Selye, Wolff, and Lazarus made major contributions to the theory of stress, thus increasing our understanding of the effects of stress on the body and mind as well as how to diminish or alleviate deleterious effects.

The biological theories contributed much to our present knowledge of the human psychic condition and mental illness. Attention is given to genetic and organic factors that contribute to mental illness.

Theories of human behavior serve as a framework for the mental health–psychiatric nurse. None of the various approaches covers all the aspects of human functioning. Thus the nurse is likely to select from several major theories and develop an eclectic approach to the study of behavior and application in her practice.

REFERENCES AND SUGGESTED READINGS

1. American Psychiatric Association: Diagnostic and statistical manual of mental disorders, ed. 3, Washington, D.C., 1980, The Association.
2. Bandura, A.: Principles of behavior modification, New York, 1969, Holt, Rinehart and Winston.
3. Beck, A.T.: Cognitive therapy and the emotional disorders, New York, 1976, International Universities Press, Inc.
4. Beck, A.T., and others: Cognitive therapy of depression, New York, 1979, The Guilford Press.
5. Berne, E.: Transactional analysis in psychotherapy, New York, 1961, Grove Press, Inc.
6. Berne, E.: Games people play: the psychology of human relationships, New York, 1964, Grove Press, Inc.
6a. Berne, E.: What do you say after you say hello: the psychology of human destiny, New York, 1972, Grove Press, Inc.

7. Burns, D.: Feeling good, New York, 1980, Signet.

8. Cannon, W.B.: The wisdom of the body, New York, 1932, W.W. Norton & Co., Inc.

9. Cannon, W.B.: Stresses and strains of homeostasis, American Journal of Medical Sciences **189**(1):1, 1935.

10. Caudill, W.: The psychiatric hospital as a small society, Cambridge, Mass., 1958, Harvard University Press.

11. Child, I.L.: Humanistic psychology and the research tradition: their several virtues, New York, 1973, John Wiley & Sons, Inc.

12. Davis, J.M.: Antipsychotic drugs. In Kaplan, H.I., and Sadock, B.J., editors: Comprrehensive textbook of psychiatry/IV, ed. 4, Baltimore, 1985, Williams & Wilkins.

13. Dollard, J., and Miller, N.E.: Personality and psychotherapy: an analysis in terms of learning, thinking, and culture, New York, 1950, McGraw-Hill Book Co.

14. Ellis, A.: The basic clinical theory of rational-emotive therapy. In Ellis, A., and Grieger, R.: Handbook of rational-emotive therapy, New York, 1978, Springer Publishing Co., Inc.

15. Erikson, E.H.: Childhood and society, ed. 2, New York, 1964, W.W. Norton & Co., Inc.

16. Erikson, E.H.: Identity, youth and crisis, New York, 1968, W.W. Norton & Co., Inc.

17. Freedman, A.M., Kaplan, H.I., and Sadock, B.J.: Comprehensive textbook of psychiatry II, ed. 2, Baltimore, 1975, The Williams and Wilkins Company.

18. Freud, A.: The ego and mechanisms of defense, New York, 1946, International Universities Press, Inc. (Translated by C. Baines.)

19. Freud, S.: The ego and the id, New York, 1962, W.W. Norton & Co., Inc. (Edited by J. Strachey.)

20. Freud, S.: A general introduction to psychoanalysis, New York, 1972, Pocket Books.

21. Fromm, E.: Escape from freedom, New York, 1941, Irvington Publishers, Inc.

22. Giovacchini, P.L.: Some elements of therapeutic actions in the treatment of character disorder. In Boyce, L.B., and Giovacchini, P.L., editors: Psychoanalytic treatment of schizophrenic borderline and characterological disorders, ed. 2, New York, 1980, Jason Aronson, Inc.

23. Goffman, E.: Asylums: essays on the social situation of mental patients and other inmates, New York, 1961, Doubleday & Co., Inc.

24. Goffman, E.: Stigma: notes on the management of spoiled identity, Englewood Cliffs, N.J., 1963, Prentice-Hall, Inc.

25. Goffman, E.: Strategic interaction, Philadelphia, 1969, University of Pennsylvania Press.

26. Greenblatt, M., Levinson, D., and Williams, R.H., editors: The patient and the mental hospital: contributions of research in the science of social behavior, Chicago, 1957, The Free Press of Glencoe.

27. Grinker, R.R., Sr.: Toward a unified theory of human behavior, New York, 1956, Basic Books.

28. Hinkle, L.E.: The concept of stress in the biological and social sciences, Science, Medicine and Man **1**:34, 1973.

29. Jones, M.: The therapeutic community, New York, 1953, Basic Books, Inc., Publishers.

30. Jourard, S.: Disclosing man to himself, Princeton, N.J., 1968, D. Van Nostrand Co., Inc.

31. Jourard, S.: The transparent self, New York, 1971, Van Nostrand-Reinhold Co.

32. Jung, C.G.: The psychogenesis of mental disease, New York, 1960, Pantheon Books, Inc.

33. Jung, C.G.: Two essays on analytical psychology, Princeton, N.J., 1966, Princeton University Press.

34. Kallman, F.: Heredity in health and mental disorders, New York, 1953, W.W. Norton & Co., Inc.

35. Karasu, T.B.: Psychotherapies: an overview, American Journal of Psychiatry **134**:851, 1977.

36. Knapp, S., and Mandell, A.J.: Effects of lithium chloride on parameters biosynthetic capacity for 5-hydroxytryptamine in rat brain, Journal of Pharmacology **193**:823, 1975.

37. Laing, R.D.: The politics of experience, New York, 1967, Ballantine Books, Inc.

38. Laing, R.D.: Knots, New York, 1972, Random House, Inc.

39. Laing, R.D.: Self and others, Baltimore, 1975, Penguin Books.

40. Langs, R.: The psychotherapeutic conspiracy, New York, 1982, Jason Aronson, Inc.

41. Lazarus, R.: Psychological stress and the coping process, New York, 1966, McGraw-Hill Book Co.

42. Leifer, R.: In the name of mental health, New York, 1969, Science House, Inc.

43. Leighton, A.: My name is legion: foundations for a theory of man in relation to culture, vol. 1, The Stirling County study of psychiatric disorders and sociocultural environment, New York, 1959, Basic Books, Inc., Publishers.

44. Lemert, E.: Human deviance: social problems and social control, ed. 2, Englewood Cliffs, N.J., 1972, Prentice-Hall, Inc.

45. Levine, S., and Scotch, N.A., editors: Social stress, Chicago, 1970, Aldine Publishing Co.

46. Levy, R., and others: Early results from a double blind, placebo controlled trial of high dose phosphatidyl choline in Alzheimer's disease, Lancet I:987, 1983.

47. Lewin, K.: A dynamic theory of personality: selected papers, New York, 1935, McGraw-Hill Book Co.

48. Main, T.F.: The hospital as a therapeutic institution, Bulletin of the Menninger Clinic **10**:66, January 1946.

49. Maslow, A.: Toward a psychology of being, Princeton, N.J., 1962, D. Van Nostrand Co., Inc.

50. Maslow, A.: Motivation and personality, ed. 2, New York, 1970, Harper & Row, Publishers, Inc.

51. Mead, G.H.: Mind, self, and society, Chicago, 1934, University of Chicago Press.

52. Moss, G.E.: Illness, immunity, and social interaction, New York, 1973, John Wiley & Sons, Inc.

53. Paul, G.L.: Insight vs. desensitization in psychotherapy, Stanford, Calif., 1966, Stanford University Press.

54. Perls, F.: The gestalt approach, Palo Alto, Calif., 1970, Science & Behavior Books.

55. Perls, F.: The gestalt therapy book, New York, 1973, Julian Press.

56. Piaget, J.: The origin of intelligence in children, New York, 1952, International Universities Press, Inc.

57. Piaget, J.: The growth of logical thinking from childhood to adolescence, New York, 1958, Basic Books, Inc., Publishers.

58. Piaget, J.: The child's conception of the world, Ames, Ia., 1963, Littlefield, Adams & Co.

59. Ruesch, J., and Bateson, G.: Communication: the social matrix of psychiatry, New York, 1968, W.W. Norton & Co., Inc.

60. Ruesch, J.: Therapeutic communication, New York, 1968, W.W. Norton & Co., Inc.

61. Rush, A.J., and others: Comparative efficacy of cognitive therapy and imipramine in the treatment of depressed outpatients, Cognitive Therapy and Research **1**:17, 1977.

62. Scott, R., and Howard, A.: Models of stress. In Levine, S., and Scotch, N.A., editors: Social stress, Chicago, 1970, Aldine Publishing Co.

63. Selye, H.: The stress of life, rev. ed., New York, 1976, McGraw-Hill Book Co.

64. Sidman, M.: Tactics of scientific research, New York, 1960, Basic Books, Inc., Publishers.

65. Skinner, B.F.: Science and human behavior, New York, 1953, The Macmillan Co.

66. Skinner, B.F.: Beyond freedom and dignity, New York, 1971, Alfred A. Knopf, Inc.

67. Sullivan, H.S.: Interpersonal theory of psychiatry, New York, 1953, W.W. Norton & Co., Inc.

68. Szasz, T.: The myth of mental illness, New York 1974, Harper & Row, Publishers, Inc.

69. von Bertalanffy, L.: General systems theory: foundations, development, applications, New York, 1968, George Braziller, Inc.

70. Waldinger, R.J.: Psychiatry for medical students, Washington, D.C., 1984, American Psychiatric Press, Inc.

71. Watzlawick, P., Beavin, J.H.; and Jackson, D.D.: The pragmatics of human communication: a study of interactional patterns, pathologies and paradoxes, New York, 1967, W.W. Norton & Co., Inc.

72. Wender, P.H., and others: The psychiatric adjustment of adopting parents of schizophrenics, American Journal of Psychiatry **127**:1013, 1971.

73. Wolff, H.G.: Life stress and bodily diseases, Baltimore, 1950, Williams & Wilkins.

74. Wolff, H.G.: Stress and disease, Springfield, Ill., 1953, Charles C Thomas, Publisher.

75. Wolpe, J.: The practice of behavior therapy, ed. 2, New York, 1973, Pergamon Press, Inc.

76. Yalom, I.: Existential psychotherapy, New York, 1980, Basic Books, Inc., Publishers.

ANNOTATED BIBLIOGRAPHY

Burton, A., editor: Operational theories of personality, New York, 1974, Brunner/Mazel, Inc.

This book provides a discussion of personality theories which deal with change in the personality and which conceives personality as a growing entity. Each theory is described by its founder, if alive, or a major apostle. The concepts and techniques of the theory are applied, using a case study.

Clausen, J.: Stigma and mental disorder: phenomena and terminology, Psychiatry **44**:287, 1981.

Although the classic approaches to stigmatizing the mentally ill have been well developed to date, this article attempts to sharpen the concept. The data and analysis indicate that self-doubt and chronicity, rather than the views of others in society, impact on the client.

Norbeck, J.: The use of social support in clinical practice, Journal of Psychiatric Nursing and Mental Health Services **20**(12):23, 1982.

This article develops the concept of *social support* and applies it to the chronically mentally ill. Part of the article can be applied to many diverse populations; however, the thrust of the content illustrates application of theory to a psychiatric population.

Sill, G., and Hall, J.: A general systems perspective for nursing. In Hall, J., and Weaver, B., editors: A systems approach to community health, Philadelphia, 1977, J.B. Lippincott Co.

This chapter, written as an overview of general systems theory, extends its discussion past that of the familiar psychiatric-interpersonal theory. It also addresses concepts that are valuable across many clinical fields.

Gambrill, E.: Behavior modification, San Francisco, 1977, Jossey-Bass, Inc., Publishers.

Although this is a very large and comprehensive work, it will be useful to the person concerned with intervention, assessment, and ethics of behavior modification. Many of the conditions encountered in the psychiatric world can be found, among them alcohol and drug abuse, depression, and self-management of stress.

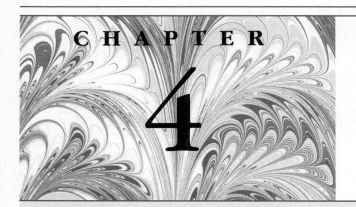

CHAPTER 4

NURSING THEORISTS' APPROACHES

Margaret T. Beard   Margie N. Johnson

After studying this chapter the learner will be able to:

Discuss key factors in the historical development of mental health–psychiatric nursing theory.

Describe the philosophical foundations and major concepts characterizing each nursing theory.

Analyze the usefulness of theoretical frameworks in providing a holistic approach to mental health–psychiatric nursing concepts.

Assess relative strengths and weaknesses of the nursing theories in guiding nursing practice.

Identify research problems to test the applicability of selected theories to mental health–psychiatric nursing practice.

Grand theories emerged as nurses began to focus on the content of their profession. A grand theory consists of broad concepts from which more specific theoretical frameworks are derived. Early theoretical writings depicted nursing as a process centered around the relationship between the client and nurse. Peplau's focus on interpersonal relationships,[31] Roger's formulation of person-environment interaction,[33] and King's view of nurse-client transaction[20] are examples of grand theories.

In the mid to late 1970s several theorists and their followers began to develop middle range theories through the testing of grand theories. A middle range theory consists of a conceptual scheme from which working hypotheses can be derived and tested. A perspective of the client constitutes middle range theory. Thus Orem's view of the client as a self-care agent,[28] Johnson's view of the client as a behavioral system,[15] and Roy's view of the client as a holistic adaptive being[35] are examples of the specificity of middle range theory.

In the past decade many writers have stressed that nursing theories should be practice oriented. A theory of practice consists of a set of interrelated theories of action that specify, according to the situation, the action that will, under the relevant circumstances, yield the intended consequences.[24] Practice theory is needed to direct nursing therapeutics and to evaluate outcomes of nursing interventions.

In the late 1960s Dickoff and James[6] influenced nursing by identifying four levels of theory: factor-isolating, factor-relating, situation-relating and situation-producing. Nursing practice theory is synonomous with situation-producing theory.

The six major theoretical nursing approaches described in this chapter are in various stages of development, but each gives some direction to practice. The work of each theorist has potential for explaining the holistic perspective of persons in a psychiatric–mental health context.

PEPLAU'S INTERPERSONAL THEORY

Hildegard Peplau's book *Interpersonal Relations in Nursing,*[31] made a major contribution to theory-based practice. Her approach, which evolved from problems in clinical situations, is process oriented and focuses on interpersonal theory as applied to the nurse-client relationship.

Major Concepts

The core of Peplau's approach is interpersonal relations. The theory comprises concepts such as communication, roles, and growth and development. All are used in expanding her conceptualization of the therapeutic

Historical Overview

DATE	EVENT
Pre-1860	Atheoretical
1860-1951	Florence Nightingale: *Notes on Nursing: What it Is and What it Is Not* (environmental theory)
1952-1960	Grand theories formulations (for example, Hildegarde Peplau)
1959-1964	Metatheoretical writings regarding the necessity of theory for nursing Grand theories Nursing science emphasized the need for a theoretical base for practice predicated on holism and the interconnectedness of person and environment
1965-1970	Nursing theory development conferences (Norris — 1969, 1970, and 1971) WICHE Conferences Dickoff and James writings
1971-1975	Conceptual frameworks for curriculums required by NLN Grand theories continue Middle range theories begin Nurse educator conferences Nursing theory conferences Theory construction writings
1978	Advances in Nursing Science (ANS) began as a forum for testing and developing nursing theory and nursing science
1980	Postdoctoral theory conferences — Clemson University Practice theory continues
1984	Nursing Science Colloquia — Boston University Practice theory continues
Future	Testing nursing theories in mental health–psychiatric nursing will contribute to their usefulness in practice

nurse-client relationship. Communication is a problem-solving process whereby the nurse and client collaborate to meet the client's needs. The position assumed by the nurse during various phases of the relationship is known as a role. In an effort to address the client's needs the nurse may assume the roles of counselor, leader, resource, surrogate, teacher, or technical expert to address the client's needs. In the therapeutic interaction these roles are designed to lead to growth and development.

A diagram of the major concepts of Peplau's theory is provided in Figure 4-1. Peplau views the therapeutic relationship as being divided into four sequential phases: orientation, identification, exploitation, and resolution. The activities involved in each of these phases are described in Table 4-1.

Holistic Perspective

The holistic approach to the person, family, and community is inherent in Peplau's theory. The nurse's approach mobilizes the person's innate capacity for self-healing and growth. Individual therapy in the interpersonal process allows the client to discover and resolve the intrapsychic and relationship patterns that tend to become chronic. Other holistic threads emphasize interpersonal relations, illness as an opportunity for discovery, and an appreciation for the quality of life and an interest in improving it. The interpersonal process affects both nurse and client, because both experience growth.

Physical dimension. The physical dimension is reflected in the clients' somatic responses to life experiences. For example, the emotional and physical dimensions are interrelated in insomnia caused by emotional trauma. Insomnia may be associated with anxiety generated by an emotional experience such as separation from a loved one, it may be an expression of hostile feelings toward certain family members, or it may be a result of physical illness. Extra attention given a client is sometimes a way of keeping the anxiety within tolerable limits. The physical dimension is reflected in Peplau's approach by the following principles:

1. Instinctual drives are imperative individual needs that lead to tension and demand tension reduction.
2. Tension can be discharged in active or passive behavior, or it may become bound within the person.
3. When the energy of tension is bound, as in a symptom, relief is felt when the tension is reduced through constructive action.

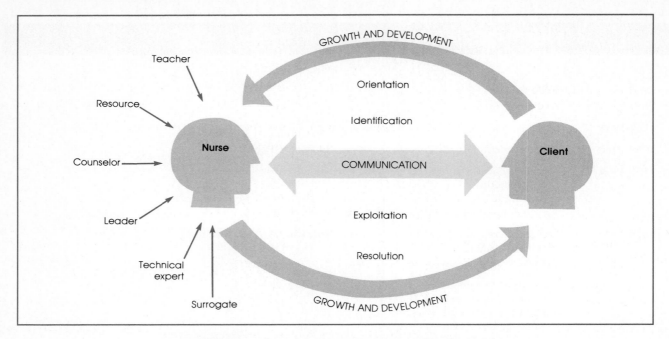

FIGURE 4-1 Peplau's nurse-client interpersonal framework.

TABLE 4-1 Activities in phases of the therapeutic relationship

Phases	Activities
Orientation	Establish need to seek professional help
	Establish working relationship
	Listen for themes that may help define problem areas more clearly
	Determine whether to continue the relationship or whether referral needs to be made
Identification	Clarify perceptions and expectations
	Identify problems more clearly
	Discuss preliminary solutions to problems
Exploitation	Work out conscious and unconscious conflicts that may not be well understood by either client or nurse
	Create a non-threatening atmosphere
	Demonstrate confidence in client's ability to become involved in problem solving
	Clarify, listen, accept, and interpret
Resolution	Determine whether client's needs have been met
	Work through difficulties in terminating the relationship
	Use bond that has developed as a positive force for the client moving into other meaningful relationships
	Assist client in setting new goals

Emotional dimension. The emotional dimension of the person is inherent in Peplau's belief that nurses face the task of assisting individuals to develop ways to convert tension and anxiety into purposeful action. Energy derived from needs, frustration, conflict, and anxiety is transformed into action. The subjectivity of the emotional responses of the client's needs requires the nurse to have a high level of self-awareness and to be in touch with various types of overt and covert actions and reactions that may be induced in the client. Mutual vali-dation of responses to experiences is a necessary and on-going aspect of the interpersonal interaction.

Intellectual dimension. The intellectual dimension is apparent in Peplau's emphasis on the capacity and responsibility of the individual for development. The person has the ability to acquire, process, and integrate information obtained in the nurse-client relationship. Through learning and memory the individual can store and recall information for problem solving in future situations. Mental organization and reorganization of information occurs as the nurse works with the client through the various stages of the relationship.

✿ *Social dimension.* In the social dimension the importance of socialization in growth and development is stressed. Nurse-client interactions may be viewed as a micromodel of general social interactions between the client and past and present relationships. Ways of functioning in society are learned over time as social exchange, values, perceptions, and behaviors are adopted. Disruptions in significant social relationships vary according to the amount of instability the individual experiences. Peplau contends that an understanding of the sociocultural context in which the client functions provides valuable information for assisting the client's return to healthy, spontaneous interactions in the social environment.

✿ *Spiritual dimension.* The spiritual dimension develops as a result of cultural forces. Infants acquire the beliefs, values, and ethics of a given culture from caretaking adults who express and exemplify them. Peplau states that clients may question their faith in others and their social and ethical beliefs. She suggests the use of a method that permits the exploration of doubts and feelings and the discovery of convictions. Peplau emphasizes the role of interprofessional relations with clergy.

Clinical Application

The following case example concerning Susan will be used to discuss the clinical application of each theorist's approach. (It will not be repeated for each section.)

Case Example

Susan, age 14, was admitted to the psychiatric unit from the emergency room after inflicting two cuts on her left arm in a suicide attempt. She stated that she had thought of killing herself by cutting her wrist but decided she did not want to die.

Two days earlier, Susan ran away with a 20-year-old female friend who was unhappy with her family situation. During the episode, Susan lost her bags that contained all her clothes when she left them unattended in a restaurant. On her return home her mother gave her money to buy more clothes. However, Susan stated, "I threw the money away also."

At the time of admission her mother reported that Susan had suffered from depression 2 years earlier. On the unit Susan was fearful and wanted her mother to remain with her; however, her mother had to return to work and could spend only a short time with Susan. After the mother returned to work Susan telephoned her several times, "just to talk."

Susan has a 22-year-old brother and a 19-year-old sister. Her father is an ex-military man who is starting his own business as a television repairman. Her mother attends school full-time in the mornings and works in the evenings. Susan's family has spent a large amount of time traveling and frequently moved from one location to another because of her father's military career. The family has been in its present residence for about 5 months.

Using Peplau's theory, the nurse establishes a therapeutic relationship with Susan. The five dimensions are explored as the nurse proceeds through the orientation, identification, exploitation, and resolution phases of the relationship. In assessing the emotional dimension, for ex-

ample, the nurse may focus on the tension and anxiety Susan is experiencing. The nurse seeks ways to assist Susan in releasing the tension through constructive channels. Through the therapeutic nurse-client relationship Susan is allowed to discover the most effective ways of releasing tension. Basic physical and safety needs are met in response to Susan's self-destructive behavior. In the intellectual dimension, the nurse views Susan as having the capacity for self-control and responsibility. Susan integrates and processes information obtained from the relationship to recall old problem-solving techniques and to learn new ones. The nurse vigilantly evaluates Susan's behavior until she can use her skills for responsible self-control.

There is considerable evidence in this case that Susan probably has some doubts about her social relationships with her family and friends. Past and present disappointments have perhaps eroded her faith (spiritual dimension) in herself and others, significantly diminishing her hope for recovery and for a meaningful existence. As the work with Susan progresses through the phases of the relationship, the nurse is alerted to indications of Susan's recovery. In some instances a lessening of anxiety may reflect Susan's decision to repeat self-destructive behavior; however, if open communication is continually encouraged, trust between Susan and the nurse may motivate Susan to move toward health rather than illness.

As described in Table 4-5, a weakness of Peplau's approach is that little attention is given to the various dimensions. In particular, the spiritual dimension can only be assumed to be present within the nurse-client interpersonal framework.

OREM'S SELF-CARE MODEL

The self-care concept of nursing as perceived by Dorothea Orem was first published in 1959.[28] Orem, like other theorists, views nursing as an interpersonal process, with nurses giving direct, necessary assistance to individuals who, because of health conditions, cannot provide self-care. Self-care is defined as the continuous contribution adults give to personal health and well-being.[29]

Major Concepts

The major concepts of Orem's theory are self-care and nursing systems (Figure 4-2). The word *self* in the term self-care is used in the sense of one's whole being. Self-care connotes "for oneself" and "given by oneself." Self-care agency is the ability to engage in self-care. The development of this ability is aided by intellectual curiosity, instruction, supervision from others, and experience in the performance of self-care measures. Self-care deficits occur when health-related problems require nursing care. Self-care requisites are universal and include health deviations and developmental processes.

Universal self-care requisites, common to persons during all stages of life, are associated with life processes and with the maintenance of the integrity of human structure and functioning. Universal self-care includes sufficient in-

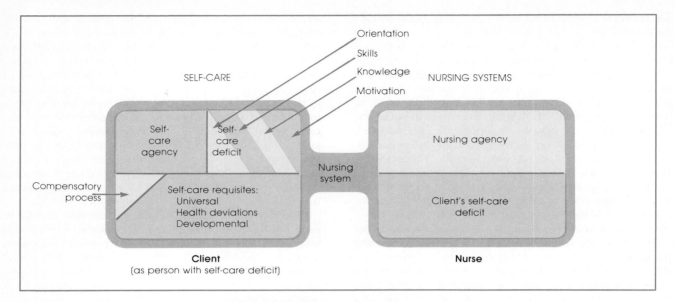

FIGURE 4-2 Orem's self-care framework.

take of air, water, and foods; care related to excrements; balance of activity and rest; balance of solitude and social interactions; and prevention of hazards to one's well-being.[30]

Self-care requisites for health deviation are associated with genetic and constitutional defects and structural and functional aberrations. The focus is on diagnosis and treatment. Health deviation self-care requisites include seeking and securing appropriate health assistance, carrying out prescribed measures effectively, and learning to live with the residual effects of illness and treatment.

Developmental self-care requisites are specialized expressions of the universal self-care requisites. They are associated with human developmental processes and with conditions and events occurring during the life cycle.

The nurse's concern is the client's self-care deficit. When helping the client address self-care deficits, the nurse considers the orientation, skills, knowledge, and motivation of the client for overcoming his deficits and improving self-care agency.

The second major concept, nursing systems, comprises the approaches nurses use to assist clients who have self-care deficits caused by health conditions. Nursing is a response to an incapacity when action is limited by health or health care needs. The system denotes a set of objects, their relationships, and their attributes, operating as a whole. Nursing systems include all actions and interactions of nurses and clients in nursing practice situations. Compensatory processes are actions performed by nurses, clients, or both to meet client's self-care requisites. These compensatory processes may be partly or wholly educational.

Nursing agency is the special ability of nurses to provide total care as a unit. Nursing agency, analogous to self-care agency, constitutes abilities for specialized types of deliberate nursing actions. Nursing agency is developed and exercised for the benefit and well-being of others; whereas self-care agency is developed and exercised for the benefit and well-being of oneself.

Holistic Perspective

According to Orem, individuals are responsible for fostering their own health. Therapeutic techniques rely on the client rather than on the nurse. The emphasis on self-care encourages approaches that mobilize the individual's innate capacity for self-healing.

Physical dimension. The physical dimension of the person, according to Orem's theory, is addressed by the following categories of universal self-care demands: air, water, food, excretion, activity and rest, and physical hazards. Assessment of subjective and objective data of each of these self-care demands assists the nurse in helping the client develop an optimal level of self-care agency. The nurse then helps the client to meet self-care demands regarding respiration, fluids and electrolytes, metabolism, excretory processes, activity and rest, and protection against hazards.

Emotional dimension. After determining the client's need, the nurse designs activities to foster self-care. The emotional dimension may be indicated by a need to foster bonds of affection, love, friendship, closeness, and management of impulses.

Intellectual dimension. The intellectual dimension involves the development of self-care agency through learning in the course of day-to-day living. The nurse intervenes to prevent disturbances in cognition, memory, and learning. Selecting activities that stimulate, engage, and balance intellectual efforts is important for optimal functioning. Orem's framework emphasizes preventive health care. The primary prevention of self-care demand includes universal and developmental self-care requisites. Secondary and tertiary prevention self-care demands include health deviation, universal, and developmental self-care requisites.

❊ *Social dimension.* Socialization is required in the nursing situation because both nurse and client are strangers entering a helping relationship. The client may need preparation for his role.[30] The ability to accept the role may be influenced by the client's temperament, self-image, and life-style. The same factors may affect the nurse's performance. The nurse may also be affected by the client's age, sex, race, culture, social status, or disease.

❊ *Spiritual dimension.* The spiritual dimension in Orem's framework is the search for a meaningful philosophy of life. The goal of health care is to enable persons to understand their illness. A meaningful philosophy is learning to live with the effects of pathological conditions and to develop a life-style that promotes continued personal development. Orem advocates that nurses, in gathering personal information about clients, determine clients' religious orientation. This information helps nurses understand how clients' religious affiliations limit or qualify the values of the nursing system variables and the operation of nursing practice.

Clinical Application

Using Orem's theory within the holistic perspective, the nurse assists Susan in optimizing the development of self-care agency (see the Case Example on p. 51). The five dimensions are explored in an analysis of self-care agency and therapeutic self-care demand. Following this analysis, Susan's self-care deficits in orientation, skills, knowledge, and motivation are identified.

The self-care agency can be understood from the description of Susan as client, a 14-year-old, and a daughter. Universal and health deviation self-care requires that Susan develop self-care agency. Susan's self-care agency deficit requires intervention in terms of coping patterns.

Suicidal behavior is a deviation from health. The necessary interventions are focused on assessing Susan's self-care demands and include guidance and the teaching of coping strategies to deal with destructive tendencies. The nurse gathers information about how Susan perceives and reacts in family or community situations. The nurse may use guided imagery as a technique to teach Susan to improve her coping patterns. The nurse may also teach Susan to tense and relax muscle groups as a method of improving coping patterns and enhancing Susan's ability to meet her self-care demands. Susan's depressed feelings, suicidal thoughts, and self-injury represent health deviations within the emotional dimension. Developmentally, Susan is experiencing a time of emotional turmoil with mood swings.

Based on the limited case example data, it is assumed that no skills or orientation deficits exist. However, Susan may have deficits in knowledge and motivation. The goal is to overcome the deficits through self-care.

To overcome deficits in knowledge, the nurse assists Susan in identifying stress as a precipitating factor for her hospitalization. The goal for Susan's self-care is to identify stressful situations. The health hazard consists of injurious behaviors as a function of stress. Intellectually, Susan is capable of understanding and learning to cope with stressful situations.

Socially, there are requisites to assist Susan in functioning optimally. Susan wants and needs guidance from a responsible adult, although she may resist these efforts from time to time. She can learn to be responsible for her health-related care.

The nurse determines and assesses deficits in motivation and implements self-care by encouraging Susan to talk about her long-term and short-term life goals. The nurse identifies and explores sources of support for Susan that are helpful to Susan spiritually as she regains faith in herself and in others.

The strengths and weaknesses of Orem's theory are presented in Table 4-5.

KING'S GOAL ATTAINMENT THEORY

The early works of Imogene King appeared in the literature in the mid-1960s. King's approach emphasizes the nursing process as a dynamic interpersonal process between the nurse and individuals in various social systems. Through reciprocal interactions, mutual nursing activities are defined to assist individuals of any age group to function in society. For King,[19,20] health is the outcome of behaviors directed toward goal attainment.

Major Concepts

King's theory of goal attainment encompasses three broad, interlocking, open systems: the personal, interpersonal, and social systems. Although the personal systems (self) and the social systems (self and society) influence the quality of care, the major elements in the goal attainment theory are contained in the interpersonal systems. In these systems two or more persons come together in a health care organization to promote an optimal state of health. The major concepts within the interpersonal systems are interaction, perception, communication, transaction, role, stress, growth and development, and time and space (Figure 4-3).

Interactions are defined as actions and reactions between persons or between persons and the environment. Purposeful interactions establish a frame of reference, and mutually agreed upon goals are developed. Interactions become increasingly complex as more individuals are involved. As diversity (for example, in background, experience, and motivation) among individuals increases, so does the complexity of the interactions. However, if the diversity is extreme, interactions may not occur at all. When interpersonal interactions are not successful, disruptive factors can usually be identified and resolved or alleviated.

Perception is defined by King as "a process of organizing, interpreting and transforming information from sense data and memory . . . . [Perception] gives meaning to

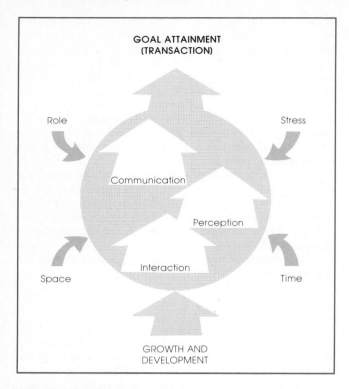

GOAL ATTAINMENT
(TRANSACTION)

Role

Stress

Communication

Perception

Interaction

Space

Time

GROWTH AND
DEVELOPMENT

FIGURE 4-3 King's goal attainment theory.

one's experience, represents one's image of reality and influences one's behavior."[19] A person's perceptual and intellectual tools are related to past experiences, concept of self, biological inheritance, educational background, and socioeconomic group. A nursing assessment takes into account the potential or actual differences between the perceptions held by the nurse and those held by the client. Accurate perception, by which both nurse and client interpret sensory data, is a primary step toward mutual goal identification and determination of strategies for goal attainment. A conflict between the nurse and client in the perception of problems and their resolution may delay the client's return to a healthy state. For example, the nurse who assesses the client's level of pain and determines that medication is needed to decrease suffering may actually do more harm than good if the client perceives the pain level as discomforting but within a personal range of tolerance. Each individual needs to be perceived as unique, with different needs, values, resources, and expectations.

The concept of communication is basic in King's framework. She defines communication as the exchange of feelings, perceptions, and values between and among individuals. Communication is the information component of interaction and may be direct (verbal) or indirect (nonverbal). Although communication is universal, the verbal and nonverbal symbols vary from one culture to another and from one person to another. Communication is further influenced by an individual's stress level, development level, prior experience, and the current context of the interaction. Communication, whether verbal or non-

verbal, is a function of the total person; the self cannot be separated from what is communicated. Any message that is conveyed has significance for the overall well-being of the individual. What an individual does not say or do is as important as what the person does say or do. Effective communication assists individuals in gaining a sense of understanding about themselves and facilitates emergence of meaningful relationships with others.

Transaction is the contractual agreement resulting from a number of interactions. Transaction is a product of communication and is influenced by individual viewpoints. Transaction is the goal of the interpersonal process between the nurse and the client.

King emphasizes the importance of transaction in a therapeutic relationship. The implication is that individuals entering the relationship take active roles in defining goals and resolving problems. Continuous give-and-take occurs as the nurse and client progress toward a transaction. Ideas, beliefs, and values are communicated between the individuals as the process evolves. The social exchange between nurse and client should always be open, honest, and mutual. Any transaction between different individuals, or between the same individuals at different times, is unique; thus transactions have temporal and spatial dimensions. The data gathered through interactions provide the nurse with the tools for implementing the nursing process.

Role and stress continuously influence interaction, perception, communication, and transactions. Role, as defined by King, is a set of observable behaviors expected of individuals in the interpersonal system. The client and the nurse have expectations of each other based on accurate or inaccurate information. When roles are misinterpreted, conflict arises. This decreases the potential effectiveness of the interpersonal relationship. Correct information about role behaviors and functions is communicated through ongoing interactions. The purpose of nursing is mutual interaction (and transaction) between persons to assess health status and promote an optimal state of health. The roles of the nurse and client are defined within this context.

Stress involves an exchange of energy for the purpose of maintaining balance and promoting growth. Stress is dynamic and continuously influences interactions. Nurses are expected to assist clients and their families in reducing the stress that interferes with optimal functioning. Just as stress affects the health status of the client, it also affects the health status of the nurse. When noxious environmental stressors influence the nurse and the client, a narrowing of perception and a decrease in interactions occur. The result is that mutual goal setting for effective nursing care is diminished, and the opportunity for growth on the part of both individuals is limited. An outside source may be necessary to assist the nurse in regaining equilibrium and increasing the effectiveness of coping skills. When equilibrium is reestablished, the nurse is able to assist the client in an examination of the negative factors that were present in the situation. The process used by the nurse in coping with stress will serve as a model for clients.

Holistic Perspective

Implicit in King's theory is a holistic orientation. Although her major focus is on the individual as a social being, she implies that persons use energy to react as whole organisms to experiences and events. Aspects of holism can also be found in King's definition of health as continuous adjustment to environmental stressors through optimal use of one's resources. King maintains that health is the way individuals deal with the stressors of growth and development while functioning in their various roles and in their various cultural environments. An analysis of the dimensions reflects King's emphasis on the social dimension of the person.

Physical dimension. The physical dimension of the person can be inferred from King's broad concept of growth and development. Growth and development represent continuous changes in individuals at the cellular and behavioral activity levels. Growth and development are life processes that help persons move from a potential achievement level to self-actualization, a critical variable.

King's concept of time may also be included in the physical dimension. Time is a continuous flow of successive events implying change, a past, and a future. It is related to rhythmicity and is observed in body temperature, elimination, sleep-wake cycles, metabolism, and fluid and electrolyte balance. Time perceptions are important in nurse-client interaction. Interactions in hospitals may occur in places that restrict space, such as a client's room. The physical area of space is territory, which is defined by behavior as well as the boundaries of actual space.

Emotional dimension. The emotional dimension is also addressed by King in her discussion of growth and development. The developing individual has the potential for achievement and self-satisfaction. Nurses and clients share information as transactions are made to meet goals. Thus individuals are helped to achieve their greatest potential for a meaningful life.

Intellectual dimension. For King the intellectual dimension may be inferred from the concept of perception. Perception is the process through which the person recalls and attributes meaning based on past experience. In assessing the intellectual dimension, the nurse can ascertain disturbances in perception such as illusions, hallucinations, and autistic thinking.

Social dimension. King addresses the social dimension more fully than the other dimensions. King views the goal of nursing as assisting the individual, a social being, to function effectively within three dynamically interacting social systems: (1) the personal system, (2) the interpersonal system, and (3) the social system. In the assessment of these systems the nurse may focus on such questions as: What stress factors interfere with the individual functioning in certain roles in society? What factors interfere with development of meaningful relationships with others?

Spiritual dimension. The spiritual dimension of the person is suggested in King's concept of health. Health relates to the way persons deal with the stress of personal, interpersonal, and social growth. One of the stressors is the maintenance of a level of health that enables a person to live a relatively useful, satisfying, productive, and happy life each day. Thus an assessment of personal, interpersonal, and social relationships as they contribute to the sense of well-being and fulfillment is an assessment of spiritual health.

Clinical Application

Use of King's theory to assist the nurse in the clinical case of Susan (refer to the Case Example on p. 51) involves the application of several concepts. Within the context of the interpersonal system, the nurse strives to develop a relationship in which both nurse and client are involved in identification of health problems and the changes needed for goal attainment. Interpersonal interactions between the nurse and Susan involve the processes of perceiving and communicating to derive a transaction, or contractual agreement, for achieving goals. The assessment is the identification of stressors, primarily in the emotional and social realms. Interactions between the nurse and Susan are influenced by the needs and past experiences that each brings to the situation. Both nurse and client have values, goals, and expectations that are also involved in the interaction. The nurse needs to refrain from making a value judgment about Susan's suicidal behavior and about the family's apparent neglect of Susan's needs; however, it may be assumed that Susan has difficulties in personal, interpersonal, and social relationships.

As described in Table 4-5, King's approach perhaps more than the other approaches discussed in this chapter emphasizes the social dimension almost to the exclusion of the other four dimensions. The specific directions for nurse-client interaction are a major strength of this approach.

JOHNSON'S BEHAVIORAL SYSTEMS THEORY

Dorothy Johnson presented her framework for nursing in 1968. Johnson's behavioral systems approach to nursing emphasizes the nurse's role in promoting optimal health for the individual. Health is maintained as the system's units (or subsystems) are kept in balance. The aim of the approach is integration of the subsystem's functions for overall system stability and growth.[11,16]

Major Concepts

Johnson's theory is based on the broad concepts of system and behavior. Individuals, as systems, are beings responding to environmental input and producing behavioral output. System units include the affiliative, dependence, achievement, ingestive, eliminative, sexual, and aggressive-protective subsystems. Behavior is linked with each subsystem in response to the subsystem's components: goals, set, choices, and action. Figure 4-4 depicts the feedback operation responsible for integration of environmental input and behavioral output. Behavior, the visible feature of the system, is the nurse's most important concern.

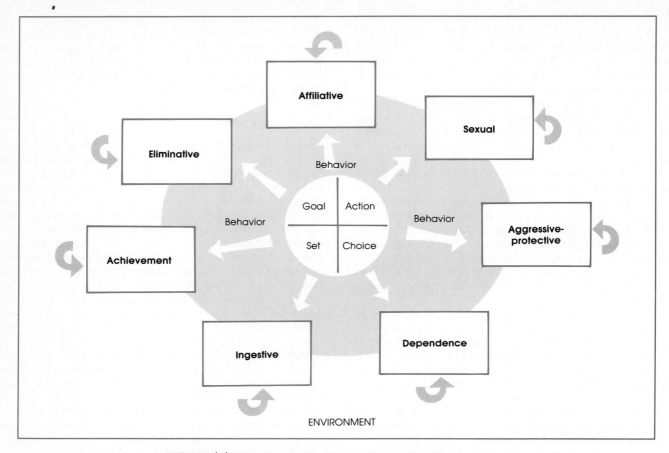

FIGURE 4-4 Basic structures of Johnson's behavioral subsystems.

TABLE 4-2 Subsystem goals

Subsystems	Goals
Affiliative	Security
Dependence	Self-dependence and interdependence
Achievement	Mastery of self and environment according to an internalized standard of excellence
Ingestive	Taking in nourishment in socially and culturally acceptable ways
Eliminative	Ridding system of waste in socially and culturally acceptable ways
Sexual	Procreation and gratification
Aggressive	Survival

The seven subsystems contribute to the functioning of the overall behavioral system. The goals of each of the subsystems are described in Table 4-2.

The components of each subsystem (goal, set, choices, and action) provide its structure. The goal is the drive or motivational aspect of the system. The set is the predisposition to act with reference to the goal. Choices are the repertoire of available alternatives. Action leads to the behavioral output of the system. Each subsystem is further guided by variables such as age, sex, motives, values, and rewards. These structural components of each subsystem give direction for nursing assessment, analysis, planning, intervention, and evaluation.

Holistic Perspective

Johnson's perspective is that the person is an open system with seven broadly defined subsystems, interacting with the environment by receiving input and displaying behavioral output. Each subsystem comprises a motivational component and a reservoir of potential behaviors, choices, and actions. The systems, which are interrelated, reflect the total person as a behavioral being. Although Johnson does not specifically address the dimensions of persons, these aspects can be inferred from the subsystems.

Physical dimension. The physical dimension encompasses the ingestive, eliminative, and sexual subsystems. Subsystem responses are affected by when, how much, and under what conditions subsystem behaviors occur. For example, in the sexual subsystem, the dual functions of procreation and gratification are considered. If a deficit exists in this subsystem, some type of sexual dysfunction may occur. Each subsystem can be assessed in terms of its behavioral response to stress within the various dimensions.

�֎ Emotional dimension. The emotional dimension may include the aggressive subsystem. For example, the nurse assesses and intervenes in problems arising when an individual responds violently to real or imagined threats.

✳ Intellectual dimension. The intellectual dimension may be assessed through an evaluation of the achievement subsystem. The consequence of the achievement subsystem includes a sense of mastery over one's environment. Mastery implies memory, learning, and growth, elements of the intellectual dimension. Stress impinging on the achievement subsystem may thwart the achievement of life goals. For example, an imprisoned individual may become intellectually dull and consequently unable to develop into a productive person. The nurse employing Johnson's theory with the intent of providing holistic mental health nursing care may find this dimension particularly useful in working with individuals in isolated situations. Finding creative and innovative ways of assisting the isolated person to achieve optimal environmental control represents a challenge to the nurse.

❀ Social dimension. Because the affiliative and dependence subsystems have the consequence of social inclusion and the formation of social bonds, both can be included in the social dimension. The nurse's goal in working with a recently widowed elderly woman, for example, may be to assist her in joining community groups in which other aged persons have regular, well-established recreational activities.

✳ Spiritual dimension. Within the spiritual dimension, an assessment of the client's relationship with self and with another person in attaining personal inclusion and evolving a meaningful existence are important. The affiliative subsystem is again used to provide the nurse with the information necessary for assessment within this dimension.

Clinical Application

Application of Johnson's theory directs the nurse to establish a data base regarding Susan's nursing care (see the Case Example on p. 51) by observing the subsystems and their structural components. The general goal of nursing intervention is to help Susan achieve balance in all systems so as to be able to function effectively again.

Susan's aggressive and dependence subsystems seem most affected. The set in the aggressive-protective subsystem, as reflected by Susan's behavior, is a predisposition to act in a self-destructive manner by cutting her arm. The choice confronting Susan is to harm or not to harm herself. Susan chose to inflict only minor injury on herself. Finally, the goal of Susan's behavior in the aggressive subsystem is to seek protection from self-destructive impulses. The extent to which Susan is able to seek protection

depends on internally and externally available resources. Thus the assessment and intervention made by the nurse in this subsystem takes into account the goal of protection. Active suicide precautions may be indicated initially, in conjunction with an opportunity to help Susan talk about her feelings of anger and hostility.

Regarding disruption in the dependence subsystem, the set exemplified by Susan is attention-seeking behavior, which has probably been present for some time. Susan's frequent telephone calls from the hospital unit to her mother exemplify her attention-seeking dependent behavior. The choice for Susan involves seeking alliance with friends or family. Susan seems to have some ambivalence regarding this choice. Observable behavior, or action, is reflected in Susan's self-destructive behavior and running away from home and school. These are responses to frustration in meeting dependence needs. The goal in the dependence subsystem is seen in Susan's seeking reassurance from her mother. The nurse's focusing primarily on the dependence subsystem will assist Susan in reestablishing appropriate trusting relationships with significant others. Family therapy, as well as individual therapy, may be indicated.

The nurse's using Johnson's theoretical approach needs to remember that disruption in one subsystem may cause disruption in one or several other subsystems. Therefore all subsystems need to be assessed for possible changes in system stability.

The strengths and weaknesses of Johnson's approach are highlighted in Table 4-5.

ROGERS'S THEORY OF THE UNITARY PERSON

Martha Rogers's conceptual orientation to a science of nursing uses terms and concepts somewhat different from those used in the other theories discussed here. Synthesizing from fields such as anthropology, sociology, philosophy, and history, Rogers[33,34] has postulated a view of the person as a continuously evolving unitary being.

Major Concepts

Two broad concepts capture the essence of Rogers's theoretical framework of the unitary person: life process and homeodynamics (Figure 4-5). Life process encompasses energy fields embedded in a four-dimensional space-time matrix that becomes increasingly complex as it evolves rhythmically along life's longitudinal axis. Life process is continuous, dynamic, and changing. It evolves irreversibly and unidirectionally along a space-time continuum. Thus a living system (a person) is an evolving process and emerges and moves continually forward from birth through death. The system is characterized by identifiable patterns and rhythms.

The energy fields of the life process are the human field and the environmental field. The human and environmental fields are open systems. The environment, external to the individual, interacts and exchanges matter and energy with the person in such a way that a pattern of wholeness emerges.

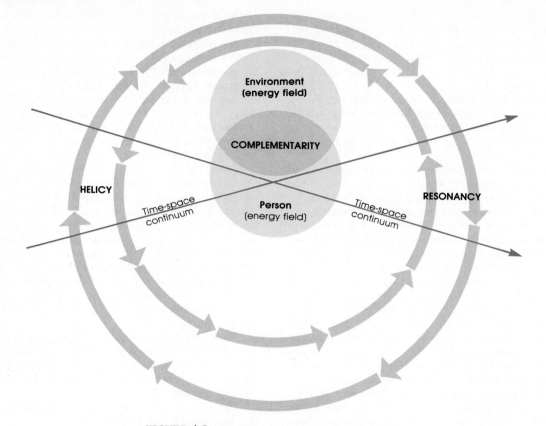

FIGURE 4-5 Rogers's unitary person framework.

Homeodynamics includes principles of complementarity, helicy, and resonancy. Complementarity recognizes life as a continuously changing process, influenced by the interaction of person and environment. Helicy refers to the direction of change—forward, nonrepeatable, irreversible, and increasing in complexity and diversity. Resonancy suggests change that increases in rate and intensity over time. Thus principles of homeodynamics are a way of viewing persons in their complex wholeness.

Holistic Perspective

The holistic perspective rests on the assumption that the characteristics of the person are wholeness and unity. A total response of the person is the focus of concern.

Self-responsibility stems from self-regulation, a dynamic quality directed toward orderly innovation and fulfillment of life's potential. Persons interacting with the environment have the capacity to arrange the environment and to exercise choice in fulfilling their potential.

Physical dimension. Rogers's approach to a unitary wholeness of persons negates viewing people in a compartmental manner. The concept of wholeness with regard to the physical dimension of the individual may be observed in sleep-wake cycles, elimination, and respiratory processes. Rogers suggests that some physiological functions are subject to conscious control.

Emotional dimension. The emotional dimension of the individual is reflected in the unique nature of persons as feeling and sensing beings. People evolve through interaction with the environment; this evolution is an expression of their wholeness. For example, pain thresholds vary greatly from one individual to another primarily as a result of the individual's emotional makeup and perception. Other feelings in the emotional dimension involve expressions of joy, sorrow, affection, and sadness. Within the emotional realm, communication is the tool for transmitting feelings.

Intellectual dimension. The intellectual dimension is based on the person as a thinking, rational being. An individual's capacity for abstraction, imagery, language, and thought are tools of the intellectual sphere. It is with these tools that the individual seeks to organize and understand experiences and the environment. An emerging understanding transcends an accumulation of facts and events.

Social dimension. Rogers's approach addresses the social dimension in the assessment of history concerning such social behaviors as smoking, drinking, and employment. Cultural attitudes toward health and illness and the use of health resources are important determinants of behavior.

The social nature of the individual is implicit in the person-environment interaction. As an open system, the individual is continually affected by environmental forces that influence the acquisition of values and attitudes. The person seeks ways to develop patterns of living that are in harmony with environmental forces. Factors such as social inequities, economic and educational deprivation, technological advances, and ecological disturbances cause disruptions in the individual's relationship with the environment. The individual is expected to participate in the evaluation of disruptive events and in the reestablishment of patterns congruent with forward movement, growth, and health. Nursing's responsibility to the individual and society is to seek means to promote the person-environment interaction to attain maximal health potential.

Spiritual dimension. In the spiritual dimension perception and thought are used as the basis for functioning. The ability of persons to perceive and transcend a present state of consciousness and find expression in reasoning and creativity may alter their perception and attitude toward their health potential.

Clinical Application

The nurse applying Rogers's framework uses the principles of homeodynamics in the assessment process with Susan (refer to the Case Example on p. 51).The nurse proceeds with an understanding that through person-environment interactions positive or negative patterns may emerge. The nurse, as a component of the environment, recognizes the influence of her behavior on Susan's behavior and the importance of both the nurse's and Susan's cooperation in identifying problem areas.

Implicit in Rogers's approach are some questions that may generate useful information. First, information about the environment and the client is collected. The nurse attempts to discover the nature of the interaction between Susan, her family, and her friends. What patterns in these interactions reflect a breakdown in perception and communication? Are the home and school environments in which Susan interacts contributing to her behavior?

Second, information about life process (historical elements) is collected. For example, what has been the nature of Susan's interaction with family, friends, and environment in the past? What factors, over time, have contributed to pattern formation?

Finally, questions such as the following are asked: Have new relationships evolved in an attempt to cope with dysrhythmic patterns? To what extent have these relationships influenced Susan's present behavior? What are the environmental factors that support or retard Susan's stability?

Working closely, both Susan and the nurse assess problems, establish diagnoses, and set goals. They establish strategies of intervention to assist Susan in repatterning her behavior.

An adherence to the unitary person framework necessitates a simultaneous assessment of all dimensions. The nurse working with Susan is likely to discover that factors in the home environment are contributing to Susan's present difficulties. Susan's patterns of coping are likely to become increasingly ineffective over time. Susan's suicidal gestures are viewed not as static behavior but rather as an evolving way of responding to her environment. Rogers's focus is on health and health potential rather than disease. Thus the goal is to use Susan's own resources and abilities to channel energy in a positive direction.

Congruence of Rogers's approach with the holistic perspective is a major strength. A significant area of weakness is a lack of direction for assessment and intervention. Other strengths and weaknesses of this approach are listed in Table 4-5.

ROY'S ADAPTATION THEORY

Sister Callista Roy placed her perspective of nursing in a systems model framework. In this model the person is viewed as an adaptive system; the need for nursing intervention arises when there is a deficit between the adaptation level and environmental demands.[35,36]

Major Concepts

The major concepts of Roy's theoretical approach are regulator, cognator, and adaptive modes (Figure 4-6). Adaptation is the process of coping with internal and exter-

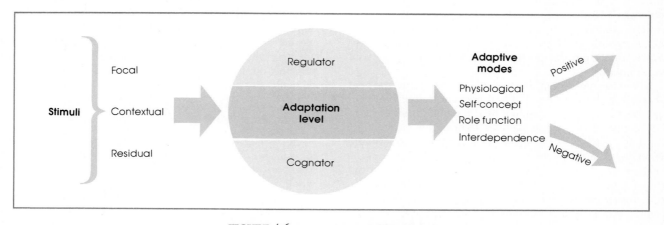

FIGURE 4-6 Roy's adaptation framework.

TABLE 4-3 Philosophical foundations and assumptions of the theoretical approaches

Theorist	Philosophical Foundations	Assumptions
Peplau	Individuals are organisms that strive to reduce tension generated by needs.	The individual has the ability to adapt to tensions created by needs.
	Need is an internal requirement that creates tension.	Both nurse and client participate in determining what each will contribute and learn in the relationship.
	Individuals are unique beings, capable of new learning and positive change.	
	Nursing is a therapeutic process.	
	Society is culture.	
Orem	An individual is an integrated whole biologically, symbolically, and socially.	Needs are adapted to the environment.
	Health is a state of wholeness.	Functioning can be altered within flexible limits.
	Nursing's concern is self-care.	Societal influence is reflected in the person-environment interaction.
King	Individuals are biopsychosocial organisms with continually evolving needs.	Behavior is understood in terms of personal, interpersonal, and social systems.
	Nursing's goal is the attainment of health.	Health is adaptation to stress.
Johnson	Individuals are an aggregate of behavioral subsystems.	An individual is a system of interrelated physiological, psychosociocultural, and mental structures and functions.
	Nursing assists individuals to develop a range of behavioral alternatives.	Persons interact with others within a group, family, and community by expressing behaviors that are intended to foster personal equilibrium and stability.
Rogers	The individual is a four-dimensional energy field evolving simultaneously with the environment.	A continuous exchange of energy and matter between a person and his environmental field results in visible behavior.
	Individuals have the capacity for abstraction and imagery, language and thought, sensation and emotions.	Individuals are capable of attaining integrity, unity, and growth.
	Individuals have self-regulating ability.	
	Nursing's responsibility is to identify evolutionary patterns.	
Roy	An individual is a biopsychosocial adaptive being.	Innate and acquired mechanisms are used to cope with a changing world.
	The level of adaptation is influenced by external and internal stimuli.	Adaptation is initiated by a stressor or focal stimulus.

nal stimuli. It is determined by the effects of three classes of stimuli: focal, contextual, and residual. Focal stimuli are those which immediately confront the person and to which an adaptive response is made. Contextual, or background, stimuli are those which contribute to the behavior as a result of focal stimuli. Residual stimuli are those which arise from the person's beliefs, attitudes, and past experiences.

The adaptive system has two main subsystems, the regulator and the cognator. Neural and endocrine body responses to stimuli are handled by the regulator subsystem. The cognator subsystem handles information processing, learning, and decision making in response to stimuli. When adaptation problems arise, the nursing process is instituted to assist the individual in one or several of the adaptive modes (physiological, self-concept, role function, and interdependence). The physiological mode encompasses needs such as circulation, temperature, activity, sleep, and nutrition. The self-concept mode is a composite of beliefs and feelings one holds about oneself at a given

time that is formed from the perceptions or reactions of others. The role function mode is the regulation of performance of duties according to expected behaviors to maintain a status in society. The interdependence mode is the achievement of harmony and balance with others by a mutual exchange of recognition, praise, and approval. The adaptive modes are patterns of responses comprising the person's coping mechanisms, which parallel the kinds of demands the person encounters.

Holistic Perspective

According to Roy, individuals have biological, psychological, and social components as well as adaptive abilities. The person is viewed from this perspective as a unified whole.

Physical dimension. The physical dimension is reflected in Roy's concept of physiological needs of persons in regard to exercise and rest, nutrition, elimination, fluid and electrolytes, and oxygen and circulation.

TABLE 4-4 Selected research studies based on theoretical approaches

Theorist	Researcher, Year	Phenomena
Peplau	Burd, 1963	Anxiety
	Clack, 1963	Aggression
	Oden, 1963	Panic
	Morris, 1967	Approach-avoidance
	Wrin, 1968	Aspiration
	Werner, 1973	Trust
Orem	Underwood, 1978	Self-care behavior in psychiatric patients
	Kearney and Fleischer, 1979	Self-care agency—instrument development
	Blue, 1982	Self-acceptance and self-care agency
	Spangler and Spangler, 1983	Self-care in the aged
	Harper, 1984	Self-care and behavior modification
	Chang, Uman, Linn, Ware and Kane, 1985	Self-care and adherence to health care regimen in the aged
King	Given, Given and Simoni, 1979	Process and outcome variables
	King, 1981	Transaction predictive variables
	Michigan State Nurses Association, 1982 (CURN Project)	Goal setting variables
Johnson	Holaday, 1974	Achievement behavior
	Majesky, Brester, and Nishio, 1978	Patient indicators of nursing care
	Damus, 1980	Post-transfusion hepatitis
	Lovejoy, 1981	Validation research
Rogers	Goldberg and Fitzpatrick, 1980	Movement group therapy in the aged
	Engle, 1981	Movement tempo and time perception
	Johnston, Fitzpatrick, and Donovan, 1982	Temporal orientation and depression
	Reed, Fitzpatrick, Donovan, and Johnston, 1982	Temporal orientation and suicide
	Floyd, 1983	Rhythmicity (sleep-wake cycle)
Roy	Roy, 1967	Role adequacy
	Idle, 1977	Self-perceived adaptation level
	Roy, 1977	Decision making and adaptation level
	Lewis, Firsich, and Parsell, 1978	Health outcomes
	Roy, 1978	Focal stimuli and distress
	Roy, 1979	Powerlessness and decision-making activities

These are handled by the regulator subsystem. Changes in mental activity (cognator subsystem) may influence physiological functions.

Emotional dimension. The emotional dimension is inherent in the self-concept mode, which involves feelings and perception. Experiences enter the self-concept through perception of past and present events. Perception of the adequacy of various experiences influences emotional adaptation. Roy emphasizes that emotional reactions may allow verbalization of fears, concerns, or anxiety. The self-concept mode also includes aspects of the intellectual and social dimensions.

Intellectual dimension. The intellectual dimension of the person is addressed in Roy's discussion of memory, information processing, and integrity. Sensory overload or deprivation can influence intellectual functioning. Maladaptive sensory responses can lead an individual to a level of disequilibrium and disorganization. Judgment is an intellectual function and is one of the psychosocial pathways of the cognator subsystem.

Social dimension. The social dimension is emphasized in the interdependence and role function modes. Social experience reflects the external stimuli that surround the individual. Roy proposes social integrity, individual adaptation, and group adaptation as system functions. Interactions and relationships develop in the social dimension as the individual adapts within the culture.

Spiritual dimension. Although not explicitly stated as a component of the theory, the spiritual dimension is among the person's innate needs. For successful adaptation, personal, social, and cultural aspects of life need to be fulfilled.

Clinical Application

In accordance with Roy's approach, the nurse establishes a data base regarding Susan's care by observing behavior in each of the adaptive modes. (See the Case Example on p. 51). The nurse then describes the focal, contextual, and residual stimuli affecting Susan's behavior. The focal stimuli requiring immediate attention are Susan's self-destructive tendencies. The contextual stimuli are Susan's relationships with her mother and possibly with other members of her family. The residual stimuli for Susan may be repressed anger and frustration in response to unmet needs.

Further, the nurse assists Susan toward health by promoting and supporting her adaptive abilities in the social and interdependence modes. From a holistic perspective, the emotional and social dimensions are the primary ones affected in Susan's care. The adaptive modes of self-concept and interdependence are patterns of behavior or re-

TABLE 4-5 Major strengths and weaknesses of the theoretical approaches

Theorist	Strengths	Weaknesses
Peplau	Emphasis on interpersonal relationship	Dimensions of persons not in sufficient detail, particularly the spiritual dimension
	Exploration of client problems in a safe, trusting relationship.	
	Guidelines for therapeutic interaction	Difficulty comparing phases of nurse-client relationship and the nursing process
Orem	Individual responsibility for self-care.	Frequent reference to the medical perspective diminishes the independent responsibility of the nurse
	Inclusion of the nursing process helpful in organizing nursing care	
King	Process delineated for nurse-client interaction	Greater emphasis on social dimension than on other dimensions
	Similarity of the nurse-client interaction process to the nursing process useful to the nurse	
Johnson	Articulation of elements constituting human behavior	Person-environment interaction not well described
	Potential for growth when system stability is achieved	Empirical indices for system stability and instability inadequately delineated
Rogers	Congruence with nursing's holistic view of persons	Rudimentary direction for assessment
	Broad conceptualization of ideas and relationships	Abstract guidelines for intervention strategies
Roy	Focus on the biopsychosocial nature of persons	Reciprocal influences of subsystems are not explicit
	Emphasis on physiological needs	

sponses that constitute Susan's coping mechanisms for demands made on her. The nurse helps Susan meet the demands to develop a positive self-concept and to achieve a balance between dependence and independence.

The assessment of focal (for example, self-destructive tendencies) contextual, and residual stimuli determines the needed intervention. The intervention directed at the stimuli constitutes the nursing action within the adaptive mode. The nurse supports and promotes Susan's adaptation. Following assessment, analysis, planning, and intervention, an evaluation is made to determine progress in adapting.

A major weakness of Roy's approach (see Table 4-5) is the lack of direction given for a meaningful, reality-based assessment.

The philosophical foundations and assumptions of each theorist are illustrated in Table 4-3. Research using each of the theoretical approaches and the phenomena studied are listed in Table 4-4. A brief summary of the strengths and weaknesses of the theoretical approaches is given in Table 4-5.

BRIEF REVIEW

The development of a theoretical base for the practice of nursing is still in its infancy. The importance of this scientific activity, however, is reflected in the serious effort put forth by nurses in research, education, and practice. A sound basis for the discipline of nursing depends on a critical examination of existing theories and conceptual models proposed for nursing practice.

In general, the six nursing theorist's approaches in their present level of development offer some degree of

direction for the practice of mental health–psychiatric nursing from a holistic perspective. The applications in some instances are minimal but demonstrate the potential of the theories for use in the practice of this nursing specialty.

Although the theories vary in strengths and weaknesses, appropriate research questions will, ideally, validate the usefulness of the theories in practice.

REFERENCES AND SUGGESTED READINGS

1. Blue, B.: Predictive potential of selected variables on self-acceptance of disabled adults, doctoral dissertation, Denton, Tx. 1982, Texas Woman's University.
2. Burd, S.F., and Marshall, M.A.: Some clinical approaches to psychiatric nursing, New York, 1963, Macmillan Publishing Co.
3. Clack, J.: Some clinical approaches to psychiatric nursing, New York, 1973, Macmillan Publishing Co.
4. Chang, B.L., and others: Adherence to health care regimen among elderly women, Nursing Research 34(1):27, 1985.
5. Damus, K.: An application of the Johnson behavioral system model for nursing practice. In Riehl, J.P., and Roy, C., editors: Conceptual models for nursing practice, New York, 1980, Appleton-Century-Crofts.
6. Dickoff, J., and James, P.: Symposium on theory development in nursing. A theory of theories: a position paper, Nursing Research 17:197, 1968.
7. Engle V.: Movement and time as correlates of health (abstract). Paper presented at the American Nurses' Association Council of Nurse Researchers Annual Meeting, Washington, D.C., 1981.
8. Floyd, J.A.: Research using Rogers' conceptual system: development of a testable theorem, Advances in Nursing Science 5(2):37, 1983.

9. Given, B., Given, C.W., and Simoni, L.F.: Relationships of processes of care to patient outcomes, Nursing Research **28**(2):85, 1979.

10. Goldberg, W.G., and Fitzpatrick, J.J.: Movement therapy with the aged, Nursing Research **29**(6):339, 1980.

11. Grubbs, J.: An interpretation of the Johnson behavioral system model for nursing practice. In Riehl, J.P., and Roy, C., editors: Conceptual models for nursing practice, ed. 2, New York, 1980, Appleton-Century-Crofts.

12. Harper, D.C.: Application of Orem's theoretical constructs to self-care medication behavior in the elderly, Advances in Nursing Science **6**(3):19, 1984.

13. Holaday, B.J.: Achievement behavior in chronically ill children, Nursing Research **23**:25, 1974.

14. Idle, B.A.: SPAL: a tool for measuring self-perceived adaptation level for an elderly population. In Bauwens, E.E., editor: Clinical nursing research: its strategies and findings, Monograph Series, Indianapolis, 1978, Sigma Theta Tau.

15. Johnson, D.E.: One conceptual model of nursing. Paper presented at Vanderbilt University, Nashville, Tenn., April 25, 1968.

16. Johnson, D.E.: The Johnson behavioral system model for nursing. In Riehl, J.P., and Roy, C., editors: Conceptual models for nursing practice, ed. 2, New York, 1980, Appleton-Century-Crofts.

17. Johnson, R.L., Fitzpatrick, J.J., and Donovan, M.J.: Developmental stage: relationship to temporal dimensions (abstract), Nursing Research, **31**:120, 1982.

18. Kearney, B.Y., and Fleischer, B.J.: Development of an instrument to measure exercise of self-care agency, Research in Nursing and Health **2**:25, 1979.

19. King, I.M.: A theory for nursing: systems, concepts, process, ed. 2, New York, 1981, John Wiley & Sons, Inc.

20. King, I.M.: Toward a theory for nursing, New York, 1971, John Wiley & Sons, Inc.

21. Lewis, F.M., Firsich, S.C., and Parsell, S.: Development of reliable measures of patient health outcomes related to quality nursing care for chemotherapy patients. In Krueger, J.C., Nelson, A.H., and Walanin, M.O., editors: Nursing research development, collaboration, and utilization, Rockville, Md., 1978, Aspen Publishers, Inc.

22. Lovejoy, N.C.: An empirical verification of the Johnson behavioral system model for nursing, doctoral dissertation, Birmingham, 1981, University of Alabama.

23. Majesky, S.J., Brester, M.J., and Nishio, K.: Development of a research tool: patient indicators of nursing care, Nursing Research **27**:6, 365, 1978.

24. Meleis, A.I.: Theoretical nursing: development and progress, Philadelphia, 1985, J.B. Lippincott Co.

25. Michigan State Nurses Association, CURN Project: Mutual goal setting in patient care, New York, 1982, Grune & Stratton, Inc.

26. Morris, K.: Approach-avoidance conflict in the orientation phase of therapy, ANA Regional Clinical Conference, New York, 1967, Appleton-Century-Crofts.

27. Oden, G.: Individual panic: elements and patterns. In Burd, S., and Marshall, M.A., editors: Some clinical approaches to psychiatric nursing, New York, 1963, Macmillan Publishing Co.

28. Orem, D.E.: Guides for developing curricula for the education of practical nurses, Washington, D.C., 1959, U.S. Government Printing Office.

29. Orem, D.E.: Nursing concepts of practice, New York, 1971, McGraw-Hill Book Co.

30. Orem, D.E.: Nursing concepts of practice, ed. 2, New York, 1980, McGraw-Hill Book Co.

31. Peplau, H.E.: Interpersonal relations in nursing, New York, 1952, G.P. Putnam's Sons.

32. Reed, P.G., and others: Suicidal crisis: relationship to the experience, Nursing Research **31**:2, 1982.

33. Rogers, M.E.: An introduction to the theoretical basis of nursing, Philadelphia, 1970, F.A. Davis Co.

34. Rogers, M.E.: Science of unitary man: a paradigm for nursing. In Laskar, G.E., editor: Applied systems and cybernetics, vol. 4, Elmsford, N.Y., 1981, Pergamon Press, Inc.

35. Roy, C.: A conceptual framework for nursing, Nursing Outlook **18**(3):42, 1970.

36. Roy, C., and Roberts, S.L.: Theory construction in nursing: an adaptation model, Englewood Cliffs, N.J., 1981, Prentice-Hall, Inc.

37. Roy, C.: Role cues and mothers of hospitalized children, Nursing Research **16**(2):178, 1967.

38. Roy, C.: Decision-making by the physically ill and adaptation during illness, doctoral dissertation, Los Angeles, 1977, University of California.

39. Roy, C.: The stress of hospital events: measuring changes in level of stress (abstract). In Communicating nursing research, vol. 11, New Approaches to communicating nursing research, Boulder, Colo., 1978, Western Interstate Commission for Higher Education.

40. Roy, C.: Health-illness (powerlessness) questionnaire and hospitalized patient decision-making. In Ward, M.J., and Lindeman, C.A., editors: Instruments for measuring nursing practice and other health variables, vol 1., Hyattsville, Md., 1979, Department of Health, Education and Welfare.

41. Spangler, F.S., and Spangler, W.D.: Self-care: a testable model. In Chinn, P.L., editor: Advances in nursing theory development, Rockville, Md., Aspen Publishers, Inc.

42. Underwood, P.R.: Nursing care as a determinant in the development of self-care behavior by hospitalized adult schizophrenics, doctoral dissertation, San Francisco, 1978, University of California.

43. Werner, A.M.: Learning to trust. In Burd, S., and Marshall, M.D., editors: Some clinical approaches to psychiatric nursing, New York, 1963, Macmillan Publishing Co.

44. Wrin, J.T.: Nurse-patient interaction: nurse's level of aspiration, In ANA Clinical Session, New York, 1968, Appleton-Century-Crofts.

ANNOTATED BIBLIOGRAPHY

Andrews, A.J., and Roy, C.: Essentials of the Roy adaptation model, Norwalk, Conn., 1986, Appleton-Century-Crofts.

The principles of Roy's conceptualization of adaptation theory for nursing practice are presented, emphasizing the nursing process. The concepts are depicted in diagrams. Individual and nursing activities are emphasized, including discussion of the person, environment, health, and nursing. The concepts are applied to common life situations with exercises for application.

Johnson, D.E.: The Johnson behavioral system model for nursing. In Riehl, J.I., and Roy, C., editors: Conceptual models for nursing practice, ed. 2, New York, 1980, Appleton-Century-Crofts.

The author discusses the basic tenets of her behavioral system framework. She includes general assumptions regarding systems theory, which form the foundation of her framework, and describes the structural and functional compontents of the concepts. The author emphasizes the responsibility of the user to seek a foundation in the natural and social sciences.

King, I.M.: A theory for nursing: systems, concepts, process, ed. 2, New York, 1981, John Wiley & Sons, Inc.

The author describes and analyzes her framework. She expands concepts of the goal attainment theory as relevant to nursing. The focus is the promotion of health practices. Of particular interest are the author's presentation and illustration of a goal-oriented nursing record that can be used to document nursing care.

Orem, D.E.: Nursing concepts of practice, New York, 1971, McGraw-Hill Book Co.

Nursing as a service to persons to promote self-reliance and responsibility is the theme of this text. The author acknowledges the absence in her book of specific solutions for health needs. Instead she describes a broad framework for the identification and search for resolution strategies.

Peplau, H.E.: Interpersonal relations in nursing, New York, 1952, G.P. Putnam's Sons.

Considered the reference source for the application of interpersonal theory to nursing. This text contains a thorough interpretation of elements of the interpersonal process and nursing's responsibility in providing a therapeutic context for meeting the needs of individuals seeking health care. Peplau consistently emphasized the use of self in promoting mutual learning and growth.

Rogers, M.E.: Science of unitary human beings. In Malinski, V.M., editor: Explorations on Martha Rogers science of unitary human beings, Norwalk, Conn., 1986, Appleton-Century-Crofts.

Rogers has further developed her conceptual system, advocating a new world view specific to phenomena of interest to nursing. Principles and theories derived from the system are validated in the real world. The three principles derived from the concept of homeodynamics are helicy, resonancy, and integrality. Roger's theory suggests a world view different from the prevailing one. Seeing the world from this view requires a creative leap with new attitudes and values.

CHAPTER 5

THERAPEUTIC COMMUNICATION

Nancy Hedlund

After studying this chapter the learner will be able to:

Give examples of three functions of communication.

Give examples of verbal and nonverbal communication, metacommunication, and structural distinctions in communication.

Discuss several theoretical approaches to communication.

Discuss techniques that facilitate therapeutic communication.

Discuss four issues in therapeutic nurse-client communication.

Explain approaches to changing behavior through communication.

Therapeutic communication in mental health–psychiatric nursing modifies ordinary communication to create client interactions that promote healing or improved mental health in two important ways. First, the nurse creates helpful client-nurse communication that addresses client difficulties with self-respect, problem solving, autonomy, and sense of purpose in life. Second, the nurse helps the client to heal through achievement of more healthy internal communication between the various dimensions of himself.

Learning effective communication in mental health–psychiatric nursing challenges the nurse to become a highly skilled listener who can plan and carry out interactions specifically designed to achieve client outcomes. Skill development includes the use of emotional and cognitive abilities in a variety of nursing interventions that include support, confrontation, trust, and affection.

DEFINITIONS OF COMMUNICATION

Verbal and Nonverbal Communication

Verbal communication refers to written and spoken messages exchanged in the form of words as the elements of language. An example of verbal communication is provided by the words "I am anxious." These are written or spoken words that convey an idea about the speaker's experience.

Nonverbal communication refers to messages that do not involve the spoken or written word and are conveyed by behavior, such as the presence or absence of body language or through any of the five senses. For example, the client's hands may tremble, accompanied by rapid breathing, gesturing, and profuse sweating. This behavior may represent the message "I am anxious." However, the person may be conveying anger or respiratory distress. The correct meaning of the message can be achieved by verbal validation with the other person.

It is possible to further distinguish between (1) communication that is the actual content of the message and (2) *metacommunication,* which is how the message is to be understood, or the intended meaning. The actual message may be a compliment, such as "You look lovely," but the metacommunication of a frown may imply the actual message is not sincere. The metacommunication tells the receiver of the message how to interpret what the sender means.

Structure of Communication

The structure of communication includes the form of language and the use of words and behaviors to construct messages. Knowledge about the structure of language provides an important way to analyze communication. Assessment of the client's communication includes analysis of

Historical Overview

DATE	EVENT
Late 1800s	With the exception of Florence Nightingale's *Notes on Nursing,* early nursing textbooks did not emphasize how to communicate effectively.
1950s	Acceptance of nurse-client communication as the core of clinical practice emerged with the publications of the mental health–psychiatric nursing theorists.
1960s and 1970s	Theories of communication formulated by nonnurses were incorporated into nursing's knowledge base and the role of nurse as therapist became well established.
Future	Nursing will continue to use technological and theoretical advances in communication to enhance its expertise in therapeutic communication.

how verbal and nonverbal modes are used to structure communication: (1) What messages are conveyed by each? (2) Are the messages congruent? (3) Are the messages consistent with the client's culturally defined and taken for granted rules? (4) To what extent are stereotypes about the self or others conveyed by the structure of the client's communication? (5) How does the structure of the client's communication contribute to the problem for which help is sought?

Analysis of the structure of nurse-client communication also includes assessment of whether the client's communication appears to be consciously intended or an unconsciously motivated message. The nurse also analyzes the degree of clarity in the message in conveying the intended information. For example, consider the following four actions:

1. Painting a picture
2. Saying, "It's good to wake up feeling ready for the day!"
3. Giving the instruction, "The normal temperature of the human being is 37° C"
4. Jaywalking

Each of the four examples of behaviors can be seen as containing an intention to create interaction. The painting of a picture may be a request to another person: "Please buy my painting." Remarking on how good it feels to awaken feeling ready for the day may imply "Don't you agree?" Instructing another about the normal temperature of human beings may imply "Do you understand?" Jaywalking may imply a request to be injured or a test of the alertness of the driver of an oncoming vehicle. Examination of the intention of a client to interact and communicate a message is best accomplished by talking about the behavior, the possible messages that may be conveyed, and the kind of response being requested.

Functions of Communication

Consideration of the *functions of communication* refers to examining what the verbal or nonverbal communication messages accomplish rather than examining how the message is structured. The two are related in that structuring the message affects the function, as in structuring a statement instead of a question:

Question: Don't you think teenagers disobey parental rules a lot?
Statement: In my opinion, teenagers disobey parental rules a lot.

One function of the question is specifically to request a response, which is not necessarily part of a declarative statement.

Another function of communication is disclosure of information or creation of a specific message about the self, others, or objects. These messages can be sent with no expectation of a response. For example, consider the four behaviors cited earlier: (1) painting a picture, (2) saying, "It's good to wake up feeling ready for the day!" (3) instructing, "The normal temperature of the human being is 37° C," and (4) jaywalking. Each behavior involves disclosure of information about an act that requests no response or interaction with others.

One important communication function is *self-disclosure,* which is communication of information or perceptions about the self. This includes intended and unintended acts that describe and evaluate the self. Through communication individuals convey what kind of person they perceive themselves to be and their level of self-esteem.

In the four examples of behavior previously listed in this chapter, creating a painting may be a way of expressing a strong image of the self. Remarking on how good it feels to awaken feeling ready for the day may be a way of describing the self as a person who happily faces each day. The instruction about normal human body temperature may be a correct response to a student's question that simultaneously conveys the speaker's sense of worth in knowing the correct information. Jaywalking may be a way of describing the self as a risk-taking person. However, an alternative analysis of the meaning of these acts could suggest that a negative self-view is inferred.

A variation on the idea of self-disclosure as a function of communication is the idea that behavior can function to communicate a symptom or mental health difficulty. Behavior that appears to communicate such symptoms is sometimes interpreted as a request for help.

Using the four previously cited illustrations of behavior, a client may paint a picture depicting impending disaster to convey a concern about his own safety. Remarks about how good it feels to awaken feeling ready for the day may express a severely depressed person's temporary optimism just before making a suicidal attempt. Instruction about normal human temperature may occur in a context in which fears of being cold and alone were being expressed. Finally, the act of jaywalking may be an expression of rebellion, lack of concern about self, or even suicidal intention. In each of these examples, the context significantly shapes the meaning of the event, which is then further clarified by validating the meaning of the behavior with the client.

Analysis of the known and unknown aspects of self as they relate to self-awareness and awareness of others can be described in a two-way matrix (Figure 5-1) known as *Johari's window.*[10] Four categories of self-awareness are shown: (1) aspects known to self and others, (2) aspects not known to self but known to others, (3) aspects known to self but not known to others, and (4) aspects not known to self and not known to others.

Johari's window can be used to organize information that the nurse acquires in the assessment process. As the nurse develops greater intimacy with the client, more information can be added to categories 1 and 2. As the client's self-awareness increases, more information can be added to category 3 and, it is hoped, to category 1. In other words, as the nurse's relationship with the client

deepens, the client will be able to share more about himself with the nurse, which is information transferred from category 3 to category 1. The developing relationship with the client also permits the nurse to learn more about the client through observation and discussion with others; this process makes it possible to add information from category 3 to category 1 as the nurse's understanding of the client grows.

THEORIES FOR ANALYZING COMMUNICATION IN NURSING
Reusch's Theory

Reusch applied knowledge of people and cultures to the analysis of communication as the social matrix of psychiatry.[11-14] Reusch proposed a general theory of communication that broadly defined communication as the full range of mechanisms or operations by which people affect one another. Communication includes written and oral speech as well as drama, dance, and the arts. The theory aims to provide a unified construct of human behavior, an understanding of psychopathological conditions such as disturbed communication, and a view of communication as a therapeutic tool.

Communication is defined as a circular process, as illustrated in Figure 5-2. A statement is the expression of internal events intended to convey information to other persons; it becomes a message when it has been perceived and interpreted by another. In other words, the message travels in a circle beginning with the internal events within one person, which are transmitted to another, and after being affected by the internal events in the other person, result in a response message back to the original sender.

Language is a collection of signs or symbols of which two or more communicators or interpreters understand the significance. Statements in the communication process contain both content and instruction. Instruction refers to the process of communication itself, including references as to how a statement is to be interpreted. This instruction is also called *metacommunication;* it is, in effect, communication about the communication. Feedback is an essential element of the system because it exerts a control or corrective effect by feeding back information about the effects of the communication activity.

Communication is described as being successful when agreement of meaning, or concordance, is established. Alternatively, the lack of agreement of meaning, or discordance, results in unsuccessful communication (Figure 5-3).

Therapeutic communication is distinguished from ordinary communication by the intent of one or more of the participants to bring about a change in the communication pattern in the system. Reusch defines a *therapist* as a person in charge of directing the change by steering communication in such a way that the client is exposed to situations and message exchanges that eventually will bring about more gratifying social relations. The nurse assumes this role in many different health care settings, in addition to traditional mental health care situations. As theories about therapeutic communication have evolved,

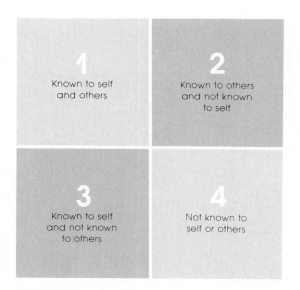

FIGURE 5-1 The Johari window.

a variety of training approaches have become available to nurses seeking to assume therapeutic roles.

Disturbed communication can originate within the individual, as well as between individuals. Nursing assessment includes looking for any of the following occurrences of disturbed communication:

1. Interference with sending or receiving messages, as may be caused by disease, trauma, or malformation of communication organs: having a speech impediment or being deaf

2. Insufficient mastery of the language: from a poor-quality education, or not speaking the same language as others in the environment

3. Incorrect or insufficient information about the self or others, as may be caused by misinterpreting a situation or having only partial information: being

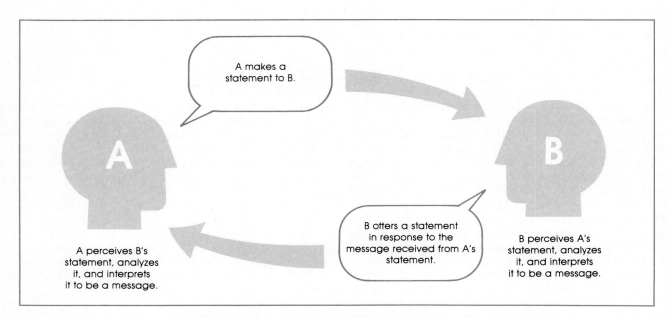

FIGURE 5-2 Reusch's feedback loop of communication.

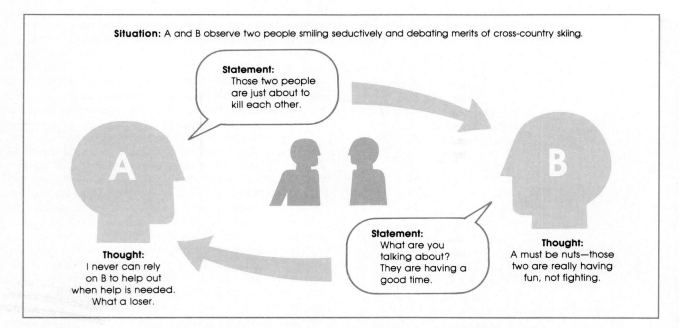

FIGURE 5-3 Unsuccessful communication produced by discordant information.

adopted and not knowing facts about one's background or not knowing there is a familial history of diabetes

4. Insufficient use of metacommunication devices, as may be caused by lack of understanding or lack of skill in interpreting one's messages to others or interpreting other's messages: misinterpreting that a slight smile meant humor when it really conveyed a sneer

5. Inability to correct information through feedback circuits, as in being unskilled in correcting information or in having obstacles in the feedback loop within a person or between persons: being unable to telephone a person or being told that the other person is not willing to talk

Figure 5-4 illustrates how these disturbances impede communication between two persons seated next to one another at a workshop. Disturbances in communication can also result from circumstances of group dynamics.

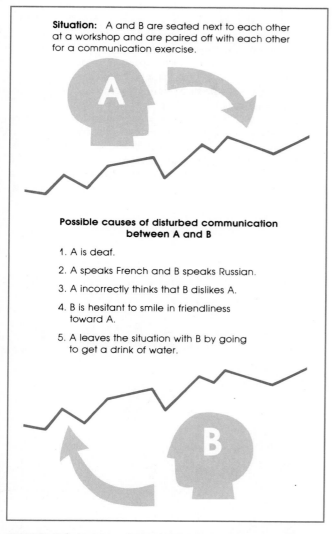

Situation: A and B are seated next to each other at a workshop and are paired off with each other for a communication exercise.

Possible causes of disturbed communication between A and B

1. A is deaf.

2. A speaks French and B speaks Russian.

3. A incorrectly thinks that B dislikes A.

4. B is hesitant to smile in friendliness toward A.

5. A leaves the situation with B by going to get a drink of water.

FIGURE 5-4 Sources of disturbed communication within the person.

Disturbed communications can also occur in large networks of people in which feedback devices are not effective. For example, when nurses work with large groups of clients as in some inpatient or day-care settings, disturbed communications can arise when the setting lacks adequate mechanisms for keeping the nurse informed about client concerns. Subgroups of clients may form to express concern to the head nurse; however, different rules of communication concerning feedback may apply in such groups. Although the norm in the institution may be that people need to express concerns openly and communicate through proper channels when they are attempting to solve a problem, a suspicious member in a newly created subgroup may lead the group to resort to extreme secrecy. As a result, a disturbed communication pattern develops that is characterized by overlooking appropriate levels of communication and going directly to the medical director of the setting.

Needs for therapeutic communication can be created by acute or long-term disturbances, such as unexpected loss of a job or a long-standing marital conflict. Crises and environmental stresses also can create situations in which participants want to initiate changes in communication behavior. Human experience is the subject of study or concern in assessing and treating communication disturbances. In such disturbances and the distressing events in human experience that cause them, anticipatory adaptation and momentary adaptation are the most powerful tools of survival of the person.

Anticipatory adaptation means that a person can begin adapting in advance of a potentially distressing situation, such as when a person tries to relax before calling to receive the results of a laboratory test. Anticipatory adaptation is one human capacity that makes therapeutic communication possible; the client needs to have the capacity to imagine events in advance and analyze how to communicate more effectively in potentially distressing situations. In other words, people needs to be able to conceptualize the future, or else they will be severely limited in their ability to solve problems that may occur in the future. *Momentary adaptation* is the ability to be effective at the moment the distressing situation actually occurs. The success of therapeutic communication also depends on the client developing this ability.

However, the therapist has an advantage in possessing a certain kind of *leverage* with the client. This leverage is developed in the process of the therapeutic relationship, and it occurs in many nurse-client communication situations. The leverage refers to the influence of the helping person on the client that adds to, but is different from, the motivation of the client to acquire or enter a state of well-being. This leverage is a kind of power or influence and is produced by the helper's efforts on the client's behalf. It refers to influence over the thoughts, feelings, and behaviors of another and is created through the processes of understanding communication, acceptance, and agreement. Figure 5-5 illustrates the three steps in developing this leverage.

First, through communication with the client, the nurse seeks to gain an understanding of the nature of the

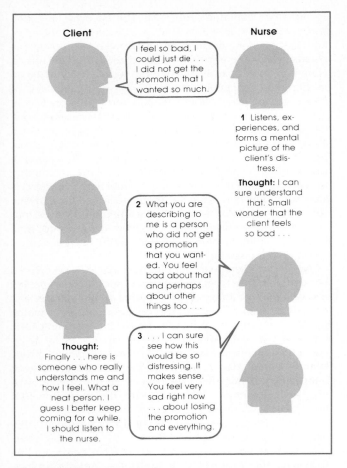

FIGURE 5-5 Steps in therapeutic leverage the nurse develops with the client.

client's distress. The nurse perceives the client's statements about himself and what needs to be changed. This first step in developing leverage—understanding—is a process that occurs within the nurse in which the client's distress becomes comprehensible. The nurse has a mental description or image of the client's distress and a cognitive acceptance of it as being the best picture of the client's reality that can be achieved at that moment.

The second step involves the nurse engaging the client in communication in which information is shared between the client and the nurse about the nurse's observations and analysis of the client's behavior. Later in this chapter, a variety of communication approaches are described to assist the nurse in developing skills in sharing information with clients, conveying acceptance, and promoting greater self-understanding.

The third step is agreement. To whatever degree possible, the nurse agrees with the client as a form of support that is relayed through communication. The agreement represents consensual validation of the client's distress and the need for improvement through change. That is, the nurse and client reach agreements about what the client is experiencing, what needs to change, and what may bring about those changes. Agreements reached through consensual validation represent a kind of negotiation, in that the nurse and patient bring their respective viewpoints to some form of similar picture of what is happening and what is to be done.

It is important for nurses to understand that for a variety of possible reasons the nurse can influence the client in some nurse-client interactions. While many approaches, such as Reusch's, perceive the therapist's leverage to have great therapeutic importance, an alternative view involved in a holistic approach encourages a balance of power in

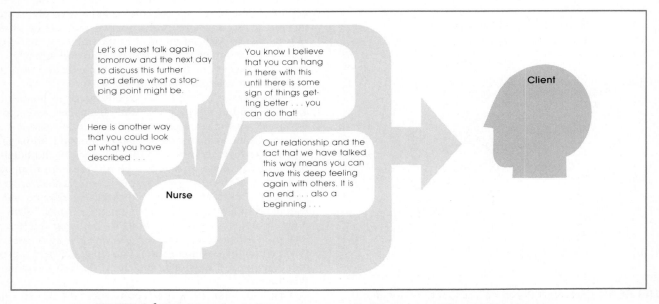

FIGURE 5-6 Helpful nurse-to-client statements using leverage to a therapeutic advantage.

which the client perceives the power of healing to reside within the self. The resolution of this balance of power in the nurse-client relationship is a function of the nurse's beliefs about practice and the specific needs of each client.

The nurse's influence or leverage can influence the client to listen to and consider new ideas and new ways of viewing experience. Figure 5-6 illustrates a nurse's use of this leverage to a therapeutic advantage. The nurse can also influence the client to continue in the therapeutic communication process, an involvement that is especially important when harm to self or others is a risk. The nurse believes in the client; by having leverage or an ability to exert influence, the nurse can help the client begin to hold more favorable views of himself or others. Finally, the leverage of the nurse creates potent learning possibilities at the time of termination of the therapeutic relationship. Through communication about the client's concerns and the influence of the nurse, the client is able to understand experientially how one person can allow another to become important and how growth can result from the therapeutic relationship and from coming to terms with the loss of the therapeutic relationship.

Double-Bind Communication

Double-bind communication is the simultaneous communication of conflicting messages. The double-bind theory, developed by the Bateson group, also called the Palo Alto group, was derived from communication theory and the analysis of communication patterns in families in which a member had developed schizophrenia. The original research addressed the analysis of family members' skills with use of various modes of communication, humor, pretending, and learning. One initial belief about the disturbed communication in persons having the symptoms of schizophrenia was that they had difficulty knowing what communication mode they or others were using. For example, they may not recognize the humor in another person's message or they may be comical without knowing it. They also may use metaphors incorrectly or fail to recognize the meaning of a metaphor used by another. A second belief about the communication problems of these persons is that they had difficulty recognizing communication modes within themselves. For example, they may have felt pain but were unsure if it hurt or tickled, or may have had an idea and not known whether other people could overhear the thought.

The essential characteristics of double-bind communication are listed in the box below.

The following examples illustrate this pattern of conflicting messages that are characteristic of double-bind communication:

Mother: *Come give mother a kiss before going out or she will be angry with you all evening.*
Adolescent: *Approaches the mother and starts to kiss her goodbye.*
Mother: *Grimaces and turns head away as if offended, and might say the youngster has bad breath or a dirty shirt collar.*

The tertiary, or third, message is implied by the expectation that the child cannot avoid the interaction with the mother, even though no response from the child can prevent the mother's anger or rejection

A more common type of double-bind communication involves conflicting messages that employ one spoken and one nonverbal message. For example, a friend might complain that no one ever calls her, but she sounds too busy to talk when someone does call. As another example, a supervisor might ask for suggestions about how to solve a problem, but frown or laugh at each suggestion.

Double-bind communication typically occurs in most types of communication situations at one time or another, so it is not necessarily associated with a disorder such as schizophrenia. Some theorists have argued that it is a necessary ingredient for the disorder but not a sufficient cause. Others suggest it results from a disturbance in communication originating in the person with the schizophrenic disorder; others simply respond to the person's disordered communication as best they can and it turns out to be a conflicting series of messages.

Assessment of this communication pattern involves analysis of the following:
1. The frequency of the double-bind communication patern
2. The importance of the relationships involved

CRITICAL INGREDIENTS OF DOUBLE-BIND COMMUNICATION

1. Two persons must be present; the person with disturbed communication assumes the role of victim or underdog.
2. The two persons engage in a recurring pattern of communication.
3. The victim or underdog receives a primary negative message or injunction, such as "don't do 'X' or I will punish you, or do 'X' or I will punish you."
4. The victim receives a secondary injunction that conflicts with the first; this is usually worded in a more abstract way so that the person might realize that there is an implied punishment for not doing "X" despite having been told to do so.
5. The individual also receives a tertiary negative injunction prohibiting escape from the situation.
6. The pattern becomes sufficiently stable and recurring that the person with the disturbed communication comes to expect the conflicting messages and prohibition of escape, even when all three types of injunction are not explicitly communicated.

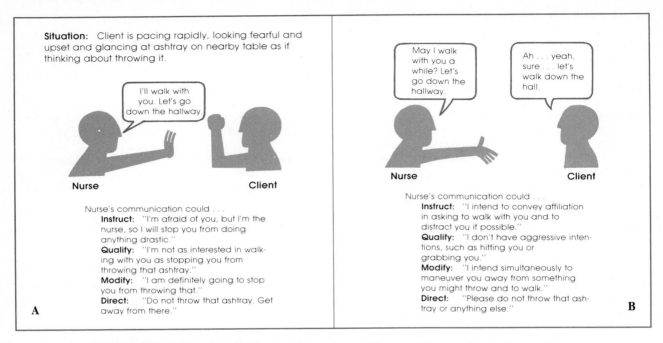

FIGURE 5-7 Metacommunication that instructs, qualifies, modifies, or directs the receiver.
A, Nontherapeutic communication. B, Therapeutic communication.

3. The seriousness of the tertiary messages prohibiting escape
4. The extent to which the victim feels either helpless or capable of coping or confronting the interactions

Kinesics

The major idea outlined in Scheflen's work on nonverbal communication[15] is that interactions, and inevitably relationships, are controlled by the nonverbal gestures and cues of communications. These gestures are called *kinesic behavior,* which is body language. An example of this anthropological approach to analyzing nonverbal behavior is kinesic reciprocals, which deal with *affiliation, dominance,* and *submission.* For example, leaning back, showing the palm of the hand, and fussing with the other person's collar are all possible courting behaviors conveying an invitation to closeness or affiliation. Reaching out in the midst of a conversation to poke the other person in the chest is a domineering behavior; laughing while being poked is a way to submit while at the same time trivializing or eliminating the other's aggressive intent. Reciprocal activities of two people are indicated by the way they place their bodies. For example, two people may lean close together to speak privately, or they may hold their arms in such a way to signal other people not to approach. Other behaviors signify awareness of passing through another's territory, such as when a person has hunched shoulders, hands to the body, and lowered head in a strange neighborhood or when visiting an unfamiliar church. Finally, two people exchanging greetings indicate through their behavior how familiar they are with one another; for example, familiarity is conveyed by a raising of eyebrows, a salutation, and a waving gesture.

Kinesic behaviors also regulate human behavior. Figure 5-7 shows how two different sets of kinesic behaviors instruct about, qualify, or direct human communication behaviors in the same hypothetical situation. This exchange of information about the communication had earlier been described by Reusch as metacommunication.

Since kinesic behaviors are body movements that convey meaning in communication, it is reasonable to expect that kinesic behaviors vary between cultures and ethnic groups just as spoken language varies.[3, 15] One frequently described variation is the use of eye contact in communication. In some cultures, maintaining the gaze for any length of time is inappropriate, whereas others use extended gazing. Typically, the British and Americans who are used to the prolonged gaze mistakenly interpret unwillingness to maintain the gaze as submissiveness or shyness when actually it can be attributed to cultural differences. Chapter 10, covering cultural diversity, discusses these cultural variations in more detail.

Proxemics

The study of *proxemics* focuses on how people use space. Investigators undertook early studies in this subject because they sought to understand how animals achieved and maintained so-called territories. In this context, territories were frequently well defined in terms of physical space. As interest in applying these ideas to human behavior took form, broader conceptions of territory emerged. For example, the definition of a person's territory at one moment may be his room, his home, or the boundaries of his farm. Alternatively, in a busy crowd or an intensely angry confrontation, a person's territory may be an intangible but real boundary surrounding the person beyond which others should not pass. Such boundaries are permeable, and they are usually flexible. More physical closeness is allowed in some instances than in others. Some of the concepts in this area of study include territoriality, social distance, personal space, ego boundaries, and crowding. People clearly are territorial (see Figure 5-8).

Four different zones of space in human interaction can be defined: intimate, personal, social, and public.[6] Perception of space is a factor in defining the boundaries of these zones. The boundaries expand or contract, depending on the context and the information the person is receiving from the situation.

The *intimate zone* within 18 inches of the body is the space in which physical activity occurs. It permits awareness of the scent and heat of another person's body. It is possible to speak in barely audible terms. Others with whom one is close are allowed into this space with ease; the entry of strangers or unwelcome others is an intrusion and creates discomfort. The practice of nursing places people in each other's intimate zone, at times, without the prior establishment of familiarity or trust. Discomfort for client or nurse can result.

From 18 inches to approximately 4 feet is the *personal zone*. It is similar to a protective zone, and it has boundaries that expand and contract according to contextual characteristics. Usually a person wants to limit entry of others into this space, so that only those with whom there is familiarity can gain entry.

Social space is about 4 to 12 feet from the person. In this zone, no touching is possible. It characterizes such situations as a group therapy session, a small group conference, or a conversation in a living room setting. *Public space* extends outward from approximately 12 feet. This space occurs in large group situations such as between a speaker and a workshop audience. These ideas can be validated by systematically observing human interaction. Behavior evoked by violations of others' boundaries varies with individuals and cultures; aggression might result in one culture and submissive behavior in another.

The use of touch in mental health–psychiatric nursing is related to the concept of space. Mental health–psychiatric nursing differs from most other arenas of nursing practice that require nurses to touch clients to change dressings, give baths, and administer injections. As a result, touch can be defined as optional rather than essential. Thus the appropriateness of touch in mental health–psychiatric nursing has aroused debate over the years.

Before the use of mental health labels, therapy roles, or psychotropic medications, touch was essential to mental health–psychiatric nursing because nurses fed and bathed their clients if necessary and administered wet-sheet packs to reduce extreme anger or anxiety. In those days, nurses did not wonder whether they should use touch in their practice. The advent of therapeutic roles in nursing meant nurse and client sat and talked in more formal and defined terms, and touching was no longer assumed to be a natu-

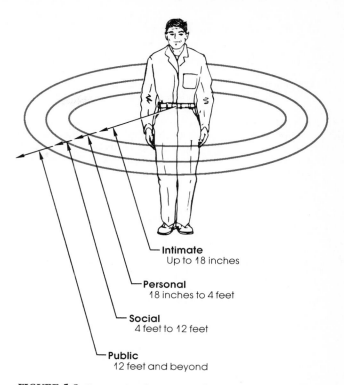

FIGURE 5-8 Proxemics focuses on four zones of space in human interaction.

ral part of practice. The relationship was differentiated as one of oral communication, not physical care and as one of therapeutic, not personal involvement. This distinction changed the way the nurse viewed her relationship with her patient and led some nurses to redefine the person as a "client."

In therapeutic interactions, the nurse can thoughtfully choose how or when to use touch to increase the effectiveness of her work with the client. Examples of touch that can be used within the context of therapeutic communication are shaking hands, touching the client's hand or arm, a back or neck rub, or a hug. In contemporary practice, even though people commonly greet parents, siblings, spouses, or close friends with a kiss and hug, nurses almost never greet a client with a kiss and hug. Kissing is not a part of therapeutic communication in our culture. Where it is culturally acceptable, it is still made absolutely clear that sexual intimacy is not intended (for example, the light kiss on one or both cheeks often shared by people of European descent).

Touch can convey many different kinds of energy or meaning, such as warmth, affection, empathy or understanding, restraint, reassurance, and emphasis. The use of touch is a conscious component of practice. Accordingly, client assessment needs to include evaluation of how the nurse may touch the client, how the client may react, and when touch is appropriate. If touch seems appropriate and consistent with the nurse's conceptual framework for practice, and if contextual factors (agency policy or an instructor's recommendation) are not prohibitive, touch-

TABLE 5-1 Communication channels: examples of function, dysfunction, and nursing intervention

Description of Channel	Example of Function and Dysfunction	Example of Nursing Intervention
Physiological	Normal gastrointestinal function versus stomachache and diarrhea in the face of distress	Discussion with client to reveal how gastrointestinal symptoms emerge in response to distress: development of stress management plan to cope with distress
Fine motor (kinesic and proxemic)	Each person in a family discussion speaks for self versus a family therapy session in which client never speaks and the mother always speaks for the child	Discussion that brings the communication pattern to the awareness of the family members; if necessary, a request that the child speak for self
Behavioral	Normal routines versus sharp deviations such as suddenly dropping out of school, marrying, or robbing a bank	If possible—if proximity with the person can be achieved—discussion about how the behavior does not fit with the "expected" routines; inquiry about possible causes
Verbal expression of behavior	Openness about behavior versus unwillingness to see or talk about behavior	Discussion of client's behavior to achieve shared awareness between client and nurse of the behavior and related problems and need for solutions
Verbal expression of thoughts, opinions, and ideas	Open discussion of ideas versus extreme shyness and reluctance to express thoughts or ideas	Discussion with client in which exploration of thoughts and ideas is pursued to determine (or correct if needed or possible), for example, distortions and error in client's perceptions
Verbal expression of feelings and emotions	Open expression of feelings, including distress, versus withdrawn and flat expression and denial of emotional pain or distress	Discussion with client to achieve openness as well as evaluation of extent of distress; effort to achieve congruence between behavior, thought, and feeling

Adapted from Longo, D.C.: In Longo, D.C., and Williams, R.A., editors: Clinical practice in psychosocial nursing: assessment and intervention, ed. 2, New York, 1986, Appleton-Century-Crofts.

TABLE 5-2 Summary of theories of communication

Theory	Dynamics	Major Concepts
Reusch	Therapeutic communication involves (1) gaining an understanding of the nature of the client's distress; (2) engaging the client in an analysis of his behavior, and (3) reaching agreement about what needs to change and what may bring about this change.	Metacommunication Anticipatory adaptation Momentary adaptation Leverage
Double bind	The simultaneous communication of conflicting messages results in the recipient's not knowing which message to respond to.	Primary, secondary, and tertiary messages
Kinesics	Behavior is regulated by nonverbal gestures and cues, also called body language.	Affiliation Dominance Submission
Proxemics	Persons have intangible but real boundaries surrounding them that they communicate to others.	Territoriality Social distance Personal space Ego boundaries Crowding Touch
Communication channels	Persons communicate through six "channels"; if one or more channels become dysfunctional, they will communicate through at least one of the other channels.	Congruence across channels

ing gestures can be incorporated into the client's care plan. Appropriate times are usually defined as special occasions that deserve the added emphasis of touch. The occasions may emerge from the client's need or the nurse's desire to emphasize a point.

Therapeutic touch, or touch with the intent to heal, is a specialized kind of touching that can be learned through training with a clinician already experienced in this approach. The nurse begins with a centering process that is similar to meditation, emphasizing awareness of one's own energies and ability to transmit these energies to other humans. The nurse's motivation is to help heal the client. This motivation creates a conscious intent to heal that combines with the ability to transmit one's energies to another person.[8]

Communication Channels

Another way to organize observations about human communication is to use the six levels of communication outlined in Longo's "channel construct"[9] of communication (see Table 5-1). The need to maintain a sense of relatedness is so great that people have evolved a kind of fail-safe system that ensures the function of at least one level of communication even if one or more of the others become dysfunctional.

Long's "channel construct" provides a focus on the process of communication, which involves the manner in which something is said or done, as in asking a direct question. Longo distinguishes the process from the content, which is the literal meaning of words and symbols, and the context, which is the setting or circumstances in which communication takes place. The construct offers a framework for assessment and intervention. The six channels provide the nurse with an outline of what to observe and how to classify the data. Evaluation of the congruence of communication across channels is an important part of clinical assessment. For example, the client who says he feels comfortable while squirming about and exhibiting a sad facial expression is demonstrating incongruence across channels.

Intervention is planned and implemented after an analysis of the following four major aspects of the communication:

1. The functional competence
2. The congruence
3. The appropriateness of the findings relative to the client's problem
4. The appropriateness of the findings relative to the context and content

Table 5-1 shows examples of functions and dysfunctions and interventions for the six channels. Table 5-2 summarizes the dynamics and major concepts of the theories of communication.

TECHNIQUES OF THERAPEUTIC COMMUNICATION

This section presents specific techniques for the use of the nurse that increase the therapeutic value of nurse-client interactions and facilitate development of learning experiences to help the client achieve greater self-awareness and a higher regard for self. Although each technique is presented separately, the techniques are typically used in combination to facilitate effective nurse-client communication. Table 5-3 provides several examples of some of the most commonly used therapeutic communication techniques. Table 5-4 gives examples of nontherapeutic techniques. A discussion of additional techniques follow.

Conveying Respect

Respect is a point of view that says to another, "You count. You have worth. You matter. You have dignity, and I will treat you in a respectful, polite manner." The nurse may convey respect to the client in several ways. By being on time for appointments and by spending the full time with the client that has been agreed upon, the nurse conveys her respect for the client's time and space. The nurse also conveys respect for the client by treating his room and belongings as private property; permission is requested to gain access to these private spaces. Some people believe that adult clients should never be addressed by first names because it conveys disrespect for their adult status. Although addressing every client with "Mr." or "Ms." may seem extreme, use of first names only when addressing all clients is also extreme and suggests that individual decisions about what to call each client are not being made.

Respect in any society is usually shown through subtle nuances in verbal and nonverbal behavior, for example, calling a person by their name. When the client is from a different social class or culture than the nurse, conscious effort permits the nurse to learn how respect is conveyed in the other person's culture and how to avoid inadvertently conveying disrespect.

Listening Actively

Listening actively implies that the nurse is an active rather than passive participant in the interaction. *Active listening* means that the nurse conveys a real desire to hear what the client has to say. Listening actively contributes to the therapeutic value of the communication process in two ways: (1) the client experiences the nurse's active interest and feels reassured of the nurse's intention to help, and (2) the nurse is likely to hear more of what the client has to say and to better understand the nature of the client's concerns.

Active listening is apparent to the client in verbal and nonverbal ways. Verbally, the nurse comments or asks questions that relate directly to what the client has been saying. The content of the nurse's questions or comments make it clear that the nurse is listening. Nonverbally, the nurse maintains eye contact (without staring), leans forward in the chair to convey interest and attention, nods to show agreement or disagreement, and frowns or smiles to convey an appropriate confusion or understanding about the client's comments.

TABLE 5-3 Therapeutic communication techniques

Therapeutic Techniques	Examples
Using silence: using absence of verbal communication	
Accepting: indicating reception	Yes.
	Uh-hmm.
	I follow what you said.
	Nodding
Giving recognition: acknowledging, indicating awareness	You're coughing and breathing deeply.
	You cleaned your house.
Offering self: making one's *self* available	I'll sit with you a while.
	I'll stay here with you.
Giving broad openings: allowing the client to take the initiative in introducing the topic	What would you like to talk about?
	What are you thinking about?
	Where would you like to begin?
Offering general leads: giving encouragement to continue	Go on.
	And then?
	Tell me about it.
Placing the event in time or in sequence: clarifying the relationship of events in time	What seemed to lead up to . . . ?
	This was before or after . . . ?
	When did this happen?
Making observations: verbalizing what is perceived	You appear tense.
	You seem uncomfortable when you . . .
	I notice you biting your lips.
	I become uncomfortable when you . . .
Encouraging description of perception: asking the client to verbalize what he perceives	When do you feel anxious?
	What is happening?
	What does the voice seem to be saying?
Encouraging comparison: asking that similarities and differences be noted	This was something like . . .
	When have you had similar experiences?
Reflecting: directing back to the client's questions, feelings, and ideas; encouraging the client to bring forth his own ideas, which the nurse thereby acknowledges	**Client:** Do you think I should tell the doctor . . . ?
	Nurse: You are wondering if it is important.
Focusing: concentrating on a single point	This seems like an area we can concentrate on.
Exploring: delving further into a subject or idea	Tell me more about that. Would you describe it more fully? What kind of work?
Seeking clarification: seeking to make clear anything not meaningful or vague	I'm not sure that I follow. What would you say is the main point of what you said? Tell me whether my understanding of it agrees with yours. Are you using this word to convey the idea of . . . ?
Presenting reality: offering for consideration what is real	I see no one else in the room. That sound was a car backfiring. Your mother is not here; I'm a nurse.
Verbalizing the implied: voicing what the client has hinted at or suggested	**Client:** My wife pushes me around just like my mother and sister do.
	Nurse: Is it your impression that women are domineering?
Encouraging evaluation: asking for appraisal of the quality of his experiences	What are your feelings in regard to . . . ? Does this contribute to your discomfort?
Attempting to translate into feelings: seeking to verbalize the feelings being expressed only indirectly	**Client:** I've been in this hospital for six weeks. I might as well be dead.
	Nurse: You feel as if you're not getting any better?
Suggesting collaboration: offering to share, to strive to work together with the client for his benefit	Maybe this is something you and I can figure out together.
Encouraging formulation of a plan of action: asking the client to consider behavioral alternatives that may be appropriate in future situations	What could you do to let your anger out harmlessly? Next time this comes up, what can you do to handle it?

Based on data from Hays, J.S., and Larson, K.H.: Interacting with patients, New York, 1965, The Macmillan Co., Publishers.

TABLE 5-4 Nontherapeutic communication techniques

Nontherapeutic Techniques	Examples
Reassuring: indicating that there is no cause for anxiety	I wouldn't worry about . . . Everything will be all right. You're coming along fine.
Giving approval: sanctioning the client's ideas or behavior	That's good . . . I'm glad that you . . .
Rejecting: refusing to consider the client's ideas	Let's not discuss . . . I don't want to hear about . . .
Disapproving: denouncing the client's ideas and behavior	That's bad. I'd rather you wouldn't . .
Agreeing: indicating accord with the client	That's right. I agree.
Disagreeing: opposing the client's ideas	That's wrong. I definitely disagree with . . .
Advising: telling the client what to do	I think you should . . . Why don't you . . . ?
Probing: persistent questioning of the client	Now tell me about . . . Tell me your life history.
Challenging: demanding proof from the client	**Client:** I feel dead all over. **Nurse:** If you don't need the surgery, then why are you here?
Defending: attempting to protect someone or something from verbal attack	This hospital has a fine reputation. No one here would lie to you. But Dr. B. is a very able psychiatrist. I'm sure that he has your welfare in mind when he . . .
Requesting an explanation: asking someone to provide reasons for feelings, behavior, and events	Why do you think that? Why do you feel this way? Why did you do that?
Indicating the existence of an external source: attributing the source of thoughts, feelings, and behavior to others or to outside influences	What makes you say that? What made you do that?
Belittling feelings expressed: misjudging the degree of the client's discomfort	**Client:** I have nothing to live for, I wish I were dead. **Nurse:** Everybody gets down in the dumps, [or] I've felt that way sometimes.
Making stereotypical comments: offering meaningless clichés and trite expressions	Nice weather we're having. I'm fine, and how are you? It's for your own good. Keep your chin up. Just listen to your doctor and take part in activities. You'll be home in no time.
Giving literal responses: responding to a figurative comment as though it were a statement of fact	**Client:** I feel like my insides are coming out. **Nurse:** Show me where they're coming out.
Using denial: refusing to admit that a problem exists	**Client:** I'm nothing. **Nurse:** Of course you're something. Everybody is somebody. **Client:** I'm dead. **Nurse:** No, you're not.
Introducing an unrelated topic: changing the subject	**Client:** I'd like to die. **Nurse:** Did you have visitors this weekend?

Based on data from Hays, J.H., and Larson, K.H.: Interacting with patients, New York, 1965, The Macmillan Co., Publishers.

Defining Boundaries

The boundaries of nurse-client communication are the social, physical, and emotional limits of the interaction. The nurse's efforts to help the client work within these boundaries create opportunities for the client to gain self-awareness. For example, the interaction is defined as therapeutic rather than social, which means it is occurring because of the client's need and is intended to benefit the client. The interaction can be friendly in spirit, but the conversation is not meant to establish friendship. The nurse assists the client to understand and accept that the nurse's purpose is to help the client learn; the client is not expected to help the nurse learn (although the nurse often learns much in working with clients). The nurse cares about the client's well-being; the client is helped to know that he is not expected to care about the nurse in a personal way. Gentle confrontation of the client's attempts to make the relationship different from the therapeutic boundaries allows the client to understand more about his own motives and to accept the nurse's intentions to be helpful.

The physical boundaries of the nurse-client communication define where the communication will and will not occur. For example, the nurse and client typically meet in a clinic or an office, and meeting in the home of the nurse or client is usually not acceptable unless the contact is structured as a home visit. Alternatively, the nurse and client may appropriately communicate in the home of the nurse if the nurse's home is a private practice setting. At issue here is that the physical space is consistent with the definition of the communication as having therapeutic not social purposes.

A further example of defining boundaries is the establishment of ground rules in the communication process. For example, the nurse can establish such rules as the following: (1) the client may not make phone calls to the nurse's home, and (2) the client may not attempt to meet the nurse in a social situation.

Defining boundaries contributes to the therapeutic potential of the nurse's communication with the client because it maintains a focus on the healing process. The structure is also useful in that the nurse can at any point remind the client about the boundaries in a gentle but firm way, stressing the value of keeping the interaction on therapeutic terms. This attention to boundaries also conveys that the nurse continues to care about the client and that the nurse remains committed to the therapeutic purposes of the relationship.

Structuring Time

The therapeutic potential of nurse-client communication can be enhanced by having the client know exactly how much time the nurse has available for the conversation. For example, a 30-minute conversation on an inpatient unit is likely to be disappointing if the client expects the nurse to stay for an hour. Alternatively, the client is likely to feel respected and cared about if the nurse agrees to meet for 30 minutes and keeps that time agreement. For the client who wants extra time, very positive effects can sometimes be achieved by the nurse's occasional decision to make available an unexpected extra half hour with the client.

Pacing

Pacing emphasizes the nurse's ability to recognize the verbal and nonverbal patterns of the client's immediate behavior and levels of tension. Pacing involves following these patterns until the nurse can take the lead in the conversation, directing discussion to needed areas of focus but doing so in a way consistent with the client's pattern of communication. Pacing also implies that the nurse has a goal. Imagine an example of a client who has been raped who needs to recount what has happened. The client may focus on extraneous information as a means of reducing tension. The nurse, by following and then pacing the client's comments and observing the client's behavioral indicators of tension, can gently lead the client into discussion about the event. The nurse's sensitivity to the client's capacity to tolerate tension is important in maintaining rapport and a sense of alliance with the client. Therapeutic communication is disrupted if the client is overwhelmed. As a client gains confidence and moves through phases of the relationship, the capacity to experience and profit from intense emotional response increases and the pace with which the nurse approaches these issues can be much faster.

Effectively Using Questions

Since the assessment process requires nurses to obtain information from clients, the habit of asking clients questions is easy to acquire. In some instances a question is an appropriate way to seek an answer. For example, the easiest way to find out a client's age might be to ask, "How old are you?" or "What is your birth date?" However, an abundance of questions about the client's background tends to make the client feel barraged. Intensive questioning can also convey the message, "You are a statistic." Learning about the effective use of questions is best achieved by examining written verbatim accounts of nurse-client interactions (also called process recordings) to see how often questions are used and what responses from clients occur. In many instances, information can also be obtained by the use of more indirect invitations to talk, such as "Tell me about your family, brothers, sisters, parents. . ."

Asking clients "Why did you do that?" or "Why?" can be especially problematic for them. Naturally the nurse wants to know why a particular behavior or event occurred, and the information would also be useful to the client. However, clients frequently do not know why they have done something or felt a certain way. They are a "client" who needs to talk about some behavior or event because they are troubled about it in some way and do not understand why it happened. Clients often say, "I don't know why I did that." When asked why, they probably have good reason to say, "If I knew why, I wouldn't be here!" If the information the nurse seeks is a description of how the event took place, that is the question to ask. For example, "Tell me how the argument got started in the first place," or "What were you doing at the time?" are effective questions. "Why did you argue?" is usually nontherapeutic for two reasons: the client is not likely to know, and the question sounds like a demand for explanation or self-defense.

Another very overused question is "How did you feel about that?" This trite question is often heard when a client's nursing care plan recommends "encourage verbalization of feelings." The incorrect belief is that expressing feelings is an end point in therapeutic intervention. However, it is really only a beginning point, and the question often leaves the client consciously experiencing a painful feeling or memory. The expression of feelings is only the first step in the "working through" process of healing or achieving resolution of painful feelings and memories. The steps include

1. Verbalization of the painful feelings or memories
2. Validation with another person (such as the nurse) that the feelings or memories are understandable human experiences and that they are acknowledged as sources of pain for the client
3. Mourning or "working through" the pain by talking about the feelings several times, leading to re-experiencing of the feelings in a less intense way, emergence of hope, and perception of new alternatives.
4. Restitution, in which the client has gained a new perspective on the painful feelings or feels relieved to a sufficient degree that they are no longer a problem

In summary, instead of directly asking the client how he feels, the nurse needs to help the client proceed through the sequence and progress beyond simply expressing and experiencing the pain to resolving the painful feelings and memories as well. As a general rule, questions can be replaced by reflection, by open-ended statements that invite the client to complete the statement, and by declarative statements of what the client may be feeling that contain a slight inflection or implication of a question. Clients can respond to these invitations if they feel comfortable, but are spared the feeling of being interrogated that can be created by a series of questions. These invitations are especially effective if they are offered with a moderate degree of warmth and spirit of understanding that carefully avoids excessively sympathetic tones of voice often heard in interactions with clients.

Restating

The client can be aided in efforts to achieve self-understanding by the judicious use of *restating,* in which the nurse repeats to the client what has been said. For example, the nurse is using restating in the following interaction:

Client: *We are really having a rough time at home.*
Nurse: *You're having a rough time at home . . . . (voice trails off)*

Client: *Well, yes. What I mean is that my teenager is really arguing with me a lot and I feel like I don't know what to say.*
Nurse: *You aren't sure what to say. . . .*
Client: *Right. I want to really come down hard and say a curfew is a curfew. Instead, I hold back. I don't know why.*

The nurse restates back to the client what has been said, using the client's choice of words. The use of restating can be in the form of a question or a statement:

Nurse: *You're having a rough time at home? (Emphasis on the word "home" and voice inflection conveys a question.)*

or

Nurse: *You're having a rough time at home. . . (Emphasis on the words "rough time" and voice inflection conveys a statement that trails off, as if waiting for the client's response.)*

The purpose of restating is to increase the client's awareness of what he is saying and how it is being said. The approach needs to be used in a calm manner without aggressively confronting the client or trying to pressure the client into greater self-awareness. The nurse needs to incorporate this approach into a larger repertoire of skills so that it is not overused; excessive reliance on restating is irritating to clients because the nurse sounds unwilling to respond or appears overly reliant on a technique.

Validating

Validating is a technique that can be valuable to therapeutic communication in two important ways: assisting the client to achieve a more realistic view of the world, and creating in the client the experience of feeling understood. *Validation* is the agreement of the nurse with certain elements of the client's communication, as in the following example:

Client: *Boy, you can't believe how bad my boss is. I get hassled all the time for things that aren't even my fault. I really think he has it in for me. Maybe he's even really completely against me because he wants somebody else in the position.*
Nurse: *Yes, it would make sense for you to feel distressed if the boss is against you. I can tell that you feel distressed—that this work situation is uncomfortable. (Pause.) I wonder if we could talk more about what he does and what he says and the circumstances so that I could get a better picture of it.*

Here the nurse has validated the appropriateness of feeling upset about the client's supervisor, although the actual story about the supervisor has not been validated. Instead, the nurse requests further exploration of the topic. The client can feel understood with regard to the distress that he has experienced on the job. The client can also sense the nurse's interest and potential acceptance because of her request to pursue the topic further. At the same time, the nurse's statement also contains a subtle suggestion that the story about the supervisor might not be completely true. Use of a subtle hint can be an important first step in casting doubt on a client's perception of experience, which may be all the doubt that is appropriate to show until more information about the situation is obtained. The client is neither totally believed nor totally disbelieved at the outset.

Asking for Demonstrations and Illustrations

Asking for demonstrations and illustrations may involve the client in giving the nurse an example, or the nurse can have the client literally show her what has gone on. For example, a client complained that her mother made her feel guilty every time she talked to her on the phone. The nurse helped the client go through a detailed demonstration of preparing to call her mother, dialing the number, repeating her lines to her mother, and then filling in her mother's responses including mimicking her tone of voice. The client laughed because she identified two aspects of her "guilt": her desire to avoid seeing her mother that day and her anger at her mother for saying it was all right yet sounding very whiny. The client was able to use this information in talking with her mother; over a period of time, her mother agreed that although she knew it was wrong, she was, in fact, attempting to make her daughter feel guilty.

Providing Information

Providing information to a client increases the client's resources for solving problems and making decisions. It also conveys the message that the nurse cares and is a giving person. Apprising the client of specific resources that match his needs provides information. Enlisting the assistance of others such as a social worker or rehabilitation counselor can also provide information needed to confront a particular problem. Another significant way of providing information is teaching the client mental health concepts, such as communication skills, to enhance the person's ability to solve problems and relate effectively to others. For example, the nurse may teach problem-solving methods as a way of tackling difficult decisions. The nurse may also teach the concepts of transactional analysis to the client and his significant others as a way to work on communication problems at home and during interactions with her.

Emphasizing Relationships Between Parts and Wholes

Therapeutic nurse-client interaction can assist clients to understand how their way of thinking about experience leads to problems or inaccuracies in perception. Some clients generalize too much on the basis of limited experience; others seem to see only discrete events and fail to learn by generalizing despite multiple similar experiences. These problems can be addressed in the nurse-client in-

teraction, using the interaction as an illustration when possible. Clients who tend to generalize on the basis of too little experience can be assisted to see the gaps in their information:

Client: I know that you don't really like me. People never do like me.
Nurse: That's a pretty big conclusion. How did you arrive at that idea?
Client: You were late today. I know what that means.
Nurse: Would you describe how it is that my being late makes it possible for you to think I don't like you?
Client: I just know. It's always been that way.
Nurse: Somebody was late whom you wanted to like you, and you felt bad because you feared they didn't?

A lengthier example relating specifics to the client's overgeneralization may be needed, but the example illustrates the point that the nurse can lead the client from the general idea (probably a distortion) to certain specifics, some of which confirm the idea and others that do not. The goal of this communication process is to teach the client that general ideas can be formed on the basis of too little or incorrect information. Strengthening skills in inductive thinking enables the client to analyze specific observations to confirm or deny general propositions in his thinking.

Clients who focus too much on specific events need assistance in developing deductive thinking skills so that general propositions (learning) can occur on the basis of discrete experiences or events. The skills of generalizing from experience require an ability to think in more abstract terms. The nurse-client communication can focus on this issue:

Client: Well, I've done it again. I had a huge fight with my wife, and I hate myself for doing it. I'm so depressed.
Nurse: This sounds familiar. I am curious about what led to the disagreement.
Client: It's the same old thing. Every time I forget to do the dishes, it's the same thing: a big fight.
Nurse: You forgot?
Client: Well, see, I was really mad about the house being a mess and having to think about all there was to do, most of which isn't my job, and I just forgot all about the dishes.
Nurse: That sounds like the other day when you were angry with me and forgot to keep our appointment. Is this a way of doing things that keeps you in trouble: you get angry and fail to do your end of things, say you forgot, and then fight and feel terrible about yourself?

The continuation of this interaction is aimed at helping the client see the relationship between the outcome of feeling bad about himself and the many separate events in which failure to fulfill an obligation is excused as forgetting and a disagreement ensues. Learning that the discrete events are related to the larger undesired outcome is the first step in creating an opportunity for the client to change. All the while, the nurse avoids the message, "You bring this on yourself," which can sound punitive and reinforces the client's self-deprecation. Instead, the nurse emphasizes the relationships between parts and whole in an objective manner.

Using Nurse-Client Communication for Experiential Illustrations

As a part of the therapeutic communication process, the nurse provides feedback to the client; this involves the nurse's sharing perceptions of what the client seems to be saying. The following example describes a nurse's response to a client who has described a conflict with a friend. The client described himself as having been unreasonable, ineffective, and overly angry:

Nurse: I have listened to you describe the situation and in my view there was good reason to feel angry. Perhaps it was not such a good idea to threaten to walk out, but the way you describe having stated your concerns sounds like a very reasonable statement.

However, when the nurse-client communication is used as illustration, the nurse provides feedback that directly relates to the communication that has occurred between nurse and client. For example, the nurse could have responded to the same client in the following way:

Nurse: You describe yourself as having been unreasonable, ineffective, and overly angry after expressing your feelings to your friend, feelings you were probably justified in having. I am thinking that may also happen when we talk. Remember the time you were irritated because I answered the phone during our talk and then later berated yourself for having an understandable reaction? (Voice trails off, leaving client the option of responding.)

The major value of using the nurse-client communication to illustrate ideas or conclusions is that both parties have shared the interaction; this means that the client will not think that the nurse failed to understand a situation that had been reported by the client. Another advantage is that this technique says to the client, "What we talk about is very important. You can learn from the way we talk about things and by going back to earlier conversations, which may help you understand yourself better."

Sharing That the Client Is Thought About

With most clients, the nurse will think about the client at times other than when the two are engaged in a therapeutic interaction. Sometimes this involves feelings about the client; at other times the nurse is attempting to understand the person or evaluate whether their interactions are helping the client. In any case, a positive statement the nurse can make to the client is "I was thinking about you." This is a common gesture of warmth in our society.

When a friend or relative calls or is encountered unexpectedly, one often says, "I was just thinking about you the other day." Often an explanation is added in which the person is complimented, such as, "I was remembering how much fun we had that time we went to the theater." With clients, a parallel message that conveys warmth and the feelings of being cared about is, "You know I was thinking yesterday about our last conversation and wondering how that family reunion went." In so doing, the nurse gives the client an unexpected gift of time (the time spent thinking about the client) and also eases introduction of communication about a potentially painful topic by the warm and caring context that has been created.

Offering Hope

Offering hope is a communication technique frequently used in day-to-day interactions with clients; the issue of hope or the lack of it can also be a major clinical problem to which the nurse addresses therapeutic efforts. (See Chapter 15 on Hope–Despair.)

Offering hope is a subtle and delicate matter. The nurse needs to simultaneously convey understanding and acceptance of the client's despair or pain. In some instances, hope is an optimistic attitude about the client's potential to return to health. In other instances, it is the belief that the client can become engaged in a therapeutic process that will permit problem-solving to begin. Hope is also related to spiritual beliefs, which for some people are directly connected to religious beliefs. Hope in these instances implies some form of faith in a higher power that will support or otherwise lend energy to the healing process. This means that the nurse will either need to support the client's spiritual beliefs or enlist the help of someone who can.

Guidelines that enhance the therapeutic potential of the nurse's offering of hope include the following:

1. Avoid a Pollyanna or overly cheerful attitude.
2. Accept the client's pain or distress as a valid part of the current experience.
3. Avoid urging the client to be more positive.
4. Offer statements calmly and with adequate opportunity for the client to respond.
5. Avoid urging the client to accept the beliefs of any specific religious faith.

Summarizing

Therapeutic nurse-client communication is aimed at creating learning opportunities for the client, and summarizing is an important way in which the nurse can reinforce important ideas or points. Summarizing also provides a check on the nurse's perceptions. By saying "Now let me try to summarize what we've talked about, and you tell me if it sounds right," the nurse can validate perceptions about the communication. In addition, this is a way of saying, "I have formed certain ideas about you and what you have said here, but I do not just assume I am correct. I value your opinions."

The nurse can also invite the client to summarize, as in saying, "Suppose you were to put what we've talked about in a nutshell. How would you say it?" This is another way to check perceptions and determine discrepancies between the views of the nurse and those of the client. It also says, "I am interested in hearing how you sum things up; your way of looking at things is important, and you are the best person to tell me about it."

ISSUES IN THERAPEUTIC COMMUNICATION

This section reviews the following issues in therapeutic nurse-client interaction:

1. How much self-disclosure by the nurse is appropriate?
2. How much energy and reactivity is appropriate for the nurse to display?
3. How much personal feedback does the client receive?
4. When or how is confrontation of the client therapeutic?
5. To what extent or in what ways is humor appropriate?

In this discussion, opposing views on the issues as well as the rationale for these views will be presented. Decisions about these issues need to incorporate the client's needs, contextual factors in the clinical setting that impinge on practice, and her informed judgment.

How Much Self-Disclosure?

Those who believe that self-disclosure by the nurse has therapeutic value argue that if the client views the relationship in personal terms, this problem can be addressed in the therapeutic interaction. Self-disclosure provides the client with an opportunity to perceive the nurse as a genuine human being rather than as a mechanical clinician. This approach is believed to be especially helpful when used to reassure the client that other people have the same or similar concerns.

Those who maintain that self-disclosure is inappropriate in nurse-client communication argue that personal disclosures on the part of the nurse encourage the client to view the relationship as one of personal friendship rather than therapeutic involvement. The nurse who uses a great deal of self-disclosure fills the conversation with talk about herself rather than the client. This limits the client's opportunity to gain self-awareness and increases the likelihood that the relationship will focus on the unresolved personal problems of the nurse rather than on those of the client.

Examples of nurse responses to a client's inquiry about where the nurse lives may include the following:

Client: I was wondering, where do you live, anyway?
Nurse: I live out in Ridgewood. (Self-disclosure.)

or

Nurse: I'm curious about your reason for asking. . .

or

Nurse: I live out in Ridgewood (pause). I'm curious about your reason for asking. (Modified self-disclosure.)

The client's question does not contain sufficient data for the nurse to make assumptions about why the question is being asked. The nurse may believe that self-disclosure is not acceptable because she perceives that the client's question expresses a wish to become more personally involved with her. If the nurse believes self-disclosure is effective, the client's question can simply be taken for its face value. If the nurse wants additional data and sees no problem in answering the question, the third response achieves both purposes.

Clients also frequently remark that the nurse reminds the client of someone, often a person in the client's past or present who is important. For example:

Client: You're just like my friend J.D.
Nurse: Well I'm certainly not J.D.! (No self-disclosure.)

or

Nurse: I wonder what about me reminds you of J.D.? (No self-disclosure but invitation to say more.)

The first response indicates surprise or anger at the client's comment; the nurse's response does not imply that any self-disclosure is likely to occur. The second response requests more information and leaves the issue of self-disclosure open.

How Much Emotion and Energy?

Strong emotion and energy conveyed in the nurse's reactions, feelings, or sentiments may have a significant impact on the client. This can be planned or accidental in nature. Examples of strong emotion or energy that the nurse can convey to the client are

1. Warmth, affection, caring, approval, and love
2. Encouragement, optimism, and hope
3. Irritation, anger, and disapproval
4. Downhearted feelings, despair, and depression
5. Touch, with or without the conscious intent to heal

Traditional approaches in therapeutic communication and psychotherapy have emphasized the importance of the clinician maintaining a neutral and objective stance in responding to the client. This approach precludes the nurse from expressing more than a very mild degree of affection and caring, encouragement, irritation or anger, moodiness, or touch. The rationale for this approach is that the nurse who expresses strong emotion or energy encourages the client to experience the relationship as a personal one, which is thought to be incompatible with the professional goals of the relationship. The client who experiences the relationship with the nurse as a personal one is more likely to misinterpret the nature of the relationship.

Advocates of the neutral or objective approach view client distortions and errors in interpretation as transference reactions. According to this view, it is nontherapeutic to communicate strong emotion and energy, thus encouraging the client to experience transference reactions. For example, the nurse's enthusiasm toward a client's report of a success may later induce the client to be frightened that a failure would disappoint the nurse. The nurse's expression of feeling downhearted can encourage the client to feel responsible, inadequate, or obligated to try to cheer up the nurse. Touching the client may cause fears that the nurse is making sexual overtures. In each of these examples, the client's untoward reaction may be related to a pattern of responding in an earlier relationship with a parent, sibling, or other significant person.

Clinicians who believe the expression of energy and emotion with the client has therapeutic value form the other extreme. They argue great therapeutic opportunities are created by provoking client reactions, such as when the nurse touches the client or expresses approval, encouragement, anger, or moodiness. The client's reactions are the focus of the therapeutic communication, which can lead to greater self-awareness for the client.

Another somewhat different argument in favor of showing emotion and energy suggests that the client will see the nurse as a more genuine person if feelings are candidly expressed when they occur. If the nurse feels happy, optimistic, angry, or downhearted or wants to touch the client, these reactions are appropriate for the nurse to share. The client has the opportunity to share in how another person experiences and talks about feeling these energies. This sharing is thought to assist the client in becoming more self-aware and better able to communicate effectively with others. When the nurse conveys strong emotion and energy, the client can experience the nurse's approval for a success or the nurse's disapproval for a failure to manage a problem effectively. Some believe that the reality-testing value of such experiences far outweighs the dangers of causing excessive transference reactions.

How Much Feedback?

In therapeutic communication, *feedback* refers to the nurse's sharing with the client (1) perceptions of the client's behavior, or (2) interpretations of the client's behavior. The client who storms into the meeting with a tense facial expression, tightened lips, and lack of verbal expressions receive one of the following responses:

Nurse: Well (softly), I see a person who is tense and not saying very much. . . .(pauses after open-ended statement).

or

Nurse: You seem upset (pauses).

In the first response, the nurse describes the observed behavior in terms that are as objective as possible. In the second response, the nurse makes no attempt to describe what is observed, instead sharing an interpretation of what has been observed.

Decisions about appropriate use of feedback include whether to use feedback at all as well as to what degree either type of feedback described should be used. Many nurses use feedback techniques extensively in therapeutic communication, believing that self-awareness is achieved as a result of helping the client learn how he is perceived by others. Assuming that the client is unaware of critical elements of behavior, especially in areas in which problems are reported, the nurse undertakes to bring these elements into the client's conscious awareness.

An alternative view is held by those who do not use feedback techniques very much or at all in therapeutic communication. The rationale is that extensive use of feedback techniques puts the nurse in an excessively directive role with the client. Instead, the nurse's role in therapeutic communication is defined as nondirective in which reflection of the client's thoughts is used to facilitate his responsibility for directing the conversation.

Feedback in which the nurse describes as objectively as possible observed behavior is generally accepted by those who advocate using feedback. However, use of interpretations of these observations is a controversial matter. Some nurses believe that the client can benefit from knowing the nurse's interpretations and conclusions. The client may then respond and offer alternative interpretations for discussion. Other nurses believe that interpretations are too directive, and that they create a risk of bringing to awareness thoughts or feelings for which the client is unprepared. They believe the nurse's role is to facilitate the client's expression of thoughts and feelings, not to impose or force these expressions before the client is ready.

How Much Confrontation?

In mental health work, *confrontation* usually refers to an encounter between two persons in which one person seeks to encourage another to face or acknowledge something presumed to be painful or objectionable. The nurse may confront a client about his resistance evidenced by missing his appointments. The plan to confront the client assumes that the client does not want to face this fact and that the nurse's role is to encourage the client to talk about it. The client may need to be made aware that he is manipulating the staff to get his way or being inconsistent in what he tells the staff are his concerns. The steps used

---

STEPS IN USING CONFRONTATION IN CLINICAL PRACTICE

1. Analyze who needs to be confronted about what.
2. Analyze the appropriate person to be the confronter.
3. Analyze the degree of resistance felt toward the person who is to be confronted.
4. Analyze the degree of defensiveness expected from the person to be confronted.
5. Develop a detailed plan for the confrontation based on specific therapeutic goals.
6. Implement the plan and evaluate the effectiveness of the nursing action.

in confrontation are outlined in the box on p. 83. Confrontation is often associated with the nurse's being angry, resulting in confrontation of the client in a way that seems to require the client to defend against the nurse's anger.

At each point in this sequence, the nurse can decide whether to implement the intervention or whether too much opposition exists for the confrontation to achieve a therapeutic purpose. Since the word "confrontation" often connotes antagonism, following the careful analysis outlined above is necessary. Deliberately antagonistic or retaliatory nursing actions are inappropriate. The potential to provoke anger in the client can create situations of real or potential danger to oneself or others. This risk is only undertaken with careful planning and anticipation of possible outcomes.

There are no rules to guide decisions about when and how much to confront clients in mental health–psychiatric nursing practice. Since there is little research or documentation in this area to guide practice, the decision is often based on the judgment of the nurse. Some nurses believe a confrontation mode should never be used because it is caused by the nurse's anger, and because it is so likely to sound punitive, provoking self-defensive or aggressive responses. Other nurses use confrontation extensively, believing that it simulates a real encounter with the added dimension of the willingness of the nurse to talk about the situation with the client (which may not always be possible in real life). Those who use confrontation in their practice believe clients can be held accountable for their behavior and that confrontation is the way to achieve this goal. Opponents of this approach usually agree that clients can be responsible for their behaviors, but they rely on gentler forms of feedback that minimize clients' needs to defend themselves or respond forcefully.

How Much Humor?

Humor contributes an essential ingredient to human interaction. It breaks the ice, smooths over stressful moments, and lightens the atmosphere in a great many situations.

The benefits of humor are many. An important consequence in the mental health arena is tension reduction and transcendance of uncomfortable moments or situations. Humor also creates a bond of shared pleasure between people, allowing for enjoyable times that contrast therapeutically with painful problems and distressing feelings that have been shared. Humor is believed to have important physiological effects as well. For example, it has been suggested that humor affects the immune system by promoting the body's ability to combat such health challenges as cancer and diseases of the connective tissue (arthritis, lupus erythematosis, and others).[16]

There is some debate about how much humor should be used in mental health–psychiatric nursing practice. Those who believe the therapist should remain neutral contend that humor is appropriate only in very limited and well-thought out situations. Others believe that whatever amount of spontaneous humor occurs is probably beneficial. This position is further reinforced by the idea that structuring or limiting humor makes the nurse-client interaction too contrived.

Consideration of why a statement or story is funny can shed light on the problem. For example, one cause of humor is incongruity in human interaction. When an event is so different from what might normally occur, it strikes people as being funny. This is why we laugh when someone loses their dentures or has unzipped pants. Children have a great sense of humor and appreciation of the incongruous, often enjoying wearing costumes with funny faces or telling jokes. These behaviors persist into adulthood in many people.

Anxiety also produces humor. An anxiety-provoking situation or conversation is often turned into a joke or something less serious. For example, late in the night at "slumber parties" or on camping trips, people often tell ghost stories and laugh at the story endings, even though they may be frightening. As another example, we often joke about death, sex, and elimination.

Hostility is a third cause of humor. We joke about things or people that evoke angry feelings, particularly when it is not socially acceptable to directly express the anger. The "left-handed compliment" is one example of this type of humor, in which a compliment is extended that clearly contains an insult. This occurs when we say, "You did pretty good for a beginner," or "That's a great-looking suit; isn't that the same one you've worn to the last few presentations?" Another form of this kind of humor occurs when someone says, "Remember when. . . . .?" to recall something uncomfortable that has happened to another person. This request typically causes the person being addressed to describe the embarrassing event, resulting in everyone having a good laugh at the person's expense. Our society seems to value the ability of people to "take a joke" or laugh at themselves, suggesting that we are more comfortable with indirect expression of anger. It then follows that if someone chooses to express anger indirectly through a joke, the other person needs to accept it with good spirit as if no hostility were involved.

The clinical use of humor in mental health–psychiatric nursing practice is usually seen to include thoughtful analysis and interpretation of what underlies the expression of humor. This analysis includes examining the nurse's motives in using humor. It also includes evaluation of how the humor—and the underlying messages—may affect the nurse-client interaction.

Laughing at the sheer incongruity of a situation may seem to be a perfectly innocent attempt to help a client develop a sense of humor. However, if calling attention to the incongruity suggests the client looks silly or is acting in a foolish manner, the nurse can reinforce an already negative self-image. In this example, the nurse can also be expressing hostility toward the client, which suggests the nurse needs to resolve some feelings about the client in a more constructive way. Encouraging laughter at incongruity or the unexpected in others may seem perfectly innocent, but it can reinforce the client's denial of anger or it may encourage derogation of others to bolster negative self-esteem.

Use of humor during anxious moments caused by self-disclosure or provocative topics can sometimes be an effective way of lessening the tension for nurse or client. This use of humor is to be carefully evaluated, however, to ensure that it does not trivialize matters that are important to the client. One problem with using humor in such situations is that communication usually has multiple levels. The nurse may be lessening tension on one level but insulting the client on another. With sensitivity and practice, the nurse can learn to use humor effectively in such moments. One important requirement is learning to avoid using humor at times when anger or disapproval toward the client is being experienced.

The nurse may share humor found in movies, books, records, and the like. These offer rich opportunities to promote laughter and a sense of humor in the client. The nurse can achieve therapeutic goals by sharing reactions to a movie, loaning a book, or sharing cartoons with the client. These behaviors provide a "personal touch" to the nurse's work with the client. They require thoughtful use to be sure that the implied friendliness is therapeutic rather than social in nature. In this way, the client knows he is special without the attendant problems of being too special or too close for the client's well-being.

FRAMEWORKS FOR MODIFYING DYSFUNCTIONAL COMMUNICATION

Effective use of paradoxical intervention, transactional analysis, or neurolinguistic programming requires careful study and systematically supervised practice. Use of paradoxical interventions is possible if the nurse acquires training in the method and receives supervision to the point of minimal to moderate proficiency in clinical practice. Clinicians who wish to use TA or NLP must obtain formal training from programs sanctioned by the organizations that credential practitioners in these methods; clinicians must be able to provide evidence of such credentials.

Use of Paradoxical Interventions

This novel framework for treating dysfunctional communication and interaction specifically addresses difficulties relating to problem formation and problem resolution. The framework deals with the concept of change by showing how changes in behavior can allow people to discover new ways to define problems and new methods for creating solutions.

This framework recommends that the practitioner distinguish between *first-order change,* which is change within a system in which the system itself remains unchanged, and *second-order change,* in which the system itself is changed. For example, imagine a family that is seeking help with making mealtimes more pleasant by avoiding the dysfunctional fighting and bickering that characterize their usual interaction. Further imagine that they do what many people do who are trying to solve a problem; they believe they are trying to solve the problem by eliminating or reducing the fighting. The problem

may well become compounded by the fact that the more they try to change, the more the arguing persists. In other words, they are trying to solve the problem with a first-order change, but this results in doing "more of the same," and it fails to solve the problem.

A second-order change involves changing the family members themselves, not just altering the frequency of a behavior. Second-order change, or change in the system itself, requires people to *reframe* the problem. Reframing, also called *paradoxical intervention,* means that a fresh and different look at the problem is sought. For example, the family members who complain about excessive bickering at mealtimes are instructed to make themselves engage in bickering for 5 minutes at the beginning of each mealtime whether they want to or not. After a few days, they typically complain that they do not want to fight any longer, and the bickering is reduced because the system has changed.

Effective use of this framework depends on the following steps:

1. In-depth study of the ideas and methods
2. Arranging supervision of clinical work by someone who has formal training experience with the method
3. Practice in analyzing human interaction problems using the concepts so as to be able to identify the following:
   a. First-order changes that have been attempted
   b. How members of the interaction system communicate the nature of their problem and how they have attempted to solve it
   c. Second-order changes that may present a solution, including paradoxical changes or interventions

Transactional Analysis (TA)

TA provides a language and theoretical framework for changing communication so a person can achieve the state of "I'm OK, you're OK" in interpersonal relationships.[3,13] The TA framework is applicable to communication within the person, between two persons, in relationships over time, and within the individual over time with regard to the life plan the person is following. The framework is based on Berne's idea that early life experiences create ego states within a person. Ego states are defined as systems of feelings accompanied by related sets of behaviors. The three ego states are presented in Chapter 3 on Theoretical Approaches.

Figure 5-9 shows a simple diagram of the three ego states, using circles to represent the three primary ego states within a person. The diagram also shows how communication has an influence on the ego states of the developing human being.

A person can develop any one of the following four life stances:

I'm OK, you're OK.
I'm OK, you're not OK.
I'm not OK, you're OK.
I'm not OK, you're not OK.

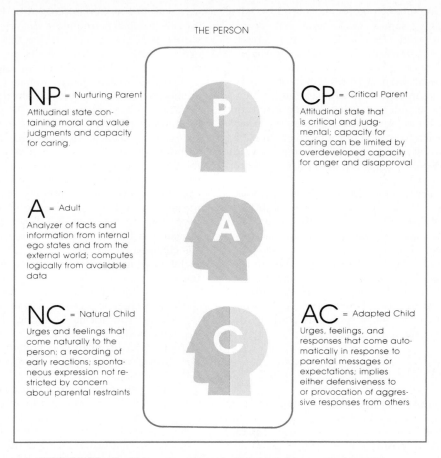

FIGURE 5-9 The three ego states depicted in transactional analysis.

Figure 5-10 illustrates interactions that come from each of these four life stances or communication stances.

Some communications between people are complementary, which means the ego states of the participants are complementary or parallel. For example, adult-to-adult interactions and parent-child interactions are complementary if both people are comfortable being in the ego state expected by the other. On the other hand, interactions are said to be crossed when there is absence of complementary or parallel interactions. For example, a teenager may whine and complain in response to a parental expectation. This reaction may be very difficult from the parent's expectation that the youngster speak from an adult ego state, process the information objectively, and understand the parental stance. In a different situation, the teenager might speak from an adult ego state to request permission to stay out past the usual curfew hour, and be met with an angry reply that "a rule is a rule." Figure 5-11 illustrates complementary and crossed interactions.

Another important aspect of communication used in the TA framework is permissions and injunctions, which are the do's and dont's that normally occur in human interaction. The TA approach guides the nurse in assessing what the client has been told to do or not to do in life, in general and/or in specific situations. Permissions and in-

junctions can also be used as intentional nursing interventions. For instance, the nurse may reassure a client by saying, "It is okay for you to talk with your spouse instead of fighting," or "Don't pick a fight when you can start out with talking." In this example, talking instead of fighting is a new behavior. The nurse gives the client permission to try something new in the first example and instructs the person not to use the old behavior in the second. These nursing actions can be helpful if the client has been taught to expect that fighting is the only way to solve problems.

Many clinicians using the TA approach strongly advocate the use of positive rather than negative messages to the client. This means they would never tell the client, "Don't do that." Instead they would offer permission. In one rather unusual example, a nurse tells about encountering a man seeking counseling who was carrying a gun because he was thinking of killing his boss. The nurse had the presence of mind to say calmly to him, "You have my permission to put that gun down on my desk right now, so I can put it in a safe place for you." The man complied.

The TA framework is as useful to the nurse in professional and personal roles. The approach can guide the nurse to more effective and satisfying communication in interactions with clients, clients' family members, peers, friends, and the general public. The approach is best

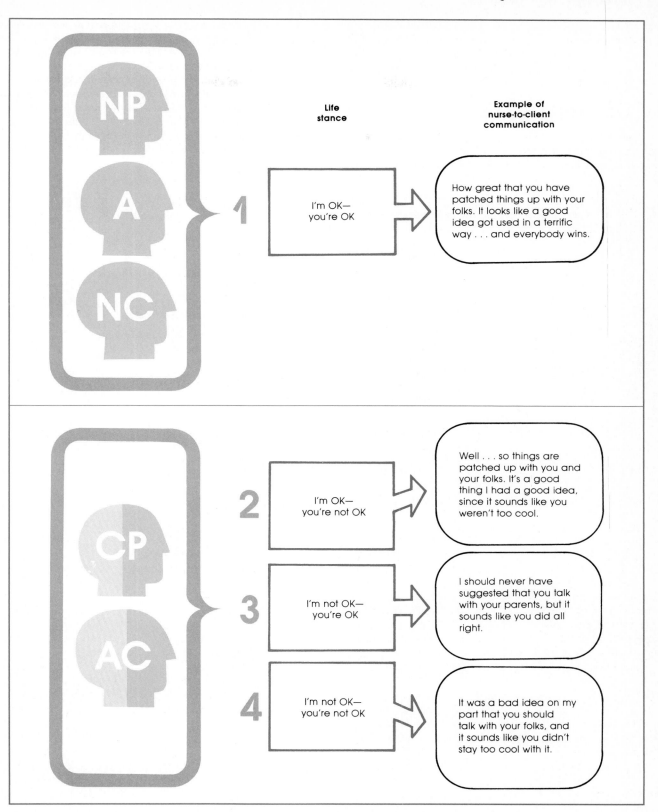

FIGURE 5-10 Communication from the four life positions of transactional analysis.

learned by having supervision or consultation from someone trained in the method. However, many useful applications can be made through independent learning. Figure 5-12 illustrates some applications of the method that may effect a change in communication.

Neurolinguistic Programming

Neurolinguistic programming is based on the idea that language is not actual experience; it is a representation of experience. Language is defined as a map of each individual person's experience.[1,4] The person is described as having multiple levels of experience, all of which become part of his communication. In this framework, language is observed and interpreted to achieve understanding of the map of the person's different levels of experience. The framework is helpful in mental health–psychiatric nursing because it provides a unique way of analyzing communication that does not assume that the client's language is necessarily a good picture of his experience.

The framework assumes that a person's experience involves three critical processes:

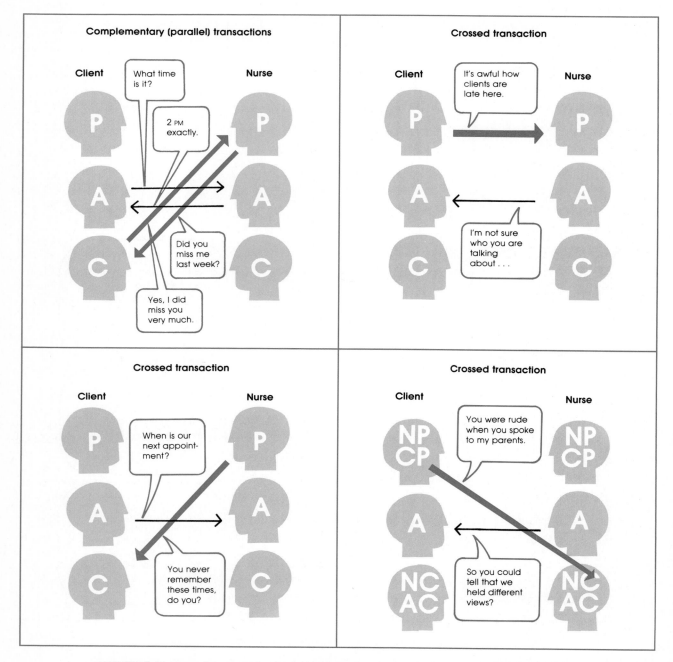

FIGURE 5-11 Complementary and crossed transactions as depicted in transactional analysis.

1. Sensory experience occurs.
2. The experience is processed through verbal patterns (called meta-programs).
3. It is then expressed as behavioral responses (called patterned operations).

These behavioral responses can be observed and used as a basis for developing ideas about the nature of the client's internal experience.

For example, imagine that a client angrily responds to a nurse's inquiry about how the day is going by saying, "You know it's a terrible day for me, so why do you keep asking?" To analyze why this happened using the NLP framework, the client's sensory experience includes what the nurse said and how it was said (the nonverbal messages). This sensory experience has been filtered or processed by the client's meta-programs (verbal patterns for expressing beliefs, values, and opinions). This processing can then be seen as having resulted in the client's response to the nurse.

The NLP framework outlines certain beliefs that are essential to the use of the NLP model:

1. People change because they are motivated to change.
2. All behavior is goal directed, which means it has a positive intention. Once the desired outcome is understood, the individual can consider whether alternative behaviors are more productive in achieving this outcome.
3. Limitations and problems are also opportunities. Every situation involving behavior represents the best a person can be at the time; every experience creates an opportunity for the individual to obtain more information about his situation.
4. The nurse can obtain important information and facilitate change by questioning the client.
5. One person cannot be responsible for the particular internal state of another person; this means that one person cannot cause another to feel or act in a particular way, since each individual has a choice about his behavior.

In the NLP framework, the use of predicates in languages is carefully analyzed. Predicates are the verbs or action words that accompany the noun in a sentence. Predicates are said to either refer to a mode of sensory experience or to be neutral. Those that refer to sensory experience include words associated with seeing, hearing, smelling, tasting, and touch. Predicates that are considered to be neutral include words that suggest thinking, knowing, being aware of, and noticing.

Examples of a person describing a worrisome situation using the various sensory modes follows:

Smell: I can smell something rotten in this deal.
Sight: This looks bad.
Hearing: It sounds like we don't have all the facts.
Touch: I get itchy just thinking about what could happen.
Taste: This gives me a bad taste in my mouth.
Neutral: I just know there's something wrong here.
Neutral: I wonder why this doesn't seem right?

This aspect of language analysis in the NLP approach further involves looking at the use of what are called the *submodalities* of the five sensory experiences. Examples of these submodalities are:

Smell: Odor, pungency, intensity
Sight: Clarity, shape, location, movement
Hearing: Pitch, loudness, location
Touch: Temperature, texture, weight
Taste: Flavor, texture, temperature

The NLP approach extends the analysis of human experience by examining how the client's nonverbal behavior relates to the sensory mode of the predicate that they

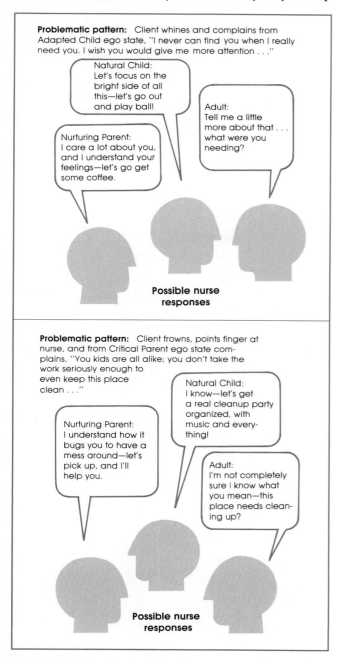

FIGURE 5-12 Use of transactional analysis to change problematic communication patterns.

are using. Eye movements are the nonverbal behaviors that are particularly significant in this analysis, since they seem specifically related to sensory modes of experience. Part of the NLP framework is based on Bandler and Grinder's observations[1] that when therapists ask clients to recall a past event visually, they often look up to their right. When asked to recall a feeling, they often look down to their right. A question about how they know something is often followed by a glance to the left. Bandler and Grinder further observed that rapport between client and therapist is enhanced when the therapist pays attention to the client's sensory experience.

The NLP framework includes the assumption that people move back and forth between paying attention to their internal self or internal cues and paying attention to external cues. Bandler and Grinder suggested that nonverbal behavior can be classified according to (1) whether it was auditory (A), visual (V), or kinesthetic (K); and (2) whether it was internal (i) or external (e).

These categories permit nonverbal behavior to be classified as one of six types of sensory experience:

Auditory—external	Visual—internal
Auditory—internal	Kinesthetic—external
Visual—external	Kinesthetic—internal

The individual moves from one system to another, and even employs two systems at the same time. A detailed list of words that are associated with auditory, visual, and kinesthetic sensory experience is found in the box below.

One way to increase rapport with the client is to ask questions or offer openings for conversation that are in the sensory system in which the client has been communicating. For example, when the client has either orally or nonverbally conveyed visual experience, the nurse can inquire what the person has seen in a particular situation or how the person imagines a situation to be. Auditory experience is elaborated by asking what has been heard or by asking the client to repeat a conversation. Kinesthetic experience can be pursued by asking about what the client felt in a particular situation. The client's internal dialogue is revealed by asking questions about what the person says to himself.

SENSORY-BASED LANGUAGE

AUDITORY (HEAR)

say	resounding
talk	tell
yell	discuss
rasp	praise
sing	purr
babble	call
whine	chant
argue	noise
tone	listen
boom	ring
chime	voice
snore	scream
quiet	sound
music	silent
describe	shout
loud	speak
clatter	whisper
aloud	grumble
shrill	lie
verbalize	harmony
clang	mellifluous
squawk	melodic
compute	staccato
debate	clamor
utter	foretell
shriek	
hiss	

VISUAL (SEE)

aim	stain
dark	diagram
sketch	look
view	picture
glow	blind
portray	clear
bright	pretty
neat	image
scan	foggy
vision	sight
hazy	survey
dull	glare
pattern	reveal
appear	shine
show	spotless
cloudy	draw
watch	peer
light	spy
reflect	view
dim	perspective
observe	colorful
ugly	glimpse
visible	stare
hide	wink
focus	overlook
brilliant	
oversight	

KINESTHETIC (FEEL)

sting	extend	smooth
point	compress	mold
fumble	trudge	support
cool	ragged	stable
unbalanced	massage	concrete
shocking	attach	clumsy
merge	warm	pushing
flat	grasp	relaxed
tender	stick	swimming
bend	shape	calm
throw	solid	lance
rough	tough	pierce
hot	attack	torn
grab	hard	sore
tension	steady	startle
push	cold	starve
reach	soft	stamp
connect	electric	grovel
jarring	firm	gird
link	stiff	fondle
cram	fasten	guzzle
tackle	handle	hammer
manipulate	twist	slug
pack	sturdy	smoky
shuffle	probe	breathless
unite	touch	heavy
catch	fall	smolder
balance	backing	stolid
take	cut	stodgy
resist	lift	forge
sharp	hurt	
twinge		

Adapted from Cameron-Bandler, L., Conwell, L., and Lebeau, M.: 22-day NLP Certification Program (handout), Boston, 1981, The NLP Center for Advanced Studies, Inc.

Nonproductive or ineffective nurse-client interactions can be analyzed by reflecting on each exchange in the interaction and noting whether the nurse responded in the mode of sensory experience conveyed in the client's verbal and nonverbal behavior.

BRIEF REVIEW

Communication is the process by which the nurse accomplishes the tasks of the nursing process. Therapeutic communication is the content of the nurse's intervention. Effective implementation of the nursing process requires the nurse to develop knowledge in the following areas: theories for analyzing communication, techniques of therapeutic communication, issues in therapeutic communication with clients, and frameworks for modifying dysfunctional communication.

Definitions of communication distinguish verbal and nonverbal forms. The structure of communication can also be analyzed with regard to sentence structure, choice of words, and content. Communication can be seen as having functions such as disclosure of information, self-disclosure, and achievement of self-awareness.

Communication has been of major interest in many pursuits since the beginning of recorded history. Nursing has formally recognized the importance of communication with the client since the days of Florence Nightingale. In more recent years, nurses in mental health–psychiatric nursing have developed important guidelines for therapeutic communication with clients in one-to-one relationships and with group and family methods of treatment.

Theoretical approaches that facilitate the nurse's understanding of communication processes include the work of Reusch, Bateson, Scheflen, and theorists studying proxemics and communication channels. Other clinically useful approaches that demonstrate how behavioral change can be effected through communication include paradoxical interventions, transactional analysis, and neurolinguistic programming.

Therapeutic communication involves mastery of techniques such as conveying respect, listening actively, defining boundaries, structuring time, using questions, restating, and validating. Other necessary skills include asking for demonstrations and illustrations, providing information, emphasizing relationships between parts and wholes, using nurse-client communication to illustrate, sharing that the client is thought about, offering hope, and summarizing.

Issues in therapeutic communication include how much self-disclosure is appropriate for the nurse, how much emotion and energy is therapeutic for the nurse to express, how much confrontation is appropriate, and how much feedback and humor to incorporate into the communication process.

REFERENCES AND SUGGESTED READINGS

1. Bandler, R., and Grinder, J.: The structure of magic, vol. 1, A book about language and therapy, Palo Alto, Calif., 1975, Science & Behavior Books.
2. Berne, E.: Transactional analysis in psychotherapy, New York, 1961, Grove Press, Inc.
3. Birdwhistle, R.: Introduction to kinesics, Louisville, 1952, University of Louisville Press.
4. Cameron-Bandler, L.: They lived happily ever after, Cupertino, Calif., 1978, Meta Publications.
5. Dilts, R., and others: Neuro-linguistic programming, vol. 1, The study of the structure of subjective experience, Cupertino, Calif., 1980, Meta Publications.
6. Hall, E.T.: The hidden dimension, New York, 1966, Doubleday & Co., Inc.
7. Harris, T.: I'm OK, you're OK: a practical guide to transactional analysis, New York, 1969, Harper & Row, Publishers, Inc.
7a. Hays, J.S., and Larson, K.H.: Interacting with patients, New York, 1965, The Macmillan Co., Publishers.
8. Krieger, D.: Therapeutic touch: how to use your hands to help and heal, Englewood Cliffs, N.J., 1979, Prentice Hall, Inc.
9. Longo, D.C.: Communications and human behavior. In Longo, D.C., and Williams, R.A., editors: Clinical practice in psychosocial nursing: assessment and intervention, ed. 2, New York, 1986, Appleton-Century-Crofts.
10. Luft, J., and Ingham, H.: The Johari window: a graphic model of awareness in interpersonal relations. In Luft, J., editor: Group processes: an introduction to group dynamics, Palo Alto, Calif., 1963, National Press Books.
11. Reusch, J.: Disturbed communications, New York, 1957, W.W. Norton & Co., Inc.
12. Reusch, J.: Therapeutic communication, New York, 1961, W.W. Norton & Co., Inc.
13. Reusch, J., and Bateson, G.: Communication: the social matrix of psychiatry, New York, 1951, W.W. Norton & Co., Inc.
14. Reusch, J., and Kees, W.: Nonverbal communication, Berkeley, Calif., 1956, University of California Press.
15. Scheflen, A.: Body language and social order: communication as behavioral control, Englewood Cliffs, N.J., 1972, Prentice-Hall, Inc.
16. Simonton, O.C., and Matthews-Simonton, S.: Getting well again, Los Angeles, 1978, J.P. Tarcher.
17. Watzlawick, P., Weakland, J., and Fisch, R.: Change: principles of problem formation and problem resolution, New York, 1974, W.W. Norton & Co., Inc.
18. Williams, H.: Humor and healing: theapeutic effects in geriatrics, Gerontion: A Canadian Review of Geriatric Care 1(3):14, 1986.

ANNOTATED BIBLIOGRAPHY

Daniel, E.J.: Any other song: a plea for holistic communication, Bowie, Md., 1980, Robert J. Brady Co.

Daniel describes one client's plea for help through conversation and inner dialogue that accompanied the helping process experienced by the client. This case study illustrates failures in communication typical of nurse-client interactions in which good intentions may fail to create adequate helping responses to the client at risk. Learning is facilitated by the description of the client's inner dialogue, which makes clear what the client is experiencing even when his words fail.

Sundeen, S.J., and others: Nurse-client interaction: implementing the nursing process, ed. 2, St. Louis, 1981, The C.V. Mosby Co.

Based on a concern about dualism in care, a holistic approach to nurse-client communication is proposed. Dualism is the result of differences in medical and nursing approaches to client care. Although dualism is less than effectively defined for the text's purposes, an excellent overview of essentials of communication is presented, including the nursing process, emergence of the self, self-growth, communication, therapeutic relationships, the helping relationship as a process, and a general basis of stress and adaptation for analyzing behavior.

DEVELOPING A THERAPEUTIC RELATIONSHIP

Jackie Coombe Moore   Carol R. Hartman

After studying this chapter the learner will be able to:

Describe the development of the therapeutic relationship in the practice of mental health–psychiatric nursing.

Discuss self-awareness and its role in the nurse-client relationship.

Identify components of the nurse-client relationship.

Describe the use of warmth, empathy, and genuineness in the nurse-client relationship.

Discuss student reaction to psychiatric nursing.

Discuss the therapeutic use of self.

Describe the phases of the therapeutic relationship.

Identify barriers to the therapeutic relationship.

Discuss aspects of the supervisory process.

The *therapeutic relationship* is the cornerstone of mental health–psychiatric nursing. Therapeutic relationships imply the establishment of a warm, trusting relationship between the nurse and client for the purpose of helping the client. It is imperative that the client trust the nurse and that the nurse accept the client.

A social norm dictates that one does not talk to strangers; however, the nurse and client enter the therapeutic relationship as strangers to discuss personal, even intimate details of the client's life, as well as thoughts and feelings, in a brief period. The limits and expectations inherent in the therapeutic relationship are discussed openly and established by mutual agreement. The focus of the therapeutic relationship remains on the mutually established goals and the activities that facilitate the achievement of these goals. The therapeutic relationship is usually brief or conducted for a limited period and progresses through defined stages. The primary responsibility for maintaining both the relationship and the focus of the relationship lies with the nurse. The principle focus addresses the needs of the client. Termination of a therapeutic relationship is planned in advance, discussed, and allotted sufficient time so that the ending of the relationship becomes in itself therapeutic.

EARLY NURSING THEORISTS

Schwartz and Shockley[34] analyzed client problems and recommended nursing care for treating those who were assaultive, demanding, withdrawn, hallucinating, and delusive, and those with eating difficulties, incontinence, sexual dysfunctions, suicidal behavior, and extreme anxiety. Case material and guidelines for creating a therapeutic relationship showed that the nursing process was the healing method and context for treating these behavioral difficulties. The approach was innovative because at no point were medical diagnoses used for identifying client problems. Instead, the authors advanced the idea that nursing practice be based on observed client behaviors.

Orlando[27] formulated her ideas about the dynamic nurse-client relationship after being coordinator of a project implementing mental health principles within a nursing curriculum. She stressed the value of the client's role in determining the adequacy of the nurse's care. She suggested that client dissatisfaction and distress were caused by (1) physical limitations, (2) adverse reactions to the setting, and (3) experiences that prevent the client from communicating his needs. For the beginning clinician Orlando recommended the following actions: (1) careful observation of the client's behavior and reactions, (2) care-

🍇 *Historical Overview* 🍇

DATE	EVENT
1900s	Until the early twentieth century the role of the psychiatric nurse was largely custodial, emphasizing care for the physical needs of the patients.
1920s	The first major emphasis on the use of interpersonal relationships and milieu as therapeutic tools came from Harry Stack Sullivan.
1950s	Discussion of the relationship between nurse and patient proliferated.
1952	Tudor discussed the influence, behavior, and role that the nurse had in relation to the patient. Peplau provided the basis for current nursing practice as she emphasized the process of nursing, the nurse's role as a participant-observer, and the importance of understanding the patient's subjective experiences.
1954	Schwing placed the nurse in the role of primary therapist and explored the power of the caring practices of the nurse in making therapeutic contact with the psychotic patient.
1960s	The concept of a more active role for both nurse and patient emerged. Orlando emphasized attention to the patient's daily living skills and gentle, consistent feedback. The concept of the mentally ill as clients rather than patients emerged. The emphasis shifted to the client as an active participant in therapy, with responsibility for personal behavior.
1980s	The current trend is to view the client holistically, emphasizing the relationship of mind and body and the need for the nurse to respect and accept the client, while using the nurse-client relationship to facilitate change.
Future	As more emphasis is placed on the biological aspects of psychiatric disorders, the value of the nurse-client relationship is being questioned. Nursing will need to develop new theories useful as a base for measuring the effectiveness of the nurse-client relationship.

ful examination of the nurse's reactions to the client and the nurse-client relationship (self-awareness), and (3) validation of the nurse's observations with the client rather than assuming that the nurse's observations are always correct. The book effectively advanced two significant concepts for the field of mental health–psychiatric nursing: the importance of the nurse's having self-awareness, and the importance of communication with the client for involvement in an evaluation of the relationship.

Ujhely[38] emphasized the nurse's potential to be a healing force, using the nurse-client relationship as the context in which healing occurs. As a Jungian psychoanalyst and a nurse psychotherapist, Ujhely's insights about mental health–psychiatric nursing and communication clearly established the reciprocal nature of the nurse-client communication in the healing process. Ujhely was one of the first nurse theorists to recognize that the nurse's involvement in the client relationship is as worthy of analysis as the client's involvement. A major component of the self-analysis required for effective communication with clients is consideration of what the nurse brings to the nurse-client relationship. The nurse's contribution to the relationship is analyzed so that the nurse's values, problems, and conflicts are not permitted to interfere with the client's work and commitment to the process of healing.

According to Ujhely, the context of the relationship also incorporates what the client brings to the relationship. For example, the client may describe an early experience of physical abuse from both parents. A nurse communicating with this patient who experienced abuse as a child may react intensely to the client's communication. The nurse-client relationship then assumes a dimension of mutuality with respect to physical abuse experienced as a child.

The nurse's subsequent effectiveness in working with this client requires exploration of how this personal experience affects communication with the client. The nurse may be tempted to communicate excessive sympathy or, alternatively, critical judgment of the client. Recognition of these and other responses that may not be helpful permit the nurse to avoid these and instead to calmly communicate understanding of the client's distress and a trust of the client's ability to learn a nonabusive parental role.

Travelbee's comprehensive approach[40] to communication in mental health–psychiatric nursing translated ideas about therapeutic communication into the context of everyday psychiatric nursing practice. For example, she dispelled the myth of "getting too involved" with clients, a traditional warning given to students who may lack the skills to deal with intense client involvement. Travelbee provided an alternative view by describing mental health–psychiatric nursing as incorporating (1) responsibility to family and the community in addition to the client, (2) prevention, and (3) support of clients and families during mental suffering. She believed that nurses are skilled in the conduct of therapeutic relationships with the clients, and her work has directly contributed to establishing that view of mental health–psychiatric nursing. She argued that the client's mental suffering provides a rationale for the nurse utilizing an empathic approach to the client.

THE NURSE'S SELF-AWARENESS

The client and nurse bring to the relationship their unique beliefs, behaviors, attitudes, intelligence, and values. How do two people, with such a potential range of diversity, come together and interact to assist the client in gaining or regaining a sense of worth, energy, and direction? The first step is for the nurse to increase her own self-awareness. This involves communication with others and self-evaluation, which reveal previously unknown aspects of one's personality. Aspects of self-awareness to be explored are self-concept, beliefs, values, and life experiences.

Self-Concept

Self-concept influences the nurse's therapeutic effectiveness. The nurse's feelings about herself influence the way she interprets the communication and behavior of the client and her ability to interact with the client. Nurses possessing a positive self-concept have faith in their competence and believe that they have something useful to offer others. This feeling of self-worth allows the nurse to accept and respect the worth of others. Positive self-worth can help a person accept criticism, ask for assistance appropriately, and think of obstacles as temporary difficulties rather than overwhelming problems.

A negative self-concept makes it difficult for the nurse "to see, hear, or think clearly, and therefore she is more prone to step on and depreciate others."[31] The nurse who is uncertain of her self-worth is afraid to be open with clients and too timid to risk finding new solutions to problems. She may find it difficult to seek help from peers or supervisors, since that may expose her inadequacy. Finally, it is difficult to convince a client that it is possible to have a positive self-concept if the nurse cannot be a role model for feelings of worth.

Beliefs and Values

Nurse-client relationships are strongly affected by the beliefs and values of the persons involved. On the basis of beliefs and values, people assume approving or disapproving stances with respect to the behavior of others. Some values lead to complete rejection of involvement with persons who have different beliefs. For example, because the nurse values nonviolence, she may not know what to say to a client who is accused of spouse beating. She may request that the case be reassigned. Other values, although important, do not prevent interaction. Still others seem insignificant in the course of relationships. A nurse may accept a client with a history of food-stamp fraud; although the nurse's values may define this behavior as objectionable, this does not prevent initiation of the therapeutic interaction.

Nurses recognize that cultural value differences exist and that misunderstandings are more likely to occur when communications do not conform to expectations about how people should think or act. Nurses and clients from different socioeconomic groups may also have differing values. The nurse's awareness of the values she has developed within her own class and culture and her awareness of the values of clients from different classes and cultures may help prevent misunderstandings that ultimately impede the therapeutic relationship (See Chapter 10.)

The nurse's beliefs about human nature affect the therapeutic relationship. Some nurses believe that human beings are inherently good. Problem behaviors, even criminal behaviors and violent crimes, are thought to be the result of misunderstanding or lack of love during critical stages of development. Nurses who believe people are inherently good tend to view clients as persons who are distrustful of others and, therefore, led to commit antisocial acts. Nurses maintaining this viewpoint may believe society needs to provide love, understanding, and retraining for these people.

Other nurses have an essentially negative view of people, regarding them with suspicion. These nurses may lack hope that clients can actually change behavior or improve themselves. This opinion may lead the nurse to believe that society as a whole needs to be protected, and individuals with inappropriate behavior need to be controlled.

Beliefs about human nature lead to ideas about what is needed for people to resolve their problems. How each nurse functions in the therapeutic relationship will be shaped by her beliefs about human nature. The more optimistic the views, the more opportunities for growth.

Life Experiences

Nurses can experience the same problems as their clients. Sometimes the nurse has successfully resolved past problems. In other instances, the nurse may be coping with life stresses and problems that are as serious as the problems faced by her clients. The therapeutic effectiveness of the nurse is enhanced by (1) recognition of her problems, (2) an underlying optimism that change is possible, and (3) a nonjudgmental attitude toward herself or the client for having problems. For example, the nurse who has become accustomed to taking diazepam (Valium) 6 to 8 times a day may not consciously admit to the seriousness of the problem; she may fear there is no way to stop or deeply disrespect herself for taking the pills. This nurse may communicate with chemically dependent clients differently from the nurse who has experienced a similar problem but became involved in a treatment program in which she was able to stop using drugs. As a result, the second nurse has a higher regard for herself for having faced and overcome the problem.

Another problem, faced most often by young or inexperienced nurses, is a lack of success in coping with adversity. A nurse who has had a sheltered life may be overwhelmed by the difficulties a client is experiencing. Consultation with a more seasoned nurse may help to ease feelings of inadequacy.

ROUTES TO SELF-AWARENESS

A variety of opportunities are available to the nurse in mental health–psychiatric nursing to facilitate the process of self-awareness. These opportunities fall into three primary categories: interpersonal relationships, reading, and writing (see Table 6-1).

Interpersonal Relationships

Involvement in relationships contribute to self-awareness. The family offers the first and probably most enduring lesson in self-awareness. These lessons are modified by subsequent life experiences that usually include other deep, personal relationships. Teachers also play a significant role in developing self-awareness. A teacher's influence is limited by the degree to which the student allows the relationship to develop.

Sometimes an instructor or supervisor becomes a mentor. A mentor is a person who guides a relationship in which the intellectual and career development of another person is supported, facilitated, and promoted. One does not make a formal contract with a mentor; rather, the relationship is a process of love and respect that has a primarily professional/intellectual focus that evolves over

---

TABLE 6-1 Example of a section of a process recording

Purpose of the Interaction: This interview was conducted primarily to explore and overcome resistance exhibited by the client 2 days earlier when he "forgot" our meeting. Based on the outcome of this interview, the contract with the client will either be reestablished or terminated.

Context of the Interaction: On the previous clinical day, the client had "forgotten" our meeting and refused to talk when he was found playing pool. Another meeting was set up for the next clinical day. The client did not show up at the time and place we agreed upon. He was found asleep in his bed. He agreed to accompany me to the courtyard near the unit. This was our fourth interaction. It was a warm, sunny day. There were few distractions.

Client Behavior	Nurse Behavior	Analysis
Client sat down on a bench, leaned forward with elbows on thighs, and stared straight ahead. He yawned several times and rubbed his eyes.		This client isn't interested in the upcoming interaction. "Metacommunication tells how verbal communication can be interpreted."
	I sat down on the bench beside the client about 2 feet away. I turned to face the client. I established eye contact. I felt my jaws tighten somewhat before I spoke. I was leaning slightly toward the client with legs uncrossed and hands on my knees. I was breathing faster and deeper than usual.	Observing personal space. Open posture for active listening. Physiological changes secondary to anxiety.
	Thought: What's the best way to approach this resistance thing? Do I ease into it or confront him with my feelings? I'm sure seeing his manipulation, now.	I wanted to reaffirm our contract by breaking down resistance but not to run him away. "Forcing him to talk about a painful area may increase the client's anxiety."
	Feeling: I felt a little frustrated and angry at the client's resistance.	My feelings of anger and frustration can become a communication barrier if left unresolved. "In an accepting relationship, an individual can deal with resisted material." I need to be more accepting—student weakness.
	"Joe, I want to talk to you about our agreement." Three second pause.	Therapeutic: Defining boundaries by reaffirming contract.
	"We agreed to meet every Tuesday and Thursday at 1 PM for an hour to talk. Today is the second time this week that you weren't where you said you'd be."	Confrontation: Pressure another person into facing something objectionable. Perhaps I got into the subject abruptly because of feelings of frustration and anxiety.

Continued.

TABLE 6-1 Example of a section of a process recording—cont'd

Client Behavior	Nurse Behavior	Analysis
	I was still in the same position except that I was gripping my knees with my hands. I quietly sighed after I spoke and relaxed my grip. I looked straight at the client with a serious expression. Thought: Well, I wonder how he's going to react to that. Feeling: I felt less frustrated and angry and a little relieved.	I relaxed some after my statement. I had vented my feelings through confrontation. "In many instances this act is associated with the nurse's being angry. . . ." The nurse is objective and neutral when confronting.
Started moving his feet up and down a little. Ducked his head down slightly. Half-chuckled when he spoke. "Well, I didn't really mean it sincerely." In a louder tone: "Sometimes I like to talk and sometimes I don't. Maybe I'd rather play pool or sleep."		Foot movement may mean he is anxious about being confronted. Lowered head seems submissive. Voice change may indicate anger.
	I straightened up a little, maintaining eye contact with client. Sighed. Rubbed my chin with right hand and squinted my eyes slightly. Thought: I think he's about to get angry. I wonder what he really thinks about me. I hope I can work this out with him. Feeling: A little anxious. "Joe, how would you feel if I broke my word to you?"	My behavior, thoughts, and feelings are centered around the client's anger, what to do about the anger, and my own anxiety. Therapeutic: Encouraging comparison, asking that similarities and differences be noted.
	I put my hand back on my knee and half-smiled. I spoke in a slow, low tone.	The smile may seem incongruent with the message, but I am trying to be nonthreatening.
Still facing me with eye contact. Serious expression.		Expression indicates that client's anger hasn't escalated. Absence of previously noted expressions of anger.

time. The mentor's expertise and caring are a powerful combination in guiding the nurse's growth in self-awareness and knowledge.

The nurse can choose to work with a therapist, counselor, or other helping person to learn how to be more effective in therapeutic relationships with clients. Through this exchange, the nurse creates an opportunity to achieve greater self-awareness and a more positive regard for self, which increases her effectiveness in working with clients. At the same time, the nurse can learn from the therapeutic methods of the counselor, observing how the counselor communicates and uses opportunities to be helpful that arise during interactions.

Reading

Through formal study of mental health–psychiatric nursing, the nurse is exposed to written ideas about clinical practice. From these sources the nurse can become aware of her personal philosophy of practice. The habit of reading, however, begins long before and, ideally, continues long after one's formal education. Reading fiction and nonfiction helps one learn more about human nature and thus about oneself. Portrayals of people's lives demonstrate the range of human emotion, the struggles, and the ways in which people relate to themselves and to others. Diaries and journals are rich sources of detail about the personal experiences of others. Many books, journals, and diaries have been written by former mental patients that detail the experience of mental illness and health caregivers from the client's point of view. In addition, professional publications provide a useful source of current information and research studies.

Writing

Writing in a diary, journal, or log is another significant route to learning about oneself. The nurse can write notes in a completely unstructured style or can answer specific questions daily or weekly. It is often helpful to review

TABLE 6-1 Example of a section of a process recording—cont'd

Client Behavior	Nurse Behavior	Analysis
"I wouldn't like it."		Client's verbal response is appropriate, an indication of the effectiveness of the question.
	"Well, I don't like it either. My job is to learn about people by meeting with a client who is willing to discuss his problems, and possibly to explore solutions to those problems."	I'm trying to establish rapport by displaying genuineness. "Being myself" is expressing to client my thoughts and feelings. My thoughts probably indicate a low level of warmth. I stated in an informative and matter-of-fact way my intentions and purpose for interaction.
	Thirty second pause. "I'd like to work with you if you would agree to meet and talk." I spoke slowly and clearly in a low tone. Thought: I hope he agrees.	Restating my purpose and recontracting.
Client turns away from me and laughs quickly, looks across courtyard. He puts his elbows on his thighs and looks down.		Behavior indicates a return to a submissive state, "lowering head."
	Feeling: I sensed the client's ambivalence and felt uneasy.	A strength: Awareness of client's feelings. A weakness: Should have communicated my understanding to client.
Client turned his head and was making eye contact. Spoke in a shaky voice.	Thought: I hope he is is not too uncomfortable. I don't want him to just "give in" because he thinks I'm in charge.	
"I want to work with you."	"Then we will meet every Tuesday and Thursday at the nurse's station at 1 PM as we had originally planned, if that is still a good time for you."	Recontracting complete.
		Client's resistance may indicate that he had been "testing" me. His behavior may indicate a trend of not fulfilling commitments and being egocentric which are characteristic of schizophrenia.

these notes with an instructor or mentor to assist the nurse in identifying patterns of behavior or feelings, biases, or hallmarks of personal growth that may not be apparent to the nurse.

Process recording is a formal method of writing that helps the nurse not only deal more effectively with clients but also learn about herself. Process recordings are descriptions and analyses of interactions with clients. The record includes a verbatim account of the nurse's and the client's communications. The word-for-word record of the interaction ensures that complete data about the interaction are available to the nurse for subsequent analysis.

Table 6-1 provides an example of a process recording. The use of process recordings facilitates identification of communication techniques, maladaptive behaviors, and beliefs and values, as well as the nurse's strengths and weaknesses. Process recordings also contribute to the effectiveness of clinical supervision by instructors, supervisors, or consultants. Over time, at regular intervals, the process recordings can be reviewed and summarized to document major patterns or themes and overall progress of the relationship. Finally, these recordings can be used for the nurse's analysis of her progress in working with clients. The instructor or supervisor can point out areas for improvement in technique or analysis, clarify behavioral concepts, and give feedback. Process recordings can be used in this way to develop insight into both client and nurse behaviors.

COMPONENTS OF THE THERAPEUTIC RELATIONSHIP
Rapport

Certain people seem to have qualities that enable them to help others. These people have the ability not only to understand what the problem is, but also to leave the people who come for help feeling good about themselves. When this happens, *rapport* has been established. Rapport is the key ingredient in the negotiation and maintenance of the therapeutic relationship.

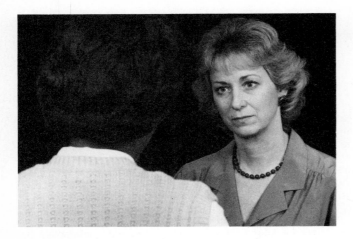

FIGURE 6-1 A therapist demonstrates active listening as she works with a nursing student.

Rapport requires a level of similarity and agreement in the language, body movement, and gestures of two people. Carefully observe the behavior of two people in deep conversation (Figure 6-1). Notice how they nod their heads in agreement on some point being made. Observe the rate of speech and tonal qualities used by both persons. Facial expressions often mirror one another. Soon you will notice that shifts in one person's body position are reflected by changes in the other person's position. The matching and mirroring of gestures and expressions are usually unconscious.

The qualities that have been found to facilitate rapport are noticeable in most helping people. These qualities are warmth, empathy, and genuineness.

Warmth. Warmth implies the ability to make the client feel cared for and comfortable. It denotes acceptance of the client as a unique individual. It involves a nonpossessive caring for the client as a person and a willingness to share the client's joys and sorrows. Warmth can be conveyed by eye contact, a tone of voice that sounds interested and caring, a touch on the arm, or a smile. Nonpossessive warmth involves permitting the client to have his own feelings and experiences and also involves appreciating the client for himself, regardless of his behaviors. On the opposite page is a scale for measuring nonpossessive warmth in which *stage 1* is the lowest level and *stage 5* is the highest level.

Empathy. The ability to sense the client's private world as if it were one's own is known as *empathy.* Beyond that, it is the ability to convey this understanding to the client. It is not necessary for the nurse to feel the same emotions the client feels. Rather, empathy is an appreciation and awareness of these feelings and an ability to communicate this awareness.

The nurse may demonstrate different levels of empathy as shown in the Case Example above. The scale on the opposite page represents nine degrees of empathy; at the lowest level the nurse may be inattentive or misinterpret the client's feelings. At the highest level, the nurse's awareness allows her to sense and respond to feelings the client has only partially revealed. The empathic nurse communicates verbally, an understanding of feelings that may be deeply hidden even to the client.

Case Example

Mrs. Jackson has met with the nurse to complete her psychosocial history and explore the recent events in her life in greater detail. She has discussed her youth and upbringing fairly calmly. She has discussed her relationship with her three children as being somewhat strained but satisfying, until her husband's death months earlier. She had sat quietly until she mentioned her husband, maintaining eye contact, speaking in a calm, somewhat low voice. As she discussed her current difficulty with her children since the death, she suddenly stopped speaking, lowered her head, and slumped into a limp position, tears running down her cheeks.

The nurse may respond with different levels of empathy. A nurse with low empathy may ignore the change in behavior and go on with history taking by asking: "Mrs. Jackson, you were talking about your children. What ages are they?" (Stage 1 empathy.) A nurse with a higher level of empathy, who is aware of most obvious feelings but is not totally accurate in identifying the hidden feelings of the client may respond by saying: "Mrs. Jackson, you seem upset right now. Would you like to end our discussion andd resume it later?" (Stage 4 empathy.) A nurse who understands the client's full range of spoken and unspoken feelings may respond by leaning toward Mrs. Jackson, speaking softly and using touch as she says, "Sometimes you feel so sad and alone. It's like you just can't go on anymore." In this manner the nurse is able to respond to Mrs. Jackson's inability to continue the conversation as symbolic of her inability to function in her life. (Stage 9 empathy.)

Genuineness. Genuineness involves being oneself. This implies that the nurse is aware of her thoughts, feelings, values, and their relevance in the immediate interaction with a client. A high livel of genuineness does not mean that the nurse expresses her feelings and thoughts at all times—only that she does not deny them. The nurse's response to the client is sincere and congruent with her internal responses; however, she may choose the internal responses she verbalizes. It is also important that the nurse's verbal and nonverbal communication be congruent. The scale on p. 100 exemplifies the levels of genuineness. The Case Example below demonstrates the use of a high level of genuineness.

Case Example

The client, Terry, and nurse have been talking quietly for a few minutes when the client suddenly becomes angry and shouts, "I don't want to talk to you! In fact I don't ever want to talk to you again! Just get away from me and leave me alone!" The nurse is surprised, hurt, and unsure how to respond. She and the client have had a positive relationship in the past. A possible response that is genuine yet therapeutic would be: "I'm sorry you feel that way. I'm also confused. I value our relationship highly and I'm puzzled that you no longer want to talk to me." (Stage 5 genuineness.)

In the example above, although the nurse felt hurt, she chose to respond by expressing her honest confusion, rather than by acting hurt, angry, or by leaving the client.

WARMTH

STAGE 1

Offers advice or gives clear negative regard

Tells the client what is "best" for him or approves or disapproves of his behavior

Makes herself the focus of evaluation

Sees herself as responsible for the client

STAGE 2

Responds mechanically indicating little warmth

Ignores the client or his feelings

Communicates no unconditional regard

STAGE 3

Indicates a positive but semi-possessive caring

Communicates that what the client does or does not do matters to her

STAGE 4

Communicates a deep interest and concern for the client

Communicates nonjudgmental and nonpossessive warmth

Maintains some conditionality in the more personal areas of the client's functioning

STAGE 5

Communicates nonpossessive warmth without restriction

Respects the client's worth as a person and his rights as an individual

Gives the client freedom to be himself, to regress, to be defensive, to dislike or reject the nurse

Cares about and values the client for his potential without allowing her feelings to interfere in evaluations of his behavior

Shares the client's joys, aspirations, sadness, and failures

Adapted from Rogers, C., and others: The therapeutic relationship and its impact, Madison, 1967, University of Wisconsin Press.

EMPATHY

STAGE 1

Is unaware of the client's feelings

Responses are inappropriate for mood or content of client's statements

May be bored, disinterested, or offer advice

STAGE 2

Shows a negligible degree of accuracy in responses to the most obvious feelings

Ignores emotions that are not clearly expressed

Is sensitive to obvious feelings but misunderstands what the client is saying

Responses inhibit or misdirect the client

STAGE 3

Responds accurately to the client's expressed feelings

Shows concern for deeper feelings that she assumes are present, although she does not sense their meaning to the client

STAGE 4

Recognizes less obvious feelings

May anticipate feelings that are not current or may misinterpret feelings

Is sensitive and aware but not entirely attuned to the client in the current situation

Desire and effort to understand are present, but accuracy is low

STAGE 5

Responds accurately to the client's readily discernible feelings

Shows awareness of feelings and experiences that are not so evident, but tends to be somewhat inaccurate in her understanding of them

Her misunderstandings may not be disruptive because of their tentative nature

STAGE 6

Recognizes most of the client's present feelings, including those not readily apparent

May misjudge the intensity of the feelings with the result that responses may not be suited to the client's mood

Deals directly with what the client is currently experiencing

Is attuned to the client, but does not encourage exploration

Understanding is limited

STAGE 7

Responds accurately to most of the client's present feelings

Shows awareness of the intensity of the client's feelings

Moves slightly beyond the realm of the client's awareness to encourage him to explore currently unrecognized feelings

Moves to more emotionally laden areas

STAGE 8

Identifies client's feelings accurately

Uncovers meanings of the client's experiences of which the client is unaware

Moves into feelings and experiences with sensitivity and accuracy

Sensitive to her mistakes and alters her responses appropriately

Reflects a rapport with the client

Tone of voice reflects a seriousness in her approach to client

STAGE 9

Responds unerringly to the client's full range and intensity of feelings

Recognizes each emotional nuance and communicates an understanding of the feelings

Attuned to the client's feelings and reflects this in her words and voice

GENUINENESS

STAGE 1

Interacts defensively

Evidences considerable discrepancy between her experiencing and her current verbalization

Makes contradictions in her statements

STAGE 2

Responds appropriately, but responses do not express what she really feels or means.

Responses are contrived or rehearsed

STAGE 3

Defensiveness is implicit

STAGE 4

Is neither implicitly nor explicitly defensive

Presence of a façade is not evident

Lack of genuineness is not shown

STAGE 5

Gives open, honest responses

Is open to feelings and experiences of all types, both pleasant and hurtful

Has no defensiveness

Verbalizations match feelings and thoughts

An honest, but more defensive and less therapeutic response is: "I don't understand why you're angry at me. I haven't done anything to you, but if you don't want to talk it's okay with me, I have other things to do." (Stage 3.)

Therapeutic Use of Self

The therapeutic use of self means going beyond the realm of learning general therapeutic techniques to discover which techniques the nurse can use well and those she cannot seem to use at all; determining which behaviors convey warmth, empathy, or genuineness, and those that are perceived as cold or unhelpful. Therapeutic use of self means individualizing the use of therapeutic techniques and using special personality characteristics to an advantage in working with clients. For example, a nurse with a fine sense of humor may be able to tease a client to encourage him to see some aspect of his behavior. On the other hand, a nurse who rarely teases will seem stilted or artificial if she attempts to use humor as a therapeutic technique.

The therapeutic use of self involves doing what one can do best. Experience reveals the strengths and limitations the nurse brings to the situation, as well as how and when clients are affected by different behaviors. The process requires extensive clinical experience, self-evaluation, and openness to the feedback of others. Trying new techniques and receiving feedback may be uncomfortable at first. In time, the ability to use oneself therapeutically becomes a more natural way of responding to clients,

without having to consciously plan each move. Therapeutic use of self involves a trust in one's instincts and a sensitivity to subtle cues about when to act in a certain way with a client.

PHASES OF THE THERAPEUTIC RELATIONSHIP

The phases of the therapeutic relationship are the *preinteraction phase,* the *orientation* (introductory) *phase,* the *working phase,* and the *termination phase.* These phases are outlined according to the tasks that are to be accomplished for each stage. This section focuses on student reactions to the phases of the relationship and strategies for the student nurse to use in achieving the tasks of each phase.

Preinteraction Phase

The preinteraction phase begins as soon as the student nurse is aware of her intent to interact with a client. For the nursing student this is often a period of anxiety and self-doubt. It is important during this phase to become aware of one's own beliefs, thoughts, and feelings. Recognizing personal values, biases, or fears gives the student the opportunity to develop a greater self-awareness and seek assistance from a more experienced nurse, thus freeing herself from feelings that may interfere with the therapeutic relationship.

The tasks of the preinteraction phase are listed in the box below.

Reactions to the preinteraction phase. Reactions that are likely to surface during the preinteraction phase include anxiety, the need to know the client's history, role threat, feelings of incompetencey, fear of being hurt or of causing distress, fear of losing control, and fear of rejection.

Everyone brings elements of his past experience into any new situation. For the student nurse, this may include rumors about the horror of mental hospitals and psychiatric clients. (Mental illness and mental hospitals are often portrayed as frightening in movies and literature.) These fears, usually of the unknown, lead to an increased anxiety that makes it difficult for the student nurse to hear instruction or accurately assess a situation.

Student nurses often feel incompetent before their first client interaction. They doubt their ability and verbalize fears such as, "How can I help a person just by talking?" The student nurse may be afraid of being asked for advice or feel ill-equipped to supply answers.

Feelings of incompetence are worsened because there

TASKS OF THE PREINTERACTION PHASE

Explore personal beliefs, feelings

Pursue routes to self-awareness

Review appropriate theory

Analyze strengths and limitations in relating to others

Plan for first interactions with client

Research Highlight

The 24-Hour Stay

S.A. Hambrick-Batler & K. Sarasin

PURPOSE

This study was designed to evaluate the usefulness of a 24-hour stay in a psychiatric unit, thus decreasing the anxiety students feel about their psychiatric clinical rotation as well as increasing the student's sensitivity to the psychiatric client.

SAMPLE

Thirty-seven nursing students entering the first day of their psychiatric clinical rotation participated in the study.

METHODOLOGY

Students met with instructors and were given guidelines for the 24-hour stay and filled out a pretest assessment form. Each student went through a regular admission procedure and was admitted to a unit in a psychiatric hospital. For 24 hours the student was expected to conform to unit policy and participate in unit activities as a client. The instructor rotated through the units assessing the students' anxiety level throughout the 24-hour stay. A discussion session was held the second clinical day to integrate the experience. Students completed a posttest assessment form.

FINDINGS

Students exhibited lower levels of anxiety toward clients after the stay. Also, students were able to focus on professional issues involved in establishing a therapeutic relationship rather than on personal anxieties.

IMPLICATIONS

The first-hand experience of 24 hours as a psychiatric client facilitates the students' empathy for clients and the transition into the professional role.

Based on data from Journal of Psychosocial Nursing 24:23, 1986.

are fewer traditional nursing tasks associated with the care of psychiatric clients. The staff often do not wear uniforms or stethoscopes or other symbols associated with the nursing role. Clients may be dressed in street clothes, out of their rooms, or off the unit or floor involved in activities. The feeling of role threat that a nurse experiences may push her to seek concrete tasks to perform. Reading the client's chart may be a task the nurse uses to decrease anxiety. Reading the chart can also become a way of avoiding the initial contact with a client.

Nursing students often express the fear that they will hurt or be hurt by the client. Students fear that clients are fragile and imagine that an inappropriate comment will send the client "off the deep end" or "set him off." Students fear that the client may do harm to himself either physically or psychologically. Moreover, students sometimes believe that psychiatric clients are volatile and may physically or psychologically hurt the nurse at the slightest provocation.

Related to the fear of hurting or being hurt is the fear of loss of self-control. The student fears that the client may say or do something that may cause an undesirable reaction in the student. The student may have a history of crying easily, blushing, or even having a quick temper, and be frightened that these behaviors may surface in the clinical setting.

Another fear often expressed by students is that of being rejected by the client: "What if no one wants to talk to me?" This fear is related to shyness or a need for approval or gratitude from the client. It is difficult to think of offering oneself as a helper, and then being rejected as unneeded or unwanted.

Strategies for accomplishing the tasks of the preinteraction phase. The student may find it helpful to ask these questions before interaction with the client: "What is my greatest fear about getting to know this client?" "What do I expect this client to be like?" "Is there any type of person or problem that I worry about working with?"

It may be helpful to review behaviors associated with the various psychiatric disorders. The nurse may know the client's diagnosis at this point and can read specifically about that disorder. Even if the diagnosis is not known, the basic concepts of anxiety, loss, self-esteem, trust, or dependency can be applied to most clients.

Self-awareness includes the analysis of personal strengths and limitations in relating to others. At this phase in the relationship the nursing student's list of weaknesses may seem to far outnumber the list of strengths. It is helpful to remember that interacting with others is not a skill unique to psychiatric nursing; rather, it is a skill that one has practiced daily over a lifetime. The nursing student is preparing to refine, improve, and expand on existing skills. A characteristic that at first glance may seem to be a liability may prove to be a strength as the nurse gains expertise.

The fears and expectations of the student nurse need to be examined before the first meeting with the client. It is sometimes helpful just to know that others have experienced similar feelings. Open discussion of fears often makes them less intense. Factual information about the nature of psychiatric illness can allay the student's fears. Another strategy for decreasing anxiety is to review situations in the past where the student has successfully dealt with problems such as rejection or a person who is tearful, angry, or easily hurt. Looking at behaviors that have been successful in the past can help prepare the student for potential situations in the clinical arena. It may be helpful for students to imagine a situation and then role play a successful resolution. The Research Highlight (p. 101) discusses a method used by one nursing school to decrease anxiety about psychiatric clients.

Knowledge of the client's history facilitates the nurse's ability to ask pertinent questions, however, beginning students tend to structure the first interview so that they obtain the same information that is in the chart, rather than the information that the client wishes to discuss. Thus it is helpful to conduct the first interview without having read the chart. This reduces the possibility of preconceived expectations on the part of the nurse and facilitates the nurse's ability to follow the client's lead during the interview.

After the nursing student has explored personal beliefs, analyzed strengths and limitations, and reviewed psychiatric disorders, it is then helpful to make tentative plans for the first meeting with the client. Tentative plans that the nursing student can make include when and where to interview the client as well as what initial approach is to be used. The student needs to be aware of the physical structure of the setting in which the interaction will take place and minimize any barriers to communication. It is also helpful to formulate several possible questions that can be asked to begin the interaction and to elicit information from the client. These questions may be as simple as, "Tell me what brings you to the hospital?" or "I'd like to get to know you. Tell me something about yourself." Even if the tentative plans cannot be implemented, having them in mind reduces the student's anxiety before the interaction.

Orientation Phase

The orientation or introductory phase begins when the nurse and client meet. It is essential for the nurse to understand and acknowledge the client's perception of the problem and reason for seeking help. Understanding the client's perception of the situation is basic to establishing rapport, gathering data, and formulating a contract.

The nurse obtains a psychosocial history, using an organized framework for gathering data and getting to know

---

TASKS OF THE ORIENTATION PHASE

Establish rapport, trust, and communication
Determine what help the client desires or needs
Gather data, including client feelings, strengths, and weaknesses
Define client's problems
Formulate a *contract*
Mutually set goals

---

and understand the client. Telling his history allows the client to describe the current situation and the events leading up to the current situation in the way the client perceives them. Discussing the past is often less threatening than discussing the present. Discussing behaviors is also less threatening than discussing thoughts and feelings. Initially the client may not be able or willing to discuss feelings; however, the nurse may surmise feelings that can be validated and discussed later in the relationship. Clients often want, even need, to discuss feelings, but hold back, waiting for assurance that the nurse is willing to listen to feelings. It is the nurse's responsibility to be open to cues about the client's willingness to discuss feelings.

During the orientation phase, the nurse and client identify the problems and the factors that lead to the difficulty; however, it is common that there may be some differences in perception at this point. While identifying the client's problems, it is also helpful to identify the client's strengths. Each client brings some strengths and assets to the situation, and it is easy for both nurse and client to overlook these when focusing on the problem.

Collecting data and identifying problems form the basis for the establishment of a mutual agreement for care: this is called a contract. The contract is a vital component of the relationship because it allows the nurse and the client to know what to expect from each other. Without the contract, the relationship lacks direction, and many misunderstandings are possible because of unmet expectations. Basic elements of the contract include lengths, location, and time of future meetings. The roles of the nurse and client are defined, including the concept of confidentiality. Later, goals for the relationship are established and criteria for terminating the relationship are discussed.

Establishment of goals for the relationship is an important task of the orientation phase. To the extent that problem identification involves both nurse and client, the goals are set mutually. For the severely distressed client, the nurse takes responsibility for goal setting until the client has progressed to a state where problems and goals can be reviewed and discussed. The role of the nurse is to nurture the collaborative relationship until there is a joint responsibility for setting and working toward treatment goals.

The tasks of the orientation (introductory) phase are listed in the box at left.

Reactions to the orientation phase. The student nurse sometimes finds it difficult to approach the client and ask to spend time just talking without having concrete tasks to facilitate the interaction. The student nurse sometimes expresses guilt about "goofing off" and yet is surprised at how exhausting the clinical day can be.

Since the client may have no obvious illness, it is sometimes difficult for students to recognize the symptoms of psychiatric problems. Student nurses may identify with the client, causing them to deny that the client has problems or even question their own sanity. There may be an uncomfortable sense that mental illness is contagious. The clients may indeed have problems similar to those of the student nurse, since psychiatric problems are not unique to hospitalized clients. For instance, both the client and student nurse may be experiencing anxiety, and at this early stage it is very difficult for the student nurse to distinguish the degree to which the anxiety affects the client.

As the client discloses his problems the student nurse may feel overwhelmed and helpless. This feeling can combine with her desire to help, causing the student nurse to rush headlong into trying to solve all of the client's problems immediately, even before the problems are accurately identified and explored. The novice also tends to "do for" the client at this time, sometimes going to the canteen, bringing small items to the client, and doing other small tasks that the client can appropriately do for himself.

In contrast with feeling overwhelmed, the nurse may resist entering the therapeutic relationship. The student nurse subconsciously fails to pick up on cues the client sends and continues with a social relationship. The communication remains superficial and often the student nurse reports that the client "doesn't feel comfortable" enough to discuss problems yet. This sometimes leads to the client's rejection of the nurse, since clients often do not feel up to embarking on new social relationships. Table 6-2 discusses the characteristics of a therapeutic versus a social relationship.

Stacklum[37] identified several stages that nursing students go through. In the orientation stage, students exhibit selective inattention, obsession with detail, dissociation of theory from practice, and avoidance behavior related to anxiety. Second, the students overidentify with their clients and are unable to correctly identify the client's problems because of the students' excessive use of denial. The students' thinking becomes concrete and they tend to keep interactions social rather than therapeutic. Finally, hostility is often directed against the staff as the students begin to question their ability and experience feelings of anger, frustration, or omnipotence. The working stage of the relationship begins as the student's anxiety decreases, allowing them to accept the client, listen actively, analyze the data in relation to theory, and plan realistic nursing actions.

Strategies for accomplishing the tasks of the orientation phase. The tasks of the orientation phase are accomplished more easily if the nurse remembers that it is a time of exploration, a time to get to know another unique individual. To decrease her anxiety about asking personal questions, the nurse needs to remember that the client, by virtue of being identified as a client, has implied the need for a helping relationship. Helping relationships by nature include disclosure of personal beliefs and feelings.

The initial interview sets the tone for the orientation phase and deserves particular attention and planning. Communication techniques that allow the client to control the interview are important. These include general leads, clarifying, accepting, and silence. It is also important that the nurse is certain that the client's communication is understood. Techniques such as encouraging comparison, paraphrasing, seeking clarification, and exploring ensure that the nurse is accurately interpreting the client's message. The amount and type of self-disclosure the nurse

TABLE 6-2 Characteristics of a therapeutic versus a social relationship

Focus	Therapeutic	Social
Purpose	Help for the client	Mutual enjoyment or need fulfillment
Values	Nurse accepts the client without judging	Often based on shared value systems
Goals	Mutually set to meet client's needs; specific and known	May not have specific goals or may be for mutual satisfaction
Meetings	Planned for regular specific dates and times	May be erratic, chance, or planned
Responsibility	Nurse keeps relationship focused on goals	Shared
Length	Time-limited based on goal attainment or number of meetings	Flexible, may last years
Self-disclosure	Nurse discloses only what will help the client; intimate details, thoughts and feelings of client discussed	Mutual and equal; sometimes remains on a superficial level
Termination	Planned and discussed; an important part of the relationship	Usually gradual and unplanned or caused by outside factors such as relocation; often not discussed

uses is limited, as is the amount and type of confrontation (see Chapter 5).

During the initial interview the nurse can expect to encounter some resistance from the client. This may come in the form of the client's doubting that he can be helped by therapy; asking more of the nurse than is appropriate in a therapy setting; showing hostility, dependence, or sexual interest in the nurse; giving standard, rote answers to questions; or revealing little if any new information. The nurse may also resist entering the therapeutic relationship, finding it difficult to empathize with the client, being irritated at the client's resistive behavior, or generally finding it difficult to respect the client as a unique individual. The issue of both client and nurse resistance will be discussed further as transference and countertransference

Once the initial assessment is concluded, the nurse determines appropriate tentative nursing diagnoses. Tentative goals are mutually established and a plan formulated. The diagnosis, goals, and plans usually change as the relationship between nurse and client changes and as the client reveals more of the problem. The nurse may find that it takes more than one interview to adequately assess the client's needs. As the nurse and client interact, the dynamics of the problem and the needs and desires of the client become more clear. The therapeutic relationship is not static. It is sometimes not clear when the orientation phase ends and working phase begins, especially since goals and plans are continually reassessed throughout the relationship. However, once a contract is established, a tentative plan formulated, and the client begins working on identified problems, the relationship can be considered to enter the working phase.

Working Phase

During the working phase of the relationship, it is necessary to maintain and strengthen the rapport that was established during the orientation phase. There are two sections of the working phase: helping the client develop insight and translating insight into behavioral change. Change is usually painful and clients often resist at this stage. Data gathering is continuous throughout the therapeutic relationship. Intervention is directed toward having the client rethink his problems and respond differently toward others and himself. The focus of the relationship is the present situation, rather than the past. Transference and countertransference are key issues in resistance. Problems and goals are evaluated and redefined, if necessary, in the light of new data.

Reactions to the working phase. During the working phase of the therapeutic relationship the student nurse's reaction seems to center around frustration at not being able to solve the client's problem, overinvolvement with the client, and other manifestations of countertransference. Many student nurses may be impatient with the client for failing to see solutions that she sees, and for a lack of willingness to change. Other student nurses become profoundly frustrated with the health care system or society for not providing the client with the material or emotional supports the student nurse perceives as necessary for the client. For instance, a student nurse may become distraught when placement cannot be found for a pregnant, runaway teenager who has no one but an abusive or rejecting family. The student nurse may focus on what cannot be done and lose sight of what can be accomplished.

Transference and countertransference reactions are likely to occur during the working phase of the relationship. *Transference* is the unconscious transfer of qualities or attributes originally associated with another, especially a parent or sibling, to the nurse. It is a deviation in the nurse-client relationship that occurs because the client tends to bring frustrations, conflicts, and feelings of dependence from a past relationship into the current one with the nurse. The client expects positive or negative responses that have been a part of the earlier relationship, even when the current relationship with the nurse does not provoke these responses or suggest that they are appropriate. The client may express feelings of affection, re-

jection, or hostility that are too intense and out of proportion for the current situation. The client may fear rejection by the nurse, or feel guilty about perceived inadequacies.

Countertransference is the reverse of transference. The nurse's unresolved problems lead her to respond to the client's transference by investing the client with certain attributes from the nurse's earlier experiences; that is, the client's transference provokes the nurse's countertransference reaction. For example, a client might sulk because of a perceived neglect on the part of the nurse and say, "You are punishing me. You hate me, and that's why you didn't stop to talk with me." This is transference on the client's part. The nurse may then become angry and say, "Your behavior is unacceptable. You are not making a satisfactory effort to get better," thinking that the client is acting just like a younger sibling acted years ago. This is countertransference on the part of the nurse.

Transference carries with it a therapeutic potential as well as a potential barrier to the relationship. Following is a list that indicates transference and countertransference experiences[43]:

1. The client expresses an unreasonable dislike for the nurse.
2. The client describes the nurse as unreal, mechanical, or depersonalized. When the nurse comments in a manner designed to gather more information, the client tends to ignore the point and responds tangentially.
3. The client becomes overinvolved with a personal trait of the nurse that has little or no bearing on the nurse's experience or skill or the client's ability to work with the nurse.
4. The client expresses an excessive liking for the nurse, thinks she is the best or only possible nurse for him, and claims that no one else in the world could assume and successfully carry out the therapeutic task.
5. The client dreads the hours with the nurse and is persistently uncomfortable during them.
6. The client finds it difficult to focus on any aspect of his reasons for being with the nurse. He is vague about them and discusses them as if he were consulting the nurse about his "case" as one professional colleague to another.
7. The client is preoccupied with the nurse to an unusual degree in the intervals between sessions and may find himself imagining remarks, questions, or situations involving the nurse. The nurse may appear in the client's dreams.
8. The client is habitually late for appointments or shows other disturbances regarding time arrangements, such as running past an agreed upon time. Any disturbance about any aspect of the arrangements, once mutually agreed upon and initiated, falls into this category.
9. The client exhibits a pattern of continually arguing, seeking love, or remaining uninvolved or indifferent about important issues in his life.

10. The client becomes defensive with the nurse and exhibits extreme vulnerability to the nurse's observations, inferences, or interpretations.
11. The client consistently misunderstands or persistently requires further clarification of the nurse's comments. If he never agrees with the nurse's comments, the possibility of transference can be tested by repeating a point made by the client, with which the client will disagree.
12. The client seeks to elicit a particular emotional response from the nurse through provocative remarks, double-edged questions, or dramatic statements.
13. The client becomes overly concerned with the confidentiality of his work with the nurse.
14. The client looks beseechingly or angrily for sympathy regarding real or imagined maltreatment at the hand of an authority figure.
15. The client praises the nurse for improvements in his life that are actually not direct results of their work together.
16. The client expresses the desire to be the nurse's only client.
17. The client reports transitory physical symptoms during contact with the nurse. These symptoms may occur only during the time the client is with the nurse or with certain other people.

The nurse can recognize countertransference in a similar manner: basically by substituting "nurse" for "client" in the preceding list. Also, if client transference is observed, it is equally necessary for the nurse to examine the relationship and her own feelings for countertransference.

The nurse may find the experience of transference and countertransference particularly difficult. Since both phenomena occur on a subconscious level, the process may develop completely out of the awareness of the novice who has no previous experience with resistance. Besides blocking the therapeutic process, the client may also be blocking the nurse's immediate goals. A goal-oriented nurse may feel successful only to the extent that client goals are met. If the client seems not to be progressing, the nurse may feel at fault or inadequate. It is especially important during the working phase for the nurse to maintain open communication with a supervisor who can facilitate the nurse's progress through the resistance.

Case Example

The nurse had been with a group of clients for the whole day. They had all been on a picnic and had returned to the ward. One of the clients, Jane, had attached herself to the nurse when going outside for this first ward outing. Frightened and unsure of herself, she would wrap her arms around the nurse when outside. As she gained confidence, she would gradually separate from the nurse and move on by herself or with other clients. When all had returned to the ward, Jane went into the kitchen with the nurse to prepare a cup of coffee. Other clients joined them in the kitchen and began to talk to the nurse. When they left, the nurse asked Jane to hand her the sugar for her coffee. Jane started to

---

TASKS OF THE WORKING PHASE

Maintain the relationship
Gather further data
Promote the client's development of insight
Facilitate behavioral change
Overcome resistance behaviors
Evaluate problems and goals and redefine as necessary

---

scream at the nurse, accusing her of cheating her, taking things from her, hating her. Jane was most distraught, and when the nurse tried to speak or move toward her, Jane yelled louder. The nurse, keeping some distance, followed Jane to her bedroom, while Jane continued to yell. Another nurse came into the room, moving closer to Jane. Jane did not yell at her and began to calm down. The nurse who was the focus of the outburst removed herself after the other nurse had stepped in. Later that day, Jane came to the first nurse and apologized for her behavior. Together they sat down and talked about what happened. Jane claimed that for a time the nurse had become her mother. In this situation the transference was most dramatic. Jane and the nurse could now talk about Jane's need to be so physically close to the nurse when they first went outside, how it made her feel like a little girl, and how she resented the other clients talking to the nurse in the kitchen.

Strategies for accomplishing the tasks of the working phase. The first portion of the working phase centers on developing the client's insight and determining the problem. Data gathering focuses on symptoms, feelings, interpersonal relationships, past history, and environmental dissatisfactions in an attempt to identify patterns of behavior.

The tasks of the working phase are listed in the box above.

People typically use certain coping mechanisms, defense mechanisms, communication, or behavior patterns in response to perceived threats. The client may not be aware that the current behavior is a pattern that has been used in the past. Once the pattern is identified, the nurse assists the client in discovering the theme underlying the perceived threat. For instance, the nurse may identify a pattern of withdrawal in a client. The withdrawal may be exhibited in response to an underlying theme of fear of rejection.

Case Example

Jean, a 39-year-old mother of three, was hospitalized for depression while going through a divorce. She was unable to work, lost interest in friends, and was having difficulty sleeping and eating. On questioning she stated that her husband no longer loved her, her friends thought she was a failure, and she believed that the people at work were laughing at her. Her response to these perceived rejections was to withdraw. When her husband was interviewed he stated that he still loved his wife and was willing to work on the marriage. Jean's fear of rejection led to her withdrawal and perpetuated the problems she dreaded most. Understanding Jean's withdrawal as a pattern enables the nurse to confront the discrepancy between Jean's perception of the situation and that of her husband, while pointing out the pattern of withdrawal.

Focusing on symptoms. A thorough analysis of symptoms is often useful in linking unconscious psychological patterns to patterns of behavior. In eliciting information from a client regarding a symptom, the nurse may recognize a connection, but this does not mean that the client does. Many possibilities exist for the client's lack of awareness; the nurse decides how and when to make the connection and how and when to use the information. The objective is for the client to have control over the therapeutic process and to function independently of the nurse. Initial efforts to focus on symptoms include introducing the client to the internal psychological processes associated with the behavior, and the possible external triggering events, as in the following example:

Client: I have this pain in my neck. It goes down my arm. (Demonstrates with left hand the pain track in right arm.) I've had an examination by a doctor, and there is nothing physically wrong with me. He sent me here. (Looks down, silent.)

Nurse: Are you experiencing the pain now?

Client (Looks at nurse, raises right hand behind neck.) Well, it hurt more in the waiting room.

Nurse: It hurt more in the waiting room than it does now—hmm. . . . Before I ask you more about this pain, what are some of your thoughts concerning the doctor's recommendations to come here?

The nurse consciously asks for the client's thoughts. At this point the nurse is operating on a hunch that the client is not used to expressing herself in emotional feeling terms.

Client: Well, I love my kids and husband, and I want to do things—if only the pain would stop. . . . (Looks at nurse, and tears come to her eyes.)

Nurse: It is the pain that stops you—it's difficult to understand how this is related to how you think and feel about things.

Client: Yes, it doesn't make sense, it's not my imagination, but I don't know what else to do. (Looks downward, defeated.)

Nurse: Well, when you have been stuck before, what have you done?

Client: Tried something new. (Looks at nurse and face becomes a bit more animated.)

The nurse has noticed the nonverbal shifts in the client. The client has become more alert, interested, and curious. The nurse decides the client is ready to explore some options.

Nurse: Can I ask you some questions now, and perhaps have you try something?

Client: Okay.

Nurse: Take a deep breath and let it out. (Demonstrates more relaxed body posture and shakes her shoulders, loosening tension in her neck.)

Client: (Mimics nurse's actions.)

Nurse: Now, how is the pain in the neck?

Client: Well, it's not there. Sometimes I'm able to do this at home, but it doesn't last.

Nurse: Sure, now think back to the waiting room. (Observes client as she thinks and remembers.)

Client: (Becomes tense and puts right hand up to back of neck.)

Nurse: What thoughts do you recall?

Client: I was nervous. I felt I shouldn't be here. I thought people would make fun of me. (Looks at nurse and realizes her hand is behind her neck.)

Nurse: How does the neck feel now?

Client: It's getting a bit tense.

Nurse: Relax yourself. (Makes relaxing body movements.)

Client: (Follows nurse's motions.) This seems too simple. It's more than will power.

Nurse: I agree with you. What is important is to appreciate that the neck pain, which is very real, is a signal to pay attention to what is going on inside. In the meantime, it's useful to know that you can do some immediate things to reduce the pain, and as you become aware of some of the thoughts and feelings, you will have more options—you won't be stuck.

Focusing on feeling states. Focusing on feeling states assists the client in unraveling the trends and patterns of interrelationships. Clients often believe that their feeling states come out of the blue or are caused by a specific event. In the following example, the client is not aware of the connection between his emotional arousal and his conscious and subconscious cognitive processes:

Client: I felt fine coming over here today, until I got caught up with all the turtles on the road.

Nurse: Turtles?

Client: Yeah, slow drivers.

Nurse: And now?

Client: I'm just getting over being mad. It was a good day, I thought I was getting a handle on this anger. (Starts to cry.) I'm fine until I get here, then it all comes out. It was a hard weekend. You know Mag and I went to the mountains for the weekend. Plans were for her mother to visit.

Mag has a degenerative brain disease. Mag and the client are in a committed love relationship not approved of by family members. The client has been assuming major responsibilities for Mag.

Client: (Face reddens, clenches fists, tries unsuccessfully to hold back tears.) I don't know how she can do this to her daughter. God, how Mag must feel! Her mother phones at the last minute (we were there Friday). Her mother says she wants to visit with a friend; she'll come Sunday some time. Goddamn her! (Full rage.) She does it all the time.

Nurse: *Terribly enraging. (Leans forward.)*

Client: *Yes, why do I expect things from her when I know they aren't forthcoming? Poor Mag, how upset she must feel.*

Nurse: *Was Mag enraged, upset?*

Client: *(Regains some emotional control.) She gets upset when I get angry . . . then she gets going a bit.*

Nurse: *Sometimes your anger gets to her.*

Client: *I almost didn't come today. I was mad at you and all the talk about my mother. I'm mad at her—there's nothing there; when it's my birthday, there's nothing, not even a card.*

Nurse: *You are mad at a lot of people. And you were angry with me and almost didn't come.*

Client: *At times I don't think you are available to me.*

Nurse: *Like in 2 weeks when I'll be on vacation.*

Client: *I know, I know, you don't have to tell me (laughing and crying).*

Nurse: *It seems that to get a handle on the rage it is important to appreciate how it builds up when you feel cut off from what you want and what you need.*

Client: *Yes, it was a hard weekend with Mag. When I get angry, she says I'm angry with her. I was looking forward to sharing the weekend with other people. I guess I was disappointed.*

Focusing on interpersonal relationships. How people approach relationships with others reflects beliefs, values, and self-esteem. When clients bring their perceptions of the personalities of others into the therapy situation, it allows the nurse access to the client's patterns of projection, expectations, and values.

Case Example

Jill, the client, and Bill married after many years of courtship. After a year and a half they separated. Bill has three teenage daughters, Jill a teenage son from previous marriages. Jill left because she believed Bill would not let her be a mother to the daughters, and that he wanted her as a housekeeper and not as a wife. Bill disagrees with this. They are trying to reconcile their relationship. The present situation involves Jill's response to Bill asking her about a blanket he was thinking of sending to his daughter, who has just started college.

Client: *Bill wanted the blanket for himself. He didn't want me to have it.*

Nurse: *How did you arrive at that conclusion?*

Client: *Well, when Bill phoned me the night before I was going away for the weekend, he asked for it.*

Nurse: *He wanted the blanket.*

Client: *Well, he said he phoned to wish me a good time, and then he asked me if I knew where the gold blanket was. I said I had it. I asked him why he was asking about it. He said that he was looking for it to give to Juliet to take with her. I asked how he had decided it should be the gold blanket. Here it goes again. He doesn't want me to have the blanket.*

Nurse: *Did he say that?*

Client: *No, but why did he phone? We said good night the night before, and he said he would see me next week.*

Nurse: *What do you think?*

Client: *Because he wanted the blanket—I know.*

Nurse: *I'm sure you have reasons for knowing that. But it would be useful to try to make them a little bit more clear.*

Jill's potential for assuming and thinking she knows what is in the minds of others is a possible pattern of projection. It is an unconscious phenomenon, and is most convincing. The nurse took care in confronting this possibility, since Jill's sense of reality may be challenged, thus provoking great anxiety and confusion.

Client: *Well, I guess it's in his tone of voice. I don't want the blanket; I don't want anything that's not mine. I just took the blanket when I left the house because my blankets were on the children's beds and I didn't want to disturb the household any more than I was doing.*

Nurse: *You are sensitive to the needs of Bill and the children.*

Client: *(Nods yes.)*

Nurse: *Bill knows this. He doesn't understand it all, but he knows it.*

Client: *(Continues to nod yes.)*

Nurse: *Bill said he didn't want the blanket.*

Client: *Yes, but I don't believe him. There must be something special about the blanket.*

Nurse: *Did you ask Bill?*

Client: *Yes. He said there wasn't.*

Nurse: *Now I'm confused.*

Client: *Bill said he asked me because he went looking for the blanket and couldn't find it. He wanted to know where it was, so he asked me.*

Nurse: *What makes it difficult to believe that?*

Client: *There has to be more to it than that.*

Nurse: *Like what?*

Client: *That he doesn't want me to have it.*

Nurse: *(Gently.) Did he say that?*

Client: *No. It's hard to believe that I'm assuming all this.*

Nurse: *It may be more difficult not to realize this. What would Bill have had to do to convince you to keep the blanket?*

Client: *Not bring it up. In other relationships in my life I don't do the assuming I do with Bill. In part, it is hard to face because it makes me feel that I'm the problem in the marriage.*

At this point Jill was beginning to recognize a pattern with Bill. Actually, she manifested this propensity at work and in social relationships. However, the breakup with Bill enabled her to begin to attend to her behavior.

Focusing on past history. Having a client recall life events not only allows for discernment of long-standing patterns of behavior, but also indicates how the individual has internalized patterns of coping. Although the client may be conscious of attitudes toward people important in the past, he may not be conscious of how this affects the present. People and events in the present may resemble those of the past, and the individual's responses may be based on these past experiences in a greater degree than is appropriate or useful in the present. The client may be aware of unreasonable reactions, but more often the client justifies the current response, thus unwittingly maintaining patterns that perpetuate limiting and defeating experiences from the past. By contrast, patterns that were important to the person in the past may no longer be necessary. Following is an example of focusing on past history:

Client: Well, when I get into these social situations, I feel I got to make up for something. I figure it isn't right to put such emphasis on dress and things like that. I keep saying I'm better than they are. (Laughs.)

Nurse: Kid from the other side of the tracks, huh? With a chip on her shoulder. Got to make up for something.

Client: (Becomes sober.) Yes. (Silent.)

Nurse: How is it possible that someone so competent is a failure and has to keep making up for something?

Client: (Thoughtful, silent, tears come to eyes.) You know, it's silly . . . (drifting) nothing ever mattered. . . . (lost in thought, tearing.)

Nurse: To whom?

Client: Nothing I ever wanted for myself meant anything to my mom. Early, I just ignored her. Now I realize I pushed her away, but there are always strings attached. . . . (Silence.)

Nurse: Go on. . . .

Client: Dad and I were close. He always stood up for me. Sure he drank, and he was terrible toward Mom. Limited her on money. Didn't get along with my sister. She just broke away.

Nurse: You were saying that your mother never thought much of what you wanted. (Therapist pulls client back to theme of not being accepted.)

Client: When I got accepted to an outstanding public school, it didn't mean anything her. Oh, I would hear her brag to her friends, or she would get mad if I got a low grade. (Silent.) One time I got an "F." I was so mad, I was going to quit that damn school. Who were they to give me an "F"? My father agreed. He was going to let me go to a private school, even though we didn't have the money. My mother said no. He and I went to make the arrangements, and the school said no because I couldn't transfer at that time of year. There we were, caught by my mother. (Laughs.)

The nurse had a choice between focusing on being in an alliance with the father or continuing with the experience of not being good enough, always having to make up for something. The nurse chose the latter.

Nurse: Sounds like your mother may have had your best interests at heart—not having you run from an "F."

Client: (Rather startled.) Well, yes, I suppose so. I know she didn't want me.

Nurse: Didn't want you?

Client: Oh, it's understandable. She had a hard time. Dad was drinking a lot. You know, she left him and then went back to him. She had Dorey, and a year later she was pregnant with me. She had to stay in bed most of her pregnancy because of her heart condition. She was in a long labor with me. I put these things together later. This is why I know she didn't want me.

Nurse: Sounds like she went through a lot to have you.

Client: She went through a lot with my father. He wasn't physically abusive. I was his "chicky"—I could have anything. (Laughs.) He never treated me like he treated my mother and sister.

Nurse: Sounds like you were very special to him.

Client: I never thought of that.

Focusing on past history reveals patterns of behavior and their psychodynamic makeup. The roots of these patterns are locked into internalized beliefs. The organization of these past experiences can be further explored, eliciting information not readily available on a conscious level. One hypothesis is that these subconscious beliefs are factors in repetitive, dysfunctional patterns in the present. Exploring and interpreting these beliefs is therapeutic. Awareness and abreaction (living through these memories), in addition to interpretation of their relevance to current defensive patterns of behavior, are the working therapeutic tasks of the client and nurse. The preceding example is a demonstration of how an internal, current state of "having to make up for something in social situations" has roots in past experiences. The first step in helping the client explore patterns of behavior is to bring these patterns into the client's awareness, and to link them with past events or internal processes such as emotional states and thought patterns.

Focusing on environmental dissatisfactions. Like feelings, interpersonal relationships, and past history, current dissatisfaction with life in general provides another source of information regarding prevailing patterns. Complaints about work, school, which course to choose, which job to take, pleasure in a job, the landlord's responsibilities, or living conditions all become relevant focuses of an interview because patterns interfering with the client's development and sense of satisfaction, control, and growth are revealed.

The first step is to find out from the client whether the attitudes and feelings expressed arise in other situations. The client is assisted in becoming aware of the fact that the attitudes and feelings are present in different situations. Having this awareness, the client is able to explore what he wants, the resources needed to get it, how to pursue what he wants, and other necessary ingredients in decision making. The dilemma regarding the life situation is, in part, perpetuated by the client not knowing what he wants. The recurrent attitudes and the emotional states block awareness, as shown in the following example:

Client: I don't know if I want to teach. For 5 years I've been administering special projects. Now I'm going back to the classroom. My wife is mad at me because I'm busy every night planning classes. I don't know if I really like teaching.

Nurse: Has there been a time when you liked teaching? (How does the client identify pleasurable experiences?)

Client: I don't know. I had taught classes for 1 or 2 years and then changed to something else. So, I never get to relax—you know what I mean—I do the hard part of organizing a class, and then I leave the next year.

Nurse: Have you ever worked in a situation in which you felt relaxed?

Client: Well, the time I left teaching for a year and worked in a collective restaurant.

Nurse: How was that for you?

Client: I liked working with the people. We worked together. You knew what to expect.

Nurse: Knew what to expect?

Client: Yeah, you know, I keep thinking I returned to teaching because my parents kept emphasizing security. Dad worked for the city. Mom worked as a nurse. They kept emphasizing, "Get a job for security, benefits, retirement. . ."

Nurse: What does this have to do with your current concerns?

Client: I don't know. I don't know if I dislike teaching because I'm doing it as a result of my parents' beliefs, or because I haven't given myself a chance to enjoy it.

Nurse: How successful are you in giving yourself a chance to enjoy what you do?

Client: Not very. That's what my wife is complaining about; it's hard to do things together that we enjoy. Oh, at times, but it's like we can't decide what to do or I'm worrying about my class preparations. I don't know—life is serious, hard. You must work; it's like there isn't much I do that I can say I really enjoy.

Nurse: It may be useful to find out what and how you do things when teaching to either experience pleasure or quench it.

Client: Yes, I'm desperate. I find myself worrying about it so much that it's driving my wife away from me.

In the preceding example the nurse agrees with the client that a lack of pleasure is being experienced in many areas of the client's life. He associates part of this pattern with parental upbringing. He is so distressed about his present reaction to teaching that the nurse encourages further exploration in this area to identify patterns of thinking and behaving that deplete the client's experience of satisfaction and pleasure in carrying out an important life activity, work. The nurse does not focus on changing jobs, but rather on identifying the theme of displeasure.

Translating insights into action. Thus far the discussion of the working phase has emphasized identifying and exploring patterns of dysfunctional behavior. How is this process employed for behavioral change? First, although it is helpful for the client to intellectually recognize that some of his behavior has childhood roots, a behavioral change toward positive goals is what counts. The process of exploration and identification results in behavioral change because it creates a challenge to nonproductive beliefs and adds the dimension of choice to the client's repertoire. Clients can expand their basis for making decisions and thus respond differently. Clients may feel less guilty and more in control of their behavior and the response of others. They are more open to feedback. They

may be more tolerant of others because they have a broader framework to use to understand themselves and others. A second dimension of the working phase is using insight and knowledge to change behavior and incorporate healthy patterns into the client's repertoire of responses.

Use of information about patterns requires a model of how, in reality, behavior can be changed. Exploration of therapeutic techniques for change reveals that regardless of the technique, one or more of the following behavioral processes are invoked: combining, separating, sorting, and altering behavioral criteria relevant to values and beliefs or rehearsing new behaviors. For example, when the nurse asks a client to notice how a past event, emotion, or relationship is related to a current behavioral response, the client is forced primarily to *combine* information from seemingly unrelated topics.

Separating occurs when the client *unlinks*: for example, a cause-effect conclusion:

Client: My mother is the cause of my problems with women.

Nurse: How's that?

Client: My mother's nagging when I was little still makes me angry with women today.

Nurse: How does this affect you today?

Client: When a woman asks me to do something, I just get mad and say she's not going to tell me what to do.

Nurse: So what you think about being asked to do something makes you mad.

Client: Well, yeah, I learned it with my mother.

Nurse: You learned that when your mother nagged you, you felt angry. Today you've discovered that when a woman asks you to do something, and you associate it with the past, you get mad.

Client: Yeah, my mother is dead; so it is the way I think.

Sorting is involved when interventions force a client to select information in a way that differs from an existing pattern. In a continuation of the preceding example of a man angry with women, the nurse may ask: "Tell me about a time that a woman asked you to do something and you didn't get mad or angry with her?" This question encourages the client to explore different experiences. If he cannot find any positive examples, the nurse can ask, "How would a woman have to ask you to do something without your getting angry?" The client may then outline the behavior necessary for him not to feel nagged.

Altering beliefs about behavior is another powerful way to change behavior. For example, the behavior of a client who is extremely intimidated by authority figures changes when he no longer believes the boss's anger is directed at him. He learns that anger comes from within and represents that person's way of expressing feelings such as frustration and anger. The client learns to replace his original response with a range of possibilities. For example a technique called "chair work" in Gestalt therapy has the client perform the following inner dialogue: the part of himself that is frightened of the boss talks with the part of himself that wants to speak up. Encouraging the client in this process encourages the client to begin to challenge and change his reasons for being frightened of the boss. Comments from the therapist are usually aimed at altering the client's interpretation of his behavior; this is called *reframing.*

Rehearsing new behaviors addresses the use of information about patterns and change. Role playing experiences in self-assertion is one way behavioral changes are accomplished and reinforced. The use of role playing as a basis for changing behavior indicates that the nurse not only uses communication techniques to focus interviews on relevant experiential areas, but also actively participates in strategies that encourage behavioral change. It is important to disrupt the client's dysfunctional behavior patterns during therapy. Disrupting the pattern jolts the client out of habitual behaviors and increases the client's insight and awareness. Experiencing new behaviors during therapy reinforces the concept that the client has control of and makes choices in his life.

During the later part of the working phase, the nurse interprets, confronts, and encourages the rehearsal of new behaviors.

Interpretations are aimed at clients who are reframing their view of what is causing distress or dysfunctional behavioral responses. For example, the client who felt something was missing in social situations and who revealed a strong belief that her mother could not possibly want her because of the difficult delivery (see p. 108), was ultimately able to connect much of this feeling to her unilateral relationship with her father, which resulted in part from a fear that he would treat her as he did her mother. Her resentment of her father surfaced, as did her jealousy and love. Her understanding of her father's fear of his children and competition with them for the mother's attention was underscored by the fact that the mother and father "made up" when the kids were out of the house. The client linked the "making-up feeling" to her desire and need to resolve within herself, and with her mother, their capacity to reject each other's loving gestures. At this point interpretation was insufficient. The daughter began to communicate with her mother and actively change her behavior toward her mother.

Confrontation involves concepts that are similiar to those of interpretation, except that it is based on the present. Because a confrontation is usually a direct encounter between nurse and client, the nurse is clear about the effect she wants; that is, the behavioral patterns she is attempting to change.

Case Example

Tabitha, a young social worker, was aware of and had explored at length a strong need to please people and to gain their approval. She had developed a strong self-defeating, self-limiting view and presentation of herself at work, in her marriage, and with her siblings. She damned herself. She recognized the secondary gain in this behavior: obtaining sympathy and attention. The pattern was often directed toward the nurse. The transference aspects were investigated. The behavior diminished but was still apparent and at times blatant. During one particular session, the client was describing her behavior in her new work setting:

Client: I don't think I'm doing very well. Oh, they like me, but the supervision isn't too good, and I don't think I put enough into my work. I'm not reading; I'm not keeping good notes. My sister, a budding, highly successful psychologist, seems more into her work than me. I don't know; I think, well, I'm doing all right, but I don't think it's as. . . good as it should be (looks at the nurse). What do you think?

Nurse: I agree with you.

Client: (Genuine surprise.) What?

Nurse: You have been telling me all the things you are not doing and how you appraise yourself. And I believe what you say.

Client: Don't you care?

Nurse: No. (Silence)

Client: (Looks stunned.)

Nurse: I only care that you care.

Client: (Silent and thoughtful.) I see what you mean—I wanted you to tell me I was okay.

Nurse: And would you believe me?

Client: I wouldn't really. It's hard to change. The responsibility. . . of caring. . . moving out on my own—taking responsibility for what I can do.

The preceding example emphasizes the fact that a client's insight into parental issues, sibling rivalry, or transference is of little value unless the client's behavior changes. The nurse's assuming a confrontational stance by saying "no" was directed at forcing the client to search for her own sense of worth, regardless of what the nurse thought of her. Any doubt concerning the client's lack of self-worth was dispelled by indications of her desire for reassurance. The next step is to have the client rehearse open, cooperative strategies. The client can now participate in exercises designed to facilitate her ability to compete more directly.

In addition to behaviors that the client reports to the nurse, problematic behavior patterns also arise within the context of the nurse-client relationship. The nurse seeks to create a balance in maintaining rapport and creating anxiety in the therapeutic process. Anxiety provokes the client to exhibit the behaviors that are used to alleviate anxiety. Patterns may also surface in relationship to others in the environment, such as staff or other clients. The nurse makes careful observations that are shared with clients to facilitate the client's understanding of their responsibility in creating and maintaining relationships. In the Case Example of Jean, who withdrew from her husband (pp. 105-106), it is likely that at some point Jean will withdraw from the nurse (being late, missing appointments, or refusing to share new information), demonstrating in the *here and now* her pattern of withdrawal. She is "transferring" her feelings and behaviors from past relationships onto her current relationship with the nurse.

Bringing old patterns of feeling and behaving into the current situation affords the opportunity to successfully alter these behaviors. Also, people who have been important and trustworthy, providing positive past experiences, influence the nurse-client relationship.

Ignoring transference can lead the nurse to behavior with the client that perpetuates the pattern; for example, being overly critical of the client, withholding information, or being overinvolved in making decisions for the client. Focusing on behavior and its immediate effect, without blame or presumption, is a constructive means for the nurse and client to mutually explore their relationship.

Case Example

When the nurse asks Jean about her missed appointments Jean becomes angry and states that she knows the nurse is "tired of her" and "really wants to terminate the relationship." After further discussion the nurse asks Jean if the current situation is in any way similar to the situation with Jean's husband or coworkers. Soon Jean develops the insight that the feeling of being unloved and the response of withdrawing is a recurrent pattern, and is not necessarily based on a realistic appraisal of the situation. Jean is then in a position to change her behavior with the nurse.

Although painful, the client's acknowledgment of personal responsibility for interpersonal relationships is the first step toward change. The client has the power to change her attitudes, feelings, and behaviors and therefore, to change other's response to her. It is the client's responsibility to risk trying new behaviors. Since behaviors that created problems for the client in the past surface in the present situation with the nurse, these behaviors can be confronted and new behaviors tried within the therapeutic relationship. Jean's fear of rejection by the nurse is not nearly as important as her fear of rejection by her husband; thus she can try being on time without missing appointments no matter what her feelings may be. Jean may learn to tell the nurse when she is feeling rejected and ask the nurse to validate her impressions by inquiring about the nurse's feelings toward her. If new behaviors can be attempted with a successful resolution of the withdrawal within the context of the therapeutic relationship, then the hope is established that change is possible in more important relationships.

The working phase comes to an end mainly when the initial goals and any intermediate goals have been addressed, and the client has developed ways of assessing and making changes for himself. If the client desires only a reduction in the symptoms, the nurse accepts this and moves to the termination phase.

Termination Phase

The termination phase begins during the orientation phase by defining responsibilities and therapeutic outcomes, and continues during the working phase as progress and outcomes are evaluated. The main objective of the termination phase is to bring a therapeutic end to the nurse-client relationship. The process of termination directs the nurse's attention toward making a potentially negative separation a positive one. When the process of termination is complete, it is known as closure.

The tasks of the termination phase are listed in the box at right.

Reactions to the termination phase. Endings are a normal part of life; however, in our society, endings are some-

times equated with failure. Since people usually attempt to avoid failure, the subject of parting is often not broached and no plans are made regarding how to successfully terminate relationships. Accordingly, many relationships end badly, leaving scars and unresolved conflicts. Many people never learn the skill of termination. This is true for the nurse as well as the client. The termination phase of the nurse-client relationship resurrects past experiences with separation and may be associated with a sense of disappointment or abandonment. Rather than feeling sad about parting, many people get angry and belittle the experience.

Another area of difficulty, particularly for the student or beginning nurse, is letting go of a close and often satisfying relationship. The intimacy and mutual acceptance found in the therapeutic relationship exemplify desirable qualities in personal relationships. During termination, both the client and nurse may be tempted to continue the relationship on a social level. This may simply be a reluctance to say "good-bye," or perhaps a lack of understanding of the nature of the relationship. Failure to terminate the relationship violates the therapy contract established by the two individuals. The nurse who experiences great difficulty in terminating a relationship can seek the advice of a peer or a more experienced nurse to sort out the ethical issues involved in converting a therapeutic relationship to a more personal one.

Student nurses who have difficulty terminating may attempt to delay termination, as discussed above, or may fail to adequately say good-bye. Students are often surprised at how difficult it is to say good-bye to clients. Student nurses sometimes fail to recognize how attached they have become to clients until the actual parting. Student nurses may protract the last meeting well beyond the time limits originally agreed upon for meetings. They may agree to have future contact with clients by phone, letter, or visit. Conversely, the student nurse may avoid saying good-bye by being overly casual with the client during the parting, avoiding discussion of termination, or avoiding the last meeting all together.

Strategies for accomplishing the tasks of the termination phase. Termination may occur before or after agreed upon goals have been met. Strategies may differ, depending on the nature of the termination. Termination is an important growth-producing experience for the client and the nurse.

Strategies for termination before agreed upon goals have been met. This type of termination is not unusual and can be precipitated by decision of the nurse, discharge of the client, or request of the client. When a client

---

TASKS OF THE TERMINATION PHASE

Bring a therapeutic end to the relationship
Review feelings about the relationship
Evaluate progress toward goals
Establish mechanisms for meeting future therapy needs

---

wishes to terminate prematurely, previous agreements expressed in the contract can do much to ensure a positive ending. It is useful for the client and nurse to agree in the beginning not to part in anger, nor to part without discussing the feelings parting evokes. Ideally three sessions are devoted to evaluating and ending the relationship. One session is the minimum time to devote to termination. This allows time for the client and the nurse to negotiate an ending to the relationship or to resolve any conflicts.

The fear of closeness can precipitate an early termination to the relationship. The implied intimacy of the therapeutic relationship can trigger the same fears for the nurse as for the client. The discussion on transference and countertransference (p. 104) highlights signs that can alert the nurse to these reactions. If the nurse finds herself too tense and unable to work through personal reactions to a client, it is best to terminate the relationship and refer the client to another therapist. This is most effectively done when the nurse assumes responsibility for her behavior and allows the client to express thoughts and feelings of rejection. The emphasis is on the best interests of the client. Often unrealistic attitudes and a sense of pride impede the nurse in making this reasonable decision; for example, the idea that the nurse can work with everyone. The presupposition is that nothing about a client detracts from productive, intimate work. This defies human existence. The mental health–psychiatric nurse constantly examines her personal beliefs and values to gain flexibility, but this does not mean that there are no limits.

Resistance from the client can be expected to surface during the termination phase. However, it is unfair to the client to treat this resistance as expected and therefore unworthy of attention. Fault finding by either party is a pattern that needs to be disrupted during the last meeting. In some cases the client states that the therapy is not beneficial, not working. The client's refusal to follow through on something that has been agreed upon may result from the client's assessment that what is going on does not coincide with his needs. The client's resistance does not mean that what is being done is not ultimately useful. It simply means that at this particular point, there has been a loss of appropriateness of therapeutic efforts for the client. The client may ask to terminate the relationship or just refuse to continue.

Resistance often comes in the form of a *flight to health*. The flight to health is exhibited by a client who suddenly declares no further need for therapy. The client claims to be "all right" and to desire to discontinue the therapeutic relationship. This may be a form of denial or fear of the anticipated grief over separation.

Whether the client resists by belittling the relationship or by claiming to be "cured," it is important for the therapist to contact the client and encourage renegotiation of the relationship. As long as the issues surrounding what needs to happen for the therapy to continue are examined, the client can decide to continue or terminate with a sense of direction for the future.

External factors can also cause premature termination, particularly for the nurse in a hospital setting. Discharge decisions may be made without considering the goals the client and nurse have set. It is helpful if discharge decisions are made known in advance so that the nurse and client have time to initiate the termination process. Discharge planning is an area for negotiation between the nurse and other health team members. The student nurse, who has a limited number of clinic hours, is particularly susceptable to a sense of loss when the client is discharged on a day the student is not in the clinic. The lack of closure is compounded if the nurse does not believe the goals that she and the client set were achieved.

Strategies for termination when agreed upon goals have been met. Painful experience with separation can be replaced by a positive experience; but even the termination of a good relationship in which therapy goals have been met can be a difficult process.

If the client or nurse has experienced the loss of an important person, the act of terminating the nurse-client relationship will ressurrect memories and feelings associated with the previous loss. Sorting the past from the present becomes a focus of therapy. Both nurse and client discuss their feelings about the separation. When the nurse is able to discuss feelings of sadness or loss about the ending of the relationship as well as her satisfactions, she is modeling an appropriate expression of feelings and encouraging the client to explore ambivalent feelings honestly. It may be helpful to discuss the grief process as it applies to the nurse-client relationship.

During the exploration of feelings about termination, it is helpful to relate those feelings to past experiences of loss, while bearing in mind that no new topics are discussed in this phase. Spiritual concerns, if not developed in the early phases of therapy, are most appropriately integrated during termination. Exploration of beliefs about the value of life and the meaning of death flow naturally from discussions of endings and beginnings. This is an extremely valuable experience for both client and nurse.

Flight to illness occurs when the client exhibits a sudden return of symptoms. This is an unconscious effort to demonstrate that termination is inappropriate and that the nurse is still needed. The client may disclose new information about himself or more problems in an attempt to delay parting. The threat of suicide is the most extreme symptom of flight to illness. The nurse has a difficult task to remain calm, sensitive, and firm in moving toward termination.

Often the client reveals a belief that he is unable to function without the nurse's assistance. The client may become increasingly dependent and appear to lose all ability to adapt. The nurse may also believe the client cannot function on his own. The nurse may have particular difficulty if the therapy has gone well. The nurse may unwittingly undermine the termination if her own personal needs, such as the need to feel helpful, cause her to overestimate her contribution and underestimate the client's contribution to the success of therapy. Both client and nurse need to examine their beliefs about the ability of individuals to control their own lives, as opposed to being controlled by outside forces. Both the client and nurse need to respect the client's role in achieving the goals of therapy.

Although the goal of the therapeutic process is for the client to continue to evolve and grow independently of the nurse, provisions are made for the client to return to therapy if the need arises. It is helpful for the client and nurse to discuss the future and anticipate possible situations the client may face. The client can project possible solutions to problems and rehearse skills learned in therapy. Client and nurse can assess the client's resources and support systems. Specific signs and symptoms that may denote a recurrence of problems are identified and a plan formulated for meeting future therapy needs. Referrals are made where appropriate.

BARRIERS TO THE THERAPEUTIC RELATIONSHIP

In the therapeutic relationship certain common problems or barriers have been identified. The nurse is alerted to the presence of these barriers by feelings of frustration, discomfort, anger, discouragement, confusion, or when the client changes suddenly by expressing hostility or withdrawal. The barriers may come from the environment, the nurse, or the client.

Environmental Barriers

Barriers to the nurse-client relationship may be external. Many of these, such as lack of privacy, inappropriate meeting place or furniture, and noise are discussed as barriers to communication. Some of the external barriers to the relationship may be within the nurse's control. The nurse may be able to find a relatively quiet, private place for a one-to-one interaction, but not be able to postpone the serving of lunch if one of her clients feels the need to interact at noon. The nurse can minimize the external barriers by paying attention to detail: wise scheduling of her time, honest discussion of her duties with each client, and effective collaboration with other team members.

Nurse Barriers

Nurses bring their previous experiences and distinct personalities to the nurse-client relationship. Some of these experiences and personal traits may create barriers to the therapeutic relationship.

Nurses, on the whole, are compassionate people, dedicated to helping clients, a quality that sometimes leads to nurses becoming too involved with clients, or "rescuing." Nurses sometimes attempt to solve all of the client's problems without allowing the client to make choices or mistakes. This discourages the client from taking personal responsibility and creates a situation where the nurse is working harder than the client to solve the client's problems. Sometimes the client resents the implication that he is not able to mutually or independently solve problems. Usually the nurse who works harder than the client finds herself becoming discouraged and worn out. Changes that the client makes are sometimes temporary since the change was the nurse's idea, not the client's. The nurse may become more frustrated as her efforts go unrewarded.

A related barrier comes from nurses who have become skeptical about the ability of clients to change. These nurses may have started as rescuers and become discouraged, or they may have begun with a pessimistic view of human nature. Such nurses tend to approach the nurse-client relationship by maintaining a certain distance from the client, using a matter-of-fact approach to the exclusion of other techniques. Inherent in this pessimistic view is the tendency to label clients either by diagnoses or as "trouble makers."

Just as nurses bring past experiences to the nurse-client relationship, they also bring current life situations to work. Like any other people, nurses experience divorce, death, sense of loss, job dissatisfaction, problems with children or peers, and other personal situations that may be difficult to ignore when establishing the nurse-client relationship. Nurses may be preoccupied, interested in socializing with each other, or just plain tired. It takes energy and dedication to switch from a social self to a therapeutic self to focus on the client.

Some nurses are not comfortable with feelings. They prefer that the client think and solve problems without becoming upset or angry. These nurses are disturbed by tears or loud voices and often fear that the client is "losing control" if he openly expresses any strong emotion. Nurses who are uncomfortable with feelings tend to discourage the client from sharing intimate details or going into depth about a problem; they claim that the client was "getting upset." The nurse who is uncomfortable with feelings is in need of considerable behavioral change to participate therapeutically in the nurse-client relationship.

Client Barriers

Most psychiatric problems can be categorized as difficulties in interpersonal relationships. It is therefore not surprising that these difficulties would surface in the nurse-client relationship. Even knowing that problems are bound to arise, there are certain client behaviors that present particular barriers to the relationship. Among these are excessive dependence, hostile aggressiveness, sexual acting out, manipulation, and self-destructive behaviors.

Excessive dependence is sometimes difficult to recognize in the early stages of the relationship because the dependent client initially appears cooperative and to be genuinely seeking help. Indications that dependence is a pattern include the client's excessive flattery of the nurse and self-depreciation. The client may compare the nurse favorably to others and feel hurt or jealous of the nurse's attention to other clients. The client may constantly ask for the nurse's opinion and advice before making decisions or may seek approval and attempt to please the nurse by excessive compliance to the nurse's suggestions or by performing small favors for the nurse.

The pattern of excessive dependence is called *learned helplessness*. It has the effect of creating secondary gains, because the client has many of his needs for attention, contact, and protection met through this behavior. Whereas the client may be initially perceived as pleasant and nonthreatening, later the nurse may become irritated with the constant, excessive demands that the dependent client makes of her. The client may harbor an underlying sense of guilt, anger, and even self-hatred at his dependence.

Hostile aggressiveness is a pattern of behavior that is particularly difficult for the nurse to tolerate. Signs may range from challenging, demeaning, and critical remarks to threats of physical violence. Swearing and lewd statements are another form of aggression. The main distinction between anger and aggression is that agression, rather than being an expression of feeling, conveys an intent to harm or destroy.

Like excessive dependence, the pattern of hostile aggressiveness is learned and creates a secondary gain for the client. The client may feel more powerful by hurting or intimidating others. The client may use intimidation to drive people away, thereby decreasing the fear associated with closeness. At times, the client is asking for external control such as medication, hospitalization, or seclusion. It is extremely important to assess the underlying reason for a client's aggressive behavior.

Sexual acting out may take the form of excessive flattery, asking the nurse for a date, suggestive remarks, or physical contact. The physical contact may range from excessive casual touching to grossly inappropriate and aggressive acts. Some of the milder expressions of sexual acting out may be a form of dependence: need for approval, attention, or a validation of the client's worth. Sexual acting out creates a powerful emotional response on the part of the nurse based on her own past experiences and value system. As with hostile aggressiveness there may be a variety of underlying reasons for the sexual acting out.

Overt sexual behavior has more in common with hostile aggressiveness and may be an attempt to gain power and control over the nurse, or to intimidate and drive the nurse away. In other instances, sexual acting out is a pattern of self-defeating behavior designed to confirm the client's feelings of worthlessness by causing the nurse to reject the client.

Manipulation is an immature pattern of behavior in which the client seeks to obtain personal goals, often without regard for the goals of others (Chapter 16). The client believes that he is entitled to have his desires met without delay and often without personal effort or sacrifice. Team members' beginning to feel protective about a client and angry toward other team members about the care a client is receiving may be an indication for the nurse that she is dealing with a manipulative client.

Secondary gains that the client receives from manipulation include having many needs met without expending much effort, distracting attention from his problems, diverting the attention of the staff, and therefore gaining the freedom to continue old, familiar patterns of behavior. Manipulation is used as a defense against anxiety and successfully decreases the client's anxiety while creating discomfort for those who are being manipulated.

Perhaps the most difficult client barrier is the threat of self-destruction. Suicide is the ultimate self-destructive act. As a barrier to the relationship it is helpful to think of the underlying motivations of self-destruction as being similar to those of other dysfunctional behaviors such as excessive dependence, hostile aggressiveness, and manipulation.

Strategies for overcoming client barriers. Perhaps the most important aspect of dealing with client barriers is for the nurse to be aware that barriers represent patterns of behaviors that the client uses to cope with interpersonal relationships. The real clues to the client's problem are often found in the behaviors the client expresses towards the nurse, rather than the client's verbalization of the problem. The barriers provide objective data to be considered along with the client's subjective perceptions. For example, a client who verbalizes the need to be close to others, yet refuses to confide in or trust the nurse, is giving the nurse two important pieces of information.

The nurse must look beyond the obvious behavior to the underlying meaning that it has for the client and the secondary gains that reinforce the behavior. For example, a client asks a nurse for a sexual favor. It is important to assess the context in which the behavior occurred: What was the previous relationship between client and nurse? Had there been any revealing topics discussed recently? Had the relationship changed? Were there any anxiety-provoking incidents in the client's life? Are the client's needs for affection and attention being met? Is the client hostile? Does the client have a history of sexual acting out? What was the nonverbal behavior and tone of voice during the conversation? Consideration of questions like these help the nurse to determine the meaning of the behavior.

The nurse also needs to assess the consequence or secondary gain that the client receives from the behavior. What does the client expect to happen as a result of his behavior? Is this a pattern that the client uses in similar circumstances? Why does the client continue to behave in this way—what does he get out of it? In assessing the consequences that the client expects from his behavior, it is sometimes helpful to ask directly, "How do you suppose I'll respond to what you just said?" It is also important for the nurse to be aware of her own feelings in response to the behavior. Chances are that the nurse's initial response will be similar to that of others in the past. For example, if the nurse finds that the client's behavior provokes feelings of pity, anger, or fear, it is probable that others have reacted or may react in the same way.

It is generally helpful for the nurse to avoid responding emotionally to the barriers the client erects. The most helpful response is one that will facilitate breaking the pattern of reinforcement that the client typically receives for the behavior. When the nurse remains calm and seeks to clarify the motivation for the behavior, this, in itself, becomes an intervention. The nurse is saying, "You matter. Your feelings matter, and I want to understand you." The client may not be aware of the behavior and its role in his problem. Gently, calmly pointing out the pattern and helping the client explore how it has been used in relationships is therapeutic. Above all, the nurse's willingness to continue to work on the relationship, in spite of obsta-

Research Highlight

A Study of the Influence of Role Modeling on Student Attitude Formation During Psychiatric Rotation

Sharon Dodds

PURPOSE

This research was designed to study the influence of role modeling by instructors and experienced nurses in the psychiatric field on the formation of positive attitudes of nursing students during their psychiatric rotation.

SAMPLE

The sample consisted of 50 white, middle-class, senior, baccalaureate-level nursing students (49 female and 1 male) attending a small midwestern private college. Each student had experienced nursing in a variety of speciality settings, including psychiatric nursing.

METHODOLOGY

Data were obtained through the use of a group administered questionnaire. Students were also asked to rate the role model with whom they had the most contact during their psychiatric rotation using the semantic differential technique. The scale ranged from 1 to 7 with 1 representing the stu-

dents' most positive perceptions of their role model and 7 representing their most negative perceptions. In addition, an open-ended question provided an opportunity for the students to explain their responses to the questionnaire.

FINDINGS

Of the students responding, 33% said that they would like to work in the field of psychiatric nursing, 26% were defined as having a positive view of their role model, and 65% of the students responded that they would not like to work in the field of psychiatric nursing. These were evenly divided between individuals who had experienced a positive role model and those who had experienced a negative role model.

IMPLICATIONS

With the promotion of positive attitudes toward psychiatric nursing, perhaps more nursing graduates will be encouraged to pursue this speciality and fulfill the public's need for more and better qualified nurses.

Based on data from Issues in Mental Health Nursing, **2:**51, June 1980.

---

cles, tells the client that he is accepted, valued, and respected. Interventions for specific problem behaviors are covered in other chapters.

THE SUPERVISORY PROCESS

Supervision involves a nurse of lesser experience working with a clinician of greater experience. Supervision is distinguished from consultation and the educational process by certain legal responsibilities of the supervisor. The objectives of supervision are to facilitate the development of the beginning nurse. The supervisor assumes an inherent responsibility that is aimed at protecting both the client and the supervisee. Consequently the supervisor has decision-making power over the work being done. The supervisor guides the selection of clients to ensure that the nurse has responsibilities and decision-making powers that correspond to her ability. Nevertheless, the authority for direct action remains with the supervisor.

The supervisory relationship provides an opportunity for growth in that it is designed to facilitate the beginning nurse's self-exploration and self-awareness. It is not a therapeutic relationship. Assisting someone in becoming self-observant and more able to process communication patterns is often perceived as confrontational and creates tension. Tension needs to be reduced to a productive level; this reduction in tension usually occurs as the supervisee alters her expectations of herself and others.

Rapport and a working alliance are as important in a supervisory relationship as in a therapeutic relationship. The phases of the therapeutic relationship present parallel experiential tasks in the supervisory relationship. Reciprocal evaluation by supervisor and supervisee enhances the relationship and facilitates goal attainment. Confusion is averted when the supervisor and the beginner adhere to meeting times and the supervisee comes prepared with notes of her work.

At times supervision may involve collaboration in joint clinical efforts by the student nurse and a more experienced clinician. This collaboration allows for open processing of information and for demonstration and assessment of effectiveness by both the supervisor-clinician and the student nurse. More importantly, it opens the door for modeling behavior. (See the Research Highlight above) This type of experience also facilitates receptiveness to feedback in the supervisory relationship. Supervision can focus on clarifying immediate client problems and decision making regarding issues that have a direct or indirect impact on the client.

BRIEF REVIEW

The historic origins of mental health–psychiatric nursing emphasize the therapeutic potential of the nurse-client relationship. The nurse's therapeutic ability is enhanced by self-awareness as well as knowledge. The nurse establishes rapport through trust, warmth, empathy, and genuineness, and creates a climate in which the client can explore personal issues to gain insight and change problematic behavior. The course of the nurse-client relationship progresses through various stages, each with tasks, difficulties, and potential rewards. The ultimate goal of the nurse-client relationship is the independent functioning of the client.

REFERENCES AND SUGGESTED READINGS

1. Abraham, I.: Support groups for nursing students in psychiatric rotation, Issue in Mental Health Nursing, 4:159, 1982.
2. American Psychiatric Association: Diagnostic and statistical manual of mental disorders (DSM-III-R), Washington, D.C., 1986, The Association.
3. Bandler, R., and Grinder, J.: Frogs into princes: neurolinguistic programming, Moab, Utah, 1979, Real People Press.
4. Bandler, R., and Grinder, J.: The structure of magic, vol. 1, A book about language and therapy, Palo Alto, Calif., 1975, Science & Behavior Books, Inc.
5. Burnard, P.: Self awareness for nurses, Gaithersburg, Md., 1986, Aspen Publishers, Inc.
6. Campbell, J.: The relationship of nursing and self-awareness, Advances in Nursing Science, 2(4):15, 1980.
7. Cameron-Bandler, L.: They lived happily ever after: a book about achieving happy endings in coupling, Cupertino, Calif., 1978, Meta Publications.
8. Coleman, E., and Edwards, B.: Brief encounters, New York, 1980, Anchor Press.
9. Colliton, M.: The history of nursing therapy, Perspectives in Psychiatric Care 3(2):10, 1965.
10. Dodds, S.: A study of influence of role modeling on students' attitude formation during their psychiatric rotation, Issues in Mental Health Nursing, 2:51, 1980.
11. Donna, M.E.: Travelbees' intervention in psychiatric nursing, ed. 2, Philadelphia, 1979, F.A. Davis Co.
12. Farrelly, F., and Brandsman, J.: Provocative therapy, Cupertino, Calif., 1981, Meta Publications.
13. Gagan, J.: Methodological notes on empathy, Advances in Nursing Science, 5(1):65, 1983.
14. Grinder, J., and Bandler, R.: The structure of magic, vol. 2, Palo Alto, Calif., 1976, Science & Behavior Books, Inc.
15. Haley, J.: Problem-solving therapy, San Francisco, 1977, Jossey-Bass, Inc., Publishers.
16. Haley, J.: Uncommon therapy, New York, 1973, W.W. Norton & Co., Inc.
17. Hambrick-Butler, S.A., and Sarasin, K.: The 24-hour stay . . . nursing students experience psychiatric hospitalization from the patient's perspective, Journal of Psychosocial Nursing and Mental Health Services, 24(4):23, 1986.
18. Hughes, C.: Supervising clinical practice in psychosocial nursing, Journal of Psychosocial Nursing and Mental Health Services, 23(2):27, 1985.
18a. Kasch, C.: Toward a theory of nursing action: skills and competency in nurse-patient interaction, Nursing Research 35(4):226, 1986.
19. Krieger, D.: Foundations for holistic health nursing: the Renaissance nurse, Philadelphia, 1981, J.B. Lippincott Co.
20. Landcaster, J.: Adult psychiatric nursing, New York, 1984, Medical Examination Publishing Co., Inc.
21. Lankton, S.: Practical magic: a translation of neuro-linguistic programming into clinical psychotherapy, Cupertino, Calif., 1980, Meta Publications.
22. La France, M., and Mayo, C.: Moving bodies: nonverbal communication in social relationships, Monterey, Calif., 1978, Brooks/Cole Publishing Co.

23. Loomis, M.: Levels of contracting, Journal of Psychosocial Nursing, 23(3):9, 1985.
24. Mellow, J.: Nursing therapy as a treatment and clinical investigation approach to emotional illness, Nursing Forum 5(3):64, 1966.
25. Mellow, J.: Evolution of nursing therapy through research, Psychiatric Opinion 4(1):15, 1967.
26. Mellow, J.: The experimental order of nursing therapy in the treatment of acute schizophrenia. In psychiatric research in our changing world: proceedings of an international symposium, Montreal, October 3-5, 1968, International Congress Series No. 187, New York, 1968, Excerpta Medical Foundation.
27. Orlando, I.J.: The dynamic nurse-patient relationship, New York, 1961, G.P. Putnam's Sons.
28. Peplau, H.E.: Interpersonal relations in nursing, New York, 1952, G.P. Putnam's Sons.
29. Rogers, C., and others: The therapeutic relationship and its impact, Madison, 1967, University of Wisconsin Press.
30. Satir, V.: Conjoint family therapy, Palo Alto, Calif., 1967, Science & Behavior Books, Inc.
31. Satir, V.: Peoplemaking, Palo Alto, Calif., 1972, Science & Behavior Books, Inc.
32. Schoffstall, C.: Concerns of student nurses prior to psychiatric nursing experience: an assessment and intervention technique, Journal of Psychosocial Nursing and Mental Health Services, 19(11):11, 1981.
33. Schroder, P.: Recognizing transference and countertransference, Journal of Psychosocial Nursing, 23(2):21, 1985.
34. Schwartz, M., and Schocrisy, E.: The nurse and the mental patient, New York, 1950, Russell Sage Foundation.
35. Schwing, G.: A way to the soul of the mentally ill, New York, 1954., International Universities Press, Inc. (Translated by R. Ekstein and B.H. Hall.)
36. Sechehaye, M.: The curative function of symbols in a case of traumatic neurosis with psychotic reactions. In Burton, A., editor: Psychotherapy of the pyschoses, New York, 1961, Basic Books, Inc., Publishers.
37. Staklum, M: New student in psychiatry, American Journal of Nursing, 81:762, 1981.
38. Sullivan, H.S.: The interpersonal theory of psychiatry, New York, 1953, W.W. Norton & Co., Inc.
39. Sundeen, S., and others: Nurse-client interaction, St. Louis, 1985, The C.V. Mosby Company.
40. Travelbee, J.: Interpersonal aspects of nursing, ed. 2, Philadelphia, 1972, F.A. Davis, Co.
41. Tudor, G.E.: A sociopsychiatric nursing approach to intervention in a problem of mutual withdrawal on a mental hospital ward, Journal of Psychiatry 15:193, 1952.
42. Witherspoon, V.: Using Lakovic's system countertransference classifications, Journal of Psychosocial Nursing and Mental Health Services, 23(4):30, 1985.
43. Wolstein, B.: Transference: its meaning and function in psychoanalytic therapy, New York, 1954, Grune & Stratton, Inc.
44. Yalom, I.: The theory and practice of group psychotherapy, New York, 1975, Basic Books, Inc., Publishers.

ANNOTATED BIBLIOGRAPHY

Coleman, E., and Edwards, B.: Brief encounters, New York, 1980, Anchor Press.
   The authors focus on the potential of short-term relationships: how to achieve meaningful brief relationships and how to terminate successfully.
Jourard, S.: The transparent self, New York, 1971, Van Nostrand-Reinhold Co., Inc.
   This book explores the hypothesis that individuals can attain

health and their fullest personal development when they have the courage to be themselves and to find goals that have meaning for them. The author focuses on self-disclosure and on the individual's purpose and meaning for existing, which arises from relationships with others.

O'Brien, M.J.: Communications and relationships in nursing, ed. 2, St. Louis, 1978, The C.V. Mosby Co.

This book is written to help nursing students consider the various tactics that contribute to effective communication and meaningful relationships in their lives and work. The nurse's self-concept, attitudes, and communication skills are explored as she forms relationships with others.

Ujhely, G.: Determinants of the nurse-patient relationship, New York, 1968, Springer Publishing Co., Inc.

This book deals with the many variables that affect the nurse-client relationship, including the data both nurse and client bring to the relationship and the context within which the relationship takes place.

CHAPTER 7

THE PROCESS OF PSYCHOTHERAPY

Ann Hutton   Bonnie Clayton

After studying this chapter the learner will be able to:

Define psychotherapy.

Trace the historical development of psychotherapy.

Analyze the role each of the twelve curative factors plays in enhancing the effectiveness of psychotherapy.

Describe the four assumptions about clients and their implications for the role of the nurse therapist.

Identify the variables that influence the clients selection for therapy.

Describe areas of competence that need to be considered in determining the nurse's qualifications as an individual psychotherapist.

Differentiate between client variables that are more likely to be associated with a "successful" outcome in psychodynamic therapy and those associated with a positive outcome in short-term or problem solving behavior therapy.

Trace the steps involved in developing short- and long-term goals in psychotherapy.

Describe the process of evaluating short- and long-term goals in psychotherapy.

The power of interpersonal influence, that is, the direct human impact of one individual on another, is the context of individual psychotherapy. Whatever the theoretical framework of the therapist, the field of action is the dynamic interaction between two people. Individual *psychotherapy* is a particular kind of constructive interpersonal relationship in which the purpose is to effect a positive change in the emotional well-being of an individual who seeks assistance through the professional intervention of another.

Psychotherapy is by definition a process deliberately designed to assist an individual who suffers from a dysfunctional condition that may be caused by disease, injury, developmental disability, or response to environmental stress from family, community, or cultural sources. Treatment can be from a wide variety of approaches given by members of any of the mental health professional disciplines. In the field of mental health, individual psychotherapy is the major modality of treatment. The term psychotherapy may or may not include other constructive interpersonal relationships, such as counseling or guid-

ance, that are designed to assist essentially healthy individuals toward personal fulfillment, a greater degree of health, self-actualization, resolution of a situational problem, or similar growth-related goals.

The goal of psychotherapy is to remove or alleviate symptoms that interfere with the person's functioning or to promote more effective coping patterns in response to developmental or situational stresses. In psychotherapy there is the assumption that the troubled individual benefits from greater understanding of himself. Intellectual and emotional reappraisal of the person's disturbed or troubled behavior is regarded as a prerequisite to positive change.

THEORETICAL APPROACHES

Fundamental assumptions regarding the nature of human beings lie behind the numerous forms of psychotherapy. The student therapist needs to develop an understanding of these assumptions and how they influence the process of psychotherapy so that, to the extent known,

❧ *Historical Overview* ❧

DATE	EVENT
Early 1900s	The "talking cure" of psychotherapy originated with Freud, who believed that symptoms of mental disorder could be cured by uncovering repressed memories of traumatic experiences in early childhood. The interpersonal relationship between the client and the analyst was a profoundly important aspect of treatment.
1930s	Following somatic treatments such as insulin and electroconvulsive therapies, clients were more receptive to individualized care. The nurse was the professional available, although she was ill prepared, to provide supportive psychotherapy.
1950	The use of chlorpromizine reduced client's violent behavior and allowed the nurse more time for caring for the emotional needs of the client.
1952	The concept of interpersonal relationships proposed by Peplau became the basis for psychiatric nursing practice. Nurses and other professionals resisted the concept of nurses as psychotherapists and use of the terms "one to one relationship" and psychotherapeutic nursing persisted into the 1970's.
1963	The Mental Retardation Facilities and Community Mental Health Act drew psychiatric nurses into staff positions in community mental health centers. This transition from hospital to community centers promoted a wider acceptance of nurses as psychotherapists. Training grants from the National Institute of Mental Health to prepare nurses at postgraduate level became available.
1980s	Growing numbers of psychiatric nurses successfully established themselves in the independent practice of psychotherapy. Emphasis has shifted from decreasing deviations based on internal drives and conflicts to increasing individuation and developing capacity to manage the stresses of everyday life.
Future	Increasing emphasis on the biological aspects of mental illness and questioning relationship therapies that are not scientifically grounded in theory will require nurses to document the effectiveness of the nurse-client relationship with further research.

the methods and techniques that best help the client can be used. Much of what is known about the success of one school of psychotherapy in comparison with another is based on therapists' claims or beliefs that their particular type of therapy is effective.

What is commonly understood is that most forms of psychotherapy are more effective than no treatment at all. A recent study comparing differences in the effectiveness of individual, group, or couple therapy demonstrated that clients as a whole were helped equally by the three modes of therapy, and when small differences did occur, they could be accounted for by how well the mode of therapy fit the client's characteristics.[70] (see the Research Highlight on p. 120.)

Since many different orientations toward therapy produce equally effective results, therapists and researchers have assumed that there are certain common or nonspecific aspects that underlie all types of psychotherapy; these common factors and not the specific techniques are related to the successful outcome of therapy.

Common Curative Factors

These common curative factors that appear to cut across all major orientations provide a way for under-

standing the healing aspects of psychotherapy. That is, in spite of differing views regarding mental functioning, human behavior, and specific techniques, these common factors may exert their influence, especially during the initial period of therapy, by setting the stage for therapy and motivating a distressed client to stay in treatment. These common factors are closely interrelated and depend for their effectiveness on the capacity of the client to trust, respond to, and be influenced by the qualities of understanding, respect, encouragement, and most important, a measure of love offered in the therapeutic relationship.[80] The capacity of the therapist to facilitate these characteristics is an essential part of the therapeutic process.

Since nurses use therapeutic models extrapolated from the major schools of psychotherapy, both the common and specific factors associated with these schools need to be understood. The twelve common factors are outlined here and on pp. 121-124.

Search for a common goal. Individuals seek psychotherapy for different and specific reasons, which may be grouped into four categories[87]:

1. Distressing symptoms such as anxiety, depression, or unrealistic fears (phobias)
2. Perceptual deficits resulting in inability to think rationally (thought disorders)

Research Highlight

A Comparative Outcome Study of Individual, Group, and Conjoint Psychotherapy

P.A. Pilkonis, S.D. Imber, P. Lewis & P. Rubinsky

PURPOSE

The purpose of this study was to compare the differential effectiveness of individual, group, and conjoint (couple) therapy in a sample of psychiatric outpatients. The study was designed to overcome methodological problems which have been presumed to interfere with demonstrating differential outcome effects in previous research.

SAMPLE

The sample consisted of 64 clients between the ages of 18 and 55 (mean age 31.7), who were suffering from an affective, anxiety adjustment, or personality disorder, and who were living with another adult who agreed to answer questionnaires, and, depending on random assignment, participate in conjoint therapy. Eight subjects were unavailable for follow-up, leaving a sample of 56. Significant others were spouses or sexual partners living in same household, mothers (N = 7), friends, relatives or roommates (N = 5). A total of 42 significant others completed the study. Exclusion criteria consisted of drug or alcohol abuse, psychosis, organic impairment, or involvement in another type of treatment. Of the 64 original subjects, 20 were accepted into the study for nonrandom assignment to one of the three treatment conditions because of their preference for a particular mode of treatment. The majority of subjects were seeking help for problems that had existed for over 2 years and were rated by their therapists as being moderately to severely symptomatic.

METHODOLOGY

A battery of assessment instruments were used to measure symptoms, adjustment, and depression at intake, after 3 and 6 months of treatment, at termination, and at the end of a follow-up period that averaged 31 weeks. In addition, measures were used that were considered to be particularly relevant to outcomes associated with the different focuses involved in individual, group, and couple therapy. Assessment questionnaires regarding the adjustment of each client were completed by the client, the therapist, and the significant other. Significant others were also asked to complete questionnaires that assessed their own adjustment, whether or not they had participated in conjoint therapy.

Therapy was conducted by nine experienced therapists (three in each mode of therapy) who were skilled in the type of treatment they provided. The mean number of sessions was 26.8.

Therapists treated subjects using their customary framework for therapy within the particular modality (that is, individual, group, or conjoint). Although most of the therapists were eclectic in their orientation, they could be classified as either cognitive-insight or affective-insight therapists.

FINDINGS

The subjects as a whole demonstrated significant improvement from intake to termination. The measures chosen because they were specific to each mode of therapy also reflected the general improvement, but not as consistently as the other outcome measures. Improvements measured at termination were maintained as a whole at follow-up, with some measures showing a gain from termination to follow-up. Status at intake was, as is usual, the best predictor of outcome, but other factors such as lower social class and longer length of treatment were also associated with poorer outcomes. Individual therapy appeared to be more effective in facilitating self-awareness for lower-class clients than group or couple therapy. More chronically distressed clients benefited most from group or conjoint therapy in lessening interpersonal problems, while older persons responded best to conjoint therapy and upper-class clients had better outcomes in group therapy. Random versus nonrandom assignment to treatment mode had little effect on the multiple measures of therapy outcomes.

IMPLICATIONS

This study supports the assumption that nonspecific factors are important in influencing therapy outcome; that is, the experienced therapists in this study, regardless of modality, all seemed to use approaches that enhanced self-understanding, reduced family conflict, and improved interpersonal functioning and morale. Of considerable interest was the finding that improvement was maintained from termination to the average follow-up time of 31 weeks. Where differences in outcome did occur, they were found to be attributed to therapist differences interacting with client characteristics rather than to differences across modes of therapy. The results suggest that lower-class, upper-class, chronic, and aged clients may differentially benefit from a particular mode of treatment. Since lower-class and chronically ill clients tend in general to have poorer outcomes, mental health workers may be of help to these refractory groups by developing techniques within the modalities that optimize the chances for a positive outcome. The public can be educated regarding the importance of finding the best fit between the therapist, the client, and the therapy mode. Finally, this study, by including measures from the client's significant others, demonstrated that the client's family has an important impact on treatment and in influencing drop-outs from treatment.

Based on data from Archives of General Psychiatry **41**:431, 1984.

3. Problems in social and interpersonal functioning that may interfere with work, marital and other intimate relationships, or school achievement
4. Feelings of dissatisfaction regarding one's life and accomplishments

Most theorists suggest that a general goal for psychotherapy is to help clients deal more effectively with their problems, interpersonal conflicts, and emotions. This has been referred to as assisting the client to gain self-control, to master unintegrated parts of the self, to recognize previously unrecognized alternatives for living, or to develop autonomy and awareness of freedom of choice, all of which constitutes "the development of *intentionality* of purpose."[36] In addition to the achievement of greater control, the client needs to modify unrealistic expectations of himself and others.[80] Other well-known theorists tend to use somewhat different terms to describe intentionality or self-mastery. Maslow[56] referred to this construct as "self-actualization," and Rogers[71] spoke of personal growth and achieving congruence between one's inner self and external experience.

Regardless of the terminology, most approaches to psychotherapy place considerable value on autonomy as a component of mental health. Psychotherapists target their interventions to assist the client in the achievement of some approximation of mental health. Freud,[24] for example, concentrated on making the client conscious of his lifelong, unconscious, distorted patterns and conflicts in living. The purpose of the uncovering process is to allow the ego to recognize these distortions and gain mastery over the impulses producing the distortions so that gratifications can be achieved in more satisfying and socially sanctioned ways. Freud's well-known dictum that mental health is the capacity "to love and to work" implies the essence of intentionality, or the freedom to act autonomously rather than in response to distortions in relationships or strivings outside of awareness.

Possessing the capacity for productive work and satisfying, intimate relationships goes beyond the notion of merely bringing into awareness the unconscious part of the mind. The individual who has not developed the capacity for initiating and maintaining meaningful interpersonal relationships often is a person who does not allow the particulars of that incapacity into full awareness. Information that generates fears of rejection or diminished self-esteem is excluded from awareness. Inattention to the anxiety that maintains loneliness or ungratifying relationships prevents learning of new skills to overcome the problem. However, one can be aware of a sense of loss or failure and still not be satisfied or considered mentally healthy.

Intentionality presupposes that the individual recognizes the need to take responsibility for his behavior. Responsibility can be defined as the ability of an individual to recognize his accountability for his thoughts, feelings, and actions. Responsible persons accept blame for their failure and credit for their successes. Responsibility also involves the recognition of some choice in terms of behavior and free will.

The extent to which some clients can become intentional, responsible, and free to choose a course of action may be limited. Individuals may suffer from impaired cognitive function or have other disorders that compromise their ability to function competently and autonomously in a number of areas. Restrictions because of age, genetic endowment, or illness are considered by the therapist; however, the therapist works with clients toward assuming responsibility for their behavior to the extent that their capabilities permit.

The notion of helplessness—being stuck or immobilized and unable to make autonomous choices—underlies most problems for which individuals seek help. Overcoming this lack of intentionality becomes the primary focus of psychotherapy. This overall, general goal is also congruent with the goals of nursing, which emphasize assisting individuals to regain health and independence and to maximize their potential. For nonpsychotic individuals, the experience of a subjective sense of free will is an almost universally perceived phenomena. There is some evidence that belief in increased internal or personal control is an indicator of improvement in therapy.[25]

The major schools of psychotherapy differ in terms of how they view individual autonomy. The existential theory sees the individual as a responsible being functioning within the laws of nature and capable of making choices. The behavioral and psychoanalytic traditions propose a more deterministic concept of individuals. The former views behavior as controlled by the external environment, whereas the latter believes mental functions are determined by both internal drives and external factors.

Both behavioral and psychoanalytic therapists rationalize the dilemma regarding determinism and free will by suggesting that during therapy, the client moves from a position of being stuck or inhibited, with relative lack of freedom of choice, to an increased sense of awareness of the factors that have been controlling his thoughts, wishes, or behaviors. In addition, the client increases his sense of self-mastery or control in dealing with the vicissitudes of life.

Interpersonal and family systems theorists combine elements of both determinism and free will. Interpersonal theorists see individuals as acting and reacting continuously with their environment. An individual's behavior is both determined by and determines the behavior of others. In this sense no one can be considered totally free to respond without being influenced by the interpersonal context in which the exchange occurs. In therapy the individual becomes more fully aware of how he influences and is in turn influenced by the characteristics of the relationships in which he is involved. The development of interpersonal insight along with feeling more in control of one's internal feelings and thoughts allows individuals to alter their behavior in interpersonal relationships and to experience a greater sense of freedom in making choices regarding the directions their lives take.

Even therapists who espouse the most ambitious of goals, for example, personality reconstruction in psychoanalysis, recognize the limits of how completely an individual's behavior and attitudes can be changed. Realistic adjustment of goals and expectations in keeping with the client's characteristics and problems at the time of his introduction to therapy is a function of the therapeutic process. No model of therapy claims complete cure or immunization from future distress.

Mobilization of the client's hope and expectancy of help. The very nature of the client's distress usually heightens susceptibility to therapeutic influence. Unless the client has experienced severe deprivation early in life, the benefits of the healing relationship with the therapist provide momentum for the therapy. During times of stress people have a propensity to reach out for help by seeking to establish relationships with others or by trying to control themselves to prevent the expression of frightening feelings or impulses. If the client has inhibited the expression of concerns, intense feelings of alienation may have been generated. A sense of relief is experienced as the therapist serves to bring hope, listen to, and communicate an optimistic yet realistic perspective that the client can be helped to make choices and to learn to cope with difficult situations. Achieving hope is more complicated for clients who may be suffering from affective disorders that involve depression. In such cases, therapeutic efforts may be directed toward clarifying the nature and source of the client's depression and assisting the client to recognize how cognitive style and emotional reactions maintain the depression.[26]

Even during the initial interview, the idea that help is available and that the therapist has confidence that the client can be helped will arouse hope and reduce anxiety and feelings of hopelessness that interfere with recovery. Activating the client's hope and expectations for help is associated with a positive therapeutic outcome.[21] Regardless of the length of therapy, initial favorable expectations correlate positively with improvement in therapy.

Anticipatory guidance and accurate expectations. Many therapists engage in what Frank[21] and his associates have termed a *role induction interview,* or role expectancy structuring, a technique of providing information in advance of how the client is expected to behave. For example, the depressed client may be advised that an aspect of therapy will reduce his need to ruminate about problems, which will reduce his insomnia and result in improved energy and ability to manage day-to-day situations. Other expectations regarding the length of treatment, the importance of keeping appointments, anticipation of negative or painful feelings, the types of techniques the therapist will be using, and expectations for how the client is to behave are all aspects of role induction. Such "induced" role behavior may have a positive influence on the course of therapy. Studies have demonstrated that having preparatory information about what to expect reduces ambiguity and anxiety during times of stress, thus freeing the individual to gain a more realistic perception of problems and the potential for solving them. Knowing not only what to expect but also the rationale for treatment is part of anticipatory guidance and contributes to increasing the client's trust in the therapist.

Use of verbal communication. Most forms of psychotherapy emphasize the importance of the verbal interaction between therapist and client. The client has the op-portunity to relate difficulties and symptoms to the therapist, who listens attentively and attempts to clarify and understand what the client has to say. Most therapeutic modalities rely predominantly on the use of verbal interaction, although experiences such as role playing, guided imagery, hypnosis, meditation, biofeedback, and other variations in techniques may be employed. Particularly in the beginning stages of therapy, the therapist's ability to demonstrate understanding and acceptance of the client through accurate empathy and well-formulated interpretations contributes to the effectiveness of therapy.

Universality. Universality as a curative factor is more likely to be associated with group than individual therapy.[92] However, one of the products of learning in any form of psychotherapy is the client's discovery that the problems experienced are not unique. Others have similar pain, need help, and experience the same kinds of difficulty. Many individuals who seek help have not been able to share their concerns and despair with others in meaningful ways. Cut off from receiving corrective feedback, they develop a tendency to think of themselves as unique in the world, with the misapprehension that they are the only ones who ever felt hatred toward their parents; felt like killing themselves; had forbidden hostile, loving, or sexual impulses; felt easily rejected or slighted; or felt shy or inadequate. The curative aspects of universality involve the individual's discovery not only of not being unique in the world but also of not being alone. The promise of the therapist's continued interest, help, and support through regular appointments decreases fears of having to face the unknown alone.

Facilitation of emotional arousal. Varying degrees of emotional arousal are a necessary component of successful psychotherapy. *Catharsis,* or the release of strong feelings, has long been considered an important, if not sufficient, component of the therapeutic process. Early in the course of his work, Freud discovered that no long-lasting benefits occurred from the mere venting of feelings. However, emotional release seems to reduce anxiety and depression and motivate the client to stay in therapy.

One way in which emotional arousal contributes to therapeutic improvement is that arousal of anger or anxiety permits the therapist the opportunity to help relieve the client of these unpleasant feelings.[34] This generates positive feelings on the part of the client toward the therapist.

The nature of the therapeutic relationship itself generates confusion and ambiguity for the client in that the relationship is unlike other relationships the client has experienced. In therapy, the refusal of the therapist to directly give advice provokes anxiety in the client. Anxiety and uncertainty motivate the client to find new ways for understanding feelings. Thus stimulation of feelings is accompanied by cognitive learning and understanding of the implications of the emotional experience.

Heightened arousal (not too little or too much) and uncertainty seem to create a climate in which the client is receptive to the meaning, attributions, explanations, or interpretations of the therapist regarding the client's difficulties. Uncertainty creates tension in the client, who in this mildly anxious state is likely to have less control and to openly express more meaningful material to find out what will reduce the tension.

Clients differ as to what constitutes emotional arousal. For example, a seemingly mild expression of emotion may signify intense arousal for an ordinarily shy or inhibited individual, whereas some individuals who are used to angry outbursts may have difficulty expressing their caring or loving feelings. As with some of the curative factors, most schools of psychotherapy emphasize the importance of emotional arousal in the beginning stages of therapy. Although emotional interactions may occur at any stage in therapy, the therapist does not usually deliberately seek to stimulate arousal unless the therapy has reached an *impasse*.

Provision of new information. Provision of new information is a component of facilitating emotional arousal. Emotional arousal without understanding the cognitive implications of the arousal experience does not contribute to lasting change. Psychotherapy is a learning process, the subject of which is the self. Self-understanding is a process whereby an individual discovers both previously unknown, often unacceptable aspects and some positive aspects of the self. Recognizing parts of the self that have existed outside of awareness leads to greater understanding of how these parts may have contributed to or maintained problems or distortions in relationships.

Two basic processes explain why provision of new information contributes to change in psychotherapy. First, humans have a need to make sense of their world. Understanding reduces cognitive uncertainty and anxiety and helps people to feel more in control of their lives. Clients in psychotherapy resist becoming more self-aware because they have learned not to give free expression to thoughts and feelings that threaten their security. The therapist needs to demonstrate through interpretations, clarifications, and other experiences in therapy that the client's suffering can be understood and brought under control. The simple act of labeling feelings often reduces anxiety.

Second, acquisition of new information helps individuals see new possibilities for solutions to their problems. In states of high anxiety, people tend to distort incoming stimuli. For example, individuals dominated by perfectionistic cognitive assumptions, such as needing to do everything right or risk feeling like a failure, react to all situations in terms of their perceived adequacy or inadequacy. In therapy, clients may test the validity of their assumptions about the world by trying out new attitudes and behaviors. As the client tries out new behaviors, information about the adequacy of the old assumptions in contrast to new behaviors and attitudes are reviewed as part of therapy. As clients begin to perceive the world and themselves differently—that is, as more capable, less helpless, and more in contol—they feel and act more in keeping with these cognitions.

Sharing in a "myth" or set of principles. Various rationales exist to explain the nature of the client's distress. What is important about the treatment is the conviction of the therapist that the rationale is meaningful and that the client accepts and believes in its effectiveness. Like the acquisition of new information, sharing a set of principles that explains the client's difficulties is reassuring. It allows the individual to make sense of disturbing experiences. The therapist's explanation may also be less judgmental than the one the client had before therapy.[31] Furthermore, explanations function as coping mechanisms. The rationale provides a framework for the transfer of understandings from the therapy setting to experiences outside of therapy. Perceiving a sense of control and mastery over troublesome behaviors helps the individual identify appropriate coping strategies.

The scientific accuracy of the rationales offered to the client does not seem to be as critical as the client's comprehension and acceptance of the explanation. In actuality, the validity of a theoretical system of therapy is impossible to document scientifically. Yalom[92] proposed that the best way to judge whether an explanatory system is correct is whether it strengthens the client's will and ability to change.

Enhancement of mastery and maintenance of improvement. Therapy needs to provide successful experiences that enhance mastery, competence, and self-esteem. Generally, the client's inability to control feelings, thoughts, and impulses undermines his self-confidence. His attention is focused on taking care of his self-esteem. This emphasis on the self leads to distortions in interpreting perceptions and experiences. The individual may ruminate about failures, going crazy, or losing control. During the course of therapy the client needs to experience success in handling problems previously avoided.

Research has demonstrated that clients who believe their improvement results from their own efforts maintain their improvement. Improvement associated with self-effort is especially true for those clients who believed themselves to be responsible for outcomes in their lives.[21] Such a belief reinforces the idea of autonomy, responsibility, and intentionality. Clients usually feel dependent on the therapist during the initial stages of therapy and fear the loss of the therapist's support. Gradually, as the therapist encourages clients' movement toward more satisfying, mature, and independent living, they begin to analyze themselves, including their behavior, to make interpretations, and thus to give up dependence on the therapist.

New social learning experiences. In all forms of therapy, the therapist has the opportunity of interacting with the client and of using positive and negative reinforcements to shape the client's behavior. The therapist selectively reinforces both what the client talks about in the therapy hour and improvement in interpersonal effectiveness in outside relationships. The relationship with the therapist becomes a powerful reinforcing agent. As such, the client can use the reassurance and support from the therapist as a basis for trying out new behaviors.

The client's acquisition of new social skills requires that the therapist respond to the client in a way that is different from what the client has generally come to expect in day-to-day relationships. For example, a "help-rejecting complainer" is an individual who gives the impression to others of being depressed, unhappy, and seeking advice. Although the client invites suggestions and reassurances, rejection is apt to occur as the client finds reasons why the suggestions do not work. Typically this self-defeating interaction pattern soon results in the individual's being rejected or alienated from others who weary of the demand for reassurance. To introduce new social learning experiences, the therapist does not respond in the usual way to the client's invitation for advice but instead will focus on the pattern of interaction and the underlying conflictual feelings of the client about feeling small, helpless, dependent, and yet distrustful of powerful authority figures. In terms of social learning theory, the therapist has failed to reward the client's maladaptive interpersonal response patterns. As the therapist declines to respond in the way the client anticipates, the client is forced to seek new ways of behaving. Failure to be rewarded for a learned behavior leads to extinction of the behavior.

Imitative behavior. Learning by imitation and identification with the therapist is perhaps the most important aspect of psychotherapy. Imitative behavior is more than mere mimicry; it involves the acquisition of values, attitudes, and modes of behavior that are of considerable value in guiding the client's actions. Many clients, successfully treated in psychotherapy, adopt the value system of their therapists. Whether the therapist acknowledges it, identification is an effective force in psychotherapy, even in brief forms of therapy.

Imitation of the therapist implies that the client is attempting to determine how the therapist is thinking, feeling, or acting and then to model his behavior accordingly. Identification suggests a more subltle, unconscious process of internalizing apects of the therapist, "trying them on," and eventually incorporating them as part of the self.

Imitation in therapy is motivated by the client's need to maintain a relationship in which dependence is felt. In addition, the therapist reinforces the client's imitative efforts that have adaptive value, such as tolerance, patience, calmness, honesty in the expression and acceptance of feelings, thoughtful decision making, care, and concern. These values are commonly recognized because of their prosocial characteristics.

Each school of psychotherapy varies in terms of how much the therapist reveals to clients. Most forms of therapy take a positive view concerning the value of therapist self-disclosure and suggest the therapist is able to model the values of honesty and openness that enhance identification. The use of self-disclosure is discussed in Chapter 5.

Intense confiding relationship. The nature of the therapist-client relationship is the most important element that catalyzes the other curative factors.

When clients sense that the therapist understands and cares about them, they are more likely to be receptive to interpersonal learning experiences, to identify with the therapist, and to risk new behaviors. In other words, therapy is apt to be effective when the nurse-client relationship is positive.

Most therapists agree that a supportive and caring attitude is probably impossible if the therapist actively dis-

likes the client. Stated positively, the client learns to care about the therapist to the extent that he feels cared about and supported. Realistically, the therapist is caring but not "all-caring"; accepting of the client's dependency needs and demands yet careful to establish appropriate limits; and consistent in demonstrating an attitude of patience in wanting to help the client, yet letting the client know that the solution to problems rests ultimately with the client rather than the therapist. This interplay between acceptance and rejection is what strengthens the emotional ties between client and therapist.

Both negative and positive reactions to the therapist need to be anticipated. Many clients who seek therapy have experienced conflicts with authority figures, and development of a trusting relationship with a therapist is a difficult and prolonged process under such circumstances. Rebelling and withholding of relevant information are ways in which the client reveals ambivalence about the therapist. These distortions in the relationship need to be openly discussed so therapy can proceed. The therapist diffuses any satisfaction the client may achieve in being negativistic by remaining attentive and accepting of the client's feelings. However, sustained, effective therapy requires a prevailing positive relationship.[21,31,90,92]

Specific Curative Factors

In contrast to the common factors that occur in virtually all models of psychotherapy, specific curative factors pertain to those techniques used by therapists of different theoretical persuasions to influence the client in bringing about change. The common curative factors establish the atmosphere for change to take place; the client feels respected and understood, trusts the therapist sufficiently to reveal his feelings and problems, and anticipates that the therapy will be helpful. The specific factors in psychotherapy involve the skill and training of the therapist in the use of specialized behavioral change techniques or in the judicious use of insight-promoting techniques such as confrontation and interpretation. The timing and proper "dosage" of interpretations, the skill and knowledge of when to reinforce a client's response or behavior, and knowing how to analyze a client's *free associations* are all aspects of specific curative factors in psychotherapy. Many of these aspects have been discussed earlier in Chapter 6.

CHARACTERISTICS OF THE THERAPIST
Qualifications

Many questions arise about who is qualified to perform psychotherapy. The Statement on Psychiatric and Mental Health Nursing Practice of the American Nurses' Association states[2]:

The nurse who practices psychotherapy must acquire appropriate preparation and be accountable for such practice. Proficiency in the art and science of psychotherapy is an outgrowth of advanced, specialized educational experiences and of ongoing efforts to refine psychotherapy skills through practice, continuing education and the use of competent supervision or consultation.

This statement lacks specificity regarding that which constitutes "appropriate preparation" and proficiency in conducting psychotherapy. The ANA Division on Psychiatric and Mental Health Nursing Practice has been encouraging psychiatric nurses practicing as psychotherapists to become certified as Clinical Specialists in Psychiatric and Mental Health Nursing as a means of ensuring that professional standards are met, that the public is protected, and as evidence of qualifications for receiving third-party reimbursement. (See Chapter 48.)

Certification is not the only issue pertinent to qualifications. Other factors that are considered under the heading of therapists' qualifications include (1) personal attributes, (2) knowledge (educational requirements), (3) skills and abilities, and (4) ethical responsibilities.

Personal attributes. Since the work of therapy is conducted through an interpersonal relationship between therapist and client, the personal attributes of the therapist as they relate to the interaction are of considerable importance.

Each school of therapy and professional discipline recommends different means by which potential therapists or students in graduate schools can acquire more self-knowledge. Anywhere from 3 to 5 years of personal analysis is required for those undergoing training in psychoanalysis; however, training in other therapies or disciplines may also recommend or require personal psychotherapy for student therapists. The rationale for requiring personal therapy for trainees is based on the understanding of how the therapist's personal conflicts and characteristc ways of responding to people may influence the therapy process. In addition therapists who have participated as clients in the process of therapy are assumed to have greater sensitivity for what their clients are experiencing.

The important issue is not personal therapy itself, but the amount of emphasis placed on the development of self-awareness. The goal of self-knowledge is for therapists to understand themselves and how they respond in the context of therapy. Beginning therapists experience how their personal values and attitudes can influence the process of therapy. The student therapist may learn to work with her personal reactions in therapy in ways other than personal therapy. Role playing, participation in groups focused on clinical issues, and individual supervision are the most common methods employed to achieve greater self understanding.

The therapist needs to become aware of the following traits[90]:

1. Tendencies to be domineering, pompous, or authoritarian
2. Tendencies toward passivity and submissiveness
3. Need to use the client for gratification of own needs
4. Inability to tolerate the expression of certain impulses or emotions
5. Conflicting attitudes toward money
6. Inability to tolerate acting out
7. Need to be liked and admired
8. Tendency to set perfectionistic goals
9. Perpetuation of a frustrating relationship with the client based on repetition of earlier unsatisfactory relationships
10. Hostility toward the client based on prejudices or bias
11. Lack of self-confidence in her ability
12. Other attributes such as lack of creativity, poor sense of humor, inability to tolerate criticism, low energy, and poor physical health

Positive, ideal attributes for persons seeking to become therapists include creativity, personal insight, industry, integrity, sense of ethical values, and ability to form relationships. The desired qualities have a great deal to do with the therapist's own personal value system, which reaffirms the importance of the therapist's ability to undertake a soul-searching of attitudes and prejudices and how these are communicated to clients.

Education. The climate for educating psychotherapists needs to be one in which the student is indoctrinated into a lifelong process of learning and openness to the possibility of change. Three primary dimensions of the educational process accommodate these principles[12]:

1. Establishing conditions that promote the student's self-development
2. Having the educators act as role models for effective functioning
3. Developing a course of study combining theory with training in the skills the student needs to acquire to become an effective therapist

Although each of the core mental health professions considers different knowledge of content areas as necessary, there is general agreement that the potential therapist needs to be acquainted with the following broadly defined theories and concepts[12]:

1. Human growth and development and personality theories, including the psychodynamics of healthy and pathological adaptation
2. Theories of therapeutic influence
3. Concepts related to prevention
4. Intervention techniques, including skills in therapeutic communication and working with resistance
5. Diagnostic and assessment skills
6. Goal-setting skills and planning
7. Legal and ethical standards
8. Research and evaluation methods
9. Social systems and cultural theories that affect human adaptation
10. Knowledge and skill in making referrals
11. Understanding of community mental health services
12. Other theories and issues that pertain to the types of therapy being studied, the populations targeted for intervention, and theories pertinent to a particular professional discipline, for example, nursing theories or frameworks

Skills and abilities. The student of psychotherapy needs to develop skill in the facilitative conditions for effective psychotherapy. These conditions include accurate empathy (ability to understand and communicate empathically), nonpossessive warmth (respect), and genuineness,

Research Highlight

Empathy and Outcome in Brief Focal Dynamic Therapy

H.K. Free, B.L. Green, M.C. Grace, L.A. Chernus & R.M. Whitman

PURPOSE

This study tested the hypothesis that the therapist's empathy is a significant variable in determining success in psychodynamically oriented brief psychotherapy. The study was based on the important role that empathy has been allocated in outcome research and the paucity of studies of its role in therapy using a psychoanalytic approach.

SAMPLE

The subjects were 59 outpatients (68% were women) from the University of Cincinnati Department of Psychiatry who met the selection criteria for exploratory and insight promoting therapy. The age was 33.2 years. Most of the subjects were well educated, white, and had affective or adjustment disorders. Almost half of the sample also had DSM III, axis II diagnoses of borderline and dependent personality disorders.

METHODOLOGY

The subjects were randomly assigned to one of 13 psychiatric residents in a well supervised, psychoanalytically oriented training program. Data consisted of case presentations based on detailed process notes. The therapy was brief, lasting 12 weeks and was based on principles of focused psychodynamic therapy. Three outcome measures were completed at the beginning and end of therapy: (1) patients' completed a symptoms checklist. (2) therapists rated symptoms, and (3) therapists rated six areas on a standardized measure of adjustment and functioning. Empathy was rated on a standardized measure by the therapists and clients after the third and sixth sessions, and by two supervisors after the case presentations of those sessions.

FINDINGS

The sample as a whole demonstrated significant improvement on three of the global outcome measures (symptom checklist, Health-Sickness Rating Scale, and target symptoms), and subjects who had the best adaptive functioning before therapy (DSM-III, axis V) showed the most improvement at termination. Empathy was rated highest by subjects, lower by therapists, and lowest by supervisors. There were no significant correlations among the three groups on ratings of empathy. Interestingly, the only empathy ratings that correlated with outcome measures were those that were made by the subjects. Two outcome measures with which empathy correlated were reduced hostility and improved interpersonal relationships.

IMPLICATIONS

An interesting result of this study is the failure to find agreement on empathy ratings between therapists, subjects, and supervisors. From the client's perspective, empathy is perceived as what the therapist communicates, not necessarily what the therapist may understand and communicate to a supervisor. Since there was high interrater agreement by the supervisors regarding the therapists' empathy ratings, the researchers noted that the supervisors had a tendency to give high empathy ratings to bright and articulate therapists who gave good case presentations. This bias suggests the importance of using audio taping or videotaping as a means of obtaining a more valid assessment of the therapy process. In spite of the limitations, this study does underscore the significance of a positive client-therapist relationship, which must be perceived as such by the client.

Based on data from American Journal of Psychiatry **142**(8):917, 1985.

authenticity, or congruence. A recent study suggests that clients who perceived their therapists as empathic experienced improvement in the quality of their interpersonal relationships.[23] (See the Research Highlight above.)

A therapist's ability to communicate empathically, respect the client, and authentically share herself are necessary but not sufficient factors to facilitate interpersonal change. Further study is needed to verify the power of these therapist skills to influence the course of therapy. Until then, emphasis needs to be on training therapists to be skilled not only in the conditions for therapeutic effectiveness but also in all aspects of therapeutic communication, including the skills of listening and attending and the basic skills for therapeutic influence (empathy, questioning, summarization, confrontation, interpretation, and reflection). All practitioners of psychotherapy have an obligation to develop their therapeutic skills through both simulated exercises and supervised clinical practice. The graduate curricula of most programs preparing nurses to practice as psychotherapists contain these two components, along with theoretical content.

Ethical responsibilities. Certain values underlie ethical practice, and each therapist needs to articulate these values as they pertain to her practice. Remaining objective yet involved and committed to the welfare of one's clients presupposes that one assumes responsibility for one's practice and adheres to a code of moral, ethical, and legal principles and standards.

Nurse therapists, like other professional psychotherapists, adhere to the standards of practice and codes of ethics representing their particular discipline. In addition to adhering to standards of practice and a code of ethics, clinicians need to be committed to maintaining and developing strong intradisciplinary and interdisciplinary relationships. Such relationships benefit the public in the dissemination of new information and make it possible for therapists to work cooperatively in achieving goals.

Role

The therapeutic situation is a formalized, structured encounter between two people, one of whom is in the position of requiring the professional services of the other. The reason for the encounter is the perceived need of the client for help. This situation affects the nature of the interpersonal relationship that is to become the context of therapy by establishing the roles of the therapist and the client. The therapist is the professional expert, possessing knowledge and expertise. The client is in a relatively vulnerable role, presumed to be lacking in knowledge and mastery of the interpersonal situation, and consequently the client is experiencing personal pain.

A nurse therapist may function in the role of psychotherapist within a wide range of levels of professional autonomy and in a variety of institutional environments. However, certain principles guide the therapist; these include the following assumptions about the client.

Assumption 1: There is a perceived need for help. In some instances, the client may not perceive the need for help or may not have initiated therapy. A parent, spouse, son, or daughter is commonly the motivating force in initiating therapy. Under these circumstances, the client may not believe that therapy is necessary, and the individual may be resentful and angry. This possibility needs to be kept in mind as a part of the initial assessment and is addressed beginning with the first interview. If motivation for change comes from someone other than the client, a different mode of therapy may be appropriate. For example, family therapy or couple therapy may be more effective in reducing the individual's anxiety and in facilitating the therapeutic process.

Even when the client believes that a need for help exists, perception of the kind of help that is needed may be quite different from that of the therapist. Expectations of a quick formula for reducing the personal pain or magical advice about managing complex interpersonal difficulties are not unusual. During the early phases of assessment, the therapist addresses what the client actually anticipates in the course of treatment, where and by whom the client believes the work of therapy occurs, and what the expectations are about the length of therapy.

The client may deny to himself or others that a need for help exists and may express that denial as anger, rejection, or hostility toward the therapist. When the therapist recognizes the dynamics of denial, the guidelines for response become more clear. Denial as a defense is not sophisticated and can be easily broken; however, an astute therapist recognizes and respects the need for the defense and acts accordingly. Confrontation may be appropriate in some circumstances, but in many instances, initiating confidence in the therapist through nonconfrontation provides the promise of reducing personal distress and allows the client to give up the defensive denial. The issue of how much confrontation to use is discussed in Chapter 5.

The possibility of finding understanding and caring assistance in a professional relationship can be reassuring to the extent that the client learns to master even the most intractable resistance.

In any event, the anger, resentment, or hostility directed toward the therapist during the early assessment phase of therapy can best be understood as a displaced expression of the client's distress. The individual often does not recognize the "true" object of anger at this time. The therapist may have insufficient information to deal directly with the content; however, the role of the therapist is to assist the client to reduce this immediate distress in order to proceed with the work of therapy.

Assumption 2: The need for help is often expressed as a symptom. People in a high-tension culture have been made increasingly aware of the impact of stress on physical and emotional well-being. As a consequence, clients often relate physiological problems such as headaches, ulcers, or hypertension to the interpersonal difficulties for which assistance is sought. The described symptom may be only remotely related to the actual need that led the client to seek assistance and may be outside awareness.

The goal of therapy may be to alleviate the symptoms, or the goal may be insight. In either event, the role of the therapist is to make it possible for the client to explore the problem. The woman who is depressed and suicidal following divorce may clearly identify the divorce as the "precipitating event"; however, she may be quite unaware that the experience of loss associated with the divorce reactivated feelings of unresolved grief and guilt over the accidental death of a parent many years earlier.

Inability to identify or describe a symptom or problem actually can be the major symptom. Confusion of thought that leads to inability to focus on any specific area of difficulty may indicate serious psychopathology, or it may simply be a measure of the anxiety level of the client. Distractability and inability to concentrate are familiar experiences to most people; however, when such patterns seriously interfere with daily functioning, they may become a symptom that indicates a need for therapy.

Assumption 3: The client is anxious. Anxiety is universally recognized as a miserable emotional state from which the individual seeks relief. Simple reassurance and explanations are rarely effective. Reduction of the client's anxiety is regarded as helpful by the client, facilitates establishing early rapport as a framework for the therapeutic alliance, and makes it possible for the client to participate most effectively in establishing and reaching the goals of therapy. The therapist helps the client to gain better control of anxiety by showing interest, openness, and confidence that therapy is helpful.

Assumption 4: The client is experiencing acute or chronic low self-esteem. Like anxiety, low self-esteem is expressed in many different ways. However, the therapist may safely assume that individuals who seek psychotherapy have a condition of low self-esteem.

In an effort to protect himself against further loss of self-esteem, the client may present an aggressive, overly assertive façade. Recognition of the dynamics of this phenomenon leads the therapist to a supportive rather than critical response. The dynamic relationship between chronic low self-esteem and depression is discussed in Chapter 14; however, probably no area of disjunctive interpersonal relationships is more susceptible to positive intervention than depressive expressions of low self-esteem. Positive relationships are ego enhancing, reinforcing, and provide assurance of personal worth and value. A major aspect of the therapist's role is to assist the client in changing low self-esteem through the therapeutic process.

Goals

Certain tasks or goals exist that, like common curative factors, transcend individual differences of clients and therapists. The following 10 goals were compiled by Perry, Frances, and Clarkin in a case book reviewing differential approaches to selecting psychotherapeutic interventions[69]:

1. To establish and maintain the therapeutic alliance.
2. To build a positive interpersonal basis for the therapeutic work that follows.
3. To provide support in keeping with the client's level of self-directedness.
4. To educate the client or family members about managing psychotropic medications or disturbing symptoms.
5. To use various intervention strategies to alleviate painful affects such as anxiety or depression.
6. To implement strategies that modify specific maladaptive behaviors.
7. To use cognitive-behavioral techniques that modify specific misconceptions, beliefs, or assumptions upon which clients base their feelings and behavior.
8. To convey understanding and facilitate insight, by using psychodynamic interpretations or explanations.
9. To help the client to expand emotional awareness and increase sensitivity to feelings.
10. To assist the client to communicate more effectively and to experience more satisfying interpersonal relationships.

Client Selection and Type of Therapy

Choosing the type of therapy that is most suitable for a client's difficulties is not facile. Client variables interact with therapist variables and availability of resources. Although the tendency has been to see insight-oriented therapy as the ideal, this is clearly not the case. Clients learn in all types of therapy: insight, supportive, or behavioral. The type of approach and the therapist's characteristics need to fit the beliefs and expectations of the client.

However, recommendation of one type of therapy over another is often made on the basis of factors other than the client's needs or characteristics. Expense, therapists' background and training, and factors related to institutional or private systems of care, also influence selection of clients and type of services offered. The question of client selection and type of treatment needs to be based on the variables in which there is relative confidence that services rendered will be helpful.

In general, clients of lower socioeconomic status may do better in short-term reality oriented or problem-solving therapy directed toward supporting the client's ego and dealing with external, situational factors. Psychotic or retarded clients may respond best to a combination of approaches such as supportive therapy, medications, and social and functional skills training. Individuals with personality problems, or neurotic conflicts may best be treated with uncovering, or psychodynamic, approaches. Depressed individuals have been reported to respond well to the use of medications in combination with cognitive psychotherapy. Clients with phobic disorders do well in behavioral therapy, often combined with medications, particularly in the case of agoraphobia. Likewise, sexual dysfunctions are treated with behavioral therapy as well as by conjoint and interpersonal techniques. Clients with anxiety reactions have been found to be helped by both psychodynamic and behavioral approaches such as systematic desensitization and progressive relaxation accompanied by medication therapy.

There are certain criteria for determining a client's suitability for an uncovering type of therapy or supportive therapy. Those clients considered suitable for uncovering therapy have the following characteristics[72]:

1. Motivation for therapy
2. Evidence of some positive achievements in the past
3. Perceptions of their symptoms as ego dystonic (alien to self)
4. Possession of ego strength sufficient to endure painful affects and having a formal diagnosis related to symptoms (anxiety, depression) or personality neurosis (hysteria, or obsessive-compulsive, narcissistic, or dependent personality) rather than somatic complaints
5. History of useful or previously satisfying interpersonal relationships
6. Maintenance of a reasonably stable life situation
7. Motivation to explore one's inner self
8. Reasonable intelligence and desire for self-improvement and personal growth

In contrast, supportive or reality-oriented therapy is recommended when the following factors exist[72]:

1. Motivation for symptom relief or environmental change
2. Pretherapy adjustment is poor to very poor
3. Perception of symptoms as either *ego syntonic* or *dystonic*
4. Possession of weak ego and a diminished capacity to endure painful affect
5. History of unsuccessful or few past relationships
6. Presence of stress or life crises

Supportive therapy aimed at bringing the client to an emotional equilibrium as rapidly as possible is useful for a wide range of difficulties either singly or in conjunction with other types of interventions. Different types of individual therapy may be classified as supportive, including reality therapy, guidance, relaxation therapy, meditation, biofeedback training, hypnosis, environmental manipulation, occupational therapy, music and dance therapies, and use of reassurance, suggestion, persuasion, ventilation, catharsis, somatic therapies, and psychotropic drugs. Situations in which supportive therapy is most beneficial include the following[90]:

1. When the primary difficulty is a conflict between realistic stresses and a basically healthy personality

2. For maintaining chronically mentally ill borderline or psychotic clients
3. As a means of supporting a client until he is ready to participate in uncovering or psychodynamically oriented therapy
4. As a temporary method during insight therapy when anxiety threatens to overwhelm existing coping capacity

THERAPEUTIC PROCESS
Assessment

After the client has agreed to enter into therapy, the nurse begins her assessment of the client. Some preliminary information about the client needs to be gathered. For example, the therapist may want to know whether or not the client had ever experienced a severe or psychotic type of emotional disturbance or been hospitalized for emotional difficulties. In addition, knowledge of the presence of suicidal or homicidal ideation, a history of impulsivity, and the client's level of social and intellectual functioning and level of self-awareness helps to determine the degree of risk involved in making interpretations and to balance that risk against the possible therapeutic gains of deepening rapport, facilitating information sharing, and validating partial hypotheses. The taking of a psychosocial history may be conducted by adhering to an outline or set of questions designed to elicit specific information about the client's past life and present circumstances, or by using the outline in a more flexible manner by adapting the interview process to the needs of the client and the interviewer's own style of investigation.

Analysis

Nursing diagnosis. In the analysis process the therapist identifies problems based on the assessment data generated in the interview process. The putting together of the interpretations with the assessment data generates what has been referred to as nursing diagnoses. The nursing diagnoses identify the client's needs, which guide the planning and implementation phases of therapy. Since nursing diagnoses are so critical in determining action, the therapist's interpretations need to be based as much as possible on concrete data that can be validated with the client.

While observing the client, the interviewer formulates tentative nursing diagnoses that are then validated with the client.

Validation involves the therapist's being able to facilitate the flow of the client's verbalizations to gain as much information regarding feelings and thoughts about the client's problem as possible. Asking the client to focus on specific examples of when the problem occurs helps to add clarity to the nature of the problem(s). A series of specific examples may begin to reflect a theme or pattern of conflict in the client's life, such as difficulty with separation and loss or with passivity versus assertiveness.

The therapist's use of interpretations aids the process of validation in four ways. First, the making of interpretations deepens rapport with the client and, if managed well, leads the client to revealing more information about the problem under discussion. Second, in the initial interview, the client's responses to interpretations may be used as a gauge of the client's capacity and motivation to make use of psychodynamically oriented therapy or to determine if some other therapy approach is needed. Third, interpretations provide the means for directly validating the therapist's hypotheses concerning the client's difficulties. Fourth, because interpretations and accurate empathy deepen rapport, they help overcome the client's initial resistance to therapy.

Since the making of interpretations is a powerful technique, the client's resistance may be aggravated early in therapy before an alliance has been developed, or in contrast, the therapist may create unrealistic hopes that all of the client's problems can be understood and solved because of the therapist's expertise.

During the analysis phase, a number of nursing diagnoses are formulated, each of which may partially account for the client's difficulties. Taken together these nursing diagnoses can be used to formulate a view of the client's situation that is as holistic as possible. Nursing diagnoses are developed based on the five dimensions and on the conceptual models for therapeutic intervention.

Planning

The treatment goals and plan of action influence each other. Goals that are specific to the client determine whether therapy is to be short- or long-term, focused on the past or present, oriented toward education or support, or to produce behavioral change or insight.

The client's problem may be an expression of an unsatisfied wish or desire. The goal becomes a statement of what needs to be adjusted (in keeping with reality) to satisfy the wish. The therapist first needs to discuss the purpose of identifying and clarifying goals with the client and then involve the client in exploring what change means to him. Most clients can identify their perceptions regarding their current level of functioning and their expectations about how they wish they were functioning. The difference between the two can be referred to as a "performance discrepancy."[15] The client may wish to change the way he thinks, feels, or behaves or the way others react toward him. Specifying outcome criteria in behavioral terms makes the goal-setting process more specific and increases the validity of the outcome evaluation. For example, a client may set as a goal "thinking more positively about myself," or "being more assertive with my spouse, mother, father, or boss." These goals can be translated into actual behaviors, which can be observed, counted, or monitored by the client and the therapist.

The second part of specifying goals involves identification of the circumstances and individuals involved in the desired change. For example, a client, Barb, may enter therapy complaining that her husband is cold, distant, and uncommunicative. The therapist in this instance wants to know the nature of the specific circumstances when the husband acts in ways that cause Barb to believe he is being cold or unresponsive.

The third component for determining goals involves looking at the feasibility of the goals. What makes it difficult for the client to change? What are the risks, for example, possible loss of relationships, suicidal impulses, or acting out behaviors, that may be precipitated by change? How are things to be different for the client if the desired change is accomplished? What are the rewards or gains that maintain the change? For example, it is unrealistic for Barb, who is dissatisfied with her husband's behavior toward her, to enter therapy believing that it will change her husband? The therapist needs to determine with the client what it may look and feel like if her husband were to change in accord with her desires. Then the therapist explores with Barb the reciprocal role she plays in maintaining her husband's behavior and what she needs to do to bring about any change. This type of exploration allows the client an opportunity to clarify and determine for herself how realistic and feasible her goals are.

The next steps in goal setting pertain to defining a level of change and defining the steps or tasks and sequence of short-term goals needed to reach the long-term goal.

Defining the level of change means determining the criteria by which progress in therapy will be evaluated and specifying the amount and direction of desired or expected change. For example, with Barb, whose complaint centered around her husband's lack of attention, several problem areas can be identified:

1. Problems with intimacy and autonomy based on past relationships with her parents (felt she could never please her father whom she felt neglected her except when she was in trouble)
2. Low self-esteem and inability to state her desires directly; use of passivity and indirect ways of eliciting desired behaviors from her husband
3. Idealistic expectations for marital relationships based on rigid views of masculine and feminine roles

The therapist's clinical judgment (experience and knowledge), in conjunction with the client's presenting problems, determines what expected level of change is most suitable. Given the variables in this equation—the client's motivation, resources available, present level of functioning, method of treatment, therapist's skill, and uncontrollable factors in the environment—determining the level of expected outcome is often a complex essential task.

The process by which long-term outcomes are achieved consists of intermediate steps that contribute to the overall goals. These short-term goals can be equated to a learning sequence, and for some goals, behavior therapists may establish specific learning hierarchies. These learning hierarchies are frequently used with phobic clients or those with approach-avoidance conflicts. Another method is to establish daily or weekly goals that can be monitored during therapy sessions. These goals may pertain to changes in, for example, life-style habits, eating, smoking, and exercise, or to changes in thoughts, feelings, and consequent behaviors. The subgoals or process goals may also involve the client's behavior and response in therapy; for example, in psychodynamic or existential therapy, the client's participation in nondefensive self-exploration regarding his behavior, feelings and thoughts in relation to salient problem areas and experiences in life is an implied process goal.

After the goals have been selected, the therapist may choose to elicit some commitment from the client about the work to be accomplished. An oral agreement or written contract is seen by many therapists as making the process of psychotherapy more explicit and engages the client in an active role in pursuit of the goals. At this time the therapist may become aware of obstacles or ambivalence on the part of the client toward change, and these issues or resistances may become the focus of the beginning stages of therapy. A flexible approach to the contract or commitment needs to be maintained so that as circumstances change in therapy, the therapy agreement can be renegotiated.

As the goals for therapy are clarified, the therapist begins thinking in terms of identifying priorities and determining methods for change. The client's expectations can be determined by asking, "How can I (we, the clinic) be of help?" The client may respond in rather vague terms or be specific in stating expectations. These expectations help to determine the intervention.

Several models of intervention are possible, and the major ones were presented earlier in this book (Chapter 3). Each of these models prescribes the use of different methods of interventions. On the basis of the client's presenting problem, level of functioning, and expectations, the therapist may determine one or more of the following to be appropriate:

1. Psychodynamic therapy or other types of uncovering, insight oriented therapy are needed.
2. Behavioral change strategies will help the client cope effectively with specific problem areas that can be concretely identified.
3. Medical or drug intervention is needed.
4. Supportive therapy, including environmental manipulation, is needed because change through insight or behavioral methods does not seem possible or warranted.
5. Cognitive therapy is helpful to alter an overly rigid or negative self-concept or to reduce anxiety.
6. Therapy oriented toward recognizing dysfunctional interpersonal patterns will benefit a client whose major difficulties reside in this area.
7. Existential, humanistic, or nondirective approaches are indicated for a client who is having difficulty with basic feelings and desires in life and who feels fragmented or alienated.
8. Further evaluation or psychological testing is needed before determining a method of intervention.

Planning for therapy is an ongoing process. The therapist needs to anticipate and reevaluate the client's needs as therapy progresses and adjust interventions accordingly. For example, a young married man became severely depressed following the unexpected death of his father. As he began to deal with his anger and grief in therapy, it became evident that he was having considerable difficulty in his marriage. His passivity and placating interaction style, a role much like the one his father had played with his mother, became apparent. As the client's depression was resolving, it seemed appropriate to reassess the need for individual therapy or to refer the client and his wife for marital therapy. Such ongoing planning and evaluation often involves other mental health professionals or community resources.

Implementation

Organizing the progression of therapy into phases from the initial contact to termination seems to imply that there is an orderly progression through the phases. For some individuals this may be the case, whereas for others the process may be more discontinuous with progressions and regressions. Implementation is similar to planning in that progression may be blocked at a particular phase of therapy. However, progression ultimately depends on successful resolution of each of the previous phases.

Orientation phase. The primary objectives for the initial interview include the following[54,87,90]:

1. To establish rapport with the client, a relationship that secures continuance of the therapeutic process
   a. By supplying the proper emotional climate for the interview (for example, accurate empathy, genuineness, warmth, respect, listening, and clarifying)
   b. By structuring the purpose of the interview
   c. By clarifying misconceptions about psychotherapy, that is, explaining how therapy works and role expectations of client and therapist
   d. By dealing with inadequate motivation
   e. By handling resistances and preparing the client for psychotherapy
   f. By using language the client understands
   g. By assessing the degree of cooperation of the client with the therapist and estimating reliability of what the client is reporting
2. To get pertinent information about the client
   a. By listening to his spontaneous account
   b. By focusing on selective data; paying attention to the process by which the client relates his story
3. To establish a tentative nursing diagnosis
   a. By developing tentative nursing diagnoses regarding each assessment dimension
   b. By using DSM-III-R
4. To estimate the tentative dynamics (in terms of inner conflicts, mechanisms of defense, interpersonal functioning, network of relationships, nature and background of presenting problem(s), and major sources of conflict)
5. To determine tentative cause
   a. By obtaining dates and circumstances of symptom onset
   b. By determining precipitating events; why client is seeking help at the present time
   c. By determining client's perception of symptoms and world view
6. To assess tentatively the actual and potential assets, strengths, and weaknesses of the client,
   a. By determining the client's coping style
   b. By identifying areas in which the client is succeeding and failing; ability to participate in goal-directed behavior
   c. By determining motivation for therapy
   d. By exploring the client's level of insight or willingness to see himself involved in difficulties versus blaming of others and willingness to express himself verbally
   e. By estimating the possible outcome
7. To make practical arrangements for a therapy-treatment contract
   a. By tentatively stating optimal goals; summarizing impressions of client's difficulties, seeking validation with the client, and mutually agreeing on goals
   b. By assessing the appropriateness of various modes of psychotherapy, that is, selection of a treatment approach geared to needs of the client
   c. By accepting the client for treatment or arranging for referral
   d. By making appropriate time and place arrangements, for example, frequency of sessions and arrangements for any contact via phone in between sessions
   e. By making financial arrangements
8. To arrange for needed consultations or psychological testing

The therapist needs to avoid the following during the initial encounter with the client.[90] (1) arguing with, minimizing or challenging the client, (2) praising the client or giving him false reassurance, (3) making false promises, (4) offering the client a diagnostic label, (5) questioning the client on sensitive areas of his life (instead, the therapist waits for an opening or for the subject to be brought up naturally), (6) trying to "sell" the client on accepting treatment, (7) joining in attacks the client makes on his family, friends, or associates, and (8) participating in criticism of another therapist.

Clients may exhibit resistance to engaging in therapy during the initial encounter by doubting that they can be helped by therapy; demonstrating difficulty in accepting the parameters of the treatment situation; showing hostility, dependence, or sexual interest in the therapist; or generally engaging in behaviors that are counterproductive to the development of a working relationship. Therapists may have countertransference problems such as finding it difficult to empathize with the client, being irritated at the client's resistive behavior, or generally being unable to demonstrate respect and genuine regard for the client and understand his distress.

Development of the therapeutic alliance. The development of a therapeutic alliance in which the client collaborates with the therapist is important in terms of the overall effectiveness of therapy. Two essential types of therapeutic relationships exist: the forms of therapy that emphasize the analysis of transference distortions and those that consider a positive relationship to be a necessary but not a sufficient component of therapy. This latter type has been referred to as developing a "helping relationship." The dimensions of the helping relationship include: accurate empathic understanding, respect or positive regard, genuineness (congruity), and concreteness or *specificity* of expression. Psychodynamically oriented therapists deem analysis of transference distortions to be important; however, they also use various dimensions of the helping relationship. In a sense, two types of relationships are said to coexist in psychodynamic therapy: (1) the transference relationship and (2) the "therapeutic" or "working" alliance, which develops out of the rational part of the client's ego. The nature of the relationship in psychodynamically oriented therapy is characterized by the therapist in the role of authority figure at least in the early stages of the therapy. As therapy progresses, the client may move from seeing himself as the recipient of the therapist's support and help toward the development of a sense of working together and a sharing of responsibility for working on treatment goals. The capacity of the client to form such an alliance and of the therapist's skill in nurturing it are important components of the therapeutic relationship.

Therapeutic communication. Through the analysis of the client's verbal and nonverbal incongruent and discrepant messages, the therapist helps the client to understand communication blockages. Clarifying dysfunctional communication frees the client to define feelings and problem areas more clearly and to apply problem-solving and decision-making methods directly to the troublesome issues. See Chapter 5 for further discussion of Therapeutic Communication.

Working phase. The working phase of therapy can be broken down into two subphases: (1) determining the nature of the client's problems through confrontation and self-exploration and (2) translating insight and understanding into corrective action, that is, facilitating the client's initiative in creating change.

Many of the general curative factors discussed earlier in this chapter relate to variables that in the orientation phase set the climate for therapy, namely, demonstrating value and respect for the client, clarifying expectations, and developing a working alliance. However, these factors are not sufficient in themselves to provoke change. Once a therapeutic alliance has been established with the client, the therapist begins to challenge the discrepancies, distortions, and games, in the client's life and in his interactions within the helping relationship itself, to the degree that it helps the client develop the kind of self-understanding that leads to constructive behavioral change.[28] This challenging process is known as confrontation. Discrepancies, incongruities and double messages, and resistances reveal areas in the client's life and relationships about which he is ambivalent, confused, or in conflict. For example:

Client: Lately I've found myself thinking that all men are rats. I think about how unfair Bob's been to me, and it reminds me of all the other hurts in my life. . . . I just can't get it out of my mind . . . and I hate him for reminding me of my past.

Therapist: I guess it seems unfair to you that you're hurting so much, and you'd like to hurt him back. What really seems unclear though is whether you want to get even with Bob or whether you keep hoping against odds that Bob will treat you better.

In this instance the therapist has chosen to point out a discrepancy between the client's expressed intention and her present behavior. She had shared with the therapist a desire to improve her life circumstances, but she remains attached to Bob because of her mixed feelings and desire to hurt him. At some point the client's generalization about all men being "rats" can also be challenged.

Confrontation needs to be balanced carefully against the client's capacity to tolerate facing painful meanings of his behavior and the degree to which the client trusts and believes the therapist. Confrontation too early, too much, or too little can inhibit the therapeutic process. Confrontation is not used to criticize or to imply fault; neither is it used as a gimmick or game. Confrontation can be seen as an extension of empathy because it requires an understanding of the client's feelings of which the client may not be entirely aware.

Confrontation demonstrates to the client that the therapist understands the nature of the client's problem and that the therapist is able to communicate this understanding to the client. Confrontation opens up new possibilities and alternative ways for viewing the world and for acting and behaving.

During this first subphase the therapist continues to use forms of intervention in keeping with the type of therapy being practiced. Interpretations, *reframing* (finding alternative ways for viewing behavior), empathy, and challenging of distortions are used with the goal of helping the client to explore ambiguities and incongruities in life.

The therapist studies and considers how the client describes both his impact on others in the social environment and the impact the client makes on the therapist. These observations are used in helping the client appreciate his role in eliciting undesirable interpersonal responses. This process is described as a sequence of events that occur as a regular part of interpersonal learning.[92] Feedback from the therapist helps clients become more self-observing and to appreciate the nature of their behavior and cognitions, the impact they have on others, and how the responses of others influence self-perceptions. As clients recognize their own responsibility in creating unpleasant interpersonal exchanges, they also gain awareness of the possibilities for changing. Thus in addition to discovering that their problems can be understood and explained, clients also gain insight about the nature of their relationships and how what once seemed automatic and unchangeable can indeed be altered. As discussed in the section on curative factors, this interpersonal learning is likely to have more impact if it takes place in the presence of an emotionally charged experience. If the client risks trying out new behaviors, these experiences and their consequences become the focus of the therapy sessions and provide the therapist with the opportunity of reinforcing adaptive, positive interactions and of further analyzing maladaptive, negative exchanges.

The impact the client has on the therapist is also used to make comparisons of how the client may provoke similar responses in those with whom he associates in the social environment. In psychoanalysis, distorted responses of the client to the analyst are the transference reactions. The distortions in the relationship with the therapist are analyzed and used to uncover repressed memories of childhood. Transference responses occur in the present relationship with the therapist but are based on frustrations or conflicts from the past. Working through these transference responses (feelings of jealousy, competitiveness, hostility, and love) allows the therapist to make connections between the client's present behavior and past events. The therapist needs to have skill and evidence to make these connections and interpretations between the client's past and present behavior.

Resistances frequently encountered during this first subphase of working through relate to (1) the client's feelings of guilt or fears of rejection about revealing difficulties and (2) difficulty in coping with the anxiety aroused when problems are uncovered. Potential countertransference problems for the therapist include (1) avoidance of problem areas that cause the therapist anxiety, (2) attempts to confront the client too soon or to probe too deeply, and (3) irritation toward the client for not gaining insight rapidly enough.[90]

The second subphase involves translating insights and understandings into action either through prescribing specific behavioral programs or through the natural consequences of the insights and learning gained by the client. In the later instance, the client takes the initiative to try out new modes of behaving or relating, and these experiences and their ramifications become the focus of the therapy sessions. This phase of therapy has been compared to movement from the developmental stage of childhood to adolescence. The client and therapist become more involved in active problem-solving.

During this subphase the therapist is concerned with promoting the factors that contribute to and maintain behavioral change, such as (1) using interpretations to develop insight, (2) creating incentives for change, (3) dealing with factors that block action, (4) helping the client to master anxieties associated with life goals, (5) reinforcing or shaping desirable and adaptive behavioral change, (6) extinguishing or frustrating undesirable behaviors, (7) helping the client to accept or adjust to environmental conditions that cannot be changed, (8) helping the client adjust to those symptoms or character patterns that cannot be altered during therapy, and (9) helping the client transfer learning to new situations.[18,90]

The extent to which *insight* is essential for change has been a source of debate among therapists of differing theoretical ideologies. Insight is not a singular concept. Instead, it can be thought of as occurring on four levels at which clients may learn (1) how they are seen by others, (2) what they are doing to others, (3) why they do what they do (motivational insight), and (4) how they become the way they are (genetic insight).[92]

Genetic insight is considered to be the deepest level of insight and is cultivated in psychoanalytic therapy; however, this depth of insight may not be necessary in order for clients to use new information to make changes. Insight is only the first step in analytic therapy. As therapy progresses, insight deepens through repeated interpretations of how childhood patterns remain operative in the client's current life. However, the important factor is not the insight itself, no matter how deep, but the client's motivation in using the insight to effect change. Insight as a

curative factor is a means rather than a goal of individual therapy.

The following list reviews the types of general insights a client may acquire in psychotherapy[79,92]:

1. The world is not such a bad place after all. One comes to recognize that although life is at times unfair and unjust, people are generally more trustworthy than the client had imagined.
2. One has to be less demanding of others. People resent and react negatively to exploitation. Expectations need to be scaled down (accept limitations in oneself and others) if one wants to be happier.
3. If one achieves something or receives pleasure out of some activity or experience, one's satisfaction is sufficient. One cannot expect the praise and adulation of others; otherwise one will be continually disappointed.
4. As a prime lesson, one learns to delay gratification. One has to learn to modify wishes and desires, endure tensions, frustrations, and disappointments.
5. One learns to live life more fully and honestly, to be less caught up in unimportant issues.
6. Separation is painful, but the pain need not last forever. The gratification that occurs from interpersonal closeness can be symbolic as well as physical.
7. If one wants to reach a goal, one has to institute realistic action. Wishing does not produce results. Effort is a component of any achievement.
8. Tension, suffering, anxiety, fear, or depression are not nearly as bad as one had considered them to be. Avoidance of painful affects does not solve problems. Ultimately, both pain in life and death are inescapable.
9. Certain interpersonal maneuvers do not work and are self-defeating. Anger and hostility in self and others do not destroy others or oneself. Feelings are not the same as acts. Ingratiation typically does not bring the approval one seeks, and if it does, it is at the cost of self-depreciation. Negativism does not coerce others into doing one's bidding. Each person stands alone; attempts to "merge" with another person do not bring security. Attempts to get even with others result in more unhappiness.
10. Cooperation generally brings the greatest returns.
11. Accepting one's feelings and motives, no matter how unpleasant or "immoral" they may seem is the best guideline. Feelings need to be acknowledged as a part of the human condition but not necessarily acted upon.
12. One needs to learn to stand up for one's rights as a way of showing respect for others and for oneself. This is also a more effective means for satisfying one's needs and desires.
13. One needs to respect, accept, and subordinate oneself to higher authority. Competing with or rebelling against persons in legitimate authority positions is generally futile. One usually has the choice of leaving the arena or of taking constructive action within the system. Accepting authority

does not mean abandoning one's own autonomy. To the contrary, it frees the individual from struggles with others.

14. One learns to accept that the past is irreversible, but some latitude exists in determining the present and future.

15. One gains a clearer understanding of one's identity and role in life than was possible before therapy. One learns to be more flexible in that one is able to assume a variety of roles when it is appropriate, for example, one may function in authoritarian or subordinate, dependent or independent, assertive or submissive, competitive or cooperative roles without undue conflict.

During this second subphase each therapist uses a different repertoire of skills to help the client translate insight into action. One method is for the therapist to use various methods of verbally rewarding the client to reinforce positive change. Simple statements of praise, such as "It seems like you made a good decision" or "It feels good to have others respond positively to you," are often effective.

Some therapists use persuasion and directives to get the client to try new behaviors, for example, being more assertive or initiating an interaction both inside and outside therapy. Therapists may also direct the client to observe and record troublesome behavioral or thought patterns to identify the connection between environmental events and the onset of difficulties. For example, a woman who found herself in frequent arguments with her husband noted that the arguments were more likely to occur when she wanted him to anticipate her needs. She quickly felt rejected and acted as if she had been treated unfairly, which she translated into angry outbursts and name calling. The next step is to have this client try out an alternative approach with her husband, such as expressing her desires and feelings more directly.

Nondirective therapists tend to use more subtle approaches by having the client focus on a specific incident; eliciting feelings about the incident; and finding out what went wrong, what the client wanted to do differently, and what kept the client from responding in accord with these desires. Through an exploration of motives and feelings, clients often come to their own conclusions about how they want to act or respond in the future to similar situations. The nondirective approach allows the client to select the time and place he will risk trying out the new behavior. This nondirective approach has the added dimension of permitting the client to maintain control and to believe that one's own efforts made change possible. The therapist is then in a position to reward the responsible and self-motivated act. Eventually, engaging in more satisfying relationships becomes its own intrinsic reward, and the therapist becomes less important as an object of reinforcement.

Clients may exhibit various types of resistances during this period. Clients may have difficulty giving up the rewards achieved through their symptoms. For instance an individual with strong dependency needs often finds it difficult to become more self-reliant because of the security that is experienced in being able to rely on someone else.

Another client threatened suicide when she reached a point in therapy at which she recognized she did not want to give up her neurotic symptoms and get better, but at the same time, she felt that maintaining her old patterns was also untenable.

In the preceding example, the therapist needs to work with the client to understand her resistance and the nature of her fears about getting better, while providing sufficient support to keep her from following through with her threat of self-harm. At the same time, the therapist needs to be concerned with the conditions that support change by reinforcing any indicators of healthy strivings.

Significant others involved in the client's life are likely to respond to changes in the client in ways that weaken the client's resolve or precipitate maladaptive but familiar interactional patterns. By discussing these possibilities ahead of time, the client can either change the anticipated behavior or plan and rehearse ways of managing the response and resist the pull to act in expected ways. Some therapists anticipate this resistance to change by talking with the client's spouse at the outset of therapy and preparing him or her in general for what to expect during the process of therapy.

If more drastic adjustments are needed in the client's environment, such as changes in living arrangements, job, or physical condition, individual therapy may need to be combined with other forms of therapy, such as family or marital therapy, or psychoeducational approaches that teach the client self-care and management skills. Some aspects of a client's environment may not be subject to change (for example, accidents, economic recessions, job layoffs, natural disasters, illnesses or deaths of friends or relatives, poor housing, or unfavorable work environments). In such instances working with the client to adjust to what cannot be altered in therapy may be a very important aspect of the therapeutic work.

Both confrontations and interpretations are used during this phase of therapy. The interpretations are focused on the issue causing the client distress, starting with what is most current and close to awareness and working back to the past to what comes more gradually and with greater effort into the client's awareness. For example, a client complained to his therapist that he was furious with his boss for expecting him to work extra hours without compensation. He expressed his anger indirectly by being late for important meetings and failing to complete his work on time. An initial interpretation made by the therapist was to point out to the client that he seemed to feel a need to try to get even with his boss, but in so doing he created circumstances in which his boss may see a need to request his staying overtime to complete his work.

Interpretations are also used during this phase of therapy to analyze the client's transference distortions and resistances. A client's casual comment that he has nothing of significance to discuss after the therapist has returned from vacation signals that the client may be feeling angry, rejected, abandoned, resentful, or jealous in response to the therapist's absence. When the client experiences these unrealistic feelings toward the therapist, his attention is being diverted from working on his problems. That is why transference phenomena are considered a form of resistance. Analyzing these transference feelings and interpreting their connections with the past are processes that lead to insight and promote change.

Through the reexperiencing of these early unresolved feelings and needs with the therapist, the client gradually gives up old patterns and learns or relearns new patterns of relating. This is called the *corrective emotional experience*. The therapist avoids repeating or gratifying needs based on the old needs and reacts to the client's often unreasonable behavior in an accepting manner. Through interpretation and by actually trying out new behaviors, the client comes to realize that anticipating rejection may cause him to act in ways that in fact elicit rejection. As the therapist fails to respond to the client in the expected way, the client feels more secure in the relationship and can use the alliance aspect of the relationship as a model for developing other satisfying interpersonal relationships and as the back-drop for facing unpleasant circumstances in his life. These *themes* or troublesome situations in the client's life may need to be played out and worked through numerous times before the client begins to experience the rewards and satisfactions that come from mastering fears and anxieties and from experimenting with new behaviors. Using role playing or assigning homework or tasks to work on that help the client to master fears or try out new behaviors is helpful during this phase of therapy.

Following are potential sources of countertransference for the therapist[90]:

1. Frustration, irritation, or discouragement that the client is not able to utilize insight to promote positive changes
2. Tendency to try to push the client too much toward achieving goals
3. Fear of being too directive resulting in passivity
4. Resentment at the client's inability to cooperate with corrective procedures

At some point, as with unalterable environmental factors, the limitations of what therapy can do are recognized and accepted by both the client and therapist. Discussing with the client the limitations of therapy at the outset and that the goals reflect these expected constraints on what can be accomplished in therapy is beneficial.

The result of the working phase of therapy is that the client begins to take more responsibility for his own life and to redefine his relationship with the therapist in more realistic terms.

Termination phase. Termination, the final stage of therapy, has been referred to as the phase of individuation. If the working phase of therapy is analogous to the developmental stage of adolescence, then the final phase represents adulthood because of the separation from the therapist and individuation of the client. Some authors have described this final phase of therapy as a part of life's continuous process of meetings and partings.

Termination is often the most difficult aspect of therapy, not only for the client but also for the therapist. This is particularly true for the beginning psychotherapist who has successfully negotiated the course of therapy with the client including the powerful, existential impact of exerting positive interpersonal influence toward the recovery of a disturbed or otherwise dysfunctional person. Termination is often characterized by angry disappointment in the client. Unless the therapist has a clear understanding of the dynamics of the situation, she may misinterpret the emotional reaction of the client and waiver in the consummation of the final goals of therapy.

Assuming realistic goals have been achieved, the process of termination can be initiated. The beginning therapist encounters challenges directly related to the termination process and may quickly discover that a poorly planned termination colors the entire program of therapy. The importance of working carefully through the painful termination process cannot be overemphasized. Yalom[93] described anxieties occurring at termination as a manifestation of the existential fear of not being, of death. Confrontation with painful separation may reawaken the ultimate problem of coping with the threat of nonexistence.

The therapist who has achieved a moderate level of self-awareness usually recognizes tendencies to rationalize faltering decisions about how and when to terminate therapy. The anticipated loss experienced by the client is only half of the dynamic process. Termination of therapy is also a genuine loss experience for the therapist, and therefore the pain of the anticipated loss may arouse defensive responses that are not really determined by the needs of the client.

A deliberate plan for separation from the therapist and the positive conclusion of a deeply meaningful relationship can be as constructive as any aspect of therapy. The experience is essentially one of loss and therefore follows the principles of allowing time for mourning, for planning to integrate the "lost object" into the self, and for planning continued growth and individuation. As mentioned earlier, the loss is not unilateral, and the therapist needs to have the opportunity to share with the client her feelings at the conclusion of the relationship. The therapist needs to recognize and share with the client that the satisfactions of accomplishment in achieving goals at whatever level of success are tempered with the pain of separation.

Termination ordinarily leads to resistance in the client. The simple and elaborate manifestations of client resistance are recognized by the therapist who is attuned to the vicissitudes of the relationship, including her own position. Resistances of the client to initiation of the termination process can be considered as being a *flight to health* or *flight to illness*. Such responses are certainly not mutually exclusive; the client may demonstrate both impulses from week to week or from moment to moment.

A precipitous, unplanned ending of the therapeutic relationship is perhaps the clearest expression of the flight to health. The client who declares he no longer needs therapy and decides not to continue, following introduction of the termination process, in a sense has declared autonomy and self-determination, that is, he will make the decision on how and when to terminate. The therapist, of course, is ill-advised to regard this as an example of early cure.

Such abrupt termination is most probably withdrawal from an anticipated painful situation—the impending separation from the therapist. People who have experienced unresolved interpersonal loss in the past may fear reactivation of the loneliness, depression, fear, and grief of that earlier trauma. Failure to mourn the loss of a loved one is common in our culture. The letting-go process required in an experience of loss is often agonizing, and the client who anticipates further unresolved grief may choose to declare a "cure" and end therapy abruptly.

Difficulties experienced in leaving home at adolescence or in having an adolescent son or daughter leave home are a variation on the theme of unresolved loss experiences that may cause serious resistance at termination. From the therapist's viewpoint, unresolved loss experiences of the client are important to be worked through in therapy. Termination provides an optimal opportunity because of the frequently increased intensity of the transference at the threat of termination.

Obviously, the client who ends therapy abruptly abandons any opportunity to manage unresolved grief; therefore the therapist needs to contact the client and encourage completion of the program of therapy. The positive aspects of concluding a meaningful relationship, with open expression of the emotional impact on both parties, can be instrumental in vicarious mourning for the earlier loss. Bringing into verbal awareness the fears associated with separation and perceived abandonment is a poignant therapeutic event made possible by the strength of the relationship with the therapist. Learning that grief can be less painful under such circumstances is often one of the most productive of outcomes.

The flight to health resistance can be exemplified in ways other than abrupt termination. Denial of all symptoms is a less drastic, dynamically identical manuever that is more amenable to intervention by the therapist. Denial is a primitive defense, common to the young child. The therapist who relates denial to initiation of termination can work with the client toward recognizing and accepting that linkage.

More discouraging to both client and beginning therapist is the regressive return of symptoms, or the "flight to illness." Dynamically this is a primitive effort by the client to demonstrate that termination is inappropriate, that the therapist cannot leave the client (he is too ill), and that the client cannot manage without further support and therapy.

Resurgence of dependence is a common conflict at termination. Whereas flight to health may be described as denial of dependence, flight to illness may appear to be a collapse of the client's adaptive ability and is an appeal for continued care. As in previous examples of resistance, this reaction needs to be dealt with directly and with sensitivity, with the objective of openly and verbally linking the recurrence of symptoms with the initiation of termination.

The literature on the necessity for the therapist to proceed with sureness, sensitivity, and wisdom during termination with the client is growing. Yalom[93] described the apprehension with which even the most experienced therapists proceed toward termination when the client protests with the most frightening of challenges, the sui-cide threat. He described a woman client who reacted to the approaching termination date with increasing preoccupation with suicide. The therapist held to the decision to terminate, and eventually the woman accepted the inevitability of the separation and worked productively through the final sessions of therapy. Yalom concluded[93]:

> It seems that one important thing for clients to learn is that though therapists can be helpful, there is a point beyond which they can offer nothing more. In therapy, as in life, there is an inescapable substrate of lonely work and lonely existence.

Whether therapy is an intensive, long-term experience or a brief encounter directed toward symptom management or crisis resolution, the termination phase affords opportunity for review, summarization of learning, and a review of goals achieved, or at least considered. The potential for the client to gain deeper understanding of his patterns of response to anticipated loss can be realized if termination is managed well.

Nurses are sometimes in organizationally determined situations that prevent them from assuming responsibility for termination of clients. For example, hospitalized clients are rarely discharged as a result of the nurse therapist's decision, and therefore termination may be abrupt, poorly executed, and not productive for either client or therapist in achieving the potential growth associated with the final phase of therapy.

Termination processes can be accomplished best when the interdisciplinary team agrees to work for the best interests of the client, that is, when discharge decisions are made known early enough for some degree of working through the termination process between nurse and client. The awareness of the nurse of the importance of the termination process, as difficult as it may be, is an important prerequisite for such a system to be successful.

Mann agrees that the client does not feel absolutely cut off from further contact, even with a carefully designed time-limited psychotherapy model. Termination is for regularly scheduled therapy sessions; however, the client is told, " 'This does not mean that you will necessarily stop seeing me altogether. You can ask to come back at any time for further occasional sessions if you feel you need further help.' "[53]

The concept of a course of therapy being an experience that has distinct phases, including a beginning and an ending, is fundamental to understanding the meaning of the termination process for both client and therapist.

Evaluation

Evaluation is an essential though often neglected component of the therapy process. To many people evaluation may precipitate anxiety over the thought of having deficiencies exposed. Actually, evaluation can be seen as an opportunity for reinforcing accomplishments and for learning and problem solving in relation to issues and skills that can be improved. For example, it is as worthwhile to determine why goals are not achieved as to know why they are. Are the goals or methods inappropriate? Is the formulation of the problem at fault?

The purposes of evaluation are to determine the extent

to which goals have been achieved and to provide data that can be used as guidelines for future action. Evaluation can be divided into two major areas: (1) the therapist's evaluation of the process and outcome of therapy, and (2) the effectiveness of psychotherapy.

Therapist's evaluation. Evaluation starts with assessment and continues through analysis of the problem, formulation of goals, and implementation of intervention strategies. In the course of the evaluation process, a number of interrelated questions need to be answered: (1) What goals can realistically be achieved, given the client's problem, level of functioning, background, and resources? (2) What impact are the intervention strategies having on the client in terms of goal achievement? To what extent is the client developing a therapeutic alliance? (3) Is there a need to alter goals? Add goals? Change strategies? Seek other resources? and (4) To what extent have the goals of therapy been achieved according to the outcome criteria? Providing answers to the foregoing questions implies that evaluation is an ongoing process in which the therapist is continually in touch with the client's progress and is evaluating the need for resetting goals or employing alternative strategies.

Session-by-session evaluation of short-term goals provides data concerning client behaviors and interactions that indicate successful achievement of outcome goals. It may be necessary to try a variety of approaches if it appears that the goals are ineffective or that a new issue or problem has emerged. In the process, the therapist is acting as a participant-observer and data collector who evaluates the effectiveness of various frameworks for generating solutions for clients' problems.

The whole evaluation process presupposes that realistic short- and long-term goals have been defined, since it is by these criteria that client progress and goal achievement can be determined. Operationalizing outcome criteria involves determining what changes in behavior, attitudes, feelings, or status are acceptable as evidence that the goals have been achieved. Whether the goals involve symptom relief (supportive therapy) or changes in ways of feeling, interacting, or behaving, if they have been defined clearly and in operational terms, evaluation of their achievement is accomplished with greater ease and validity.

Goals are realistic to the extent they are based on an accurate determination of the client's needs. Evaluation during therapy and at termination can thus be based on what is pertinent for a particular client to achieve. It is thus possible on the basis of individually developed goals to evaluate the client's progress so that even dysfunctional clients may reach the expected level of goal achievement.

Effectiveness of psychotherapy. During the past decade questions regarding the risk, cost effectiveness, and efficacy of various types of psychotherapy have generated considerable interest in the results of research studies designed to answer these basic questions. Unfortunately, studies that adhere to the tenets of research design and methodology are so lacking in sufficient numbers as to make most generalizations suspect. However, given this caveat, three generalizations are usually made by authors who have attempted to review and summarize the current status of psychotherapy outcome studies[22,26,63]: (1) When data from a number of studies are pooled and evaluated, it appears that almost all forms of established psychotherapy are equally effective for approximately 60% to 70% of the clients in comparison with either untreated controls (clients on a waiting list) or unplanned help. However, the evidence varies from one study to another according to the type of evaluation criteria being used, the type of therapy employed, the skill and training of the therapist, and characteristics of the client. (2) Behavior therapy in terms of short-term benefits appears to be superior for treating phobias, compulsions, obesity, and sexual problems, and cognitive therapy or antidepressant drug therapy is equally effective with depressed clients. However, for the vast majority of clinical syndromes, no one form of therapy has been demonstrated to be significantly more effective than any others in the long run. (3) Follow-up studies demonstrate that regardless of the type of therapy, clients who show initial improvement tend to maintain it. Also, in studies comparing the effectiveness of one type of therapy with another, any significant differential effects favoring one therapy at the termination of treatment over another seem to disappear with time. Further, it appears that this loss of a significant difference can be accounted for by clients who received the less successful approach catching up to those who initially were exposed to the more successful type of therapy. This result has suggested to some that the main benefit of therapy may be to accelerate improvement that, given time, might have occurred naturally anyway.

The profusion of new treatment methods and practitioners has compounded the problem of evaluating efficacy. There is no clear agreement among practitioners and researchers about what variables or aspects of therapy need to be studied. For a particular type of psychotherapy to be considered efficacious, "it must be measurably equal to or better than other treatments and better than nontreatment by standards that permit independent observers, using the same methods, to disconfirm the results of the original investigator."[46] According to this definition, all forms of existing psychotherapy would have to be tested against each other under controlled conditions. Given that there are some 150 to 250 different types of psychotherapy and 150 discrete diagnostic categories of mental disorders according to the DSM-III-R, Parloff[63] pointed out that 4.7 million separate comparison studies would be needed, an obviously unrealistic task.

With the current emphasis on cost containment, funding for research studies may become increasingly scarce. Some argue that psychotherapy, because it is more art than science, need not be subjected to research. However, as Parloff[63] pointed out, classifying something as art does not preclude evaluation of quality, worth, and impact. Psychotherapy remains to some extent a clinical art, "but at its best it is an art in the hands of a highly skilled expert."[81] While some of these skills remain difficult to operationalize, research studies to date have informed clinicians of certain universal therapeutic techniques and common curative factors on which no school of psychotherapy has exclusive claim. Further elucidation of the aspects of psychotherapy that enhance efficacy, including the study of the influence of the therapist's characteristics on therapy outcome, can be of value to all in the helping professions who hope to influence individuals in distress.

BRIEF REVIEW

In this chapter psychotherapy is broadly defined as any intervention which uses the psychological processes inherent in the professional helping relationship to influence clients to change in ways that alleviate their symptoms, overcome interpersonal problems, or generally improve functioning. The form of the relationship has become specialized as mental health–psychiatric nurses have expanded their role to include that of nurse psychotherapists.

Historical events and trends have influenced the inclusion of psychotherapy as one of the competencies of nurses. Of significant importance was the adoption of theoretical frameworks from other disciplines and adaptation of those theories into the practice theory of nursing. The impact of psychotropic drugs in controlling aberrant behavior of the mentally ill was of particular importance in making the client psychologically available for treatment programs.

Twelve common curative factors are used as the basis for the development of a general framework for the practice of psychotherapy. Each school of psychotherapy differentially weights the importance of the common curative factors. In addition to the common factors, emphasis is placed on the contribution strategies and techniques specific to a particular school of therapy have in influencing the course of therapy.

Nurse psychotherapists function in a variety of settings both within the community and in institutional settings, in private practice, or as collaborative members of the health care team. The nurse therapist starts with certain basic assumptions about the client that provide the frame of reference for the processes involved in assessment and in establishing a working alliance with the client.

Not everyone seeking help is necessarily a suitable candidate for individual therapy. Certain variables appear to influence the selection process, whether or not clients stay in therapy or terminate prematurely, and the nature of the therapeutic outcome. Motivation, willingness to be introspective, and having a neurotic conflict are considered key factors in being an appropriate candidate for uncovering or psychodynamic therapy. Behavioral therapy has broader applications in terms of both the types of clients and types of problems considered suitable for intervention than does psychodynamic therapy. Supportive therapy may be recommended for clients who are experiencing temporary life stresses, for the chronically mentally ill, as a precurser to uncovering therapy, or as an adjunct to other types of therapy.

The assessment and planning phases of psychotherapy require considerable training and knowledge of factors that predispose to emotional illness. During the early phase of implementing therapy, the development of the therapeutic alliance through listening and influencing skills and other common curative factors is especially significant. As therapy progresses during the working phase, the focus of the therapy and the techniques used vary according to the particular theoretical orientation of the therapist, and the needs or problems presented by the client.

The value of therapeutic goal setting and evaluation transcends any particular school of therapy. Increasing emphasis on research in psychotherapy underscores the growing awareness that the effectiveness of psychotherapy depends on being able to specify what aspects of therapy are universally helpful and what aspects or techniques are effective with particular types or characteristics of clients. The importance of understanding and working through the dynamics of termination is a key factor in the outcome of therapy.

REFERENCES AND SUGGESTED READINGS

1. Abramson, L.Y., Garber, J., and Seligman, M.E.P.: Learned helplessness in humans, an attributional analysis. In Garber, J., and Seligman, M.E.P., editors: Human helplessness: theory and applications, New York, 1980, Academic Press, Inc.
2. American Nurses' Association, Division on Psychiatric and Mental Health Nursing Practice: Statement on psychiatric and mental health nursing practice, ANA Publication Code PMH-3 10M, Kansas City, 1982, The Association.
3. American Nurses' Association: Certification catalog, Kansas City, Mo., 1983, The Association.
4. American Psychiatric Association: Diagnostic and statistical manual of mental disorders (DSM-III-R), Washington, D.C., 1987, The Association.
5. Auvil, C.A., and Silver, B.W.: Therapist self-disclosure: when is it appropriate? Perspectives in Psychiatric Care 22(2):57, 1984.
6. Beck, A.T., and others: Cognitive therapy, New York, 1979, The Guilford Press.
7. Beck, A.T., and others: Treatment of depression with cognitive therapy and amitriptyline, Archives of General Psychiatry 42:142, 1985.
8. Berger, D.M.: On the way to empathic understanding, American Journal of Psychotherapy 38(1):111, 1984.
9. Bockrath, M.: Your patient needs two diagnoses—medical and nursing, Nursing Life 2:29, 1982.
10. Burgess, A.W., and Lazare, A.: Community mental health: target populations, Englewood Cliffs, N.J., 1976, Prentice-Hall, Inc.
11. Burns, D.D.: Feeling good: the new mood therapy, New York, 1980, William Morrow & Co, Inc.
12. Charkhuff, R.R., and Berenson, B.G.: Beyond counseling and therapy, ed. 2, New York, 1977, Holt, Rinehart & Winston, Inc.
13. Carpenito, L.J.: Is the problem a nursing diagnosis? American Journal of Nursing 84:1418, 1984.
13a. Cattell, R.: Psychotherapy by structured learning theory, New York, 1986, Springer Publishing Co., Inc.
14. Chessick, R.D.: Psychoanalytic listening II, American Journal of Psychotherapy 39(1):30, 1985.
15. Cormier, W.H., and Cormier, L.S.: Interviewing strategies for helpers: a guide to assessment, treatment, and evaluation, Monterey, Calif., 1979, Brooks/Cole Publishing Co.
16. DeLeon, P.H., Vanden Bos, G.R., and Cummings, N.A.: Psychotherapy—is it safe, effective and appropriate? American Psychologist 38(8):907, 1983.
17. Doona, M.E.: Travelbee's intervention in psychiatric nursing, ed. 2, Philadelphia, 1979, F.A. Davis Co.

17a. Durham, J., and Hardin, S.: The nurse psychotherapist in private practice, New York, 1986, Springer Publishing Co., Inc.

18. Egan, G.: The skilled helper: a model for systematic helping and interpersonal reading, Monterey, Calif., 1975, Brooks/Cole Publishing Co.

18a. Ellis, A.: Overcoming resistance, New York, 1985, Springer Publishing Co., Inc.

19. Foreman, S.A., and Marmar, C.R.: Therapist actions that address initially poor therapeutic alliances in psychotherapy, American Journal of Psychiatry 142(8):922, 1985.

20. Frances, A., Sweeney, J., and Clarkin, J.: Do psychotherapies have specific effects? American Journal of Psychotherapy 39(2):159, 1985.

21. Frank, J.D.: Therapeutic components of psychotherapy, Journal of Nervous and Mental Disease 159:325, 1974.

22. Frank, J.D.: The present status of outcome studies, Journal of Consulting and Clinical Psychology 47:310, 1979.

23. Free, N.K., and others: Empathy and outcome in brief focal dynamic therapy, American Journal of Psychiatry 142(8):917, 1985.

24. Freud, S.: Analysis terminable and interminable. In Strachey, J., editor: Sigmund Freud: collected papers, vol. 5, New York, 1959, Basic Books, Inc., Publishers.

25. Furlong, F.W.: Determinism and free will: review of the literature, American Journal of Psychiatry 138:435, 1981.

26. Garfield, S.L.: Psychotherapy: an eclectic approach, New York, 1980, John Wiley & Sons, Inc.

27. Giberson, D., and Larson, L.: Factors that affect patient compliance with psychiatric follow-up therapy after hospital discharge, Nursing Research 30:373, 1981.

28. Gordon, M.: Nursing diagnosis, New York, 1982, McGraw-Hill Book Co.

29. Griffith, J.W., and Christensen, P.J., editors: Nursing process: application of theories, frameworks, and models, ed. 2, St. Louis, 1986, The C.V. Mosby Co.

30. Hagerty, B.K.: Psychiatric-mental health assessment, St. Louis, 1984, The C.V. Mosby Co.

31. Halleck, S.L.: The treatment of emotional disorders, New York, 1978, Jason Aronson, Inc.

32. Hardin, S.B., and Durham, J.D.: First rate: a survey of clients and nurse psychotherapists, Journal of Psychosocial Nursing and Mental Health Services 23(5):9, 1985.

33. Hays, J., and Larson, K.: Interacting with patients, New York, 1965, Macmillan Publishing Co.

34. Hoehn-Saric, R.: Emotions and psychotherapies, American Journal of Psychotherapy 31:83, 1977.

35. Horowitz, M.J., and others: Brief psychotherapy of bereavement reactions, Archives of General Psychiatry 41:438, 1984.

36. Ivey, A.E., and Simek-Downing, L.: Counseling and psychotherapy: skills, theories, and practice, Englewood Cliffs, N.J., 1987, Prentice-Hall, Inc.

37. Jourard, S.: The transparent self: self-disclosure and well-being, Princeton, N.J., 1964, D. Van Nostrand Co., Inc.

38. Karasu, T.B.: Recent developments in individual psychotherapy, Hospital and Community Psychiatry 35(1):29, 1984.

39. Kim, M., McFarland, G., and McLane, A., editors: Pocket guide to nursing diagnoses, ed. 2, St. Louis, 1987, The C.V. Mosby Co.

40. Kopp, S.: If you meet the Buddha on the road, kill him: the pilgrimage of psychotherapy patients, New York, 1972, Bantam Books, Inc.

41. Koss, M.P., and others: Outcome of eclectic psychotherapy in private psychological practice, American Journal of Psychotherapy 37(3):400, 1983.

42. Krikorian, D.A., and Paulanka, B.J.: Self-awareness—the key to a successful nurse-patient relationship, Journal of Psychiatric Nursing and Mental Health Services 20(6):19, 1982.

43. Kute, I., Borysenko, J.Z., and Benson, H.: Meditation and psychotherapy: rationale for the integration of dynamic psychotherapy, the relaxation response, and mindfulness mediation, American Journal of Psychiatry 142(1):1, 1985.

44. Lefcourt, H.M.: Personality and locus of control. In Garber, J., and Seligman, M.E.P., editors: Human helplessness: theory and applications, New York, 1980, Academic Press, Inc.

45. Lego, S.: The one-to-one nurse-patient relationship. In Huey, F., editor: Psychiatric nursing: 1946-1974—a report on the state of the art, New York, 1975, American Journal of Nursing Co.

46. London, P., and Klerman, G.L.: Evaluating psychotherapy, American Journal of Psychiatry 139:709, 1982.

47. Luborsky, L.: Helping alliances in psychotherapy. In Claghorn, J.L., editor: Successful psychotherapy, New York, 1976, Brunner/Mazel, Inc.

48. Luborsky, L., and others: Predicting the outcome of psychotherapy: findings of the Penn Psychotherapy Project, Archives of General Psychiatry 37:471, 1980.

48a. Luborsky, L., and others: Do therapists vary much in their success? Findings from four outcome studies, American Journal of Orthopsychiatry 56(4):501, 1986.

49. MacHovec, F.J.: Current therapies and the ancient East. American Journal of Psychotherapy 38(1):87, 1984.

50. Maholick, L.T., and Turner, D.W.: Termination: that difficult farewell, American Journal of Psychotherapy 33(4):583, 1979.

51. Malan, D.H.: Individual psychotherapy and the science of psychodynamics, London, 1979, Butterworth Publishing, Inc.

52. Malan, D.H.: Toward the validation of dynamic psychotherapy, New York, 1980, Plenum Press.

53. Mann, J.: Time-limited psychotherapy, Cambridge, Mass., 1973, Harvard University Press.

54. Marguiles, A., and Havens, L.L.: The initial encounter: what to do first, American Journal of Psychiatry 138:421, 1981.

55. Marguiles, A.: Toward empathy: the uses of wonder, American Journal of Psychiatry 141(9):1025, 1984.

56. Maslow, A.: The farther reaches of human nature, New York, 1971, The Viking Press.

57. Morrison, E., and others: NSGAE nursing adaptation evaluation: a proposed Axis VI of DSM-III, Journal of Psychosocial Nursing and Mental Health Services 23(8):10, 1985.

58. Murphy, G.E., and others: Cognitive therapy and pharmacotherapy, Archives of General Psychiatry 41:33, 1984.

59. Murphy, P.O., Cramer, D., and Lillie, F.J.: The relationship between curative factors perceived by patients in their psychotherapy and treatment outcome: an exploratory study, British Journal of Psychology 57:187, 1984.

60. Muslin, H., and Val, E.: Supervision and self-esteem in psychiatric teaching, American Journal of Psychotherapy 34(4):545, 1980.

61. Nadelson, C., and Notman, M.: Psychotherapy supervision: the problem of conflicting values, American Journal of Psychotherapy 31(2):275, 1979.

62. Neill, J.R., and Ludwig, A.M.: Psychiatry and psychotherapy: past and future, American Journal of Psychiatry 34(1):39, 1980.

63. Parloff, M.B.: Psychotherapy research evidence and reimbursement decisions: Bambi meets Godzilla, American Journal of Psychiatry 139:718, 1982.

63a. Parloff, M.B.: Frank's common elements in psychotherapy: nonspecific factors and placebos, American Journal of Orthopsychiatry 56(4):521, 1986.

64. Peitchinis, J.: Therapeutic effectiveness of counseling by nursing personnel: review of literature, Nursing Research 21:138, 1972.

65. Pelletier, L.R.: Nurse-psychotherapists: whom do they treat?, Hospital and Community Psychiatry 35(11):1149, 1984.

66. Peplau, H.E.: Interpersonal relations in nursing, New York, 1953, G.P. Putnam's Sons.

67. Peplau, H.E.: Therapeutic concepts. In National League for Nursing: Aspects of psychiatric nursing, League Exchange No. 26, Sec. B, New York, 1957, The League.

68. Peplau, H.E.: In defense of nursing diagnosis (letter to editor), Nursing Outlook 32:240, 1984.

69. Perry, S., Frances, A., and Clarkin, J.: A DSM-III case-book of differential therapies: A clinical guide to treatment selection, New York, 1985, Brunner/Mazel, Inc.

70. Pilkonis, P.A., and others: A comparative outcome study of individual, group and conjoint psychotherapy, Archives of General Psychiatry 41:431, 1984.

71. Roger, C.: On becoming a person, Boston, 1961, Houghton Mifflin Co.

72. Rosenbaum, C.P., and Beebe, J.E., III: Outpatient therapy: an overview. In Rosenbaum, C.P., and Beebe, J.E., III: Psychiatric treatment: crisis/clinic/consultion, New York, 1975, McGraw-Hill Book Co.

73. Schramski, T.G., and others: Factors that contribute to posttherapy persistence of therapeutic change, Journal of Psychology 40(1):78, 1984.

74. Schroder, P.J.: Recognizing transference and countertransference, Journal of Psychosocial Nursing, 23(2):21, 1984.

75. Shapiro, S.A.: Contemporary theories of schizophrenia, New York, 1981, McGraw-Hill Book Co.

76. Shepherd, G.L.: Formats for peer review of dynamic psychotherapy, Hospital and Community Psychiatry 36(5):517, 1985.

77. Sifneos, P.E.: The current status of individual short-term dynamic psychotherapy and its future: an overview, American Journal of Psychotherapy 38(4):472, 1984.

78. Simons, A.D., Garfield, S.L., and Murphy, G.E.: The process of change in cognitive therapy and pharmacotherapy for depression, Archives of General Psychiatry 41:45, 1984.

79. Strupp, H.H.: Toward a specification of teaching and learning in psychotherapy. In Barten, H.H., editor: Brief therapies, New York, 1971, Behavioral Publications, Inc.

80. Strupp, H.H.: Psychotherapy: clinical, research, and theoretical issues, New York, 1973, Jason Aronson, Inc.

81. Strupp, H.H.: Themes in psychotherapy research, In Claghorn, J.L., editor: Successful psychotherapy, New York, 1976, Brunner/Mazel, Inc.

82. Strupp, H.H., and Hadley, S.W.: Specific vs. nonspecific factors in psychotherapy, Archives of General Psychiatry 36(10):1125, 1979.

82a. Strupp, H.H.: The nonspecific hypothesis of therapeutic effectiveness: a current assessment, American Journal of Orthopsychiatry 56(4):513, 1986.

83. Travelbee, J.: Intervention in psychiatric nursing: process in the one-to-one relationship, Philadelphia, 1969, F.A. Davis Co.

84. Tudor, G.E.: Sociopsychiatric nursing approach to intervention in a problem of mutual withdrawal on a mental hospital ward, Psychiatry 15:193, 1952.

85. Ujhely, G.: Determinants of the nurse-client relationship, New York, 1968, Springer Publishing Co., Inc.

86. Vandenbos, G.: Psychotherapy: practice, research, policy, Beverly Hills, Calif., 1980, Sage Publications, Inc.

87. Weiner, I.B.: Individual psychotherapy. In Weiner, I.B., editor: Clinical methods in psychology, New York, 1976, John Wiley & Sons, Inc.

88. Widiger, T.A., and Rover, L.G.: The responsible psychotherapist, American Psychologist 39(5):503, 1984.

89. Williams, J., and Wilson, H.: A psychiatric nursing perspective on DSM-III, Journal of Psychosocial Nursing and Mental Health Services 20(4):15, 1982.

90. Wolberg, L.R.: The technique of psychotherapy, vol. 2, ed. 3, New York, 1977, Grune & Stratton, Inc.

91. Wolberg, L.R.: The practice of psychotherapy, 506 questions and answers, New York, 1982, Brunner/Mazel, Inc.

92. Yalom, I.: The theory and practice of group psychotherapy, New York, 1975, Basic Books, Inc., Publishers.

93. Yalom, I.: Existential psychotherapy, New York, 1980, Basic Books, Inc., Publishers.

94. Zahourek, R.P., and Crawford, C.M.: Forced termination of psychotherapy, Perspectives in Psychiatric Care 16(4):193, 1978.

ANNOTATED BIBLIOGRAPHY

Carpenito, L.J.: Nursing diagnosis: Application to clinical practice, Philadelphia, 1983, J.B. Lippincott Co.

This book is a detailed guide to the use of nursing diagnosis as a guide to clinical nursing practice. It describes the most highly developed approach to operationalizing a conceptual framework for nursing process to date. Beginning with a historical perspective on nursing process, the author proposes a method for distinguishing between nursing diagnoses and other problems in which nurses intervene. The steps of the nursing process are described as they relate to the topic. The major portion of the book is devoted to a manual of nursing diagnoses consisting of forty-three diagnostic categories. Each category is described according to definition, etiological and contributing factors, defining characteristics, focus assessment criteria, nursing goals, and principles and rationale for nursing care.

Herron, W., and Rouslin, S.: Issues in psychotherapy, Bowie, Md., 1982, Robert J. Brady Co.

The authors present issues commonly encountered in the practice of psychotherapy and in need of attention by therapists of all disciplines. Written to be provacative, the authors hope therapists will think more about how they use themselves in therapy.

Nemiroff, R., and Colarusso, C.: The race against time, New York, 1985, Plenum Press.

This book applies psychodynamic theory to the clinical practice of psychotherapy with older adults. Focusing on the older adult, the relationship between theory and therapy is demonstrated and detailed case histories are presented.

Peterson, C.: Theories of counseling and psychotherapy, New York, 1986, Harper & Row Publishers, Inc.

The author presents comprehensive summaries of the major theories of psychotherapy to provide the student with a grasp of the structure and organization of each theory and to use as a basis for practice. Included in the discussion are cognitive, learning, psychoanalytical, phenomenological, extential, and eclectic approaches.

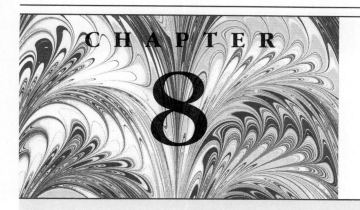

CHAPTER

8

THE NURSING PROCESS

Carolyn Shannon   Patricia Wahl

Martha Rhea   Janice Dyehouse

After studying this chapter the learner will be able to:

Discuss historical influences on the development and use of the nursing process in mental health–psychiatric nursing.

Define the components of a nursing assessment within the holistic nursing framework.

Describe the process of analysis and nursing diagnosis.

Define the elements and purposes of the therapeutic plan.

Discuss holistic considerations and intervention in health and acute and chronic illness.

Discuss the evaluation process.

Mental health–psychiatric nursing is an interpersonal and helping service in which the nursing process is used to provide care to the individual, family, and community in various states of mental health. The nursing process focuses on the client. To the extent that the client's psychopathology allows, he is an active participant in the nursing process with some degree of control over his problem resolution. The nurse needs to be cognizant of the extent to which the client can maintain autonomy and self-responsibility in the nursing process.

The nursing process has a particular importance to the practice of mental health–psychiatric nursing. Since information about the client's emotional and behavioral responses are often elusive, the nurse frequently infers from the client's perception and behavior the most effective manner in which to proceed in facilitating his growth and resolution of health concerns. These inferences are used as a basis for decision making. The mental health–psychiatric nurse continually reviews data, searching for cues that provide greater understanding to maladaptive client patterns and relationships.

Effective use of the nursing process requires the adoption of a conceptual framework within which to view the data. One of the numerous models from which to choose is that of holistic nursing. The purpose of this chapter is to develop the nursing process within the holistic conceptual approach.

NURSE-CLIENT COLLABORATION

A basic premise held by mental health–psychiatric nurses is the importance facilitating client self-responsibility. One approach that aids in developing client self-responsibility is nurse-client collaboration. Inviting the client to participate in his care may enhance his motivation for change and growth. Collaboration with the client also conveys respect for the client and his thoughts, feelings, needs, and wants.

With client input and feedback, the nursing process is more effective; priority problem areas are identified with greater precision; goal incongruence is detected quickly; interventions are often of higher quality; the accuracy of evaluation is improved; and the degree of professional satisfaction is broadened.[6]

In numerous instances client disturbances or disrupted functioning will limit the individual's collaboration. The nurse needs to adjust the type of collaboration according to the client's ability. The nurse continually assesses client readiness for collaboration and progressively involves him in decision making.

PHASES OF THE NURSING PROCESS
Assessment

Assessment involves the collection of data that reflect the mental health status of the client in relation to all di-

Historical Overview

DATE	EVENT
Pre-World War II	Mental health–psychiatric nurses depended mainly on experience, rote procedure, and intuitive judgment as a basis for nursing care.
1940s	Mental health–psychiatric nurses had some awareness of theory but still provided primarily custodial care with no attention to a systematic approach to nursing care.
1950s	Psychiatric nurses were using nursing care plans as a tool for communicating their practice. Peplau[35] developed a model of nursing care that emphasized a systematic approach to the nurse-client relationship.
1960s	Orlando[33] was among the first to describe nursing as a deliberative process with a focus on the interpersonal relationship.
1970s	Psychiatric nursing texts included the nursing process as a method for organizing nursing care within a conceptual framework.
1980s	Mental health–psychiatric nurses continue to refine their use of the nursing process.
Future	With increased understanding, the mental health–psychiatric nurse will more deliberately apply the nursing process.

mensions of the person: physical, emotional, intellectual, social, and spiritual. (For a more detailed description of the five dimensions see Chapter 9.) Clients are the primary sources of data. Other sources include the significant others who make up clients' interpersonal network, written records, and other health care personnel. The use of a variety of sources strengthens the assessment by expanding and validating the nurse's perception of the clients and their situations. Data are gathered from these sources through (1) interviews with the client and significant others, (2) physical and mental status examination of the client, and (3) diagnostic tests, including psychological tests.

Interaction, observation, and measurement are the three primary methods used to gather data. Data gathered by interaction and observation are collected during the interviews, mental status, and physical examination. Measurement involves the use of instruments to quantify data. The effects of three methods of collecting data during the nurse-client admission interview are summarized in the Research Highlight on p. 143.

The assessment data collected during the first nurse-client interaction are important because they provide a baseline of information against which subsequent data may be compared. By making these crucial comparisons, the nurse may more easily determine whether changes occur in the client's condition. This initial information also provides a basis for making sound clinical judgments rather than random interpretations of a single piece of data. Comparison of subsequent data to the baseline provides a vital feedback mechanism that links the steps of the nursing process and provides essential continuity.

For the assessment data to make sense to the nurse they need to be organized in some way, usually grouped into categories. An assessment format is commonly used to display the data in this way. The design of the format depends on factors such as the client being assessed (individual, family, or community), the scope of the assessment (limited or comprehensive), and the nurse's level of autonomy (agency or private practice setting). The organization of the format reflects a concept of "the client." In an agency setting where a predetermined assessment format may be required, the nurse decides whether additional information is needed to satisfy her concept of nursing practice and sense of accountability. This chapter includes a format for comprehensively assessing the individual client from a holistic nursing perspective. The holistic nursing assessment format is constructed according to the five dimensions of the person.

Making a holistic assessment involves all the attending skills of the nurse to encourage the client to relate his story without the use of intrusive or interfering measures. The nurse strives to gather data without bias or prejudice. This is difficult to do, since the interviewer to some extent leads the client to explore certain aspects of the story in more detail on the basis of the conceptual framework (such as holistic nursing) being used.

Physical dimension. Clients who have been diagnosed as mentally ill need to have thorough physical assessments, since they may have both related and unrelated medical problems that need care. Often changes in behavior are the first signs that something is physically wrong. These changes may be associated with physical conditions such as brain tumors or metabolic disturbances

The Effects of Three Methods of Collecting Information During the Nurse-Patient Admission Interview

C. Lindeman

PURPOSE

This study was designed to compare the effects of three methods of collecting information during the admission interview procedures. Based on analysis of the literature and clinical observation, the admission procedure was determined to be a potentially stressful experience for patients and one in which the nurse could influence the patient's well-being through effective nursing practice. The three methods of interview were (1) structured verbal, (2) structured nonverbal and (3) unstructured verbal. The dependent variables or effects on patient well-being that were measured included anxiety (blood pressure, pulse, and respiration rate), patient satisfaction with care, and nursing personnel's ability to identify the relative importance ascribed by a patient to specific aspects of hospital care.

SAMPLE

The sample consisted of 92 patients admitted for surgical procedures to Luther Hospital in Eau Claire, Wisconsin.

METHODOLOGY

Patients were assigned to one of the three types of admission procedure in order of admission. The hospital's admission interview form was used either by the nurse or by the patient for the structured verbal and nonverbal procedures, respectively. The unstructured verbal interview did not make use of an interview form. Patients' vital signs were recorded at the time of admission, before surgery, and numerous times after surgery. Correspondence between the patient and the nurse as to relative importance of aspects of care was measured by using a card-sorting procedure. Various aspects of care were listed on cards. Each patient and a nurse caring for that patient separately sorted the cards in order of importance, and their responses were compared. A patient satisfaction survey was mailed to patients after discharge.

FINDINGS

The method of admission interview did not produce systematic differences in patients' blood pressure, pulse, or respiration rates, which were all used as indicators of anxiety. The method of collecting data also failed to produce any differences in patients' reports of satisfaction with care, based on the survey mailed after discharge. However, the method of collection did produce a difference in accuracy of nursing personnel's identification of the relative importance ascribed by a patient to specific aspects of hospital care. That is, the structured verbal interview was more effective than the structured nonverbal interview but was not significantly more effective than the unstructured verbal interview.

IMPLICATIONS

For nursing practice the major implication of the results is that verbal communication in face-to-face interactions is more effective in learning about what patients value in their care than is a nonverbal procedure in which the patient completes the interview form privately. The increasing importance of matching nursing care to patients' concerns means that effective communication must characterize nursing practice.

Based on data from Krampitz, S.D., and Pavlovich, N., editors: Readings for nursing research, St. Louis, 1981, The C.V. Mosby Co.

such as hyperthyroidism and hypothyroidism. Such conditions are often overlooked when the predominant symptoms are related to a mental illness. Nurses on inpatient units have the opportunity to observe symptoms and subtle changes in behavior that can contribute to the diagnosis, which could have tremendous consequences for the client. Assessment of the physical dimension focuses on genetic factors, physiological processes, and body image using data gathered from the history and physical examination.

A genetic history is the first method of assessment and reveals a profile of the genetic strengths and risk factors for the client. The client is questioned about illness in family members, both living and deceased. Information is elicited to determine the presence of stress disorders, psychoses, substance abuse, mental retardation, depression, and suicide in the client's family history.

Assessing physiological processes is the second major concern in the physical dimension. At the time of data collection, the determination of whether a physical examination is done and who does it depends on the clinical setting and the role of the nurse. In some instances, the physical examination data are gathered from written records or through consultation with a physician or other health care professional.

The objective findings of a physical assessment need to be compared with the client's perception of the problem. Discrepancies between the findings and the client's reported symptoms may indicate a need for further evaluation and validation either with other health professionals or through more comprehensive medical testing. Inconclusive findings also require further evaluation and monitoring.

The client's health and medical histories are explored to include an overview of the client's growth and developmental history and a chronological record of illnesses, injuries, and medical care received.

When all systems function smoothly, the client takes

them for granted. One may abuse the systems for some time without getting into difficulty. Thus a careful review of daily health practices may elicit the potential for future trouble. This review may also yield clues contributing to the present problem if there is one. These practices include food preferences and eating patterns, sleep patterns and cycles, daily or weekly drug use, smoking habits, and exercise routines.

If the client's current problem focuses on somatic symptoms, questions are asked to determine whether the client perceives the somatic difficulties as the primary source of the problem or as an associated factor of the problem.

Many clients who are anxious or depressed search for the source of their discomfort in somatic problems. Many clients needing psychiatric treatment are first seen by their family physician or in a medical clinic. Specific physical complaints that are associated with emotional distress include chronic fatigue, diarrhea, allergic symptoms, constipation, emesis, enuresis, loss of appetite, weight loss or gain, impotence, frigidity, decreased or increased sexual interest, increased or decreased amount of sleep, early morning awakening, restless sleep, and repetitive or disturbing dreams.

Assessment of physical appearance is one aspect of the physical examination that is performed even when a complete examination is not done. This general survey reflects first impressions of the client's overall appearance.

The final component of the physical dimension to be assessed is body image. Body image is the mental image of one's physical body that forms part of the larger self-concept. The body image is relatively fixed by the end of adolescence. Determination of the client's body image provides the nurse with information on which an assessment can be based concerning the congruence of this mental image with reality.

Sexuality is a human aspect that is encompassed in multiple dimensions of the person. However, sexuality is assessed in this section on body image, since the person's sexual identity is so intricately entwined with the body image.

Emotional dimension.
The emotional status of the client is assessed in terms of affect, appropriateness of affect to the situation, quality and stability of mood, physical signs of emotion, and emotional response patterns. Affect is determined by those observable characteristics of a client that usually indicate an emotional state. It includes facial expression, posture, body movements, and physical signs of emotion such as crying. It is the emotional picture that the client presents to observers. The appropriateness of affect to the situation is based on the congruency between the affect the client is displaying and the culturally expected affective response in a particular situation. Both affect and appropriateness of affect are culturally determined in part, and this is considered in any interpretation by the nurse.

Mood is a state of feeling and is not directly observable. Mood includes both the particular emotional state being experienced, such as anxiety, anger, or euphoria, as well as the range and intensity of the emotional experience. Stability of mood simply refers to the degree of constancy or fluctuation in mood. When the mood changes very abruptly and suddenly it is considered labile. When the mood continues with little change over time it is considered constant.

Physical signs of emotion include observable signs indicating autonomic nervous system (ANS) activity such as flushing, sweating, and tachycardia. These signs merely indicate ANS activity and are not conclusive evidence of a particular state of emotion.

Patterns of emotional response include the client's most common or prominent emotional experiences and how the client deals with and expresses emotions. If a particular emotional response pattern such as anxiety, anger, guilt, or despair is established, further exploration of the depth, intensity, and persistence of this emotional re-

TABLE 8-1 Disorders of perception

Disorder	Definition	Example
Illusions	Common experiences everyone has at one time or another when they misinterpret a sensory experience. A stimulus in the environment sparks the experience, but the person does not interpret it correctly.	An elderly client mistakes a chair for a person. An inebriated client mistakes cracks in the floor for snakes.
Hallucinations	False sensory perceptions that have no identifiable source outside the individual.	A client sees doors, hears voices, or sees snakes where none exist.
Delusions	Fixed false beliefs out of keeping with reality or the client's level of knowledge, and not shared by their subculture. The beliefs are "fixed" in that they are not amenable to reason and do not change.	A client insists that a general in the Pentagon has been telephoning him and accuses the nurse of not calling him to the phone when, in fact, the client has recieved no telephone calls.
Déjà vu	The sensation that what one is experiencing has been experienced before. The experience is paradoxical, since the client cannot recall any previous experience that corroborates the feeling of recognition.	A client enters a room for the first time and remarks that it seems as though an identical experience has happened before.

action is pursued. Clients may be asked to describe their feeling tone as it exists for that moment and to compare it with how they have felt in the past. In this way the nurse gets a glimpse of the client's baseline before seeking services.

Emotional status is commonly altered in acute illness. The entire range of affect may be encoutered, both qualitatively and quantitatively. Exhilaration, giddiness, and an exaggerated sense of well-being are displayed in mania; melancholy and despondency are seen in depressive states; the organic brain syndromes are generally characterized by lability; "flat," "uncanny," and "bizarre" are terms used to describe schizophrenic affect.

The emotional dimension of the person is open to inaccurate interpretations by others. Because of this possibility, it is imperative that the nurse exercise great care to avoid interpretations based on incomplete data. Interpretations of data that occur during assessment can be considered tentative and recalled during analysis when a more complete understanding is possible.

✳ ***Intellectual dimension*** Assessment of the intellectual dimension includes observing the client's perception, memory, cognition, communication, and flexibility-rigidity.

Because perception is the process by which the client makes meaningful and adaptive interpretations of sensory, emotional, and intellectual stimuli, perceptual disorders markedly affect the individual's ability to function. Disorders of perception commonly include illusions, hallucinations, delusions, and déjà vu. Table 8-1 presents the definitions and examples of these disorders. Table 8-2 describes the various kinds of hallucinations and common organic causes.

Memory is divided into three areas: immediate, recent, and remote. Immediate memory affects the client's ability to attend and retain information presented in the current situation, such as the inteview. Mental retardation, high levels of anxiety, or organic brain syndromes may contribute to difficulties with immediate memory function.

Recent memory reflects the client's ability to recall

TABLE 8-2 Organic causes of hallucinations

Nature of Perception	Common Causes	Nature of Perception	Common Causes
Visual hallucinations		**Auditory hallucinations—cont'd**	
Simple lines, dots, and flashes of light	Psychedelic drugs Epilepsy Migraine headaches Tertiary syphilis Retinal disease or damage	Multisensory	Structural abnormalities of the brain, e.g., temporal lobe epilepsy
Insects, bugs, spiders, or small rodents (rats) usually accompanied by fear and suspicion	Delirium tremens (alcohol withdrawal)	Hearing one's thoughts spoken (clear sensorium)	Schizophrenia
		Gustatory/olfactory hallucinations	
Miniature people in entertaining scenes	Organic toxic states Delirium	Unpleasant odor (often smoke, feces, or perspiration), isolated or in conjunction with salivation, chewing, and sniffing	Migraine headaches Temporal lobe epilepsy
Scenes and panoramas (often accompanied by auditory hallucinations and a religious theme or messasge)	Temporal lobe epilepsy		
		Other sensory hallucinations	Organic lesions Schizophrenia
Autoscopy (mirror images; seeing of one-self)	Most frequently epilepsy, focal lesions, and brainstem infections Less frequently depression	Ill-defined	Depression
		Tactile and somatic sensations (hallucinations of pain, touch, or deep sensation)	
Auditory hallucinations		Pain such as twisting and tearing	Schizophrenia Epilepsy Migraine headaches
Noise such as buzzing or ringing	Salicylism Middle ear infection Auditory nerve injury Delirium Schizophrenia	Tactile zoopathy (insects crawling over body)	Toxic states, especially drug and alcohol intoxication
		Somatic zoopathy (infestation of body by insects)	Delirium Schizophrenia
Voices	Delirium	Phantom limb pain	Amputation
Clouded sensorium		Epigastric distress (feeling of fullness, pain)	Migraine headaches Temporal lobe epilepsy
Clear sensorium—often full sentences and abusive or sexual content	Functional psychosis such as psychotic depression, schizophrenia, and drug-induced psychosis		

Based on data from Devaul, R., and Hall, R.: In Hall, R., editor: Psychiatric presentations of medical illness, Jamaica, N.Y., 1980, Spectrum Publications, Inc.

events of the past few days, such as those leading up to the need for service. The inability to give a coherent picture of these events suggests a recent memory problem. Remote memory involves the client's ability to recall events of the distant past and can be assessed by asking about life milestones, such as birthdate. The inability to give an answer is highly suggestive of memory dysfunction. When it is difficult to determine the actual dates of occurence, outside information such as a relative or an old medical chart may be consulted for validation. When there are discrepancies between reports by the client and other sources, additional observation and information are needed to determine the status of memory.

Cognition includes the functions of orientation, fund of knowledge, judgment and insight, abstract or concrete thinking, and attention. Orientation encompasses the clarity of the client's conscious processes and his ability to ascertain the significance of his present situation. Orientation is tested for person, self, place, and time. Orientation to person and self is judged on the basis of whether the person knows who he is and can identify others. Orientation to time includes knowing the year, month, season, day, date, and time of day. Does he know how old he is or his birthdate? Orientation to place is judged by whether the client knows where he is.

The client's general fund of information will optimally include commonly known facts. This is somewhat determined by the person's educational experience and interests and may be influenced by gender and culture. Modification of the traditional testing procedure is advisable to ascertain this. For instance, a person with little formal education from a rural subculture may not respond to questions of a political or geographical nature but may have a considerable knowledge of herbs and gardening.

Judgment is the end result of the client's ability to assess a situation, analyze it, come to an appropriate conclusion, and make sound decisions. Judgment can involve decisions in the areas of social, family, financial, and employment situations. Judgment is a sensitive area of functioning, since it is so complex.

Insight enables clients to understand and relate the significance of their symptoms and illness. It is common for clients to initially have limited, if any, insight into their problems. For some, the development of insight becomes a focus for treatment; for others, it is of a secondary nature. However, it is useful for the nurse to establish a baseline with which to measure change in insight.

Abstract reasoning involves the ability to think beyond a concrete level. Many factors can influence the client's ability to abstract. Communication is severely affected when the client thinks in mostly concrete terms. Questions and comments need to be phrased so that abstraction is not relied on. Patient education is planned, keeping in mind that the client will take what is said literally. In one example of concrete thinking, a client who was preoccupied with the effects of his medication inquired about the term "half life" of the drug by asking if it meant that half his life was gone.

Abstract reasoning is tested by the interpretation of proverbs or the identification of similarities between items. The person is asked to restate a common saying in general, nonpersonalized terms. Any number of proverbs can be used. Following is an example of a proverb and possible interpretations, both abstract and concrete:

PROVERB	INTERPRETATION
"Don't cry over spilled milk."	*Concrete:* Persons shouldn't cry if they spill some milk.
	Abstract: Persons should not waste time regretting what has already happened.

Other commonly used proverbs are:

"People who live in glass houses shouldn't throw stones."
"A rolling stone gathers no moss"
"Rome wasn't built in a day."

The ability to abstract is also tested by asking the client to identify similarities between items, for example, oranges and apples, a coat and a dress, and a table and a chair. If he cannot respond, the client needs to be given the answer as an example and then asked about another set of items. This is a test of the client's ability to consider general relationships as opposed to dealing at a sensory level.

Attention refers to the degree of distractibility that the client shows during the interview. If his attention is drawn easily from the conversation by unimportant or irrelevant stimuli, it may indicate a high level of anxiety, a response to illusion or hallucinations, or an inability to focus or process material because of organic defects.

Communication is assessed by focusing on the client's manner of speaking, writing, and drawing. The manner in which the client speaks can reveal almost as much as what he says. Besides the qualities and quantity of the speech, careful attention needs to be paid to the content of the thoughts. This component of assessment focuses on thought processes the client expresses. People under stress typically are preoccupied by intrusive thoughts. Does the client describe any major preoccupations? What is he thinking about? The following lists a number of thought disturbances that the client may communicate:

Blocking is a sudden cessation of a train of thought that occurs in the middle of a sentence. Blocking happens to everyone occasionally and was described by Freud in 1901 as one form of the psychopathological aspects of everyday life. Its clinical significance, however, is seen when the person repeatedly blocks on the same theme.

Tangentiality is the loss of goal direction in communication; it is a failure to address the original point by digressing to another end point. It differs from circumstantiality in that the person with the latter problem eventually comes to the point but takes a long, circuitous route.

Circumstantiality occurs when the person includes nonessential details in a message.

Fragmentation is the communication of incomplete ideas. Thinking is disrupted, and thoughts are scattered. However, fragmentation is not associated with rapid or pressured speech, as is the case with flight of ideas.

Autistic thinking is highly individualized and self-centered; the client attaches individualized meanings to the words he uses. Such meanings are not usually related to ethnic or cultural variation.

Confabulation involves fabrication of experiences, often recounted in a detailed and plausible way to fill in and cover up gaps in memory. The client realizes to some extent that he cannot remember but tries to cover up the problem to save face.

Clang associations are characterized by rhyming of words. For example, the client may say, "Goose, loose, moose."

Perseveration involves involuntary and pathological persistence of an idea or response. For example, one client repeatedly said, "Ring a bell doggie" regardless of what was said to him. No one knew what the phrase meant to the client. The only change that ever occurred in this individual's speech pattern was an addition: "Ring a bell doggie, I won't wake everybody up." The client added this phrase because he often shouted "Ring a bell doggie" at night and woke other clients. The other clients and the staff members repeatedly told him not to wake everybody up. He did not change his behavior, but he modified his speech.

Ideas of reference involve incorrectly interpreting incidents as having direct reference to oneself. The client who watches television and thinks the news announcer is reporting a story about him is demonstrating ideas of reference.

Paranoid ideation involves the belief that one has been singled out for unfair treatment.

Depersonalization is the loss of one's identity as a person or the feeling that one does not occupy one's body.

Grandiosity is an overappraisal of one's worth and ability.

Unworthiness is an underappraisal of one's worth and ability.

Religiosity refers to excessive concern with spiritual and religious matters.

The client's ability to communicate in writing can be assessed from samples already available, or the client can be asked to write a brief autobiographical sketch or a creative story. The writing sample is examined for flow, order, and thought content.

Finally, the client may be asked to draw himself, his family, his home, or something abstract such as a feeling or his illness. The drawing is examined for form, color, and dimension.

The final area of assessment in the intellectual dimension is that of the client's degree of flexibility-rigidity. Flexibility-rigidity involves the clients ability to respond to change and to accommodate behavior as new conditions arise. Refer to Chapter 15 for a thorough discussion of this concept.

✻ ***Social dimension.*** Assessment of the social dimension involves the client's self-concept, interpersonal relationships, socialization, cultural factors, environmental factors, and location of the client on the trust-mistrust and dependence-independence continuums. It is helpful to gather information from both the client and persons who are important to the client. These two sets of data can be compared to detect areas of conflict or agreement.

Self-concept is assessed on a continuum from positive to negative. Self-esteem is assessed on a continuum from high to low. After adolescence, self-concept is less amenable to change and is more constant than self-esteem. However, in general self-concept and self-esteem are correlated. That is, a person with a positive self-concept usually has a high level of self-esteem, while the person with a negative self-concept has a low level of self-esteem. Based on the client's description of himself, and the nurse's observations of the clients grooming, body language, and other pertinent data, the nurse formulates an idea of how the client views himself and to what degree he values himself. The extent to which the client's views are realistic and congruent with other's perceptions influences the assessment.

It is important to explore the client's interpersonal relationships in all social groups—family, school, work, community. These relationships are examined in terms of compatibility-conflict, trust-mistrust, dependence-independence, congruence of expectations, and level of support afforded the client.

Throughout the collection of data about the client's significant interpersonal relationships, clues to the related areas of culture and environment may emerge. It may be pertinent to develop a picture of the various environments in which the client lives, works, studies, and plays. Sources of stress and support can be identified in these areas. It may also be helpful to know about the cultural influences from the client's early development.

Regarding the client's level of socialization, the nurse notes the degree to which the client conforms to the norms and values of both the family of origin and the larger society. Because of changing sex roles and alterations in norms for social behavior, socialization is a significant area for assessment. The nurse needs to be alert to the fact that clients experience conflict in their social environments because of these changes. For example, the woman who is socialized to the traditional female role but who needs to enter the job market, may experience considerable conflict in adjusting to the new role.

The nurse looks for clues about the client's level of trust-mistrust and dependence-independence. The level of trust-mistrust can be assessed by determining whether the client is excessively naive or suspicious. The level of dependence-independence can be assessed by determining how the clients are able to function emotionally and behaviorally with regard to their support system.

Acutely ill clients may experience severe disturbances in their ability to communicate with and relate to others. The desire to express needs and feelings and to participate in social interactions may remain intact, although ability to do so may be impaired. Some clients may exhibit pervasive mistrust that contributes to impaired interpersonal relating.

Throughout the interview, clients display certain attitudes toward the interviewer. The nurse notes these attitudes, since they offer clues as to how the client relates to other people as well. Some individuals appear to be indifferent toward the nurse. They may simply lack any interest in those around them. Some are passive: they take no part in the process, offer no opposition, and act submissive. Other clients may be aggressive, using direct physical assult or verbal aggression. Some clients are hostile, unfriendly, and antagonistic; some are suspicious and will not trust the interviewer. They check around the room and challenge the motives of the interveiwer. Others are seductive and flirtatious; some try to manipulate the interview, redirect it, focus on the interviewer, or give false information. The antiauthoritarian person expresses contempt for parents, legal authorities, or social organizations and is likely to include the interviewer in his put-downs. Other clients are dramatic, telling vivid tales in the history they give and finding satisfaction in the effect they achieve. Finally, the nurse needs to note any changes in the attitude that occur during the course of the interview. Clients are typically nervous at the outset, as they become more comfortable, their behavior may change.

�֎ ***Spiritual dimension.*** The term *spiritual* refers to the search for a meaning in life and a belief in powers greater than oneself. In the past, assessment of the individual's spiritual dimension was not systematic. The information that was sought regarding the client's spirituality was often limited to their religious affiliation. However, to participate in providing holistic health care, the nurse needs to assess the individual's spiritual needs and incorporate them in the nursing plans.

In assessing the spiritual dimension, the nurse uses all of her interpersonal skills: listening, communication, observation, and interviewing. Because spiritual needs are often expressed subtly instead of overtly, the nurse is sensitive to their expression. Clients may express cues to indicate their need and readiness to talk about spirituality such as references to religious affiliation or spiritual practices. Individuals' spiritual lives are a subject that is sometimes laden with emotion. Thus the spiritual dimension may best be addressed at the end of an interview.

Four aspects of spiritual dimension are assessed, as discussed in Chapter 9. First, the nurse needs to assess the extent to which the individual's need for a meaningful philosophy of life is being met. Within this area an assessment is made of the individual's perception of the meaning of life. Clients may be unable to verbally express what they are experiencing, but they can give clues that enable the nurse to begin an assessment. An exploration of the values and beliefs that guide the individual's behavior may provide useful data. The individual's concept of illness may be a relevant area for focus.

A second aspect to explore is the need for a sense of the numinous and transcendent. This need is conveyed through hope or hopelessness and a perception of faith. Determining a person's beliefs about obtaining his goals in life is essential to an assessment of attitude. The person's hope is assessed in terms of its past, present, and future orientation and whether it is grounded in reality or in magic.[40] Without sources of hope, persons lose their will to live.

In assessing the need for a trusting relationship with a deity, other people, and nature, the nurse determines who or what the clients worship and how they describe their concepts of a deity.

Clients may conceptualize a deity as one who is loving and giving, as one who punishes, or as one who controls the person's life. Whether a client turns to the deity for support needs to be explored. Clients who believe in a punitive deity may not expect divine support.

An assessment of the practices in which individuals engage to worship a deity provides essential data. Religious practices such as prayer, reading the Bible, confession, and meditation may be stabilizing forces in the person's life.[40] The nurse needs to understand and respect cultural and subcultural differences in spiritual practices.

Spiritual beliefs may be sorted into three categories of influence[8] inspiring, ineffectual, and deleterious. Inspiring beliefs lead to growth, peace of mind, and strong inner force. Ineffectual beliefs are colorless. They do no harm, but neither are they of much use as a source of support. Deleterious beliefs cause distress because they are associated with emotions such as fear, anger, guilt, and anxiety or physical and interpersonal disturbances. Through the spiritual assessment, the nurse must distinguish beliefs that sustain the client from those that are a source of conflict.

Problems with one's deity may be a sign of other problems with authority. People may form an alliance with their deity that is used to set them above other mortals, thereby giving them some distance from people whom they fear. At the same time, the alliance gives them the illusion of powers greater than those of other people. The clearest example of this phenomenon can be seen in clients who claim to be the Messiah.

Psychiatric clients whose maladaptive behavior involves religiosity are attempting to resolve intrapersonal conflicts through spiritual or religious practices. Close inspection of the way such persons use or even abuse their religions usually reveals that they are not on any better terms with their deity than with other significant people in their lives. The spiritual dimension of their illness then becomes a central focus in their treatment.

The box on pp. 149-152 shows the tools and format used for giving a comprehensive holistic assessment.

Analysis

Analysis is the step of the nursing process in which the nurse uses diagnostic reasoning to analyze and synthesize the data collected during assessment. For the first time in the nursing process the data are considered as a whole body of information. The end result of analysis is the nurse's clinical statement of the client's health status. This clinical judgment is known as the nursing diagnosis.

Within the holistic framework, illness, health, and dysfunction are seen as having multiple causative factors. No single event causes the current dysfunction or illness; rather, a series of events, each influencing the other, leads to the present situation. For the nurse, the task is to inter-

HOLISTIC NURSING ASSESSMENT FORMAT

PHYSICAL DIMENSION

Genetic History

Has any member of the family had any of the following problems?

Physical illness that seemed to be influenced by the person's emotional states, such as stomach ulcers or asthma

Excessive use of drugs or alcohol

Mental retardation

Schizophrenia or other psychoses

Depression

Suicide

For each "yes" response, inquire about details such as the relation of the family member to the client and the onset and progression of the illness. A multigenerational family tree or genogram may be constructed as a tool for detecting patterns of mental illness in a family. (See Chapter 29 for example).

Health History

Describe illnesses, injuries, surgeries, and hospitalizations. Include the dates of onset, duration, resolution, and any sequelae. Note the following:

Do patterns emerge such as recurrent illnesses or accident?

Were the illnesses mild or serious? Acute or chronic?

Were there any sequelae?

What is the pattern of the client's use of health care services: routine, episodic, frequent?

Are any of the incidents related to developmental stages?

Growth and Developmental History

Explore chronologically the sequence and content of this history, noting points that clients perceive as significant. One approach is to ask clients to describe themselves at typical developmental stages: What were they like? What was the family like? What was it like at school during kindergarten, elementary, junior high, high school, and college? What were their friends like? Construct an image of this person's life.

Activities of Daily Living

Construct an image of how the client spends a typical 24-hour period. Elaborate as necessary to refine the image of the client's life-style. Focus on the following areas:

Diet and Elimination

Describe appetite. Any recent change in either weight or appetite?

How much and over what period of time? Any food restrictions?

If yes, are these self-imposed or prescribed by someone else? Food allergies?

Describe any use of over-the-counter drugs to affect diet or elimination. How much fluid does the client drink each day? What kind of fluids?

Describe the pattern of diet and elimination for a 24-hour period.

Exercise and Activity

How often does the client exercise?

What kind of exercise?

How long are the exercise periods?

What effect does it have?

Sleep and Rest

Describe typical sleep pattern, including hours of sleep (time of retiring and time of awaking), quality of sleep (how the client feels on waking), any difficulties falling asleep or staying asleep, or daytime napping.

Tobacco, Drugs, and Alcohol

Describe use, including kind, amount each day or week, time of day, length, any efforts to stop, and interference with everyday functioning.

Leisure Activities

Describe what the client does for relaxation, pleasure, or peace of mind; include how often, how long, and what effect it has.

Review of Body Systems

Head, eyes, ears, nose, throat (HEENT); integument; breasts; cardiovascular; respiratory; gastrointestinal; renogenitourinary; reproductive; nervous; musculoskeletal; hematopoietic; and endocrine systems.

Conduct the usual analysis of a symptom for positive responses. It may be helpful to inquire about how the client perceives the symptom and its possible relationship to other factors.

Physical Examination Findings

Report significant findings from the physical exam including those that are within normal limits and specifically describing those that are outside the normal limits.

Examine Diagnostic Test Results

Laboratory, x-rays, psychological.

General Appearance

What are the client's general physical characteristics, especially unique or unusual features?

Is the client's style of dress neat, untidy, gaudy, or eccentric?

Is the client's posture relaxed, rigid, anxious, or worried?

Does the client sit on the edge of the chair as if he might bolt at any minute?

Does the client assume unusual postures? If the client demonstrates only usual movements, are they held as is posed for any length of time?

Does the client avoid direct eye contact or stare off into space?

Does the client's motor activity seem to involve excessive or very few body movements?

Does the client pace during the interview? Is the client unable to refrain from getting up from the chair?

Does the client wring hands or clothes during the interview?

Does the client perform repetitive acts? (These acts may be monotonous acts that accomplish nothing, or they may be purposeful.)

Does the client have any mannerisms such as a gesture, grimace, or other nonverbal forms of expression?

Does the client have any unusual motor behaviors that suggest a neurological disorder such as static or intention tremors, athetosis, chorea, or dystonia?

Does client have any noticeable deformities?

Does the client appear to be the stated age?

Continued.

HOLISTIC NURSING ASSESSMENT FORMAT—cont'd

Is the client well-groomed, dirty, or unkempt?
Are there any detectable odors?

Body Image

Ask the client:
"How would you describe your appearance to me?"
"How do you feel about your body?"
What do you like and dislike about your body?
What do you value most about your body?
If you could change your body in any way, what, if anything, would you change?

Another method for assessing a client's body image is to provide him access to a full-length mirror and ask him what he sees. An assessment is then made as to whether the client is viewing himself realistically.

Sexuality

Ask the following as a screening question—"Do you have any sexual complaints?" If further information is needed the following may be considered:
How do you see yourself as a woman/man?
Have you ever wished you were the opposite sex? If yes, why?
Has the problem that brought you here interfered with the sexual aspect of your life?
Are you satisfied with your sex life?
Do you have any worries concerning sex?
Are your needs and those of your partner compatible?
If not, how do you deal with the problem?
How do you express yourself sexually (touching, fondling, intercourse, masturbation)?
Do you have any difficulty in the performance of sexual activities?
Is your preference for a sexual partner a person of the same or opposite sex?

EMOTIONAL DIMENSION
Affect

Observe the following:
Facial expression: Smiling? Frowning? Scowling? Mask-like? Fearsome? Anxious?
Motor behavior: Restless? Lethargic? Bizarre posturing? Mannerisms? Gait?
Physical signs: Tears? Flushing? Sweating? Tachycardia? Tremors? Respiratory irregularities? Tics?

Appropriateness of Affect to the Situation

What is the relationship between the client's mood and thought content?
Is there a wide variation between what the client says and his emotional state as expressed in his face or behavior?
What is the client's affect in relation to different topics of discussion? Does the client show flattening of affect in association with ideas or situations that normally call for a more intense response?
Is there disharmony between the client's affect and thought content as indicated by an inappropriate response such as smiling or silly behavior when the expected attitude should be one of concern or sadness?
Does the client demonstrate a tendency to cover up a deep depression by feigning cheerfulness and high spirits?

Does the client convey *ambivalence* expressed in simultaneous, contradictory feelings directed toward the same object?

Mood
Quality of Mood

Is the client apprehensive? Anxious? Fearful?
Is there a blunted, apathetic quality to the client's affect—an impoverished, constricted, or flat feeling?
Does the client describe an elevated or depressed mood?

Stability of Mood

Is the client's affect labile during the interview? That is, do his emotions shift from moment to moment?
How easily do the client's emotional changes occur in response to pleasant or unpleasant stimuli?
Does the client have periodic mood swings from elation to depression or vice versa?
Does the client report having a hard time getting started in the morning but perks up emotionally as the day goes on or vice versa?

Emotional Patterns

Which emotions predominate in the client's life? How does the client express these emotions? Ask for examples that show how the client deals with anxiety, anger, guilt, or despair. Note the client's level of emotional awareness. Specific areas for assessment are discussed in the related chapters.

INTELLECTUAL DIMENSION
Sensation and Perception

Do you ever see or hear things that other people say are not really there?
Do you ever smell or taste things that other people say are not real?
Do you ever have thoughts about something that you believe but that no one else does?
Do you ever believe that your thoughts or actions are under outside control or influence?
Do you ever feel you have been singled out for special attention by others?

Memory
Immediate Memory

Give clients three items of information such as a name, an object, and a color. Instruct them to remember these things as you will be asking them to recall the information later in the interview. Continue the interview for 3 to 5 minutes before asking for recall.

Recent Memory

Ask for the sequence of events leading up to the client's seeking services. If this information was supplied by the client in relating the history of present illness then it can be used for this assessment and not repeated.

Remote Memory

Note the client's ability to accurately relate past events in sequence with appropriate descriptive detail. As with recent memory, check with other sources of information to validate the accuracy.

HOLISTIC NURSING ASSESSMENT FORMAT—cont'd

Cognition

Orientation

Can the client correctly identify the following: Current time? Place? Other persons? Self?

Fund of Information

Ask client to name the five largest cities in the United States or the names of the last three presidents.

Judgment

Social judgment: To what extent is the client aware of social norms and the need for compliance with them or the law?

Family judgment: To what extent does the client appreciate how his behavior affects his family or vice versa?

Financial judgment: Does the client manage money effectively?

Employment judgment: Does the client have unrealistic job expectations or aspirations or fail to recognize his responsibilities to his employer? To what extent does the client plan for the future? Are the plans inappropriate or realistic?

Insight

Does the client recognize that he is ill or that he has emotional problems or symptoms?

To what extent does the client recognize his own contribution to the problem?

Does the client blame other people or circumstances for his difficulties?

Does the client recognize his need for help?

Has the client any desire for help or treatment?

Is the client willing to assume self-responsibility for changing his behavior?

Abstract Thinking

Ask for interpretation of proverbs, such as Rome wasn't built in a day, or for identification of similarities between items, such as oranges and apples.

Attention

Observe for degree of distractibility, and ability to concentrate and cooperate with instructions during the interview. Testing for digit span recall can also be used. Ask the client to repeat some series of digits after you say them. Begin with a series of 3 numbers such as 8,4,1, reading them at the rate of about 1 per second, then allowing the client to repeat them. If the client succeeds, increase the number in the series by 1 until the client fails. When this occurs give the client another series of the same length to try again. Stop when the client is unable to succeed in two tries. Do not choose consecutive numbers or numbers that form easily recognized dates such as 1,9,8,8.

Communication

What is the client's rate of speech? Is it slower or faster than average?

Is the client mute?

Is the speech volume higher than normal conversation, or is it lowered to a whisper?

Does the client speak in a monotone (without any fluctuation in intonation)?

Is the client's speech clearly enunciated, or are some words slurred?

Does the client have noticeable speech impediments?

Does the client use *neologisms?*

Does the client talk freely, or does he respond to questions in monosyllables?

Is the client's speech pressured (rapid-fire) or *circumstantial* (roundabout)?

How well are the client's thoughts organized?

Are the client's thoughts coherent? Are the ideas logical, disorganized, or only loosely associated?

Flexibility-Rigidity

Does the client seem open to ideas different from his own?

Does the client become overly upset when his normal routine is disrupted, or does he adjust with relative ease to change?

Is the client able to make decisions based on logical reasoning, or is he unable to make up his mind on any issue?

Does the client seem too easily influenced by the ideas of others?

SOCIAL DIMENSION

Self-Concept

Describe yourself as a person, including your strengths and limitations.

Describe the kind of person you would like to be.

How do you compare in relation to other people?

If you could change something about yourself, what would it be?

Interpersonal Relations (family, work, school, community)

How and where does the client fit into these groups?

What roles does the client assume within these groups?

What are the role expectations placed on the client by the others in the groups?

Does the client measure up to the expectations?

How does the client feel about the expectations?

What are the client's expectations of himself in the various roles?

Is the client overextended or underachieving in these roles?

Who makes up the basic family unit?

Does the family contain the client's "significant other" relationships, or does the client consider people outside the family to be more important?

Within the family, who is supportive of the client? Competitive? Demeaning?

Who interacts with whom in the family? What is the nature of these interactions?

What is the pattern of communication within the family?

What role does the client play within the family? What roles do the other family members play?

How is conflict handled within the family?

What is the level of trust between family members?

How is the balance of dependence-independence distributed within the family?

Cultural Factors

Is the client a member of an identifiable ethnic group?

From an urban or rural background?

Continued.

HOLISTIC NURSING ASSESSMENT FORMAT—cont'd

Does the client observe traditions or customs? Describe them.
Does the client maintain a life-style congruent with the dominant societal culture? With the culture in which the client grew up?

Environmental Factors

Have client describe factors in his home, work, school, neighborhood, and community that contribute to his enjoyment and well-being. Have him describe those that contribute to his stress level.

Level of Socialization

Is the client overconforming to the point of sacrificing individuality?
Is the client nonconforming to the point of provoking society's intolerance?
Is the client experiencing difficulties such as legal problems or domestic violence?

Trust-Mistrust

Does the client appear to be generally or unusually naive about life, considering his age and developmental level?
Does the client seem to be vulnerable or easily taken advantage of?
Does the client describe a need for self-protection that seems out of proportion to the degree of threat that exists in the client's environment?
Does the client make statements about not trusting anyone?
Does the client seem to be suspicious of the interviewer?

Dependence-Independence

Does the client make statements like "I don't need anyone but myself"?
Does the client behave as though he has everything under control?
Does the client profess to be unable to make it through even minor stresses without the presence of certain people or things?
Does the client behave in a clinging manner toward other people?
Does the client frequently resort to whining?
Does the client give the impression of being either more or less dependent than would be expected for his age or developmental level?

SPIRITUAL DIMENSION
Philosophy of Life

Ask the client:
What meaning does life have for you?
What is important to you in life?
What do you believe about illness in general? For instance, do you believe you have any control over it?
Do you have any beliefs of a religious or spiritual nature about treating illness?
What do you believe about death?

Sense of Transcendence

Would you describe yourself as a pessimist or an optimist?
Do you think your life has become better or worse as you have grown older? Why?
Do you foresee that your life will be better or worse in the future?
Do you view the world as a generally friendly place or a hostile place?

Concept of Deity

Do you engage in any spiritual or religious practices? Describe them.
Are they the same practices you grew up with? If not, does this create any conflict for you?
Do you believe in any power greater than yourself? Describe your belief.
What is your relationship to the greater power?
Do you feel your spiritual beliefs provide you with support? Do they cause you any conflict?

Spiritual Fulfillment

How much control do you believe you have over what happens to you in life?
To what extent do you believe other forces play a role in what happens to you in life?
What are your special creative abilities?
Tell me what beauty means to you. What is there in the world that you consider beautiful?
Do you have a personal means for meeting your inner spiritual needs? Describe it.

---

pret the data to understand the dynamic relationships and patterns within the client's world. For example, the nurse will note that the lack of appropriate nutrition can influence the client's ability to tolerate stress, the client's developmental phase influences his response to hospitalization, the client's aging process influences his ability to benefit effectively from medication, the client's lack of spiritual identity or direction influences his ability to cope with the grieving process, and that the client's poor communication patterns influence his effectiveness in the work setting. Thus, by reviewing the data holistically, the nurse comes to an understanding of the client's needs and

concerns. These identified health concerns form the basis of the nursing diagnosis.

Analysis is the newest and least understood step of the nursing process. During the past 15 years, nursing leaders have invested considerable energy in developing a base of understanding for analysis. Their focus has been the development of a classification system of nursing diagnoses.

The work of two groups is of primary importance at a national level. The first is the North American Nursing Diagnosis Association (NANDA), originally called the National Group for the Classification of Nursing Diagnosis. The group has held a series of national conferences on nursing diagnoses since 1973. The work of this group has focused on the development of a basic taxonomy of nursing diagnoses without regard to specialty areas. The second is a task force appointed by the American Nurses' Association Council on Psychiatric and Mental Health Nursing to study and make recommendations on the Phenomena of Psychiatric and Mental Health Nursing. The task force is, at this time, working on a taxonomy of phenomena called Psychiatric Nursing Diagnosis I (PNDI).

The psychiatric nursing diagnosis is a two-part statement that describes the quality, content, and context of the client's health concern and its relationship to contributing factors. The first part of a nursing diagnosis, the stem, describes the broad category of the client's health concern and may apply to any number of clients. The statement, for example, "Spiritual Distress," is a nursing diagnosis stem. The second part of the diagnosis describes the relationship of the health concern to those factors that are related or contributing to it. The second part of the nursing diagnosis individualizes the diagnosis to a particular client. For example, "Spiritual distress related to loss of hope." Sample nursing diagnoses that are useful to psychiatric nurses are categorized according to the five dimensions of the person in the box below.

SAMPLE NURSING DIAGNOSES

PHYSICAL DIMENSION

Alteration in health maintenance
 (related to impaired judgment)
Sleep pattern disturbance
 (related to depressed mood)
Alteration in bowel elimination: diarrhea
 (related to ingestion of prescribed Lithium regimen)
Alteration in nutrition: less than body requirements
 (related to persistent self-induced vomiting)
Self-care deficit: feeding, bathing/hygiene, dressing/grooming
 (related to cognitive impairment)
Impaired physical mobility
 (related to perceptual impairment and body image disturbance)
Sexual dysfunction
 (related to trauma of childhood sexual abuse)
Disturbance in body image
 (related to unrealistic spatial perceptions)
Ineffective breathing pattern
 (related to hyperventilation associated with anxiety)

EMOTIONAL DIMENSION

Anxiety
 (related to situational crises)
Fear
 (related to phobic stimulus of closed spaces)
Dysfunctional grieving
 (related to persistent unresolved feelings of guilt about spouse's chronic illness)

INTELLECTUAL DIMENSION

Diversional activity deficit
 (related to lack of motivation and initiative associated with depression)
Sensory-perceptual alterations
 (related to narrowed perceptual fields associated with severe anxiety)
Alteration in thought processes
 (related to memory deficit and impaired judgment)
Impaired verbal communication
 (related to psychotic thought process)
Knowledge deficit
 (related to denial of a need for and refusal to accept information about prescribed medication)

SOCIAL DIMENSION

Social isolation
 (related to atypical social behavior and avoidance of interpersonal interactions)
Disturbance in self-esteem
 (related to perceived loss of status)
Disturbance in role performance
 (related to conflict about the demands and expectations of multiple roles)
Ineffective individual coping
 (related to separation from established support system)
Ineffective family coping: disabling
 (related to highly ambivalent family relationships)
Ineffective family coping: compromised
 (related to exhaustion of supportive capabilities from prolonged chronicity of mental illness)
Family coping: potential for growth
 (related to acceptance of need for psychiatric treatment)
Alteration in parenting
 (related to deterioration of marital relationship)
Impaired home maintenance management
 (related to impaired cognitive functioning)
Potential for violence: directed at others
 (related to overt expression of rage through physical aggression)
Noncompliance
 (related to basic mistrust of caregivers)
Powerlessness
 (related to physical deterioration and resulting increased dependency)

SPIRITUAL DIMENSION

Spiritual distress
 (related to loss of hope as a response to intense suffering)
Potential for violence: self-directed
 (related to a perceived helplessness and hopelessness)

The conceptual framework forms the basis for analysis just as it does for the other steps of the nursing process. The conceptual framework determines the categories in which the data are organized. The holistic model provides this framework for understanding the relationships among the data and for developing the nursing diagnoses.

Once the data are categorized, the nurse examines them to determine patterns. Gaps in data collection areas in which the information is insufficient to make an interpretation are identified. Data are compared with standards, norms, values, and expectations to identify the existence of actual or potential health concerns. At this point the nurse gives priority to the client's wishes, values, and culture in determining what data need to be taken into account or emphasized and what action needs to be considered. Once health concerns are identified, the nurse establishes a causal, or etiological, relationship by exploring the factors that are influencing or contributing to the client's health concerns.

As nursing diagnoses are developed for each client, they are listed in order of priority. As the client and nurse interact, more information becomes available and new insights and patterns emerge. What initially seemed like a minor problem may assume higher priority as the full implication of its relationship to the client's current concern emerges.

Mental health–psychiatric nurses use nursing diagnoses to provide direction for therapeutic nursing interventions and evaluation. They encounter the use of the DSM-III-R Classification system of psychiatric diagnoses in clinical practice and thus need to understand how it is used. The essential features of the disorder described in the DSM-III-R contribute to the nurse's understanding of the psychiatric diagnosis. These features are required to make the specific diagnosis. The psychiatrist uses the DSM-III-R as a guide to psychiatric diagnosis and treatment of the client. The psychiatric nurse can make a contribution to the psychiatrist's diagnostic process by communicating clinical observations and other relevant information collected about the client. The nurse can benefit from the psychiatrist's diagnosis by using the information and implications it has for developing nursing diagnoses and care plan. The client's diagnoses may provide the nurse with a substantial body of information, but it is an incomplete base of information for the nursing process. The practice of psychiatry and psychiatric nursing are different but complementary. The client benefits from a coordinated interface of the two disciplines.

DSM-III-R diagnoses. The psychiatric diagnoses for the client are identified according to the guidelines of the revised edition of the *Diagnostic and Statistical Manual of Mental Disorders* (DSM-III-R). Published in 1987 by the American Psychiatric Association, the DSM-III-R is the most current classification system for mental disorders in clinical use. The most outstanding feature of the DSM-III-R is the multiaxial approach to classification of mental disorders, in which each client is assessed on each of five different axes.

The five axes are briefly described here, and examples of each are given in Appendix A, but the DSM-III-R manual offers a more thorough explanation of the system and how it is used. Axis I describes the clinical syndrome or illness and conditions not attributable to mental illness that will be the focus of treatment or attention. Axis II describes the personality disorder or specific developmental disorder. Axis III describes possible physical disorders and conditions. Axis IV describes the severity and type of psychosocial stressors that the client has experienced within the past year or that pertain to the mental disorder. Axis V describes the global assessment of functioning.

Following are some of the advantages of the DSM-III-R over previous classification systems.[43]

1. It is compatible with a holistic view of the client, and it represents a more comprehensive approach to the biological, social, and psychological aspects of the client.
2. It promotes interdisciplinary communication.
3. It allows consideration of the clients strengths and problems.
4. It uses a descriptive phenomenological approach to assessing each client.

Planning

Purposes of the therapeutic plan. The plan of care guides the nursing-client action. It sets forth the goals to be achieved and defines the goals in terms of the behavior that will help achieve them. It also defines the priorities that pertain to various goals and actions. Just as the assessment experience can be therapeutic for some clients, the process of planning and working through the decisions to be made can also be helpful

Planning offers an opportunity for the client to learn about his personal health and behavior. The nurse's expectations for client participation in the plan needs to take into consideration the client's strengths and resources, coping mechanisms, and adaptive skills as well as his maturational and intellectual abilities. The extent to which the client is in contact with reality determines the degree to which he can participate in the planning process. Some clients with psychiatric problems may choose not to participate in defining goals for treatment because they believe they are not ill. Throughout the planning process the nurse needs to involve the client, his family, and other health team members.

The ultimate purpose of the plan is to guide the proposed intervention. In situations involving a number of staff members, the plan coordinates efforts and protects the client from random or conflicting interventions. The plan also provides the baseline for evaluation, which will be considered in more detail later in this chapter. The short-term goals, long-term goals, and outcome criteria need to be individualized, taking into consideration whether the client's problem is acute or chronic. To be realistic, nursing goals (1) are formulated from well-grounded nursing assessments and diagnoses, (2) are stated clearly in terms of client behaviors, (3) arise from an awareness of current client coping deficits, and (4) from an awareness of the client's potential for growth, ability to integrate gained insight, and need for behavioral

TABLE 8-3 Examples of nursing diagnoses, long-term and short-term goals, and outcome criteria

Goals	Outcome Criteria

NURSING DIAGNOSIS: ANXIETY RELATED TO FEAR OF DISAPPROVAL

Long-term goal

The client will verbally express his opinions in interpersonal situations without experiencing a sense of internal panic within 3 months.	Client will begin the assertiveness training workshop on 6/17. Completion date is 7/30. Client will make one comment to a stranger in the office coffee shop every morning about the weather, from 6/18 through 6/22. Client will attend and participate in the bimonthly meetings of the local Toastmasters Club, beginning 6/26.

NURSING DIAGNOSIS: POTENTIAL FOR VIOLENCE DIRECTED AT OTHERS RELATED TO OVERT EXPRESSION OF RAGE (THROUGH PHYSICAL AGGRESSION)

Short-term goal

The client will not exhibit acts of physical aggression for 48 hours.	Client will tolerate the presence of other persons in the dayroom for four periods of 15 to 30 minutes each day without exhibiting acts of physical aggression. Client will engage in verbal interaction with a selected client for two 5-minute periods without exhibiting physical aggression within the next 48 hours.

changes. Examples of nursing diagnoses, goals, and outcome criteria are presented in Table 8-3.

Completeness of goal statements. A nursing goal is a statement of a desired, achievable outcome to be attained within a predicted period based on the current situation and resources.[28] Without realistic and attainable goals, direction is lost, purpose for intervening is obscured, and evaluation of effectiveness is rendered impossible.

For ensured completeness in composition of goal statements, realiance on the investigative process is warranted. This process involves finding the "who, what, when, where, and how" of the situation.

Who is *always* the client. Nursing goals are stated in terms of the client; nursing interventions are the measures undertaken by the nursing staff to facilitate client goal attainment. Stating goals using the clients name reminds the nurse to ask the following questions:

1. Is it, in fact, a goal for the client?
2. Is it, in fact, individualized for this specific client? This facile safeguard is one small way to mobilize or to maintain actively practiced theoretical principles.

What is the action verb used to specify the behavior to be undertaken by the client. These verbs need to be carefully chosen to minimize subjectivity that increases the risk of variability and ineffectual evaluation. Especially to be avoided are the nonspecific verbs of "will understand" and "will know." Objective action verbs permit evaluation based not on beliefs or guesswork but on observable behavior.

How and *how much* refer to the verb modifier, reflectig the manner in which the client will carry out the behavior. The modifier allows for greater accuracy and precision by identifying, if necessary, any conditional requirement or restriction of the behavioral outcome. Type, degree, or amount are the usual considerations to further describe the action verb, for example: Client will walk _____ briskly, or client will drink _____ 1,500 ml.

It is important to remember to include the verb modifier only if it adds clarity and enhances the meaning and focus of the action. It will only confuse the caregiver if the goal is stated, "Client will eat heartily." Does the nurse then concentrate efforts on the client's food intake or the client's mood or affect during mealtime? Perhaps more helpful would be the statement, "Client will eat three fourths of all food served at mealtime." This modifying clause clarifies the behavioral outcome to be measured.

Where also serves the purpose of clarifying specific restrictions or requirements of the designated client behavior. Again, this may not always add relevance to the goal statement; therefore consideration is given to the reason for these types of modifiers. Client will sing a solo _____ in the music room, or client will initiate one 5-minute conversation _____ in the meeting room.

When represents specification of the time interval or target date for completion of the client behavior indicated by the action verb. It may also provide information about the action to be taken by the client, for example: "The client is to take Haldol, 10 mg p.o., at 9 AM and 6 PM daily."

The *when* serves a dual purpose in the following goal: "Client will take Haldol, 5 mg p.o., at 9 AM and 6 PM daily, without staff reminders, by 8/14." The two time specifications in this goal statement (9 AM and 6 PM, and 8/14) represent two very different types of *when* considerations. The date, 8/14, specifies the target date for completion of the goal. However, the times, 9 AM and 6 PM, specify instructions for the client action to be taken in pursuing the goal. *When* specifications may not always be used but need to be given consideration.

Short-term goals, long-term goals, and outcome criteria. Goal statements are generally divided into two categories: short term and long term. Short-term goals are typically considered to be more immediate, of smaller proportion, and the sequential steps necessary for achievement of the broader long-term goal. Months and years are usual measurement intervals for long-term goals, the directional indicators for the more tangible short-term goal statements. Goals that delineate target dates for the shift, the day, or the week are thought of as being short term in nature. Outcome criteria are the most definitive statements of the steps leading to the accomplishment of the short- and long-term goals (Table 8-3).

Reliance on sound problem-solving techniques adds credence to goal formulation. However, one of the most frequently committed errors of ommission in the practical application of the problem-solving approach to client care is this essential step of goal setting. For example, if the nurse assesses the client to be disoriented regarding time and place, the goal may be stated as:

Goal A: The client will respond correctly when questioned regarding time and place by 3/19.

or

Goal B: The client will locate the orientation board when questioned regarding time and place by 3/19.

The subtle difference between the preceding goal statements clearly reinforces the need for accurate identification of a nursing diagnosis based on nursing assessment. If the client's *disorientation* is a transient or acute condition rather than the result of a chronic brain syndrome, goal A obviously is a more reasonable statement of direction. Goal B would be more appropriate for the client whose recall and retention are more severely impaired. This example clearly depicts the necessity of goal setting to the entire directional process inherent in the therapeutic plan and in the provision of care.

Nursing goals frequently are not written in a realistic fashion. The goal will not facilitate client growth if it is conceived in unrealistic terms or negates current client functioning. The following example depicts the essential nature of discerning client ability before goal setting:

NURSING DIAGNOSIS	SHORT-TERM GOAL
Alteration in the thought processes related to depressive ideation	A. *Unrealistic:* The client will participate in dialogue with nurse for 15 minutes within 24 hours.
	B. *Realistic:* The client will participate in occupational therapy working on assigned project for 10 minutes daily within 24 hours.

Chronicity of illness has limited the client's ability for acquisition of age-appropriate socialization skills. Thus goal A clearly is unrealistic according to the baseline conversational skills of the client. It would serve only to increase the client's sense of frustration and inadequacy as he faced this insurmountable goal.

Goals need to be relevant to the pace set by the client for acquisition of desired behaviors. Conveyed expectations often influence the rapidity or retardation of the demonstration of gain. In the following example the nurse underestimates the client's ability for self-care, as well as minimizes his fairly immediate reliance on routine, by setting a 6-day deadline for achievement. Based on historical data and awareness of the client's strength in this area, the client will most realistically achieve the goal within 2 days.

NURSING DIAGNOSIS	SHORT-TERM GOAL
Self-care deficit related to depressed motivational level	A. *Unrealistic:* The client will shave, shower, and brush teeth daily before 9 AM without prompting within 6 days.
	B. *Realistic:* The client will shave, shower, and brush teeth daily before 9 AM without prompting within 48 hours.

A nursing goal, in essence is an up-to-date target for the client and nurse. Timing is indicated by the goal statement, which reflects an individualized, directional course of action. The desired behavior is identified, and all measures are geared toward attainment of the specified behavioral outcome. The nurse's ability to conduct a triage of client problems greatly aids in the maintenance of current goals and the pace at which the therapeutic efforts proceed, for example:

NURSING DIAGNOSIS	SHORT-TERM GOALS
Ineffective individual coping related to knowledge deficit about stress reduction techniques	A. *Unrealistic*
	1. The client will use autogenic relaxation exercises immediately after recognizing anxiety symptoms by 6/20.
	B. *Realistic*
	1. The client will participate twice daily for 3 days (6/20, 6/21, 6/22) in scheduled autogenic relaxation training workshops.
	2. The client will identify two prodromal symptoms, experienced repeatedly before onset of severe anxiety states, in discussions on 6/21.
	3. The client will use autogenic relaxation exercises immediately after recognizing anxiety, symptoms of restlessness, and tremulousness by 6/22.

The preceding exemplifies the obvious way in which nursing goals have an impact on the pace and currency of therapeutic endeavors. Goal A represents an overwhelming abstract conglomeration of several concrete, sequential goals, whereas goal B specifically defines a pace and course of action and increases the chance of accomplishment for the client.

The type of clinical setting influences the formulation of goal statements. The acute care facility uses time intervals from a much different perspective than does the extended care facility or the outpatient clinic. The average length of hospitalization on an acute care unit may be 3 to 7 days, whereas the length of stay in an extended care facility may average 3 to 7 years.

The focus of the setting affects the content and direction of the goal statement. Stabilization of a client experiencing a psychotic state or crisis is often the primary aim in an acute care unit, whereas the maintenance of optimal functioning, although at a reduced level, may be the focus in the long-term facility.

The cultural and social framework of the individual client influences the formulation and design of goals. Congruence with cultural expectations and norms is essential for effective action. For expample, many Native Americans avoid eye contact when conversing. Without consideration for their traditions and culture, the novice may assess this downward casting of eyes as indicative of low self-esteem. A goal or expected outcome may then be devised related to increased eye contact and social interaction as two behavioral indicators of an improved self-concept. However, in reality this custom conveys respect to the person with whom the conversation is being held. The appropriateness of goal statements clearly depends on the cultural values of the society in which the client was reared or currently resides.

Discharge planning. Discharge planning is a special area of planning that begins during the assessment phase of the nursing process with the first nurse-client contact. The assessment data that are important for discharge planning include:

1. The client's prognosis for recovery
2. The clients' mental status and current level of functioning in activities of daily living.
3. The client's DSM-III-R Axis V diagnosis. This information reflects the clients's highest level of adaptive functioning during the past year. These data can also be used as a baseline in determining a realistic goal for the clients level of functioning at discharge or postdischarge
4. The client's resources and potential resources (personal, social, community, economic)
5. The client's perception of their problems, needs, and resources
6. The client's expectations of health care providers
7. The client's plans for discharge or their expectation of the outcome of treatment.

Using the assessment data outlined in the previous list, the nurse collaborates with the client to establish realistic goals for discharge. Early nursing interventions increase the client's level of functioning and make his search for needed resources more successful. Later nursing interventions focus on need for referral and postdischarge treatment.

In any setting where multiple disciplines are involved in client care, multidisciplinary involvement in discharge planning is important. The nurse may assume responsibility for the coordination of this multidisciplinary activity. Conferences may be held for the purposes of sharing input or for group discharge planning.

Implementation

Nursing interventions are directives for specific behavior on the part of the nurse based on scientific rationale. Psychiatric nursing interventions are highly individualized and well grounded in the theories of human behavior. When the planning process for nursing strategies includes the client, shared knowledge and the quality of interaction are enhanced. Other basic considerations for design of nursing actions include restrictions in the setting supplies, and resources. The best-laid plans are of little relevance if the equipment or personnel necessary are not available, or if costs are too prohibitive to implement them.

Nursing is a unique practice that can be demonstrated through concise and well written intervention statements. Nursing orders are statements of nursing intervention.

Documentation of the intervention statement requires as much attention to composition and descriptiveness as is necessary for the goal statement. Each nursing order is dated and initialed by the nurse when added to the therapeutic plan. The following questions are helpful for the nurse to keep in mind when composing nursing interventions:

Does the intervention address *who, what, how, where,* and *when?*

Is the intervention written specifically so that another team member is able to carry out the action effectively?

Is a target date for completion indicated?

Does the intervention allow for evaluation?

Does the nursing intervention facilitate client goal attainment?

Have other interventions been reviewed, revised, and updated?

Considerations of the five dimensions of the person and age-specific tasks for the individual client are inherent in all nursing actions. To increase the chance of success and provide positive reinforcement, maximization of individual strengths and effective coping skills are built into the strategy from the onset.

Evaluation

Evaluation begins in the assessment phase of the nursing process, where it focuses on comparing the client's health status against criteria for "normal" functioning and development. It continues when the goals are established for the client's care. The monitoring of changes in the client's behavior and the effect these changes have on the client's overall health status continues in everyday practice.

The nurse begins to evaluate how the client responds to professional attention—the opportunity to be heard and to vent feelings. The client, too, is involved in the evaluation process from the start. The individual's subjective experience of changes in mood or thoughts serves to corroborate observations the nurse or others may make of his behavior.

Changing behavior is usually a slow process. In a real sense, only the client can change his behavior. Sometimes, as in crises, the changes in the client's behavior are quick and dramatic. Nurses depend on client feedback to evaluate how well the nursing care plan is working.

The evaluation includes data from many sources, including the client and the family. The family has the advantage of knowing the client over time. They frequently can detect the small differences that are a sign of significant progress.

Two types of evaluation are particularly pertinent in clinical practice: formative evaluation and summative evaluation. *Formative evaluation* describes judgments made about the effectiveness of the nursing interventions as they are implemented. These judgments are used to make immediate modifications in nursing care of the client, when necessary. *Summative evaluation* involves judgments about the effectiveness of nursing care when it is terminated. It involves a retrospective review of the entire course of care, and it measures the extent to which the goals for the client's care were achieved. Summative evaluation requires the establishment of outcome criteria for the client's care.

In general the purpose of all evaluation is the improvement of nursing service to the client. As psychiatric nursing continues to expand its range of practice, it must address the issue of accountability and increase the evaluation skills of its practitioners. Beginning skills in evaluation are learned through use of the nursing process. If applied diligently, they will provide a strong impetus to improving nursing practice.

RECORDING

Documentation is a written record of the nursing process and an important tool for the nurse. The recording provides a visible baseline and feedback mechanism for the nurse engaged in using the nursing process. It also offers the nurse a means of communicating about nursing practice with other professionals involved in the client's care.

Many methods and formulas have been designed for recording, including the nursing care plan, the narrative record, and the problem-oriented record (POR). Factors such as setting, role function, and client population determine which method the nurse uses. Whichever one is used, each component of the process—assessment, analysis, planning, implementation, and evaluation—is addressed.

Narrative Record

The narrative record is constructed according to chronological order beginning with an admission entry and continuing with entries that are written at least once each shift or after any significant occurence. The notes include observations or other important client data collected, nursing interventions that are implemented, and client responses to the interventions. The narrative record is contained within the client's larger chart in a section commonly entitled "nurse's notes." A major disadvantage of this approach is the lack of structure and organization of information to facilitate the recording of the nursing process. In recent years, the narrative record has been replaced by the more structured problem-oriented record.

Problem-Oriented Record (POR)

The problem-oriented method of recording is being used more frequently as a method for documenting nursing care. Following are the primary advantages of the POR:

1. It complements use of the nursing process.
2. It provides organization and coordination of information.
3. It facilitates evaluation of the quality of care.

Regardless of variance in terms and organizational detail, the POR has four basic components. The components parallel the five steps of the nursing process and are as follows:

1. The *data base* comprises the information collected during the assessment step of the nursing process. The assessment data may be compiled in the format of the holistic nursing assessment tool composed of the five dimensions of the client (see the box on pp. 149-152).

2. The *comprehensive problem list* is formulated during the analysis step of the nursing process. Each entry on the list is dated, numbered, and titled. The problem titles form the nursing diagnoses, which represent a more thorough process of analysis.

DATE	NUMBER	TITLE
2-25-87	1	Depressed mood
2-25-87	2	Anxiety
2-25-87	3	Ineffective individual coping

3. *Initial plans* reflect the planning step of the nursing process. The plans are written for each problem on the problem list. Each entry is dated, numbered, and titled to match the corresponding problem in the problem list. The initial plan for each problem is subdivided into five parts:

a. Subjective data include verbal information from the client and significant others. The data are recorded as direct quotes or as paraphrases with the source of the information indicated. The letter *S* is used to index the entry of subjective data:

   S *Client states, "I feel so nervous and shaky inside."*

b. Objective data include information about the client collected through observation, measurement, and sources such as written rocords of other health care workers. The source of the data is indicated. The letter *O* is used to index the entry of objective data:

   O *Client is observed to be fidgety and restless with shortened attention span and narrowed perceptual field during the initial interview.*

c. Assessment statement is a succinct analysis of the subjective and objective data. The most concise form of assessment statement is the nursing diagnosis. It may also include more detail, such as the reason for the problems and interpretation of the data. The letter *A* is used to index the entry of the assessment statement:

   A *Client's anxiety is related to his inability to express feelings and is exhibited as constricted, controlled affect.*

d. Plans include the long-term goals and the short-term goal statements with accompanying outcome criteria and planned nursing interventions. The letter *P* is used to index the entry of the plans.

4. *Progress notes* reflect the implementation and evaluation steps of the nursing process as well as a recycling to earlier steps of the process such as further assessment, analysis, or revision of plans as they pertain to a particular problem. The entry of each progress note is dated, numbered, and titled to correspond with the matching problem from the problem list and initial plans. Progress notes consist of four parts, which are titled and indexed in a form identical to that of the initial plans—SOAP.

> **S** *Update on subjective data included in the initial plans or new subjective data pertaining to the problem*
>
> **O** *Update on objective data included in the initial plans or new objective data pertaining to the problem*
>
> **A** *Substantiation of the analysis included in the initial plans, revision of the analysis, and factors such as interpretations of the effects of medication, nursing interventions, and progress or prognosis of the client*
>
> **P** *Intent to follow the plans as outlined in the initial plans or a revision or proposal of plans*

The format of a progress note is as follows:

DATE	NUMBER	TITLE
2-25-87	2	Anxiety

> **S** *Client states, "I don't feel quite so nervous and shaky today."*
>
> **O** *Client was observed to engage in a 30-minute period of task-oriented activity without notable restlessness. Attention span and ability to perceive the requirements of the task were adequate.*
>
> **A** *Client's anxiety level is beginning to decrease. As yet, there is no indication of any change in client's inability to express other emotional states.*
>
> **P** *Continue with nursing care as outlined in initial plans.*

BRIEF REVIEW

The nursing process is a systematic problem-solving method used within the framework of the nurse-client relationship. The problem-solving method and the interpersonal relationship comprise the foundation of nursing practice. Nurses have developed and refined the nursing process over the past 30 years. Concurrently psychiatric nurses have been in the forefront developing the concept of the nurse-client relationship. More recently the concept of holistic nursing has emerged on the nursing frontier.

The nursing process begins with assessment. Assessment involves the collection of data from the five dimensions of the client—physical, emotional, intellectual, social, and spiritual—as seen through the holistic nursing model. The data from these dimensions are categorized and collated for the purpose of analysis, the second phase of the process.

During analysis, the data are examined to determine gaps, incongruities, patterns, associations, and relationships. This is repeated for all five dimensions. Next, areas of concern are identified that reflect problems with the client's health status. Nursing diagnoses are then formulated as statements of the client's health concerns.

Based on the analysis and nursing diagnoses, the planning phase of the process begins. The purposes of the plan are to provide communication, individualization, and continuity of nursing care. The direction of the plan is determined by the goal statements: short-term goals, long-term goals, and outcome criteria. These goals outline sequential behavioral steps that lead to the accomplishment of the desired outcome. From the goal statements nursing interventions are derived. These nursing interventions define the action of the nurse in assisting the client to accomplish the goal. Implementation of nursing care follows planning. In this phase of the process, the planned nursing interventions are enacted.

The final phase of the nursing process is evaluation. At this point, the nurse compares the actual outcome with the projected goals. However, evaluation is more pervasive than this. Since the nurse is constantly using current feedback to determine the effectiveness of the process and the dirdection in which to proceed, evaluation is actually a thread through all the other phases. Throughout the nursing process, the nurse and client interact, collaborate, and animate this dynamic problem-solving system within the interpersonal space they share.

REFERENCES AND SUGGESTED READINGS

1. American Psychiatric Association: Diagnostic and statistical manual of mental disorders (DSM-III-R), Washington, D.C., 1987, The Association.
1a. Austad, C.S., and others: Treatment implication of the post discharge contact, Hospital and Community Psychiatry **37**(8):839, 1986.
2. Barry, P.D.: Psychosocial nursing assessment and intervention, Philadelphia, 1984, J.B. Lippincott, Co.
3. Bauer, B.B., and Hill, S.S.: Essentials of mental health care: planning and intervention, Philadelphia, 1986, W.B. Saunders, Co.
4. Blattner, B.: Holistic nursing, Englewood Cliffs, N.J., 1981, Prentice-Hall, Inc.
5. Bockrath, M.: Your patient needs two diagnoses—medical and nursing, Nursing Life **2**:29, 1982.
6. Boettcher, E.: Nurse-client collaboration: dynamic equilibrium in the nursing care system, Journal of Psychosocial Nursing and Mental Health Services **16**(12):7, 1978.
7. Bower, F.L.: the process of planning nursing care: nursing practice models, ed. 3, St. Louis, 1982, The C.V. Mosby Co.
8. Brallier, L.: Transition and transformation: successfully managing stress, San Francisco, 1982, National Nursing Review Inc.
9. Carnevali, D., and others: Diagnostic reasoning in nursing, Philadelphia, 1984, J.B. Lippincott Co.
10. Carnevali, D.: Nursing care planning: diagnosis and management, Philadelphia, 1983, J.B. Lippincott Co.
11. Carpenito, L.J.: Nursing diagnosis: application to clinical practice, Philadelphia, 1983, J.B. Lippincott Co.
12. Carpenito, L.J.: Handbook of nursing diagnoses, Philadelphia, 1984, J.B. Lippincott Co.
13. Carpenito, L.J.: Is the problem a nursing diagnosis? American Journal of Nursing **84**:1418, 1984.

14. Carpenito, L.J.: Actual, potential, or possible? American Journal of Nursing, **85**:458, 1985.

15. Carpenito, L.J., and Duespohl, T.A.: A guide for effective clinical instruction, ed. 2, Rockville, Md. 1985, Aspen Systems Corp.

16. Flynn, P.: Holistic health, Bowie, Md., 1982, Robert J. Brady Co.

16a. Fraser, R.: The nursing process—a core concept for mental handicap nursing, Nursing 2(37):1096, 1985.

17. Geach, B.: The problem-solving technique, Perspectives in Psychiatric Care **12**:9, 1974.

18. Gordon, M., and McKeehan, K.: Nursing diagnosis: looking at its use in the clinical area, American Journal of Nursing, **80**:672, April, 1980.

19. Gordon, M.: Nursing diagnosis, New York, 1982, McGraw-Hill Book Co.

20. Griffith, J.W., and Christensen, P.J., editors: Nursing process: application of theories, frameworks, and models, ed. 2, St. Louis, 1986, The C.V. Mosby Co.

21. Johnson, D.: The behavioral system model for nursing. In Riehl, J., and Roy, C. editors: Conceptual models for nursing practice, ed. 2, New York, 1980, Appleton-Century-Crofts.

21a. Johnston, J.: The nursing process and psychiatry, Nursing Mirror **158**:1, 1984.

22. Kim, M., McFarland, G. and McLane, A.: Pocket guide to nursing diagnoses, ed. 2, St. Louis, 1987, The C.V. Mosby Co.

23. Kim, M., McFarland, G., and McLane, A.: Classification of nursing diagnoses: Proceedings of the fifth conference, St. Louis, 1984, The C.V. Mosby Co.

23a. Kitson, A.: Standard of care in psychiatric nursing, Nursing Times 82(52):51, 1987.

24. Krall, M.L.: Guidelines for writing mental health treatment plans, American Journal of Nursing **76**:236, 1976.

25. Krieger, D.: Foundations for holistic health nursing practices: the Renaissance nurse, Philadelphia, 1981, J.B. Lippincott Co.

26. Lancaster, J.: Adult psychiatric nursing, Garden City, N.Y., 1980, Medical Examination Publishing Co., Inc.

27. Larkins, P.D., and Backer, B.A.: Problem-oriented nursing assessment, New York, 1977, McGraw-Hill Book Co.

28. Little, D.E., and Carnevali, D.L.: Nursing care planning, ed. 2, Philadelphia, 1976, J.B. Lippincott Co.

29. McFarland, G.K., and Apostoles, F.E.: The nursing history in a psychiatric setting: adaptations to a variety of nursing care patterns and patient populations, Journal of Psychosocial Nursing and Mental Health Services **13**:12,1975.

29a. McFarland, G., and Wasli, E.: Nursing diagnoses and process in psychiatric mental health nursing, Philadelphia, 1986, J.B. Lippincott Co.

30. Mundinger, M., and Jauron, G.: Developing a nursing diagnosis, Nursing Outlook 23(2):94, 1975.

31. Newman, M.: Theory development in nursing, Philadelphia, 1979, F.A. Davis Co.

32. Newman, M.: Nursing diagnosis: looking at the whole, American Journal of Nursing, **84**:1496, 1984.

33. Orlando, I.J.: The dynamic nurse-patient relationship: function, process and principles, New York, 1961, The Putnam Publishing Group, Inc.

33a. O'Sullivan, A., and others: Discharge planning for the mentally disabled, Quarterly Review Bulletin 12(3):90, 1986.

34. Parsons, P.J.: Building better treatment plans, Journal of Psychosocial Nursing and Mental Health Service, 24(4):8, 1986.

35. Peplau, H.E.: Interpersonal relation in nursing: a conceptual frame of reference for psychodynamic nursing, New York, 1952, The Putnam Publishing Group, Inc.

36. Peplau, H.E.: In defense of nursing diagnosis (letter to editor), Nursing Outlook **32**:240, 1984.

37. Rittman, M.R, and others: Nursing diagnosis in psychiatric nursing, Florida Nurse 34(9):16, 1986.

37a. Robitaille-Tremblay, M.: A data collection tool for the psychiatric nurse, Canadian Nurse 80(7):26, 1984.

38. Schaffer, K.R.: Sex-role issues in mental health readings, Reading Mass., 1980, Addison-Wesley Publishing Co., Inc.

38a. Stanley, B.: Evaluation of treatment goals: the use of goal attainment scaling, Journal of Advances in Nursing 9(4):35, 1984.

39. Steele, S.: Educational evaluation in nursing, Thorofare, N.J., 1978, Slack, Inc.

39a. Stephenson, M.: Problem remains . . . trying to implement the nursing process in an acute area of psychiatry, Nursing Mirror **158**:1, 1984.

39b. Stockwell, F.: The nursing process in psychiatric nursing, London, 1985, Croom Helm Ltd.

40. Stoll, R.: Guidelines for spiritual assessment, American Journal of Nursing **79**:1574, 1979.

40a. Stone, K., and others: Making decisions . . . difficulties in applying the nursing process when trying to work with chronic problems, Nursing Mirror 158(1):2, 1984.

41. Thomas, M.D., Sanger, E., and Whitney, J.D.: Nursing diagnosis of depression, Journal of Psychosocial Nursing and Mental Health Services, **24**:6, 1986.

42. Watson, A.C.: Use of nursing diagnosis in group work with vietnam veterans, V.A. Nursing **54** (1):34, 1986.

42a. Whyte, L., and others: The nursing process in the care of the mentally ill, Nursing Times, 80(5):49, 1984

42b. Willard, C.: The story of John . . . how the nursing process can be applied to psychiatric illness, Nursing Mirror **158**:1, 1984.

43. Williams, J., and Wilson, H.; A psychiatric nursing perspective on DSM-III, Journal of Psychosocial Nursing and Mental Health Services 20(4):15, 1982.

44. Yura, H., and Walsh, M.: The nursing process, ed. 4, New York, 1983, Appleton-Century-Crofts.

ANNOTATED BIBLIOGRAPHY

Carnevali, D., and others: Diagnostic reasoning in nursing, Philadelphia, 1984, J.B. Lippincott Co.

A distinctive and concrete domain for nursing that has been field-tested is described. The authors then detail the diagnostic reasoning process developed by nurses at varying levels of expertise. A description of practicing clinicians applying the diagnostic reasoning process from a purely nursing perspective is given. The final sections deal with major professional issues involving the development of taxonomic structure and methods for studying the diagnostic reasoning process. Implications for nursing after diagnostic reasoning has become an explicit skill in professional nursing are outlined.

Carpenito, L.J.: Nursing diagnosis: application to clinical practice, Philadelphia, 1983, J.B. Lippincott Co.

The book is a detailed guide to the use of nursing diagnosis in clinical nursing practice. It describes the most highly developed approach to implementing a conceptual framework for nursing process. Beginning with a historical perspective on nursing process, the author proposes a method for distinguishing between nursing diagnoses and other problems in which nurses intervene. The steps of the nursing process are described. The major portion of the book is devoted to a manual of nursing diagnoses consisting of 43 diagnostic categories. Each category is described according to definition, etiological and contributing factors, defining characteristics, focus assessment criteria, nursing goals, and principles and rationale for nursing care.

Rawlins, R.P., and Heacock, P., editors: Psychiataric nursing: a manual for clinical practice, St. Louis, 1987, The C.V. Mosby Co.

This manual is a clinical guide to use in writing psychiatric nursing care plans. It includes 34 plans for a variety of behaviors that are seen in a psychiatric setting, and guidelines for taking a history. Case examples also depict the various behaviors.

CHAPTER 9

THE PERSON AS A CLIENT

Peggy A. Landrum   Ruth P. Rawlins

Cornelia Kelly Beck   Sophronia R. Williams

After studying this chapter the learner will be able to:

Discuss the historical development of the holistic approach to the person.

Describe the qualities of each dimension of the person.

Describe the person-environment relationship.

Describe the nature of stress and adaptation within each dimension of the person.

Discuss the impact of self-responsibility on health status.

The primary goal of nursing care is to assist the client in developing strategies to achieve harmony within himself and with others, nature, and the world. Emphasis is placed on the integrative functioning of the client's physical, emotional, intellectual, social, and spiritual dimensions. Each person is considered as a whole with many factors contributing to health and illness.

This chapter presents an overview of the person within the framework of holistic philosophy. The following general concepts of the holistic approach to health care are explored: (1) human dimensions, (2) relationship of the person with the environment, (3) stress and adaptation, and (4) self-responsibility. The chapter is intended to challenge the learner to consider the highly interactive nature of human functioning in relation to both health and illness.

HOLISTIC HEALTH CARE CONCEPTS

Several concepts are generally accepted as premises of a holistic orientation to health care. The general concepts discussed in this chapter are shown in Table 9-1.

Dimensions of the Person

The recognition of all human dimensions encourages a balanced and whole view of a person. Each facet of an individual is important and contributes to the quality of life experience. If either the person or others ignore any

facet, the person is less able to live in a balanced state. When this happens, fewer options are available to the individual. For instance, people who ignore their physical aspect probably are not able to take advantage of exercise as an outlet for emotional stress. If people do not develop their intellectual capacities, they may lack the knowledge and cognitive skills necessary for problem solving. If they do not recognize their spiritual component, they may be limiting their ability to construct meaningful life goals. Individuals create options for themselves by respecting their needs in each dimension and by developing each dimension as fully as possible. To the extent that they are willing to do this, they increase available alternatives regarding any life situation.

Although the dimensions are separated here for exploration purposes, we recognize that this is an artificial separation that can occur only in an analysis. In reality they are intricately interwoven, and the person as a whole functioning organism is more than the simple combination of dimensions.

Physical dimension. The physical aspect involves everything associated with one's body, both internal and external. Inputs to the body (such as food, water, and air), transformation of these inputs within the body, and outputs from the body (such as waste products, energy for exercise, and energy for healing) are included in the physical dimension.[11] Some issues related to this dimension are genetics, nutrition, breathing, touching, rest, body weight, the sleep/wake cycle, autoimmunological func-

DATE	EVENT
Ancient Times	Primitive people perceived their body as a dwelling place of the soul, and illness was seen as the result of malevolent spirits projecting some noxious object into the body.
	Indian and Chinese philosophers saw all of life as a whole, and the spirit was unseparated from the rest of the person.
400-300 BC	Plato contended that human beings possess a spirit with direct access to the realm of the nonphysical, seen in prophesy and healing.
	Aristotle distinguished between experiences that involved physical activities (sensations, appetites, passions) and those that involved activity of the soul (thinking).
1600s-1700s	Descartes suggested the body and mind were two different entities encouraging the establishment of medical systems in which physical problems were solved by dealing exclusively with the body and mental problems were approached by dealing with the mind.
	Repressive measures by the Church of England led a small religious group to separate from the main church and seek religious freedom. This group of separatists, or Puritans, believed that an austere life released their soul from bondage to the body and permitted union with a devine being.
1800s	William James proposed relationships between experiences that involved emotional stimulus, emotional behavior (visceral reactions and overt actions) and emotional experience.
1960s	The emergence of mass society identified by such factors as depersonalization, mechanization, and loss of individuality and privacy has promoted the view that people are a mass target of influence rather than individual human beings.
	The women's movement contributed to altering sex role differentiation particularly in areas of work and education.
	Dramatic changes were seen in childrearing practices, male and female roles, and concerns about the environment and the structure of society.
1980s	Research indicates that intellectual capacity is not predetermined, that individuals use less than half of their brain and that the decline in intellectual functioning can be prevented.
	Current health care models recognize the interrelationships of the mind, body, and environment.
Future	As the elderly population increases, nurses will need to provide holistic care to this population in an era of decreased funding.

tioning, energy, fitness, movement, body image, healing capacity of the body, stress reduction through physical activity and relaxation, and the physical environment. In this section genetics, physiological processes, and body image are selected for discussion because of the relevance of these concepts to mental health–psychiatric nursing.

Genetics involves a complex process through which individuals inherit particular characteristics, potentials, predispositions, and limitations. Hereditary factors in mental illness are typically investigated by twin studies, genetic marker studies, and adoption studies. Evidence of a genetic influence on psychiatric dysfunction is continually increasing. The contribution of heredity to the development of alcoholism, the major affective disorders, and schizophrenia have most often been studied, with some attention to the role of genetics in the development of

antisocial personality disorder. All of these disorders show tendencies to cluster in biological relatives, even when the related individuals do not grow and develop in the same family environments. Studies on familial clustering of various disorders support genetic theory.[55]

Currently, evidence supports the theory that heredity contributes to the potential for such disorders. However, the manifestation of symptoms and specific behaviors is then triggered by physiological, social, and environmental forces. Mental health–psychiatric nurses recognize that genetic influence is not absolute. Such risk can be modified or counteracted by other forces.

Sleep is necessary for good health, and sleep alterations can be one of the earliest indicators of behavioral and somatic disturbance. Two types of sleep occur: NREM (non-rapid eye movement) is a quiet sleep that encompasses

TABLE 9-1 Holistic health care concepts

Concept	Assumptions
Multidimensionality	Interaction and balance of the physical, emotional, intellectual, social, and spiritual dimensions is evident. Emphasis is on respect of needs and development of potential in each dimension.
Relationship with the environment	The person-to-environment interaction is a crucial factor in determining the quality of life experiences in both health and illness.
Self-responsibility	Each person is an active participant in the maintenance of optimal health status. The health care system cannot "make" people healthy; individuals choose their own life-styles and directions.
Life cycle development	Each person progresses through stages of life with particular needs, issues, feelings, and behaviors affecting that person at different times. It is helpful to realize that growth and development at any one stage affects later stages.
Stress and adaptation	An individual's ability to cope with stressful events is a primary factor in each person's experience of health and illness. Stressful conditions are unique to each person, may be experienced throughout the life cycle, and affect the whole person.

THE STAGES OF SLEEP

Stage 1	Twilight phase: person is easily aroused; lasts up to 30 minutes
Stage 2	Sound sleep, but person is aroused with ease
Stage 3	Deep level of sleep; strong stimulus is needed to wake person
Stage 4	Deepest phase of sleep, reached approximately 30 to 40 minutes after beginning stage 1
REM	Final stage of sleep cycle; person is difficult to arouse; dreaming and nightmares occur

the first four stages of sleep, and REM (rapid eye movement) is the active final stage of sleep, characterized by extremely rapid eye movement (see box at right.)

REM sleep is necessary for mental restorative processes, including learning, memory, and psychological adaptation. Emotional and mental stress increases the need for REM sleep. Decreased sleep time results in loss of REM sleep, for which the body tries to compensate by increasing REM sleep during the next sleep period. Chronic disruption of REM sleep interferes with healthy psychological functioning. Lack of sleep for prolonged periods can produce psychosis. Dysrhythm of sleep-rest activity can severely tire individuals and contribute to the experience of illusions and hallucinations.

Stage 4 sleep is necessary for physical restorative processes; thus strenuous physical activity creates additional need for Stage 4 sleep. Integumentary cellular renewal occurs during the deepest sleep period, usually midnight to 4 AM; constant disruption can significantly extend healing time.[27] Mental health–psychiatric nurses recognize the important role of adequate sleep cycles in overall functioning of their clients.

Body image is a significant aspect of the physical dimension. Body image addresses how the person views himself. This view of self is fairly well established by the end of toddlerhood and relatively fixed by the end of adolescence. Messages youngsters are given as they are maturing lay the foundation for the development of body image. Words such as "cute," "ugly," "strong," "weak," "awkward," "good," and "bad" are incorporated into an internalized visualization, the body image. Ideal body image and perceived body image constitute the physical aspect of the total self-concept. The body is considered by some to be the most significant avenue for expression of the total self.[42] It is the body that others see, that acts and demonstrates competencies, and that in these acts reveals emotions.

The way people perceive their physical bodies may also have important emotional consequences. A realistic body image may significantly enhance one's potential for successful achievement throughout life. When body image is not distorted, a correlation exists beween self-perception and the perception of others. Individuals who incorporate into their belief system a consistent, realistic, and stable body image are demonstrating their ability to appropriately assess reality.

One's body image—shape, size, mass, structure, and function and the significance of the body and its parts—is dynamic and open to change. Body image may change as alterations occur in the individual's anatomy or personality. For example, an adolescent girl may gain extra pounds if she constantly snacks on high-calorie foods to relieve anxious feelings. As she becomes aware of tight clothing, she may also become acutely aware of her excess body bulk and withdraw from selected social contacts until she returns to her original weight and shape.

The idea that personality is correlated with body build was introduced in the 1920s and further refined in the 1940s. Three basic body types were described: endomorph (pyknic), mesomorph (athletic), and ectomorph (esthetic).[64] The term *endomorph* denoted a round, soft body frequently associated with an affectionate, sociable personality, subject to mood swings. Traits attributable to the endomorph included love of comfort and eating, sociability, politeness, tolerance, and complacency. The athletic *mesomorph* was one of average size with a muscular build who preferred physical activity and displayed traits of assertiveness, love of adventure, courage, callousness, ruthlessness, and indifference to pain. Finally, the *ectomorph* was a tall, thin, fragile person, tending to possess a withdrawn temperament and demonstrating traits of restraint, privacy, secretiveness, and introversion. This system of correlating personality and body build is not universally accepted. However, there are different social reactions to these different body builds. The components of a person's body structure set up expectations about the person's abilities and greatly influence what the person can do.

The various aspects of the physical dimension interact constantly with each other. For instance, a person's nutritional status directly affects other areas such as energy, weight, and physiological processes. Eating excessive amounts of sugar is known to decrease energy levels and cause fatigue and shakiness. Heredity establishes certain parameters for physical growth and development. Exercise leads to better eating habits, better ability to sleep, weight control, improved cardiovascular and pulmonary functioning, joint flexibility, fewer injuries, faster healing response, fat reduction, increased energy, and stamina.

A person's physical dimension affects emotions, intellectual functioning, social experiences, and even spirituality. Physical fitness is associated with an improved body image, positive attitudes, self-confidence, a decreased number of periods of depression, greater ability to relate to other people, increased assertiveness, and an increased number of spiritual experiences. Physical activity is an effective way of counteracting emotional stress and tension. Factors such as body image, physical energy, and sexuality affect social interactions. In general, when people neglect themselves physically, they limit their potential in other areas as well; everyone has experienced how difficult it is to be sociable, to have fun, to think clearly, or to laugh and play when not feeling well physically.

The degree to which people experience physical well-being is an indicator of how effectively they are taking care of their total selves, as well as how effectively they are integrating the healthy aspects of their other four dimensions—emotional, intellectual, social, and spiritual.

❋ *Emotional dimension.*

Terms such as mood, emotion, and affect are used interchangeably by professionals and lay persons. Dozens of instruments are designed to measure emotional states, and a multitude of descriptive terms are used to describe moods and emotions. This richness of language reflects the importance of this dimension to our culture. In this book, the term "emotional" rather than "psychological" is used to describe this dimension. "Psychological" implies a combination of emotional and intellectual components, whereas "emotional" refers to affective states and feelings. In general, *emotion* refers to a fleeting feeling, *mood* refers to a prolonged feeling, and affect represents the observable manifestation of a person's feelings. Some terms commonly used to describe mood include those in the box at upper right.

The various theories of emotion attempt to integrate three components: the motor behavior associated with emotion (what is expressed), the experienced aspect

TERMS USED TO DESCRIBE MOOD	
Angry	Lonely
Anxious	Mad
Bored	Mean
Calm	Miserable
Cheerful	Outraged
Confused	Pained
Despairing	Pleasant
Distraught	Relaxed
Enraged	Remorseful
Exasperated	Sad
Fearful	Scared
Frightened	Solemn
Furious	Stunned
Grieving	Terrified
Happy	Worried
Infuriated	

(what is felt), and the physiological mechanisms that underlie emotions (what happens inside the body). Although emphasis varies, each of the components receives attention in most existing theories of emotion.

All theories of emotion accept the idea that the activation of the physiological systems (the parasympathetic and sympathetic nervous systems, the limbic system, and the reticular formation) is correlated with emotional experiences and that cognitive processes mediate emotional experiences. A second characteristic of most theories of emotion is the concept of an adaptation level, described as a physiological or cognitive state that assists the individual in maintaining homeostasis. A third common element suggest that a social, related event can elicit and define the nature of a particular emotional experience, such as fear in response to a loss of power. None of the theories of emotion views individuals as passive receptacles of emotional experiences.

Emotional experiences are actively constructed by *appraisal processes;* some emotional experiences are actively sought, and others are avoided. These appraisal processes are determined partially by learned patterns of response. One person may react to a particular situation with fear, whereas another reacts with anger. A final persistent theme in theories of emotion is the idea that control plays a role in determining emotional experiences. Individuals can maximize positive feelings and minimize negative feelings by exercising control, whether over social events or the rate of stimulation.

Emotion is defined in the following manner for purposes of this book: (1) emotion is affective and includes a feeling element or awareness; (2) the central nervous system and the autonomic nervous system are involved in emotion by producing motor, glandular, and visceral activities; and (3) emotion is related to motivation as an energizer of behavior.[35]

The first component of emotion is the affective property. *Affect* is the individual's observable manifestation of

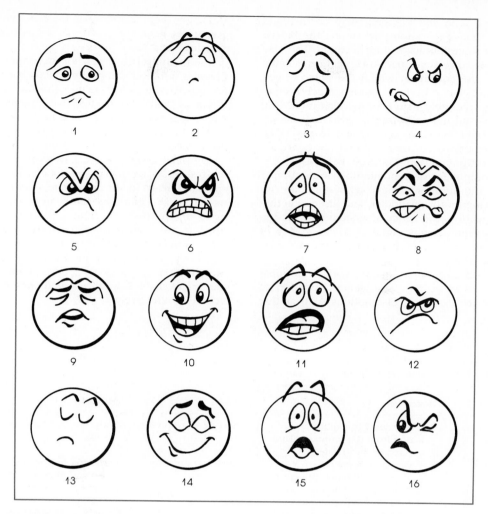

FIGURE 9-1 Facial expressions that demonstrate mood. *1,* anxious; *2,* arrogant; *3,* bored, *4,* concentrating; *5,* disapproving; *6,* enraged; *7,* frightened; *8,* frustrated; *9,* grieving; *10,* happy; *11,* horrified; *12,* negative; *13,* prudish; *14,* satisfied; *15,* surprised; *16,* suspicious.

his feelings. Observation of behavior, including posture, facial expressions (Figure 9-1), tone of voice, gestures, crying, sweating, and clenched fists, provides objective data about one's affect.

The feeling element, or awareness of feeling, is perhaps the most commonly recognized aspect of the emotional dimension. Feelings may be more difficult to conceptualize than the physical realm because they are less tangible, but they are still a vital part of each person. Feelings such as joy, anger, sadness, and fear occur most naturally in young children, who are not yet restricted by many *should's* and *should not's* regarding the experience and expression of feelings. Adults, however, often attach judgments to their feelings, and consequently ignore the ones with which they are uncomfortable. Certain cultures are more likely to label particular feelings as good or bad, but all feelings are subject to being ignored at one time or another. For example, a person may not feel joy if it seems

"undeserved." Anger may be ignored because it is considered "impolite." Sadness, or grief, may not be acknowledged when it "makes someone else uncomfortable." Fear may be suppressed because of a need to "be strong." Feelings in themselves are neither good nor bad; they simply are a part of human experience. Because each individual has the capacity to experience the entire realm of feelings, they are meant to be experienced, not ignored. In ignoring or suppressing feelings, people limit their opportunities to function as whole persons.[53]

Feelings provide people with a way of staying in touch with themselves, with what pleases them and what does not. Often they may be one's first source of information about what is going on and about how one is responding or wants to respond to a situation. The emotionally aroused person generally has an awareness of his own feelings; excited, afraid, angry or joyful.

Individuals learn at an early age how to express feelings. Words, voice tone and volume, body posture and movements, and facial expressions are among the behaviors people use to communicate their feelings. The way that an individual expresses a particular feeling is influenced greatly by the culture in which the person lives. Studies have found that American women receive emotional cues more accurately than do American men. One explanation is that during socialization girls are encouraged to express their emotions openly and to pay close attention to the emotions of others, whereas boys are actively discouraged from engaging in these behaviors.[1]

The second component of the definition of emotion is that the central and autonomic nervous systems are involved in producing motor, glandular, and visceral activities. During stimulation, the reticular system and the hypothalamus send simultaneous impulses to the cortex of the brain and to the viscera; these impulses result in physiological changes (Table 9-2).

Physiological changes that occur with emotional arousal are referred to as the "emergency" function of emotions. The physical aspects of emotions such as fear and anger seem to help individuals survive in case of danger. Stress responses such as increased heart rate, blood pressure, and rate of breathing make available an increased supply of oxygen for strenuous muscle activity. Changes in blood composition make more sugar available for quick energy and cause clotting in case of injury. Blood is taken from digestive organs and distributed where it is needed most. Pupil response produces greater visual acuity. Increased perspiration carries away waste products of intense muscle action.

The final component of emotion is its relationship to motivation as an energizer of behavior. The Latin word *emovere* means to stir up, agitate, excite, and move. To be moved in an emotional sense means to "stir up oneself" or to be "pushed." At times, emotion not only stirs one up, but also causes one to push (motivate) oneself.[48] When a person experiences emotions such as fear and anger, body resources are mobilized to meet emergencies. Mobilization of resources as described in the preceding paragraph enables the threatened person to either fight or flee more effectively.

TABLE 9-2 Summary of physiological changes that may occur with emotional arousal

Change	Description	Change	Description
Increase in heart rate	The increased epinephrine released from the pituitary gland accelerates heart rate.	Increase in respiration	Both rate and depth of breathing accelerate
Increase in blood pressure	The increased heart rate may cause a rise in blood pressure. Other changes take place in the distribution of blood. A greater volume is made available to the lungs and muscles, and internal organs receive less. Flushing of the face and neck during anger and blushing during embarrassment result from these changes in blood pressure and circulation.	Gastrointestinal changes	Peristaltic movements of the stomach and intestines may cease. The flow of digestive juices, including saliva, decrease, producing feelings of dry mouth and being "sick to the stomach" and a lack of appetite.
Muscle tension tremor	Muscle tone is increased. Tremor ("knocking of the knees") often occurs when opposing groups of muscles are contracted simultaneously.	Galvanic skin response (GSR)	Minute but detectable changes occur in the electric properties of the skin. These can be recorded and measured by means of an instrument called a galvanometer. An electrode is attached to the skin, usually the palms of the hands. A swing of the instrument's needle indicates a GSR. GSR is a sensitive indicator of changes in emotional state and is used as one component of the lie detector test. Blood pressure and rate of respiration also are monitored in persons taking a lie detector test.
Changes in blood composition	The amount of blood sugar, the acid-base balance, and the epinephrine (adrenalin) content of the blood are significantly increased.		
Increase in perspiration	Shaking hands with a person provides a quick and fairly reliable indication of the degree of emotional tension the person is experiencing by the presence or absence of perspiration.	Pilomotor response	This is the technical term for "goose pimples": the small hairs on the skin rise.
		Pupil response	The pupils of the eye tend to dilate.

Emotional states are significantly determined by cognitive factors. When individuals are physiologically aroused, they label, interpret, and identify their stirred-up state according to the precipitating situation. What is perceived in the immediate situation is interpreted through past experience; this provides the means by which a feeling is labeled and understood. The same increase in heart rate, rapid breathing, and trembling can be experienced as "joy" or "anger" depending on the perception of the immediate situation. For example, parents send their estranged adolescent a letter. The boy is aware of his trembling hands and pounding heart while holding the envelope. When he opens the envelope, he finds that it contains an airplane ticket to return home. The adolescent may feel anger or joy, depending on whether the gesture is interpreted as manipulative or caring.

Mild emotions may be constructive in their overall effect by energizing one's actions toward worthwhile goals. Once an emotion has become attached to an object or situation, one's behavior is directed toward reaching the goal. College students who love the color and excitement of football games are not likely to stay home when invited to go. Mild anxiety sharpens a student's cognitive abilities and facilitates the achievement of educational goals.

As emotions reach the intermediate range of intensity, they may prompt a person to take action, such as leaving an unhealthy situation; conversely the intensity of the emotion may be detrimental to problem solving and task performance. When people do not adequately cope with a highly intense emotion, it becomes increasingly disruptive to organized behavior. Severe emotional upheavals actually defeat their emergency function, and prolonged emotional mobilization produces physiological changes that are not only useless but are actually harmful to the person.[63] For example, when fear is aroused in situations requiring struggle or escape, the accompanying physiological conditions may provide incredible energy and lend "wings to our feet." However, if emotional activation is too intense, the fear may paralyze our action, "rooting us to the spot" or "freezing us in our tracks."

The way a person expresses or ignores feelings and copes with emotional stress has implications for the whole person. When emotionally aroused, the person undergoes changes that affect every activity. Emotional reactions are altered, thoughts and actions are affected, and overall adjustment may be disturbed. Physical manifestations of feelings are constantly present. Consider, for example, the tingling and expansive sensation of joy, the tight muscles and clenched body posture of anger, the gut-level sickness of grief, and the rapid heart rate and breathing associated with fear. Although these reactions vary from one person to another and from one situation to another, every person's body and emotions are always interacting in some way. Receptors, muscles, internal organs, and nervous mechanisms interact, resulting in changes in brain waves, physiological reactions, and behaviors. When not coped with adequately, emotional stress can contribute to physical discomfort and illness, ranging from muscle tension, general fatigue, and mild aches to cardiovascular disorders, cancer, rheumatoid arthritis, and migraine headache.[52] The emotional dimension also affects intellectual functioning; the ability to evaluate new ideas and to make effective decisions is influenced by feelings. When emotionally aroused, one may say or do something one would not normally say or do, such as threaten or attempt suicide. Feelings and emotional stress influence how individuals fulfill social roles and relate to other people, both personally and professionally.

Intellectual dimension. A variety of definitions of the intellectual dimension have been developed. The one chosen for this discussion divides intellectual functions into four main classes: 1) *receptive functions*, which involve the abilities to acquire, process, classify, and integrate information; 2) *memory and learning*, by means of which information is stored and recalled; 3) *cognition*, or thinking, which concerns the mental organization and reorganization of information; and 4) *expressive functions*, through which information is communicated or acted upon.[41] Although each function represents a distinct set of behaviors, they normally operate cooperatively.

The two main receptive functions are sensation and perception. Although sensory reception is classified as an intellectual function, it is actually a physiological arousal process that triggers the central registering and integrating activities. The individual receives sensation passively and shuts it out only by voluntary actions, such as holding the nose to avoid an unpleasant odor.[41] The sensory processes include vision, hearing, smell, taste, and touch.

The receptive function of perception involves active knowing of an object. For example, as sound waves cause movement of the tympanic membrane, auditory sensation occurs. As the impulses transmitted by the tympanic membrane are organized, a sound is heard. The same sound, such as thunder, ocean waves, or a slamming door, can be perceived in many different ways with a variety of meanings attached to it. Thus perception provides a bridge between the reception of stimuli by all of the senses and the integration of these sensations into meaningful data; these data are then organized within the context of the person's experience and used for adaptive functioning.

Memory and learning comprise the second main class of intellectual functions. Preceding any memory or learning is the process of registration, in which perceptions are selected, recorded, and programmed in the memorizing centers of the brain. The attention focusing components of perception and the individual's emotional state play an important role in the registration process. For example, two people experiencing the same sensory event may register completely different information depending on their selective attention and their emotional state.

Three types of memory are clinically distinguished by the length of time information is retained: immediate memory, recent memory, (both of which are types of short-term memory), and long-term, or remote memory. *Immediate memory* involves the fixation of information that is selected for retention during the registration process. It lasts from about 30 seconds to several minutes, unless sustained by rehearsal. With repetition or rehearsal, a memory trace of registered information can be maintained for hours.[41] *Recent memory* involves the retention of information for an hour or so to 1 to 2 days; this is longer than information could be maintained by conscientious repetition, but the information is not yet fixed in long-term storage as learned material. *Long-term memory,* or learning, is the individual's ability to store information. The process of storage begins as early as ½ second after information enters short-term storage and lasts as long as the information remains in long-term memory. Information that was recently learned can be disrupted or dissipated more easily than older memories because traces become progressively strengthened with time. Evidence exists that information in short-term storage is organized on the basis of contiguity and sensory properties, such as similar shapes, colors, and sounds, whereas information in long-term storage is organized on the basis of meaning.[41]

The third class of intellectual functions is thinking, or cognition, which is defined as any mental operation that relates two or more bits of information. Cognitive operations may be defined by the nature of the information being manipulated (numbers, words, designs, concepts) and the actual operation (comparing, compounding, abstracting, ordering, judging). For example, the operations of "distance judgement" involve abstracting and comparing ideas about space, whereas "computation" may involve the operations of ordering and compounding numbers.

Thinking processes also can be hierarchically arranged according to the degree to which the concept being considered is concrete or abstract.[41] In concrete thinking, focus is on a particular aspect of an object or situation, such as the idea of "a round table." Concrete thinking, although useful in focusing on particulars, binds the person to immediate experience. Abstract thinking involves making generalizations about a category of objects or drawing relationships between situations, such as the idea that "knowledge is power." Abstract thinking considers the past and the future in responding to situations. In essence, it frees the person to think and act based on the construction of possibilities.

The nature of one's thoughts, positive or negative, influences the quality of one's experience by affecting the judgments one makes about the experience. Through thoughts and beliefs, individuals create their own experience of reality. They "program" themselves with the information that they acquire and by the way that they process and organize it.[58] When people give themselves positive messages, they are more likely to proceed in a positive manner. When they maintain thoughts of failure, they increase the probability of failure.

The fourth class of intellectual functions is expression, which includes activities such as speaking, drawing, writing, facial expressions, and physical gestures and movements. These activities comprise the observable behavior from which all other mental activity is inferred. Language is particularly important because it influences the way people perceive, interpret, and respond to their world.

In general the intellectual dimension makes possible such processes as acquiring information through the senses of vision, hearing, smell, taste, and touch; filtering and integrating incoming stimuli; sorting and recalling information; organizing information; and communicating information through activities such as words, gestures, facial expressions, and movements.[41] Using these intellectual processes, one is able to engage in such activities as goal setting, problem solving, and decision making.

The intellectual dimension interacts with and influences the other human dimensions. Any thought or message one communicates to oneself can induce physical changes. Thoughts of stressful or relaxing conditions affect heart rate, respiration rate, skin temperature, and other physiological functions. Mental images affect one's body in much the same way that equivalent events in the external world affect it; for example, visualization of running creates muscle contraction, and images of danger elicit autonomic nervous system responses such as increased pulse rate and sweating.[59] Many civilizations throughout history have used visualization techniques to affect physical healing. Today mental imagery is being incorporated successfully in the treatment of conditions ranging from headaches to cancer.[65]

The effect of intellectual functioning on the emotional dimension is evident when one judges one's feelings as right or wrong, expects that one should or should not feel certain emotions, and is able or not able to communicate emotional experiences to oneself and others. The intellectual dimension also influences one's relationships with other people. For instance, positive or negative thoughts about a relationship contribute to the actual evolution of the relationship. If people think that they have no friends or that they have lost intimacy with someone, they tend to selectively gather and organize information from the environment to support the thought. Ultimately individuals communicate based on this selected information, resulting in the exact situation that they believe has occurred. Intellectual functioning also contributes to the nature of one's spiritual dimension through such processes as visualization, meditation, creative thinking, ability to communicate, and ability to develop meaning in one's life. Finally, one's thoughts are influenced by environmental factors, such as people and places; conversely, people influence their surroundings by what they think and communicate.

Social dimension. The social dimension comprises the aspects of individuals that enable them to function in society. Intrinsic to the social dimension are interactions and relationships with others. People constantly interact with the social system (society) in which they live, and through the socialization process acquire the knowledge, skills, and dispositions that allow them to function in their society. As individuals are socialized, they experience dependence, independence, and interdependence in their interactions. Their relationships with others contribute to the development of self-concept and varying degrees of trust and mistrust. The interrelationship of society, the environment, culture, and the individual evolves from continuous social interaction.

Social interaction is action that mutually affects two or more individuals. A *social relationship* is a continuing pattern of social interaction. Basic human needs can be satisfied only by interaction with other people. Through these interactions, social relationships are established in the family and in the larger community. Individuals who have had satisfying social interactions in early life are usually comfortable both in social interaction and with being alone in the adult years. When an individual's needs for social interaction have not been met during early development, it may be difficult to successfully interact in the adult years.

A group of people who engage in interaction and maintain relationships over time is referred to as a society. A link exists between the health of the individual and the health of the society, each simultaneously affecting the other. The society encompasses several generations of individuals at any given time. Because of varying views and perceptions, a generation gap may lead to stress as these different generations engage in social interaction.

Two mechanisms hold society together.[13] The first is mutual interdependence, which refers to reciprocal interaction between individuals to promote survival. In mutual interdependence, members of society adapt to the needs and interests of others. At particular times, individuals depend on others for survival; at other times, independence is an essential aspect of survival. Dependence and independence constitute the extremes on either end of the continuum of interdependence. Throughout life, individuals progress through various stages of dependence and independence, with a goal of establishing a balance between the two.

The second mechanism that contributes to the cohesiveness of society is the internalization of common norms. *Norms* are rules that govern social behavior in a wide variety of situations. Without norms as a guide to behavior, every situation would be problematic, and individuals would spend much time deciding how to behave in a given situation. Individuals are unaware of the norms that govern a great deal of their behavior; they simply have learned appropriate responses in given situations and automatically behave according to the norms.

The process by which norms are internalized is *socialization.* Socialization is the basic process by which a person becomes a functioning member of society. Persons are continually integrated into groups by acquiring as their own the norms, values, and perspectives of such groups.[46] Socialization influences people in areas such as beliefs, attitudes, values, habits, customs, motives, and behaviors. Individuals learn through socialization how to interact with other people and how to behave in interpersonal relationships. The process of socialization, which begins at birth and ends only at death, consists of deliberate as well as unconscious activities.

The family is one of the primary mechanisms of socialization. The family provides the setting for an individual's initial experiences of social interaction and relationships, as well as exposure to social norms, values, and perspectives. Within the family framework, individual members learn socially acceptable attitudes, values, behaviors, and expectations. Healthy families facilitate growth and development of their members throughout the life cycle, whereas maladaptive families may restrict individual functioning in one or more dimensions.

The community also represents a major socializing force. Each community adopts variations of the more general norms that are prevalent in a given society. Community attitudes and values, as well as physical restrictions and resources, directly and indirectly influence the individual. (Chapters 25 and 29 of this text provide in-depth discussions of the family and the community, respectively.)

Socialization prepares individuals for the roles they assume in society. *Social roles* are patterns of attitudes, values, goals, and behaviors that are expected of individuals by virtue of the position they occupy in society. Society defines a number of social roles that influence the individual's relationship with others. A concept related to role is status. A *status* is a position in society, and a role is the behavioral counterpart of a position. For example, nurse is a status, and provision of care for clients is the role. Statuses and role characteristics may be achieved, ascribed, or assumed. Individuals occupy achieved statuses, such as educational and occupational statuses, as a result of their own motivation, efforts, and competence. Ascribed statuses, such as family of origin, sex, age, and ethnicity, are socially assigned.

Throughout the life cycle, individuals assume numerous social roles with corresponding sets of expectations. Each person occupies several interacting role positions at any given time in the life cycle, such as parent, child, student, friend, and spouse. *Role transitions* occur when statuses are acquired or discarded. The student status, for example, is discarded once the individual graduates. In other situations the role changes. *Role change* refers to situations in which status is retained while role expectations change. Occupation of any particular role entitles a person to certain privileges and imposes certain limitations. The ability to enter into and enjoy a variety of roles increases one's options and allows optimal development of one's capabilities.

During the process of socialization the individual develops a *self-concept.* The self-concept consists of the individual's ideas, feelings, values, and beliefs about himself that result from social interactions with others. Cooley[14] coined the phrase "looking-glass self" to describe an individual's perception of himself as a reflection of how he thinks others perceive and evaluate him. Thus children learn to think of themselves as good because they perceive that others evaluate them as good. Generally, factors influencing the development of self-concept are expectations of and evaluation by significant others, genetic and environmental factors, and developmental tasks and crises. Redefinition of oneself in response to developmental and situational crises occurs throughout the life cycle.

Self-concept may be positive or negative. A positive self-concept implies acceptance of oneself as a person with strengths and weaknesses, and it enhances self-confidence in one's social interactions. A negative self-concept is reflected in feelings of worthlessness and lack of respect for oneself and one's abilities.

Self-esteem is a major component of self-concept. Self-esteem is judgment or evaluation of one's own worth in relationship to one's ideal self and to the performance of others. Self-esteem may be high or low. Individuals with positive self-concept and high self-esteem tend to be autonomous and to display a basic trust of themselves and other people. Mistrust of oneself and others is manifested by persons with a negative self-concept and low self-esteem. In general, self-concept and self-esteem influence how one relates to others.

Personal identity is the component of self-concept that allows an individual to maintain a sense of continuity, or sameness, over time, and thus enables the individual to occupy a stable position in the environment. Personal identity is based on one's overall pattern of qualities. These patterns are known and considered to be personal and distinctive. It provides a reference point from which to monitor and evaluate one's own thoughts, feelings, and behavior—in any given moment and over time—in relation to the environmental reality that surrounds a person. To a large extent, personal identity regulates and coordinates one's view both of outside reality and of oneself within that reality. A large amount of information is available from oneself and from the environment at any given time; personal identity is a primary factor in a person's determination of what information is relevant. For example, an individual whose personal identity includes self-competence may view a potentially difficult situation as easily manageable; an individual who views himself as incapable could view the same situation as threatening or impossible to resolve. People tend to interpret information so that it confirms their own theories of reality based on their own personal identities. One person may interpret benign comments as critical, whereas another may not perceive intended criticism. Although personal identity forms the basis for a sense of continuity, feedback from ongoing self-perception, self-evaluation, and interaction with the environment allows continuous development over time.[26]

Human *sexuality,* an important aspect of all dimensions, is influenced significantly by the social dimension. Sexuality refers to human qualities that are associated with one's expression of oneself as either male or female. Thus sexuality encompasses a broad spectrum, ranging from attitudes, beliefs, and feelings to social roles and actual behaviors. People learn to identify and value their maleness or femaleness largely through interacting with other people. Sexuality is interdependent with one's self-concept, self-esteem, and personal identity. People with a positive self-concept and high self-esteem are likely to feel comfortable with the experience and expression of their sexuality. A positive attitude toward and acceptance of one's sexuality can also enhance self-esteem and strengthen personal identity.

Social norms that govern the expression of sexuality are learned primarily through the socialization process and can differ greatly among societies. Social norms determine the acceptable sexual roles in any society. The norms are used to establish the attitudes, values, and behaviors that are expected of people by virtue of their sexual identity. Sexual role behavior includes all behaviors that express or disclose oneself as male or female. As with deviation from other social norms, individuals who choose nontraditional sexual roles may be considered aberrant. In recent years, sexual roles have become less restrictive in this society.[32]

The social dimension interacts with and influences each of the other human dimensions. Social interaction makes possible meeting physical needs, such as nourishment, touch, clothing, shelter, and health care. The social and emotional dimensions are intertwined, as witnessed by the feelings elicited and experienced in any kind of relationship. Social roles also assist people in meeting their emotional needs: a maternal role may allow the expression of tenderness; a child role may encourage playfulness. The interrelatedness of the social and intellectual dimensions is evident in communication. Socialization allows a person to develop communication skills, and communication is a primary factor that makes socialization possible.

Both verbal and nonverbal communication are primary factors in interpersonal relationships; in addition, social interaction is the primary framework in which communication skills are learned. Through communication individuals share experiences, thoughts, feelings, and information; express and meet their needs; make teaching and learning possible; and develop social support systems.[58] Through social contact people learn either basically positive or negative thought patterns. Social roles influence attitudes toward learning and thus educational and career choices. Society influences the particular way in which spirituality is expressed and consequently affects a person's individual spiritual experience.

Spiritual dimension. Spirituality is at the core of the individual's existence, integrating and transcending the physical, emotional, intellectual, and social dimensions. Frequently, spirituality is defined as sensitivity or attachment to religious values. Religion refers to an organized system of faith, worship, and prescribed rituals and observances, that serve as a medium for the expression of one's spiritual needs. Organized traditional religions tend to adhere to the revelations of one or more persons that are passed along to those who follow.[19] A person's spiritual dimension encompasses much more than these revelations, more than established doctrine introduced by others. This dimension allows one to experience and understand the reality of existence in unique and direct ways that go beyond one's usual limits. Hence spirituality is not synonymous with religious beliefs.

The spiritual dimension is the most elusive for many people because of the individual nature of spirituality and because of a tendency, particularly in Western culture, to emphasize what is tangible. The spiritual dimension deals with a reality that is more than tangible. Spiritual needs permeate an individual's life principles and incorporate his total being. When spiritual needs are met satisfactorily, the person is free to function with a meaningful identity and purpose and to relate to reality with hope and confidence. Needs related to the spiritual dimension are experienced throughout the life cycle, and these needs are basic to the individual's inner strivings toward goals in life that hold the deepest values for the individual. The extent to which the spiritual needs are met directly affects feelings of hope.

Some needs that are related to the spiritual dimension include[12]:

1. A meaningful philosophy of life
2. A sense of the *numinous* and *transcendent*
3. A deep experience of trustful relatedness to God, a supreme being, or a universal power or force
4. A relatedness to people and nature
5. Self-actualization

All individuals have a philosophy of life of which they may or may not be consciously aware. A philosophy of life is a set of standards and ideals that guides individuals in decision making about their goals and that largely determines the meaning which they attribute to their lives. Beliefs, values, morals, and ethics are essential components of an individual's philosophy of life. A belief is a conviction in the truth or existence of something or someone, a state of mind in which confidence or trust is placed in some person or thing. An individual's beliefs are influenced by society and by cultural belief systems. Through the socialization process, beliefs are internalized and modified throughout the life cycle.

Values are a class of beliefs shared by members of a society that determine what is desirable or what ought to be. Values are positive and negative; positive values indicate what is desirable, and negative values demonstrate what is undesirable. In the process of socialization, individuals learn the dominant values of a society; however, individuals also develop personal values.

Morals relate to the individual's conception of what is right and wrong in behavior. Kohlberg[37] formulated and validated stages of moral development that begin in childhood and continue into adulthood. The stages are defined by ways of thinking about moral issues and by choices. He believed that morality represents a set of rational principles of judgment and justice that are valid for every culture. An individual's value judgment system and philosophy determine the level of moral development attained. Moral development is also influenced by reasoning abilities, problem-solving experiences, and the type of knowledge used in thinking. Individuals who receive little or no information regarding cultural and personal morality develop uncertainty because they have to work out so many answers for themselves. While morals relate to the concept of what is right and wrong, *ethics* are the specific set of values, moral codes, and rules of conduct by which an individual's morals are implemented.

One's values, beliefs, and goals are based largely on the meaning, or purpose, that one attributes to one's life. People play an active role in the choice and development of giving their life meaning and purpose.

A sense of the numinous and transcendent is the second spiritual need. Numinous refers to an appeal to the higher emotions, such as awe or reverence. Transcendence involves the ability to go beyond one's ordinary everyday limits, to experience more than one's usual existence. Transcendence involves moments of enlightenment: "Oh, I see!" "Aha! This is it!" "Now it all fits!" These moments may be as simple as viewing another person, a flower, or a mountain in new ways and as mysterious as psychic healing or a strong feeling of oneness with the universe.[58] While searching for a meaning in life, individuals may attempt to transcend the limitations of their human condition or try to forget unpleasant human experiences such as loneliness, restlessness, dissatisfaction, and aloneness. The stamina that enables individuals to persist until they arrive at a purpose to which they can commit themselves is determined by hope and faith. Hope, which is discussed in Chapter 14, is basic to survival in health and illness. Faith is a firm belief in something and always involves certainty, even where there is no evidence or proof. The difference between life and death may be the presence or absence of hope and faith. For example, nurses encounter critically ill clients who recover against all expectations because they have hope and faith. Hope and faith are evident in the specific, personal meaning that motivates individuals to continue life and survive in the most unfavorable conditions.

One way of describing the third spiritual need—a deep experience of a trustful relatedness to God, a supreme being, or a universal power or force—is in terms of the individual's religion. The concept of a deity refers to the meanings, ideas, thoughts, and expressions individuals have for a supreme being or universal power or force; these are determined primarily through culture. Several human behavior patterns are related to the concept of a deity. These behaviors are the tendency to congregate, the tendency to imitate, and the desire to appeal to a higher force when one's own resources fail. The need for a trustful relatedness to the object of worship can be met through the belief that the object is loving and active in one's life. With this belief, there is reassurance that life has meaning and that one can appeal to power outside one's personal realm.

The concept of a deity is closely related to worship, which is the reverent love and allegiance accorded a deity, idol, or sacred object. Each religious group subscribes to a particular form of worship within an institution such as a church, temple, synagogue, or other designated space. Worship involves a connectedness with a deity or power that may result in a spiritual relationship with others in the group. This spiritual relationship is expressed in love and care for other persons. Love is defined in this sense as intense concern for another person. Care is compassion as opposed to tolerance, tenderness as opposed to a sense of duty, and respect as opposed to obligation.

Attitudes of peace, dignity, and belonging are often communicated through an individual's own sense of accountability to a higher spiritual authority or deep sense of commitment to others. The presence of God, the integration of the universe, and the meaning of life are often evoked through continued participation in familiar religious rituals and ceremonies.

A relatedness to people and nature is a fourth spiritual need. Some individuals may not experience a trustful relatedness to a deity; however, they may have a meaningful relatedness to other people and to nature that enables them to grow spiritually.

Research Highlight

Nurses' Attitudes About Spiritual Care

K. Soeken & V. Carson

PURPOSE

The purpose of the research was to examine the relationship between the spiritual well-being of the nurses and nursing students and their attitudes toward providing spiritual care for clients.

SAMPLE

The sample consisted of 29 senior baccalaureate nursing students and 24 graduate nursing students enrolled in a public institution. Average ages were 22.3 and 29.4 years. All but three participants were women. The majority considered themselves to be a member of a religious group.

METHODOLOGY

The spiritual well-being (SWB) scale was developed as a general measure of religious well-being (RWB) and existential well-being (EWB). The "health professional's spiritual role" scale was developed to measure attitudes about the health professional's role in meeting clients' spiritual needs. Questionnaires were administered in two regularly scheduled classes.

FINDINGS

The possible range of scores for RWB and EWB was 10 to 60 with a midpoint of 35. Scores tended to be in the upper range indicating positive religious and existential well-being. On the HPSR Scale the mean was 105.2 out of a possible range of 25 to 150, indicating an overall positive attitude toward providing spiritual care.

IMPLICATIONS

The ability to measure spiritual well-being could be used by nurses to assess client's spiritual needs, to evaluate outcomes of spiritual nursing interventions, and to determine which outcomes are most effective. An additional benefit is the ability to provide experiences that will increase the nurse's own spiritual well-being. Nurses with a high level of spiritual well-being and motivation can be trained as spiritual specialists.

Based on data from Health Progress **67**(3):52, 1986.

Nurses can facilitate a person's spiritual as well as physical and social well being through their role as an "advocate." (See the Research Highlight above.) True advocacy involves more than speaking up for or speaking in behalf of another. An often neglected or forgotten meaning of the term advocate is the notion of walking along with or accompanying another on their journey through life.[12a] Such sharing is not an easy or objective task because it opens the advocate to more anxiety and pain as well as more satisfaction and joy. Through such relationships, individuals often have the opportunity to experience another's core or centeredness. It is no longer necessary, maybe even impossible to treat that person as an object which one needs to manipulate.

Spirit has been viewed throughout history as the force by which humans are related to the universe, to nature, and to other people. The spiritual dimension enables us to connect with a positive universal energy that makes it possible to "more fully develop our courage, our ability to genuinely love, our wisdom, and our compassion."[4] This sense of relatedness, or connectedness, is an important aspect of the spiritual dimension. A relationship with nature may evoke humility, respect, courtesy, and sometimes fear. Events that seem coincidental or accidental, such as psychic healing, encountering an old friend who recently appeared in a dream, or suddenly "knowing" that

a family member is in danger, may exemplify a universal relatedness. This seems feasible in view of the thesis that the universe is one energy.[58] Without this sense of connectedness, an individual may experience isolation, hopelessness, and purposelessness.

Self-actualization, the fifth spiritual need, is the epitome of spiritual experience but is a need that is met less often than the others. Individuals who achieve self-actualization have transcended their limitations and realized their highest potentials. The self-actualized person has experiences that are described as "limitless horizons opening up to the vision, the feeling of being simultaneously more powerful and also more helpless than one ever was before, the feeling of great ecstasy and wonder and awe, the loss of placing in time and space with, finally, the conviction that something extremely important and valuable has happened, so that the person is to some extent transformed and strengthened even in his daily life by such experience."[45] Maslow believes that, to attain self-actualization, individuals need to be free of mundane worries, especially those related to survival. Once individuals experience self-actualization, they may develop an esthetic sense that enables them to create and appreciate beauty in painting, sculpture, music, and nature (see Figure 9-2).

Figure 9-3 shows the interrelationships of the five dimensions of the person and the components within each

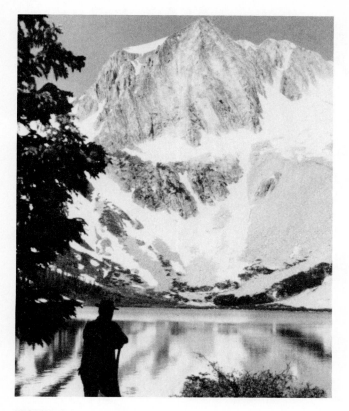

FIGURE 9-2 An individual's spirituality is enhanced by viewing the wonders of nature.

dimension. The components within each dimension form the basic framework for the five dimensions throughout this text.

Relationship with the Environment

The environment is an irrevocable aspect of human existence. As indicated in the discussion of systems theory (see Chapter 3), every living organism is interdependent with its environment. In addition, each individual organism constitutes an environment for the smaller systems within itself. Just as a person is multidimensional, each individual's environment is composed of a multitude of factors that are influential in the person's life—people, places, things, events. At any moment and in any situation, one is in dynamic relationship both with one's immediate surroundings and with more distant environmental factors. An ongoing pattern of adapting occurs as person and environment contribute to the nature of each other.

Continual energy exchanges between people and their environment occur on many levels. In all exchanges between the person and environment, one takes in energy from outside sources, processes and uses it, and then returns some form of energy to the environment. Thus individuals are simultaneously affected by input from their surroundings and through their output, contribute to environmental characteristics. As a person's outputs are pro-

cessed by and incorporated into the environment, they become new inputs that affect the person. Because of this ongoing relationship between people and their environment, one cannot fully understand individuals in isolation from their surroundings. People feel, think, and behave differently in various environmental settings.

Regardless of the actual content of the environment, one's interaction with it contributes significantly to who one is, how one lives, what one does, and certainly to states of health and illness.

A person relates to the environment through all dimensions, often simultaneously, both satisfying personal needs and helping satisfy the needs of various environmental entities. As a result of the interdependent nature of the person-environment relationship, people need to deal with their surroundings in ways that promote coordination and synchrony rather than conflict and chaos. Mutual adaptation is necessary. Environmental factors may act as both resources and stressors; they can provide security and excitement or they can contribute to hardship and obstacles.

The physical environment may contain elements that facilitate meeting one's needs in all dimensions, needs such as adequate living quarters, a safe neighborhood, availability of cultural events, and opportunities for spiritual growth. Conversely, the physical environment can inhibit a person's overall development through crowded living conditions, excessive crime, and unavailability of various resources.

Emotional needs frequently are met through environmental interaction. One's environment is conducive to health when emotional support is readily available and when one has a number of avenues for expression of feelings. Such an environment encourages development in all dimensions.

Intellectual development is closely related to environmental situations. A healthy environment provides opportunities for intellectual growth and development and adequate stimulation and encouragement to learn. In turn, such an environment facilitates the ability to get one's needs met in other areas.

By definition the social dimension is closely entwined with the environment. People are simultaneously dependent parts of society and independent wholes within society. Through resources of the environment, a person is able to meet physical needs such as food, shelter, and health care. Primarily through the social dimension one is able to create caring relationships in which one fulfills many basic needs. Thus one's environment is a crucial aspect of healthy development; when possibilities for social contact are limited or when the contacts are primarily negative, people find it more difficult to function optimally in all dimensions.

Spiritual beliefs and experiences are greatly affected by the beliefs of the society in which a person lives. A rich environment offers many opportunities for personal exploration and expansion, which enhances one's ability to cope effectively with stressors in all other dimensions as well.

When one considers the person-environment interrelationship, it is crucial to remember that each individual

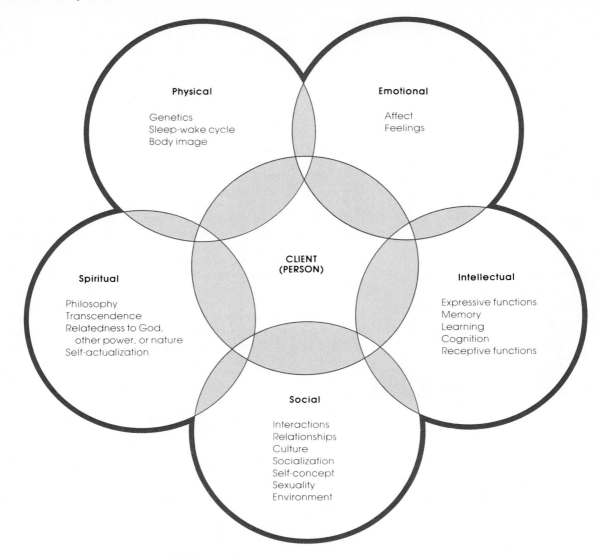

FIGURE 9-3 Integration of the five dimensions of the person.

interacts with the environment based on subjective experience as well as actual external stimuli. One's perceptions of and responses to the environment are largely determined by one's attitudes, values, feelings, and beliefs. Past experience, attributed meanings, and expectations of the future contribute to an inner reality; from this reality, one interacts with and adapts to the environment.[10]

Self-Responsibility

Holistic health philosophy maintains that people are ultimately responsible for their own lives. They continually make choices and decisions that determine who they are, what they experience, and how they live. Although many factors contribute to the nature of these choices and decisions, individuals are responsible for those which they make. Even when options seem limited or nonexistent, people still choose among alternatives.

Self-awareness is a prerequisite to the genuine acceptance of responsibility for oneself. To be aware implies that one is able to focus attention on a particular experience in a way that promotes individual "knowing" of the experience. Awareness is a kind of "tuning in to" and willingness to recognize what is currently significant. Experiences that have occurred in the past or that are anticipated in the future are meaningful only as they relate to the present and as they influence current choices and decisions.

As a whole person, one needs to develop as much awareness as possible; of oneself, including strengths and weaknesses, feelings and behaviors, attitudes and beliefs, social patterns, and a sense of meaning; of one's environment, including people, places, objects, and energy; and of one's connections with the environment, including expectations, energy exchange, nature of interactions, and boundaries between oneself and the environment. As people develop a sense of awareness, they are able to recognize the reality of their life situations. Only then can they begin to identify their contributions to life events, acknowledge the choices they make, and fully assume responsibility for themselves.

Locus of control indicates how individuals perceive a sense of personal responsibility in life. Basically, locus of control is related to whether individuals perceive that they have power over events that affect them. Internal locus of control, or internality, means that an outcome is a consequence of the individual's own actions and is thus under personal control. External locus of control, or externality, refers to the belief that an outcome is determined by fate, chance, or powerful others and is thus beyond personal control.[3] If people can develop a locus of control that is more internal than external, they may learn to acquire more responsibility for their own health.[62]

The concept of locus of control, or self-responsibility, affects each person in all dimensions. For example, physically, people believe either that they can control their actions and general nutritional and fitness status or that outside circumstances make it impossible for them to change their patterns. Emotionally, some people assume responsibility for their own feelings, whereas others believe that something or someone else can cause them to feel a particular way. Intellectually, individuals believe either that they choose their thoughts or that they learned them long ago and cannot change them. Socially, people may see how they contribute to the success and failure of interactions and relationships, or they may attribute outcome to the other person(s) involved. In the spiritual dimension, people believe either that they create meaning for themselves or that meaning is revealed to them by outside forces.

A holistic approach to living is based on the assumption that the individual exerts primary influence in all areas. People are, in fact, responsible for the sum of their life experiences. In contrast to a sense of responsibility for oneself and control over one's own life, people occasionally—or often—believe and act as if other people, circumstances, or fate exerts more influence over their life situations than they do. Phrases such as "I have to . . . ," "I should . . . ," "I can't . . . ," and "I couldn't help it" indicate a sense of helplessness, or a belief that one is not in control of oneself. People who feel responsible for themselves generally use more powerful phrases, such as "I choose to . . . ," "I want to . . . ," "I won't . . . ," and "I contributed by. . . ." The difference in the two sets of phrases reflects two distinct approaches to living. The former represents feeling at the mercy of outside force (external locus of control); the latter (internal locus of control) allows people to assume both the power and the responsibility of directing their own lives.

Historically the U.S. health care system has encouraged specific and restricted roles for both health care professionals and clients. Those who represent the system often are expected to behave "professionally" rather than authentically, to act in a kind but detached manner rather than with true caring, and to view themselves as authorities rather than as coparticipants. In contrast, consumers of health care services are expected to comply with instructions rather than to understand the rationale behind them, to allow others to make health decisions for them rather than participating in decision making, and to view health care professionals as authorities rather than as consultants.

In the realm of personal health, self-responsibility means that individuals view themselves as active participants in their health status, including the occurrence of illness and accidents. They are not victims or passive recipients of any outside force, including the health care system; they maintain their sense of personal power rather than believing that others exert control over them. Self-responsibility includes the recognition that people in some way participate in or contribute to their illness and accidents. Therefore individuals need to seek information about this participation and reevaluate the choices they make. For example, if people determine that they have contributed to the development of a cold by insufficient rest, an ulcer by inadequate relaxation, or a state of depression by lack of assertiveness, they may want to make different choices that are more likely to contribute to a healthier status. In general, individuals who assume responsibility for their health status actively strive toward effective coping with stressors, reaching their own potentials, and maintaining balance within their lives.

As one develops a greater sense of responsibility, one is less able to accept the "fix-it" attitude that many people learn as children; that is, if something goes wrong, someone else will fix it. Although the health care system in many cases can effectively treat illness or injury, it cannot be responsible for the ways in which people contribute to their state of health, to illness, or to an accident. Only the individual can, for instance, maintain fitness levels, or wear seat belts, or deal effectively with stressors. As one assumes greater responsibility for one's health, one chooses healthier behaviors. In this way, each person retains personal power and integrity rather than relinquishing control to someone else.

For most people, the prospect of responsibility for their health and illness is exciting and powerful. However, responsibility also contains an awesome and at times frightening element. People can no longer blame other persons or things for "making them" ill, "leading" them in a certain direction, or "running" their lives. An attitude of helplessness is replaced by resoluteness. These transitions are not always easy.

In considering self-responsibility for participation in illness or an accident, it is important that the concept of responsibility not be confused with guilt, self-blame, or self-criticism. When people accept responsibility for illness, they are able to view their current situation as a starting point, explore how they contribute to the situation, determine the message or meaning, and choose a new direction. However, when individuals distort responsibility into guilt, they inhibit personal growth. Self-blaming and self-critical attitudes limit people. Self-responsibility means not that a person becomes paralyzed with guilt and self-blame but that the person learns from illness and continually strives to make healthier choices.

Life-Cycle Development

Holistic concepts are applicable as an individual proceeds through all stages of the life cycle. (Part 4 of this text provides an in-depth discussion of life-cycle development.) The dimensions of the person and the environment are interdependent at every age. Each stage of life is typically accompanied by particular kinds of stressors that require different kinds of coping mechanisms. Self-responsibility, recognizing one's needs and making choices to obtain what one wants, is an important component at every stage of life.

Stress and Adaptation

Holistic health philosophy recognizes stress as a primary factor in all states of health and illness. Basically *stress* is the body's arousal response to any demand, change, or perceived threat, and a *stressor* is the circumstance or event that elicits this response. Selye[63] has described a generalized response to stressors that involves the autonomic nervous system and the endocrine system. This general adaptation syndrome (GAS) has three states: (1) an alarm reaction, (2) resistance, and (3) exhaustion. The apparent purpose of the GAS is to assist the individual in resisting the stressor as efficiently as possible and in maintaining a state of equilibrium. When stressors (real or perceived) are chronic and there is no opportunity to regain equilibrium, the exhaustion state may lead to illness or death. (See Chapter 3)

Stress is neither inherently good nor bad; it produces positive and negative effects. Stress is healthy when it facilitates stimulation and alertness, contributes to personal growth and development, or assists individuals in meeting their needs. Life is not very challenging and people accomplish little if demands are not made on them. However, stress is not healthy when it creates a sense of helplessness, leaves one feeling tired and apathetic, inhibits optimal functioning, or predisposes one to illness. These conditions occur when a person does not create opportunities to regain equilibrium.

A stressor can be anything that elicits the stress response of physiological and biochemical change. Like the effects of stress, stressors may be positive or negative. On a physiological and biochemical level, the body does not seem to distinguish between positive and negative stressors. Both elicit the same responses, and both can have positive or negative consequences. Although negative stressors often are more intense and of greater concern, events such as marriage, job promotion, moving to a new home, vacation, and graduation are demanding and require change. These positive life changes elicit the same basic stress response as situations like divorce, loss of job, or academic failure. One factor that can make a negative stressor more harmful is the tendency to prolong the arousal associated with it. A person does this by continuing to worry or maintain other strong feelings long after the actual stressor is gone, as in the case of prolonged concern following an examination or reliving an argument a month after it has happened.

The range of events or circumstances that can act as stressors is wide and varied and can affect all dimensions of the person. Examples of negative stressors include physical deprivation or injury, emotional strain or loss, self-defeating thoughts and beliefs, social isolation or overextension, and spiritual conflicts. Examples of stressors that are generally thought of as more positive include athletic contests, emotional commitments such as marriage or parenthood, intellectual stimulation or accomplishment, expansion of social involvement, and spiritual enlightenment. Examples of environmental stressors include pollution, weather conditions, lack of personal space, physical surroundings, and occupational settings.

An event or circumstance becomes a stressor to a particular individual when the person consciously or unconsciously perceives it as such. What is stressful for one person may not be for another. For example, someone who enjoys the sun and water may perceive an ocean beach as a relaxing place; the same setting can be stressful for someone who is afraid of the water and is hypersensitive to the sun. A new assignment at work or graduation from school may be perceived as exciting by one person but frightening by another. An individual also perceives potential stressors differently according to particular life situations. For instance, divorce may be experienced primarily as relief at age 30 but overwhelming to the same person at age 60. The role of parenthood can be perceived as a welcome challenge at one point in life but an unwelcome obstacle at another. Many variables determine a person's perception and experience of stressors including age, sex, physical condition, personality, learned attitudes and beliefs, family situation, cultural background, social support system, spiritual beliefs, and environment.

Over time, every individual develops coping patterns, which are behaviors used to maintain a sense of equilibrium when faced with stressful situations. Coping behaviors are numerous and may be adaptive or maladaptive. Adaptive coping behaviors enable an individual to change or reinterpret a stressful situation, or to control stress resulting from a situation, without adverse effects in other aspects of life. Examples include hobbies, conflict resolution, building relationships, time management, relaxation strategies, and exercise. Maladaptive coping occurs when the behaviors used to respond to stressors produce negative side effects and may be harmful or produce additional stress when used often or over a long period of time. Examples of maladaptive coping are drug abuse, overeating, tantrums, and social isolation. People tend to use coping behaviors that have worked in the past. If adaptive, the person can become stronger with each stressful situation; when maladaptive, the person may become more vulnerable to the effects of stress over time.

Approaches to *stress management* are numerous and varied. The first step of stress management is the identification of stressors in one's life. These stressors may be major events, such as marriage or moving to a new city, or daily occurrences, such as traffic or constant worry about a particular issue. They may originate outside oneself (the cranky boss, the alcoholic spouse, or depressed economic conditions) or within the individual (self-critical thoughts, poor nutritional habits, lack of assertiveness, or anxiety about the future). The stressors can affect any dimension of the individual.

To identify personal stressors, individuals examine how they react to what occurs in their particular situation. The following reactions indicate at least some degree of stress: feelings of helplessness or hopelessness, perceived loss of control, chronic anxiety and worry, a "knot" in the stomach, continual frustration, increased heart and respiration rates, cold hands and feet, neck and shoulder muscle tension, clenched jaw, feeling overwhelmed, excessive or constant fatigue, and nervous laughter. Once aware of one's physical and emotional reactions, one often can locate the stimulus of the reaction, that is, the stressor.

The second step of stress management is to determine which, if any, stressors one wishes to eliminate, those with which one simply wants to reduce contact, and those to which one would like to diminish one's response. A person who is retaining beliefs and attitudes from the past that are now acting as stressors may wish to replace these with constructive, reinforcing thoughts. One may be able to make relatively simple changes in a home or work environment to make it less stressful; for example, furniture arrangement, new color scheme, sharing chores, or creating a private space. If one determines that a particular person is acting as a stressor, one may choose to become less involved or to detach oneself completely.

As people consider which stressors they wish to eliminate, an important point to remember is that it is neither possible nor desirable to completely empty their lives of stressors. The removal of certain stressors may be impractical, and the removal of others simultaneously deprive the person of challenge and personal growth opportunities. Positive attitudes and the willingness to cope in healthy ways with stressors are much more critical to health than is the quantity of stressors that people encounter.

The third and crucial step of stress management, then, is to develop effective coping mechanisms so that one is able either to counteract one's own stress response when it occurs or to use the response constructively. Stress is a problem only when the body initiates physiological and biochemical activity in preparation to deal with the stressor and then does not experience any release. This can easily occur as a person faces one stressor after another without any recovery time; the person's body stays in a constant state of readiness, which leads to the destructive effects of stress. Ultimately individuals are in charge of whether they choose to counteract or use the stress response.

Physical dimension. Stressors related to genetic factors, physiological processes, and body image are listed in the upper right box. The reader is referred to other texts on physical health and illness for a further discussion of physical stressors and the individual's responses to them. Stressors affecting body image are discussed briefly in this section because of their impact on a person's mental or emotional health.

Stressors that threaten one's body image are those which are perceived to alter, actually do alter, or contribute to the alteration of the individual's physical structure,

---

EXAMPLES OF STRESSORS AND MALADAPTIVE RESPONSES TO STRESSORS

Physical Dimension

STRESSORS	MALADAPTIVE RESPONSES
Genetic dysfunctions	Congenital abnormalities
Nutritional deficiencies	Physical defects
Drug use	Physical diseases
Disease, illness, injury, pain	Withdrawal symptoms
Aging process	Negative body image
Sensory deprivation	Sleeplessness
Environmental factors	Restlessness
Inadequate or excessive physical activity	Decreased energy
Body image alterations	Fatigue
Sleep disorders	Impaired growth
	Hyperalertness
	Metabolic disturbances
	Gastrointestinal disturbances
	Sexual dysfunction
	Cardiovascular deterioration
	Self-destruction

---

such as changes in body appearance, size, or shape. A person's perception determines reality for the person; thus a perceived alteration in body image can be as stressful as an actual one. For example, adolescents may perceive themselves as "fat" if they exceed their personally defined ideal weight, regardless of how others perceive them. Personal definitions of "ideal weight" are partially determined by cultural standards; staying thin may be a desirable goal if the adolescent's culture places a premium on this characteristic. Threats to body image are stressful because the ability to relate in meaningful ways to others or develop a satisfactory sexual identity are related to the concept of self and body image. Major stressors to body image fall into six categories: (1) normal maturation, (2) elective surgical procedures, (3) disease or other disorders, (4) surgery or trauma, (5) drugs, and (6) social influences.

Norris[50] identified four factors that influence an individual's adjustment to alterations in body size, function, or structure: (1) the meaning the stressor has for the individual; (2) the extent to which the individual's pattern of adaptation is interrupted; (3) the support system and patterns of adaptation available to the individual; and (4) the nature of the threat, degree of change, and rate at which it occurs. The person's level of growth and development influences the significance of the loss.

Reactions to body image changes vary greatly as individuals attempt to handle threats to loss of self-control or control of their immediate space. Such responses are not uncommon when clients are faced with potentially threatening nursing procedures, such as enemas, catheterizations, and other restrictions that immobilize them so that they are dependent on others to care for intimate needs. Denial can lead to restlessness, fatigue, vulnerability, intractible pain, nervousness, insomnia, and phobias. Adaptation occurs more readily when the person is encouraged to express feelings, allowed time to develop healthy coping mechanisms, provided support from meaningful others, and assisted in lowering the anxiety level.

✳ *Emotional dimension.* Any situation that elicits an emotion from the individual and generates a physiological response has the potential for producing stress. Stressors in every dimension may elicit strong emotions and place demands on one's emotional coping capacity.

Emotional health and illness can be viewed along a continuum. At any time, a person's state of health can be reflected at a specific point on the continuum. The intensity and duration of the emotion determine where one is placed on the continuum.

One's position on the continuum is determined by one's ability to satisfy needs and to fully experience and constructively deal with one's feelings. Some healthy emotional responses include laughing, crying, loving, anger, trust, fear, hopefulness, and powerfulness. Unhealthy emotional responses may include excessive guilt, hurt, long-term resentment, and helplessness. Researchers are beginning to explore the interactive effects of various expressions of emotion; examples include biochemical changes which may occur in the brain during laughter, and differing content of tears when shed due to emotion rather than to physical irritation.

One's position on the emotional continuum changes as one responds to stressors in healthy or unhealthy ways. There is no state of absolute emotional health or of absolute emotional illness. Emotional health is an evolving process in which people are able to have their needs met, are willing to recognize and accept their feelings, and choose to use their emotional energy to enhance their life situations. A sense of emotional health is maintained when harmony exists within oneself, with others, and in inter-actions with the environment. Emotional distress results when basic needs are not met, causing disruption, disorganization, and dysfunction in one's emotional equilibrium. See the box at lower left for examples of stressors and responses in the emotional dimension.

✳ *Intellectual dimension.* Stressors in the intellectual dimension may be any factor of either internal or external origin that interferes with receptive functions, memory and learning, cognitive functions, or expressive functions.

The complex processes of sensation and perception employ many aspects of the central nervous system; consequently proper functioning is largely dependent on good physical health.

The healthy person has good recall for immediate, recent, or remote events and thus is able to learn what is meaningful. Such a person also employs internal and external strategies for enhancing memory, such as increasing study time or tying a string around a finger. Although moderate levels of anxiety can enhance memory and learning, high anxiety levels often lead to forgetfulness or the inability to learn.

The inability to recall specific information such as a friend's name or a significant historical date is an indication of memory loss. Defects of memory also can affect motor skills, conceptual relationships, or speech patterns, and each may be affected differentially. For example, the motor speech habit of organizing sounds into a word may be retained and the ability to organize words into meaningful speech lost. Similarly, sensory modalities and output mechanisms involved in stored memories are also differentially affected. For example, a person may retain the ability to recognize a picture but not be able to recognize numbers or letters.[11]

Long-term memory storage is impaired in some brain disease. The time of onset of the memory loss can be approximated by eliciting the most recent of the remote memories, since all events preceding the disease onset may be poorly remembered or not remembered at all. In other types of brain injury or disease, only specific bits of remote memory are lost. An alteration in level of consciousness usually accompanies a global loss of long-term memory.[41]

Persons who have adapted well to stressors have attained the cognitive developmental level of formal operations;[54] they are realistic, rational, and logical; consider a range of differing viewpoints; and use their imagination to solve problems in a creative manner. In addition, they are able to maintain basically positive thoughts that enhance growth. Poor adaptation to stressors results in a disintegration of cognition. Such disintegrations may occur in the form, the content, or the flow of thought.

In response to stressors the form of thought may become unrealistic, irrational, or illogical, as in dereistic and autistic thinking. In *dereistic thought,* the laws of logic, experience, and reality are not followed. An extreme example is the person who jumps off a 12-story building, not "knowing" that death will occur. Autistic thinking focuses on internal processes; fantasy life becomes reality. *Symbolic associations* and concrete associations are other

---

EXAMPLES OF STRESSORS AND MALADAPTIVE RESPONSES TO STRESSORS

Emotional Dimension

STRESSORS	MALADAPTIVE RESPONSES
Anxiety	Crying
Anger	Restlessness
Depression	Substance abuse
Hopelessness	Isolation
Guilt	Aggression
Elation	Suicide
Fear	Homocide
Grief	Helplessness
	Hopelessness
	Feelings of worthlessness
	Hostility
	Addiction

types of disintegrations of the form of thought. In symbolic associations, words or other symbols that have a common meaning take on specific meanings known only to the individual. In concrete associations, the individual is unable to generalize or to make abstract associations.

The thought content of a person who has adapted to stressors is oriented to reality and under the person's control. Unhealthy adaptation to stressors may be reflected in chronically negative and self-defeating thoughts or even in a person's inability to maintain a realistic orientation or control the content of thought. This lack of control is reflected in delusions—false beliefs that are seen as reality by the individual. These beliefs may be classified as bodily delusions or delusions of persecution, control, influence, infidelity or grandeur. A characteristic of delusions is their inability to be corrected by reason, argument, or logic.

The flow of thoughts in a person who has adapted well to stressors is characterized by a regularity and evenness. An unhealthy adaptation to stressors may result in the inability to regulate and pace the flow of thoughts, such as occurs in flight of ideas, thought retardation, or blocking. With flight of ideas, the person's thoughts rapidly digress from one idea to another, although some connecting train of thought is usually apparent. In thought retardation, thoughts form at a very slow speed. Blocking is the spontaneous loss of a train of thought.

Healthy individuals possess all of the physical capabilities for using their expressive functions and are able to express both their ideas and feelings. Their verbal and nonverbal communication is organized, consistent, and a true expression of themselves. They have a variety of channels for self-expression, including speech, dance, and other artistic forms. An unhealthy response to stressors, particularly emotional stressors, can be manifested in pressured speech, tangential speech, circumstantial speech, or muteness.

Like other disturbances in the intellectual dimension, expressive and receptive disabilities have been associated with particular anatomical lesions. Specific sensory impairments can result in disturbances called *apraxias, aphasias,* and *agnosias.* (See Table 9-3). Language disturbances usually appear in clusters of related dysfunctions. Impairment of any intellectual function essential to language processes is usually reflected in more than one language modality. Likewise the impairment of any language modality often reflects involvement of more than one of the functions in the intellectual dimension. For example, *agraphia* (literally, no writing) and *alexia* (literally, no reading) only rarely occur alone; they usually occur together, often with other language disturbances.[41] See the box at upper left on p. 180 for examples of stressors and responses in the intellectual dimension.

❀ *Social dimension.* Meaningful relationships in which people experience nurturance and support are crucial factors in one's ability to cope with all types of stressors. Social stressors arise from a number of different sources, for example, the family, the work place and the social class position. Potential stressors include family conflict, living or working in a hostile environment, poverty, unemployment, and social isolation. Because people

TABLE 9-3 Common expressive and receptive disturbances

Category of Deficit	Specific Deficits
Agnosia	
Sensory interpretation deficits characterized by an inability to recognize objects through the use of a particular sense.	Spatial agnosia: disorder of spatial orientation; inability to recognize spatial relationships
	Autopagnosia: inability to locate and name parts of own body
	Finger agnosia: inability to recognize own fingers
	Tactile agnosia: inability to recognize objects by touch
	Auditory agnosia: inability to identify common environmental sounds without looking; inability to recognize sounds
	Visual agnosia (very rare): inability to recognize objects by sight or their pictoral representation
Apraxia	
Loss of previously possessed ability to perform skilled acts	Motor or kinetic apraxia: usually affects finer movements of the upper extremities and is believed to be caused by loss of kinesthetic memory traces
	Audiomotor apraxia: difficulty in carrying out an action on verbal command
	Ideational apraxia: in ability to formulate plan of action successfully
	Constructional apraxia: inability to put parts together to make a whole
	Dressing apraxia: inability to dress properly
Aphasia	
Impairment in the reception, manipulation, or expression of the symbolic content of language	Expressive aphasia: trouble initiating speech
	Auditory receptive aphasia: trouble understanding speech
	Visual receptive aphasia: impaired ability to understand written language (dyslexia, alexia)
	Expressive writing aphasia (dysgraphic): inability to initiate written communication
	Amnestic or nominal aphasia: inability to identify people and things by their proper names

often depend on families as a primary source of nurturance and support, familial conflict can be particularly stressful. The effects are compounded when the individual has not developed a social support system outside the family, such as close friends or trusted associates. When families cannot adapt to the normal growth and develop-

EXAMPLES OF STRESSORS AND MALADAPTIVE RESPONSES TO STRESSORS

Intellectual Dimension

STRESSORS	MALADAPTIVE RESPONSES
Brain dysfunction	Perceptual disturbances
Limited intelligence	Thought disintegration
	Disorientation
Inability to express self	Loss of contact with reality
	Decreased cognitive functioning
Altered level of consciousness	Loss of memory
	Impaired judgment
Brain lesions	Impaired concentration
	Impaired decision making
	Delusion
	Illusions
	Hallucinations
	Forgetfulness
	Inability to learn
	Negative thinking
	Irrational thinking
	Illogical thinking
	Inability to speak (mute)
	Pressured speech
	Tangential/circumstantial speech
	Blocking
	Language disturbances

EXAMPLES OF STRESSORS AND MALADAPTIVE RESPONSES TO STRESSORS

Social Dimension

STRESSORS	MALADAPTIVE RESPONSES
Family conflict	Withdrawn behavior
Hostile environment	Alienation
Poverty	Criminal behavior
Unemployment	Impaired relationships
Social isolation	Sexual acting out
Threat to self-concept	Addiction (alcohol and drugs)
Threat to sexual role	Aggressive behavior
Role dysfunction	Low self-esteem
	Identity confusion
	Dependence
	Abusive behavior

ment of individual members, crises occur that are stressful to both the family member and the family as a unit.

Social isolation is an interpersonal stressor because it denies satisfaction of certain kinds of social needs and distorts certain social processes. Social interaction, the basis of social relationships, is a kind of stimulation with an optimal level; too much or too little is a stressor. Too much social interaction infringes on the individual's life space, whereas too little may be experienced as social isolation or deprivation.[40]

Any circumstance that adversely affects one's self-concept can be stressful. Situations in which a person is subjected to chronic criticism and devaluation can contribute to a low self-esteem and to a sense of worthlessness. Behavior that is incongruent with one's personal identity can be stressful, causing a sense of conflict and anxiety. Any event that necessitates a sudden change in self-concept is especially stressful because of minimal time for adaptation; examples may include an accident that results in disfigurement, death of a significant other, loss of a job, and a natural disaster.

Various experiences related to social roles, such as conflicting pressures and strains, may be stressors. An individual may feel role stress when a social structure creates very difficult, conflicting, or impossible demands for his position within the structure. The following are various types of role stress:

Role conflict—enactment of roles that conflict with one's value system or multiple roles that conflict with each other

Role ambiguity—enactment of roles that are not clearly defined in terms of expected behavior

Role incongruity—transition to a role that requires a significant modification in attitudes and values (for example, conflict between personal and professional values)

Role overload—enactment of role in which excessive demands are made and insufficient time is available to fulfill obligations (for example, student, worker, parent, spouse); most likely in highly industrialized societies and in higher-level positions[28]

Role incompetence—inability to fulfill role obligations associated with any given role (for example, inadequate occupational knowledge or expertise)

Role overqualification—enactment of a role which does not require full use of a person's resources (e.g., experienced professional working in position designed for new graduate)

Many roles are temporary, existing for the individual only for a given age or status. The roles of children are replaced by a different set when they reach young adulthood and by still another when they reach later years. One problem many individuals face is the transition from old to new roles; it is difficult to leave the familiarity of settled positions and face the uncertainty of new ones. Such stress normally accompanies developmental changes, such as the transitions from childhood to adolescence, high school to college, single to married, and working to retirement.

Experiences that threaten an individual's sexual identity or interfere with sexual role behaviors may be stressors. When one's attitudes, beliefs, or preferences regarding sexual behavior differ greatly from one's peer group, social isolation and self-doubt may occur. The inability to

TABLE 9-4 Social Readjustment Rating Scale

Life Event	Mean Value
1. Death of spouse	100
2. Divorce	73
3. Marital separation from mate	65
4. Detention in jail or other institution	63
5. Death of a close family member	63
6. Major personal injury or illness	53
7. Marriage	50
8. Being fired at work	47
9. Marital reconciliation with mate	45
10. Retirement from work	45
11. Major change in the health or behavior of a family member	44
12. Pregnancy	40
13. Sexual difficulties	39
14. Gaining a new family member (e.g., through birth, adoption, older person moving in)	39
15. Major business readjustment (e.g., merger, reorganization, bankruptcy)	39
16. Major change in financial state (e.g., a lot worse off or a lot better off than usual)	38
17. Death of a close friend	37
18. Changing to a different line of work	36
19. Major change in the number of arguments with spouse (e.g., either a lot more or a lot less than usual regarding childrearing, personal habits)	35
20. Taking out a mortgage or loan for a major purchase (e.g., for a home, business)	31
21. Foreclosure on a mortgage or loan	30
22. Major change in responsibilities at work (e.g., promotion, demotion, lateral transfer)	29
23. Son or daughter leaving home (e.g., marriage, attending college)	29
24. Trouble with in-laws	29
25. Outstanding personal achievement	28

Reprinted with permission from Journal of Psychosomatic Research **11**:213, Holmes, T.H., and Rahe, R.H., The Social Readjustment Rating Scale, Copyright 1967, Pergamon Press, Ltd.

meet one's sexual needs may result from internal or external obstacles and can act as a stressor; examples include illness or injury that affects some aspect of sexuality, conflict between personal and societal values, excessive guilt regarding sexual expression, and low self-esteem with perceived sexual inadequacy. Stressors that affect sexuality can also limit a person's capacity to develop intimacy within significant relationships.

Responses to social stress are determined by the individual's cultural values, past experiences with similar conditions, adequacy of coping mechanisms, and attribution of meaning. The failure to master social stress may lead to mental illness, physical illness, addiction, and criminal behavior.

Conditions of complex urban life, crowded living arrangements, and disruptions in social relationships have been identified as possible determinants of physical illness. These conditions often require excessive adaptation to change in a short period and create the experience of chronic frustration, both of which elicit prolonged physiological arousal. Studies concerning diseases such as tuberculosis and other respiratory disorders concluded that individuals deprived of meaningful social contact are more likely than others to develop these conditions. Social factors have also been shown to be important determinants in rheumatoid arthritis, hypertension, and coronary heart disease. These latter diseases may indicate the individual's lack of preparedness for new and unfamiliar situations. (See the box at right on p. 180 for examples of stressors and responses in the social dimension.)

Many events in a person's life contribute to social stress. Some of the life events cited in the Social Readjustment Rating Scale developed by Holmes and Rahe[34] are social stressors that may result in mental or physical illness. (See Table 9-4.) These events require a high level of adaptation and elicit a stress response.

Spiritual dimension. Stressors to the spiritual dimension can be any factors that interfere with an individual's ability to meet spiritual needs. Challenge to an individual's beliefs may be a stressor, particularly when these beliefs and values are unclear. Similarly, actions that transgress a person's values or moral code can be stressors. For instance, a woman who firmly believes that it is wrong to interfere with her body in any way but finds it necessary to have a hysterectomy may experience stress. A less severe stressor is a contradiction between a person's values and life-style. When people consistently find themselves spending time and energy in ways that do not fit with their values and beliefs, conflict arises and stress increases. Another stressor is the situation in which an individual is faced with choosing between two values that are in conflict. An example is the nurse who must choose between the rights of clients to know their diagnoses and possible concern for their fragile emotional conditions.

When two such values are in conflict, the person experiences stress until one value is affirmed as a priority and the other is surrendered, at least temporarily.[69]

Spiritually healthy or unhealthy persons can be distinguished by their responses to stressors on their philosophy of life. Spiritually healthy persons have clarified their goals and values, are decisive, spend their time and energy in reaching their goals, and are able to make moral and ethical judgments based on these beliefs and values. Persons who have not adapted well to stressors may respond by wishing to undo, redo, or relive the past. They may express shame, regret, or guilt; relate their illness to their guilt for failing to meet some standard of conduct; be unable to forgive themselves or receive forgiveness; project blame onto others or engage in self-destructive behavior.[9]

Events that precipitate a struggle with the meaning of life can serve as stressors. Such events may involve an anticipated role change, the loss of a meaningful relationship, personal illness, illness or death of a family member or close friend, or any kind of intense suffering. During such crises people are brought face-to-face with the ultimate issues of life, such as immortality, personal limitations, loss of control, and suffering in relation to the purpose of their lives.[67]

Spiritually healthy persons have found a reason for being that gives meaning to their existence. This meaning can be found in an organized religion involving the worship of a deity, in relationships with other persons, in a relationship with nature or the surrounding world, or in nonspiritual goals such as money. These persons have a sense of hope, a fundamental sense that things can work out and difficulties, including illness, can be overcome.

In contrast, spiritually unhealthy persons feel a sense of meaninglessness or purposelessness that may be characterized by questioning the meaning of their own existence, by hopelessness or despair, by feelings of uselessness, or by a sense of abandonment. In a situation of intense suffering, these persons may question the meaning of the suffering; doubt their ability to endure the suffering; question the credibility of their belief system; express that suffering is a necessary reparation; or become withdrawn, irritable, restless, self-pitying or fatigued. Unresolved feelings about death can be manifested in fears of darkness, being alone, or going to sleep; disturbing dreams; demanding behavior; or avoidance, preoccupation, or joking about death. Chronic feelings such as these act as stressors and decrease an individual's ability to adapt.

Disruptions in relationships, including a sense of isolation from others, can elicit a chronic stress reaction. A sense of relatedness or connectedness with others contributes to feelings of courage and hope, which help one continue even when the "odds" seem unfavorable.

Individuals require a certain amount of private time and space in which they can develop their own sense of meaning and relatedness, and in general recharge themselves. When this time is unavailable because of external obligations or by choice, people experience stress. The need for self-actualization with its accompanying aesthetic sensitivity cannot be met when people are constantly entrenched in the external world.

EXAMPLES OF STRESSORS AND MALADAPTIVE RESPONSES TO STRESSORS

Spiritual Dimension

STRESSORS	MALADAPTIVE RESPONSES
Challenge to personal beliefs or morals	Hopelessness
	Despair
Value conflicts	Decreased self-value
Loss of health, general well-being	No pleasure
	Decreased quality of life
Struggle with meaning, purpose in life	Meaninglessness
	Fragmentation or loss of sense of continuity
Fear of death or dying	Alienation
Lack of faith	
Abandonment	Isolation

Spiritually healthy persons have a keen sense of awareness of the world about them and allow a variety of experiences to enter their consciousness. They have a sense of freedom and harmony and have developed their potential for creativity. Spiritually unhealthy persons block out events or distort them before they are allowed to enter consciousness. These persons feel little control over what happens to them or over their own response to events. (See the box above for examples of stressors and responses in the spiritual dimension.)

BRIEF REVIEW

Five major concepts are generally accepted premises of holistic health care philosophy. First, each person is multidimensional; one's physical, emotional, intellectual, social, and spiritual dimensions are in constant interaction with each other. Historically, interest has been shown in all five dimensions; however, Eastern views of human dimensions have typically been more holistic than Western views. The physical dimension involves everything associated with one's body, both internal and external. The emotional dimension consists of affective states and feelings, including motor behavior associated with emotion, the experienced aspect of emotion, and the physiological mechanisms which underlie emotion. The intellectual dimension includes the receptive functions, memory and learning, cognition, and the expressive functions. The social dimension is based on social interaction and relationships as well as the more global concept of culture. The spiritual dimension is that aspect of a person from which meaning in life is developed and through which transcendence over the ordinary is possible.

The second premise of holistic health care philosophy is that the environment makes significant contributions to the nature of one's existence. Each person's environment consists of many factors which are influential in that person's quality of life. Consequently, people cannot be fully understood without consideration of environmental factors such as family relationships, culture, and physical surroundings. Individuals interact with their unique environments through all dimensions, based on subjective experience as well as external stimuli.

The third premise is that each person experiences development across his life cycle; in each stage of life, the individual experiences and confronts different issues or similar issues in different ways. One's experience of each stage of life forms the basis for further development as one moves through the life cycle.

Fourth, the holistic health care provider maintains that stress is a primary factor in health and illness. Any event or circumstance can act as a stressor. Regardless of the source, stress has an impact on the whole person. Stressors directly affecting the physical dimension are numerous; examples include stressors associated with genetic factors, physiological processes, and body image. Emotional stress may result from any experience or situation, related to any dimension that elicits an emotion from the individual and generates the physiological stress response. Examples include poor physical conditions, perceived social inequities, a significant loss, intellectual incompetence, and a sense of meaninglessness. Stressors affecting the intellectual dimension may be any factors that interfere with receptive functions, memory and learning, cognitive functions, or expressive functions. Social stressors may arise from interactions and relationships with other people, as well as from more general societal and cultural factors. Stressors affecting the spiritual dimension may be any factors which interfere with one's ability to meet spiritual needs. Value conflicts, perceived loss of meaning, and a sense of isolation are examples of stressors to the spiritual dimension.

Fifth, people are ultimately responsible for the directions and the life-styles they choose. Locus of control is a concept that indicates the extent to which individuals perceive a sense of personal responsibility in life. Within a holistic framework, people are viewed as active participants in and contributors to their health status; they are willing to learn from illness and to strive toward healthier choices.

REFERENCES AND SUGGESTED READINGS

1. Baron, R.A., and others: Psychology: understanding behavior, Ed. 2, New York, 1980, Holt, Rinehart & Winston General Book.
2. Barr, W.: Pyridoxine supplements in the premenstrual syndrome, Practitioner **228:**425, 1984.
3. Blankstein, K. and Egner, K.: Relationship of the locus of control construct to the control of heart rate, Journal of General Psychology **97:**291, 1977.
4. Brallier, L.W.: Stress management as a path toward wholeness. In Krieger, D.: Foundations for holistic health nursing practices: the Renaissance nurse, Philadelphia, 1981, J.B. Lippincott Co.
5. Brallier, L.W.: The nurse as holistic health practitioner, Nursing Clinics of North America **13:**643, 1978.
6. Brodsky, C.: A study of norms for body form-behavior relationships, Washington, D.C. 1954, The Catholic University of America Press.
7. Burkhardt, M.: Dealing with spiritual concerns of clients in the community, Journal of Community Health Nursing **2(**4**):**191, 1985.
8. Cadoret, R.J., and King, L.J.: Psychiatry in primary care, ed. 2, St. Louis, 1983, The C.V. Mosby Co.
9. Campbell, C.: Nursing diagnosis and intervention, New York, 1977, John Wiley & Sons, Inc.
10. Capra, F.: The turning point: science, society, and the rising culture, New York, 1982, Simon & Schuster, Inc.
11. Clark, C.C.: Enhancing wellness: a guide for self-care, New York, 1981, Springer Publishing Co., Inc.
12. Clinebell, H.: Basic types of pastoral counseling: new resources for ministering to the troubled, New York, 1966, Abingdon Press.
12a. Colston, L.: The handicapped. In Wicks, R., Parson, R., and Capps, D., editors: Clinical handbook of pastoral counseling, New York, 1985, Integration Books.
13. Cole, S.: The sociological orientation: an introduction to sociology, Chicago, 1975, Rand McNally & Co.
14. Cooley, C.: Human nature and the social order, New York, 1902, Charles Scribner's Sons.
15. Craig, W.J.: Caffeine update, Adventist Review **158(**35**):**3, 1981.
16. Davis, G.: The hands of the healer: has faith a place? Journal of Medical Ethics **6:**185, 1980.
17. Denver, G.E.A.: Community health analysis: a holistic approach, Germantown, Md., 1980, Aspen Systems Corp.
18. Dunn, H.L.: High level wellness, Thorofare, N.J., 1961, Slack, Inc.
19. Ferguson, M.: The aquarian conspiracy: personal and social transformation in the 1980's, Los Angeles, 1980, Jeremy P. Tarcher, Inc.
20. Flynn, P.A.R., editor: The healing continuum: journeys in the philosophy of holistic health, Bowie, Md., 1980, Robert J. Brady Co.
21. Garsee, J.: The development of an ideology. In Schuster, C.S., and Ashburn, S.S.: The process of human development: a holistic approach, Boston, 1980, Little, Brown & Co., Inc.
22. Girdano, D., and Everly, G.: Controlling stress and tension: a holistic approach, Englewood Cliffs, N.J., 1979, Prentice-Hall, Inc.
23. Goe, J.: Psychophysiological disorders. In Lancaster, J., editor: Adult psychiatric nursing, Garden City, N.Y., 1980, Medical Examination Publishing Co., Inc.
24. Gordon, J.S.: The paradigm of holistic medicine. In Hastings, A.C., Fadiman, J., and Gordon, J.S., editors: Health for the whole person, Boulder, Colo., 1980, Westview Press, Inc.
25. Greenspan, S.: Intelligence and adaptation, New York, 1979, International Universities Press, Inc.
26. Guidano, V.F. and Liotti, G.: Cognitive processes and emotional disorders: a structural approach to psychotherapy, New York, 1983, The Guilford Press.
27. Guyton, A.C.: Textbook of medical physiology, ed. 6, Philadelphia, 1981, W.B. Saunders Co.
28. Hardy, M.: Role strain and role stress. In Hardy, M. and Conway, M.: Role theory: perspectives for health professionals, New York, 1978, Appleton-Century-Crofts.
29. Hayter, J.: The rhythm of sleep, American Journal of Nursing **80(**3**):**457, 1980.
30. Heiniger, M.C., and Randolph, S.L.: Neurophysiological concepts in human behavior: the learning tree, St. Louis, 1981, The C.V. Mosby Co.
31. Highfield, M.F.: Oncology nurses' awareness of their patients' spiritual needs and problems, master's thesis, 1981, University of Arkansas for Medical Sciences.
32. Hogan, R.M.: Human sexuality: a nursing perspective, Norwalk, Conn., 1985, Appleton-Century-Crofts.

33. Hollen, P.: A holistic model of individual and family health based on a continuum of choice, Advances in Nursing Science 3(4):27, 1981.

34. Holmes, T.H., and Rahe, R.H.: The social readjustment rating scale, Journal of Psychosomatic Research **11**:213, 1967.

35. Kaluger, G., and Kaluger, M.F.: Human development: the span of life, ed. 3, St. Louis, 1984, The C.V. Mosby Co.

36. Kaplan, H., and Sadock, B.: Comprehensive textbook of psychiatry IV, ed. 4, Baltimore, 1985, Williams & Wilkins.

37. Kohlberg, L.: Development of moral character and moral ideology. In Hoffman, M.L., and Hoffman, L.W., editors: Review of child development research, vol. 1, New York, 1964, Russell Sage Foundation.

38. Lancaster, J.: Adult psychiatric nursing, New York, 1980, Medical Examination Publishing Co., Inc.

39. Leininger, M.: Transcultural nursing: concepts, theory, and practice, New York, 1978, John Wiley & Sons, Inc.

40. Levine, S. and Scotch, N.: Social stress, Chicago, 1970, Aldine Publishing Co.

41. Lezak, M.: Neuropsychological assessment, New York, 1976, Oxford University Press, Inc.

42. Lugo, J. and Hershey, G.: Human development: a multidisciplinary approach to the psychology of individual growth, New York, 1974, Macmillan Publishing Co., Inc.

43. Malasanos, L., and others: Health assessment, ed. 3., St. Louis, 1986, The C.V. Mosby Co.

44. Maslow, A.H.: Motivation and personality, ed. 2, New York, 1970, Harper & Row, Publishers, Inc.

45. Maslow, A.H.: Toward a psychology of being, ed. 2, New York, 1968, Van Nostrand Reinhold Co., Inc.

46. McKee, J.: Introduction to sociology, ed. 2, New York, 1974, Holt, Rinehart & Winston, Inc.

47. Menninger, W.: A psychiatrist for a troubled world, New York, 1967, The Viking Press. (Edited by B. Hall.)

48. Munn, N.: The fundamentals of human adjustment, Boston, 1961, Houghton Mifflin Co.

49. Norman, S.: Diagnostic categories for the patient with a right hemisphere lesion, American Journal of Nursing **79**:2126, 1979.

50. Norris, C.: The professional nurse and body image. In Carlson, C., coordinator, Behavioral concepts and nursing intervention, Philadelphia, 1970, J.B. Lippincott Co.

51. Nowakowski, L: Health promotion/self-care programs for the community, Topics in Clinical Nursing 2(2):21, 1980.

52. Pelletier, K.R.: Mind as healer, mind as slayer: a holistic approach to preventing disorders, New York, 1977, Dell Publishing Co., Inc.

53. Perls, F., Hefferline, R.F., and Goodman, P.: Gestalt therapy, New York, 1951, Bantam Books, Inc.

54. Piaget, J.: The growth of logical thinking from childhood to adolescence, New York, 1958, Basic Books, Inc., Publishers.

55. Rainer, J.: Contributions of the biological sciences. In Kaplan, H. and Sadock, B.: Comprehensive textbook of psychiatry, ed. 4, Baltimore, 1985, Williams and Wilkins.

56. Rew, L.: Exercises for spiritual growth, Journal of Holistic Nursing 4(1):20, 1986.

57. Robins, L., Clayton, P., and Wing, J., editors: The social consequences of psychiatric illness, New York, 1980, Brunner/Mazel, Inc.

58. Ryan, R.S., and Travis, J.W.: The wellness workbook, Berkeley, Calif., 1981, Ten Speed Press.

59. Samuels, M. and Bennett, H.: The well body book, New York, 1973, Random House, Inc.

60. Saxton, D.F., and Haring, P.W.: Care of patients with emotional problems, ed. 4, St. Louis, The C.V. Mosby Co., 1984.

61. Schuster, C.S., and Ashburn, S.S.: The process of human development: a holistic approach, Boston, 1980, Little, Brown & Co., Inc.

62. Segal, J.: Biofeedback as medical treatment, Journal of the American Medical Association, **2232**:179, 1975.

63. Selye, H.: The stress of life, ed. 2, New York, 1978, McGraw-Hill Book Co.

64. Sheldon, W., Stevens, S., and Tucker, W.: The varieties of human physique: and introduction to constitutional psychology, New York, 1941, Harper & Brothers.

65. Simonton, O., Mathews-Simonton, S. and Creighton, J.: Getting well again, New York, 1978, Bantam Books, Inc.

66. Stein, J.: Supergene, Omni **3**(3):81, 1980.

67. Stoll, R.I.: Guidelines for spiritual assessment, American Journal of Nursing **79**:1574, 1979.

68. Sun, M.: FDA caffeine decision too early, some say, Science **209**:1500, 1980.

69. Tubesing, D.A.: Stress skills, Oakland, Ill., 1979, Whole Person Associates, Inc.

70. White House Conference on Aging: Spiritual well-being, Washington, D.C., 1971, Department of Health, Education, and Welfare, U.S. Government Printing Office.

71. Wolanin, M.O., and Phillips, L.R.: Confusion: prevention and care, St. Louis, 1981, The C.V. Mosby Co.

ANNOTATED BIBLIOGRAPHY

Baron, R.A., and others: Psychology: understanding behavior, ed. 2, New York, 1980, Holt, Rinehart & Winston General Book.

This comprehensive book includes a framework for understanding maladaptive behavior, details causes and treatment of maladaptive behavior, and discusses areas of assessment and prevention. Emphasis is given to the latest research findings on biological factors in the cause of disorders.

Kaluger, G., and Kaluger, M.F.: Human development: the span of life, ed. 3, St. Louis, 1984, The C.V. Mosby Co.

This book presents the basic universal principles of growth and development while emphasizing the significance of individual differences and recognizing the environmental influences in creating differences.

Kreiger, D.: Foundations of holistic health nursing practice: the Renaissance nurse, Philadelphia, 1981, J.B. Lippincott Co.

This book focuses on the healing of the whole person and discusses human embryologic development on a continuum through death. From prehistoric time to the present, it lays the foundations for modern holistic health nursing. The content includes clinical articles covering therapeutic touch, imagery, stress management theories, and the holistic conceptual framework as it is used in the nursing process. Emphasis is placed on revitalizing humanism in nursing within the philosophy of holism.

CULTURAL CONSIDERATIONS IN THERAPY

Toni Tripp-Reimer   Sonja H. Lively

After studying this chapter the learner will be able to:

Trace the historical relationship of culture to mental health–psychiatric nursing practice.

Define the concept of culture.

Discuss dysfunctional aspects of either positive or negative stereotyping.

Distinguish between the concepts of ethnocentrism and cultural relativity.

Identify important cultural variables in mental health–psychiatric nursing.

Describe cultural influences on values and patterns of communication in the nurse-client relationship.

Identify culturally sensitive intervention strategies.

A case of suspected child abuse was reported recently to the staff of a county mental health facility. The case involved a Vietnamese refugee family newly arrived in the United States. The referral was made by a school nurse who, while conducting routine physical assessments, identified long bruised areas on the chest and back of a girl in the second grade. However, rather than being caused by incidents of child abuse, the marks were the results of the lay practice of dermabrasion *(cao gio),* a standard home treatment for the symptoms of fever, chills, and headaches that accompany "wind illness." This practice consists of applying oil to the back and chest of the child with cotton swabs. The skin is massaged until warm and then rubbed with the edge of a copper coin until marks (bruises) appear. Thus the parents had not been abusing the child but rather were following a culturally prescribed and sanctioned mode of folk therapy.

In a neighborhood mental health clinic a nurse therapist misread a Navajo client's body language. The nurse knew that good counseling skills include direct eye contact. She had been taught that clients desire this and that when clients do not engage in direct eye contact they are disinterested or have something to hide. In fact, this Navajo client was being polite by averting his eyes, as might a person from Asia or Appalachia.

These two vignettes illustrate the importance of knowing about the client's culture in mental health–psychiatric nursing. The potential for misunderstanding is accentuated when the nurse and recipient are from different cultural or ethnic groups. Misunderstandings may arise from variations in values, beliefs, and customs or patterns of behavior. Sensitivity to these cultural variables is a requisite for quality health care in multiethnic situations.

THE NATURE OF CULTURE

Culture is defined as learned patterns of values, beliefs, customs, and behaviors that are shared by a group of interacting individuals. Rather than material objects, culture is a set of rules or standards for behavior. The sharing of a common culture is important because it allows members of the group to predict each other's actions and react accordingly.

Culture is learned; it is not genetically inherited. Although all humans have basic biological needs (such as elimination and safety), they respond to these biological needs in cultural ways. For example, every individual has a need for nutrients, but culture determines the patterns of behavioral responses to this need, including what, where, when, and with whom one eats. Culture is transmitted from one generation to the next by the process called *enculturation.* It may be learned formally, as in Lamaze prenatal classes, or informally by observing the behaviors of various individuals within the culture. By

Historical Overview

DATE	EVENT
1910s	Emil Kraepelin traveled to Indonesia, found that the frequency of mental disorders in Java differed from that of his native Germany, and attributed this difference to heredity rather than culture. He is considered one of the earliest pioneers in the study of the relationship between culture and mental disorder.
1914	In his book *Totem and Taboo*,[20] Freud attempted to use anthropological sources to substantiate his psychoanalytic theories. Using cultural data, Freud erroneously argued that the Oedipal complex is universal.
1927	Malinowski[46] studied natives of the Trobriand Islands in the Pacific Ocean and convincingly demonstrated the errors in Freud's theory of a universal Oedipal complex.
1928	In her hallmark book *Coming of Age in Samoa*,[48] Mead documented that the adolescence experience is largely influenced by one's culture.
Late 1920s-Early 1930s	The culture and personality school in anthropology, was founded by Margaret Mead, Ruth Benedict, Ralph Linton, Clyde Kluckhohn, Gregory Bateson, and Irving Hollowell, who initiated extensive investigations of psychiatric problems in a cross-cultural perspective.
1934	In the book *Patterns of Culture*, Benedict[2] noted that mental health practitioners need to define behavior as normal or abnormal only within the particular cultural context in which they are working.
1930s-1940s	Transcultural data highlighted the effects of culture on psychopathology, and there was an overemphasis on the exotic manifestations of psychopathological conditions among Third World peoples.
1952	Peplau introduced the idea that culture is an important client variable in mental health–psychiatric nursing.
1960s	Transcultural nursing was established as a legitimate field of study. The civil rights movement led many nurses to emphasize the necessity for specialized knowledge and skill in providing care for minority clients.
1962	In a review article, King[34] concluded that psychopathology is universal, its prevalence across culture groups is similar, but manifestations of psychopathological behaviors differ among cultures.
1969	The Council on Nursing and Anthropology was established to investigate the integration of cultural content into nursing practice.
1970s	A new perspective emerged that identified the ways in which culture influences mental disorders and characteristics of health systems.
1974	The Transcultural Nursing Society was established.
1970s-1980s	Investigators in the field of mental health began to identify methods for working with culturally distinct clients in pluralistic societies.
1981	The American Nurses' Association Council on Cultural Diversity in Nursing Practice was initiated to promote minority rights and improve care for minority clients.
Future	Because the United States is a pluralistic society and continues to have high rates of immigration, cultural variables will increasingly be viewed as crucial factors in holistic assessment of and intervention with clients in mental health settings.

watching different persons, modeling their behavior, and observing the reactions of others to this behavior, appropriate and acceptable behavior is learned.

Individual behavior is not necessarily representative of the culture. The culture defines dominant patterns of values, attitudes, beliefs, customs, and behaviors but does not determine all the behaviors in any group. There will be variation from the dominant pattern. If this variation is encountered in one individual, it is called idiosyncratic behavior. Depending on the meaning of this idiosyncratic behavior to the group, the individual may be called eccentric or deviant or he may fall within the normal range.

However, a group of individuals within a society who share values, beliefs, and behaviors that differ from those of the dominant society is referred to as a *subculture*.

The term cultural group is sometimes used imprecisely. People who share some common characteristics do not necessarily share a culture. Rose[62] and Sullivan[79] have argued that American elderly people constitute a subculture; this is an inappropriate designation of the term subculture, since they erroneously categorized the elderly after observing life patterns that only superficially indicate homogeneity. In fact, their "shared" characteristics do not represent an aged subculture but only features that are dictated by specific life circumstances, such as mandatory retirement laws and declining physical integrity. Similarly, socioeconomic level or social class does not determine a cultural group. Consequently the "culture of poverty" is a misnomer.

Integration is the tendency for all aspects of a culture to function as an interrelated whole. Because cultures fulfill certain common functions, they resemble each other in basic domains. Universal aspects of culture include kinship, education, diet, religion, art, politics, economics, health, and patterns of communication. It is difficult to study only one aspect of a culture because these categories are so closely interrelated.

Culture contains both ideal and real components; that is, the way people think they should behave often differs from their actual behavior. Every society has ideal cultural patterns, *norms,* that represent what most members of the society say they ought to do in a particular situation. These norms may be enforced through legal or social means. However, real behavior may differ from the ideal and still be acceptable.

Cultural identity differs from race. Cultural identity concerns shared values, beliefs, and patterns of behavior within a group of people, whereas racial identity refers to biologically inherited characteristics that are transmitted through genetic mechanisms and may be observed in physical traits.

Because each individual tends to view his culture as correct, many people have the misconception that only other people have a culture. Although it is difficult to determine the effect of culture on one's behavior, it is important to remember that all people are under the influence of their own culture system. The box below summarizes what culture is and what it is not.

STEREOTYPING

Because each client is approached on an individual basis, it is imperative not to overgeneralize or stereotype on the basis of cultural or ethnic affiliation. Sensitivity to cultural differences in clients is essential, but ethnic affiliation serves only as a clue to assist in assessment and intervention in mental health–psychiatric nursing, and cultural affiliation gives only background data.

Most stereotyping is the result of believing ideas thought to be known about another culture. For example, among members of the dominant American culture, Anglos* the Hispanic concept of *machismo* is surrounded by misconceptions. In Hispanic cultures machismo is a combination of the culturally desirable traits of courage and fearlessness in a man. The man is the head of his family and the protector of his honor. As an authority figure the man must be just and fair; misuse of authority results in loss of respect. The machismo ethic also allows a father to be more openly expressive of his love for his children than is generally seen in Anglo culture. However, the dominant American culture has generally emphasized the dysfunctional aspects of machismo (heavy drinking, seduction of women, and domineering and abusive spouse behaviors). These aspects of machismo have also been overemphasized by health care workers.

Even stereotypes that characterize people in a positive way may be misleading. For example, there is evidence that Anglos stereotype blacks as providing more care for the elderly than is true.[29] Similarly, investigations of the elderly in San Francisco's Chinatown have revealed a serious erosion of Chinese patterns of kinship and community.[8,32] These findings contradict stereotypes of the Asians as always revering their elders. As a result of this "positive" stereotyping, actual problems of elderly blacks and Chinese-Americans may be overlooked.

*The term "Anglo" is used throughout this chapter to refer to Americans of northern European descent. This use of the term is a purposeful strategy to highlight the point that all people, not only members of minority groups, are influenced by their culture.

WHAT CULTURE IS AND WHAT IT IS NOT

CULTURE IS	CULTURE IS NOT
The total way of life of a people	Genetically inherited or determined
Values, beliefs, and norms of a population	Individualistic, ideosyncratic behavior
Learned, regulated, shared	Racial or biological characteristics
Transmitted from generation to generation	Deterministic
Stored in memories, books, and objects of the people	Easily changed
Exhibited in actions	Static
Dynamic, constantly changing, adaptive	
Ideational and real	
Integrative	

Indiscriminately characterizing all members of minority populations as traditionalists leads to another stereotype. All members of the subculture may be stereotyped as maintaining traditional ethnic values, beliefs, and customs; however, each ethnic group has members who are more or less acculturated to the dominant society. An exception is a tendency for more adherence to tradition by certain ethnic or racially distinct groups, because economic, religious, political, and social acculturation may be restricted in American society, especially among recent immigrants. Furthermore, every ethnic or minority group has a historical memory of prejudice that is evident in all immigrant experiences. This memory affects even second- and third-generation members so that they never feel quite comfortable with the dominant cultural group in America.[21,22,74,76,91]

The degree to which any one individual in a subculture adheres to the traditional culture depends on a number of different factors, including age, sex, education, and generation of immigration. The Research Highlight below demonstrates the importance of not assuming that traditional health beliefs and behaviors are retained, even in individuals with high ethnic affiliation.[7,88]

ETHNOCENTRISM AND CULTURAL RELATIVITY

Ethnocentrism and *cultural relativity* are complementary concepts. Each denotes the perspective from which cultural characteristics are interpreted. The distinction between them concerns whether the data are interpreted from the perspective of the health professional's culture or that of the client. From an ethnocentric perspective a nurse judges the behaviors of clients of a different culture by the standards of her own culture. From a culturally relativistic perspective the nurse attempts to understand the behavior of transcultural clients within the context of their culture. In application, cultural relativity can be considered an intervention strategy that stresses cultural acceptance over cultural imposition.

Sometimes sterotyping is done unconsciously, simply because client behaviors are interpreted within the health professional's own value system. This practice, documented in a study concerning health professionals working with Appalachian migrants, is reported in the Research Highlight on p. 189.

CULTURAL VARIABLES IN MENTAL HEALTH–PSYCHIATRIC NURSING

Knowledge of cultural variables are important for the practice of mental health nursing for three major reasons. First, culture patterns the ways in which mental illness is defined, influences the perception of the mentally ill by their reference groups, and identifies appropriate health-seeking behaviors. Second, culture itself may act as a stressor for the client. Third, cultural differences between the

---

Research Highlight

Retention of a Folk Healing Practice (Matiasma) Among Four Generations of Urban Greek Immigrants

T. Tripp-Reimer

PURPOSE

The purpose of this study was to delineate specific facets of *matiasma*, the configuration surrounding the evil eye, and to trace the retention of knowledge and use of this configuration over a four-generation population.

SAMPLE

The study sample included 328 individuals of Greek descent from 102 extended family units living in Columbus, Ohio.

METHODOLOGY

Data were collected during a field investigation over an 11-month period through the use of semistructured interviews and participant observation.

FINDINGS

The data yielded results indicating the Greek community's beliefs and practices concerning the cause, prevention, diagnosis, and treatment of the evil eye. Although the Greek community was politically, economically, and geographically integrated into the larger metropolitan community, it remained culturally distinct. However, the retention of beliefs and practices concerning the evil eye varied dramatically by generation of immigration. In the first generation, virtually all the members knew about the evil eye and nearly 90% had used practices concerned with the evil eye. However, by the fourth generation, although 46% were still knowledgeable about the evil eye, none had actually used practices concerning it.

IMPLICATIONS

This study demonstrates the importance of the generation depth as a variable in the health beliefs and behaviors of clients. It points out the importance of not stereotyping individuals on the basis of their cultural background.

Based on data from Nursing Research **32**:97-101, 1983.

Research Highlight

Barriers to Health Care: Perceptual Variations of Appalachian and Non-Appalachian Health Care Professionals

T. Tripp-Reimer

PURPOSE

The purpose of this study was to identify the way in which health professionals characterized Appalachian clients.

SAMPLE

The study sample included health professionals who worked in a variety of clinical settings with a high proportion of Appalachian migrant clients.

METHODOLOGY

The health professionals were asked to identify and interpret characteristic Appalachian behaviors. Subsequent analysis was conducted that divided the professionals into two groups: those who grew up in Appalachia and those who grew up elsewhere.

FINDINGS

Both groups generally identified the same five areas of Appalachian behavior: (1) Appalachians tend to have large families, (2) Appalachian migrants tend to move back and forth between the urban areas and the "hills," (3) Appalachian migrants tend to quit school at an early age, (4) many Appalachians use welfare services, and (5) Appalachian migrants tend to be oriented to the present.

Although the same objective facts were noted by both groups, there was a dichotomous interpretation of the behavior based on the background of the health professional. Non-Appalachians tended to view the behaviors negatively, from an ethnocentric perspective, whereas Appalachian professionals generally interpreted the same behavior as adaptive, from a relativistic perspective.

IMPLICATIONS

This study illustrates the difference beetween a culturally relativistic and an ethnocentric perspective. Mental health nurses need to understand client behavior in the context of the client's culture and not to interpret client behavior from personal standards.

Based on data from Western Journal of Nursing Research 4:179-91, 1982.

nurse and client may lead to misunderstandings and a nontherapeutic relationship.

Influence of Culture in Mental Illness

The definition of mental illness is part of a belief system and is largely determined by cultural factors. In particular, there is wide variation in the way mental disorders are defined and identified. These differences can be better understood by using the framework that distinguishes *emic* and *etic* perspectives devised by Pike.[47] This framework differentiates how members within a culture group define normal and abnormal behavior (emic) as opposed to the way individuals outside that culture group define the same behavior (etic).

An emic definition is culturally specific; that is, an emic analysis seeks to discover the perspective of individuals within a particular culture. The main aim of emic study involves the discovery of native principles of classification and conceptualization. The emic approach yields a definition of mental disorder from inside the client's cultural perspective. The result is sometimes called "subjective culture."[3,19,69,77]

Etic categories are culturally universal. An etic analysis generally includes observing behavior without learning the viewpoint of those being studied. Using externally derived criteria, the etic investigator examines and compares several cultures.[3,19,57,58,69] Because these etic categories can be applied across cultures, Pike calls them culture-free features of the real world. The categories of mental disorder in the scientific diagnostic system (DSM-III-R) can be viewed as an etic classification system according to which data from individual clients are analyzed. This etic approach imposes a classficiation system that may be external to that of the client.

The client and the nurse may come to the health care setting with different belief systems of how mental disorder is defined, how it is caused, and how it can best be treated. The question that emerges is "What do we mean when we say that behavior is abnormal or pathological?" A nurse whose client indicates that he has been in contact with a dead relative or that he has been possessed by a spirit may consider this to be a sign of mental disorder, without recognizing that it may be an accepted occurrence in his culture.

Many culture groups encourage altered states of consciousness that initially may appear to indicate mental disturbance to a Western nurse. As described by Bourguignon,[4,5] altered states of consciousness are universal phenomena that are experienced in at least a number of forms by all humans. In addition to normal waking consciousness, there are other states of consciousness, such as dream states and states of alcohol or drug intoxication. Mental health–psychiatric nurses recognize some of these states. However, other altered states of consciousness are less familiar to nurses but are found in the majority of the world's societies.

Two other states of consciousness are *trance* and *possession trance*. Trance is generally interpreted as soul absence of some kind and is frequently linked to hallucinations or visions. Possession trance, on the other hand, involves the belief that the body has been taken over in its functions by a spiritual entity. These two altered forms of consciousness are generally considered sacred, ritual states by members of cultures with these beliefs. They involve cultural patterning and therefore are influenced by learning and tradition. In an ethnographic sample of 488 societies, 90% of the societies had one or both of these institutionalized ritual types of altered states of consciousness. The incidence of societies with altered states of consciousness ranged from 97% in North American Indian groups to approximately 80% in the Mediterranean area. These findings led to the conclusion that trance and possession trance are universal human capacities.[4]

The idea of possession may be familiar to health professionals from Biblical scripture. In Matthew 12:22, Jesus "drove out devils and healed possessed persons." Among American Pentecostal groups, and more recently the charismatic religious movements, the Holy Ghost is believed to possess individuals. This possession is sometimes called "baptism of the Holy Spirit."

From an etic perspective a client who indicates that he has been possessed by a spirit may be seen as expressing symptoms of mental disorder. From an emic perspective the client may be seen as engaged in normal, culturally sanctioned behavior.

Emic and etic definitions of mental disorder involve factors other than altered states of consciousness. A study of Indo-Chinese refugees in Los Angeles found that only psychotic, endangering behaviors were regarded as requiring professional help and other problems, such as depression, were not defined as needing professional help.[94] Similarly, a recent study[13] found significant differences between Appalachians and mental health professionals in their identification of problematic behaviors. Behaviors that were identified as indicative of mental illness by the mental health professionals were labeled as lazy, mean, immoral, criminal, or psychic by Appalachians. The study concluded that nursing can provide a better framework for understanding client behavior by incorporating the study of culture as a concept central to determining which behaviors indicate mental disorders and which do not.[16]

In Western scientific practice there is generally a split or dichotomy between mental and physical symptoms. However, many other cultures view the mind and body more holistically: mental distress may be expressed through somatization. For example, Arce and Torres-Matrullo[1] point out that "Hispanics tend to conceptualize mental illness as a physical disease of the nervous system . . . . Affective responses such as anxiety or depression are reported in psychophysiological concomitants—dizziness, fatigue, headaches, and various gastrointestinal disturbances." Similarly, Chinese people also tend to express their emotional distress in somatic rather than emotional terms and this is reflected in their language, which is rich in body metaphors.[92] Instead of identifying stress or tension, Chinese may speak of headaches, dizzy spells, stomach troubles, or insomnia, the key symptom of a serious problem.[55] In discussing problems with emotions, Greeks refer to "nerves." This Greek relationship is also mirrored in their clinical practice in which most Greek psychiatrists are also neurologists. Consequently, Greek psychiatrists' clients usually experience neurophysiological symptoms.[66]

There are many instances in which emic and etic classification systems may not be congruent, as when the emic classification systems attributes mental disorder to nonscientific causes. Illnesses that are attributed to nonscientific causes are generally termed *folk illnesses*. Folk illnesses have been divided into two major categories: naturalistic and personalistic illness.[17]

Naturalistic illnesses. Naturalistic illnesses are caused by impersonal factors; that is, entities without regard for the individual. Generally, naturalistic illnesses are based on an equilibrium model; when the balance is disturbed, illness results. The equilibrium theory is common throughout the world. Three of the most prevalent examples are the yin and yang model of Chinese culture, the Navajo model of balance and harmony with nature, and the hot and cold model of Hispanic cultures.

Among the traditional Indo-Chinese, health is based on the balance of yin and yang forces. Yin forces are characterized as cold, weak, female, and small. Yang forces are characterized as hot, strong, male, and large. An excess in normality of biological or emotional states is a yang illness. A deficiency results in a yin illness. Treatment for yin and yang conditions occurs by the principle of opposition. Yin illnesses are treated by yang foods, medications, or techniques; yang illnesses are treated by yin foods, medications, and techniques. Examples of cold, or yin, treatments are acupuncture and consumption of herbal teas and vegetables. Examples of hot, or yang, treatments are moxibustion (burning a cone of mugwort on the skin) and consumption of foods that are spicy or high in protein or fat content. Lin and Lin[44] have identified one Chinese theory of mental illness as resulting from the imbalance of yin and yang. Mental illness may be attributed to harmful emanations affecting yin and yang: numbness, insanity, disturbance of speech, and anger. Excesses or deficiencies in physiological functions are thought to affect the balance of yin and yang, leading to mental illness. For example, sexuality, climatic changes, diet, and exercises are implicated in manic excitement, which is referred to as "peach blossom insanity" and is believed to occur commonly in the spring among the young.

Personalistic illnesses. Personalistic illnesses result from punishment or aggression but are specifically directed toward an individual. Two personalistic beliefs are evil eye and witchcraft.

The evil eye, discussed in the Research Highlight on p. 188, is a pervasive folk illness known throughout Mediterranean and Spanish-speaking cultures. The evil eye is usually unintentionally caused and may result simply from envy or admiration. For example, a woman may unintentionally cast the "eye" simply by admiring another woman's child. The child may later feel lethargic, have a headache, or be irritable. Cultural groups differ in the way they determine if the eye has been cast. Among Mexican-Americans, casting of the eye (*mal ojo*) is detected by rubbing a raw, uncooked, unshelled egg over the abdomen of the affected individual. The egg is then broken into a glass of water; if it assumes a sunny-side up position, it indicates that the eye has been cast. Greeks determine whether the eye (*matiasma*) has been cast by dropping oil into a glass of water; dispersion of the oil over the water indicates presence of the evil eye. Generally, diagnosis of the eye is sufficient to remove the affliction.

Groups with belief in the evil eye also have methods of protecting against it. For example, Hispanic girls may wear gold crosses or have tiny spiders embroidered on their dresses. Greek children may wear a blue stone to "reflect" the eye. In addition, after complimenting a child, the Hispanic admirer may touch a child gently on the forehead to thwart any unintentional effects of envy. Greeks may invoke the name of the Virgin Mary after admiring a child.

Belief in witchcraft as a cause of illness also falls into the personalistic category. Snow[73] found this belief widespread among Puerto Ricans, Haitians, and American blacks. She estimated that a third of black clients treated at a southern psychiatric center believed that they were victims of witchcraft. Among blacks the terms commonly used to describe such occurrences are roots, root work, witchcraft, voodoo, a fix, a hex, and mojo. Regardless of the term used, the common theme is that someone has done something to cause another person illness, injury, or death.

In summary, there is wide variation in the ways different culture groups define mental disorder. It is important to understand, in addition to the etic Western diagnostic systems, the client's emic perspective in defining normal and abnormal behavior.

Influence of Culture on Illness Behaviors

A number of investigators have studied illness behaviors across cultures. From these studies it can be concluded that cultures differ in the expression of symptoms and in perception and treatment of the ill person by others.

Psychotic disorders are found in every culture, and primary manifestations of these disorders are common to people in any culture. On the other hand, secondary features of these disorders are highly conditioned by culture. For example, in many groups guilt and suicidal ideation do not accompany depression. In addition, somatic rather than emotional symptoms may be most dominant, as with the Chinese expression of depression. Finally, the content of delusions and hallucinations are largely culturally patterned.[33]

There is also wide variation in the way that clients with the same disorder may be perceived and treated by their cultural group. This variation is most evident in tracing the treatment of individuals with one disorder from culture to culture.

Influence of Culture on Health-Seeking Behaviors

For a variety of reasons, consulting mental health professionals may not be the first or only course of action by minority clients seeking mental health care. Mental health services may be seen as inaccessible, for reasons of distance, finances, or language, or inappropriate by minority groups.

A study of traditional Chinese on the west coast of the United States revealed that the majority of families made early, intensive, and prolonged efforts to cope with members having psychiatric difficulties. These efforts included advice, diet and herbal therapies, and faith healing. Secondarily, community leaders and family physicians were called in for consultations. Only as a last resort did these traditionally oriented families turn to social service agencies. This delay in asking for psychiatric help was in large part the family's genuine concern for the well-being of its sick members.[34]

Among groups with beliefs in folk illness, mental health professionals may not be immediately sought for treatment of a disorder. In these instances clients may first seek assistance from a person trained in the use of folk treatments. For example, depending on their specific cultural background, Hispanic clients may use the services of a *curandero, santero,* or spiritist. Blacks who believe they have a folk illness may use the services of a root worker or spiritualist. Similarly, Navajo clients may first use the services of a hand trembler, who diagnoses the client's problem, and then a medicine man, who uses chants, songs, and sand paintings to affect a cure.

It is also important to know that the client may have used the services of a folk practitioner before or in conjunction with mental health therapy. Wintrob[87] promotes the idea that individuals with a belief in folk remedies such as root-work may regard biomedical treatment as only palliative because curing the total condition requires the neutralization by a specially skilled folk healer.

Influence of Culture on Client Stress

All societies have systems of classifying persons according to age and sex. Each society ascribes differential status and norms of behavior in terms of this classification. That is, people are expected to behave and to be treated differently on the basis of their age and their sex. It appears that every society places stress on its members at one or more stages in the life cycle. Knowledge of these high-stress periods may assist mental health nurses in anticipating client problems.

For example, although all societies define a certain group as elderly, there is wide variation in the way members of the society perceive the aged person. The aged as a group may be highly regarded or largely disvalued. In some societies old age is a time of high prestige and power, whereas in others it is a period of insecurity, alienation, and high stress. Old age may be when people enjoy the greatest respect or when they endure emotional and physical abandonment.

In the United States the aged are typically stereotyped as nonproductive, physically and mentally deteriorating, poverty stricken, disengaged, and burdensome. Among other culture groups the aged may be the most powerful, the most engaged, and the most respected members of the society. Jackson, Bacon, and Peterson[30] conducted a study of 102 noninstitutionalized retired urban blacks. Their findings suggest that emotional adjustment to aging may be easier for blacks than for white middle-class Americans. Nobles,[52] McAdoo,[49] and Jones[3] described the role of the elderly black woman in black families as a source of love, strength, and stability. Often black grandmothers share in the responsibility for child care or informally adopt children whose parents are experiencing economic hardship or are temporarily seeking employment opportunities away from home. This ability of elderly black women to maintain the family unit provides them with a functional role and assists in promoting a positive aging experience.

Similarly, adolescence seems to be an especially troubled time for most Americans. This has been viewed as stemming from a number of factors[61]:

1. The lack of a clear termination point of adolescence
2. The prolongation of the education process and subsequent social role fulfillment
3. The variety of cultural choices open to the adolescent in the areas of life-style, occupation, and religion

On the other hand, compared to these dominant American cultural norms, old-order Amish adolescents have fewer stressors. The adolescent's education is finished when the eighth grade is completed and the choices available to the Amish adolescent are limited. It is likely that the adolescent boy will become a farmer like his father and that the adolescent girl will become a mother and homemaker like her mother.

Sex role differences may also lead to differential stress periods. Schlegel[62] investigated situational stress among the Hopi. She concluded that the role of the adult Hopi woman and the socialization she undergoes for this role places the adolescent Hopi girl in a position of high stress, since the tribal arrangement is matrilineal. Historically Hopi women were farmers owning their own land and passing it from mother to daughter.[15] These activities required a great deal of skill and role development that may have been stress producing. On the other hand, for the Hopi male the major period of developmental stress comes later, in young adulthood.

As previously noted, cultures are not static; they evolve through time. However, when culture change is rapid and extensive, the change may produce stress. Culture change may occur when an individual from one culture moves into another, as has occurred recently in the United States for persons from Southeast Asia, Cuba, and Haiti. The immigrant undergoes acculturation, which has been defined as the process in which the "customs, knowledge, attitudes, values and material choices of one culture or way of life become adopted in whole or in part by the people of another."[42] A number of stressors have been identified for new immigrants; these correspond to the several meanings of the concept of culture shock[13]:

1. The strain involved in expending effort on adaptation, speaking a new language, abiding by unfamiliar customs, and following a variety of new rules of behavior
2. A sense of loss at being uprooted, which is particularly prevalent among involuntary or forced migrants such as refugees
3. The rejection of the newcomer by the host population
4. The confusion of one's roles, values, and feelings
5. Rejection of the host's culture by the newcomer with accompanying feelings of discomfort, anxiety, or disgust
6. The feeling of helplessness in dealing with the new culture

A national study of the mental health needs of Southeast Asian refugees found a high incidence of mental health problems.[56] Data from more than 1,000 agencies working with refugee populations indicate that the age group 19 to 35 years is most at risk. This group contains the majority of single adults who are most excluded from the traditional family support system. The next age group (36 to 55 years) is the second most frequently reported group at risk. Stress for this group tends to result from the loss of traditional roles and status and a marked degree of intergenerational conflict. Common mental health problems of Southeast Asian refugees are, in descending order of importance: depression, anxiety, marital conflict, intergenerational conflict, school adjustment, psychophysiological illnesses, thought disorders, suicide, violence, and child abuse. The study also indicated that all smaller ethnic groups that lacked an ethnic community support system were more at risk of mental health problems than those with community support.

Role of the Nurse

To be effective, the nurse needs a clear, solid understanding of the client's culture. Because role expectations of the nurse vary from one culture to another, the nurse needs to be alert to different world views and preferred behavior styles.

The middle-class, white, American client characteristically views a helpful nurse as democratic, passive, and concerned with emotions. Clients with other backgrounds, such as Asian and Hispanic, may expect the nurse to be an authority figure who is active in providing interpretations and suggestions for problem solutions.[12] In the latter two groups, nurses may be perceived as persons who warrant respect and deference: an expert who will provide answers. Out of respect for authority, clients such as Native Americans do not speak until spoken to and expect the therapist to be directive and provide solutions to their problems.

Values and Health Behaviors

A variety of approaches have been used to compare the values of different cultural groups. One of the most basic is simply to describe the dominant values of a specific group. For example, Hicks[26] identified a dominant value of Appalachians as the ethic of neutrality. He found that mountaineers typically demonstrate this value, which is composed of four behavioral imperatives:

1. One must not be assertive or aggressive.
2. One must avoid argument and seek agreement.
3. Unless otherwise requested one should mind one's own business. Asking direct, personal questions is taken as an attempt to interfere in a person's private matters.
4. One must not assume authority over others. To do so would violate the presumption of equality.

This ethic of neutrality has important implications for mental health nurses working with Appalacian clients. In a study investigating traits that made practitioners unsuccessful with Appalacian clients, it was noted that those who were rough and domineering had little success with Appalacian clients.[85] Counseling and health teaching given in an authoritarian manner are not readily accepted. Appalacians tend to disapprove of answering questions that may be used against them in agency reports. The following topics are generally avoided by successful Appalacian practitioners:

1. Income and how it is spent. (This can be used against the client by welfare agencies.) One successful practitioner in a clinic noted that "we can overburden clients by asking too much and too often about welfare. If some individuals are unable to pay, the clinic does not press them. We don't try to worry much about the financial aspects; some pay and some don't."
2. Questions about how often their children go to school. (This can be used by truant officers.)
3. Questions about who is living with the Appalachians. (This can be used by welfare workers and landlords.)
4. Questions about their neighbors. (This can get the neighbors into trouble.)

If the information listed above is absolutely necessary, successful practitioners suggest approaching sensitive topics with indirect questions and refraining from using coercion. Finally, they emphasize that the Appalachian client may be sensitive to perceived criticism.

A second approach to value orientations is to compare several cultures along a number of dimensions. Kluckhohn and Strodtbeck identified various problems with which all societies must cope. They considered the way that humans organize their thinking about time, personal activity, interpersonal relations, and their relation to nature.

Temporal orientation. The temporal orientation is divided into three time frames: past, present, and future. Although all societies deal in all three time domains, cultures differ in their emphasis. While peasant, agricultural cultures tend to emphasize a present orientation, highly industrialized cultures tend to have a future orientation.

Activity orientation. The activity orientation identifies whether a given culture is primarily oriented toward the "doing" (achievement) mode of action or the "being" mode. Middle-class America has been characterized as having an achievement mode of activity; that is, each person is valued for accomplishments, not for his inherent existence. On the other hand, in societies with a being orientation, each person is valued for his very existence, not for his accomplishments. The being pattern is typical of lineage societies (such as Chinese) in which the person is valued as a link in the chain of continuity between generations.

Relational orientation. The relational orientation distinguishes among interpersonal patterns and is concerned with the ways in which the society sets goals for its individual members. It is characterized by collateral, lineal, and individualistic modes.

When the collateral principle is dominant, the goals and welfare of the laterally extended groups (siblings or members of the same age group) are of prime importance. Collectivistic societies such as Russia and Israel typically demonstrate a collateral orientation in the ideal. In these societies, the goals of the individual are subordinated to those of the group, and the group maintains responsibility for all its members.

When the lineal mode is dominant, group goals and welfare have primary importance. However, with the lineal orientation, continuity of the group and ordered succession within the group through time are important issues. In virtually all societies with emphasis on lineality, as in Samoa, kinship is the basis for maintaining the lineage.

When the individualistic principle is dominant, individual goals have primacy over the goals of specific collateral or lineal groups. Each person's responsibility to the total society and his place in it are defined by autonomous goals. Most industrialized Western societies, including the United States, emphasize the individualistic orientation. The individual alone is held responsible for personal behavior and is judged on the basis of personal accomplishments.

People-to-nature orientation. The orientation of people to nature identifies whether humans dominate nature, live in harmony with nature, or are subjugated to nature.

The dominating nature orientation holds that humans can master or control natural events. This is the leading middle-class American orientation to nature; given sufficient time, science and technology will prevail. The orientation of harmony with nature gives a sense of holism among humans, nature, and the universe. Many Native American and Asian philosophies promote this integrated approach. The orientation of subjugation to nature is often presented as fatalism. Among many Moslems, one simply accepts one's ultimate fate as inevitable, often as the will of Allah.

Because it contains diverse ethnic populations, the United States exhibits greater heterogeneity than most other Western cultures; it does not exhibit a uniform, dominant value system. Although a dominant orientation can be identified for middle-class Americans of northern European descent, members of other American culture

TABLE 10-1 Dominant value orientations of selected American ethnic groups

Ethnic Group	Temporal Orientation	Activity Orientation	Relational Orientation	People-to-Nature Orientation
Dominant American	Future over present	Doing	Individualistic	Over-with-subjugated
Southern black	Present over future	Being	Collateral-lineal	Subjugated-over-with
Puerto Rican	Present over future	Doing	Individualistic	With-subjugated-over
Southern Appalacian	Present	Being	Lineal-collateral	Subjugated
American Indian	Present	Being	Collateral-lineal	With
Mexican-American	Present	Being	Lineal-collateral	Subjugated
Traditional Chinese-American	Present	Being	Lineal	With

From Tripp-Reimer, T.: In nursing assessment: a multidimensional approach, by J. Bellack and P. Bamford. Copyright © 1984 by Wadsworth, Inc. Reprinted by permission of the publisher, Wadsworth Heath Sciences Division, Monterey, California.

groups may have dominant value orientations that vary considerably from this. Table 10-1 illustrates the diversity in dominant value orientations of selected American ethnic groups.

Values and Mental Health Nursing Practice

Clients' behaviors are generally consistent with their cultural values. To illustrate this point, the potential influence of value orientations on client behaviors is presented in the following discussion.

As illustrated in Table 10-1, the dominant American culture perceives the relationship of people to nature as one of control. Clients with this dominant culture orientation believe that humans, through science and technology, can control nature. These clients tend to actively seek the assistance of mental health practitioners with the belief that these practitioners can, through the application of scientific knowledge, alleviate their problems. On the other hand, Appalachian clients tend to feel subjugated to nature. This may result in a fatalistic approach to mental disorder. Consequently they may be less optimistic about the benefits of counseling.[90] In contrast, Navajos have been identified as feeling in harmony with nature, society, and the world of the supernatural; this, in fact, is the core and essence of Navajo myths and belief systems. Correspondingly the Navajo religion is a design in harmony, a striving for rapport between humans and every phase of nature.[67] This orientation has been generalized to the majority of native Americans who hold that there is a common order to the universe and to people's state of mind and being.[23] Thus health care may be seen as a religious activity and scientific mental health practitioners as adjuncts to a more holistic therapy.

In the relational value orientation, middle-class Americans tend to be individualistic, seeking self-actualization through vocational and personal improvement. This contrasts with the traditional Asian relational orientation, in which the lineal mode is dominant. The welfare and integrity of the family is of prime importance to traditional Asian-Americans. Family members may be expected to submerge behaviors and feelings to further the welfare of the family. Furthermore, the behavior of an individual member of the family is expected to be a credit to the entire family. Socially acceptable behavior is therefore expected both for the individual's and family's self-respect. Similar qualities of the Hispanic culture are (1) family being one of the most proud and valued aspects of life, and (2) the need for preserving the family's unity, respect, and loyalty.

A number of studies have indicated that traditional Asian-Americans prefer to use family or friends as a primary source of help for mental health problems. Families may deny that members have emotional problems until they become unmanageable. This results, in part, because mental disorders are viewed as shameful.[94] In these cultures, for example, extreme psychotic symptoms are tolerated if there is no destructive behavior.[44] Mental health nurses working with traditional Asians may find that their clients experience strong feelings of guilt and shame when admitting that problems exist. Because of this, issues of confidentiality are crucial in dealing with traditional Asian clients. Furthermore, in counseling traditional Asians it may be the relatives, more than the clients, who need to be convinced before the client can start or continue a therapeutic progarm.[83] In some instances, greater benefit may be derived from family therapy, instead of individual therapy. Thus, an Asian or Hispanic client may need to be viewed as an integral member of the family constellation. The family is included in the therapy plan and treatment goals.

In temeral orientation, middle-class Americans tend to be future oriented. This future orientation may be seen in examples of deferred gratification, such as an emphasis on the importance of extended education. In addition, members of the dominant American culture tend to structure time rigidly. Adhering to time schedules is a way of life. Both work and leisure are time-structured. In a clinical setting this may mean that they will be punctual and may carefully watch the clock during therapy. In contrast, individuals with a present time orientation may have a more flexible adherence to schedules. An Anglo nurse should avoid immediately labeling missed appointments or tardiness as signs of disrespect, laziness, or lack of interest. In studying Mexican-Americans, Hoppe and Heller[28] proposed that time orientation may be one reason Hispanic clients may be late for appointments. Carter[9] stressed awareness of differences in values regarding time for the blacks from low socioeconomic groups. Instead of labeling tardiness as blatant disregard of time, problems of health, economics and transportation need to be considered. The Native American's fluid time consciousness contrasts starkly with the dominant middle-class American cultural value of strict adherence to time schedules. The Native American is better able to focus on the present and enjoy it rather than being bound by time constraints. In mental health practice a focus on the present may result in a crisis orientation rather than a preventive approach. It also promotes a more flexible adherence to schedules. Consequently mental health nurses need to be aware that clients with a present orientation who are deeply engaged in a counseling situation may be reluctant to leave the appointment simply because "the time is up."

Patterns of Communication

Communication of emotional states is strongly influenced by culture. Many Indo-chinese emphasize self-control because they believe it is one's duty to maintain an even temper. Hostility is not expressed toward persons who are considered "superior," such as parents, elders, or health professionals. A client's smile or "yes" may not necessarily indicate compliance or agreement as much as it indicates an unwillingness to be disrespectful or impolite. An authoritarian manner by a health professional may elicit only token verbal agreement from the Indo-Chinese client.

Volume, speed, and directness in conversation is influenced by cultural values. Health practitioners may be viewed as loud and boisterous by minority clients. Likewise, the softer volume of Asian or Native American speech may be interpreted by the mental health nurse as shyness.

Many cultures value indirectness and subtlety in speech. The frankness of the American mental health professional may alienate minority clients. For example, Asian clients may interpret this communication style as rude, immature, and lacking finesse. On the other hand, Asian clients may be labeled as evasive and afraid to confront their problems by Anglo health professionals.[78]

Nurses need to be aware of the role of language in intercultural therapy. In working with Hispanic groups, Delgado[11] noted that "group process is greatly facilitated when members and leader can speak both English and Spanish." Yamamoto and Acosta[88] likewise believed that with both Asians and Hispanics language is a vital issue. Treatment in the native language is essential when working among unacculturated groups. Being fluent in the client's native language greatly facilitates discussion and understanding of emotionally charged topics. Clients would then be able to spontaneously express feelings in words that are most comfortable to them. However, when a bilingual nurse is not available, interpreters can be used effectively.

The meaning of silence may also vary considerably among various cultures. For some groups silence is extremely uncomfortable, and they attempt to fill every gap in the conversation. In contrast, many Native Americans often consider silence essential to understanding: a person needs to fully consider what another has said before giving a response. Silence by traditional Chinese and Japanese clients does not necessarily indicate that they have completed talking; it may mean they wish the nurse to consider the content of what they said before continuing. Other cultures may use silence much differently; the English and Arabs use silence for privacy, and the Russians, French, and Spanish may read it as a sign of agreement among parties. Asian cultures may view silence as a sign of respect for an elder.

Many ethnic groups, such as Native Americans, Southeast Asians, and Appalachians, may view direct eye contact differently than do Anglos. For example, Navajos tend to use more peripheral vision and avoid direct eye contact, because direct eye contact is considered hostile. Lack of eye contact among Japanese and Mexican-Americans is a sign of politeness and respect, not one of lack of interest, low intelligence, or shyness. This nonverbal behavior may be misunderstood by professionals.

Cultural norms dictate differences in personal space. Hall,[24] in his research on territoriality, identifies four interpersonal distance zones used by middle-class adults from the northeastern United States:

Intimate	Contact-1½ feet
Personal	1½ feet-4 feet
Social	4 feet-12 feet
Public	Greater than 12 feet

Nurses and clients from the population group that includes Native Americans, Appalachians, Japanese, and Mexican-Americans, would comfortably position themselves between the personal and social distance. This positioning is done unconsciously: "It just feels right." The counselor may feel uncomfortable with Latin Americans, Africans, black Americans, or Indonesians whose cultures generally dictate closer personal space.[78] Blacks engage in eye contact more often than whites when they are speaking, and they have a closer personal space and greater body activity. Thus, nurses working with black clients may misinterpret their clients' nonverbal behaviors as indicating anger or aggression.[78] Also, black clients may be uncommunicative, not because of an inability to deal with their feelings but because of their distrust of the dominant American culture.

The psychotherapy situation is often ambiguous and unstructured. Consequently a number of cross-cultural therapists* have suggested that many minority clients prefer a logical, rational, structured approach over an affective, reflective, ambiguous one. They further point out that nondirective, client-centered approaches may not work well with many minority clients. They recommend that the nurse use a directive approach that is highly goal

*References 7, 35, 65, 78, 80, 81, 84.

oriented. For example, short-term therapy that deals with immediate concrete concerns is preferable to the long-term insightful approach. Behavioral therapy, such as contracting for targeted problems and goals or teaching assertiveness or relaxation can be most helpful.[97]

However, it is crucial to remember that the client's cultural background serves only as a cue for assessment and intervention. For example, "talk therapy," acceptable to a client from the dominant American middle-class, is an enigma for the client who is action oriented and whose locus of control is external. As a general approach to therapy with minority clients, Draguns noted the following[12]:

> Be prepared to adapt your techniques (general activity level, mode of verbal intervention, content of remarks, tone of voice) to the cultural background of the client; communicate acceptance of and respect for the client in terms that are intelligible and meaningful within his cultural frame of reference; and be open to the possibility of more direct intervention in the life of the client than the traditional ethos of the counseling profession would dictate or permit.

Culturally Sensitive Intervention Strategies

For a nurse involved in transcultural counseling, a variety of treatment approaches need to be explored depending on the characteristics of the client. There is an increasing acceptance of the efficacy of specific therapeutic modalities for clients with certain behavioral characteristics.

Ethnotherapy (family therapy and ethnicity). As previously stated, the family unit of varying ethnic groups may be the cornerstone to individual behavior. Restoring a greater sense of identity may require resolution of cultural conflicts within the family, between the family and the outside community, or in the larger society in which the family exists. Nurses may need to coach families to sort out strong convictions from values asserted for emotional reasons. Often families need to differentiate those traditional ethnic values they wish to retain or delete. Those ethnic values retained play a significant role in family life and personal development throughout the life cycle by influencing family patterns and belief systems.[51]

Families who are experiencing cultural transition when migrating to the United States, for example, Vietnamese, Hispanics, and Haitians, may experience numerous stresses, such as loss of support systems, decrease in health status, or economic stressors. These factors lead to isolation (fear of new environment), enmeshment (imposing strict traditional values, avoiding any support in adapting to new demands), and disengagement (no longer accepting family values and life-style, vulnerability to new environmental stressors).[40] However, some families may negotiate the acculturation process without difficulty if adaptation factors are positive.

For those families seeking assistance, there are several approaches to cultural transition in a new environment.

Transitional mapping. During the first interview, the nurse needs to establish which phase of the migration process the family is experiencing and their previous experiences in migration phases. A comprehensive map is created that includes the position of each family member, the entire family's life-cycle stages, cultural origin, family form, and current status with other family members and the community. Factors supporting adaptation and rates of adaptation by family members as a whole are considered. If differential adaptation rates exist, the impact of transitional conflict can be assumed and therapy begun.[71]

Link therapy. This therapeutic process involves having a single family member represent the "link" between the mental health nurse and the extended family. This is not characteristic of family therapy approaches; however, it may be appropriate for East Indians, Africans, or Iranians, in whose cultures parents cannot discuss issues in the presence of children. The family member acting as the link therapist is trained to initiate interventions with guidance and supervision of the family counselor. The most successful link therapist is a person experiencing unresolved transitional conflict, because a fully acculturated or entrenched traditionalist would dictate the transitional direction to be taken by the family.[39]

The key to treating families who are in cultural transition is to recognize that their problems arise because different family subsystems adapt at different rates. Transitional therapy clarifies the differential rates of adaptation and facilitates the family's resolution of transitional conflict. The nurse must not presume that the values of the new or dominant American middle-class culture are right for everybody and that a nuclear family structure is the correct family system. Ethnic families need to be encouraged to make their own choices, facilitated by the mental health nurse.

BRIEF REVIEW

Culture includes the learned patterns of values, beliefs, customs, and behaviors that are shared by a group of individuals. Knowledge of the client's culture assists the nurse in predicting the client's actions and acting accordingly; it allows her to assume a culturally relativistic perspective. At the same time, it is important not to overgeneralize or stereotype clients on the basis of cultural or ethnic affiliation.

The definitions of mental illnesses, the perceived role of the mental health nurse as well as the secondary characteristics of these illnesses are largely determined by cultural factors. The client's culture itself can serve as a stressor to the individual.

When the client and the nurse are from different cultural groups, misunderstandings can arise from differences in values and patterns of communication. Thus a key component is to assess and treat the client from his ethnic perspective. This involves assessment of cultural variables related to illness behaviors and health seeking behaviors. It is important for the nurse to develop culturally sensitive interaction strategies that focus on immediate, concrete solutions to mental health problems. Emphasis is on family involvement as a major asset to supporting the client's acceptance of clinical interventions. It is also crucial for nurses to assess their own cultural background and how it influences therapeutic interventions with ethnic minority clients. The preferred outcome is to have both the nurse and client be enriched from the cultural interaction.

REFERENCES AND SUGGESTED READINGS

1. Arce, A., and Torres-Matrullo, C.: Application of cognitive behavioral techniques in the treatment of Hispanic patients, Psychiatric Quarterly **54**:230, 1982.
2. Benedict, R.: Patterns of culture, Boston, 1959, Houghton Mifflin Co. (Originally published in 1934.)
3. Berry, J.W., and Dasen, P.R., editors: Culture and cognition: readings in cross-cultural psychology, London, 1974, Methuen & Co., Ltd.
4. Bourguignon, E.E.: Culture and varieties of consciousness, Reading, Mass., 1974, Addison-Wesley Publishing Co., Inc.
5. Bourguignon, E.E.: Possession, San Francisco, 1976, Chandler & Sharp Publishers, Inc.
6. Bryde, J.: Indian students and guidance, Boston, 1971, Houghton Mifflin Co.
7. Bush, M., Ullom, J., and Osborne, O.: The meaning of mental health: a report of two ethnoscientific studies, Nursing Research **24**:130, 1975.
8. Carp, F., and Kataoka, E.: Health care problems of the elderly of San Francisco's Chinatown, Gerontologist **16**:30, 1976.
9. Carter, J.: Frequent mistakes made with black clients in psychotherapy, Journal of the National Medical Association **71**:10, 1979.
10. Chang, B.: Asian-American patient care. In Henderson, G., and Primeaux, M., editors: Transcultural health care, Reading, Mass., 1981, Addison-Wesley Publishing Co.
11. Dancy, J.: The black elderly: a guide for practitioners, Ann Arbor, 1977, Institute of Gerontology, University of Michigan.
12. Delgado, M.: Hispanics and psychotherapeutic groups, International Journal of Group Psychotherapy **33**:4, 1983.
13. Draguns, J.: Common themes and distinct approaches. In Pedersen, P.B., and others, editors: Counseling across cultures, Honolulu, 1981, University of Hawaii Press.
14. Eaton, J., and Weil, R.: Culture and mental disorders: a comparative study of the Hutterites and other populations, Chicago, 1955, Free Press.
15. Farris, L.: The American Indian. In Clark, A.L., editor: Culture, childbearing, and health professionals, Philadelphia, 1978, F.A. Davis.
16. Flaskerud, J.: Perception of problematic behavior by Appalachians, mental health professionals and lay non-Appalachians, Nursing Research **19**:140, 1980.
17. Foster, G., and Anderson, B.: Medical anthropology, New York, 1978, John Wiley & Sons, Inc.
18. Foulks, E.F.: Anthropology and psychiatry: a new blending of an old relationship. In Foulks, R.F., and others, editors: Current perspectives in cultural psychiatry, Jamaica, N.Y., 1977, Spectrum Publications, Inc.
19. French, D.: The relationship of anthropology to studies in perception and cognition. In Kotch, S., editor: Psychology: a study of science, New York, 1963, McGraw-Hill Book Co.
20. Freud, S.: Totem and taboo, standard edition of the complete psychological works of Sigmund Freud, vol. 13, London, 1914, The Hogarth Press. (Edited by J. Strachey.)
21. Giordano, J., and Giordano, G.P.: The ethnocultural factor in mental health: a literature review and bibliography, New York, 1977, Institute on Pluralism and Group Identity.
22. Greely, A.M.: Why can't they be like us? New York, 1969, Institute of Human Relations.
23. Hahn, R.: Aboriginal American psychiatric theories, Transcultural Psychiatric Research Review **15**:29, 1978.
24. Hall, E.: The hidden dimension, New York, 1969, Doubleday Publishing Co.
25. Harwood, A.: Ethnicity and medical care, Cambridge, Mass., 1981, Harvard University Press.
26. Hicks, G.: Appalachian valley, New York, 1976, Holt, Rinehart & Winston.
27. Hoffman, L.: Foundations of family therapy, New York, 1981, Basic Books, Inc.
28. Hoppe, S., and Heller, P.: Alienation, familism, and the utilization of health services by Mexican-Americans, Journal of Health and Social Behavior **15**:304, 1974.
29. Jackson, J.S.: Aged Negroes, their culture departures from statistical stereotypes and rural-urban differences, Gerontologist **10**:140, 1970.
30. Jackson, J.S., Bacon, J., and Peterson, J.: Life satisfaction among black urban elderly, Journal of Aging and Human Development **8**:169, 1971.
31. Jones, F.C.: The lofty role of the black grandmother, The Crisis **80**:19, 1973.
32. Kalish, R., and Yuen, S.: Americans of East Asian ancestry: aging and the aged, Gerontologist **11**(suppl.):36, 1971.
33. Kiev, A.: Transcultural psychiatry, New York, 1972, Free Press.
34. King, S.: Perceptions of illness in medical practice, New York, 1962, Russell Sage Foundation.
35. Kitano, H., and Matsushima, N.: Counseling Asian-Americans. In Pedersen, P.G., and others, editors: Counseling across cultures, Honolulu, 1981, University of Hawaii Press.
36. Kleinman, A.: Major conceptual and research issues for cultural (anthropological) psychiatry, Culture, Medicine and Psychiatry **4**:3, 1980.
37. Kluckhohn, F., and Strodtbeck, F.: Variations in value orientations, Evanston, Ill., 1961, Row, Peterson & Co.
38. Knab, S.: Polish Americans: historical and cultural perspectives of influence in the use of mental health services, Journal of Psychosocial Nursing and Mental Health Services **1**(24):31, 1986.
39. Landau, J.: Link therapy as a family therapy technique for transitional extended families, Psychotherapeia **7**:382, 1981.
40. Landau, J.: Therapy with families in cultural transition. In McGoldrick, M., Pearce, J.K., and Giordano, J., editors: Ethnicity and family therapy, New York, 1982, Guilford Press.
41. Lazarus, A.: The practice of multidimensional therapy, New York, 1981, McGraw-Hill, Inc.
42. Leighton, A.: Mental illness and enculturation. In Galdston, I., editor: New York Academy of Medicine: Lectures to the laity: medicine and anthropology, Freeport, N.Y. 1971, Books for Libraries, Inc.
43. LeVine, E., and Franco, J.: Effects of therapist's gender, ethnicity and verbal style on client's willingness to seek therapy, The Journal of Social Psychology **121**:51, 1983.
44. Lin, T., and Lin, M.: Service delivery issues in Asian-North American communities, American Journal of Psychiatry **135**:454, 1978.
45. Lin, T., Tardiff, K., Donetz, G., and Goresby, W.: Ethnicity and patterns of help-seeking, Culture, Medicine and Psychiatry **2**:1, 1978.
46. Malinowski, P.: Sex and repression in savage society, New York, 1970, Meridian Books. (Originally published in 1927.)
47. Martin, E.P., and Martin, J.M.: The black extended family, Chicago, 1978, University of Chicago Press.
48. Mead, M.: Coming of age in Samoa, 1920.
49. McAdoo, H.P., editor: Black families, Beverly Hills, Calif., 1981, Sage Publications.
50. McAdoo, H.P.: The impact of upward mobility of kin-help patterns and the reciprocal obligations in black families, Journal of Marriage and the Family **4**:761, 1978.

51. McGoldrick, M., Pearce, J.K., and Giordano, J.: Ethnicity and family therapy, New York, 1982, Guilford Press.

52. Nobles, W.: African philosophy: foundations for black psychology. In Hones, R., editor: Black psychology, ed. 2, New York, 1980, Harper & Row, Publishers.

53. Orley, J.: Culture and mental illness: a study from Uganda; Nairobi, Kenya, 1970, East African Publishing House.

54. Padilla, A., and Ruiz, R.: Latino mental health: a review of the literature, U.S. Department of Health, Education, and Welfare Pub. No. 76-113, Washington D.C., 1973, U.S. Government Printing Office.

55. Pedersen, P.B., and others, editors: Counseling across cultures, Honolulu, 1981, University of Hawaii Press.

56. Pennsylvania Department of Public Welfare, Bureau of Research and Training, Office of Mental Health: National mental health needs assessment of Indochinese refugee populations, Harrisburg, 1979, The Bureau.

57. Pike, K.L.: Language in relation to a unified theory of the structure of human behavior, Glendale, Calif., 1954-1955, Summer Institute of Linguistics.

58. Pike, K.L.: Language in relation to a unified theory of the structure of human behavior, ed. 2, 1967, New York, Humanities Press International, Inc.

59. Reeves, K.: Hispanic utilization of an ethnic mental health clinic, Journal of Psychosocial Nursing and Mental Health Services 24(2):23, 1986.

60. Richardson, E.: Cultural and historical perspectives in counsleing American Indians. In Sue, D., editor: Counseling the culturally different: theory and practice, 1981, New York, John Wiley & Sons, Inc.

61. Ridley, C.: Clinical treatment of the nondisclosing black client, American Psychologist 39:11, 1984.

62. Rose, A.: The sub-culture of the aging. In Rose, A., and Peterson, W., editors: Older people and their social world, Philadelphia, 1965, F.A. Davis.

63. Ruiz, M.: Open-closed mindedness: intolerance of ambiguity and nursing faculty attitudes toward culturally different patients, Nursing Research 30:177, 1981.

64. Ruiz, R.: Cultural and historical perspectives in counseling Hispanics. In Sue, D., editor: Counseling the culturally different: theory and practice, New York, 1981, John Wiley & Sons, Inc.

65. Ruiz, R., and Cassas, J.: Culturally relevant and behavioristic counseling for Chicano counseling students. In Pedersen, P.B., and others, editors: Counseling across cultures, Honolulu, 1981, University of Hawaii Press.

66. Samouilidis, L.: Psychoanalytic vicissitudes in working with Greek patients, The American Journal of Psychoanalysis 38:223, 1978.

67. Sander, D.: Navajo medicine, Journal of Human Nature 1:54, 1978.

68. Schiamberg, L.: Some sociocultural factors in adolescent-parent conflict, a cross-cultural comparison of selected cultures. In Zsze, W.: The human life cycle, New York, 1975, Jason Aronson, Inc.

69. Segall, M.: Human behavior in cross-cultural psychology: global perspectives. Monterey, Calif., 1979, Brooks/Cole Publishing Co.

70. Silver, M.: Focus on health care: Vietnamese in Denver. In Van, P., Arsdale, P., and Pisarowicz, J., editors: Processes of transition: Vietnamese in Colorado, Austin, Tx., 1980, High Street Press.

71. Sluzki, C.E.: Migration and family conflict, Family Process 18:379, 1979.

72. Smith, E.: Cultural and historical perspectives in counseling blacks. In Sue, D., editor: Counseling the culturally different: theory and practice, New York, 1981, John Wiley & Sons, Inc.

73. Snow, L.: Sorcerers, saints and charlatans: black folk healers in urban America, Culture, Medicine and Psychiatry 2:69, 1978.

74. Sowell, T.: Ethnic America, New York, 1981, Basic Books, Inc.

75. Spiegel, J.: An ecological model of ethnic families. In McGoldrick, M., Pearce, J.K., and Giordano, J., editors: Ethnicity and family therapy, New York, 1982, Guilford Press.

76. Stein, H.F.: The Slovak-American "swaddling-ethos": homeostat for family dynamics and cultural persistence, Family Process 17:31, 1978.

77. Sturtevant, W.: Studies in ethnoscience, American Anthropologist 66:99, 1964.

78. Sue, D.: Counseling the culturally different: theory and practice, New York, 1981, John Wiley & Sons, Inc.

79. Sullivan, T.: Values, beliefs, and practice of the elderly in the United States, implications for health and nursing care, Transcultural Nursing Care 2:13, 1977.

80. Sundberg, N.: Research and research hypothesis about effectiveness in intercultural counseling. In Pedersen, P.B., and others, editors: Counseling across cultures, Honolulu, 1981, University of Hawaii Press.

81. Toupin, E.: Counseling Asians: psychotherapy in the context of racism and Asian-American history, American Journal of Orthopsychiatry 50:76, 1980.

82. Tousignant, M., and Mishara, B.: Suicide and culture: a review of the literature from 1969 to 1980, Transculture Psychiatric Research Review 18:5, 1981.

83. Triandis, H., and Draguns, J.: Handbook of cross-cultural psychology, vol. 6, Psychopathology, Boston, 1980, Allyn & Bacon, Inc.

84. Trimble, J.: Value differentials and their importance in counseling American Indians. In Pedersen, P.B., and others, editors: Counseling across cultures, Honolulu, 1981, University of Hawaii Press.

85. Tripp-Reimer, T.: Appalachian health care: from research to practice, Proceedings of the Fifth National Transcultural Nursing Conference, 48, 1980, Salt Lake City, University of Utah.

86. Tripp-Reimer, T.: Ethnomedical beliefs among Greek immigrants: implications for nursing intercention, In Morley, P., editor: Developing, teaching and practicing transcultural nursing, Proceedings of the Sixth National Transcultural Nursing Conference, 126, 1981.

87. Tripp-Reimer, T.: Barriers to health care: perceptual variations of Appalachians and non-Appalachian health care professionals, Western Journal of Nursing Research 4:179, 1982.

88. Tripp-Reimer, T.: Retention of a folk healing practice (matiasma) among four generations of urban Greek immigrants, Nursing Research 32:97, 1983.

89. Tripp-Reimer, T.: Cultural assessment. In Ballack, J., and Bamford, P., editors: Nursing assessment: a multidimensional approach, Monterey, Calif., 1984, Wadsworth Publishing Co.

90. Tripp-Reimer, T., and Friedl, M.: Appalachians: a neglected minority, Nursing Clinics of North America 12:41, 1977.

91. Tseng, W.S., and McDermott, J.F.: Culture, mind, and therapy: an introduction to cultural psychiatry, New York, 1981, Bruner/Mazel.

92. Tung, M.: Life values, psychotherapy and East-West integration, Psychiatry **47**:8, 1984.

93. Tung, T.: The family and the management of mental health problems in Vietnam. In Lebra, W., editor: Transcultural research in mental health, Honolulu, 1972, University of Hawaii Press.

94. Van Deusen, J.: Health/mental studies of Indochinese refugees: a critical overview, Medical Anthropology **4**:231, 1982.

95. Weldman, H.H.: Implications of the culture broker concept for the delivery of health care. A paper presented at the Annual Meeting of the Southern Anthropological Society, Wrightville Beach, S.C., 1973.

96. Weiss, M.S.: Research experience in a Chinese-American community, Journal of Social Issues **33**:120, 1977.

97. Yamamoto, J., and Acosta, F.: Treatment of Asian Americans and Hispanic Americans: similarities and differences, Journal of the American Academy of Psychoanalysis **10**:4, 1982.

98. Yuki, T.: Cultural responsiveness and social work practice: an Indian clinic's success, Health and Social Work **11**(3):223, 1986.

ANNOTATED BIBLIOGRAPHY

Pedersen, P.B., and others, editors: Counseling across cultures, Honolulu, 1981, University of Hawaii Press.

This book is an edited volume of articles that deal with a variety of aspects of cross-cultural mental health. Specific chapters address issues concerning racial and ethnic barriers in counseling, themes and approaches in cross-cultural counseling, and special considerations for working with the following minority clients: foreign students, native Americans, Asian-Americans, and Chicano college students.

Sue, D.: Counseling the culturally different: theory and practice, New York, 1981, John Wiley & Sons, Inc.

This book presents a more unified approach to cross-cultural counseling. The book is divided into three parts. Part One deals with broad concepts and theoretical foundations that serve as a base for counseling minority clients. It covers politics of counseling, barriers to effective cross-cultural counseling, value differences between health professionals and clients, and issues such as whether a counselor who is culturally different can work effectively with a minority client. Part Two focuses on issues and techniques when working with specific ethnic populations including Asian-Americans, blacks, Hispanics and American Indians. Part Three, presents a series of case studies depicting a variety of cross-cultural counseling situations. These vignettes reveal how traditional mental health approaches may be at odds with cultural values and suggest alternative ways of dealing with the critical incident.

pelled or safely contained. The significance and meaning of anxiety depend on the nature of the underlying conflict. The conflict may be a legacy of the individual's experiences during early stages of growth and development. It is the stimulation from his adult environment that activates the conflict.

Phobias are fears that are disproportionate to the demands of the situation and cannot be explained or reasoned away. A phobia leads to avoidance of the feared situation. The feelings are profound, reaching panic proportions, with physiological symptoms such as palpitations, sweating, rapid breathing, diarrhea, and urinary frequency in the presence of the phobic stimulus.

Simple phobias are the most common type of phobias and are often reported by the general population. A specific object or situation is irrationally feared; for example, fear of snakes. Simple phobias often arise in childhood and seldom persist beyond adolescence. When they continue into adulthood, they usually require treatment if the person is to be free of the fear. The degree of impairment depends on how often the individual comes in contact with the phobic stimulus. For someone living in a small town, the fear of elevators may be a minor problem, but it could drastically restrict the person who lives and works in a city with tall buildings. The list of official names for specific fears is lengthy. Table 11-1 is a partial list of types of phobias.

TABLE 11-1 Formal names of some phobias and their meanings

Name	Meaning (fear of. . .)
Acrophobia	Height
Agoraphobia	Open spaces
Ailurophobia	Cats
Arachnophobia	Spiders
Anthophobia	Flowers
Anthropophobia	People
Aquaphobia	Water
Astraphobia	Lightning
Brontophobia	Thunder
Claustrophobia	Closed spaces
Cynophobia	Dogs
Dementophobia	Insanity
Equinophobia	Horses
Herpetophobia	Lizards, reptiles
Keraunophobia	Thunder
Mikophobia	Germs
Murophobia	Mice
Mysophobia	Dirt, germs, contamination
Numerophobia	Number
Nyctophobia	Darkness
Ophidiophobia	Snakes
Pyrophobia	Fire
Thanatophobia	Death
Trichophobia	Hair
Xenophobia	Stranger
Zoophobia	Animal

According to psychoanalytic theory, phobias originate in the oral stage of development. Intense conflicts give rise to basic impulses that need to be repressed and denied conscious expression. As repression fails, the original source of the anxiety is displaced to some other object, person, or situation. This source of anxiety is outside the self and may be only loosely or indirectly related to the original conflict. Freud's classic case of Little Hans typifies the dynamics of displacement. Freud treated a 5-year-old boy for a phobia of horses. The boy's fear of his father was displaced to horses, a symbolic object that he could avoid. Freud determined that Hans's aggressive feelings toward his parents, especially his father, were repressed, resulting in a mental conflict that emerged as a fear of horses.

Displacement is an essential dynamic in phobias. Displacement allows conscious impulses such as forbidden aggressive or sexual needs to be denied in the self and placed on other objects or persons. Displacement thus keeps the relationship between the self and the forbidden impulse out of awareness. If displacement does not succeed in binding all of the anxiety, the range of fears may increase so that more phobias appear or more complicated defenses are employed.

Several different forms of anxiety described by Freud are listed in the box on p. 206.

Interpersonal

Karen Horney and Harry Stack Sullivan share the beliefs that (1) social interaction is imperative in human development, (2) the origin of anxiety lies in interaction with others, and (3) the development of a self-system serves to provide security and to protect the person from anxiety.

Horney[18] believed that there are multiple adverse factors in the environment that can produce insecurity in the developing child, resulting in basic anxiety. Basic anxiety is a profound insecurity and vague apprehensiveness. Because the world is viewed as hostile, the pressure from basic anxiety prevents children from relating spontaneously. The child is forced to find ways to relate to others that can allay basic anxiety. In doing so, the child develops coping strategies: Moving toward other people for fulfillment of dependency needs, moving away from other people because of the need for independence, and moving against people through the need for power. These needs for relating to others become the basis for inner conflict.

TABLE 11-2 Sullivan's states of anxiety

State	Description
Primitive	A fearlike state induced by the anxiousness of the mothering person
Mild	An uneasy, uncomfortable state commonly occuring in interpersonal relationships
Severe	State in which the individual negates aspects of himself and attunes to disapproving comments from important people

FORMS OF ANXIETY DESCRIBED BY FREUD

Primary Anxiety	The sudden stimulation and trauma of birth is the first experience of anxiety. The environment is perceived as threatening and this threat predisposes the person to anxiety later in life.
Subsequent anxiety	Emotional conflicts depend on the maturation of the ego and the superego. As the ego develops it protects the individual from instinctual demands of the id, from attack and frustration by the external world, and from rebuke by the superego.
Reality anxiety	Often equated with fear and is based on the perception of danger in the environment. Either some important object is absent or the person's existence is threatened.
Neurotic anxiety	Arises when the perception of danger is from the instincts of the id. The anxiety is based on the fear that the ego is unable to prevent an instinctual urge from getting out of control, and that the person will engage in acts for which he will be punished. The ego then resorts to maladaptive defense maneuvers.
Free-floating anxiety	A type of neurotic anxiety characterized by general apprehensiveness and pessimism.
Phobic anxiety	A type of neurotic anxiety that is an intense reaction to fear of some object that can be avoided.
Panic state	A type of neurotic anxiety accompanied by acute anxiety, intense physiological arousal, and disorganization of personality and functional abilities.
Moral anxiety	Fear of the superego; danger to the ego coming from the superego is experienced as guilt or shame. The ego is punished for doing or thinking something that is contrary to the parental standard or moral code.
Castration anxiety	Refers to a variety of anxieties having in common a fear of bodily damage or of some kind of diminuation of one's capacities. Confusion about sexual identity is often associated with castration anxiety.
Separation anxiety	Represents the fearful anticipation of the loss of significant person.

Normally a person can resolve these conflicts with adaptive coping strategies; however, the neurotic person develops irrational solutions because of intense basic anxiety. The neurotic person creates an idealized image, and unrealistic view of the self, and attempts to live up to this self-image. His pride reinforces the basic anxiety and leads him to overvalue other people (to help to maintain the idealized image) and to self-hate or self-contempt. Basic anxiety and the resulting conflicts can be avoided if the child is raised in security, respect, warmth, and love.

Sullivan[55] makes distinctions between several states of anxiety, (see Table 11-2).

Sullivan believes that severe anxiety produces confusion, forgetfulness, and inhibits learning. Less severe anxiety or mild anxiety promotes learning.

Although fear and anxiety may be experienced in much the same way, Sullivan makes a distinction between these two states. *Fear* comes about because of tension arising from the danger of actual physical harm to the person. Fear is an adaptive response that heightens the individual's sensitivity, resulting in increased alertness and increased energy available for bodily responses for self-preservation.

Sullivan believes that all human behavior is oriented toward the pursuit of satisfaction and security. The attainment of satisfaction is closely related to the physical exigencies of the human body and includes meeting the needs of sleep, food, and sexual fulfillment. The feeling of security arises from fulfillment of these biological needs according to culturally approved patterns. An individual experiences intense and painful uneasiness, insecurity, and anxiousness when he meets his needs through culturally disapproved means.

Otto Rank[46] believes that the central problem in human development is individuation and the repeated separations that occur throughout a person's life. Each separation creates not only greater independence for the person, but also produces an increase in anxiety when conditions of relative security and unity are disrupted. In Rank's view anxiety is also experienced because of the ensuing threat to autonomy when the individual refuses to separate. There is the continually revolving dilemma of fear of becoming an individual and fear of losing individuality. This view is poignantly represented in adolescent struggles with authority.

Alfred Adler[2] sees anxiety as arising from feelings of inferiority. In his view, anxiety provides the means for adopting a helpless stance and a basis for avoiding decisions and responsibility. In addition, anxiety can be an aggressive weapon or a means of dominating others. This use of anxiety provides a means of controlling others in an attempt to rid oneself of basic feelings of inferiority. For example, a wife has anxiety attacks as a means of controlling her husband and decreasing her feelings of inferiority.

Learning

In the learning theorist's view, anxiety can motivate behavior. For example, if a student is anxious about the consequences of failing a test, the anxiety may motivate studying behavior. Anxiety may also be a response to an unpleasant experience; for example, when a child, after touching a stove and getting burned, becomes anxious about exposure to hot objects. Anxiety also may be the

BEHAVIORAL REACTIONS TO CONFLICT	
CONFLICT	**BEHAVIORAL REACTIONS**
Approach to approach	The individual is motivated to pursue two equally desirable but incompatible goals
Approach to avoidance	The person wishes, at once, to obtain and avoid a goal
Avoidance to avoidance	The person must choose between two undesirable goals
Double approach to avoidance	The person sees the desirable and undesirable aspects of either alternative *(ambivalence)*

predominant feeling accompanying a behavorial sequence. For example, a person who wants to stop smoking may become very anxious when reaching for a cigarette.

In this theory the development of fear and anxiety as learned drives are based on the primary drive of pain. Dollard and Miller[9] believe that fear and anxiety are learned because (1) neutral cues can evoke feelings associated with pain, (2) fear and anxiety can motivate the person to avoidance behavior, and (3) fear and anxiety can be reinforcers to behavior because their reduction calls forth similar behavioral responses to eliminate pain in the future. An example may be found in a child's fearful response to taking injections. Originally the needle is a neutral cue, but after the first injection the child's behavior alters. The sight of the needle (stimulus cue), previously associated with pain (innate drive) and now fear (learned drive), evokes crying, running, or combative behavior (responses) that serve to reduce fear (reinforcement). If the behavior is successful, the learned response becomes a learned drive as well, and the child will habitually experience fear and engage in avoidance thoughts or actions at the sight of a needle.

Conflicts occur when a stimulus evokes competing behavioral reactions (see the box above).

Dollard and Miller view the resolution of conflicts as entailing several outcomes. The individual usually makes choices easily between desirable alternatives and can resolve avoidance conflicts by escape or by lessening the negative aspects of one of the choices. Approach to avoidance conflicts appear to cause the greatest indecision and ensuing anxiety. When a person is far from the goal, the tendency to approach is stronger, but as the goal is approached, the avoidance desires increase and the person is immobilized through the indecision evoked by the competing tendencies. For example, a child feels hungry and sees a cookie jar. As he approaches the container he remembers that he is not allowed to eat cookies before meals. The child may stop movement toward the cookies because his desire to eat cookies and to please his mother are equally strong; he is indecisive. Should he satisfy himself and risk punishment? He can talk himself into taking the cookies anyway, feeling he deserves them and thus increasing the approach tendencies or he may try to reduce his fear of punishment by asking permission and negating avoidance tendencies and thus be able to take the cookies. He may also develop symptoms, such as a stomachache that would protect him from the original conflict. Usually resolving the conflict through increasing

one's motivation to approach the goal ("I'll take the cookies anyway") results in increased anxiety. Attempts to reduce the avoidance tendencies, the fearful aspects of the situation, usually result in less painful alternatives than attempting to increase motivation to approach.

Dollard and Miller identify four basic assumptions in analyzing conflict behavior: (1) the nearer a person is to a goal, the stronger the tendency to approach it, (2) the nearer a person is to a feared goal, the stronger the tendency to avoid it, (3) avoidance desires increase more rapidly nearer the goal than do approach desires, and (4) whether the tendency to avoid or approach is stronger depends on the strength of the drive. For example, a very hungry man may approach dangerous situations more readily to fulfill this drive.

Existential

According to existentialist writers, anxiety is a fact of life. It arises from being situated or thrust into the world as a finite being who is faced with eventual death or nothingness. Anxiety is an underlying current throughout life and is faced continually. Anxiety becomes more evident in certain situations: in confrontation with one's values, freedom and authority, other persons, one's need to be authentic and death.[25]

May[33] defined anxiety as apprehension caused by a threat to some value that an individual holds essential to his existence. Situations that precipitate anxiety usually have an aspect of choice involved. Individuals choose what they value. This freedom to choose can precipitate anxiety because of the possibility of erring or choosing unwisely.

Consideration of others is important in making choices; anxiety can result from the tension between personal freedom and commitment to the group or social context of one's life. To become oriented primarily to the group may mean the individual becomes authentic or loses the self. The anxiety arising from an inauthentic existence comes from the inability to face and accept oneself. Ultimately the greatest anxiety comes from the threat of nothingness, death, and the realization of life's limitations.

Table 11-3 reviews the main theories of anxiety, illustrating the meanings attached to its causes as well as the different dynamics involved when a person is anxious. These theories orient the nurse to differing observational data and suggest a variety of models for nursing intervention for anxiety states.

TABLE 11-3 Theories of anxiety

Theorist	Types of Anxiety	Source of Anxiety	Dynamics	Observational Cues	Nurse's Role in Anxiety
INTRAPSYCHIC					
Freud	Developmental anxiety Primary Subsequent Ego anxiety Realistic Neurotic Moral	Ego overwhelmed by excessive stimulation; biological and instinctual needs paramount	Development of defensive mechanisms—unconscious maneuvers related to repression of instinctual demands	Development of symptoms	Sounding board or screen for projection of transference feelings
INTERPERSONAL					
Horney	Basic anxiety	Hostile environment	Development of coping strategies and idealized self-image	Patterns of behavior in relation to others	Passive participant in experience; a source of support and approval
Sullivan	Primitive anxiety Mild anxiety Severe anxiety Fear	Interpersonal relations and fear of disapproval by significant others	Development of security operations	Areas of vulnerability in interpersonal relations	Reflective participant-observer in experience of anxiety to provide security base
LEARNING-BEHAVIORAL					
Dollard and Miller	Fear Anxiety	Learned drive acquired by association with a primary drive	Development of strategies in response to conflict	Antecedent environmental stimulus; consequent behavioral response	Active reinforcer; model of response options, cognitive reframer
EXISTENTIAL					
Kierkegaard and May	Lived anxiety (normal and basic)	Conditions of life; threat of nothingness; threats to something valued	Development of accepting attitude, leading to authenticity, freedom, and taking responsibility for one's choices; or nonaccepting attitude, leading to inauthenticity and despair	Inability to live with uncertainty or ambiguity, to flee situation; refusal to actively participate	Active participant in dialogue regarding fears, uncertainties, and values; makes assessment of life review and encourager of client decision making

RELATING TO THE CLIENT

Initial interactions with clients create a certain amount of anxiety in both client and nurse. Because anxiety is communicable and easily transferred from client to nurse and nurse to client, it is essential that the nurse be aware of her anxiety as she begins a therapeutic relationship with an anxious client. An awareness of her feelings, particularly anxiety, and their effect on the client enables her to prevent her feelings of anxiety from interfering in the relationship.

Some questions that the nurse can ask herself to promote self-awareness include the following:

1. Do I recognize when I am becoming anxious?
2. What is contributing to my anxiety about this client?
3. What are the symptoms of my anxiety?
4. How do I handle anxiety?
5. How do I respond when I meet anxious people?
6. What are some other ways I can respond to anxious people?

During the orientation phase of the relationship the nurse identifies anxiety through awareness of her verbal and nonverbal communication with the client. Monitoring rate, tone, and pitch of speech as well as her breathing and posture has a calming effect, provides information and projects self-confidence. Behaviors that indicate the nurses anxiety may include responding defensively, rationalizing, denying, projecting, avoiding the client, or overloading herself with task-oriented activities.

During the working stage of the relationship anxiety is

increased as the client deals with emotionally charged issues. The nurse may feel unsure about how to relieve the client's distress. She may have a sense of hopelessness or inadequacy, undermining her self-esteem and coping abilities. If anxiety increases it is communicated between the client and nurse and a reciprocal pattern of escalating anxiety ensues.

Termination may also increase anxiety whether the relationship has progressed well with resistance lessened, intimacy deepened, and positive outcomes achieved or problems remain unresolved. As the client prepares for termination, the nurse may attempt to hold on to the relationship and fail to acknowledge that it is ending, thus increasing anxiety about termination. It is important that the nurse recognize the value of sharing her anxieties with a supervisor or other trusted person when a relationship terminates uneasily.

NURSING PROCESS
Assessment

✦ *Physical dimension.* Clients experiencing anxiety can be assessed in three primary systems: musculoskeletal, cardiovascular, and gastrointestinal. Table 11-4 lists characteristics of responses in each system.

There may also be a direct relationship between the increase in physiological responses to anxiety and the intensity of a person's emotional state. For example, in a client experiencing a significant loss physiological responses will be evident such as flushing, irritableness, headache, and fastidiousness about his surroundings, clothing, and other personal items—denying that there are any concerns or anxious feelings. If the source of stress continues or increases, additional symptoms may become manifest as the client's threshold for anxiety continues to be tested, requiring more defensive maneuvers. Clients may exhibit a particular sequence of symptoms in stressful situations.[29] Knowledge of the client's symptom pattern is helpful in planning interventions as well as providing knowledge of the levels of defense that are called into play for the anxious client. The symptom pattern for this client involves personal and physical changes and develops into compulsive behavior and use of denial as defense mechanisms. The nurse may expect the client to reenact this sequence of symptoms when he experiences anxiety in the future.

The environmental stressors that can precipitate or exacerbate the physiological symptoms of anxiety include caffeine consumption, use of opium and hallucinogenic drugs, reaction to an epinephrine medication, loss of sleep, fatigue, premenstrual edema, poor nutrition and hypoglycemia, threats to body integrity as a result of surgery or injury, blood loss, hyperthyroidism, and hyperventilation.

Anxiety can appear after ingestion of 500 to 600 mg of caffeine; this is the equivalent of 5 or 6 cups of coffee per day. Caffeine can produce symptoms indistinguishable from anxiety, such as nervousness, irritability, agitation, tremors, rapid breathing, palpitations, and dysrhythmias. In addition, even a brief abstinence from caffeine by per-

TABLE 11-4 Physical characteristics of anxiety

System	Characteristics
Musculoskeletal	Increased tendon reflexes
	Rigid, tense muscles
	Knee and ankle clonus
	Muscular tremors
	Increased generalized fatigue
	Increased weakness
	Clumsiness
	Jerking of limbs
	Tics
	Unsteady voice
	Tightening of throat
	Unsteadiness
	Inability to move
Cardiovascular	Palpitations
	Precordial pressure
	Throbbing sensations
	Increased pulse, respiration, blood pressure
	Flushing and heat sensations
	Cold hands and feet
	Sweating
Gastrointestinal	Nausea
	Belching
	Heartburn
	Cramps
	An "empty stomach" feeling
	Bad taste in mouth
Others	Difficulty sleeping
	Dilated pupils
	Urinary urgency
	Urinary frequency

sons who are moderate users may produce anxiety. It is important to review the use of caffeine by anxious patients.[44] Foods high in caffeine include coffee, tea, cola drinks, cocoa, over-the-counter analgesics, stimulants, and appetite suppressants.

Psychophysiological disorders can be viewed as a group of illnesses in which the dominant feature is emotinal maladaptation that leads to irreversible organ or tissue damage. The emotional disorder leaves the person vulnerable to severe physiological dysfunction. These disorders are different from the commonly occurring response of increased susceptibility to illness as a result of an emotional upset and from the emotional turmoil resulting as a reaction to disease.

A hypochondriacal response is distinct from psychophysiological reactions and may occur as a response to anxiety. The client's excessive anxiety is displaced from its unconscious origins to one or more body organs that become the center of preoccupation. Frequent complaints include insomnia, irritability, and alternating aches and pains. The clients with a hypochondriacal response focuses on these body sensations that are often unique to this anxious state. The worry and preoccupation distract

FIGURE 11-1 Anxiety during test taking is often expressed as seen in this illustration.

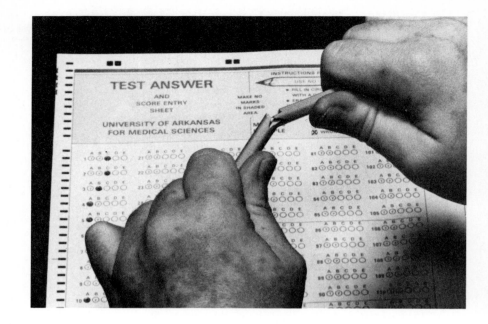

TABLE 11-5 Levels of anxiety

Severity of Anxiety	Physical	Intellectual	Social and Emotional
MINIMAL (near 0)	Basal levels of: Blood pressure Pulse Respiration rate O_2 consumption Pupillary constriction Muscles relaxed; little or no resistance to passive range of motion	Cognitive activity minimal Disregard for external environmental stimuli; no attempt to actively process information Focus typically on single, non-threatening mental image States of altered consciousness	No social interaction No attempt to deal with environmental stimuli Minimal emotional activity Feelings of indifference, invulnerability, and contentment prevail
MILD (+1)	Low-level sympathetic arousal Moderate to low skeletal muscle tension Body relaxed; movements smooth, directed, and purposeful Makes and holds eye contact easily Voice calm, well-modulated	Perceptual field open; able to shift focus of attention readily Passively aware of external environment Self-referent thoughts positive; low concern for unexpected or negative outcomes	Behavior primarily automatic; habitual patterns and well-learned skills Positive feeling of security, confidence, and satisfaction dominate Solitary activities
MODERATE (+2)	Sympathetic nervous system activation ↑ Blood pressure ↑ Pulse rate ↑ Respiratory rate Pupillary dilation Sweat glands stimulated Peripheral vascular constriction Increased muscular tension, mixed sense of tension and excitement; may experience "jitters" Heightened performance of well-learned skills	Narrowing of perception; attentional focus on specific internal or external stimuli Conscious effort in processing of information; optimal level for learning Self-referent thoughts ± mixed; some concern about personal ability or available resources necessary to solve problems; probability of positive outcomes increasingly uncertain	Increased skill in learning and refining of skills; analyzing problematic situations; integrating cognitive and motor domains Feelings of challenge; drive to resolve problems or dilemmas Mixed sense of confidence/optimism with fear, lowered self-esteem, and potential inadequacy

TABLE 11-5 Levels of anxiety—cont'd

Severity of Anxiety	Physical	Intellectual	Social and Emotional
	Voice suggests interest and concern with problem analysis; rate of speech increased, pitch heightened Increased alertness		

SEVERE (+3)	Fight-flight response
	Generalized sympathetic nervous system discharge
	Stimulation of adrenal medulla
	  ↑ Catecholamines, accelerated heart rate, palpitations
	  ↑ Blood glucose
	  ↓ Blood flow to digestive system
	  ↑ Blood flow to skeletal muscles
	Muscles extremely tense, rigid, fixed
	Hyperventilation
	Physical actions increasingly agitated, random, and disorganized; pacing, wringing of hands quivering, fidgeting, trembling, immobilization
	May experience loss of appetite, nausea, "cold sweats"
	Verbal effects: stammering, blocking, rapid, high-pitched speech, fragmented sentences, hesitations
	Facial expression: poor eye contact, fleeting eye movements; may fix gaze if preoccupied with internal thoughts; gnashing of teeth, jaw clenching
		Perceptual capacity restricted; exclusive attention to singular stimuli (internal or external) or multifocal, fragmented processing of stimuli
		Problem solving inefficient, difficult
		Some threatening stimuli disregarded, minimized, denied
		Disorientation in terms of time and place
		Expected likelihood of negative consequences or outcomes high; estimates of personal self-efficacy low
			Flight behavior may be manifested by withdrawal, denial, depression, somatization
			Feelings of increasing threat, need to respond to situation are heightened
			Dissociating tendency; feelings are denied

PANIC (+4)	Continued physiological arousal Actions disorganized, directionless; unable to execute simple motor tasks; fumbling, gross motor agitation, flailing May strike out verbally or physically; may attempt to withdraw from situation Eventual depletion of sympathetic neurotransmitters Blood redistributed throughout body Hypotension May feel dizzy, faint, or exhausted Appears pale, drawn, weary Facial expression: aghast, grimacing, eyebrows raised, mouth agape, eyes fixed; may hide face Voice louder, higher pitched; may ramble incessantly; may falter or be speechless; gasping	Perception severely restricted, may be impervious to external stimuli Thoughts are random, distorted, disconnected, logical processing impaired Unable to solve problems; limited tolerance for processing novel stimuli (verbal, auditory, or visual) Preoccupied with thoughts of highly probable negative outcomes; conclusion may be drawn, negative consequences seen as inevitable	Emotionally drained, overwhelmed Reliance on earlier, more "primitive" coping behaviors: crying, shouting, curling up, rocking, freezing Feelings of impotence, helplessness, agony and desperation dominate; may be experienced as horror, dread, defenselessness; may be converted to anger, rage

Adapted from Longo, D., and Williams, R.: Clinical practice in psychosocial nursing: assessment and intervention, N.Y., 1986, Appleton-Century-Crofts.

the client's attention from unpleasant anxiety-producing feelings. (See Chapter 34.)

✳ *Emotional dimension.* Anxiety includes a mixture of feeling states with negative feeling components, such as fear, distress, shame, shyness, guilt, and anger and positive components such as joy, love, and excitement. (See Figure 11-1). An assessment of the level of a person's anxiety is a priority in working with anxious clients (see Table 11-5). The nurse collects data about the duration, intensity, and appropriateness of the anxiety. Because anxiety interacts with other dimensions of the person, the physical, intellectual, and social responses are also included in the assessment.

✳ *Intellectual dimension.* Anxious persons are usually preoccupied by an anticipation of unpleasantness; they fear that a dreaded event is about to happen or may happen, although it is not occurring presently. There appear to be exceptions to this future time orientation in clients experiencing anxiety after involvement in such traumatic situations as combat, rape, or close avoidance of actual physical danger. However, when the anxiety response recurs, the person, on recalling the event, appears to experience the trauma in the present through a flashback process.

Interference with realistic thinking can be readily observed in the anxious person, as reflected in (1) repetitive thinking or rumination about the danger, (2) reduction in the ability to reason and to objectively evaluate and reappraise one's thoughts (see the Research Highlight on p. 213), (3) overreaction to stimuli that are perceived as dangerous, (4) difficulty with short-term recall and blocking on words, (5) difficulty in concentrating on immediate tasks, and (6) *hypervigilance* to dangerous stimuli. In addition, anxious persons who concentrate and dwell on negative outcomes may see every situation as catastrophic; they assume that potential threats are actual threats. They are not able to discriminate and the tendency to avoid the threat does not lead to increased confidence or ability to cope.

A person can attach dangerous meanings to the experience of anxiety itself. In this situation a vicious cycle of escalation can occur, in which a thought that is threatening produces anxiety that in turn causes the person to evaluate the situation as even more threatening; this produces even more anxiety. Anxiety becomes a type of preoccupation characterized by increased self-awareness, self-doubt, and self-depreciation. This preoccupation with self interferes with attention to environmental cues and information processing; the person may respond with irrelevant responses pertaining mainly to himself. The worry that arises from this self-focus interferes with problem solving because attention is diverted to emotionally demanding self-issues. Highly anxious clients appear to be nondiscriminatory in terms of the situations to which they respond with anxiety and tend to be inferior in learning complex and difficult tasks. For example, overhearing nurses talking about a blood transfusion, the client assumes it is for him, even though plans are being made for his discharge.

Three conditions are necessary for anxiety to occur.

The nurse may observe that the client is (1) overstimulated by his thoughts or by environmental cues, (2) the client may have expectations that are incompatible with his abilities and, (3) the client may be completely unable to act. Anxiety continues because of this inability to engage in purposeful action. Indecision, conflict, and external restraint thwart the person's behavioral options, make them unclear, and contribute to an anxious reaction.

Anxiety that is aroused internally may be expected to evoke responses that are different from behavior precipitated by an external danger. When anxiety arises from a thought or internal cue, its reduction depends on avoidance of this thought or memory. This is a *defense mechanism.*

There are four levels of defense against anxiety. The individual's first line of defense is considered normal and involves conscious efforts at maintaining control over anxiety by changing the environment or one's perspective. Ways of coping include removing oneself from stressful situations, indulging in physical satisfactions such as eating or sex as escape routes, use of social or recreational pursuits to divert one's attention from problems, daydreaming and fantasizing as substitute satisfactions.

The second line of defense against anxiety involves character changes and manipulation of relationships with others. These defenses may lead to personality disorders if prolonged or exaggerated and to difficulties in the interpersonal areas of work, marriage, and parenting.

The third line of defense comprises the repressive defenses, which involve changes in the intrapsychic process. These repressive defenses fall into four main categories, (1) those aimed at keeping conflicting ideas out of one's awareness; (2) those aimed at inhibiting attention, concentration, conscious awareness, memory, emotions, sensory stimulation, and motor and visceral functioning; (3) defenses of displacement and phobic avoidance; and (4) *undoing* through compulsive rituals.

The fourth line of defense is seen in the use of the regressive defenses and involves a return to a state of helplessness, withdrawal from reality through psychotic manuevers, internalization of hostility with suicidal thoughts, and acting out of repressed sexual or hostile impulses (see Table 11-6).

✳ *Social dimension.* Anxiety arising from social situations appears to be related to loss of self-esteem and affection and fears of rejection in highly valued social settings.

Anxiety during the development stages can be viewed in many ways, but essentially it is related to changes in individual and environmental expectations as the person develops. These changes can lead to anxiety because the person faces an uncertain future and unknown outcomes from the growth process. Generally, developmental anxiety is referred to particularly stressful stages such as adolescence and the separation and stranger anxiety behavior of the young infant. When assessing an anxious person, it is important to consider normal life crises that may last for several weeks or months as possible sources of anxiety.

Anxiety is often generated in the child by an empathic

Research Highlight

Anxiety, Critical Thinking, and Information Processing During and After Breast Biopsy

Diane W. Scott

PURPOSE

This exploratory study examining the variables of anxiety level, critical thinking ability, and capacity to process information (time perception) was undertaken to further knowledge about ways people cope with stress. The goal of the study was to determine the relationship between these three variables during and after the acute life crisis of a breast biopsy to ascertain a possible cancer diagnosis.

SAMPLE

The sample population consisted of selected women admitted to a large, urban cancer center for surgical biopsy to determine the presence of carcinoma of the breast. Eighty five women between the ages of 18 and 60 with educational levels ranging from high school through college and representing various socioeconomic levels, volunteered for participation in the study. Subjects were afebrile on both testing occasions and had no previous diagnosis of cancer. The surgical biopsy procedure was performed under general anesthesia.

METHODOLOGY

Participants were tested by the State-Trait Anxiety Inventory (STAI), the Watson Glaser Critical Thinking Appraisal (CTA), and by time perception Judged Duration [JD] of a previously experienced interval.

Testing occurred on two occasions: on admission to hospital, before biopsy and knowledge of diagnostic results; and 6 to 8 weeks after the procedure and having been informed that the biopsy indicated a nonmalignant condition. Temperatures were taken orally with an IVAC digital thermometer to control for the effect of body temperature on time perception. After collecting sociodemographic information in an initial interview, the tests were administered in the same sequence: STAI, CTA, and JD. To measure JD, subjects pressed a button to activiate an electronic timer at the beginning and end of the CTA test. Subjects were asked for an estimation of elasped time immediately after deactivation of the timer. This was contrasted with the actual time obtained from the digital read out. Retesting at the 6- to 8-week interval occurred most often in the subject's home; debriefing followed the second round of testing.

FINDINGS

Critical thinking ability was substantially reduced at the time of hospitalization. State anxiety and judged duration were found to be significantly related during the postcrisis testing, and the high anxiety subgroup tested during the acute crisis period showed a diminished reasoning ability. The anxiety levels of clients were extremely high before they were informed of the diagnostic results. The group average was above that of acutely ill psychiatric clients, and one third of the group scored one standard deviation above the norm for medical-surgical populations. State anxiety levels were significantly reduced 6 to 8 weeks after biopsy.

All variables changed as predicted, with anxiety decreasing significantly between acute and postcrisis phases and critical thinking improving. Time estimation did not change significantly.

IMPLICATIONS

Nurses need to address and respond to the decreased reasoning ability of the clients when requesting their participation in such critical decisions as informed consent, choice of surgical procedure, and adjuvant therapy at admission. Those clients having high anxiety levels and diminished reasoning ability appear to be a high-risk group requiring special nursing consideration.

Clients who overestimate time appear to have difficulty in adjusting to the fast-paced, intense, sensory stimulation of the hospital routine. They also may need special consideration in terms of lessening their distractibility by pacing stimuli and allowing for slower decision making and opportunities for concentration. Clients with varying levels of anxiety, critical thinking ability, and time estimation may constitute groups differing in coping abilities, and thus requiring different nursing considerations. A series of studies has been designed as a follow-up to this study, which will lend increased understanding of behavior of people experiencing anxiety and lead to better nursing identification and follow-up on high-risk groups.

Based on data from Nursing Research **32**(1):24, 1983.

response or emotional contagion from the parent. This learned response can be repeated later in life when the person identifies with and reacts to the emotional responses of another person.

Social anxiety refers to the discomfort experienced in the presence of others. This discomfort creates uncertainty regarding the scrutiny or remarks of others. Social anxiety is caused by specific characteristics of social situations as well as the behavior of others.

It is important for the nurse to assess social contexts that can cause anxiety for the client, such as (1) the number of persons present, (2) the amount of attention offered by others as well as that expected from the client when in a large group, (3) familiarity with the persons

TABLE 11-6 Defense mechanisms

Defense Mechanism	Purpose	Definition	Example
FIRST LEVEL: CONSCIOUS ATTEMPTS AT COPING			
Suppression	Helps keep forbidden drives and wishes out of one's conscience	Voluntary and intentional exclusion from conscious level of ideas, feelings, and situations that produce anxiety	A student receives a poor report card and "forgets" to give it to his parents
Substitution	Helps reduce frustration by disguising motivations	Replacement of an unacceptable need, attitude, or emotion with one that is more acceptable	A woman feels unattractive physically, so she puts her energy into sports and competitive trials
Rationalization	Helps raise self-esteem and social approval by disguising motivations	An attempt by the ego to make unacceptable feelings and behavior tolerable and acceptable	A nurse fails to do a procedure correctly and justifies her feeling of incompetence by stating that there is too much work on the ward
Fantasy	Provides a way to resolve conflict and meet needs in a symbolic way	A conscious creation or distortion of unacceptable fears, wishes, and behaviors	A nurse fails an important test and daydreams about her heroic attempts to save a client
SECOND LEVEL: CHARACTER DEVELOPMENT AS A WAY OF COPING			
Identification	Helps preserve the ego of the person while allowing concealment of inadequacies	An attempt to emulate oneself to resemble an admired, idealized person	A little girl dresses like her mother and mimics her behavior
Internalization or introjection	Attempts to deny or disguise by changing the ego to avoid threat	Assimilation (often symbolic) of loved or hated wishes, values, and attitudes	A child scolds his toys while playing, similar to the prohibitions of his parents
Restitution	Attempts to assuage guilt feelings by making reparation	Going back or attempting to resolve unconscious guilt feelings	A boss is short tempered with an employee and then gives her the rest of the afternoon off
THIRD LEVEL: REPRESSIVE ATTEMPTS AT COPING			
Compensation	Helps relieve fears of failure in one activity by emphasizing another can result in one-sidedness caused by overcompensation	An attempt to make up for real or imagined deficiences	A girl feels socially unattractive or inept, is responded to this way by peers, and becomes an honor student
Reaction formation	Serves as a protective device to prevent painful or unacceptable attitudes from being expressed	The assumption of attitudes, motives, and needs that are opposite those repudiated consciously	An adolescent struggles with hostile feelings, but presents herself in an ingratiating way
Sublimation	Helps channel forbidden instinctual impulses into constructive activities	Diversion of unacceptable instinctual drives into personally and socially accepted areas	A young man who struggles with rebellion against authority becomes a policeman who enforces law and order
Displacement	Helps the person disguise feelings by using a less threatening object to release feelings	Redirection of an emotional feeling from one idea, person, or object to another	A physician berates a nurse, and, when a guest enters the client's room, the nurse harshly tells the person to wait for visiting hours
Projection	Helps the person avoid awareness of his undesirable impulses	Rejecting and imputing to others unpleasant aspects of one-self; attributing intolerable wishes, feelings, and motivations to others	A student suspects other classmates of being jealous of her good grades and thereby avoiding her
Symbolization	Serves to help compensate for and disguise true feelings	Disguisement of an object as a representation of a hidden idea	In a busy family, a child creates a picture of all family members on a Ferris wheel
Conversion	Channels and contains unbearable feelings through body expression	Symbolic expression of intrapsychic conflict through physical symptoms	A student develops headaches before taking an important test for which she feels unprepared

TABLE 11-6 Defense mechanisms—cont'd

Defense Mechanism	Purpose	Definition	Example
Repression	Helps provide a forgetting and protective function for the ego	Involuntary and automatic regulation of unbearable ideas and impulses; submersion of these to subconscious realm	After the recent death of a spouse the surviving spouse cannot remember the marriage date
Undoing	Disguises and attempts to repair feelings or actions that have led to anxiety or guilt	An attempt to actually or symbolically take away a previously intolerable action or experience	A mother who has just lost her temper and beaten her children develops compulsive hand-washing and child-checking behaviors
FOURTH LEVEL: REGRESSIVE ATTEMPTS AT COPING			
Denial	Helps the person escape unpleasant reality	Disownment of intolerable ideas and impulses; refusal to perceive conflict	A terminal cancer client appears not to be aware of impending death
Dissociation	Helps the person put painful feelings aside and isolate, compartmentalize them	Separation and detachment of emotional significance and affect from an idea or situation	A client relates a tale of victimization on the street in a matter-of-fact manner, even jokingly at times
Regression	Helps the person retreat from the present situation and become dependent and less anxious	Retreat to an earlier and more comfortable level of adjustment	A wife refuses to drive a car even though it causes the family much disorganization; her refusal necessitates that her husband take her everywhere

present, (4) the degree of informality in the social exchange, and (5) the expectation of evaluation by others. Large groups of people and being the focus of attention make most individuals nervous. New people or situations as well as highly formal situations that require attention to social details raise anxiety.

Overattentiveness or underattentiveness by others can affect a person's social anxiety. Socially anxious persons may withdraw and inhibit their social behavior when they are ignored. Statements that direct attention to the socially anxious person may induce shyness. Intrusions into the domain of another person, such as too much self-disclosure, overhearing private conversations, or witnessing private acts can also lead to social anxiety. Conspicuousness, novelty, disclosure, and fear of evaluation all contribute to the experience of social anxiety.

Sociocultural variables related to anxiety are important to consider during assessment. Women have scored higher than men in general anxiety, and the sex differences appear to be even more pronounced when considering women in lower class and minority groups.[43] Similarly, lower-class children appear to be more anxious than middle-class children. In his study of Scandinavian countries, Kata[22] found that there were lower levels of anxiety in persons working in high prestige occupations; anxiety also decreased with an increase in family and individual income.

Other social stressors that can lead to anxiety include decreased self-esteem through job loss, change in social status through retirement, and loss of love relationships through death of a significant person, separation, or di-

vorce. In addition, unexpected events such as illness, changes in living conditions or financial status, loss of control in ability to care for oneself, and threats to independence increase anxiety. Highly anxious family members or significant others, a lack of supportive relationships, an inability to meet the expectations of important others, and their nonacceptance of the person's emotional needs can also cause anxiety.

When a person has an organized, well-thought-out plan for alleviating his distress and this plan is interrupted with no available alternative to the original plan, helplessness and anxiety may result.[31] For example, an ailing elderly person desires to stay in his own home to remain among familiar and important belongings and has made arrangements for a relative to visit and check on him daily. When the family is transferred because of the father's job, the elderly client becomes extremely anxious and feels helpless, unable to focus on ways to maintain his independence and plan for overseeing of his health needs.

Spiritual dimension. The values one holds become important sources of support and self-definition. Throughout life, normal growth as well as crises provide the opportunity to reassess values, to give up old ones, and aspire to new ones. Relinquishing old values, and the creativity needed to view things differently can generate anxiety. Commitment to values such as freedom, autonomy, and equality may ward off despair and provide purpose and motivation for life.

Love entails being able to give as well as receive, and the autonomous, mature adult chooses, affirms, and participates in the experience of love. Anxiety can arise when the person is cut off or denied the opportunity to give love to a valued partner.

Fear and guilt about the ethical nature of one's actions may also lead to anxiety. For example, a client, being respectful of his wife's anger and rejection of the son, may not make attempts to relate to his son. The father experiences anxiety about this choice because he has strong beliefs about the value of parental support.

The nurse is concerned with assessing the client's search for meaning in life and overcoming alienation through communication with others. The client's capacity to be true to himself and to respect his individuality and uniqueness and that of others will help him face the normal anxieties of life and live with commitment, love, and hope. A significant source of anxiety in the spiritual dimension is the person's fear and distrust of himself and his abilities. No matter how extreme situations may be, if the nurse sees that the client is maintaining faith in himself and courage in terms of his convictions, anxiety will be more bearable. This belief in oneself and one's capacities can be facilitated by caring environments and is particularly important to preserve in nursing situations.

Measurement tools. Several scales are available to assess anxiety. The oldest and most widely used test for anxiety is the Manifest Anxiety Scale.[55a] The S-R Inventory of Anxiousness assesses the proneness to anxiety as it relates to interpersonal, dangerous, or ambiguous situations.[10a] The S-R Inventory of General Trait Anxiousness measures anxiety in innocuous, daily routines.[10b] This scale asks the client to imagine being in a situation in which physical danger may be encountered; for example, speeding on a curve. The client is then asked to indicate on a 5-point Likert scale the intensity of reactions to potentially dangerous objects or things. Examples of the 15 items in the physical danger subscale include:

	NOT AT ALL				VERY MUCH
Perspire	1	2	3	4	5
Feel tense	1	2	3	4	5
Heart beats faster	1	2	3	4	5

The State Trait Anxiety Inventory asks persons to identify how they generally feel (trait) and how they feel at a particular moment (state) in time.[54a] Following are examples of items from this 40-item self-evaluation questionnaire:

	NOT AT ALL	SOMEWHAT	MODERATELY	VERY MUCH
I feel calm	1	2	3	4
I am tense	1	2	3	4
I am jittery	1	2	3	4
I am worried	1	2	3	4

Several scales have been developed to assess levels of anxiety before, during, or after exposure to fearful events.

ANXIETY

DEFINITION

A vague, uneasy feeling whose source is often nonspecific or unknown to the individual.

DEFINING CHARACTERISTICS

Physical Dimension
Increased heart rate
Elevated blood pressure
Insomnia
Fatigue and weakness
Increased respirations
Diaphoresis
Dilated pupils
Voice quivers
*Hand tremors
Palpitations
Nausea and vomiting
Flushing
Dry mouth
Body aches and pains
Urinary frequency
Restlessness
Faintness
Paresthesias
Poor eye contact

Emotional Dimension
Apprehension
Nervousness
Feelings of inadequacy
Fear
Tension
Irritability
Crying
Uncertainty
Rattled
Overexcited
Distressed
Jittery
Shakiness

Intellectual Dimension
Inability to concentrate
Lack of awareness of surroundings
Rumination
Orientation to future
Self-focus
Inability to remember
*Blames others
Criticizes self and others
Loss of control
Regretful
Worried
Social Dimension
*Helplessness
*Lack of self-confidence
*Withdrawal
Spiritual Dimension
Decreased self-worth

Adapted from North American Nursing Diagnosis Association Classification of Nursing Diagnosis: Proceedings of the seventh conference, St. Louis, 1987, The C.V. Mosby Co.

*Indicates characteristics in addition to those defined by NANDA.

These scales include the Affect Adjective Check List, Today Form,[61] and the Fear Survey Schedule,[2a] which looks at fears associated with small animals, death, physical pain and surgery, aggression, and interpersonal events. The fear thermometer[58] is administered by asking the client to place a mark on a scale from 1 to 10 to indicate the level of anxiety. This form of measurement is particularly adaptable to clinical situations in which the nurse can ask the client to rate his level of anxiety:

Indicate your anxiety on a scale from 1 to 10.
Is 10 the highest level?
Is this the highest it has ever been in a specific situation?
What was it yesterday?
Has anything helped to lower your anxiety?
What would help?

Analysis

Nursing diagnosis. Anxiety, sleep pattern disturbances, and post-trauma response are three of the nursing diagnoses approved by the North American Nursing Diagnosis Association (NANDA) that apply to the anxious person. The defining characteristics of these nursing diagnoses are listed in the boxes on the opposite page and below.

The following list provides examples of NANDA-accepted nursing diagnoses with causative statements.

1. Severe anxiety related to irrational thoughts of guilt
2. Ineffective individual coping related to altered ability to constructively manage stressors secondary to marital discord
3. Ineffective individual coping related to irrational avoidance of objects
4. Ineffective individual coping: irritability related to anxiety about surgery
5. Social isolation related to irrational fear of social situations

The following Case Example illustrates the nursing diagnosis anxiety.

SLEEP PATTERN DISTURBANCE

DEFINITION
Disruption of sleep time causes discomfort or interferes with desired lifestyle.

DEFINING CHARACTERISTICS
Physical Dimension
Difficulty falling or remaining asleep
Awakening earlier or later than desired
Dozing during the day
Urinary frequency
Pain
Lack of exercise
Pregnancy
*Caffeinated beverages
Noise
Hand tremors
Ptosis of eyelid
Dark circles under eyes
Frequent yawning
Thick speech
Lethargy
Restlessness
Listlessness
Emotional Dimension
Agitation
*Anger
Fear
Depression
Irritability
Intellectual Dimension
Verbal complaints of difficulty falling asleep
Verbal complaints of not feeling well rested
Nightmares
*Preoccupation
*Worrying
Social Dimension
Presence of a roommate
*Loss of spouse

POST-TRAUMA RESPONSE

DEFINITION
The state of an individual experiencing a sustained painful response to an unexpected extraordinary life event(s).

DEFINING CHARACTERISTICS
Emotional Dimension
Emotional numbness
Confusion
Irritability
Explosiveness
Guilt about behavior required for survival
Phobias
Intellectual Dimension
Reexperience of the traumatic event (flashbacks, intrusive thoughts, dreams, nightmares)
Excessive verbalization of traumatic event
Verbalization of survival guilt
Amnesia
Vagueness about traumatic event
Social Dimension
Altered life-style (self-destructiveness, substance abuse, suicidal behavior)
Difficulty with interpersonal relationships

Adapted from North American Nursing Diagnosis Association Classification of Nursing Diagnosis: Proceedings of the seventh conference, St. Louis, 1987, The C.V. Mosby Co.

Adapted from North American Nursing Diagnosis Association Classification of Nursing Diagnosis: Proceedings of the seventh conference, St. Louis, 1987, The C.V. Mosby Co.
*Indicates characteristics in addition to those defined by NANDA.

Case Example

Gary has been preparing for an upcoming exam for several months and is confident that he will do well. As the date of the exam approaches, the possibility that he will not do well enters his mind. The exam begins to pose a serious threat to him as he considers the consequences of failure: a blow to his self-esteem, an obstacle to future plans, personal defeat, disgrace in the eyes of his friends, and a disappointment to his family. He then turns his attention to possible weaknesses, omissions in studying material, deficits in comprehension, and difficulty in expressing what he has learned. These flaws tend to overshadow his previous accomplishments and abilities. On the day of the exam he is concerned about his weaknesses and the possibility of exam questions that he may be unable to answer. As he looks at the exam his mind goes blank and his reasoning ability seems paralyzed. He is unable to recall information. The test becomes overwhelming and he further berates himself.

The following Case Example illustrates the nursing diagnosis sleep pattern disturbance.

Case Example

Leslie, 31 years old, has recently been promoted to an executive position in a small, but growing investment agency. Having functioned at a high level in her previous position, she is now increasingly anxious about dressing appropriately for her new position, making a mistake, and being fired. These fears interrupt her sleep at night, lead to increased fatigue during the day, and increase her anxiety about making mistakes. She drinks several cups of coffee each day to help combat the fatigue that, in turn, intensifies her inability to sleep at night.

The following Case Example illustrates the nursing diagnosis of post-trauma response.

Case Example

Marty, 17 years old, witnessed the death of her father during a robbery of their family-owned store. Since that time she has been unable to sleep and has recurring nightmares about the robbery. Much of her day is spent replaying over and over what she might have done to prevent her father's death. In addition to blaming herself, she feels that she is being punished for not having done things during the robbery that could have saved her father's life.

DSM-III-R diagnosis. The DSM-III-R classifications for pathological conditions related to anxiety are listed in the box at right. The essential features and manifestations of the features of agoraphobia, depersonalization disorder, and post-traumatic stress syndrome according to the DSM III-R are listed in the boxes on p. 219.

Planning

Table 11-7 lists examples of long-term and short term goals and outcome criteria related to anxiety. These serve as examples of the planning stage in the nursing process.

Implementation

✦ ***Physical dimension.*** Simply encouraging the client to pay attention to what his body is experiencing and to verbalize his self-observations can be a form of support in anxiety-related disorders. The client can be reassured that the symptoms are related to anxiety and are not the result of a physical disease after physical factors are ruled out. The lower left box on p. 219 gives helpful steps in working with an anxious client.

Helping clients find palliative relief through natural sources of anxiety reduction are also important nursing interventions. Activities that focus the client's attention on self-help include a warm bath, back rub, a walk, or a regularly scheduled workout.

Physical means of anxiety reduction also include emphasis on slower breathing, meditation, and relaxation techniques. Relaxation procedures can be either passive or active. In the passive approach the client is encouraged to relax completely as a means of becoming receptive. It is an attempt to encourage the client to let his defenses down, open his mind, and become receptive to suggestions about how to deal with stressors. Active relaxation, as in the Lamaze method and systematic desensitization procedures, involves a conscious and deliberate relaxation of one muscle group after another, while the mind remains alert. This procedure works by attempting to occupy the mind with relaxing, rather than anxious thoughts.

In *desensitization* an important part of the therapy is the use of the relaxation response as a counter response to stimuli that previously elicited anxiety. This is accomplished through (1) relaxation training, (2) construction of a hierarchy of situations that elicit anxiety, and (3) working through each situation in the hierarchy by main-

---

DSM III-R CLASSIFICATIONS RELATED TO ANXIETY

ANXIETY DISORDERS

300.21	Panic disorder with agoraphobia
300.01	Panic disorder without agoraphobia
300.22	Agoraphobia without history of panic disorder
300.23	Social phobia
300.29	Simple phobia
309.89	Post-traumatic stress disorder
300.02	Generalized anxiety disorder
300.00	Anxiety disorder not otherwise specified

SOMATOFORM DISORDERS

300.81	Somatization disorder
300.11	Conversion disorder
300.70	Hypochondriasis

DISSOCIATIVE DISORDERS

300.14	Multiple personality disorder
300.13	Psychogenic fugue
300.12	Psychogenic amnesia
300.60	Depersonalization disorder
300.15	Possession/trance disorder

Adapted from American Psychiatric Association: Diagnostic and statistical manual of mental disorders (DSM-III-R), Washington, D.C., 1987, The Association.

300.21 PANIC DISORDER WITH AGORAPHOBIA

ESSENTIAL FEATURES

The individual has an intense fear of being in public places such as busy streets, stores, elevators, crowds, or bridges from which escape may be difficult or help may not be available. The initial phase of the disorder consists of recurring panic attacks.

MANIFESTATIONS
Physical Dimension

Shortness of breath
Smothering sensation
Increased pulse rate, respiration
Sweating
Choking
Palpitations
Dizziness
Chest pain
Nausea
Tingling sensations

Emotional Dimension

Intense anxiety
Fear of dying
Fear of going crazy

Social Dimension

Fear of being alone
Fear of public places
Constricted life-style
Desire for companion when outside the home
Avoidance of crowds, bridges, public transportation

Adapted from American Psychiatric Association: Diagnostic and statistical manual of mental disorders (DSM-III-R), Washington, D.C., 1987, The Association.

HELPFUL STEPS IN WORKING WITH THE ANXIOUS CLIENT

Steps	Rationale
Observe for behaviors characteristic of anxiety	To identify anxiety
Ask: "What are you feeling?"	To help client name the feeling
Connect the feeling with behavior	To help client understand that when he gets anxious, he behaves in a characteristic way
Explore with client what happened prior to his feeling anxious	To discover the cause
Discuss alternatives for dealing with the situation (cause)	To improve patterns of handling anxiety

309.89 POST-TRAUMATIC STRESS SYNDROME

ESSENTIAL FEATURES

The individual experiences symptoms of distress following a psychologically traumatic event that is generally outside the range of usual human experience. The trauma may be experienced alone (rape or assault) or with groups of people (military combat or natural disasters).

MANIFESTATIONS
Physical Dimension

Exaggerated startle response
Sleep disturbance
Avoidance of activities that arouse recollection of the traumatic event
Sudden acting as if the traumatic event were recurring because of an association with an environmental stimulus
Diminished interest in usual activities

Emotional Dimension

Feeling of detachment or estrangement from others
Constricted affect
Guilt

Intellectual Dimension

Recurrent and intrusive recollections of the event
Recurrent dreams of the event
Numbed responsiveness
Hyperalertness
Memory impairment
Difficulty concentrating
Intensification of symptoms by exposure to events that resemble or symbolize the event

Social Dimension

Reduced involvement with the world
Behaves as though experiencing the event

Adapted from American Psychiatric Association: Diagnostic and statistical manual of mental disorders (DSM-III-R), Washington, D.C., 1987, The Association.

300.60 DEPERSONALIZATION DISORDER

ESSENTIAL FEATURES

The individuals perception of self or experience is altered so that the usual sense of one's own reality is temporarily changed.

MANIFESTATIONS
Emotional Dimension

Experience of being as if detached from and an outside observer of one's mental processes or body
Experience of feeling mechanical or as if in a dream
Marked distress

Adapted from American Psychiatric Association: Diagnostic and Statistical manual of mental disorders (DSM-III-R), Washington, D.C., 1987, The Association.

TABLE 11-7 Long-term and short-term goals and outcome criteria related to anxiety

Goals	Outcome Criteria

NURSING DIAGNOSIS: SEVERE ANXIETY RELATED TO LOSS OF SPOUSE

Long-term goals

Goals	Outcome Criteria
To develop interests outside of self	Seeks new activities and friendships
To develop a sense of autonomy	Exhibits new behavior in group situations; does not isolate himself
To increase reality perception and problem-solving ability	Is able to discuss ways to face problems
	States awareness of difference between present situation and past events
	Talks about what frightens him
	Identifies the concerns that are primarily self-originated and less likely to have drastic outcomes
	Decides which aspects of situations he can overcome
	Talks about pleasant memories of spouse
To identify values	Discusses his life and looks for things of importance and value
To emphasize a positive outlook	Can identify conflict presented by differing environmental, social, and personal expectations
	Deliberately engages in other activities or talks himself out of fears
	Speaks of good and bad aspects of interpersonal and social situations
	Aware of feelings of disappointment on sadness

Short-term goals

Goals	Outcome Criteria
To prevent anxiety from mounting and becoming uncontrollable	Although anxious, exhibits some control and can accept nurse's help
To enhance security and esteem	Identifies important objects and focuses attention on present situation: makes fewer statements of feeling helpless
To accept a warm, caring environment	Demonstrates willingness to accept nurse's help; makes fewer complaints of hopelessness
To develop ability to relax	Engages in activities other than ruminating or worrying
To express somatic concerns	Decreased somatic complaints
To achieve comfort and relief from physical symptoms	Is able to sleep and feels less restless

NURSING DIAGNOSIS: MODERATE ANXIETY RELATED TO PREOCCUPATION WITH IMAGINED ILLNESS

Long-term goals

Goals	Outcome Criteria
To identify emotional conflicts that are avoided	Can state his typical response to conflict and identify how his symptoms are generated
To increase feelings of independence	Engages in arguments or battles for control in an overt way, not through symptoms
To develop mature ways of meeting needs	Seeks appropriate help from family members and can ask for needs to be met
	States awareness of how family members or caretakers respond to his complaints and take care of him

Short-term goals

Goals	Outcome Criteria
To alleviate acute physical symptoms	Uses appropriate aids for relief of symptoms
To express feelings (anger, fear)	Recognizes his anger and fear and expresses them verbally
To identify sources of stress	Avoids known irritants
To increase knowledge of physiology, bodily sensations, and anatomy	Can state correct information about body and seeks clarification
To enhance feelings of acceptance and self-esteem	Relaxes; talks about self in ways other than through symptoms

taining relaxation until the most anxiety-producing situation can be approached and relaxation maintained. The anxiety hierarchy may be approached through imagery or in real-life situations. Another form of desensitization involves the use of a model who the client observes approaching the feared object. The model assists the client's approach and then gradually leaves as the client approaches the feared object on his own. Implosive therapy or flooding avoids the use of relaxation; rather the client is presented with the stimulus at the top of the hierarchy. The client is shown that the resulting anxiety is not unbearable by repeated exposure to the feared object.[35]

If symptoms do not abate through any of these means, antianxiety medication may be used as needed. Medications need to be discussed with the treatment team and is based on the client's level of anxiety. The use of a one-to-one relationship with the caregiver, seclusion, or restraints may be indicated to provide a safer, less stimulating environment.

Emotional dimension. One of the most important contributions the nurse can make is encouraging the open expression of feelings. Clients can be coached to distinguish anxiety from sadness, guilt, or anger; to recognize precipitants to their anxiety; and to identify the sequence of emotions they may experience when exposed to anxiety-producing situations.

Elimination of unnecessary sources of anxiety can occur by including the client in treatment plans and by providing necessary information about matters that affect care. In addition, the nurse can model appropriate behavior, demonstrate decisive behavior without being coercive, and provide encouragement and support by changing the environment for clients with disabling anxieties.

Intellectual dimension. Guidance and education are nursing interventions that help promote adaptive and growth experiences for the anxious individual. The educational approach uses supportive coaching as a means of enhancing the person's coping abilities. *Anticipatory guidance* involves helping individuals to anticipate vivid details of an expected challenge and to consider the accompanying unpleasant emotions and fantasies. Support and guidance regarding the stress are given at the same time. This approach is based on (1) provision of knowledge regarding stressful situations to reduce the part of the threat stemming from uncertainty and (2) provision of coping techniques to enable the person to actively and constructively deal with the stressful situation. Both aspects of this approach help reduce the anxiety of stressful events.

Other coping strategies that have been identified include the *work of worrying* and *positive thinking*. Worrying can help to relieve the painful effects of anxiety, warding off an anticipated trauma or reliving a recent trauma. Positive thinking, as a defense against environmental obstacles and as a pursuit of happiness, can lead to excessive generality and ineffectiveness as a coping tool. However, the encouragement of repetitive "good thoughts" can be a way of inhibiting and thwarting nega-

---

RELAXATION EXERCISE

Before proceeding with this exercise, provide for the following four conditions:
1. A quiet environment
2. A passive attitude
3. A comfortable position
4. A mental device to control distracting thoughts, such as "one" or "breathe in, breathe out"

1. *Hands.* First the fists are tensed and relaxed, then the fingers are extended and relaxed.
2. *Biceps and triceps.* These muscles are tensed and relaxed.
3. *Shoulders.* The shoulders are pulled back and relaxed and then pushed forward and relaxed.
4. *Neck.* The head is turned slowly as far to the right as possible and relaxed, turned to the left and relaxed, and then brought forward until the chin touches the chest and relaxed.
5. *Mouth.* The mouth is opened as wide as possible and relaxed. The lips form a pout and are then relaxed. The tongue is extended as far as possible and relaxed, and is then retracted into the throat and relaxed. It is pressed hard into the roof of the mouth and relaxed and then is pressed hard into the floor of the mouth and relaxed.
6. *Eyes.* The eyes are opened as wide as possible and relaxed and then closed as tightly as possible and relaxed.

7. *Breathing.* The person inhales as deeply as possible and relaxes and then exhales as much as possible and relaxes.
8. *Torso.* The buttock muscles are tensed and relaxed.
9. *Back.* The trunk of the body is pushed forward so that the entire back is arched, and then it is relaxed.
10. *Thighs.* The legs are extended and raised about six inches off the floor and then relaxed, and backs of the feet are pressed into the floor and relaxed.
11. *Stomach.* The stomach is pulled in as much as possible and relaxed and is then extended and relaxed.
12. *Calves and feet.* With legs supported, the feet are bent with the toes pointing toward the head and then relaxed. The feet are then bent in the opposite direction and relaxed.
13. *Toes.* The toes are pressed into the bottom of the shoes and relaxed. They are then bent to touch the top of the shoes and relaxed.

The final part of the exercise involves becoming completely relaxed, beginning with one's toes and following the sensation up through the body to the eyes and forehead. When learning the procedure, the person can eliminate some of the exercises and employ them only on the muscles that usually become tense. The muscle groups involved (shoulders, forehead, back, neck) depend on the individual.

Adapted from Rimm, D., and Masters, J.: Behavior therapy, New York, 1974, Academic Press, Inc.

tive, anxiety-producing thoughts. This technique can be illustrated by statements such as "I can do it," or "I did that well."

A cognitive approach to anxiety reduction essentially involves the following stages: (1) recognizing ideas that are irrational and that lead to anxiety, (2) establishing a relationship between thoughts and the anxiety attack, (3) distancing by viewing one's thoughts objectively and not as identical to reality, (4) testing the validity of one's thoughts in actual situations, (5) identifying the assumptions that lie behind the thoughts, and (6) reviewing the belief system underlying the ideas and changing the rules that have evolved from the irrational, incorrect beliefs.[5]

Another cognitive approach that is helpful in dealing with anxiety related to situational crises is the use of the problem-solving method. The aim of this approach is to help clients recognize that problematic situations are a normal part of life, and that a person can attempt to cope with the situation.

In defining the problem the nurse attempts to help the client identify the various issues involved in the situation. This aids in determining a focus and direction for the problem solving. In generating alternatives, clients need to be encouraged to defer immediate judgment and to identify as many options as possible. The nurse can help the client identify which course of action will be more likely to resolve the problem. This review can lead to further problem solving or to resolution of the disturbing situation.

Stress inoculation procedures have been developed to help the client control physiological responses and to substitute positive coping statements that bring about anxiety. Education and rehearsal are used as part of the technique. During the education phase the client is alerted to body reactions, thoughts, and images associated with emotional arousal. The client is encouraged to view the reaction in phases; these include preparing for a disturbing event, confronting or handling the situation, possibly being overwhelmed, and, finally, reinforcing oneself after dealing with the situation.

During rehearsal the client is provided with a variety of coping strategies that can be employed in each of the

---

Research Highlight

Therapeutic Touch As Energy Exchange: Testing the Theory

Janet F. Quinn

PURPOSE

This study was designed to provide a beginning inquiry into the effects of therapeutic touch. This initial research was viewed as an important step in explaining, describing, and predicting the energy exchange phenomenon of therapeutic touch. Specifically, the study was designed to investigate whether noncontact therapeutic touch would have the same effect on anxiety as therapeutic touch with physical contact.

SAMPLE

The sample group for the study consisted of 37 men and 23 women who were hospitalized in the cardiovascular unit of a medical center. The ages of the subjects ranged from 36 to 81 years, with a mean age of 59.4 years and a standard deviation of 9.8. Only subjects who could complete the English Version of the Self-Evaluation Questionnaire developed by Spielberger to test state/trait anxiety were included in the study.

METHODOLOGY

Subjects were randomly assigned to experimental and control groups. In the experimental group (noncontact therapeutic touch), four nurses administered therapeutic touch as taught by Kreiger, but hands were not placed on the subjects. The intervention involved the nurse being centered; making the intention to help the subject, moving the hands over the subject's body, redirecting areas of tension in the subject's body through hand movements, concentrating attention on the direction of excess energy, and directing energy to the subject through the hands placed 4 to 6 inches from the subject's solar plexus area.

In the control group (noncontact) the nurse mimicked the movements of the nurse in the experimental group, but there was no attempt to center, or intention to assist the subject, no attuning to the subject's condition, nor direction of energy to the subject.

The State Trait Anxiety Inventory was administered to subjects in both groups.

FINDINGS

A greater decrease in posttest anxiety scores was found in subjects treated with noncontact therapeutic touch than in those treated with therapeutic touch with physical contact. This difference was found to be significant to the .005 level.

IMPLICATIONS

The effectiveness of therapeutic touch as an intervention to aid in the reduction of state anxiety in hospitalized cardiovascular patients is becoming evident. Healing energy is the exchange that takes place between the nurse and the subjects, but it cannot be tested directly or even observed. However, presently "50% to 80% of all human illness is attributed to psychophysiological stress-related origins." A noninvasive, natural intervention, such as therapeutic touch, that can decrease anxiety appears to have important implications for holistic–comprehensive nursing care.

Based on data from Advances in Nursing Science 6(2):42, 1984.

preceding phases. These include relaxation, designing escape routes, and collecting more information about the feared objects and situations. Statements are generated to help the client relabel the experience, motivate himself for successful coping, and reinforce himself after coping successfully with the situation. Imagery procedures can be used to help the client develop a model of behavior, rehearse responses to self-doubt, and serve as a cue to initiate coping statements.

Social dimension. The nurse becomes important in the world of the client and can serve as a role model to demonstrate effective coping skills. By providing information and calm reassurance, the nurse can help the client reengage in social situations and also learn to tolerate his fears in the unfamiliar setting of the clinic or hospital. Through involvement with the nurse the client's attention can be redirected from excessive rumination to engagement in grooming, games, reading, or social activities. Clients often need guidance in focusing attention on new ways of responding to events and people, and in identifying satisfying activities and avoiding stressful ones. As noted by Quinn (see the Research Highlight on p. 222) the nurse has an additional intervention that is effective for anxiety that is based on the relationship and energy exchange between the nurse and the client.

The key aspect of the self-management approach is the development of a sense of responsibility in the client for his behavior, for changing the bothersome or worrisome aspects of his environment and for planning for his future. This participant model relies on the client's motivation to accept a program for change and involves his active cooperation in defining treatment objectives. Emphasizing self-help skills places the burden of engaging in the process of change on the client; the nurse provides only as much assistance as needed to enable the client to gain control over his life. Within this model the role of the nurse becomes that of an instigator or motivator to help the client start a program for change. The nurse also participates as a consultant and expert adviser who negotiates ways of changing and defines the goals of treatment with the client. Through modeling, work assignments, and helping the client to analyze problems and determine their solution, the nurse actively engages the client in a learning process that is future oriented and focused on the development of behavioral repertoires for dealing with anxiety. Attention is also given to the transfer of new behaviors to the environments of home, work, and social situations so that the learning has immediate applicability and the results of intervention can extend beyond the immediate treatment situation with the nurse.

Several steps are involved in establishing a self-regulation process: (1) standard setting or identification of performance criteria, (2) a self-monitoring or self-observation phase, in which clients are encouraged to attend carefully to their behavior, (3) self-evaluation, in which the information obtained from self-observation is compared to the identified standards, and (4) self-reinforcement.

Spiritual dimension. One of the main interventions that the nurse can make with the anxious client is to instill hopefulness and a sense that the anxiety can be mastered. The nurse can help accomplish this by permitting expression of negative feelings and by helping the client plan future outcomes and alternatives. One way for a person to find relief from anxiety is to transcend everyday life and find importance in objects or events outside himself, for example, doing something for others such as volunteer work or becoming politically active. This ability to transcend the mundane aspects of life provides the client with the opportunity to entertain new life choices and to create new possibilities.

The nurse can help the client find meaning in his life and his problems; the client can thus be helped to acknowledge things of importance and to commit himself to chosen values. Facilitating the resolution of conflict in values may help reduce anxiety as well as help the client meet ethical and moral obligations. Open, frank discussion of religious and spiritual needs and attitudes can facilitate the client's use of spiritual beliefs as a means of coping with anxiety.

Preparation for anticipated, dreaded events, such as loss of love relationships and death, can provide a source of strength and protection against anxiety in the face of the unknown.

INTERACTION WITH AN ANXIOUS CLIENT

Client: *I'm choking. I can't breathe. I think I'm having a heart attack.*

Nurse: *Relax. Take some deep breaths. Breathe in. Breathe out. Slowly. Breathe in. Breathe out.*

Nurse: *(Ater a brief period of time.) What is happening now?*

Client: *I'm okay. I guess I'm not having a heart attack. But I keep getting this picture of myself having a heart attack.*

Nurse: *What happens after you have the heart attack?*

Client: *I see myself helpless and dying. That's all I can see. I feel it is a premonition or ESP. Something like that.*

Nurse: *You have these pictures and nothing happens?*

Client: *Yes, I have them all the time and nothing happens.*

Nurse: *This is not unusual, Yet the imagined event rarely takes place. You might keep a record of your images of having a heart attack and see what happens.*

Client: *But what if it does happen?*

Nurse: *The fantasy is usually worse than the reality. You may want to work at not treating the fantasy as an actual event.*

The nurse initially intervenes to relieve the client's acute anxiety by helping him to relax with deep breathing exercises. Once the acute phase has subsided she asks the client to describe his feelings. This helps the client to identify his relaxed state, acknowledge that he is alive and well, and indicates his readiness to go on and discuss the incident further. The nurse pushes the client to describe the most extreme aspect of his feared image, that he is dying. She then guides him through a discussion that helps him see that the outcome of each incident is less catastrophic than he imagined.

The nurse understands that the anxious person's image

usually stops at the point when the feared image occurs. He tends to exaggerate the event and believes it is real, that he will die. The nurse does not attempt to dissuade the client from his prediction that he will die. She conveys a belief that the discomfort, however intense, does not last long, is tolerable, and that he has some choice regarding the outcome of the situation.

Evaluation

Several criteria can be applied to evaluate the process as well as the specific interventions employed. Following are some of these criteria:

1. *Adequacy.* Did the interventions mainly provide relief of symptoms or did they also include self-learning and management of anxiety?
2. *Appropriateness.* If the client was in severe anxiety, was intervention started immediately, with formal data gathering suspended until the client could participate? Did the client agree on the goals? Were the interventions relevant for the identified level of anxiety and problems arising in the five dimensions?
3. *Effectiveness.* This criterion addresses questions related to the degree to which anxiety is assuaged, behaviors altered symptoms relieved, and self-learning accomplished. Were the goals and interventions specifically related to anxiety?
4. *Efficiency.* Were interventions enough to assuage anxiety? Were sources of help and support coordinated to increase the impact on the client's problem with anxiety?

The client needs to be included in evaluation throughout the assessment and treatment phases because this aids in the teaching-learning and process for the anxious client and provides important information for the nurse's growth in her caregiving activities.

NURSING PROCESS SUMMARY: ANXIETY

ASSESSMENT

Physical Dimension
- Shallow breathing
- Breath holding
- Sighing
- Jitteriness
- Restlessness
- Pacing
- Trembling
- Tense, rigid muscles
- Flush face
- Palpitations
- Increased heart rate
- Increased blood pressure
- Gooseflesh
- Sweating
- Disturbed vision
- Upset stomach
- Gas
- Nausea
- Vomiting
- Diarrhea
- Dilated pupils
- Decreased coordination
- Insomnia
- Dizziness
- Unsteady voice
- Urge to urinate

Decreased sex drive
Amenorrhea
Chain smoking
Overeating
Alcohol or drug abuse
Psychophysiological
  illnesses:
  Ulcer
  Colitis
  Asthma
  Hypertension
  Headaches
  Eczema
  Rheumatoid arthritis
  Sexual dysfunction
  Diabetes

Emotional Dimension
- Irritability
- Pressured feeling
- Fear
- Agitation
- Frenzy
- Guilt
- Suspiciousness
- Desperation
- Uncertainty
- Distress
- Misery

Intellectual Dimension
- Confusion
- Talkativeness
- Rumination
- Rationalization
- Making excuses
- Selective focusing
- Lashing out
- Delusions
- Increased awareness
- Alertness
- Obsessive behavior
- Use of defense mechanisms
- Blocking
- Stammering
- Preoccupation
- Difficulty concentrating
- Indecision
- Inability to learn
- Blaming of self

Social Dimension
- Poor self-concept
- Decreased productivity
- Isolation
- Limited support systems
- Attention-seeking behavior
- Demanding behavior
- Withdrawal
- Aggressiveness

Spiritual Dimension
- Fear of damnation
- Doomed feeling
- Powerlessness
- Fear of death
- Fear of insanity

NURSING PROCESS SUMMARY: ANXIETY—cont'd

ANALYSIS

See "Nursing Diagnosis," p. 217.

PLANNING AND IMPLEMENTATION

Physical Dimension

Give information on the physiological responses that accompany anxiety.

Provide self-help measures: warm bath, walk, glass of wine, exercise.

Teach meditation

Teach relaxation

Provide biofeedback

Provide antianxiety medications

Use restraints or seclusion if necessary

Emotional Dimension

Encourage expression of anxious feelings.

Use client's words for expression of feelings; for example, "scared," "jittery," "nervous"

Allow client to set the pace for interaction

Use a nonjudgmental attitude.

Allow client to cry, express anger.

Intellectual Dimension

Use supportive coaching.

Use anticipatory guidance

Promote positive thinking

Encourage the "work of worrying"

Teach problem solving

Use stress inoculation

Help client become aware of anxiety and give feedback based on observations

Suggest new ways of handling anxiety

Redirect attention from ruminations to tasks and activities

Social Dimension

Promote interaction with others

Reduce secondary gain received from symptoms

Provide behavior modification

Use desenitization

Promote self-management approaches useful in school, work, and home situations.

Spiritual Dimension

Instill hopefulness that anxiety can be mastered

Help client find importance in events outside of self

Help client entertain new life choices

Use value clarification to resolve conflicts and reduce anxiety

Prepare client for death, dreaded events, or loss of love relationships

EVALUATION

Progress is seen when the client can identify his feelings of anxiety and some of the causes becomes aware of his responses to anxiety-producing events or situations, and uses adaptive coping methods to handle the anxiety. Using relaxation techniques and seeking help when anxiety increases also indicate progress or the lack of it. Involving the client in the evaluation aids the client's learning process; anxiety is lessened when the client has increased feelings of control, self-esteem, and confidence.

BRIEF REVIEW

Anxiety is a common experience among the general population, with physical manifestations being easily identified by the individual and others observing the anxious person. Nurses have studied the concept as an aspect of normal development and life crises and as a reaction to procedures, and treatments of caregiving.

Biological, psychoanalytical, interpersonal, learning theorists', and existential frameworks provide definitions of anxiety and identify the source, dynamics, and observational cues of anxiety and the role of the nurse. These frameworks provide a means for specifying clinical activities.

Self-reports, nursing observation, and standardized tests aid in identifying anxiety leading to a nursing diagnosis and subsequent care plan. In her assessment it is important for the nurse to identify the level of anxiety that the individual is experiencing. These levels range from mild anxiety to panic.

Anxiety is distinguished from fear because the source of anxiety is nonspecific whereas fear has an identifiable source.

Anxiety affects the intellectual capabilities of the individual by distorting perception, concentration, recall, and reasoning. Helplessness may result from these intellectual changes. The individual develops ego defense mechanisms to protect himself from the experience of anxiety.

Anxiety arising in social situations appears to be related to a loss of self-esteem and affection and fear of rejection. Families develop characteristic means of dealing with anxiety individually and in groups. Certain sociocultural variables appear to be related to the development and level of experienced anxiety.

Anxiety appears to be related to maturation of conflict in values, a lack or loss of love relationships, commitments, and self-definition and autonomy.

Measurement tools are primarily based on the use of self-reports and ask the client to rate his present and usual feeling states and to identify the descriptive aspects of being anxious. Measures have been developed to identify fears associated with death, physical pain, surgery, aggression, and interpersonal events.

Analysis involves coordinating observational, self-reported, and standardized measures with the duration of the anxiety response and the effect on the life adjustment of the client. The DSM-III-R categories provide a means of classifying the anxiety-related illnesses. Nursing analysis takes into consideration the level of anxiety and assessment data from the five dimensions of the person. During the planning stage the short-term and long-term goals are established according to the specific nursing diagnoses.

Implementation of goals is effected by application of specific interventions, with consideration for the client's readiness to learn. Suggestions for intervention in each of the five dimensions are discussed.

REFERENCES AND SUGGESTED READINGS

1. Adams, Margaret F.: Post traumatic stress disorder, American Journal of Nursing. **82:**1704, 1982.
2. Adler, A.: The practice and theory of individual psychology, Totowan, N.J., 1959, Littlefield, Adams & Co. (Translated by P. Radin.)
2a. Akutagawa, D.: A study in constant validity of the psychoanalytic concept of latent anxiety and a test of projection distance hypothesis, doctoral dissertation, Pittsburgh, 1956, University of Pittsburgh.
3. Allekian C.I.: Intrusions of territory and personal space: an anxiety-inducing factor for hospitalized persons—an exploratory study, Research **22:**236, 1973.
4. Beck, A.: Cognitive therapy and the emotional disorders, New York, 1976, International Universities Press, Inc.
5. Beck, A., and Emory, G.: Anxiety disorders and phobias, New York, 1985, Basic Books, Inc., Publishers.
6. Breeden, S.A., and Kondo, C.: Using biofeedback to reduce tension, American Journal of Nursing **75:**2010, 1975.
7. Campbell, C.: Nursing diagnosis and intervention in nursing practice, New York, 1978, John Wiley & Sons, Inc.
8. Caplan, G.: Opportunities for school psychologists in the primary prevention of mental disorders in children. In Lambert, N., editor: The protection and promotion of mental health in schools, Mental Health Monograph No. 5, Washington, D.C., 1965, U.S. Government Printing Office.
9. Dollard, J., and Miller, N.E.: Personality and psychotherapy: an analysis in terms of learning, thinking and culture, New York, 1950, McGraw-Hill Book Co.
10. Eaton, W.N., and others: Consumption of coffee or tea and symptoms of anxiety, American Journal of Public Health **74:**66, 1984.
10a. Endler, N., Hunt, J., and Rosenstein, A.: An S-R inventory of anxiousness, Psychological Monographs, **76:**536, 1962.
10b. Endler, N. and Okada, M.: A multidimensional measure of trait anxiety: the S-R inventory of general trait anxiousness, Journal of consulting and Clinical Psychology, **43:**319, 1975.
11. Erikson, C.W.: Cognitive responses to internally cues anxiety. In Spielberger, C.D., editor: Anxiety and behavior, New York, 1966, Academic Press, Inc.
12. Erikson, E.: Identity and the life cycle, New York, 1959, International Universities Press, Inc.
13. Freud, S.: Inhibitions, symptoms and anxiety. In Standard edition of the complete psychological works of Sigmund Freud, vol. 20, London, 1959, The Hogarth Press, Ltd. (Translated by J. Strachey.)
14. Friedman, S.B., and others: Behavioral observations on parents anticipating the death of a child, Pediatrics **32:**610, 1963.
15. Furey, Joan A.: Post traumatic stress disorders in Vietnam veterans, American Journal of Nursing **82:**1694, 1982.
16. Gomez, E.A., and others: Anxiety as a human emotion: some basic conceptual models, Nursing Forum **21:**38, 1984.
17. Horney, K.: Our inner conflicts, a constructive theory of neurosis, New York, 1945, W.W. Norton & Co. Inc.
18. Hull, C.L.: A behavior system, New Haven, Conn., 1952, Yale University Press.
19. Huppenbauer, Sandra L.: PTSD: A portrait of the problem, American Journal of nursing **82:**1169, 1982.
20. Kanfer, F.H.: Self-management methods. In Kanfer, F.H., and Goldstein, A.P., editors: helping people change, New York, 1980, Pergamon Press, Inc.
21. Kanfer, F.H.: and Goldstein, A.P.: Helping people change, ed. 2, New York, 1981, Pergamon Press, Inc.
22. Kata, K.: On anxiety in the Scandinavian countries. In Sarason, I.G., and Spielberger, C.D., editors: Stress and anxiety, vol. 2, New York, 1975, Halstead Press.
23. Kelly, D.: Anxiety and emotions, Springfield, Ill., 1980, Charles C Thomas, Publisher.
24. Kelly, W.: Post-traumatic stress disorder and the war victim, New York, 1985, Brunner/Mazel, Inc.
25. Kierkegaard, S.: The concept of dread, Princeton, N.J., 1944, Princton University Press. (Translated by W. Lowrie.)
26. Kim, S.: Preparatory information, anxiety and pain, doctoral dissertation, Boston, 1978, Boston University.
27. King, I.: Toward a theory for nursing, New York, 1971, John Wiley & Sons, Inc.
28. Kyes, J.J., and Hofling, C.K.: Psychosomatic medicine and nursing: psychophysiologic disorders. In Kyes, J.J., and Hofling, C.K., editors: Basic psychiatric concepts in nursing, ed. 4, Philadelphia, 1980, J.B. Lippincott Co.
29. Lesse, S.: Anxiety: its components, development, and treatment, New York, 1970, Grune & Stratton, Inc.
30. Levinson, H., and Carter, S.: Phobia free, New York, 1986, M. Evans and Co., Inc.
31. Mandler, G.: Helplessness: theory and research in anxiety. In Spielberger, C.D., editor: Anxiety: current trends in theory and research, vol. 1, New York, 1972, Academic Press, Inc.
32. Marinelli, R.P.: Anxiety. In Woody, R.H., editor: Encyclopedia of clinical assessment, vol. 1, San Francisco, 1980, Jossey-Bass, Inc., Publishers.
33. May, R.: The meaning of anxiety, rev. ed., New York, 1977, W.W. Norton and Co., Inc.
34. May, R.: Value conflicts and anxiety. In Kutash, I.L., and others, editors: Handbook on stress and anxiety, San Francisco, Jossey-Bass, Inc., Publishers.
34a. McNally, R.: Preparedness and phobias: a review, Psychological Bulletin **101(**2):283, 1987.
35. Mikulas, W.: Behavior modification: an overview, New York, 1972, Harper & Row Publishers.
36. Morgan, J.A., and Morgan, M.D.: Manual of primary mental health care, Philadelphia, 1980, J.B. Lippincott Co.
37. Mowrer, O.H.: Pain, punishment, guilt, and anxiety. In Hock, P., and Zubin, J., editors: Anxiety, New York, 1950, Grune & Stratton, Inc.
38. Mowrer, O.H.: the basis of psychopathology: malconditioning or misbehavior? In Spielberger, C.D., editor: Anxiety and behavior, New York, 1966, Academic Press, Inc.
39. Nemiah, J.: Anxiety states. In Kaplan H., and Sadock, B., editors: Comprehensive textbook of psychiatry, ed. 4, Baltimore, 1985, Williams and Wilkins.
40. Norman, Elizabeth M.: Post traumatic stress disorder, American Journal of Nursing **82:**1696, 1982.
41. Pasnau, R.: Diagnosis and treatment of anxiety disorders, Washington D.C., 1984, American Psychiatric Press, Inc.
42. Peplau, H.: Interpersonal relations in nursing, New York, 1972, G.P. Putnam's sons.
43. Phillips, B.N., Martin, R.P., and Meyers, J.: Interventions in relation to anxiety in school. In Spielberger, C.D., editor: Anxiety: current trends in theory and research, vol. 2, New York, 1972, Academic Press, Inc.

44. Pilette, Wilfrid L.: Caffeine, Journal of Psychosocial Nursing **21:**19, 1983.

45. Quinn, J.F.: Therapeutic touch as energy exchange: testing the theory, Advances in Nursing Science **6:**42, 1984.

46. Rank, O.: Will therapy, New York, 1936, Alfred A. Knopf, Inc.

47. Runck, B.: Biofeedback—issues in treatment assessment, NIMH Science Monograph, U.S. Department of Health and Human Services, Washington, D.C., 1980, U.S. Government Printing Office.

48. Saarni, C., and Azara, V.: Anxiety (developmental). In Woody, R.H., editor: Encyclopedia of clinical assessment, vol. 2, San Francisco, 1980, Jossey-Bass, Inc., Publishers.

49. Scott, D.W.: Anxiety, critical thinking and breast biopsy during and after breast biopsy, Nursing Research **32:**24, 1983.

50. Sczekalla, R.: Stress reactions of CCU patients to resuscitation procedures on other patients, Nursing Research **22:**65, 1973.

51. Shimko, Carole: The effect of preoperative instruction on state anxiety, Journal Neurosurgical Nursing **13:**318, 1981.

52. Slater, E., and Shields, J.: Genetical aspects of anxiety. In Lader, M., editors: Studies of anxiety, Ashford, Kent, England, 1969, Headless Brothers.

53. Sobel, E.F.: Anxiety and stress in later life. In Kutash, I.L., and others, editors: Handbook on stress and anxiety, San Francisco, 1980, Jossey-Bass, Inc. Publishers.

54. Solomon-Hast, Anne: Anxiety in the coronary care unit, Critical Care Quarterly **4:**15, 1981.

54a. Speilburger, C., Gorsuch, R., and Lushene, R.: State trait anxiety inventory: a test/manual test form, Palo Alto, Calif, 1970, Consulting Psychologists Press.

55. Sullivan, H.S.: The interpersonal theory of psychiatry, New York, 1950, W.W. Norton & Co., Inc.

55a. Taylor, J.: A personality scale of manifest anxiety, Journal of Abnormal and Social Psychology **48:**235, 1953.

56. Volicer, B.: Patients' perception of stressful events associated with hospitalization, Nursing Research **23:**235, 1974.

57. Volicer, B., and Burns, M.: Preexisting correlates of hospital stress, Nursing Research **26:**408, 1977.

58. Walk, R.: Self-rating of fear in a fear-invoking situation, Journal of Abnormal and Social Psychology **52:**171, 1956.

59. Wilson-Barnett, J.: Patients' emotional reactions to hospitalization: an exploratory study, Journal of Advanced Nursing **1:**351, 1976.

60. Wolfer J., and Visinitainer, M.: Pediatric surgical patients and parents stress responses and adjustment, Nursing Research **24:**244, 1975.

61. Zuckerman, M.: The development of an affect adjective checklist for the measurement of anxiety, Journal of Consulting Psychology **24:**456, 1960.

ANNOTATED BIBLIOGRAPHY

Handly, R., and Nett, P.: Anxiety and panic attacks: their cause and cure, New York, 1985, Rawson Associates.

   The author discusses basic principles for handling anxiety with case examples. He outlines a five-point program for conquering fear. Recognition is given to physical, mental, and spiritual goals.

Peplau, H.: A working definition of anxiety. In Burd, S., and Marshall, M., editors: Some clinical approaches to psychiatric nursing, New York, 1963, The Macmillan Co., Publishers.

   The author defines anxiety and discusses how anxiety is experienced as well as the causes of anxiety. She describes the effects of anxiety on behavior.

Vose, R.: Agoraphobia, Boston, 1981, Faber & Faber.

   This book discusses the onset, characteristics, treatment and conventional, alternative, and new approaches to the treatment of agoraphobia. Phobia clinics in the United States are also listed.

Wolpe, J., and Wolpe, D.: Our useless fears, Boston, 1981, Houghton Mifflin Co.

   The author, a well-known authority on anxiety, describes techniques for eliminating useless fears in this book targeted for the general population. He discusses how people develop fears and ways behavioral therapy helps in common life situations.

CHAPTER 12

ANGER

Ruth P. Rawlins   Sharon L. Thomas

After studying this chapter the learner will be able to:

Define anger.

Trace the historical perspectives of anger.

Describe theories of anger.

Use the nursing process in caring for angry clients.

Identify current research findings related to anger.

---

nger, a strong feeling of annoyance or displeasure, is part of each person's everyday life. Words such as *indignation, wrath, ire, frustration, hostility, resentment, aggression, fury,* and *rage* all describe feelings of anger. Viewing *anger* on a continuum with mild irritation at one end and rage at the other assists the nurse in determining the point at which the person feeling anger moves from health to illness or from constructive to destructive behavior.

When angry, people momentarily lose their intellectual clarity and feel consumed by the emotion. Not only does anger prohibit sensitivity to the environment, but it also pushes people away from each other and can leave one feeling vulnerable and alone. However transitory the experience, anger can be frightening.

Anger is a warning. The anger needs attention. For many reasons people have learned to reject, mistrust, and deny this warning device. They look on it at best as a suspect part of themselves and at worst as a sinful, destructive element. People learn to couch their anger in euphemisms: "out of sorts," "put out," "frustrated," "insulted," and countless other socially acceptable ways that attempt to describe the inner experience. Many learn to label the inner experience of anger as something completely different, such as anxiety or dread, because the label anger is so objectionable.

Viewing anger as a natural and valuable aspect of each person is a relatively new concept. To see anger in this light, anger needs to be separated from its violent counterpart, rage. Rage results when the natural pathway to a spontaneous expression of anger has been cut off. Rage is a physical experience and requires a physical release like pounding, hitting, banging, running, or pushing. It is intent on destruction and interested only in its own reduction. Anger can be expressed verbally, and its *catharsis* propels the individual toward a creative solution. Anger provides the cement for relationships, whereas rage destroys them.

All persons become angry; the nurse needs to understand the dynamics of this emotion and how to deal with it in herself and her clients.

THEORETICAL APPROACHES
Biological

Recent studies of the anatomy of the brain identify the limbic system as the regulator of aggression. Any lesion of the hypothalamus and amygdala may increase or decrease aggressive behavior. Advances in neurophysiology and neuroanatomy are identifying specific areas of the brain that may be responsible for particular emotional responses. Areas have been identified that, when stimulated, cause aggressive outbursts. Areas have also been identified that inhibit these emotional responses.

Biochemical studies suggest that the release of norepinephrine by the adrenal medulla is directly related to aggressive behavior. Modification of the aggressive behavior can be achieved by adjusting the rate of metabolism of the biogenic amines norepinephrine, dopamine, and serotonin. Other chemical and endocrine disorders such as hypoglycemia and allergies may lead to aggression. Studies of in-

Historical Overview

DATE	EVENT
Early 1900s	Institutions (prisons and mental health facilities) were created that removed people from the mainstream of life because of their violent and aggressive behavior.
1950s	The introduction of psychotropic medications reduced angry behavior in clients in inpatient settings; thus they were able to more easily learn new coping methods.
1960s	The civil rights movement erupted out of anger about segregation of blacks in schools, jobs, housing, and public facilities.
1980s	Violence is pervasive today. Increasing numbers of children and elderly are being abused, and wives battered. Murders, rapes, and suicides are increasing in number. Nuclear weapons are readily available to several nations.
	Nursing offers many opportunities for helping clients channel their anger into constructive activities. Today community mental health programs offer workshops and seminars that focus on the management of stress and prevention of violence.
Future	Because of the increase in violent acts, nursing will need to become more politically involved with prevention of violence in individuals, families, communities, and nations. In addition, more concern for the victims of assault and violence will provide new challenges for nursing.

creased blood levels of male sex hormones, particularly testosterone, correlate with increased aggressiveness. In women, premenstrual decrease in the blood levels of progesterone result in irritability and increased hostility.[30a]

Lorenz,[33] a physician and naturalist, perceived aggression as an inborn response pattern originating from a type of instinctual force similar to that of animals. He suggests that the energy of aggression develops internally without an external influence. The mechanism is contained within one's genes; when an appropriate stimulus occurs, the individual's instinctual response is to fight. He sees individuals as suffering from inability to discharge aggressive drives. This inability to release aggression may result in such self-destructive behavior as accidents and suicide.

Psychoanalytic

Freud[20] described aggression as evolving from thanatos, the death wish. According to Freud, individuals are born with a given amount of death drive (aggression) that seeks expression. Because of the strength of the death drive, individuals are prone to behave destructively. When the death drive predominates destructive behavior such as suicide occurs.

Aggression is hostile, destructive behavior. The energy of aggression is diminished through direct expression (catharsis). When direct expression is blocked, indirect expression may result and the person directs the anger toward himself. Depression, for example, is anger directed against oneself. Some diseases are indications of internal-

ized anger. These include rheumatoid arthritis, asthma, ulcers, migraine headache, hypertension, angina, and chronic backache. Disowning or behaving the opposite of what is expected is another form of inwardly expressed anger. Being overly polite, sugary, exceptionally kind or "killing with kindness" are examples of disowning. Withdrawal may be an avenue to escape from one's anger. Substance abuse in the form of drugs or alcohol provide an escape from reality. Running away, overeating, and inappropriate silence are also forms of escaping reality and withdrawing from anger.

Anger also may be displaced onto an object resembling the original object of anger. Safe objects that lack authority or power to retaliate are generally selected. For example, the worker who cannot express his feelings to his boss will vent his anger on his wife. She, being unable to talk to her husband, may yell at her child, and the child, in frustration, may kick the door. Passive aggression, is another indirect expression of anger. The individual is inhibited from expressing his actual feeling.

Case Example

Pat is angry with her husband for his preoccupation with activities outside the home. Instead of directly confronting him, she responds with sugary sweetness and indicates she "doesn't mind" his involvement elsewhere. However, she expresses her resentment by such actions as taking the car when she knows he needs it and leaving him with the children when he is busy at home. These subtle acts are substitutes for the direct expression of anger.

Interpersonal

Sullivan[52] believed that people use anger to avoid experiencing anxiety. An angry response pushes the threat away; that is, anger is used in an attempt to destroy the object or situation that produced the anxiety. Any threat to self-esteem or security results in frustration, and one feels inadequate and anxious. Anger is the emotion that wards off anxiety. A person experiences a situation in which his expectations of himself or others are not met. The resulting anger gives him a feeling of power that compensates for the underlying anxiety (Figure 12-1).

The following Case Example demonstrates frustration and anger.

Case Example

Four-year-old David sits helplessly clutching the tiny bridle of his new toy stallion, Silver. He has managed to put on the saddle

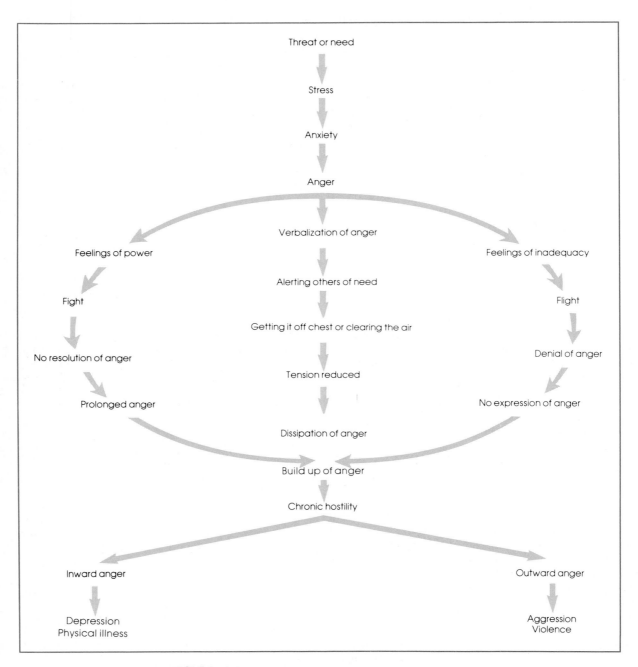

FIGURE 12-1 The development and expression of anger.

but has trouble buckling the strap. He screams, "Silver, stand still, you dumb horse!" and, even louder, "Silver!" Mother, trying to rest in the next room, screams, "David, that's no reason to get mad! Now, if you can't buckle the bridle, bring it here!" David promptly bursts into tears and throws Silver against the wall. Mother puts a pillow over her head and prays for him to grow up; then she screams, "Your temper really bugs me!" Her response only escalates David's rage, and he starts kicking and pounding the floor.

Sullivan[52] states that when the expression of anger is not allowed, there are three probable outcomes: conforming, rebelling, or malevolent behaviors. For example, David may conform to his mother's expectations. (After his mother screams, he may pick up his horse, smile sweetly, hand her the horse, and ask her if she is tired.) The behavior does not represent his real self, but it alleviates the interpersonal threat with his mother. David then learns to deny his anger and develops a behavioral pattern based on pretense. David may, however, choose to become enraged and rebel. He may throw the horse and scream at his mother. The pattern can persist into adulthood. David will then deal with his anxiety by becoming enraged. The third alternative is to neither rebel nor conform but to develop a malevolent or evil disposition. In response to his mother's scream, David may stare coldly at her, pick up his horse and go outside to play with 3-year-old Michelle in her sandbox. David may then sneak up behind Michelle, hit her on the head with the horse, grab her shovel and bucket, and run away laughing.

Behavioral

Dollard and Miller,[13] in their development of the frustration-aggression theory, suggest that all aggression results from an experience of frustration. Frustration occurs when the individual is blocked from attaining a desired goal. This leads to anger, which produces an aggressive drive leading to aggressive behavior. Today's world of change and stress is charged with frustrating events and situations, inevitably leading to a buildup of the aggressive drive. The aggressive drive is reduced by an act of belligerence. When the goal is highly valued, the sense of frustration and the ensuing aggression increases.

The social learning theorists believe that the impulse to behave aggressively is subject to the influence of learning, socialization, and experience. According to Bandura,[2] aggression is learned behavior under voluntary control. The learning of aggressive behavior occurs by observation. For example, a child watches an angry parent strike out at another person. Learning aggressive behavior also takes place by direct experience. The person feels anger and behaves aggressively. If behaving aggressively brings rewards, the behavior is strengthened.

Modeling also demonstrates aggression and can be purposeful or unintentional. Purposeful modeling of aggression occurs when the nurse indicates her angry feelings by such statements as, "I get upset when you let others continue to tell you what to do about your problems." Aggression is unintentionally demonstrated when a physi-

cian yells at a nurse in the presence of interns and clients or when a parent spanks a child while angry.

Moreno[37] believed that anger is a natural by-product of the learning process; it is the signal that a person needs to learn something. The more inadequate a person feels, the more anger may be present.

He also believes that anger is spontaneous energy that propels an individual into new learning. Those who have learned a wide variety of adequate responses to anger value their anger, express it, and see it as an emotion that promotes greater feelings of adequacy. The expression of anger frees one to reach out, to love, and to remain connected to vital people.

A basic premise of Moreno states that the emotion of anger requires a *warm-up*, a creative experience (*catharsis*), and an *integration*.

The warm-up involves a person's preparation to respond to a situation that is likely to cause anger. The process occurs swiftly and often unknowingly. Frequently attention is paid to the end product of the process and not to how it developed. Catharsis is the spontaneous expression of thoughts and feelings. Integration is the phase in which the individual can begin to understand the ingredients of the process that stimulated the anger. The release of anger allows new thoughts, feelings, and behaviors to emerge. The self feels a restoration with itself and with the other person (Figure 12-2).

The following Case Example illustrates some of these concepts.

Case Example

Nineteen-year-old Sally rushes home because she expects a call from her new boyfriend, John, at 5 PM. He is free from 5 to 5:15 and is calling to let her know if he can go out that night. Once inside the front door, she hears her 16-year-old brother David talking to his girlfriend, Jane, and she glances at the kitchen clock; it is 4:55. She whispers to her brother that John is calling at 5 o'clock, and he annoyingly nods back. With tears in his eyes, he angrily retorts into the phone. Sally realizes that David is having a fight with Jane. Sally knows that Jane is on the verge of breaking up with David and that he has been extremely

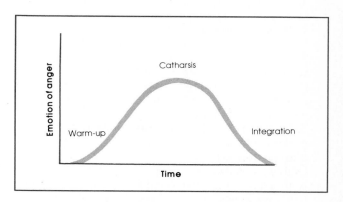

FIGURE 12-2 Components of anger.

upset about it. Sally glances a the clock again; it is 4:58. She is worried that this fight could go on for another half an hour.

Sally feels a stirring inside her stomach, the flushing of her face, and the sweating of her underarms and palms. She feels fidgety and says to herself, "Oh, damn, I've got to know if we're going out tonight! But David looks terrible. He simply has got to talk this through; he's been waiting to talk with Jane about this for 3 days." Sally paces around the living room, frequently glancing at the clock; it is 5:06. She remembers other times when David has been furious, and she is a little afraid to invite him to unload all this on her. She gets David's attention and points to the clock; he is unimpressed with her dilemma. The excited feeling she had when she came home has completely vanished, and a burning pressure is building inside her. The thought comes that John will think she is talking to someone else! Finally, her own concerns and needs overshadow her concern for her brother and she screams, "I want to talk to John, David—get off the phone!" David hollers, "I had the phone first, get lost. Who do you think you are, coming in like this?"

David swears, tells Jane he will call her back in 10 minutes, and turns to Sally and says, "Get off my back! I hate it when you pull stuff like this!" He hands her the phone and storms out of the room. Sally feels immediate relief, and, after she talks with John, she finds her brother in his room. There is a heavy silence before she says, "Things are pretty bad between Jane and you—huh?"

David: (Nods.) *You could have waited. I was on the phone first.*
Sally: *No . . . John could only call between 5 and 5:15.*
David: *You shouldn't count on the phone being free.*
Sally: *Yeah—I suppose I got mad when you ignored me* (Pauses, notices the tension is gone, and smiles.) *Sorry and good luck!*
David: (Smiles and shakes his head.) *I'm going to call her now.*

Sally tousles his hair, and they both grin. Sally walks away reflecting, "Sure feels good to clear the air, and it was a little presumptuous of me to believe that in a family of five the phone would be free for those 15 minutes. I sure love my brother."

The preceding is an example of a spontaneous, creative, and integrated expression of anger. Sally felt anger, expressed it, and made sense out of the experience. In fact, it brought her closer to her brother and taught her something about herself. Sally's warm-up proceeded in the following stages:

Excitement about having a boyfriend
Uncertainty as to whether she was going out that night
Relief at getting home before 5 PM
Disappointment that David was on the phone
Panic that David would not get off the phone in time
Perspiring, flushing, stirring in stomach
Concern and empathy for David's pain
Fear of incurring David's anger
Anger that David was ignoring her
Thoughts that John might misunderstand
Panic that John might get angry
Burning pressure inside
Outburst—verbal exchange

Any of the following beliefs could have cut off the process of Sally's warm-up:

1. David would never get off the phone no matter what she did.

2. Girls should not raise their voices.
3. David, who is bigger, would hit her if she interrupted him.
4. David does not care what happens to her.
5. David would get back at her next week.
6. She had no right to want the phone.

The catharsis of anger is the spontaneous expression of angry thoughts and feelings. Sally and David spontaneously yelled and angrily talked to one another with little forethought. Thoughts, feelings, expression, and actions occurred simultaneously, and time seemed to "stand still." Each was completely attuned to the self. The atmosphere was electric as Sally and David creatively expressed feelings and content congruently. The integration occurs after the "air has cleared."

Sally (1) once again reaffirmed the benefits of getting angry through experiencing the relief, (2) acknowledged her part in the conflict—that is, checked the assumption that she made regarding the phone and how her younger brother should accommodate her, and (3) reaffirmed her love for her brother with a gentle touch and grin.

Role reversal is vital to a successful integration of any expression of anger, since it cements the relationship and allows people to learn together. To put oneself into the role of others is to experience their reality from its most intimate perspective. It is to appreciate how another person feels, perceives, and behaves in relationship to oneself and others. It allows one to see oneself through the eyes of another.

When anger is not managed well, it is wise to examine what occurred during the warming-up process. Incomplete warm-ups leave incomplete expressions, a lack of catharsis, which leave incomplete integrations. Incomplete integrations interfere with the subsequent warming-up.

Existential

According to Frankl,[18] people need to find meaning in and from their suffering. Suffering includes the emotion of anger and gives people the choice to take the opportunity to develop deeper meaning in the life that fate has presented.

Frankl draws from his experiences as a German prisoner in a concentration camp during World War II to explain his theory. He witnessed that the men who lost hope for a future, who occupied themselves with memories of the past and ignored the present, were angry people. They could find no meaning in their suffering, and they became aggressive toward fellow inmates. Those who kept themselves alive by creating dreams of a future with family, friends, and job were more sensitive to others and better adjusted.

Frankl believes that humans are truly free to choose their attitudes when confronted with infuriating situations. People can transcend these situations with humor and curiosity. They can develop more encompassing meanings of situations and finally activate thoughts and images that produce love. Frankl sees anger as a vehicle to new understanding, meaning, and love.

Theories of anger are summarized in Table 12-1.

TABLE 12-1 Summary of the theories of anger

Theories	Theorist	Dynamics
Biological		
Biochemical		Lesions or disease in the limbic system (which regulates aggression) may cause aggressive acts. Chemical imbalances and endocrine disorders may lead to aggression.
Genetic	Lorenz	Aggression is an inborn response pattern and is genetically influenced.
Psychoanalytic	Freud	Anger is instinctual and seeks expression through aggressive acts or self-destruction. Anger may be displaced onto an object resembling the original object of anger. Some disease conditions are indications of internalized anger.
Interpersonal	Sullivan	Any anxiety producing situation has the potential for evoking anger and aggression. The emotion of anger gives one a feeling of power that compensates for an underlying anxiety. Anger attempts to destroy the object or situation that produced the anxiety.
Behavioral	Dollard and Miller	Aggression results from frustration of a desired goal.
	Bandura and Moreno	Anger is learned through the socialization process, by observation and modeling. Anger is energy that propels people to new learnings, thus enhancing feelings of adequacy as a person.
Existential	Frankl	Anger in suffering gives people an opportunity to find new meanings in life.

RELATING TO THE CLIENT

Working with angry or aggressive clients is a great challenge for nurses. It is a natural response for the nurse to be angry or distressed, to feel inadequate and helpless, to withdraw and avoid, or to respond in other ways that limit effectiveness in giving care to the angry client.

Before interacting with an angry client the nurse needs to examine her present feelings because impatience, annoyance, or irritability may be communicated to the client and escalate his anger. The nurse's cognizance of ways she handles her own anger as well as her level of confidence, self-assurance and self-esteem, influences her care of an angry client. Nurses can become more aware of their anger by examining patterns of handling anger in their family. Questions such as the following provide some self-awareness for the nurse:

Was the overt expression of anger allowed?

Was the expression of anger rewarded or punished?

Was anger a taboo topic?

How do I express anger?

How can I tell I am angry?

What anxieties lead to my anger?

Are there some people to whom I am afraid to express anger?

When am I likely to disown my anger?

Initial reactions of the nurse during the orientation phase include fear, anxiety, defensiveness, retaliation and vindictiveness. The nurse who can identify, understand, and manage similar feelings and responses to anger in herself is better equipped to accept the angry verbalizations of her client without defensiveness or increased anger.

Responding to anger with anger usually escalates the aggressive encounter. Frequently nurses respond defensively to expressions of anger by explaining or justifying the situation. Avoiding the client who verbally attacks or threatens the nurse is an additional, ineffective way that nurses deal with angry clients. Although no one wants to be the target of anger, the nurse who can accept another's anger with calmness and confidence can help the person regain control. Nurses with high self-esteem and a sound knowledge of the dynamics of anger can be effective in working with angry clients.

When the nurse is frequently the subject of angry verbal attacks, she may need to examine the possibility that her behavior is provoking the attack without her being aware of it. Reflecting on such behaviors as inconsideration, disrespect, inattention, strong opinions, and condescension may reveal a basis for the client's angry behavior.

Clients frequently experience increased anxiety during the termination phase and thus may respond with an increase in anger. The nurse knowledgeable in the phases of the nurse-client relationship is aware of this behavior and can avoid becoming threatened. Gentle confrontation about what the client is experiencing demonstrates to the client a constructive way to deal with anger.

NURSING PROCESS
Assessment

Physical dimension. The nurse assesses the client's overall posture and appearance. Nonpurposeful motor symptoms such as agitation and pacing may indicate increasing tension. A flushed face, tightened jaws, flared nostrils and protruding neck veins show intense efforts of control. The fists may be clenched, posture tense, and the voice louder. Eye contact that is direct and glaring or staring is also indicative of anger.

Physiological responses to anger result primarily from the action of the autonomic nervous system in response to the secretion of epinephrine. Blood pressure increases, and tachycardia is present. Blood composition is altered with increased fatty acids and fewer lymphocytes. Gastrointestinal changes include nausea, increased salivation, increased hydrochloric acid secretion, and decreased gas-

MESSAGES OF ANGER

SIGHT

Body tense	Lowered eyebrows
Shaking fist	Shoulders tight
Right fist hitting left hand	Pounding
Kicking	Flushed face
Stomping	Hands on hips
Slashing	Arms crossed
Holding breath	Pacing
Index finger pointed	Direct, glaring eye contact
Eyes staring	Turning away
Nostrils flared	Throwing objects
Tight lips	Accidents

TASTE

Dry Mouth	No taste to food

TOUCH

Pushing	Slapping
Hitting	Tight fist
Shoving	Elevated body temperature

HEARING

Change in voice quality	Chewing food loudly
Accusing words	Deep sighs
Statements of anger	Breaking of objects
Slamming doors	Pounding
Heavy footsteps	Hitting
Drumming of fingernails	

tric peristalsis. Changes in electroencephalograms occur. Symptoms similar to anxiety are noted, such as increased alertness, increased muscle tension, and rapid reflexes. Urination is frequently increased, pupils are dilated, and the person has difficulty relaxing and sleeping.

Disorders known to have an anger-related source include hypertension, rheumatoid arthritis, ulcers, colitis, asthma, migraine headaches, angina, and chronic backaches. It is equally important for the nurse to be aware that trauma or brain lesions may be a contributing factor in explosive, violent behavior. Because of the relationship of these conditions to anger, the nurse collects data regarding the client's past and present illnesses.

Acting-out behavior that attracts the attention of other persons and represents the inner conflicts of the person feeling anger needs to be assessed. Running away, truancy from school, stealing, setting fires, drug and alcohol abuse, and sexual promiscuity are examples of acting-out behavior.

The sensory receptors receive messages of anger, such as those listed in the box above.

People sometimes use their bodies to make a defiant statement to the world. Angry people may purposely dress unlike others or exaggerate a particular style. The "I don't care what you think" attitude can be conveyed through clothes, jewelry, and hairstyles.

Laboratory tests are scheduled to rule out a physical basis for the angry behavior. These include X-ray examinations of the skull; computerized axial *tomography* (CAT scan); arteriography; lab tests for metabolic abnormalities, chemical imbalances, endocrine disturbances; and electro-encephalogram (EEG). Genetic studies may be helpful to determine whether or not others in the family have had similar behavior.

Emotional dimension. Expressions like the following describe the discomfort of anger. "I feel . . ."

Out-of-sorts	Upset	Enraged
Disappointed	Hurt	Like breaking
Annoyed	Angry	Like hitting
Irritated	Furious	Like killing
Bad		

The nurse is alert to the many expressions of anger, depression, anxiety, withdrawal, and fantasizing. Other feelings that the nurse may observe in an angry person include powerlessness, annoyance, frustration, resentment, belligerence, rage, fury, hostility, hurt, humiliation, vengeance, defensiveness, domineering, blaming, and demanding. For some, the loss of control and negative effects felt with the expression of anger produce guilt or embarrassment. The nurse needs to be sensitive to the influences that affect the person's expression of anger and look for signs of guilt or embarrassment. For others, a sense of power comes with anger. The energy released in anger may create additional problems such as greater tension rather than relief.

In despair and depression, anger is denied and turned inward on the self. The energy of anger is used to maintain the depression. Further assessment of anger as it relates to depression is found in Chapter 14.

It is important that the nurse assess the intensity of the client's expression of anger. In addition, the appropriateness of the anger to the anger-provoking situation provides data about the client's anger threshold. A person with a low tolerance for frustration is easily provoked to anger. One with a high tolerance demonstrates self-control and adequacy in handling anger.

Intellectual Dimension. At first glance, it seems that intellect plays little or no role in the emotion of anger. The emotion itself seems to push aside rationality and any semblance of an orderly progression of thought. The strength and intensity of the anger may cause a person to misinterpret information that affects perceptions, conclusions, memory, judgment, and actions.

Long after anger dissipates, *ruminations* about the incident often regenerate the anger. Individuals can work themselves into a rage without the presence of the original stimulus. Repetitive thoughts keep the anger flowing. By listening the nurse can determine the amount of anger present through repetitive thoughts and ruminations. The following example shows one way of keeping anger alive with repetitive thoughts:

Case Example

Daniel sits slumped in his third-grade arithmetic class shortly after recess. His best friend, Steve, did not choose him for the recess soccer team, and he is scheming how to get even. He certainly is not going to walk home from school with Steve; he will walk right past his friend, pretending not to see him. He doesn't need him, anyway. His mind flashes on how he had stood there as the teams were being chosen. So what if he can't play soccer? Steve could have chosen him anyway. The big-shot soccer captain, he'd show him! He glares at the back of his friend's head. He imagines himself the captain of the soccer team choosing his friend last. By the end of the arithmetic class Daniel's stomach is in a knot, and he is convinced that Steve is a stupid slob. He believes Steve doesn't want to be his friend any more, so he marches straight up to him after class and says, "I think your mother eats worms!"

The boy kept the anger alive by ruminating about it for an hour.

The nurse assesses the methods the client uses to express his anger. Some persons deny their feelings of anger. Although the behaviors of anger are present, the individual denies the feeling. Forgetting appointments, being late, misunderstanding, procrastinating, and failing to learn are ways people deny their anger. Others displace their anger onto an object or person other than the target of their anger. Some persons express anger by scolding, sarcasm, humor, and gossiping.

The associative processes influence the development and expression of anger. People conceptually link cause to effect. For instance, because most parents are angry when punishing children, people learn to associate anger with punishment. They learn to associate anger with bad and wrong. Peoples' beliefs dictate their experience; if they believe anger is wrong, an experience involving anger will be blocked from expression as in the following example.

Case Example

June, a 29-year-old teacher, mother, and wife, came for help when she could not generate the optimistic and loving feeling that she had once possessed for her family. The family had recently moved into a new community because of her husband's promotion. John's job now entailed 2 weeks of travel every month, and the isolation of staying home with the 5-year-old boy, Jacob, and the 2-year-old twin girls in a rural neighborhood was defeating for June. She had not wanted the house in the country, but it had been a dream of her husband for years. She also had not wanted John to take the job because of the travel, but she understood the potential promotions that would be available for him in a couple of years. She always had been one to "make do" and not cause a fuss. She could not remember having a fight with anyone, but now it concerned her when she would yell at the children for the "smallest things," kick the cat when it got underfoot, and be visibly irritated at John if he was 10 minutes late. She did not like herself this way. She asked the therapist to help her be more loving and accepting. When asked how she felt about anger, she replied, "I really don't think it's right. John gets mad at me and the kids, and it just makes us feel bad. Jacob gets mad back, which makes matters worse. I think people should try to be positive if they do get annoyed and keep it to themselves until it passes. There's no sense in making other people feel bad, too; they generally do not mean to insult you. When I find myself blaming John for putting me and the kids in the country, I just tell myself to be positive—John's doing the best he can—but I'm finding it very hard to do."

In therapy, June revealed that when she was young her mother had angrily accused her of being bad and evil whenever she did something wrong. June then felt as if she were completely evil and bad. She paired anger with evil and wrongdoing. As an adult she had to learn to separate these two and to slowly learn to voice her frustrations to her husband.

People who have verbal and social skills are less likely to resort to physical means of expressing anger. An individual may preserve self-esteem by using such verbal skills as pacification, persuasion, and humor. The mind can be used to consider alternative actions and consequences of the situation. If individuals have learned to perceive the situation from a number of vantage points, they are less likely to physically attack. The presence of verbal skills implies a cognitive process. The nurse needs to assess clients' verbal skills to determine their ability to perceive situations and to consider options for dealing with the situation.

If people can develop beliefs that stimulate and initiate a new learning process, they are less likely to live in a state of anger. A flexible belief is, "If I express my anger directly, some people will interact with me directly, some will retreat for a short time and re-engage later, and some will terminate the relationship entirely. Each person has a belief about and a style of expressing anger, and I will just have to get to know the person and find out what it is. One thing is sure—we all have anger." People who develop fixed, rigid views of the world that do not allow for growth are often angry. Fixed beliefs do not allow people to accommodate to change and thus lead to frustration. A rigid belief is, "People will abandon me if I express my anger, and I will end up all alone. I must not express anger."

✳ **Social dimension.** The nurse assesses the client's patterned responses to the anger of others. Does he generally respond passively or aggressively? The following table indicates behaviors that are typically passive or aggressive (see Table 12-2).

Anger often triggers anger in others and brings the threat of rejection or abandonment. Thus a client with a high level of dependence may deny anger as an acceptable emotion. The nurse can determine the degree of dependence in a client by listening for the theme of rejection or abandonment.

TABLE 12-2 Behaviors indicating patterned responses to anger

Passive	Aggressive
Self-denying	Self-enhancing at expense of another
Inhibited, hurt, anxious	Expressive, depreciates others
Allows others to choose for him	Chooses for others
Does not achieve desired goal	Achieves desired goal by hurting others

Some people express anger in such a way that it stimulates rejection. They say to themselves, "It is not fair that I should have to feel this." They channel their anger into judgments and look for someone to blame. They angrily critique the behavior of others that stimulated the pain as wrong, unfair, or unethical and expect the other to do penance. This process alienates the individual from himself and from others. The individual loses the opportunity to learn because the original source of anger is no longer the focus. People react negatively to the critique and distance themselves from the angry person.

The following are ways of expressing anger that distance others:

Projecting self-anger onto another ("I know you hate it when I feel inadequate.")

Blaming another for pain that resulted from a prior nonassertive stance of self ("You made me cook this meal for you, and you had better enjoy it.")

Being consistently late

Screaming and shouting at others' mistakes

Belittling and ridiculing

Using sarcasm

Rejecting (A person may "say," through nonverbal behavior, "You were supposed to be home half an hour ago, so I won't talk to you for a day.")

Being angry at one incident and reiterating past grievances

Talking to another (An angry person talks to John about anger at Bill, so both are angry at Bill.)

Breaking or throwing objects, or hitting a wall

Moralizing or preaching

Covering anger with sweetness

Hitting a person

Some individuals need a relationship in which the other person serves specific, seemingly vital, functions. Because these relationships seem vital to one's sense of well-being, anger is a threatening emotion to experience and express openly. To maintain these relationships, people are likely to lie about their anger, sacrifice their integrity, and pretend. Pretense kills the essence of the vital relationship. Fear of anger and its consequences can be overwhelming, since the threat of being bereft of important people is powerful. Isolation can be devastating to some, no matter how brief the period.

Other people take more risks with their anger. The number of risks differs for each person. Some people maintain social relationships through intimidation, and the emotion of anger is more available than any other. Their love, sexuality, joy, and sadness are minimally acknowledged, and they berate these emotional experiences in others. The availability of their anger makes them appear strong. However, their fragility is evident when one sees how limited their emotional repositories actually are. Thus is essential to assess the client's self-esteem, self-concept, and feelings of adequacy.

Anger plays a vital role when terminating significant relationships. It can be used constructively to let go, or it can be used destructively to cling. Anger allows one to focus on the self in a new light. It encourages separateness. When disentangling from people, places, and roles, a person, through anger, considers new perspectives and alternatives. When new people, places, and roles are required to facilitate a change, the old ends as the new begins. However, beginnings are difficult because they highlight people's inadequacies. Often people angrily cling to the memories of more fulfilled times and do not trust the process of letting go. Clinging is a form of anger that says, "I don't want change in my life. I'm angry about it, and so it's not going to happen!"

The emotion of anger is expressed in different ways in various cultures. In some cultures to express anger is to risk rejection and isolation, in others it brings favor. When assessing cultural differences of anger, one needs to consider the influence of prejudice and fear. Groups with a minority status may fear the intensity of anger generated from the prejudice they encounter in their daily lives. They develop norms for its expression in public life that differ from those used within their own subculture. In public life they may fear that direct expression of anger may worsen their situation. Therefore they may indirectly or passively express anger, as through overly compliant or passive-aggressive behavior; directed anger against themselves; or aggression directed into creative outlets, such as sports, music, and art.

Anger is culturally defined as part of certain roles; that is, people in some roles have the right to be angry, and people in other roles do not. The boss can express anger toward an employee, but the employee cannot express anger toward the supervisor. Mothers can express anger at their daughters, but if daughters express anger at their mothers, it is disrespectful. The client can express anger at a nurse, but the nurse cannot to a client.

People develop expressions of anger that reflect the culture in which they live. All interactions play their part in conveying appropriate expressions of anger. People learn about their anger from those around them. They are socialized to behave in such a way to fit the pattern developed by their family and culture. The messages may be contradictory; for example, the family may yell at each other, and the teacher may teach polite behavior. The individual quickly becomes socialized to behave accordingly in the various contexts.

The language used when one is angry is another reflection of the socialization process. Teenagers delight in "four-letter words"; mothers may say, "You've disappointed me"; and the screams of the toddler reverberate through the house.

Anger is also expressed differently at different ages. Infants' rage can be heard loudly and clearly when needs are unmet. The toddler's tantrums and the loud "no's" from 3- and 4-year-olds are age appropriate. Table 12-3 lists age-appropriate expressions of anger that reflect the norms of the United States for persons from birth to age 16. The expressions of anger progress from physical to verbal and decrease in frequency as the child matures. Adult expressions of anger reflect this trend; that is, typically the adult expresses anger verbally or indirectly.

It is also important for the nurse to see that the client's behavior is, in part, a reflection of a life situation and the present interaction. If someone appears angry "all the

TABLE 12-3 Age-appropriate expressions of anger

Age (Years)	Expression
Birth to 1	Crying, flailing of body, pounding, and kicking
1½	Tantrum, throwing self on floor, screaming, crying
2	Same as 1½ years, plus yelling "mine" adamantly
2½	Height of tantrums
3	Greater degree of compliance; if overstimulated or tired, physical aggression (for example biting or kicking)
3½	Rebellion and refusal; loud noises; verbal aggression
4	Physical and verbal aggression; breaking toys; excluding others from play
5	Aggression not characteristic; slamming doors; verbal aggression
5½	Verbal and physical aggression; destruction during play; rebellion
6	Extremely argumentative behavior and physical abuse; rebellion; destruction of property
7	Less aggression; verbal aggression, for example, threats and leaving room; indirect expressions, such as lateness, forgetting, and accidents
8	Greater degree of withdrawal; direction of anger toward self; hurting others; verbal aggression; indirect expressions
9	Physical aggression; criticalness of others; verbal aggression
10	Competitive behavior; keeping anger to self; possible sudden eruptions—physical and verbal—and leaving room; indirect expressions
11	Increase in arousal; physical expression common, for example, slamming doors and fighting; pouting and plotting revenge common
12	Physical striking out; increased number of verbal responses; saying "drop dead"; sitting and seething
13	Leaving the situation; sarcasm and retorts; some swearing; making faces; directing anger toward self; some crying; sitting and thinking about it
14	Sitting and taking it; reduced number of angry responses; yelling, swearing, talking back; leaving the situation; taking it out on someone else
15	Reduced number of angry responses; leaving the room; sarcasm; trying to ignore or suppress anger; cold looks
16	Reduced number of angry responses; trying not to show anger; silence; sitting and glaring; slamming doors

Based on data from Gesell, A.L., Ilg, F.L., and Ames, L.B.: Youth: the years from ten to sixteen, New York, 1956, Harper & Brothers; Gesell, A.L., and others: Infant and child in the culture of today: the guidance of development in home and nursery school, rev. ed., New York, 1974, Harper & Row, Publishers; Gesell, A.L., and others: The child from five to ten, New York, 1977, Harper & Row, Publishers.

time" and is disagreeable to be around, it may be a response to a status of isolation or rejection in a primary group. Anger may be the energy that helps the person survive.

✂ *Spiritual dimension.* Clients have beliefs about anger that are integral to their philosophy of life and spirituality. If they belong to an organized religion, the nurse needs to investigate how the religion views anger. If it is seen as sinful and the nurse is encouraging its expression, clients may experience considerable turmoil.

The absence of a meaningful philosophy engenders frustration and anger. People who have no framework within which to act are left to make their way through life impulsively, much like a boat in a storm. People who lack a meaningful framework may value neither their acts nor ultimately themselves. They feel disparaging toward life's demands and resent giving to others. People may experience a lack of meaning at transition points in their lives, for example, as they are changing their focus from school to employment or from employment to retirement. What once felt vital now has little or no significance, and yet nothing else has filled the void; irritation and frustration are present. For others, finding a meaningful existence has been a continual problem, and they feel enraged. They believe they are justified in spewing their venom on the world, either openly or privately.

Beliefs about oneself evolve from one's concept as to how one has met the challenges of life. Some people are angry and disappointed about their performances. They have been unable to meet their or others' expectations and direct their anger against themselves.

A person cannot simultaneously be angry and transcend the limitations of human experience. To transcend is to leave the self behind and identify with the whole, knowing that the self will continue to exist and that it has value. In these moments there is no need for the emotion of anger.

The spiritual self is geared to move onward, to create and to objectify sensed inner realities. People strive to be spontaneous and creative beings and to develop meaningful existences. Anger is a symptom that the creative path is blocked and that clearing is needed to reroute energies to a new path of greater self-actualization.

Spiritual conflicts, absence of a meaningful philosophy, and contradictory beliefs may generate anger. The following questions can serve as a guide in determining the effects of a client's spiritual life on dealing with anger.

As an adult, what is the role of anger in your spiritual development?

How do you value anger?

In your current situation, what strong beliefs seem contradictory of one another?

POTENTIAL FOR VIOLENCE

DEFINITION
State in which an individual experiences behaviors that can be harmful either to oneself or others.

DEFINING CHARACTERISTICS

Physical Dimension
Clenched fists
Tense facial expression
Rigid posture
Tautness indicating intense effort for self-control
Increased motor activity; pacing, agitation, excitement
Overt aggressive acts
Destruction of objects in the environment
Possession of destructive weapons; gun, knife
Substance abuse/withdrawal
*Temporal lobe epilepsy
*Toxic reaction to medication
*Progressive physical deterioration; organic brain disease, brain tumor
Self-destructive behavior; suicidal acts

Emotional Dimension
Anger
Irritability
Suspiciousness
Rage
Increasing anxiety level
Fear of self or others
Depression

Intellectual Dimension
Hostile, threatening verbalizations
Boasting to or prior abuse of others
Paranoid ideas, delusions, hallucinations
Inability to verbalize feelings
Repeated complaints, requests, demands
*Dysfunctional communication patterns

Social Dimension
*High situational stress factors
*Antisocial character disturbance
Provacative acts
Argumentation
Hypersensitivity
Overreaction
Dissatisfaction
Vulnerable self-esteem

Spiritual Dimension
*Devalues self and others

From North American Nursing Diagnosis Association Classification of Nursing Diagnosis: Proceedings of the seventh conference, St. Louis, 1987, The C.V. Mosby Co.
*Indicates characteristics in addition to those defined by NANDA.

At what time in your life have you felt resentment and alienation from God, a supreme power, or other persons?

When have you expressed the need to suffer as reparation?

Measurement tools. Buss and Durkee[7] developed an inventory for assessing different kinds of hostility. Examples of statements related to different kinds of hostility include the following:

1. Assault
   a. I get into fights about as often as the next person.
   b. If I have to resort to physical violence to defend my rights, I will.
2. Indirect hostility
   a. I sometimes slam doors when I am mad.
   b. I sometimes pout when I don't get my own way.
3. Irritability
   a. It makes my blood boil when people make fun of me.
   b. Sometimes people bother me just by being around.
4. Negativism
   a. Unless somebody asks me in a nice way, I won't do what they want.
   b. When people are bossy, I take my time just to show them.

5. Resentment
   a. Other people seem to get the breaks.
   b. At times I feel I get a raw deal out of life.
6. Suspicion
   a. I know people tend to talk about me behind my back.
   b. My motto is "Never trust strangers."
7. Verbal hostility
   a. When I disapprove of my friend's behavior, I let him know it.
   b. When I get mad I say nasty things.
8. Guilt
   a. The few times I have cheated I have suffered unbearable feelings of remorse.
   b. It depresses me that I do not do more for my parents.

Analysis

Nursing diagnosis. Potential for violence is a nursing diagnosis approved by the North American Nursing Diagnosis Association above. (NANDA) that applies to the angry client. The defining characteristics are listed in the box above. The following list provides examples of NANDA-accepted nursing diagnoses with causative statements.

1. Ineffective individual coping: inappropriate anger related to loss of job
2. Ineffective individual coping: anger related to anxiety over financial problems
3. Potential for violence related to delusions of persecution
4. Impaired social interactions related to hostile, threatening statements
5. Noncompliance related to anger over physical limitations
6. Sleep pattern disturbance related to anger
7. Alteration in parenting: child neglect related to frustration and dissatisfaction of parenting role

DSM-III-R-diagnosis. The DSM-III-R-diagnoses related to anger are listed in the box at upper left.

The essential features of intermittent explosive disorder and passive-aggressive personality disorder and manifestations of these features according to the DSM-III-R are listed in the boxes on this page.

Planning

Table 12-4 lists examples of long-term and short-term goals and outcome criteria related to anger. These serve as examples of the planning stage in the nursing process.

Implementation

⊹ ***Physical dimension.*** Interventions for anger include providing constructive outlets for the energy of anger. Physical activity is helpful. The nurse can encourage jogging, swimming, weight lifting, competitive sports, dancing, and activities that allow large muscle involvement and socially accepted expressions of aggression.

Other activities often offered in occupational therapy include sanding and hammering to offset the energy of

TABLE 12-4 Long-term and short-term goals and outcome criteria related to anger

Goals	Outcome Criteria
NURSING DIAGNOSIS: INEFFECTIVE COPING: ANGER RELATED TO DISSATISFACTION WITH LIFE	
Long-term goals	
To develop more positive feelings toward self	Makes positive statements about self
To establish meaningful relationships with friends and family	Has relationships that reinforce positive self-image
To establish meaningful roles in which client can express himself creatively	Can express emotions with others and solve problems when stressed
	Has reciprocal relationships; that is, others can share with him
	Has two or three roles in which he feels productive and creative
	Accepts change as a viable aspect of his life
Short-term goals	
To establish rapport with nurse	Talks spontaneously to nurse and expresses anger
To express anger and increase availability of all emotions	Values the expression of anger, sadness, warmth, sexuality, and joy
To verbalize reasons for dissatisfaction with self; disparity between potential and reality, conflicting values that perpetuate anger, and lack of meaning	Has values that are congruent with behavior; life has established meaning
To work through unfinished business from the past that engenders and perpetuates anger in the present	Accepts past events and relationships without malice
To terminate past events that perpetuate a negative self-image and anger	Confronts existing relationships honestly; learns about self and others
To discuss the aging process and its effect on feelings of inadequacy and low self-esteem	Confronts roles honestly
To undergo physical examination to determine adequacy of health	Has a physical examination
To renegotiate or terminate relationships that perpetuate a negative self-image	Creates new relationships and roles that support growth
To establish more adequate responses to life situation	Is more spontaneous in interactions with others

anger. Use of a punching bag may dissipate feelings of anger. Providing distraction and channeling angry behavior through mildly competitive games like cards, checkers, and chess are therapeutic. Constructive tasks and challenging activities at which the client is proficient also serve to dilute anger and to provide socially acceptable outlets for expressing anger. In addition, feelings of self-esteem are fostered, and feelings of accomplishment and independence are promoted. External controls can be applied as a last resort by medicinal or mechanical restraints, or with a quiet room to provide protection and control until the client is able to gain self-control. Isolation may be required when the client becomes out of control. The nurse maintains appropriate spatial distance between herself and the client to prevent the client from feeling overpowered or dominated by the presence of authority. The Research Highlight on p. 241 explores patterns of assaultive behavior in clients.

Psychotropic medications such as chlorpromazine (Thorazine), trifluoperazine (Stelazine), and thioridazine (Mellaril) are sometimes prescribed to reduce the belligerence and aggression of angry psychotic clients. (See Chapter 22 for discussion of psychotropic medications.)

✳ *Emotional dimension.* Reducing sources of undue anxiety or high levels of anxiety is a way of preventing anger from developing or escalating. Frequently hospitalization removes the client from overwhelming stress and anxiety and the subsequent anger and allows the person time to place life situations in a more tolerable perspective.

The nurse can help angry clients by observing and acknowledging their anger. Empathic statements such as "You're upset" or "You're angry" provide validation for observations and help the client recognize the feeling of anger. If the client denies the anger, the nurse can rephrase the statement by saying, "You sound annoyed" or "You look distressed." Statements like these clarify and verify observations about the behavior and facilitate recognition of angry feelings. Encouraging description of the feelings prevents the client from avoiding or denying the feeling. "What do you mean when you say you're frustrated?" or "Tell me some more about your disappointment" focuses attention on the feeling. The nurse needs to communicate to the client that it is normal to feel angry and that the expression of the feeling can be constructive or destructive. Constructive expressions of anger in-

Research Highlight

Assaultive Behavior Among Psychiatric Outpatients

K. Tardiff & H. Koenigsberg

PURPOSE

The study was designed to assess the patterns of assaultive behavior in clients coming to outpatient clinics.

SAMPLE

The sample included 2,916 clients seen by psychiatric residents during a 1½-year study. Two private psychiatric hospitals were used in the study.

METHODOLOGY

All clients were evaluated by psychiatric residents at two large teaching hospitals. A research assistant reviewed the hospital records of all clients evaluated by the residents in the outpatient settings during the study period. Data were recorded on a worksheet developed as part of an effort to evaluate the clinical experiences of residents who cared for clients at these hospitals. Clients were classified only in regard to the presence or absence of assaultive behavior toward other persons. Diagnoses were based on DSM-III criteria.

FINDINGS

Clients who had demonstrated recent assaultive behavior toward other persons numbered 3%. In half of the cases the target was a family member (spouse). Clients were likely to be young, 20 and under, male, and had a diagnosis of childhood or adolescent disorder or personality disorder.

IMPLICATIONS

Although the rate of assaultive behavior among clients who came for evaluation in outpatient settings was lower than those among clients in state hospitals, the fact that many were seen in outpatient treatment settings underscored the need for preparing the treatment team to manage potentially violent clients. Therapists need to be concerned about the physical setting of the office as well as the availability of a mechanism by which persons outside the office can be alerted to an episode of violent behavior.

Based on data from American Journal of Psychiatry, **142**(8):960, 1985.

---

clude talking about the feeling or withdrawing until some of the anger is dissipated and then talking about it. Time can be crucial when anger is intense; for example, a period of withdrawal can provide a cooling-down time until the person regains control.

Feelings associated with anger, such as guilt and despair, need exploration also. Interventions for guilt and despair are addressed in Chapters 13 and 14.

✳ *Intellectual dimension.* When people are enraged, they require limits, a here-and-now orientation to circumstance, and people who can facilitate a more adequate response. Following is an example of setting a limit.

Case Example

It is 4 PM, time for change of shift. John has just been told he must receive 24-hour care because he is suicidal. He is 50 years old, 5 feet 10 inches tall, and 175 pounds.

John paces down the hall hitting his fist into the palm of his hand. Periodically he strikes the wall, obviously injuring his hand, but he feels no pain. He swings around and heads toward the dayroom. The other people stop talking and remain motionless. John kicks a metal trash can and swears. He looks menacingly at the nurse who has just told him he will have to remain on 24-hour care.

The nurse elicits the support of two male employees and alerts the reporting staff members to stand by. She approaches but maintains a safe distance from John.

Nurse: (Loudly and firmly.) *Get control of yourself, John. We will not let you hurt yourself.*
John: (Stops and trembles as face turns ashen.)
Nurse: (Firmly.) *What are you angry about? Use your words. I want to hear from you.*
John: You bitch, what do you know? (Turns to walk away.)
Nurse: Nothing until you tell me. Now talk about how you feel.
John: (Stops and screams.) *I feel like going home, and I don't want to be here!*
Nurse: (Loudly.) *I know. So say it again.*
John: (Looks at nurse, not trusting what he has heard.)
Nurse: I'm serious—say it again.
John: (Shouts.) *I don't want to be here. I want to go home, and I don't want to live!*

John bursts into tears, falls to his knees and covers his face with his hands. The three staff members slowly move toward him and stand close by. When the nurse sees John's body relax and soften, she gently places a hand on his shoulder and tells him that she can feel how hard the struggle is for him. He nods, and the nurse suggests that he stay in the dayroom with the others. She motions for others to come over and stands by as they invite him to join them in a conversation. She joins the conversation.

In this incident, the nurse (1) established the limits while protecting herself, (2) encountered the client's intensity, (3) encouraged the client's verbalization of feelings, (4) made physical contact with the client and, (5) integrated the client with the group.

Anger is aroused when conflicts between persons are encountered. The following steps assist in conflict resolution.

1. State, "I have a problem or I am feeling . ."
2. Describe the situation and areas of conflict.
3. Tell the person what you need from him.
4. Ask the person if he is willing to give you what you need.
5. If the answer is no, ask him what he is willing to do. Acknowledge the other person's response and thank him for feedback.
6. Listen to what the other person is willing or not willing to do. You do not have to agree to accept thoughts and feelings.
7. State what you are willing to do to reach a workable compromise and give feedback about the other person's communication.
8. The process of communication has begun, and you are now in negotiation for the resolution of the conflict. Repeat your needs as often as necessary. Keep your communication honest, direct, and free from attempts to manipulate and control.

Social dimension. Because anger is a response to a threat to the self-concept, it is essential to help the client identify the source of the threat, as well as his feelings of inadequacy, and deal with the accompanying anxiety. See Chapter 11 for interventions for anxiety.

The nurse assists the client to see the consequences of his angry behavior: rejection, abandonment, alienation, and isolation. The client is helped to explore other options he has for handling anger that do not result in rejection and alienation from others. Withdrawing from others temporarily may help prevent harsh words or actions that are regretted later. Physical activity dilutes the intensity of the emotion, and talking with another person may relieve some of the anger. However, it is important to return to the person to whom the anger was initially directed and discuss the situation when thinking is more rational.

Since dependence on others may create anger by fostering resentment toward the person being depended on, the client can be assisted to function more independently. Ways to facilitate independence include learning a skill, becoming financially independent, moving out of the home, redefining life goals more realistically, becoming less dependent emotionally on another, and learning problem-solving skills. When the client is dependent with clearly no other options, the nurse assists him to accept the situation without anger and resentment and to develop attitudes that enhance his personality and promote relationships with others.

Role-playing allows clients to explore their anger by acting out a realistic problem situation. The role playing process includes providing the leadership that allows those involved to feel spontaneous. The nurse:

1. Suggests a structure or focus that will provide the *parameters* to ensure safety
2. Keeps the focus in the *here-and-now*
3. Ensures that the focus is in keeping with the norms and purposes of the group; that is, it is *adequate*
4. Establishes a permissive atmosphere that encourages experimentation within the parameters and supports *novelty;* suspends judgments and criticisms
5. Sets the expectation that the goal of the experience is to be *creative*

Immediately following the role playing, the process is analyzed. Emotions do become highly charged during role playing, because of this, it is essential that the nurse be sensitive to both the topic and the topic's effect on the client(s).

The nurse can model how to express and resolve anger. Styles of expressing anger that are likely to allow people to stay and hear the anger and engage in dialogue are exemplified in the following: (See the Research Highlight on p. 243.) Make "I" statements about the feeling, for example:

"I feel angry because I wanted breakfast ready on time."
"I feel angry because I don't think you love me."
"I feel angry when you are late."
"I feel angry and I don't know why; I just do."

Feel the anger, express it, and verbalize the nature of the inadequacy, for example, "I feel so angry when I can't make myself understood to you."

Role playing helps the client experience the anger, withdraw, and come back to report what was learned to another. Clients often need to talk with a nurse about anger directed at others. The nurse encourages catharsis and understanding of the anger with the client. She then supports the client in expressing the anger and understanding the other person.

Spiritual dimension. Clients need to clarify their values and beliefs about anger in their lives. When anger is directed toward God or a supreme power, as sometimes happens when illness is viewed as punishment, the nurse helps the client identify the resentment, hostility, and alienation. Encouraging the client to talk about the feelings or calling in a religious leader when the nurse feels inadequate can be spiritually uplifting to the client. Clients can move beyond the anger and resentment and learn from the experience of anger. An accepting attitude on the part of the nurse is essential to helping the angry person who is questioning the meaning of illness or suffering. Attentive listening and skillful communication facilitate a discussion of spiritual values that include how well one has fulfulled life goals, the loss of significant people, and beliefs about one's own life and death.

INTERACTION WITH AN ANGRY CLIENT

Client: (Loudly.) *Someone stole my cigarettes!*
Nurse: *Your cigarettes are missing?*
Client: *No.* (Louder.) *Someone stole them. I had them on my table, and now they are gone.*
Nurse: *I'll go back with you to be sure you haven't misplaced them.* (Walks toward bedroom.)
Client: *No, I didn't misplace them. I told you someone stole them. Rodney did; he's always after me for a cigarette.*

Research Highlight

Learning a Verbal Response to Anger

M. Gluck

PURPOSE

The study was designed to determine nursing assistants' responses to angry clients before attending a class on learning verbal responses to anger and following attendance at the class.

SAMPLE

The sample consisted of 35 nursing assistants from 15 medical and surgical wards. Five assistants did not complete the assignment. Of those who did complete the assignment, 29 were women and 1 was a man. The mean age was 38 years, and the average length of experience was 10 years as a nursing assistant.

METHODOLOGY

Nursing assistants were asked to write their own responses to situations with the following types of angry behavior; demanding, verbally abusing, refusing treatment, threatening violence, and criticizing. Following completion of the free responses, the nursing assistants were asked to choose from a forced choice response to the same situations. The same test was given after completing the class to determine if instruc-

tion influenced their choice of responses for the better. The forced choice responses to each situation were designed to fit the five categories of emotion-ladened situations developed by Methven and Shlotfeldt.

FINDINGS

The findings were divided into two categories of responses, those that were aimed at reducing the client's stress and those aimed at reducing the nursing assistant's stress. The nursing assistants gave more responses to reduce their own stress (65%) than the client's stress (25%). There was a significant difference between the pretest (3.5) and the posttest (4.2) scores.

IMPLICATIONS

Persons without the verbal skills needed to handle anger who work with angry clients are more likely to intensify the client's anger than to resolve it. It is important that those responsible for education consider teaching verbal skills for dealing with anger to all levels of nursing staff so that caregivers can recognize and choose more therapeutic responses to anger.

Based on data from the Journal of Psychiatric Nursing **19**:9, 1981.

(Sees Rodney.) *Give them back to me, you thief!* (Starts toward Rodney angrily.)
Nurse: Stop! Jeff. (With authority.)

Two other staff personnel hear the interaction and enter the room. They calmly and quietly walk Jeff to another room where no others are present. Rodney sits down.

Nurse: We cannot let you hurt anyone, Jeff.
Client: I wasn't going to hurt him. I just want my cigarettes back. (Voice is calmer, appears less tense.)
(Silence.)
Nurse: What are you feeling now, Jeff?

Jeff is convinced that Rodney stole his cigarettes. Aware of this, the nurse refrains from further discussion and offers to help him look for them. On seeing Rodney, Jeff becomes increasingly angry and heads for him in a threatening manner. The nurse, with a strong and authoritative voice, tells Jeff to stop. She is aware that a short command works better with an angered client than a lengthy explanation of what he can or cannot do. Two other staff members, enter having heard the commotion, and escort Jeff from the room to eliminate further stimulation, to help

decrease his anger, and to prevent him from losing control and perhaps hurting another person. A calm statement from the nurse that he cannot hurt anyone helps Jeff to understand why he was removed from the room with assistance. After a period of time, when Jeff is calmer, he is asked to describe his feelings. It will then be important to help Jeff talk about the incident and ways he can channel his anger that are more healthy and constructive. Timing is crucial, because the angry client cannot talk about his anger while he is angry. It is after the episode that the feelings can be discussed more rationally.

Evaluation

Evaluation focuses on the expression and appropriateness of anger, the congruence between the feeling expressed and the situation, and the client's awareness of the process. When clients are involved in learning the techniques for expressing anger and problem solving and when feedback is provided by the nurse, the client is helped to learn new ways of dealing with anger. Reports from the client himself and observations by the nurse and the family provide a basis for evaluating the healthy expression of anger.

NURSING PROCESS SUMMARY: ANGER

ASSESSMENT

Physical Dimension

Acting-out behavior such as running away, truancy from school, stealing, setting fires, and sexual promiscuity
Playing competitive games
Piercing stares, glares, and hateful looks
Flushed face
Tightened jaws
Flared nostrils
Protruding neck veins
Clenched fists
Tense posture
Increased blood pressure
Tachycardia
Increased number of fatty acids
Fewer lymphocytes
Nausea
Increased salivation
Increased hydrochloric acid secretion
Decreased gastric peristalsis
Increased alertness
Increased urination
Dilated pupils
Substance abuse
Being constantly late
Accident-proneness

Emotional Dimension

Depression
Powerlessness
Annoyance
Frustration
Resentment
Belligerence
Hostility
Hurt
Humiliation
Vengeance
Defensiveness
Rage
Fury
Guilt
Disappointment
Feelings of inadequacy

Intellectual Dimension

Scolding
Sarcasm
Faultfinding
Blaming
Forgetfulness
Ruminations
Fixed, rigid beliefs
Projection
Ridiculing
Argumentativeness

Social Dimension

Poor self-concept
Disowning, as in being overly polite, sugary, or exceptionally kind or "killing with kindness"
Withdrawal
Being domineering
Making demands
Intimidation
Similar patterns of handling anger in client's family
Overreactivity
Hypersensitivity
Inability to terminate relationships

Spiritual Dimension

Absence of a meaningful philosophy of life
Blocking of spontaneity and creativity
Religious view of anger; a sin or inappropriate to express
Contradictory beliefs

ANALYSIS

See the nursing diagnosis section on p. 238.

PLANNING AND IMPLEMENTATION

Physical Dimension

Provide constructive outlets for energy of anger.
Provide protection and control until client is able to exert self-control.

Emotional Dimension

Reduce sources of anxiety.
Acknowledge client's anger with empathic statements.
Help client recognize the feeling of anger.
Encourage client to describe angry feelings.

Intellectual Dimension

Help client identify alternate methods of expressing anger.
Help client examine verbal expressions of anger.
Help client accept limited setting.
Help client learn conflict resolution.

Social Dimension

Increase client's self-esteem.
Role-play situations in which client is angry.
Practice expression of anger in a nonthreatening situation.
Teach assertiveness skills.

Spiritual Dimension

Assist clients in clarifying values and beliefs about anger.

EVALUATION

Evaluation focuses on the client's method of expressing anger, the appropriateness, the congruency between the feelings of anger and the precipitating event, and the client's awareness of the feelings of anger. Reports from the client about his responses to situations that provoke anger and from members of the family provide further evaluative data.

BRIEF REVIEW

Anger is a natural response to provocative situations or events. It has both constructive and destructive components. Because anger is a frightening emotion, people tend to deny, devalue, and avoid its expression. The adequate expression of anger promotes and adds depth to relationships; inadequate expression of anger destroys relationships.

Several theorists explain the dynamics of anger. Biologically anger may result from brain impairment or may be genetically influenced. Psychoanalytic theorists suggest that anger is inborn and seeks expression through aggression and self-destruction. Those with an interpersonal approach describe anger as a response to anxiety. Behaviorists view anger as resulting from frustration when goals are blocked or as being learned from observations or the modeling of others. The existentialists approach anger as a way to find new meanings for life or as a signal that the individual is inadequate and in need of learning.

Working with the angry client offers the nurse many challenges. Using the nursing process she assesses the client's anger and plans actions that help the client manage his anger in socially acceptable ways. Research findings provide a sound basis for the assessment and management of violent clients.

REFERENCES AND SUGGESTED READINGS

1. Babich, K., editor: Assessing patient violence in the health care setting, Boulder, Colo., 1981, Western Interstate Commission for Higher Education (WICHE).
2. Bandura, A.: Aggression: a social learning analysis, Englewood Cliffs, N.J., 1973, Prentice-Hall, Inc.
3. Barile, L.: A model for teaching management of disturbed behavior, Journal of Psychosocial Nursing and Mental Health Services 20(11):9, 1982.
4. Beatty, J., and others: Anger generated by unmet expectations, Matenal-Child Nursing Journal 10(5):324, 1985.
5. Burrows, R.: Nurses and violence . . . psychiatric ward, Nursing times 80(4):56, 1984.
6. Bushman, P.: Anger in the clinical setting, Maternal-Child Nursing Journal 10(5):313, 1985.
7. Buss, A., and Durkee, A.: An inventory for assessing different kinds of hostility, Journal of Consulting and Clinical Psychology 21(4):343, 1957.
8. Carlson, N.R.L.: Physiology of behavior, Boston, 1977, Allyn & Bacon, Inc.
9. Clunn, P.: Nurses' assessment of violence potential. In Babich, K., editor: Assessing patient violence in the health care setting, Boulder, Colo., 1981, Western Interstate Commission for Higher Education (WICHE).
10. Coutant, N.L.: Rage: implied neurological correlates, Journal of Neurosurgical Nursing 14(1):28, 1982.
11. Csernansky, J., and others: Pharmacologic treatment of aggression, Hospital Formulaiy, 20(10);1091, 1985.
12. Davidhizar, R.E.: Managing the passive-aggressive student nurse, Nurse Education 8(2):34, 1983.
13. Dollard, J., and Miller, N.: Frustration and aggression, New Haven, Conn. 1939, Yale University Press.
14. Duldt, B.W.: Anger: an occupational hazard for nurses, Nursing Outlook 29:510, 1981.
15. Dunne, K.: Anger: normal, appropriate, and justifiable, Maternal-Child Nursing Journal 10(5):316, 1985.
16. Ferguson, M.: The aquarian conspiracy, Los Angeles, 1980, Jeremy P. Tarcher, Inc.
17. Fernandez, T.: Classic: how to deal with overt aggression, Issues in Mental Health Nursing 8(1):79, 1986.
18. Frankl, V.E.: Man's search for meaning, New York, 1959, Pocket Books.
19. Frankl, V.E.: The will to meaning: foundations and applications of logotherapy, New York, 1969, The New American Library, Inc.
20. Friedman, M., and Rosenman, R.H.: Type A behavior and your heart, New York, 1981, Fawcett.
20a. Freud, S.: Mourning and melancholia. In the complete works of Sigmund Freud, vol. 14, London, 1957, The Hogarth Press, Ltd. (Translated by J. Strachey and A. Tyson.)
21. Gesell, A.L., Ilg., F.L., and Ames, L.B.: Youth: the years from ten to sixteen, New York, 1956, Harper & Row, Publishers, Inc.
22. Gesell, A.L., and others: Infant and child in the culture of today: the guidance of development in home and nursery school, rev. ed., New York, 1974, Harper & Row, Publishers, Inc.
23. Gesell, A.L., and others: The child from five to ten, New York, 1977, Harper & Row, Publishers, Inc.
24. Gluck, M: Learning a therapeutic verbal response to anger. . .interactions with patient, Journal of Psychiatric Nursing 19:9, 1981.
25. Goldstein, M.J., Baker, B.L., and Jamison, K.R.: Abnormal psychology experiences, origins, and interventions, Boston, 1980, Little, Brown & Co., Inc.
26. Golub, Z., and others: The ripple effect of anger, 10(5):333, Maternal Child Nursing Journal, 1985.
27. Heck, P: How to keep your poise under pressure, RN 49(6):15, 1986.
28. Herbener, G.: How to control anger, your own and other's, Nursing Life 2(6):42, 1982.
29. Holden, R.: Aggression against nurses, Australian Nurses Journal 15(3):44, 1985.
30. Hollander, S.L.: Spontaneity, sociometry and the warming-up process in family therapy, Psychodrama and Sociometry 34:44, 1981.
30a. Johnson, R.: Aggression in men and animals, Philadelphia, 1972, W.B. Saunders Co.
31. Johnson-Saylor, M.: An exploratory study of the experience of resentment, Western Journal of Nursing Research 8(1):49, 1986.
31a. Lee, I.: Getting things under control: angry nurses, Nursing Life 5(4):26, 1986.
32. Lindgren, K., and others: Avoidance of anger, Maternal-Child Nursing Journal 10(5):320, 1985.
33. Lorenz, K.: On aggression, New York, 1966, Harcourt Brace Jovanovich, Inc.
34. Madow, L.: Anger, New York, 1972, Charles Scribner's Sons.
35. Millon, T.: Disorders of personality: DSM-III: axis II, New York, 1981, Wiley-Interscience.
36. Moran, J.: Aggression management, responses and responsibility, Nursing Times (Part 1) 80(4):28, 1984.
37. Moreno, J.L.: Who shall survive? New York, 1953, Beacon House, Inc.
38. Moreno, J.L.: Sociometric school and science of mankind. In Moreno, J.L., editor: Sociometry and the science of man, New York, 1956, Beacon House, Inc.
39. Moreno, J.L.: The sociometry reader, Chicago, 1960, The Free Press of Glencoe.
40. Moreno, J.L.: Psychodrama, vol. 1, New York, 1970, Beacon House, Inc.
41. Mullahy, P.: Psychoanalysis and interpersonal psychiatry:

the contributions of Harry Stack Sullivan, New York, 1970, Science House, Inc.

42. Needs, A.: Making sense of violence, National Association of Theatre News **23**(1):19, 1986.

43. Neizo, B. and others: Post violence dialogue: perception change through language restructuring, Issues in Mental Health Nursing **6**:245, 1984.

44. Pisarcik, G.: Danger: you are facing the violent patient, Nursing '81 **11**(9):63, 1981.

45. Rubin, T.L.: The angry book, New York, 1969, Macmillan Publishing Co.

46. Sadalla, E., and Burroughs, J.: Profiles in eating, sexy vegetarians and other sex-based social stereotypes, Psychology Today **15**(9):10, 1981.

47. Sanford, K.: How to cope with verbal abuse, Nursing Life **5**(5):52, 1985.

48. Scott, J.: Aggression, Chicago, 1975, The University of Chicago Press.

49. Smeaton, W.: The nature and management of hostility, Nursing **2**(35):1033, 1985.

50. Smitherman, C.: Anger in nursing actions for health promotion, Philadelphia, 1981, F.A. Davis Co.

51. Stuart, R.: Violent behavior: social learning approaches to prediction, management and treatment, New York, 1981, Brunner/Mazel, Inc.

52. Sullivan, H.S.: The interpersonal theory of psychiatry, New York, 1953, W.W. Norton & Co., Inc.

52a. Tardiff, K. and Koenigsberg, H.: Assaultive behavior among psychiatric outpatients, American Journal & Psychiatry, **142**(8):960, 1985.

53. Tarvis, C.: Feeling angry? letting off steam may not be enough, Nursing Life **4**(5):58, 1984.

54. Throwe, A.: Families and alcohol, Critical Care Quarterly **8**(4):79, 1986.

55. Valzelli, L.: Psychology of aggression and violence, New York, 1981, Raven Press.

ANNOTATED BIBLIOGRAPHY

Hamburg, D. and Trudeau, M.: Biobehavioral aspects of aggression, New York, 1981, Alan R. Liss, Inc.

This book presents many perspectives on aggression: biochemical, pharmacological, genetic, psychoendocrinological, as well as views concerning adolescent violence and violence in mental illness and alcoholism.

Lanza, M.: Origins in aggression, Journal of psychiatric nursing and mental health services **21**(6):11, 1983.

The author discusses various theories of aggression and develops a model suggesting that both innate and environmental factors interact to contribute to a person's potential for aggression.

Munns, D.: A validation of the defining characteristics of the nursing diagnosis "potential for violence", Nursing Clinics of North America **20**(4):711, 1985.

This descriptive survey attempts to provide validation for the list of characteristics that define the nursing diagnosis, "potential for violence." The study validates seven of the defining characteristics.

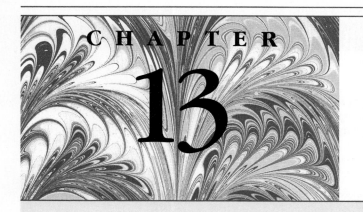

CHAPTER

13

GUILT

Louise Truex Bradford

After studying this chapter the learner will be able to:

Define guilt.

Discuss historical perspectives of guilt.

Describe theories of guilt.

Apply the nursing process to clients with guilt.

Identify current research findings related to guilt.

Guilt is the emotion that occurs when a person does something wrong and expects to be punished or expects that someone will be displeased. It is an internal process used by the mind to ensure that a person behaves in ways consistent with his internal value system. As a voice within the conscience, guilt signals the person that a behavior needs correcting. It is accompanied by a sudden rush of pain that flows inside a person and can range from a mild affect to an intense feeling.

Guilt can be appropriate to the situation and thus be healthy, or it can be absent or excessive for a given situation and thus be unhealthy (Figure 13-1).

Guilt occurs before, during, and after events inconsistent with one's value system. It may be brought on by one's thinking, acting, or feeling. The following common situations represent people experiencing the emotion of guilt:

A couple divorces after their child dies from sudden infant death syndrome.

A family spends their entire savings for the care of a son who became disabled as a result of a car wreck that happened while the father was driving.

A middle-aged recovered alcoholic works for years in Alcoholics Anonymous helping others stay sober.

In these situations, the prevailing theme is people feeling guilt about something they should not have done or something that happened. Each person has a sense of remorse about the past while living in the present.

Many situations evoke strong feelings of guilt, including ill health, sexual activity, abortion, giving birth to a child with birth defects, and surviving a person who has committed suicide or a tragedy in which others died. Nurses are challenged to identify the disruptions this feeling may cause and help the client learn to forgive himself and others and move forward with renewed enthusiasm for life without the intrusion of unhealthy guilt.

THEORETICAL APPROACHES
Psychoanalytic

Freud[15] believed the unconscious superego uses guilt or anxiety from guilt in the conscious mind to limit the individual's immoral behavior. The superego can be harsh, punitive, and blaming, or mild, lenient, and assuming no responsibility. A harsh, punitive superego can ultimately lead to the extreme punishment of the self through various behaviors, such as placation, self-deprecation or self-destruction.

The superego functions within the person as a special "internal monitoring agency." The agency is responsible for self-regulation of behavior to maintain some sort of balance, or equilibrium. The superego houses the internalized parental and social standards of behavior and uses guilt to cause the person to act in accordance with this internalized standard of behavior. If this internalized standard of behavior is extremely rigid and punitive, the person's response to violations of the standard may be guilt out of proportion to the act. If the person has no internalized standard of behavior, the person feels no guilt.

In the psychoanalytic schools, guilt is seen as a signal

🍇 *Historical Overview* 🍇

DATE	EVENT
Ancient times	In the biblical account of the Garden of Eden, Adam and Eve hid their nakedness as a result of shame regarding their bodies and experienced guilt at transgressing God's law.
	Early philosophers referred to guilt as a judgment resulting from violating a law, as well as an internal state.
	Christian religions introduced the concept of grace to deal with guilt from transgressing laws or violating standards of behavior.
1800s	Freud identified guilt as a key concept in psychiatric theory.
1953	Peplau adapted Freud's ideas about guilt and incorporated them into her interpersonal theory of psychiatric nursing by emphasizing the impact of guilt on people's lives.
1970	Guilt, as a motivator of the bargaining stage of death and dying, was incorporated into Kübler-Ross's theory of death and dying.
1980s	Guilt is now recognized as a predominant feeling in many life situations.
Future	The challenge for nursing is to further recognize the disruptiveness of guilt and promote ways to channel it into adaptive behaviors.

that alters instinctual (id) behavior. It is used by the superego to alter the activity of the person's instincts. When guilt is out of proportion to the transgression, it is called "neurotic" guilt. A person who is guilt ridden displays certain behaviors to rid himself of guilt. To deal with a "guilty conscience" a person may accept or provoke abuse or in some way seek rejection. Some people relieve a sense of guilt by giving things or time to others, by trying to please others, or by exhibiting a strong need to be liked. Another response to guilt is "emotional blackmail," in which the individual acts as a target for exploitation by others.

Two types of guilt have been identified: *leftover guilt* and *self-imposed guilt.*[6] Leftover guilt results from early parental conditioning and is shaped by emotional patterns of thinking, feelings, and behavior within the family. For example, a mother pilfered from her husband extra allowance for her son, who knew this. As an adult, the son believed he could not indulge himself and felt inferior and guilty toward his father and toward other honest, hardworking men. He struggled between indulging himself as his mother had done and being the responsible worker and family man his father was.

Self-imposed guilt can be seen in the young, anxious wife who is unable to enjoy her child and husband, feels restricted in her activities, and experiences difficulties in the homemaker role. Both her husband and friends sense what is happening, as does the young woman herself. They urge her to obtain some help with the house and baby, to go out more, and to achieve more balance in her life. She reacts by denying herself the relief from the very responsibilities she protests, generating guilt and a need for self-punishment. She becomes caught in a vicious cycle of self-imposed frustration, anger, and guilt.

During the phallic stage of psychosexual development,

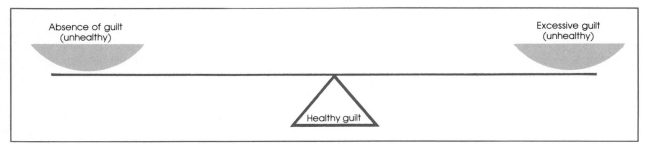

FIGURE 13-1 Guilt continuum.

the child fantasizes vividly and harbors many wishes and desires that are beyond the child's capacity to understand. The male child fears castration and the female child fears retaliation for fantasies, desires, and wishes. If the child demonstrates self-control, a sense of moral responsibility or superego develops. Once the superego is developed, it uses guilt to keep the child's behavior consistent with the intended behavior.

Testing out the environment with improper parental guidance can lead to a superego with an overdeveloped or underdeveloped conscience. The danger in this stage is for the child to control himself to an excessive degree and develop a superego (conscience) that is cruel, lacks compromise, and overuses guilt feelings. The child with an overdeveloped conscience is overly sensitive to parental desires. The child who overregulates himself to comply with parental wishes experiences much guilt. With extremely harsh or permissive parental conditioning the conscience may not develop freely, and the child may become either overly or underly permissive with himself and experience little or no guilt. A moral sense is lacking or is painfully present. A harsh moral sense may lead to varying degrees of guilt.

A healthy conscience motivates the child to control primitive emotions and desires within the norms of society, and guilt is developed in healthy degrees. An excessively tormenting, tyrannical, or punishing conscience limits the child and may not be effective in helping the child change undesirable behavior. Instead, the child may feel extreme guilt and may use ineffective behaviors in dealing with the underlying feelings.

Erikson[11] presented a developmental approach to guilt. In the developmental stage of autonomy versus shame and doubt, from 18 months to 3 years of age, the child internalizes a standard of law and order of family and society. During his quest for autonomy, a beginning conscience emerges. If the child develops a conscience that is oversensitive during this time, it may lead to shame and doubt within the child.

Guilt can be differentiated from shame. When a person is found out and exposed to other people while doing something inconsistent with his self-concept, the resulting feeling is *shame*. Experiences of shame are experiences of exposure of peculiarly sensitive and vulnerable aspects of an individual. Shame, then, is external exposure of one or more aspects of oneself to others. Shame supposes that one is exposed and conscious of being looked at—self-conscious. Shame promotes an increasing sense of being small and is related to feelings of inadequacy and insecurity. Shame is the threat, as well as the exposure, of being found out by others; although it is an individual experience within the person, shame has external consequences accompanying it. Shame reflects the character of the person; that is, what one is. A lack of shame is referred to as unfeeling, brazen, unblushing, or insensitive to oneself and others, whereas guilt feelings tell people that their own internal code of behavior has been transgressed. Both shame and guilt serve to assure society of acceptable be-

---

Research Highlight

Contrasting Experiences of Shame and Guilt

J. Lindsey-Hartz

PURPOSE

This study was designed to differentiate the experience of shame and guilt from each other and from other similar emotions.

SAMPLE

The sample was composed of 19 people, 10 females and 9 males. Ages ranged from 18 to 65 and subjects were of Jewish, Catholic, and Protestant backgrounds.

METHODOLOGY

During individualized interviews, subjects were asked to describe an experience of shame and of guilt. Subjects were given unlabeled descriptions of characteristics of shame and guilt mixed with descriptions of anxiety and depression and asked to select the description that fit their experience of shame and guilt. Four characteristics of shame and four of guilt were tested in this manner. Validity was tested by a second interview using 12 subjects.

FINDINGS

Characteristics of shame included desiring to hide or get out of the situation, feeling small and worthless, having a reticence to talk about the situation, and experiencing a change in one's identity. Characteristics of guilt included needing to talk about and confess the experience, making amends, feeling like a bad person, and experiencing an unsettling of one's identity with violation of a moral code.

IMPLICATIONS

Exploring individual experiences of shame and guilt help identify the positive and negative roles these emotions play in an individual's life. Also, an understanding of these two emotions can enrich an understanding of other emotions such as anxiety and depression and facilitate the integration of these emotions into each person's life.

Based on data from American Behavioral Scientist **27**(6):689, 1984.

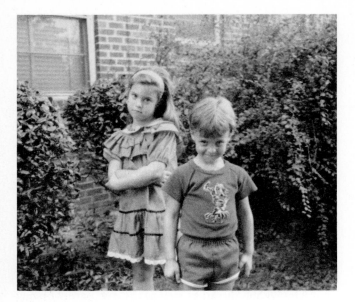

FIGURE 13-2 Children experiencing guilt.

havior from its members.[17] (See the Research Highlight on p. 249.)

Embarrassment is an emotion that is usually incorporated within shame. It is the initial feeling of shame before the person deals with the shame. The physiological reactions of blushing, feeling warm, and feeling as if the heart has skipped a beat are reactions to embarrassment. Situations that produce embarrassment can be explored to help the person identify embarrassing situations and gain a better understanding of himself.

Guilt is distinct from worry. Guilt is occupying present moments by thinking about the past. *Worry* involves being concerned in the present about something in the future. The central factor in each is that the person is not living each day to the fullest extent because of preoccupation with the past or the future.

Guilt can be distinguished from guilty fear.[17] *Guilty fear* is the intense flood of feeling that occurs when the individual is in the process of doing something disapproved of, illegal, or immoral. The feeling of guilty fear is associated with the fear of getting what is deserved. Guilty fears seeks to avoid punishment, whereas guilt needs forgiveness, exposure, and exoneration. However, guilt can promote self-hate to such a degree that forgiveness by punishment does not eliminate the feeling.

In the stage of initiative versus guilt, from ages 3 to 6, the child begins to be curious about the surrounding world. The child seeks new experiences and explores new situations. If guilt does not dominate this stage, successful development of initiative occurs. Mastering the initiative stage produces a child who can cooperate, plan, solve problems, and relate to other people. Guilt occurs when the child does something for which he can be punished or incur parental displeasure (Figure 13-2). For example, if the child wants to please his parents but soils his pants, guilt results.

Table 13-1 summarizes various terms related to guilt.

TABLE 13-1 Various terms related to guilt

Term	Definition
Guilt	The feeling evoked when one does something wrong, is possibly going to be punished, or provoke another's displeasure
Leftover guilt	The feeling of guilt shaped from patterns of behavior as a result of early parental conditioning
Self-imposed guilt	A feeling of guilt a person brings on oneself
Shame	The feeling of exposure of one or more aspects of oneself to others
Embarrassment	The initial feeling of shame that produces a behavior such as blushing or feeling warm all over
Worry	A concern in the present about something in the future
Guilty fear	An intense flood of feeling when one is in the process of doing something immoral, disapproved of, or illegal

Interpersonal

In his interpersonal theory Sullivan[46] said that guilt follows a violation of one's moral code or ideal system. Sullivan viewed guilt as a conscious process. Guilt is in the person's awareness and occurs when the person knows what he is doing or at least knows soon afterward what he has done. It is a form of anxiety. A person's internal regulating system is the "ideal system"; it houses the standard of behavior and functions as a policeman.

Sullivan described "crazy guilt" as a form of anxiety used to escape one's conscious awareness and thus the pain of anxiety. With crazy guilt, through the process of rationalizing one's behavior to oneself, the person avoids the anxiety that accompanies guilt. The antisocial person fits the category of crazy guilt. Antisocial persons, whose disorder may be the result of improper (too harsh, too little, or inconsistent) discipline, have failed to develop a conscience. These people manipulate and use others for personal gain. They are lacking an appropriate internal value system and sense of responsibility. Guilt is not a motivator to regulate their behavior in accordance with society's norms.

Unhealthy guilt can range from mild to severe. A person may seek some form of punishment that ranges from inciting verbal abuse from significant others to suicide. People who feel guilty may see their wrongdoings and shortcomings as deserving punishment. A strong need for punishment may lead clients to do anything to invite people to punish them. Self-punishment may lead to self-destruction. Guilt may become a self-defeating spiral, and the person may attempt suicide if the nurse cannot successfully intervene in this unhealthy spiral and help the client lessen the amount of guilt.

Cognitive

According to Piaget,[41] moral judgment goes through a series of stages. An internalized standard of behavior develops during these stages. Moral values from the parents are internalized by the child, and conscience develops. As cognitive processes develop, the adolescent and young adult examine their own moral sense of right and wrong and go through the process of choosing values for themselves. Meanwhile, the trained or overtrained conscience is at work within the person keeping behavior in line with one's moral values.

Guilt is both a motivator and a product. It can motivate one to behave in certain ways, and it can be the resultant emotional state produced by certain events. For example, a teenage girl's anticipation of guilt for violating her internal moral standard of behavior during dating can cause her to act in harmony with her values. Guilt occurs if she violates her standard of behavior. Conflicts may also occur for her if she does not know what her beliefs are. In the process of discovering her beliefs, she may act in a way that is inconsistent with her beliefs and may not discover until afterward that she holds a particular belief. Regardless of whether she thinks beforehand that her actions will bother her or becomes aware of the conflict between her values and her behavior only when she violates her values, the resultant painful feeling is guilt.

As a motivator guilt has healthy and unhealthy components. Healthy guilt can keep one's behavior in line with one's value system. Guilt can signal violations of conscience. Like anxiety, healthy guilt can motivate one to certain actions that may be viewed as positive depending on one's life orientation. Healthy guilt may cause one to visit a sick friend, go to school, study for a test, go to church, or speak when spoken to in a social situation. A person wanting to be liked by other people may be motivated by feelings of guilt.

Ellis theorized that people can organize and discipline their thinking to make inner thoughts more rational.[8] Individuals feel the way they think. The person's internal feeling state can be influenced and changed by changing the way a person thinks about situations and events. For example, a nursing student who makes a medication error may feel certain emotions, possibly shame and guilt. The student nurse may feel shame when her instructor becomes aware of her error and guilty because of her error and the possibility of punishment. Every time she is asked to give medicine after this incident, the student may feel guilt associated with making the first medication error. However, the student may also think through the problem and thus relieve her guilt by the cognitive process. Four things may happen: (1) the medication error occurs, (2) the student internally evaluates the event, (3) her evaluation results in the emotion of guilt, and (4) the guilt is relieved by reexamination of irrational thoughts about the error (Figure 13-3). The resultant emotions are individual reactions. In the same situation, some student nurses may have felt anger at the instructor for allowing the error to be made, disgust with themselves for the error, or worry over their progression in the nursing program. Each student has a characteristic response according to the student's personality and life experience.

Communication

Transactional analysis, developed by Berne,[4] depicts the person as having three ego states: (1) the Parent, (2) the Adult, and (3) the Child. The Parent ego state stores all of the messages a child receives from the family, such

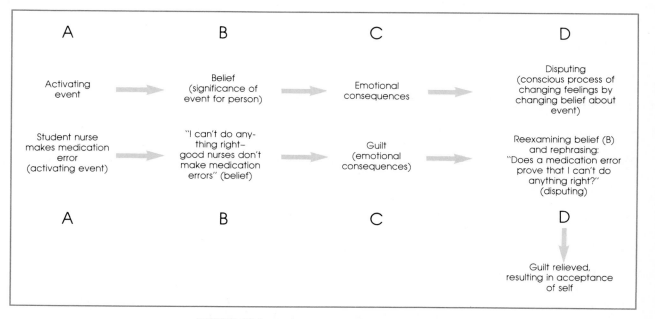

FIGURE 13-3 Application of Ellis' theory of guilt.

as "Do this," "Do that," "Hurry up," and "You should." Parents set the parameters of behavior for children by telling them what they "should" and "should not" do. These messages register in the child's mind and are rehearsed. As the child encounters situations, these *should*'s and *should not*'s are recalled. If the person has excessive "should" or "should not" messages stored up, the person may have a rich source for the origin of guilt feelings. Critical messages come from the part of the parent called the Critical Parent.

The Child ego state is the part of the personality responsible for free feelings and primitive emotions. Anger, sadness, gladness, and fear are examples of feelings arising from the Child ego state.

The Adult ego state is the center for regulation, mediation, and decision making between the Child and Parent ego states. It is like a computer processing center with information from the Parent and Child coming in and going out. The Adult takes the *should not*'s from the Parent and the *go ahead*'s and feelings from the Child and renders a decision about the person's behavior.

Guilt is self-punishment and represents a trial between the Parent and the Child. The Parent functions as the judge and the Child functions as the defendant as if a trial were going on in the person's head.[23] Guilt may also be a result of parental programming to live out one's life in a certain way. This life script guides the actions of a person.[3]

Guilt may be based on a script in which a person feels responsible for other people.[45] This person rescues people rather than allowing others to solve their own problems or care for themselves. For example, a mother may rescue her son in a divorce. She may bail him out of financial trouble or take care of his home, meals, and laundry. Her actions may be motivated by feeling guilty that she did not give her son what he needed while growing up or that in some way she was responsible for the divorce because of her nonparental guidance.

Table 13-2 summarizes various theories of guilt.

RELATING TO THE CLIENT

Nurses need to develop a sensitivity in relating to the person who feels embarrassed, shamed, or guilty. One of the most difficult aspects of dealing with guilt is the private nature of the things one feels guilty about. They are the very things one wants to hide, not talk about. Respect, acceptance, and empathic understanding on the part of the nurse help the client establish contact with and confidence in the nurse, which enables the client to discuss his guilt feelings openly.

In the working phase of the relationship, the nurse considers that guilt is often a lifelong pattern and one that is not easy for clients to change. The nurse may become frustrated and needs to recognize that change is slow. Clients who feel excessive guilt can be difficult to deal with, especially if they refuse to give up ingrained guilt responses. Often the nurse becomes insensitive and frustrated and feels helpless. Responding to the helplessness, the nurse may flee the situation and avoid the client.

Self-awareness can help the nurse deal constructively with her own responses to clients experiencing guilt. Sad stories and woeful tales may promote a feeling of sadness or pity in the nurse. Awareness of these feelings is essential to prevent the nurse from withdrawing from the client or from responding with pity or sympathy.

The nurse may attempt to force the client to react to guilt as the nurse herself may. The nurse needs to guard against this tendency when relating to the client experiencing guilt, since it may serve to increase the client's feeling of guilt. She does not force her values in dealing with guilt on the client.

While interacting with the client, the nurse may feel guilt kindled within herself. Often *overidentification* with the client can produce this feeling. For example, a divorced nurse during an interaction with a client who is in the process of divorce listens. The client express guilt about his part in contributing to the divorce. As the client discusses the situation, the nurse finds it difficult to concentrate on the client's conversation, since her mind drifts

TABLE 13-2 Summary of theories of guilt

Theory	Theorist	Dynamics
Psychoanalytic	Freud	Healthy guilt motivates one to control primitive emotions and drives. Guilt is used by the superego to alter instinctual activity and limit the individual's behavior.
	Erikson	Successful completion of the initiative versus guilt stage of development results in a person who is curious, can solve problems, and can relate to others without excessive guilt.
Interpersonal	Sullivan	Guilt occurs when a person does something for which he can be punished or receive parental disapproval. Some persons with guilt have a need to be punished. Those without guilt are seen as persons with antisocial behavior.
Cognitive	Piaget	Guilt follows a violation of one's moral code or ideal system. Guilt motivates one to behave in certain ways.
	Ellis	The person's internal feeling state (guilt) can be influenced by changing the way a person thinks about events or situations.
Communication	Berne	Guilt may be the result of parental programming to live one's life in a certain way. Parental messages of "should" and "ought" act as one's conscience and an internalized standard of behavior.

to her own marriage that failed and her feelings of guilt about the divorce. The nurse's effectiveness is hampered by her overidentification with the client. The nurse who uses active listening skills to understand the situation from the client's viewpoint can set limits on her own identification. The nurse monitors her own empathetic response, searches within herself to allow full understanding of the client's problem, and prevents her own feelings from unduly influencing her response.

The client experiencing guilt may be acting in such a way as to seek punishment from others. The nurse resists the tempation to punish the client.

Perhaps the most difficult situation of all is working with the client who experiences no guilt or remorse for harmful acts of wrongdoing. Remaining nonjudgmental and accepting the client as a human being worthy of care regardless of his behavior can tax the essence of a nurse's being. A strong self-concept, feelings of high self-esteem, and a strong support system as well as knowledge and understanding about the psychopathological condition involved prepare the nurse for dealing with the client who has no guilt feelings.

At the termination stage of the relationship the nurse may reflect on her work with the client and think that she did not do enough to help the client, particularly when the client continues to have distressing symptoms. She may feel guilt regarding what she did or did not do to help the client ease his distress. At this point, the nurse needs to accept herself and acknowledge that she provided the best care of which she and other team members were capable at the time. If she continues to be bothered by these feelings it is helpful to discuss them with another professional.

NURSING PROCESS
Assessment

Physical dimension. The physical manifestations of guilt are much like those of anxiety. Guilt may produce changes in physiological processes such as tachycardia, palpitations, dry mouth, sweaty palms, loss of appetite, nausea, fainting, nervousness, hyperventilation, diarrhea, and urinary frequency and urgency. (See Chapter 11.)

The person who feels guilty may avoid eye contact, fidget, sit motionless, stare, shuffle feet, or blush. Some phrases the client may use to describe the somatic symptoms associated with guilt are "tightness in the chest," "chest pain," "heart flip-flops," "butterflies in the stomach," "heart feels like it's running away with me," "can't sit still," and "skin feels like it's crawling."

Guilt may trigger the stress ("fight or flight") response in the body.[43] In response to a threat to the person, such as guilt, the general adaptation syndrome is activated to help the body deal with stress. To handle stressors, the sympathetic nervous system prepares the person to take action in dealing with the stressor. Thus the sympathetic nervous system is responsible for the physical manifestations of guilt. Guilt may be accompanied by symptoms in the intestinal region and disturbances of circulation and breathing that are similar to those produced by anxiety.

The person who feels guilty may use drugs and alcohol to decrease the intensity of the guilt feelings.

Emotional dimension. The client may describe guilt as a vague, diffuse, uncomfortable feeling (the pangs of conscience) much like anxiety. He may simply look, act, and state that he is not happy. The individual may describe feelings of heaviness or burden commonly seen as a significant aspect of the grieving process. (See the Research Highlight on p. 254.)

The client may report feeling ashamed, embarrassed, or indicate a lack of self-forgiveness and a feeling of unworthiness and self-condemnation. The affect may be subdued, depressed, or inappropriate, or it may be intensified. Flooded with internal feelings, the client may cry a lot. Internally the person may experience pain from an unknown source and describe it as "just not feeling right." Disguised forms of guilt are sadness, despair, hopelessness, helplessness, and limited capacity to enjoy life.

Anger or aggression may be a disguised form of guilt. The open expression of aggression serves as a release of the guilt feelings.

Feelings of inferiority may indicate guilt feelings within the client. Both are related to anxiety and represent tension between the ego and superego. Guilt, as discussed earlier, relates to wrongdoing, whereas feelings of inferiority relate to weakness and inadequacy. Guilt feelings may lead to submission, subordination, and dependence. With shame, the person may feel a tendency to hide his face or flee the situation.

Intellectual dimension. Individuals experiencing guilt are usually preoccupied with the guilt-producing situation and cannot forgive themselves. This preoccupation produces a shortened attention span and a decreased capacity to learn new things. The person may block intellectual content from conscious awareness and be forgetful and confused. The person's decision-making and problem-solving skills are less effective.

Preoccupation with guilt alters the person's perception into "tunnel vision," in which perception of the world is narrowed. Instead of seeing the world through rose-colored glasses, the person sees the world through the gray tint of guilt.

With selective inattention, the person perceives negative feedback as acceptable, processes this sensory information, and ignores additional sensory input. Compliments add to the feelings of guilt, increasing the need for punishment for wrongdoing. Thus compliments are filtered out or ignored as a protective mechanism. For example, if a man feels guilt about the care he is giving his elderly parents, he may not accept any compliments that he receives about the care.

Guilt may also cause obsessive thoughts, which result in compulsive acts to cancel the obsessive thoughts. A high degree of punctuality, rigid adherence to rules, and orderliness are all compulsive behaviors that the person uses to undo guilt. Compulsive actions are used by the mind to cancel out obsessive thoughts. For example, a woman who thinks sexual thoughts and feels guilty about them may keep her house excessively clean. This can be a symbolic way of cleaning up her thoughts. The obsessive

Counseling Families Experiencing Guilt

S. Johnson

PURPOSE

The study was implemented to test the author's proposed model for assessing grief in couples who experienced the death of their child.

SAMPLE

The sample consisted of 14 couples who had a child die during the previous 12 months. The parents' ages ranged from 24 to 54. All were white, middle-income families. All couples professed Christianity, as their religious preference except one couple who said they were atheists.

METHODOLOGY

Eight of the couples had 2 weeks or less warning that the child's death was imminent and were placed in a short prep-aration group (SPG). Six of the couples had 15 days or more warning and were placed in a long preparation group (LPG). Three structured interviews were conducted on each group.

FINDINGS

Through the interviews, a total of 451 guilt statements evolved from both groups. Every parent in the SPG expressed guilt feelings, as did all but one man in the LPG. The SPG had significantly more guilt statements than the LPG and the women had significantly more than the men.

IMPLICATIONS

If guilt is a factor in a parent's physical or mental health, then the SPG parents may be at a higher risk than the LPG parents. To prevent the destructive potential of guilt to the person and family it is essential that nurses recognize guilt reactions and channel them toward effective ways of dealing with them.

Based on data from Dimensions in Critical Care Nursing 3:238, 1984.

thought motivated by guilt is cancelled by the actions of cleanliness. Defense mechanisms such as undoing, displacement, regression, protection, reaction formation, rationalization, and somatization may be called on by the mind to handle guilt.

Perfectionism is another characteristic that may result in guilt feelings. It is the obsessive desire to maintain high standards that the person has set for himself. Guilt results when the person cannot live up to his own high standards. The client may limit his striving for perfectionism to himself or he may impose his own standard of perfectionism onto others. Guilt arises when the standard is violated.

A guilt-ridden person may wish for self-punishment. Ways in which a client's need for punishment is expressed include recriminating statements such as "It's my fault" or "I'm to blame" and statements containing "should" and "should not" or "ought to" or "ought not to." A client may also communicate a sense of disgrace as well as an invitation to criticism from others by behavior that seeks negative statements as punishment for feelings of guilt. Other indicators of guilt may include a tendency to argue one's point, blaming or unjustly criticizing another, being rude or defiant, and offering excuses or explanations for failures or forgetfulness.

A person may also show guilt by defending a friend or a cause. Whatever is defended is tantamount to the person's admitting that he is sensitive to just such an attack.

Kidding, a mild form of criticism or making fun of another person, may represent something to which the kid-

der himself is sensitive and hence may also be an expression of guilt.

❀ *Social dimension.* Interactions and relationships with others are disrupted for the person with guilt feelings. Some clients act as if they are seeking pity or sympathy from the nurse. This is exemplified in the "poor defenseless me" attitude or "I feel sorry for myself" attitude. Arguing with others may be an attempt to cover up guilt, and withdrawing from others a device used to avoid and deny one's guilt.

The client with excessive guilt feelings may demonstrate dependence in relationships. The overreliance on others to meet one's needs, both physical and emotional, can be seen as a manipulative attempt to compensate for one's inadequacies. The assessment of anger, hostility, resentment, and ambivalence about the relationship is essential in determining whether the client has underlying guilt feelings.

An assessment of family relationships and child-rearing practices may provide data about the client who feels guilty. In general, parents assume moral responsibility for their children, punishing them for disapproved acts and rewarding approved acts. A child may show guilt by submitting without protest to the wishes of his parents.

The child learns guilt as a result of transgressing the parent's standard of behavior. Through adherence to limits set by the parents, the child gives up self-will and manipulation and learns that his behavior has limits. As a result of this process, the child adopts an internal standard

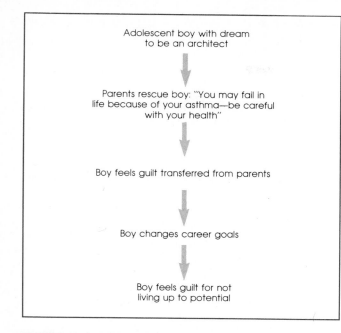

Adolescent boy with dream
to be an architect

↓

Parents rescue boy: "You may fail in
life because of your asthma—be careful
with your health"

↓

Boy feels guilt transferred from parents

↓

Boy changes career goals

↓

Boy feels guilt for not
living up to potential

FIGURE 13-4 Adolescent boy experiencing guilt.

of behavior and the locus of control moves from outside (parental) to internal (the child's).

People who are ridden with guilt may not fully develop their potential. They may have jobs with less responsibility than their abilities indicate because feelings of guilt are holding them back. For example, an 18-year-old boy with asthma goes to a vocational school to study drafting rather than to a college to study architecture, which is his lifetime dream. His family has overprotected him because of the physical illness and tried to rescue him from failure in life by telling him he could not do things because of his numerous asthmatic attacks. Although the message from the family was "If you fail, it is because of your physical limitations; be careful with your health," the adolescent heard the message as "You can't do anything." The guilt felt by the parents in producing an unhealthy child was transferred to the boy and incorporated as his own feeling of guilt. The boy's guilt was manifested as lowering of his goal in life. The boy now feels further guilt for not living up to his potential. (See Figure 13-4).

✂ *Spiritual dimension.* The nurse also looks at the client's personal philosophy and spiritual and religious beliefs. The nurse observes for any discrepancies and conflicts between the client's beliefs and behavior as a potential source of guilt. Persons who lead highly moral and religious lives or who are overly polite, courteous, and proper may have put aside tendencies to resist, to rebel, or to defend against attacks of others. The purer the life, the more painful are the feeling of guilt associated with backslidings from the set of high moral standards. The perfectionist must hold himself to his high standards to avoid feelings of guilt that may result were he to relax or fail.

The person's level of self-forgiveness needs to be assessed. Lack of self-forgiveness may be observed as constant helplessness, doing religious or volunteer work in an attempt to undo some feelings of guilt, berating oneself as unworthy, leaving the religious group if one's level of guilt feelings becomes too high, and self-destructive behavior such as suicide.

The nurse inquires about the client's religious beliefs and practices to identify tension or conflict between the beliefs and the client's practice of the beliefs. For example, the hospitalized client with a strong religious faith may feel guilty about his lack of participation in a religious activity or ritual, such as communion, prayer, or eating kosher food.

Behaviors that demonstrate guilt and shame include

SPIRITUAL DISTRESS

DEFINITION

Disruption of a person's life that pervades their entire being and which integrates and transcends their biological and psychosocial nature.

DEFINING CHARACTERISTICS
Physical Dimension
Unable to participate in usual religious practices
Sleep disturbances or nightmares
Emotional Dimension
Anger toward God or other supreme power
Anger
Crying
Anxiety
Hostility
Apathy
Discouraged
Intellectual Dimension
Questions meaning of suffering
Verbalizes inner conflict about beliefs
Verbalizes concern about relationship with deity
Rejects humor
Displacement of anger toward religious representatives
Unable to forgive and be forgiven
Preoccupation
Social Dimension
Withdrawal
Feels alienated or ostracized
Separation from religious or cultural ties
Spiritual Dimension
*Expresses concern over meaning of life, death, and belief system
Questions meaning of own existance
Seeks spiritual assistance
Questions moral and ethical implications of therapeutic regimen
Challenges belief and value system
Hopelessness

Adapted from North American Nursing Diagnosis Association Classification of Nursing Diagnosis: Proceedings of the seventh conference, St. Louis, 1987, The C.V. Mosby Co.
*Indicates characteristics in addition to those defined by NANDA

wishing to undo, redo, or relive the past; expressing regret, sinfulness, bitterness, or recriminations, viewing one's illness as a punishment from God, or devaluing self. Persons experiencing guilt limit their ability to enjoy and appreciate life. The burden of negative feelings of guilt leaves the client with little energy to create satisfactions in day-to-day living and in life in general. It becomes essential that the nurse explore with the client at an appropriate time his views about how life in general has treated him.

Measurement tools. The Mosher Forced-Choice Guilt Scale can be given to measure feelings of guilt. The test determines whether subjects have guilt and can quantify the guilt level as high or low.[30]

Analysis

Nursing diagnosis. Spiritual distress is a nursing diagnosis approved by NANDA that applies to the person with guilt. The defining characteristics of the nursing diagnosis are listed in the box on p. 255.

The following list provides examples of NANDA-accepted nursing diagnoses with causative statements.
1. Ineffective coping: guilt related to inability to live up to own expectations
2. Ineffective coping: guilt related to error in judgement
3. Ineffective coping: guilt related to excessive drinking
4. Alteration in thought processes: guilt related to preoccupation with guilt
5. Powerlessness related to self-defeating pattern of guilt
6. Spiritual distress related to guilt about past life experiences
7. Disturbance in self-concept: low self-esteem related to guilt associated with feelings of inadequacy

The following Case Example demonstrates the characteristics of the nursing diagnosis spiritual distress.

Case Example

Ada Stephensen, a 51-year-old woman, recently placed her mother, age 73 in a nursing home. Her mother lived with her until 3 months ago when her mother underwent exploratory surgery and was found to have cancer. Her mother returned home after the surgery. In the last month, her mother's condition has become worse. She is now bedfast and requires constant and total care. During her daily visit to her mother Ms. Stephensen expresses to the nurse feelings of guilt at placing her mother in a nursing home. The nurse observes Ms. Stephensen wringing her hands as she speaks and notices her loss of weight. She states that her mother took good care of her when she was a child and now she has abandoned her when she needed her most.

Ms. Stephensen's belief that she should care for her mother has been violated. She feels guilty about placing her mother in a nursing home as evidenced by her body language, weight loss and daily visits to see her mother. While the care of her mother is too complicated for her

to manage, she feels like she is letting her mother down in her time of need.

Planning

See Table 13-3 for examples of long-term and short-term goals and outcome criteria. These serve as examples of the planning stage in the nursing process.

Implementation

Physical dimension. Because the physical characteristics of guilt are similar to those of anxiety, interventions aimed at reducing anxiety are helpful for the client experiencing guilt. (See Chapter 11.)

The nurse points out the presence of physical symptoms (avoiding eye contact, fidgeting, restlessness, staring, blushing, and nail biting) to help the client identify his feelings of guilt, promote awareness, and gain some insight about the cause of the feelings.

Shame associated with perceived unpleasant or unattractive aspects of one's physical appearance can be alleviated by use of empathic statements that communicate understanding of the problem. Helping the client realistically appraise the aspect of himself that causes shame or embarrassment and focus on attractive aspects of his body fosters positive attitudes about body image and over time may lessen the shame or embarrassment.

For the client with excessive guilt who may be self-destructive hospitalization with suicide precautions is indicated. Removing sharp objects and monitoring possessions is essential for the client who is considered self-destructive. (See Chapter 14.)

Emotional dimension. Encouraging the client to express feelings of embarrassment, shame, and guilt is essential. Gradually, as the intensity of the feelings diminishes and the client accepts the feelings as appropriate and realistic for the situation, other positive areas of the client's life can be emphasized. The nurse's acceptance of the client who cries or expresses anger and resentment indicates that this is an appropriate response to the situation.

The nurse works with the client to increase feelings of adequacy. Ways in which feelings of adequacy are increased include seeking out the client, spending meaningful time with him, helping him identify his strengths and positive aspects, providing positive reinforcement, and providing diversionary activities. The nurse may also elevate the client's feelings of adequacy by helping him learn a new skill or by being part of the client's achievements.

Intellectual dimension. The preoccupation some clients have with guilt about past experiences traps them into being unwilling and inflexible about learning new ways of coping. They believe they have no choice about the situation and that guilt about the past cannot change. The nurse helps these clients understand that they can choose to change and thus free themselves from guilt feelings about the past, as in the following Case Example.

TABLE 13-3 Long-term and short-term goals and outcome criteria related to guilt

Goals	Outcome Criteria

NURSING DIAGNOSIS: INEFFECTIVE COPING: GUILT RELATED TO PAST UNACCEPTABLE BEHAVIOR

Long-term goals

Goals	Outcome Criteria
To develop satisfying relationships with people free of excessive guilt	Makes statements that are positive toward significant others Has no preoccupation with guilt in conversations Exhibits no evidence of self-criticism in statements to others Engages in no observable self-destructive behaviors Appropriately verbalizes guilt to others
To accept self and past behavior	Verbalizes acceptance of self Makes statements of feeling accepted States that past behavior is a part of self Engages in no self-destructive behaviors Verbalizes that self is forgiven for past behavior Appears comfortable with present behavior Uses eye contact while interacting with people

Short-term goals

Goals	Outcome Criteria
To examine and clarify past situation	Discusses past situation Acknowledges consequences to the self of past behavior Verbalizes what past behavior means to him Expresses feelings that come into awareness Expresses feelings related to guilt Verbalizes realistic elements of past behavior
To examine beliefs and values and their relationship to past behavior	Discusses beliefs and values Verbalizes how past behavior fits in value system Engages in problem solving about beliefs and values to determine their relevance Makes statements that reflect self-awareness
To forgive self for past behavior	Verbalizes forgiveness of self Exhibits no self-destructive behavior Makes no verbal statements of self-criticism Uses eye contact when discussing past behavior Makes no complaints of physical symptoms of anxiety Acknowledges wrongs that have been done Makes statements that reflect self-acceptance
To deal constructively with the truth	Verbally admits feelings of guilt Makes statements about guilt feelings that are appropriate to the situation Acknowledges own responsibility in situations that happen Uses physical activity to drain off tension produced by inner feelings Verbalizes own limitations Demonstrates no physical symptoms from feelings of guilt
To profit from experience caused by past behavior	States what has been learned from past experiences Predicts new behavior for future to ensure alternative ways of dealing with similar situations Uses problem solving to develop new behaviors for the future Acknowledges consequences for self that past experiences have produced Verbalizes awareness of consequences of behavior Makes statements attempting to predict consequences for behavior before it occurs Verbalizes feelings of guilt appropriate to the situation
To establish a satisfactory nurse-client relationship	Discusses thoughts and feelings freely Opens up and shares feelings with the nurse Keeps appointments, is punctual, and shares personal information

Continued.

TABLE 13-3 Long-term and short-term goals and outcome criteria related to guilt—cont'd

Goals	Outcome Criteria

NURSING DIAGNOSIS: INEFFECTIVE COPING: GUILT RELATED TO LOSS OF VALUED OBJECT

Long-term goals

Goals	Outcome Criteria
To establish realistic acceptance of loss	Discusses loss realistically Makes statements reflecting acceptance of loss Shows no evidence of unusual emotionality while discussing loss
To develop satisfying relationships with people	Makes positive statements about significant others Interacts regularly with significant others Makes statements that reflect a realistic view of the loss Exhibits no observable signs of excessive guilt Discusses loss without excessive emotion Makes eye contact while discussing the loss

Short-term goals

Goals	Outcome Criteria
To identify feelings of guilt related to loss	Verbalizes awareness of feelings of guilt Associates guilt feelings with loss when appropriate
To examine feelings associated with loss	Verbalizes feelings about loss Discusses loss
To seek relationships with people	Makes an effort to be with people Talks with people Makes eye contact with people

NURSING DIAGNOSIS: INEFFECTIVE COPING RELATED TO A LIFELONG PATTERN OF GUILT FROM OVERLY SENSITIVE CONSCIENCE

Long-term goals

Goals	Outcome Criteria
To adopt healthy coping mechanisms	Makes verbal statements of methods of handling guilt Reports being able to handle guilt Tries new coping styles and behavior
To exhibit satisfaction with self	Makes statements that reflect self-acceptance Asserts self Makes positive statements about self
To enjoy life	Laughs and smiles appropriately Verbalizes enjoyment of life Shows no self-destructive behavior Shows no preoccupation with guilt in conversation Pursues hobbies

Short-term goals

Goals	Outcome Criteria
To intervene in own pattern of guilt	Makes no verbal statements reflecting guilt Makes eye contact Avoids words like "should" and "ought" Lacks complaints of physical symptoms Shows no preoccupation with guilt in conversation
To accept self	Makes statements that reflect self-acceptance Does not allow others to take advantage of self Buys things for self States that he is able to spend time alone Makes positive statements about self

Case Example

Jeannie came to counseling because she was nervous and anxious and could not get through a day without blaming herself for her parents' divorce 8 years ago. She was now 45 years old, and both parents were dead. By examining the futility of blaming herself during the course of therapy and being helped to see her ineffective coping behaviors, Jeannie began to believe in her own ability to choose other ways of coping with the guilt. Rather than continuing to feel guilt, she chose to believe she was not the cause of her parents' divorce and left guilt feelings in the past.

Persons feeling guilt label themselves negatively, for example, "I'm at fault" or "I'm to blame." The nurse can help the client promote realistic expectations for himself by exploring with the client the reasons for the self-blame, what he thinks causes it, whether others important to him would agree with the negative label, and whether it is realistic. Through cognitive restructuring the nurse can assist the client change negative "self talk" and form positive perceptions of himself. Skillful communication techniques

Adapted from Fensterheim, H., and Baer, J.: Stop running scared! New York, 1977, Dell Publishing Co., Inc.

such as validation and clarification assist the client in discussing his self-criticisms. In addition, behavior modification in the form of *thought stopping* helps the client limit negative thoughts about himself. The box above gives the techniques of thought stopping.

Disputing[9] involves the nurse confronting the client with the irrational idea upon which he has formed his conclusion. For example, the mother of a retarded child may feel guilt because she believes she caused the child to be retarded. The nurse confronts her belief and assists her in exploring more rational explanations of her childs retardation.

Imagery is a therapeutic technique for use with clients experiencing guilt. The nurse finds out if the client can imagine how it would be and what it would feel like to be free of excessive guilt. The nurse also explores what the client would like to feel. Then the nurse helps the client relax and gives him suggestions that facilitate the client's experiencing freedom from excessive guilt. A tape can be made of the session, and the client is given the homework assignment of listening to the tape.

Some persons are unable to free themselves from guilt produced by an action or situation. They do not have the conscious ability or will to choose another course of action. The nurse can help these persons by acknowledging their guilt without minimizing the intensity of the feeling or denying the feeling and by asking how long they intend to continue punishing themselves.

Social dimension. Interventions in the social dimension focus on relationships and methods of interrupting patterns of withdrawal, dependence, and alienation or isolation that characterize persons who feel guilty. When a person avoids a friend because he owes the friend some money, simply paying back the money provides restitution and can relieve one of feeling guilty. The estrangement of the two friends may also be restored. The nurse assists the client by showing him how to make restitution. The nurse rehearses with client what he would like to say and prepares the client for possible responses from the other person. The client may write a letter, pro-

vide monetary compensation, or make an apology to rectify the situation that has contributed to the client's feeling of guilt. In other situations, in which the guilt feelings are more intense and the person isolates himself from others, the nurse becomes a support system for the client until supportive members of the family can be identified and assisted in understanding the person and his problem with guilt.

Clients who have excessively dependent personalities and at the same time resent the dependence harbor feelings of guilt over the anger and resentment. The nurse can help the client by facilitating the expression of his feelings of anger and resentment. (Chapter 12 discusses interventions for anger.)

The client who feels no guilt and who has committed a criminal act is usually placed in a psychiatric hospital for evaluation of his behavior or in a prison for punishment. In either of these cases, he is socially isolated until he is found competent to stand trial or is determined to be mentally ill.

Assertiveness helps the person who feels guilt by restoring control and power within his relationships. In addition, the person who can assert himself strengthens his self-concept. (Chapter 16 discusses ways in which clients can become assertive.)

Spiritual dimension. Interventions for clients experiencing guilt primarily promote a sense of being forgiven for wrongdoings. For many persons, the church performs the role of forgiver; members can confess, chant, pray, or repent and have their transgressions forgiven. Not only does the church forgive, but it also is seen as a deterrent for wrongdoings. The fear of punishment of God's wrath for disobeying the Biblical teachings is emphasized in many religions.

Clients who experience guilt and have no ties to organized religion are asked by the nurse to explore what they have stopped doing because of guilt feelings and to what their self-imposed punishment is related. Thus the nurse helps the client forgive himself; make restitution, if appropriate; and be more forgiving of others.

The experience of guilt is a separating experience. Interventions are aimed at identifying values and reconciling the estrangement so that the person can be relieved of guilt, can learn to live with his guilt, or can transcend the discomfort and conflict and become a more fully functioning, creative, whole person.

INTERACTION WITH A CLIENT EXPERIENCING GUILT

Nurse: (In nurse's office counseling a college student.) *Connie, what's on your mind today?*

Client: I've lost my boyfriend. I really can't believe that I said what I said. It's just not like me at all.

Nurse: Connie, tell me what happened.

Client: Well, I told him he wasn't good enough for me and I would always have a better job than him and other things. Now, after being away for the summer, I realized that it was wrong, especially after seeing him with someone else. I can't believe that I was so cruel to him.

Nurse: It sounds like you are feeling some guilt and are ashamed of your treatment of your boyfriend.
Client: Oh yes, I'm feeling guilty. I'm having trouble getting it off my mind.
Nurse: It sounds like you haven't forgiven yourself.
Client: Oh no! How can I forgive myself for being so cruel?
Nurse: Connie, what you did comes from a side of you that you are not proud of; nonetheless, it is a part of you. All of us have those things in our lives that we are not proud of. The past cannot be changed. Perhaps, when you've had a chance to talk with him and make your peace with him, you will be able to forgive yourself.
Client: I'd like to forgive myself if I could.
Nurse: It sounds to me like you are saying, "I'd like to forgive myself if I 'should'."
Client: Yes, I guess I am.
Nurse: It's OK to forgive yourself. Would you do the same thing today?
Client: No.
Nurse: Then, you've learned from the situation.
Client: Yes, I have. I've learned that I feel awful when I hurt people. I just don't know what to say to him.
Nurse: Let's take some time to practice talking to him.

The nurse deals with guilt by helping the student express her feeling and deal with it realistically. The nurse helps the student accept the feeling as a part of herself within the context that other people have similar guilt-producing experiences. The nurse also verbalizes the unspoken "should" on which the student is operating and gives the student permission to forgive herself.

One of the most powerful tools used by the nurse is acceptance. The student reveals the experience to the nurse and through the nurse's acceptance, the student can accept and forgive herself.

Finally, the nurse does not allow the student to dwell on the past and helps the student summarize what she has learned from the situation. The nurse then helps the student rehearse what she will discuss with her boyfriend.

Evaluation

To evaluate the effect of nursing interventions, the nurse assesses the client's level of guilt. The nurse also assesses the methods used by the client to cope with guilt and evaluates their effectiveness in lessening the guilt feelings. The client may still have feelings of guilt, but these feelings are in proportion to the situation and do not severely limit the person.

Interventions are successful when the client makes positive statements about himself and is free of excessive preoccupation with guilt in his conversations. Use of words like "should" and "ought" is minimal. Self-critical statements and self-destructive behavior are limited. The client verbalizes self-acceptance and self-forgiveness. The person identifies feelings of guilt as his own and deals with them in a positive way.

Other criteria indicating that interventions have been therapeutic include eye contact, less spontaneous crying, an ability to enjoy life, creative endeavors, minimal blushing episodes, and the ability to relax and to view situations realistically.

NURSING PROCESS SUMMARY: GUILT

ASSESSMENT
Physical Dimension
  Avoidance of eye contact
  Restlessness
  Nail biting
  Shuffling of feet
  Blushing
  Tachycardia
  Palpitations
  Sweaty palms
  Need for physical punishment
  Physical defects
  Somatic illnesses
  Galvanic skin responses (GSRs) during a lie detector test
  Self-destructive acts
Emotional Dimension
  Shame
  Embarrassment
  Regret or remorse
  Lack of regret or remorse

Inappropriate affect
Crying
Inability to experience pleasure
Resentment
Anger
Depression
Feelings of inferiority
Feelings of inadequacy
Intellectual Dimension
  Preoccupation with "should" and "ought"
  Self-punishing thoughts
  Selective inattention
  Forgetfulness
  Defense mechanisms: undoing, regression, reaction formation, denial
  Offering of excuses
  Arguing
  Criticizing
  Kidding

NURSING PROCESS SUMMARY: GUILT—cont'd

Social Dimension
   Poor self-concept
   Withdrawal
   Alienation
   Isolation
   Dependence
   Submission
   Lack of interest
Spiritual Dimension
   Lack of self-forgiveness
   Unrelatedness to God and others
   Noncompliance with beliefs
   Lack of creativity
   Wish to relive life
   Perfectionism
   Inability to participate in religious activities

ANALYSIS

See "Nursing Diagnosis" on p. 256

PLANNING AND IMPLEMENTATION

Physical Dimension
   Reduce physiological symptoms of anxiety through use
      of the following:
      Information on physiological responses to emotions
      Self-help measures
      Exercise
      Relaxation
      Music
   Promote a positive body image
   Identify action or event that caused guilt feelings
   Hospitalize if self-destructive
Emotional Dimension
   Encourage expression of guilt feelings
   Promote feelings of adequacy
   Encourage expression of resentment, anger, or depres-
      sion

Intellectual Dimension
   Promote idea that client can change his way of think-
      ing
   Limit self-punishing statements
   Promote rational thinking in problem solving and de-
      cision making
   Provide guided imagery
   Promote thought stopping
   Focus on the present, not the past
   Provide cognitive restructuring
   Teach assertiveness skills
Social Dimension
   Enhance self-concept
   Encourage restitution
   Listen to client nonjudgmentally
   Provide a supportive relationship.
   Enlist support of family
   Provide family therapy, group therapy, or individual
      therapy to assist with realistic expectations for self
      and others
Spiritual Dimension
   Refer to appropriate clergy or supportive person for
      forgiveness
   Help client forgive self
   Examine moral codes or value systems transgressed
   Help client experience pleasure

EVALUATION

Evaluation is based on the degree of life disruption that the client's guilt is producing and ways he has learned to cope with the guilt. Progress is indicated when he frees himself from the preoccupation with guilt, when he makes fewer self critical statements about himself, when he can accept himself with imperfections, and forgive himself and/or others for imperfections. The client's ability to explore values and moral codes and adjust self-expectations to healthy levels is further evaluative data.

BRIEF REVIEW

Guilt is an emotion that occurs when a person does something wrong and expects to be punished. Guilt arises in people when their actions conflict with their internalized value system. Guilt can be healthy, which means that it is appropriate for a given situation, or it can be unhealthy, as when it is excessive or absent.

The experience of guilt is central to human experience. It is like anxiety: it can cripple a person for life if it is not dealt with appropriately. Guilt has far-reaching and devastating consequences; therefore the nurse needs to recognize guilt in clients and help them successfully deal with feelings of guilt.

The nurse functions with clients experiencing guilt to help them express their guilt and deal with it realistically and successfully. The experience of guilt can be painful.

The nurse assesses the client to determine how the experience feels and what caused the feeling. Through establishing and building a therapeutic nurse-client relationship, the nurse sets goals, plans, and intervenes with clients to help them deal with feelings of guilt. Nursing interventions are evaluated by measuring their effectiveness in lessening guilt feelings.

REFERENCES AND SUGGESTED READINGS

1. American Psychiatric Association: Diagnostic and statistical manual of mental disorders, ed. 3, Washington, D.C., 1980, The Association.
2. Berger, L.: Parental guilt, Clinical Pediatrics **19:**499, 1980.
3. Berne, E.: Beyond games and scripts, New York, 1976, Grove Press.
4. Berne, E.: Transactional analysis in psychotherapy, New York, 1961, Grove Press.

5. Campbell, F.: The concept of shame, Perspectives in Psychiatric Care **22**:62, 1984.
6. Dyer, W.: Your erroneous zones, New York, 1976, Funk & Wagnalls, Inc.
7. Ebmeier, C.: Manifestations of guilt in an immobilized school age child, Maternal and Child Nursing Journal **11**:109, 1982.
8. Ellis, A., and Harper, R.: A guide to rational living, Englewood Cliffs, N.J., 1971, Prentice-Hall, Inc.
9. Ellis, A.: Reason and emotion in psychotherapy, New York, 1962, Citadel Press.
10. Engle, G.: Psychological development in health and disease, Philadelphia, 1962, W.B. Saunders Co.
11. Erikson, E.H.: Childhood and society, ed. 2, New York, 1964, W.W. Norton & Co., Inc.
12. Feinstein, A.: Self-responsibility in illness and the issue of guilt, Journal of American Society of Psychosomatic Dentistry and Medicine **28**(4):109, 1981.
13. Fensterheim, H., and Baer, J.: Stop running scared, New York, 1977, Dell Publishing Co., Inc.
14. Francis, B.: One reaction to guilt, Journal of Practical Nursing **31**(1):26, 1981.
14a. Freeman, L., and Stean, H.: Guilt: letting go, New York, 1986, John Wiley & Sons, Inc.
15. Freud, S.: Mourning and melancholia. In The complete works of Sigmund Freud, vol. 14, London, 1957, The Hogarth Press, Ltd. (Translated by J. Strachey and A. Tyson.)
16. Frosen, M., and others: Guilt and conscience in major depressive disorders, American Journal of Psychiatry **140**:839, 1983.
17. Gaylin, W.: Feelings: our vital signs, New York, 1979, Ballantine Books.
18. Gerrard, M.: Sex guilt and attitudes toward sex in sexually active female college students, Journal of Personality Assessment **44**:258, 1980.
19. Gerrard, M., and Gibbons, F.: Sexual experience, sex guilt and sexual moral reasoning, Journal of Personality **50**:345, 1982.
20. Glasser, W.: Reality therapy, New York, 1965, Harper & Row, Publishers, Inc.
21. Harris, T.: I'm OK—you're OK, New York, 1969, Avon Books.
22. Jampolsky, G.: Good-bye to guilt, New York, 1985, Bantam Books, Inc.
23. James, M., and Jongeward, D.: Born to win, Reading, Mass., 1980, Addison-Wesley Publishing Co., Inc.
24. Johnson, M., and Werner, C.: We had no choice: a study of familial guilt feelings surrounding nursing home care, Journal of Gerontological Nursing **8**:641, 1982.
25. Johnson, S.: Counseling families experiencing guilt, Dimensions in Critical Care Nursing **3**:238, 1984.
26. Johnson, S.: The guilt trip: why parents blame themselves . . . or others, Journal of Practical Nursing **31**(1):25, 1981.
27. Keith, C.: A paradoxical effect of guilt in the psychotherapy of children, American Journal of Psychotherapy **35**:16, 1981.
28. Keller, J., and Sack, A.: Sex guilt and the use of contraception among unmarried women, Contraception **25**:387, 1982.
29. Kessler, S., Kessler, H., and Ward, P.: Psychological aspects of genetic counseling: management of guilt and shame, American Journal of Medical Genetics **17**: 673, 1984.
30. Klenke-Hamel, K., and Jarda, L.: The Mosher Forced-Choice Guilt Scale as a measure of anxiety, Journal of Personality Assessment **43**:150, 1979.
31. Knowles, R.D.: Dealing with feelings: overcoming guilt and worry, American Journal of Nursing **81**:1663, 1981.
32. Knowles, R.D.: Dealing with feelings: worry journal and guilty time, American Journal of Nursing **81**:2035, 1981.
33. Kubler-Ross, E.: On death and dying, New York, 1970, Macmillan Publishing Co.
34. Leckman, J., and others: Appetite disturbance and excessive guilt in major depression, Archives of General Psychiatry **41**:839, 1984.
35. Lewis, H.: Shame and guilt in neurosis, New York, 1971, International Universities Press, Inc.
36. Lindsay-Hartz, J.: Contrasting experiences of shame and guilt, American Behavioral Scientist **27**(6):689, 1984.
37. Menninger, K.: Whatever became of sin?, New York, 1973, Hawthorn Publishing Co.
38. Mosden, P., O'Grady, K., and Katz, H.: Hostility-guilt, guilt over aggression, and self-punishment, Journal of Personality Assessment **44**:34, 1980.
39. Morrison, A.: Working with shame in psychoanalytic treatment, Journal of The American Psychoanalytical Association **32**:479, 1984.
40. Peplau, H.: Interpersonal relations in nursing, New York, 1952, G.P. Putnam's Sons.
41. Piaget, J.: The moral judgment of the child, New York, 1955, Macmillan Publishing Co.
42. Piers, G., and Singer, M.: Shame and guilt, New York, 1971, W.W. Norton & Co., Inc.
43. Selye, H.: The stress of life, New York, 1956, McGraw-Hill Book Co.
44. Shane, P.: Shame and learning, American Journal of Orthopsychiatry **50**:348, 1980.
45. Steiner, C.: Scripts people live, New York, 1974, Bantam Books, Inc.
46. Sullivan, H.: The interpersonal theory of psychiatry, New York, 1953, W.W. Norton & Co., Inc.
47. Wanlass, R., and others: Effects of sex education on sexual guilt, anxiety and attitudes: a comparison of instruction formats, Archives of Sexual Behavior **12**:487, 1983.
48. Wertheim, E., and Schartz, J.: Depression, guilt and self-management of pleasant and unpleasant events, Journal of Personality and Social Psychology **45**:884, 1983.

ANNOTATED BIBLIOGRAPHY

Gaylin, W.: Feelings: our vital signs, New York, 1980, Ballantine Books.

This book outlines various human feelings. Guilt is referred to as a feeling that needs forgiveness and is differentiated from guilty fear, a feeling of wanting to avoid punishment.

Gedan, S.: Say good-bye to guilt, **15**(7):30 Nursing 30, 1985.

The author discusses how to keep the burden of guilt from slowing recovery. Four steps useful for helping the client and family manage guilt are described.

CHAPTER 14

HOPE–DESPAIR

Ruth P. Rawlins

After studying this chapter the learner will be able to:

Define hope, despair, manic behavior, and suicide.

Discuss historical perspectives of hope and despair.

Describe theories of depression, manic behavior, and suicidal behavior.

Apply the nursing process to clients with depression, manic behavior, and suicidal behavior.

Identify current research findings on depression, manic behavior, and suicidal behavior.

With *hope* a person acts, moves, and achieves. Without hope one becomes dull, listless, and despairing. Hope defends against *despair;* it enables an individual to tolerate difficult situations and maintain motivation. However, hope also has the potential for decreasing a person's contact with reality. With despair there is a loss of hope and confidence. A sense of entrapment and futility prevails, convincing the person that what he wants is beyond reach. Energy for thinking and acting is lacking, and a passiveness immobilizes the individual. The hopeless individual feels like giving up and sometimes does. A decision is made that there is no use, no good, no sense to life.

The idea of hope and despair as a continuum is useful in discussing these entities. On one end of the continuum is hope, including confidence, faith, inspiration, and determination. At the other end of the continuum is despair, including helplessness, hopelessness, doubt, grief, apathy, sadness, *depression,* and *suicide.*

The hope-despair continuum is discussed in this chapter with a focus on the concept of loss. This concept includes any experience that evokes sadness in the individual. When the sadness of grief is resolved, the person integrates the experience into his life. When the grief is not resolved, he feels anger, helplessness, and guilt. The person may express these feelings adaptively and resolve the grief or may develop maladaptive behaviors, such as homicide or suicide. Internally expressed, the feelings may result in depression. (See Figure 14-1.)

Depression is a pathological state experienced by everyone to some degree at times. Infants, when neglected, become depressed and fail to respond to the environment. Adolescents are known for their recurring spells of gloom and self-hate. Women, before menstruation, after childbirth, or at menopause, may experience depression. Men and women, even those who are successful and in their prime, have times when life seems empty. Perhaps the elderly know depression best, since losses frequently occur in this age group.

Hope–Despair

THEORETICAL APPROACHES
Biological

There is some agreement among theorists that both heredity and environment play a role in depression. Studies have shown that depression is more likely to occur in a person with a family history of depression.

With the expansion of knowledge in neurophysiology, a biochemical model of depression has been proposed. This model concerns physiological chemical changes that take place during depressed states. Whether these chemical changes cause depression or are a result of depression is not clearly understood. However, significant functional abnormalities have been found in several body systems during a depressive illness. Studies of biogenic amine metabolism have indicated that a deficiency of particular bio-

🍃 *Historical Overview* 🍃

DATE	EVENT
600 BC	Early chronicles describe Nebuchadnezzar as suffering from wild, erratic moods (probably manic activity), followed by profound depression.
460 BC	Hippocrates related depression to the humidity of the brain. His theory of body substances, called humors, determined physical and mental health. Depression was blamed on a surplus of melancholy (black bile).
300 BC	Early Greek philosophers viewed fate as unchangeable and hope as an illusion or curse distorting reality, prolonging agony, and promoting a reliance on faith rather than action.
5 AD	Attitudes about hope changed with the spread of Christianity when St. Paul declared hope stands with love.
1500s	During the Elizabethan period people prided themselves on being melancholic and came to view it as a superior malady and mark of refinement among those deeply touched by the pathos in life. The writings of Shakespeare and Robert Burton included depressive themes.
1800s	Dostoevski, Poe, and Hawthorne expressed some of their inner anguish and despair in their writings. Later poets such as Shelly accepted the fatalistic cynical view of the Greeks. Nietzsche wrote "Hope is the worst of evils, for it prolongs the torment of man."
1900s	Winston Churchill, by frequent referral to his "black dog" of depression, suggested how familiar a companion was his despair.
1980s	An age of depression exists, generated by the rising expectations of standards of living after World War II, coming up against the harsh realities of the population explosion, limited resources, inflation, unemployment, and the possibility of nuclear warfare. The anxieties of the mid-1960s have given way to despair as a dominant mood. Suicide is a major health problem in the United States today.
Future	Increasing research, new medical technology, holistic nursing care, and increased public awareness will continue to advance the knowledge and treatment of depression.

genic amines at receptor sites in the brain may be related to depression. For example, norepinephrine has been found at lower levels in depressed persons. Serotonin, another biogenic amine that has been studied extensively, also is deficient in depressed persons. Measurement of the concentration of the amine metabolites in the urine of depressed clients helps determine the relationship between biogenic amines and depression. However, it is important to remember that variables such as diet, activity, endocrine factors, and anxiety levels may alter the excretion rates of amines and their metabolites.

Steroid metabolism in depression has also held researchers' interest. Investigations indicate that there is an increased steroid output in depression. Electrolyte metabolism studies showed increased sodium levels in depression and a lowering of sodium levels after recovery. Other electrolytes, including potassium, magnesium, and calcium, have been examined, with no definite conclusions reported at this time. Recent research has also indicated that depression may be related to a defect in the body's immune system. Although research in the biochemical model is inconclusive, there is evidence that a variety of factors can produce changes in body chemistry that may contribute to depression.

Psychoanalytic

A sense of hope develops from early childhood experiences, especially those related to formation of trust. According to Erikson,[25] hope emanates from a successful resolution of the conflict between trust and mistrust. The child learns to hope if the environment is suitable to the development of trust. Children first learn to trust from the mothering person. The probable basis of trust is the knowledge that help is forthcoming when needed. Hope in this framework, then, is not a solitary activity but is related to the expectation of assistance from other people.

Freud[30] viewed depression as the turning inward of the aggressive instinct. The anger is not directed at the appropriate object; it is displaced onto the self and is accompanied by feelings of guilt. Initially there may be a loss of a loved person or object. The person feels both angry and loving toward the lost object (ambivalence) but is unable to express his angry feelings because of repression, thinking that these feelings are inappropriate or irrational, or having developed a pattern throughout life of containing feelings, particularly negative ones. The individual then directs his angry feelings inward.

Bibring[11] believed that the ego may fail to achieve its narcissistic goals at any stage of development, and this fail-

TABLE 14-1 Bibring's model of depression

Developmental Stage	Ego Ideals	Characteristics of Depression
Oral	To be loved, taken care of, to get affection, to be worthy	Excessive hunger for love, affection, warmth, appreciation
Anal	To be obedient, good, kind, humane, clean, loving	Guilt, weakness, lack of control
Phallic	To be strong, secure, superior	Inadequacy, inferiority, helplessness
Latency	To be valued, important, to achieve	Powerlessness, low self-esteem

ure impairs the development of self-esteem. Low self-esteem, helplessness, and powerlessness are the most characteristic features of depression. Because infants are helpless and dependent on others to meet their needs, it was suggested that many depressions have their predisposing roots in trauma during the oral phase of development. As a result of early trauma, the individual has an excessive hunger for affection, warmth, and appreciation. A loss of affection and being loved reactivates earlier feelings of helplessness. This theory explains depression as also having predisposing roots in other stages of development (see Table 14-1).

Behavioral

Lewinsohn's behavioral model[47] proposes that a low rate of reinforcement predisposes to depression. Two variables are important in this model: (1) the individual may fail to initiate the appropriate responses to receive positive reinforcement, and (2) the environment may fail to

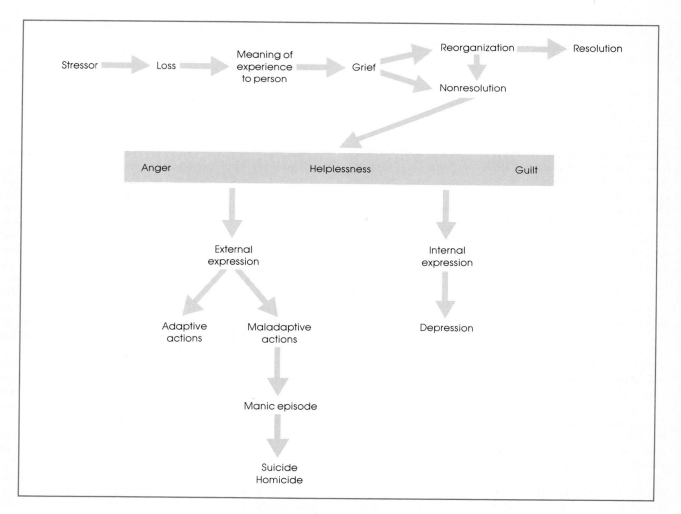

FIGURE 14-1 Concept of loss.

provide the reinforcement. These variables may occur when people find the behavior of the depressed person distressing, negative, or offensive.

The model of *learned helplessness* described by Seligman[63] proposes that it is not the situation itself that produces depression but the belief that one has no control over the situation. He defines *helplessness* as a belief that no one will do anything to aid you and *hopelessness* as a belief that neither you nor anyone else can do anything. Learned helplessness is both a behavioral state and a personality trait of persons who believe that they have lost control over their environment. These negative expectations lead to hopelessness, passivity, and an inability to assert oneself.

The object loss model of depression proposed by Bowlby[14] referred to the traumatic separation of the person from significant objects of attachment. Two factors are important in this theory: (1) a loss during childhood predisposes to adult depression and (2) a loss or separation in adult life acts as a stressor in depression. A child ordinarily has formed a bond to a mothering person by 6 months of age. Once this bond is broken, the child experiences separation anxiety and grief. According to Bowlby, unfavorable personality development is often attributed to unsatisfactory responses to loss during infancy and childhood, with a resulting predisposition to respond to all losses in a similar way.

Cognitive

Beck[6] described depression as an altered style of thinking characterized by negative expectations. This approach emphasizes the role that disturbances in thinking play in determining emotional states. Hopelessness and helplessness represent the central features of depression and reflect a negative conception of self, negative interpretation of one's experiences, and a negative view of the future. The depressed person finds that the world presents insurmountable obstacles to carrying out goals, views the self as helpless to surmount these obstacles, and has given up any hope of exercising future control over his life.

Sociological

Becker[8] defined depression as a social phenomenon. He proposed that the ego, unlike the id, is rooted in social reality and the ego ideal is composed of socially learned symbols and motives. Becker stated that a breakdown of self-esteem may involve, in addition to object losses, the individual's symbolic possessions such as power, status, roles, identity, values, and purpose for existence. Particularly susceptible to depression are individuals with upward social mobility and women who strongly identify with the role prescribed to them by their culture. The rigid sex role stereotyping that characterizes a woman as a faithful and loyal wife, a dedicated and loving mother, a competent and diligent housewife, and a supporter of moral and religious values effected through the socialization process may be detrimental to women's emotional health and personal growth. One study of female depression indicates that conflicts inherent in the changing roles of women increase their chances of experiencing depression during role transition periods.[70]

Holistic

Holism's focus on promoting health and preventing health disruptions provides a fresh approach to depression. The approach emphasizes hope as a positive life force rather than as a preventive measure to keep loss from absorbing the person. For the depressed person action is directed toward self-learning, self-motivation, and self-care within a participatory and reciprocal nurse-client relationship. Through self-responsibility, self-care, and stress management, clients can make choices and learn to control depressive thoughts, feelings, and behavior.

No one theory sufficiently explains depression. An integrated approach reflects aspects of each previously described model.[1] Here depression is described as the interaction of three sets of variables: chemical, experiential, and behavioral. Impairment of one variable affects the other two. Thus any one of the three sets of variables can contribute to depression and produce changes in the other two areas. For example, a chemical imbalance can result in distorted perceptions or a major loss can cause a chemical imbalance.

Table 14-2 summarizes the different theoretical approaches to depression.

RELATING TO THE CLIENT

Relating to the depressed client is difficult and can be deenergizing. Anger, depression, insensitivity, avoidance, withdrawal, as well as feelings of inadequacy, helplessness, and guilt are often generated in the nurse in response to depressed clients. Many of these behaviors and feelings may result partly from the nurse's perception of her inadequacy in dealing with depressed clients and partly from her personal beliefs as to how grief should be expressed by the client in a particular situation. The nurse's personal assessment of the value of the client's loss may influence the degree to which the nurse believes the client needs to grieve. Insensitivity may surface when the nurse's perception of grief behavior and the client's expression of the behavior are in conflict. Thus self-awareness—as well as knowledge of the dynamics of the illness and skills for intervening therapeutically—is an essential ingredient for the nurse in working with depressed clients.

In the preinteraction stage the nurse explores her thoughts and feelings about the depressed client. Negative reactions, such as anger and frustration or boredom, need to be identified, since these feelings may influence the relationship even before the client is seen.

During the orientation phase, establishing trust and acceptance requires patience and perseverance by the nurse. The client may reject the nurse's attempts to interact or may respond with silence and withdrawal. Short, frequent approaches to the client provide the message that the nurse cares. Sitting with the client in silence when he declines to interact indicates the nurse's interest

TABLE 14-2 Summary of theories of depression

Theory	Theorist	Dynamics
Psychoanalytic	Freud	Depression originates as a response to a loss, disappointment, or failure. Anger is displaced and turned inward on the self. Depression is masked by somatic complaints. Inability to mourn or grieve for a loss results in depression.
	Bibring	When the ego fails to achieve goals during developmental stages, loss of self-esteem, helplessness, and powerlessness may result.
Biological		Heredity influences the predisposition for depression. Chemical imbalances may cause depression such as deficiencies of biogenic amines at receptor sites in the brain.
Behavioral	Lewinsohn	Failure to receive positive reinforcement from others and from the environment predisposes to depression.
Cognitive	Beck	A negative conception of self, experiences, others, and the world contributes to depression.
	Seligman	The belief that one has no control over a situation contributes to depression.
	Bowlby	Loss during childhood predisposes to adult depression.
Sociological	Becker	Loss of power, status, identity, values, and purpose for existence creates susceptability for depression.
Holism	Akiskal and McKinney	Depression is the result of the interactions of chemical, experiential, and behavioral variables.

and availability. The nurse needs to be comfortable with the silence and accept the rejection as part of the client's illness. Gradually he will begin to trust the nurse as her commitment to the relationship is tested and validated. Demonstrating an understanding of the client's anger, sadness, or ambivalence is crucial.

Dealing with the client's negativism and resistance to change during the working phase can drain the nurse physically, emotionally, and spiritually. A nurse without a support system of her own and a strong sense of esteem is vulnerable to depression. Knowing she is a person of value and ability will fortify her against depression and help her to take the discouragement and failure that may go with working with depressed clients.

Clients may become dependent on the nurse during the working stage. Knowing when to make decisions for the client and when to encourage the client to make decisions so as to promote independence requires sensitivity and knowledge about the disease process. Themes of loss, fear of loss, control of emotions, and ambivalence predominate. Countertransference issues may be related to the nurse's own losses, her attitudes about anger, guilt, sadness and despair, her ability to identify these emotions, and her own conflicts about loss and death. Problems with any of these issues are seen in avoidance behavior, preoccupation with fantasies, blocking or denying feelings, or shortening sessions. The nurse's care of the depressed client will be more effective if she is aware of these issues and sensitive to her own feelings about loss.

As the depressed client improves and termination is pending, the nurse withdraws slowly to prevent a return to dependence and feelings of helplessness. She leaves the client with specific resources on which he can call if needed. Unfortunately depression tends to recur, and the nurse may become angry and discouraged with the repetitive behavior. She may be caught in the trap of feeling responsible for the client's depressive behavior. Knowing she has given her best nursing care may be all she can do for the client. She can not change the client's life situation. She can help change the client's attitudes toward life situations. Termination of the relationship may be difficult if the client experiences it as another loss. If the depressed client returns, the process is reinitiated with an attitude of hope that perhaps this time the client will learn, grow more, and become better able to cope with losses.

A few depressed clients reject treatment and fail to cooperate in their health regimen. The nurse may feel anger, frustration, guilt, and failure. It is helpful to permit clients to discuss their refusal for treatment without making judgments. Asking the client to help the nurse understand the reasoning behind the refusal keeps the discussion open, with a possibility that the individual may eventually decide to accept treatment. And, when the client does not accept treatment, the nurse assures him that help is available if a different decision is made. If the nurse can manage feelings of anger, guilt, and rejection so that the depressed client is not regarded as a hopeless case, some depressed clients may change their minds.

NURSING PROCESS
Assessment

✦ Physical dimension. In general, an individual who demonstrates a sense of hope has energy and drive and generates *joie de vivre.* There is a projection of overall well-being and optimism. An assessment of the

client's general health, including nutrition, exercise, habits such as smoking and alcohol intake, and self-care can determine the quality of overall health. Personality traits such as assertiveness and love of adventure, frequently are seen in these individuals.

The identification of hope in an individual includes observing facial expression (affect) and behavior in general. Persons with a sense of hope feel and look vital, vibrant, and alert.

Skilled observation provides clues as to whether the client is depressed (Figure 14-2). Sitting slumped with eyes lowered, quietly and alone, and looking sad and dejected are characteristics associated with the depressed person. The face may appear tired and drawn, with deep circles under the eyes, and with little change in expressions. The client may appear disheveled and unkempt. Hair is uncombed, and clothes may be worn several days without a change. Motor activity is decreased. The person moves as if each action requires a special effort. Walking, talking, and activities of daily living are greatly slowed down. Because of the reduced activity level (*psychomotor retardation*) and the slowing down of body processes, a cluster of symptoms called *vegetative symptoms* can be identified, which include weakness and fatigue, insomnia, anorexia and weight loss, gastrointestinal disturbances (commonly constipation), and a lack of interest in food, sleep, activities, and sex. These symptoms are the classic manifestations of depression.

Psychomotor agitation, which includes restlessness, sobbing, and excessive verbalizations, is seen in some depressed clients. Recognition of the agitation, which resembles anxiety, is crucial because the client may be at high risk for attempting suicide. In agitated depression, motor activity is seen as pacing in a given route, and movements such as hand wringing are repetitive. In anxiety, motor activity proceeds in random, unpredictable movements.

In depression, as the physiological processes are slowed down, body responses are altered. Metabolism is decreased. The depressed client complains of a loss of appetite and weight. A loss of 15 to 30 pounds is not uncommon in a 2 to 3 month period. Epigastric distress, nausea, vomiting, indigestion, and constipation occur frequently.

Depressed persons have sleep disturbances. Determining sleep habits is essential. Some wake early, between 4 and 5 AM, and cannot go back to sleep. Others sleep only for short periods. For some who sleep long periods of time, sleep is neither restful nor refreshing. Severely depressed clients who have a pattern of early morning wakefulness combined with despondency may be at risk for attempting suicide.

Neurological symptoms include headaches, dizziness, and blurred vision. Occasionally clients complain of cardiovascular symptoms such as mild chest pain, dyspnea, and palpitations. Alterations in the reproductive system include amenorrhea, impotence, and a decreased sex drive. Alterations in the immune system lead to increased susceptibility to illnesses. Illnesses such as colds, urinary tract infections, viral infections, and pneumonia are common. Thus frequent infections may be a clue to a depressed state.

Hypochondriacal complaints that have no organic basis but mimic a physical illness may be present. This morbid preoccupation with one's state of health can range from a series of minor complaints to the conviction that one has some serious disease. Minor complaints include frequent headaches, gastrointestinal disturbances, constipation, and vague aches and pains. Other complaints may involve the client's belief that he has a serious physical illness and needs to be taken seriously and evaluated medically, because the complaint may be masking depression.

Certain medications are often responsible for the development of depression, the aggravation of a preexisting depression, or the production of depressive-like symptoms such as sedation, apathy, and lethargy. Medications that may produce depressive symptoms include digitalis, antihypertensives, anti-Parkinson medications, estrogens, neuroleptics, hypnotics, sedatives and cortisones.

Because it has been concluded that there is a genetic predisposition to affective disorders, it is essential to determine the presence or absence of depression in other family members.

Symptoms of depression may accompany physical illness. The box on p. 269 lists illnesses that frequently coexist with depression.

✳ *Emotional dimension.* The nurse assesses the client's state of contentedness and optimism. With hope, there is inner buoyancy, internal peace, harmony, serenity, and a general freedom from overpowering anxiety, anger, guilt, and despair. The individual feels relaxed, secure, and safe. Tensions and conflicts are lessened and life is worth living. The individual is confident and feels an inner strength.

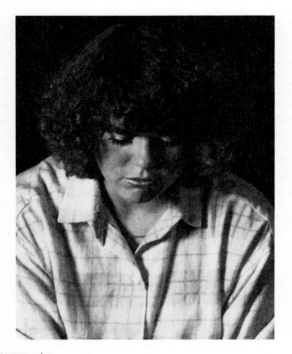

FIGURE 14-2 A depressed young woman.

PHYSICAL ILLNESSES FREQUENTLY ASSOCIATED WITH DEPRESSION

Addison's disease
Amyotrophic lateral sclerosis
Brain tumors
Cancer
Cardiac illnesses
Brucellosis
Diabetes
Hepatitus
Lingering influenza
Subacute bacterial endocarditis
Tuberculosis
Cushing's disease
Diseases of the pancreas
Diseases of the parathyroid glands
Failure to thrive
Hypothyroidism
Leukemia
Lupus erythematosus
Multiple sclerosis
Parkinson's disease
Pernicious anemia
Renal diseases

In depression, sadness is the major affect. Other characteristics to look for include irritability, agitation, hostility, anger, guilt, and lack of pleasure *(anhedonia)*. Feelings of emptiness, worthlessness, and a lack of self-respect and confidence can be identified. The client may be emotionally labile, crying easily one moment and laughing the next. Determining how the client feels early in the morning provides clues about the type of depression. Generally the client with a major depression feels worse early in the morning and improves as the day goes on. The client with dysthymia may begin the day optimistically but feel progressively worse as the day wears on.

Anxiety frequently accompanies and may mask the depression. (See Chapter 11 for further assessment of anxiety.)

The depressed person may be angry. However, the anger may not be clearly observable, because it commonly is turned inward on the self. When anger is repressed, physical symptoms such as headaches, backaches, and diarrhea may be present. (See Chapter 12 for further assessment of anger.)

Ambivalence is found in depression. Clients display mixed feelings when relating to others. They may simultaneously want and not want interaction.

In depression, persons frequently express feelings of guilt. The guilt may be related to a real situation, such as being fired from a job for drinking, or to an imagined situation. For example, a mother may feel guilty for the wrongdoing of her adult children. In either situation the expressions of guilt are reiterated over and over to anyone who will listen. The client is seen as inappropriately feeling guilt. (See Chapter 13 for further assessment of guilt.)

An assessment of depression needs to include whether the client feels a sense of powerlessness, helplessness, or hopelessness. Powerlessness is seen when the client feels no control over life events and remains unmotivated and passive. A fatalistic viewpoint is taken—what happens, happens; the harsh, rigid thinking of the despairing person allows no way to change or take control of events. Helplessness is identified in the client by lack of energy and staunch pessimism. Clients are convinced that everything that can be done has been done and will attempt to convince others as well as they have themselves. Hopelessness may accompany helplessness in a client. The client is seen as accepting the fact that it is of no use to continue treatment. There is no hope of ever feeling better. Feelings of futility, entrapment, and the impossible are expressed when the client is without hope.

Intellectual dimension. Positive experiences remembered from earlier times and reinforced through the process of learning generate optimism and hope. The person with hope is oriented, exercises reasonable judgment, explores alternatives, and generally understands the situation realistically.

Assessing hope means looking at the individual's motivation and determination. That the client did not deny the problem or run away from the difficulty is a source of comfort and hope; in the future perhaps another obstacle can be conquered. Armed with this knowledge, clients will not lack courage when they again need this sustaining quality.

Closely related to motivation is one's ability to set or change goals when the original goal is no longer feasible. A person with the ability to be flexible and adapt to changes is more likely to maintain hope against overwhelming stress. He sees alternatives to the situation. Having other options in a difficult situation gives a person a sense of autonomy. Although the choices may not be directed toward the desired goal, the person retains the freedom to decide for himself. This can provide a feeling of control.

Hope differs from wishing on the basis of the probability of attaining the object of one's desire. A wish is closely related to "magic hope." A person using magic hope realizes that the possibility of obtaining the wish is highly improbable, such as wishing for a million dollars. The person knows he is not likely to ever have the million dollars, but the fantasy is a pleasant one. The person who hopes has a strong sense of possibility that he will obtain what he hopes for. The hoping person makes concrete plans to gain what is desired, while the person who wishes (for example, for the million dollars) does not because it is so unlikely that the wish can be achieved.

In summary, an optimistic outlook, motivation to change, ability to think of options, and recognition of freedom to choose alternatives are indicators of hope within the individual.

Depressed persons have little interest in activities around them. Because thay are preoccupied with their own unhappy condition, their minds are filled with unrelenting thoughts about their misery. Negativism permeates their thinking about themselves, others, and the world. Ruminating over past events and self-blame leaves no time for communication with others.

Cognitive abilities are impaired. The client has difficulty concentrating and making decisions. Judgment, insight, and memory are also impaired. Thoughts may become rigidly fixed and expressed over and over, particularly critical, self-blaming, or self-accusing thoughts about personal failure and guilt.

The thought processes of the depressed client may be distorted, and misinterpretation of reality is evident at times. It is essential to determine the presence of delusions or hallucinations in a depressed client (see Chapter 17).

Social dimension. Assessment of hope includes observations of individual's interactions with others and their involvement in life experiences. Persons with hope are gregarious and actively involved with others. For some, approaching others who have had a similar loss may indicate hope within the individual. For example, a woman who has had a mastectomy may want to talk to others who have had mastectomies, or parents who have lost children to sudden infant death may spend time with other parents who have lost children under similar circumstances. The nurse observes whether the client reaches out to initiate interactions and notes the amount of touching, holding, and wanting to be close to another person. What is the depth of the interaction? Is it shallow and superficial, or does the interaction proceed at a deeper level with ideas and feelings being discussed? When interactions are maintained over time, relationships become meaningful and the individual receives a positiveness from the relationship and a sense of hope that this is a person who can be counted on in times of distress. Hope, then, is related to the expectation of assistance from others at a time when the person's resources are inadequate or diminished. When ill, a person depends on others and hopes for help from them. Trust generated from meaningful relationships between persons enhances hope. Thus it is vital to identify significant persons in the client's life.

Through the process of socialization, attitudes are developed. Nurturing families tend to foster positive, optimistic attitudes toward life. Assessment of family attitudes toward life events such as marriage, child rearing, male and female roles, education, work, and the larger society is useful in determining hope in an individual.

The depressed person withdraws from interactions with others and from life experiences, resulting in a self-imposed isolation. The nurse determines the nature and severity of the withdrawal and isolation by observing his participation in social interactions and activities. Which persons and activities are resources for interactions and relationships that can be strengthened? Because of increased preoccupation with oneself *(narcissism),* the client's withdrawal may be self-perpetuating and may increase distancing within the family. Data regarding the client's feelings of relatedness to family members are helpful, as many feel alienated even though family members take an active interest and show caring.

The nurse determines the degree of dependence and helplessness the client demonstrates. Are basic activities of daily living met? Does the client need assistance with appropriate dress and grooming, with hygiene, meal preparation, and personal safety?

The nurse identifies the client's needs for reassurance, support, and acceptance from others. Persons who have not had basic needs met in childhood tend to lack inner strengths and resources for trusting their own abilities and decisions. A thorough history of the client's infancy, childhood, and early school years yields information on how well his needs were met, or remain unmet.

Being emotionally needy, the depressed client may be demanding. When needs cannot be met or satisfied, more demands are made, resulting in further rejection by others. The client sees others as unable or unwilling to meet demands and becomes distrustful and passive in relationships. Assessment of the reasonableness and kinds of demands will provide information about the client's unmet needs.

Some depressed clients obtain *secondary gains,* such as additional attention, from their symptoms of depression. If they get narcissistic gratification from their disorder, clients may exploit the kindness and attentiveness of others, shirk responsibilities, and avoid the demands of interpersonal interactions. The nurse carefully assesses whether the client is receiving secondary gains from the depression.

Assessing cultural background adds important information about the client's roles and functions. Within some cultures women are expected to be subordinate and passive. Depressive symptoms may occur when individuals are in conflict with the roles and functions assigned them by the culture, as may occur, for example, when a woman chooses a career that is heavily male dominated, such as medicine. Identifying conflicts in roles and functions of the client provides valuable information in the assessment of depression.

Spiritual dimension. A client with hope has a meaningful philosophy of life and feels a purposeful sense of direction. The individual demonstrates courage to face up to the unexpected no matter how grievous or disastrous and feels a sense of challenge that provides the stamina to survive disaster and resist despair. Hope is a sense of the possible. The person believes that if the object of his desire is obtained, life will be changed in some way; be more comfortable, meaningful or enjoyable. Hope is future oriented. Feelings of satisfaction, security, and serenity emanate from the individual who hopes. Questions such as "How satisfied are you with your life right now?" and "What are your feelings about your life situation?" may determine how meaningful the person's life is at present.

A person who hopes, perseveres. Perseverance is the ability to keep on working toward solutions that will ease distress or change one's condition. Perseverance enables one to confront a difficult situation over a long period without losing courage or giving up. To persevere requires strength of will. Related to perseverance is courage, the ability to persist toward a goal even though there is no certainty the goal will be reached.

Assessment of the client's religious beliefs and values is essential. Participation in usual religious activities may strengthen hope in some clients. Questions such as "Who comforts you, or what is it that sustains you, when all else fails?" will elicit information about the individual's spiritual beliefs.

A person with hope receives strength from a relationship with God, a supreme being, or other people and nature. Assessment of the nature of these relationships provides data for determining the client's strengths and resources. A person with hope is in the process of becoming a fully functioning human being. One sees in this person a blending of inner peace as a result of his sense of purpose and a conscious recognition of his ability to live life fully. Observation and sensitive listening reveal the client's sense of hope in difficult life situations.

Measurement tools. Two commonly used tools for measuring depression include Beck's Depression Inventory[6] and Zung's Self-Rating Depression Scale.[72]

The Beck Depression Inventory (BDI)[6] (pp. 271-272) measures the kinds of feelings and behaviors demonstrated by clinically depressed persons. Beck's research established how each symptom is related to overall levels of depression.

BECK DEPRESSION INVENTORY

Read over the statements grouped with each letter, *A* through *U*. Pick out the statement within each group that best describes the way you feel today, that is, right at this moment. Circle the number next to the statement that you have chosen in each group. If two or more statements in a group describe the way you feel equally well, circle each one. Be sure to read over all of the statements in each group before you decide on one.

A. (Sadness)
  0 I do not feel sad.
  1 I feel blue or sad.
  2a I am blue or sad all the time and I can't snap out of it.
  2b I am so sad or unhappy that it is quite painful.
  3 I am so sad or unhappy that I can't stand it.

B. (Pessimism)
  0 I am not particularly pessimistic or discouraged about the future.
  1 I feel discouraged about the future.
  2a I feel I have nothing to look forward to
  2b I feel that I won't ever get over my troubles.
  3 I feel that the future is hopeless and that things cannot improve.

C. (Sense of failure)
  0 I do not feel like a failure.
  1 I feel I have failed more than the average person.
  2a I feel I have accomplished very little that is worthwhile or that means anything.
  2b As I look back on my life all I can see is a lot of failures.
  3 I feel I am a complete failure as a person (parent, husband, wife)

D. (Dissatisfaction)
  0 I am not particularly dissatisfied.
  1a I feel bored most of the time.
  1b I don't enjoy things the way I used to.
  2 I don't get satisfaction out of anything anymore.
  3 I am dissatisfied with everything.

E. (Guilt)
  0 I don't feel particularly guilty.
  1 I feel bad or unworthy a good part of the time.
  2a I feel quite guilty.
  2b I feel bad or unworthy practically all the time now.
  3 I feel as though I am very bad or worthless.

F. (Expectation of punishment)
  0 I don't feel I am being punished.
  1 I have a feeling that something bad may happen to me.
  2 I feel I am being punished or will be punished.
  3a I feel I deserve to be punished.
  3b I want to be punished.

G. (Self-dislike)
  0 I don't feel disappointed in myself.
  1a I am disappointed in myself.
  1b I don't like myself.
  2 I am disgusted with myself.
  3 I hate myself

H. (Self-accusations)
  0 I don't feel I am any worse than anybody else.
  1 I am critical of myself for my weaknesses or mistakes.
  2 I blame myself for my faults.
  3 I blame myself for everything bad that happens.

I. (Suicidal ideas)
  0 I don't have any thoughts of harming myself.
  1 I have thoughts of harming myself but I would not carry them out.
  2a I feel I would be better off dead.
  2b I feel my family would be better off if I were dead.
  3a I have definite plans about committing suicide.
  3b I would kill myself if I could.

J. (Crying)
  0 I don't cry any more than usual.
  1 I cry more now than I used to.
  2 I cry all the time now. I can't stop it.
  3 I used to be able to cry but now I can't cry at all even though I want to.

K. (Irritability)
  0 I am no more irritated now than I ever am.
  1 I get annoyed or irritated more easily than I used to.
  2 I feel irritated all the time.
  3 I don't get irritated at all at the things that used to irritate me.

L. (Social withdrawal)
  0 I have not lost interest in other people.
  1 I am less interested in other people now than I used to be.

From Beck, A.T.: Depression: causes and treatment, Philadelphia, 1967, University of Pennsylvania Press.

Continued.

BECK DEPRESSION INVENTORY—cont'd

2 I have lost most of my interest in other people.
3 I have lost all my interest in other people and don't care about them at all.

M. (Indecisiveness)
   0 I make decisions about as well as ever.
   1 I try to put off making decisions.
   2 I have great difficulty in making decisions.
   3 I can't make decisions at all anymore.

N. (Body image change)
   0 I don't feel I look any worse than I used to.
   1 I am worried that I am looking older or unattractive.
   2 I feel that there are permanent changes in my appearance and they make me look unattractive.
   3 I feel that I am ugly or repulsive looking.

O. (Work retardation)
   0 I can work about as well as before.
   1a It takes extra effort to get started at doing a task or job.
   1b I don't work as well as I used to.
   2 I have to push myself very hard to do anything.
   3 I can't do any work at all.

P. (Insomnia)
   0 I can sleep as well as usual.
   1 I wake up more tired in the morning than I used to.
   2 I wake up 1-2 hours earlier than usual and find it hard to get back to sleep.
   3 I wake up early every day and can't get more than 5 hours sleep.

Q. (Fatigability)
   0 I don't get any more tired than usual.
   1 I get tired more easily than I used to.
   2 I get tired from doing anything.
   3 I get too tired to do anything.

R. (Anorexia)
   0 My appetite is no worse than usual.
   1 My appetite is not as good as it used to be.
   2 My appetite is much worse now.
   3 I have no appetite at all anymore.

S. (Weight loss)
   0 I haven't lost much weight, if any, lately.
   1 I have lost more than 5 pounds.
   2 I have lost more than 10 pounds.
   3 I have lost more than 15 pounds.

T. (Somatic preoccupation)
   0 I am no more concerned about my health than usual.
   1 I am concerned about aches and pains or upset stomach or constipation.
   2 I am so concerned with how I feel or what I feel that it's hard to think of much else.
   3 I am completely absorbed in what I feel.

U. (Loss of libido)
   0 I have not noticed any recent change in my interest in sex.
   1 I am less interested in sex than I used to be.
   2 I am much less interested in sex now.
   3 I have lost interest in sex completely.

Zung's Self-Rating Depression Scale (p. 273)[72] is useful in measuring the level and pervasiveness of feelings of depression. Knowing the difficulty involved in getting verbal responses from depressed persons, Zung found depressed persons cooperative in responding in writing to the questions on his scale, particularly when they thought it would help determine what was wrong with them.

Other scales for measuring depression include:
1. Minnesota Multiphasic Personality Inventory (MMPI)
2. Lubin Depression Adjective Check List (DACL)
3. Hamilton Rating Scale
4. Grinker Feelings and Concerns Check List
5. Assessment of Overt Verbal Behavior
6. Assessment of Overt Motor Behavior
7. Continuous Telemetric Measuring
8. Pleasant Events Schedule

Analysis

Nursing diagnosis. The following list provides examples of NANDA-accepted nursing diagnoses with causative statements that are related to depression.
1. Ineffective coping: depression related to loss of job
2. Alteration in bowel elimination: constipation related to depression and medications
3. Sleep pattern disturbance: early morning awakening related to depression
4. Spiritual distress: lack of purpose in life related to depression
5. Powerlessness: unable to make decisions related to depression
6. Sexual dysfunction: lack of desire related to depression
7. Self-care deficit: lack of grooming related to depression
8. Impaired social interaction: loss of pleasure from relationships related to depression
9. Diversional activity deficit: loss of interest in activities related to depression

Disturbance in self-concept, self-care deficit, and hopelessness are three of the nursing diagnoses approved by NANDA that apply to the depressed client. The defining characteristics of these nursing diagnoses are listed in the boxes on pp. 274-275.

The following Case Example demonstrates the characteristics of a client with a disturbance in self-concept.

Case Example

Nancy Ellis, 46, has been depressed since her youngest child left for college 2 months ago. She has little to do at home now that all her children are away. Her husband works long hours at

ZUNG'S SELF-RATING DEPRESSION SCALE

Below are twenty statements about feelings each of us has at one time or another. Read each one and place a check in the box which best describes how you are feeling at this time.

	A LITTLE OF THE TIME	SOME OF THE TIME	GOOD PART OF THE TIME	MOST OF THE TIME
1. I feel downhearted and blue.				
2. Morning is when I feel best.				
3. I have crying spells or feel like it.				
4. I have trouble sleeping at night.				
5. I eat as much as I used to.				
6. I still enjoy sex.				
7. I notice that I am losing weight.				
8. I have trouble with constipation.				
9. My heart beats faster than usual.				
10. I get tired for no reason.				
11. My mind is as clear as it used to be.				
12. I find it easy to do the things I used to do.				
13. I am restless and can't keep still.				
14. I feel hopeful about the future.				
15. I am more irritable than usual.				
16. I find it easy to make decisions.				
17. I feel that I am useful and needed.				
18. My life is pretty full.				
19. I feel that others would be better off if I were dead.				
20. I still enjoy the things I used to do.				

his business and is inattentive to her when he is home. Her children have been an important part of her life for the past 20 years; she feels unimportant and unneeded now as she perceives that her homemaking skills and child-rearing responsibilities are over. She lacks confidence in herself and her ability to participate in community activities. She sees herself as having no job skills and her husband is not supportive of her working outside the home.

The following Case Example demonstrates the characteristics of the nursing diagnosis self-care deficit.

Case Example

Ted Young, 64, recently lost his wife after a brief illness. They had been married 42 years and had no children. He was quite dependent on her for care and for his day-to-day activities since his retirement 2 years ago, even though he was in good physical health. After her death he became despondent, having no appetite, extreme fatigue, and difficulty sleeping. He stopped shaving, forgot to change his clothes, and made no attempts to clean his home or care for his yard and garden, which had been a source of great pleasure to him before her death.

DISTURBANCE IN SELF-CONCEPT

DEFINITION

Disruption in the way one perceives one's body image, perception of self-esteem, and/or personal identity.

DEFINING CHARACTERISTICS

Physical Dimension
Inability to look at or touch body
Inability to look at self in mirror
Inability to participate in self care
*Lack of eye contact
Self-neglect
*Physical complaints
Self-destructive acts (substance abuse, risk taking activities)

Emotional Dimension
*Anxiety
Despair
Helplessness
Anger, resentment, hostility
*Fear of rejection
*Fear of failure

Intellectual Dimension
*Preoccupation with physical complaints
*Unrealistic perception of self
*Delusional thinking
Denial of existence of problem
Inability to accept positive reinforcement
*Verbal statements about actual or perceived changes

Social Dimension
Dependence
Withdrawal
Unaccepting of offers of help from others
Low self-esteem
Impaired role functioning

Spiritual Dimension
*Hopelessness
*Powerlessness
*Meaninglessness
*Decreased value in self-worth

Adapted from North American Nursing Diagnosis Association Classification of Nursing Diagnosis: Proceedings of the seventh conference, St. Louis, 1987, The C.V. Mosby Co.
*Indicates characteristics in addition to those defined by NANDA.

SELF-CARE DEFICIT

DEFINITION

State in which the individual experiences impaired ability to perform or complete bathing, feeding, dressing, or toileting self.

DEFINING CHARACTERISTICS

Physical Dimension
*Decreased strength and endurance
Lack of coordination
Motor weakness
Decreased vision
Pain
Inability to manipulate clothing

Emotional Dimension
Anxiety
Depression

Intellectual Dimension
*Cognitive impairment including memory and judgment
Perceptual impairment
*Speech impairment

Social Dimension
*Dependence
*Mistrusts caregiver
*Negative self concept
*Lack of resources
*Inadequate environment
*Low self-esteem

Spiritual Dimension
*Perception of life/death, may have chosen to die
*Decreased value of self

Adapted from North American Nursing Diagnosis Association Classification of Nursing Diagnosis: Proceedings of the seventh conference, St. Louis, 1987, The C. V. Mosby Co.
*Indicates characteristics in addition to those defined by NANDA.

The following Case Example illustrates characteristics of the nursing diagnosis hopelessness.

Case Example

Chris, 26 years old, lost his wife of 7 months in an automobile accident. He has been despondent since her death and unable to be consoled by friends or parents. He neglects his personal care and becomes less and less involved in his usual activities. He thinks life no longer has any meaning for him and he feels hopeless about it ever improving.

DSM-III-R diagnoses. The pathological conditions related to mood disorders are listed in the box at right.

DSM-III-R CLASSIFICATION RELATED TO MOOD DISORDERS

BIPOLAR DISORDERS

296.6x	Mixed
296.4x	Manic
296.5x	Depressed
301.13	Cyclothymia

DEPRESSIVE DISORDERS

Major depression

296.2x	Single episode
296.3x	Recurrent
300.40	Dysthymia

Adapted from American Psychiatric Association: Diagnostic and statistical manual of mental disorders (DSM-III-R), Washington, D.C., 1987, The Association.

HOPELESSNESS

DEFINITION

A state in which an individual sees limited or no alternatives or personal choices available and is unable to mobilize energy on his own behalf.

DEFINING CHARACTERISTICS

Physical Dimension
Sighing
Closing eyes
Turning away from speaker
Decreased appetite
Increased sleep
Failing or deteriorating condition

Emotional Dimension
Decreased affect

Intellectual Dimension
Decreased verbalizations
Despondent verbalizations

Social Dimension
Passivity
Lack of initiative
Decreased response to stimuli
Lack of involvement in care
Abandonment

Spiritual Dimension
Lost belief in transcendent values/God

Adapted from North American Nursing Diagnosis Association Classification of Nursing Diagnosis: Proceedings of the seventh conference, St. Louis, 1987, The C.V. Mosby Co.

The essential features and manifestations of the features of major depression, according to the DSM-III-R, are listed in the box at right.

The diagnosis of *dysthymia* is made when symptoms of depression are present but not of sufficient severity and duration to be diagnosed as a major depression.

Dysthymia and major depression are compared in Table 14-3.

Planning

See Table 14-4 for examples of long-term and short-term goals and outcome criteria related to depression. These serve as examples of the planning stage in the nursing process.

Implementation

Physical dimension. A healthy life-style that provides for sound nutrition, adequate sleep, exercise and activity, sexual needs that are satisfactorily met, and appropriate management of stress contributes to a sense of well-being and a joie de vivre, essential components in hope. Diet and health counseling by the nurse may contribute to the client's sense of well-being, but generally the client assumes responsibility for maintaining a healthy life-style when hope and optimism are present.

Genetic counseling for couples choosing to have chil-

MAJOR DEPRESSION

296.2x   Single episode
296.3x   Recurrent

ESSENTIAL FEATURES

Depressed mood or loss of interest or pleasure in almost all activities for at least 2 weeks. The symptoms represent a change from previous functioning and are relatively persistant.

MANIFESTATIONS

Physical Dimension

Loss of appetite
Change in weight
Sleep disturbance
Psychomotor agitation or retardation
Decreased energy
Fatigue

Emotional Dimension

Dysphoric mood
Guilt
Feelings of inadequacy
Loss of pleasure in usual activities

Intellectual Dimension

Difficulty concentrating
Slowed thinking
Indecisiveness
Excessive concern with physical health
Memory difficulties
Brooding
Loss of interest in surroundings
Delusions
Suicidal thoughts

Social Dimension

Loss of interest and pleasure in activities
Withdrawn from friends and family

Spiritual Dimension

Feelings of worthlessness

Adapted from American Psychiatric Association: Diagnostic and statistical manual of mental disorders (DSM-III-R), Washington, D.C., 1987, The Association.

dren may be indicated when there is a family history of depression, to help couples determine whether to have children.

Helping the depressed client with activities of daily living is essential, because the client has little energy or interest in caring for himself. Although interest in appearance and hygiene is negligible during depression, feelings of esteem and worth are related to appearance and cleanliness. Encouraging a neat, clean appearance seems to enhance the recovery process.

Attractively served meals with small portions may help stimulate the client's appetite. For the hospitalized client, between-meal feedings provide additional nourishment and indicate a caring attitude when served unhurriedly with time taken to sit with the client. Having relatives

TABLE 14-3 Comparison of types of depression

Cause	Dysthymia	Major Depression
	Exhaustion of adaptation; severe or prolonged stress; inadequacy in achieving goals; unresolved conflicts; chronic anxiety, fear, anger	A primary disturbance in the structure and function of brain and nervous system; toxicity, infection, injury, unresolved grief
History of depression in family	Illness can sometimes be related to depression in the family	Commonly, other family members have had depression
Onset	Gradual, over several weeks; seems to build up slowly	Fairly rapid (1 to 4 weeks) and seems to come from nowhere
Level of activity	Mixed; sometimes slowed, other times agitated	May be agitated type with restlessness and "nervousness," or psychomotor retardation
Intensity of depression	Fluctuates from mild to severe	Most often severe
Duration of depression	Varies, depending on personality; many remain chronic with periods of improvement	If untreated, may last 3 to 24 months, then improve; but can remain chronic indefinitely
Tendency to recurrence	Frequent relapses and remissions	Common, with varied periods of remission
Sleep	Fitful; awakens readily, sleeps, reawakens; morning sleep is deep	Falls asleep easily but awakens at 4 to 5 AM and cannot fall asleep again
Arising	Awakens with a heavy head, but hopes for a good day	Awakens tired and jittery, with no sense of rest; feels miserable in the morning
Eating	Varies; some show loss of appetite; others are compulsive eaters and gain weight	Little interest in food, and rapid weight loss
Crying	Some crying spells; or may say: "If I could cry I'd feel better."	Intense, spontaneous, and agitated crying spells
Self-esteem	Fluctuates between high and low	Completely lost; feeling of emptiness
Tendency to alcoholism	Strong tendency to drown sorrows in drink	Strong, especially if illness is prolonged
Fatigue	Feelings of no pep but occasional bursts of energy	Chronically tired, but shows some energy when agitated
Reserve of strength	Very little, but may "push" for brief intervals	Little to none
Physical symptoms	Innumerable vague complaints such as headache, tightness in chest, indigestion, cramps	Many complaints about stomach, bowel function, chest pains, headache
Attitude toward fatigue	Feels shame; embarrased at failure to mobilize self	Does not care
Emotional control	Varies from well-controlled to unmanageable	Generally none; needs to be managed most of the time
Mood	Unpredictable; usually optimistic in morning and depressed toward evening	Worse in the morning and tends to be better in the evening
Anxiety	Constantly present and may rise to panic states	Present, and may increase as illness progresses
Expressions of fear	Multiple fears about present and future constantly voiced	Usually intense; mostly fear of being alone
Ability to make decisions	Indecisive on important matters, positive decisions on minor matters	Absent, almost totally indecisive
Ability to concentrate	Varies, but mostly poor	None, especially when agitated
Memory	Variable and unreliable	Poor
Contact with reality and surroundings	Varies; judgment colored by level of hysteria and perceptual distortions	Usually poor; distorted judgment, lack of orientation, and inadequate perceptions are common
Delusions	Varies; if present, usually of persecution, oppression, or guilt; occasionally of unworthiness.	Common; mostly paranoid; guilt; ideas of poverty, self-deprecation, unworthiness
Sense of responsibility	Usually diffused	Mostly lost
Hallucinations	None	Uncommon but may be present

TABLE 14-4 Long-term and short-term goals and outcome criteria related to depression

Goals	Outcome Criteria

NURSING DIAGNOSIS: INEFFECTIVE INDIVIDUAL COPING: DEPRESSED MOOD RELATED TO FEELING DISCOURAGED AND HELPLESS

Long-term goals

Goals	Outcome Criteria
To develop a realistic and positive perception of self	Makes positive statements about self
	Accepts positive statements from others
	Makes positive statements about others
	Identifies positive attributes and skills in self
To be able to cope with sad situations without becoming depressed	Identifies situations that cause sadness
	Identifies ways sad situations are handled
	Explores alternative ways of dealing with sad situations
	Identifies possible consequences of alternative ways of dealing with sad situations
	Uses a new method of handling a sad situation

Short-term goals

Goals	Outcome Criteria
To deal with painful feelings by sharing and expressing them	Accepts the nurse's presence, 5 to 10 minutes twice daily, and increases time as tolerated
	Identifies and shares feelings
	Explores alternative ways of expressing feelings: for example anger—uses a punching bag, sings, plays the piano, tears up phone books; guilt—explores situations and persons with whom guilt is associated, substitutes "resentment" for "guilt"; hopelessness—states two positive statements about self and/or situation
	States that it is okay to have painful feelings
To be able to carry out activities of daily living	Improves personal appearance: bathing, care of hair, skin, nails, clothes
	Establishes acceptable eating patterns
	Establishes favorable sleeping habits
	Participates in a work assignment
	Initiates a pleasurable activity
	Drinks sufficient fluids and eats roughage foods to prevent constipation
	Describes AM-PM variations in mood and plans activities and therapy when mood is elevated
	Exercises daily
To increase and strengthen social relationships	States problem areas in social relationships
	Identifies situations that push people away
	Identifies situations that pull people together
	Initiates an activity with another person or small group of persons
	Listens to another person's problem sharing
	Expresses pleasure about the interaction or activity
To increase feelings of esteem and value	Makes decisions about planning activities, treatment, meals and visitors
	Successfully completes an activity or project
	Makes positive statements about self
	Accepts positive statements when made by others
	Does something for another person

bring favorite foods from home may increase the pleasure of eating. Active research is being conducted to relate diet to depression. Some vitamin deficiencies are produced by certain long-term medication therapy. For example, isoniazid and cycloserine, used to treat tuberculosis, can bring on a pyridoxine deficiency and produce symptoms of euphoria or depression. Women taking oral contraceptives that contain estrogen sometimes exhibit low levels of vitamin B_6, and supplements of B_6 relieve the symptoms of depression. A balanced diet is the best treatment to prevent vitamin deficiencies related to depression.

Physical symptoms need to be relieved promptly. Providing laxatives for constipation and medications to relieve headache assures the client that the nurse cares and promotes physical comfort. Because of the client's body preoccupation, the nurse does not become overly concerned with the complaints. The nurse evaluates the validity of the complaint, relieves it when possible, and does not focus on it.

Disturbances in sleep patterns are treated with comfort measures such as warm baths, quiet music, back rubs, or a glass of warm milk. A few minutes with a concerned and attentive person at bedtime to talk of events of the day, with a focus on pleasant happenings, may promote sleep.

When the client is agitated, the nurse needs to initiate regularly scheduled contacts to demonstrate acceptance of the client as a person, regardless of behavior. Providing distraction and channeling the agitated behavior through activities or constructive tasks such as housekeeping or physical exercise is helpful. Challenging activities at which the client is proficient promote the constructive expression of aggressive behavior. As a last resort, applying external controls such as seclusion in a quiet room, medications, or restraints may be necessary.

Exercise is recognized as vital in the treatment of depression. Research shows that depressed persons become more responsive if they exercise every day or participate in some noncompetitive sport (see the Research Highlight below). Developing an exercise program is effective in treating depression because it represents an achievement and success for many people. Running or swimming improves one's physical health and appearance, consequently increasing self-acceptance. In addition, depressive thoughts are difficult to maintain during exercise. If the individual is not inclined to physical sports, some other strenuous activity, such as washing the car or kitchen floor or raking leaves, has similar benefits.

A change in the environment may be indicated to reduce stress and tension, particularly when the individual is unable to perform activities of daily living. A leave of absence from work or school and the milieu therapy offered in hospitalization are often indicated during the acute phase of depression. The structured daily activity program provided in the hospital leaves the depressed

Research Highlight

Are Physical Activity, Self-Esteem, and Depression Related?

C. Parent & A. Whall

PURPOSE

This study was done to determine the relationship between physical activity, self-esteem, and depression in older adults. Two hypotheses were addressed: (1) older adults who participate daily, weekly, or monthly in a physical activity will demonstrate greater self-esteem than those who do not, and (2) older adults who participate in a daily, weekly, or monthly activity will demonstrate a lower depression score than those who do not.

SAMPLE

Thirty people 60 years of age and older from a senior citizen housing complex and participants at a neighboring senior citizen center were studied. To be included in the study, persons had to be oriented and had to be able to speak and understand, make judgments about physical activity, complete the study scales, and understand informed consent.

METHODOLOGY

Physical activity was measured in terms of the Functional Life Scale (FLS) and an activity scale created by the researchers. Self-esteem was measured by Rosendale's Self-Esteem Scale. Beck's Depression Inventory Scale was used to measure depression. Data were analyzed with the use of totals for the activity scales, the self-esteem scales, and the depression inventory.

FINDINGS

A strong correlation was found between self-esteem and physical activities performed on a monthly basis, supporting the hypothesis of a relationship between the number of activities performed monthly and self-esteem. Other findings indicated that self-esteem and depression are negatively and strongly correlated.

IMPLICATIONS

Activities, hobbies, and recreation that require physical exertion have a positive relationship to self-esteem and an inverse relationship to depression. Nurses working with depressed persons need to incorporate a physical activity into the individual's nursing care plan.

Based on data from the Journal of Gerontological Nursing **10**(3):8. 1984.

client with little time to brood over problems. It also prevents the client from sleeping during the day and thus promotes sleeping at night.

Touching has therapeutic value. A handshake or touch on the shoulder establishes contact and promotes a sense of worth and acceptance.

Medications also are frequently used for depressed clients (see Chapter 22).

Electroconvulsive therapy (ECT) is found to help some depressed clients. Because symptom reduction from antidepressant medications generally requires 2 to 4 weeks and responses to ECT are often effective in a short period of time, ECT may be the treatment of choice, particularly when the risk of suicide is high.

Emotional dimension. Promoting healthy feelings contribute to a person's sense of hope. The nurse promotes the expression of feelings by encouraging the client to share both postitive and negative feelings in a healthy manner. The following statement shows the healthy expression of a positive feeling: "I feel good knowing my daughter wants me to stay with her after I leave the hospital." The healthy expression of a negative feeling is demonstrated in the following example: "I resent it that my kids don't want me involved in their lives." Expressing feelings about disappointments, losses, and death can be influential in helping the client accept a situation that cannot be changed.

Interventions for depressed clients include helping them unburden themselves of feelings associated with a loss. Some of the feelings are anger, anxiety, guilt, loneliness, worthlessness, uselessness, powerlessness, and despair. Expression of these feelings helps a client to develop an awareness and understanding of his predominant feeling. The nurse facilitates the expression of feelings with statements that communicate empathy and understanding, such as "You're feeling angry," "You're anxious," "You think maybe you are a burden to your family," or "You wish you could be more useful at your son's house." Willingness to listen, nonjudgmental acceptance, and support are essential. Once the feeling has been identified and acknowledged, other ways of coping with the situation can be explored. While the client cannot change the situation, he can be helped to change his feelings about it.

Because severely depressed clients often feel powerless, assisting them to achieve a degree of control by making decisions about their treatment procedures, food choices, self-care, schedules, and activities helps restore feelings of power and significance.

Intellectual dimension. Interventions that promote hope include providing the individual with information about depression, its incidence, causes, signs and symptoms, and prevention. Knowledge about depression gives the individual power to make choices, to think positively about himself, to be able to assume responsibility for himself among available options, and to maintain a sense of hope and optimism.

Motivating individuals toward some positive action is conducive to maintaining hope; for example, encouraging the individual to participate in a satisfying activity or event such as competitive sports.

For the depressed client, interventions include allowing time for the client to respond. The psychomotor retardation and verbal inactivity require that the rate of conversation be slowed down to give the client time to think and respond.

The nurse can help depressed clients to distinguish between thoughts and feelings, thus permitting them to analyze their perceptions of an experience and make them more tolerable. A feeling can be explained to the client as an emotion, such as sadness or anger; thoughts use such phrases as "There is no hope," or "I am doomed." Once the distinctions are established, the client can proceed to the next step, which is identification of the facts leading to a cognitive conclusion such as "There is no hope." Usually the only facts are the client's severely painful emotions. Emotions as such, however, are not facts. Painful feelings are real and the pain is acknowledged, but the pain is not accepted as a sufficient cause for concluding that all is hopeless. That is to say, the feelings are indeed painful but the conclusion is not logical. By leading the client through these steps, it is possible to provide a way of recognizing the nature of the pain, tolerating the pain, and avoiding illogical or irrational conclusions.

The negative thinking of depressed clients, which includes self-doubt, self-pity, resentment, worrying, self-criticism, and self-accusations, can be altered to more positive thoughts by having the client focus on personal strengths and assets. The nurse can ask clients to list positive attributes about themselves to enhance positive thinking. Negative thinking can be controlled by the client's consciously stating, "I am going to stop thinking about that now." Another technique involves wearing a rubber band around one's wrist. As soon as the client is aware of a negative thought, he snaps it. Doing this consistently promotes awareness of the negative thought. Studies show than an act that is punished consistently will show a reduction frequency. When the act is a negative thought, punishment is a snap of the rubber band.

For clients who worry excessively, setting aside a pricise time for mulling over negative thoughts helps. The client decides when is the best time to devote to this negative thinking. The client may say, for example, "My worrying time will start at 11:00 and last 20 minutes." Clients are not avoiding worrying—they are deciding how long to worry. It is agreed that the client will not worry at other times.

Visualization and *guided imagery* are other interventions that help when the client is preoccupied with negative thoughts. Clients are helped to focus on happier times or peak experiences, to imagine they are in a place they love, such as the beach or the mountains or wherever they feel fully alive, comfortable, and healthy. They are asked to imagine the area is filled with bright, clear light and to let the light flow into their body, making them brighter and filling them with the energy of health. Or they can visualize drawing a heavy black magic marker circle around their negative thoughts so that the negative thoughts are contained. Visualization and imagery are both healing and liberating. They help the person let go of negative thinking.

The ability to make decisions is a difficult problem for depressed clients. The nurse can limit the clients' choices to simple ones, such as what suit or dress to wear. The nurse makes decisions for the client in more complex situations. If the problem of choosing between the plaid dress and the green dress is too difficult, the nurse simply hands the client the dress of her choice to prevent the client from being overwhelmed by the decision.

Judgment in the depressed client may be impaired. Being subject to extreme pessimism, a client may be convinced of the need to liquidate a business or quit a job. For example, helping the family assume responsibility for business affairs while the client is recovering from depression is appropriate. Clients also need protection, since many are accident prone because of their decreased concentration and poor judgment.

When delusions or hallucinations are present, the nurse helps orient the client to reality. Because depressed clients often tend to be perfectionistic, rigid, and compulsive, the nurse helps them accept flaws, in themselves and others without persecuting and blaming.

Social dimension. Nursing behaviors that foster meaningful relationships and promote independence are essential. Support persons are important in maintaining an attitude of hopefulness. Involving family members or friends and neighbors in the client's care enlarges the client's social network, a vital ingredient of hope.

Hope is fostered when the nurse helps the client successfully adapt or adjust to changes. The client comes to trust the nurse, and the feelings of trust and safety enhance hope and optimism.

A healthy environment free from pollution, excessive noise, overcrowding, and undue violence also assists in maintaining a sense of hope. Encouraging personality traits such as assertiveness, love of adventure, and risk-taking promotes hope and optimism.

Promotion of active involvement in life activates a sense of hope for the future. For example, a person who actively campaigns for conservation of natural resources demonstrates hope that the efforts are not futile. Generally people who demonstrate hope and optimism assume responsibility for creating situations that foster such attitudes.

Interventions for depressed persons include preventing them from being alone. The nurse needs to seek out the client, since depressed people tend to withdraw from others. An initial approach that does not pressure the client to talk is an important step in building trust. Short, frequent interactions exemplify a caring attitude and produce less anxiety than do longer interactions. In a one-to-one relationship, security, trust, and support are given until the client's own support system is reestablished. Activities that allow the client to interact with others, such as cards, puzzles, crafts, or small group projects, prevent further preoccupation with self. Group therapy provides interactions with others and promotes a sense of belonging as well as gives time to solve problems. Encouraging family members to stay in contact with the client is essential. Frequently depressed persons view the family as hostile

and uncaring, when actually the family is caring and concerned about the client but at a loss as to what to do.

Working with the family to rebuild broken relationships can be a rewarding experience for the nurse. When the nurse can help families enjoy life more fully and without guilt about the depressed member, satisfaction is achieved by the nurse, the client, and the family.

Encouraging interdependence, whereby the client reaches out to others to give or receive help, is therapeutic for the depressed person. For example, a client's pushing another client confined to a wheelchair to meals each day may increase the depressed client's sense of independence and feelings of being needed and important. Assertiveness training provides the dependent client with the skills to become independent. Learning how to ask for what one wants, to take risks, and to gain confidence in oneself are skills that the depressed person can learn in an assertiveness course.

Because despair over loss and death is expressed differently in some cultures, the nurse needs to be knowledgeable about the client's cultural background. It is important that she refer the client to a more knowledgeable person when she lacks the resources to deal with responses to losses, separations, and death.

Occupational therapy, activity therapy, and music therapy are effective treatment modalities for the depressed client. Activities that clients find pleasurable, as well as those that foster interactions with others, are beneficial. It is important for the nurse to strongly encourage depressed clients to participate in these activities. In addition, actively involving the client in activities is important as a way of increasing self-esteem and fostering responsibility for personal health care. Other interventions that enhance the client's self-esteem and help alleviate depression include exploring clients' feelings about themselves, identifying where the feelings may have come from and whether they are realistic, and helping the client choose between continuing to have these miserable feelings or focusing on finding more positive feelings.

Assisting clients to identify sources of pleasure and planning activities that provide pleasure and success are vital in increasing their self-esteem. For some depressed persons, working in the kitchen provides pleasure if a sense of worth and competence is felt in this area. For retired office workers, an assignment in the greenhouse may enable them to learn a new skill, thereby increasing their self-esteem. Such diversional activities also prevent brooding and self-centeredness and promote self-confidence.

Spiritual dimension. The person with hope and optimism needs minimal support and encouragement from the nurse. Reinforcing inner strengths such as courage and self-worth is a primary intervention within the spiritual dimension. With inner strengths identified and reinforced, individuals are free to strive for maximum potential and creativity. If individuals can be freed from inner conflicts, opportunities for them to grow in hope, to create, and to become more self-actualizing persons can result. Clarification of values contributes to a person's feelings of hope by reducing conflicts within that value system. For some individuals, belief in life after death is a vital component in sustaining a sense of hope. Encouraging and providing ways for clients to attend worship may fulfill the need to demonstrate and practice their beliefs.

Listening attentively to cues may tell the nurse when the depressed client is willing to discuss his hopelessness and his belief that there is no way that his life will get better. He may see death as a relief from despair and unbearable guilt and may consider suicide. The nurse, alert to the possibility of suicide, initiates a one-to-one relationship so that close observation can be maintained. The services of a chaplain, minister, or other religious leader are helpful for the client who needs assistance in forgiving himself or others.

Through opportunities to be creative in art, poetry, sculpture, or music, clients can move away from their self-centeredness toward the freedom often experienced in these pursuits and learn to value themselves as unique individuals.

When depressed clients question the meaning of their suffering and the purposelessness of their lives, the nurse needs to encourage and facilitate further expression of feelings. Once the client's feelings have been identified, the nurse can assist the client to consider other options available, and the client can move beyond the pain of depression with integrity, a greater awareness of self, personal value, and a relatedness to another. The helpless, despairing client may find meaning in or accept suffering when the nurse is available, accepting, and empathic. This satisfies the need for relatedness in such a way that the client finds the strength to come to terms with life, gain confidence, and live a more enriched life.

INTERACTION WITH A DEPRESSED CLIENT

Nurse: Betty, it's time to go to O.T.
Betty: I'm not going today.
Nurse: You're not going?
Betty: No.
Nurse: You seemed to enjoy working on your cup yesterday.
Betty: No, I didn't.
Nurse: It was beginning to look real pretty.
Betty: I didn't like it.
Nurse: (Pause.) Betty, you may not feel like going to O.T., but I would like for you to go for a short time. It is part of your treatment plan to participate in activities while you are here.
Betty: (Silence.)
Nurse: I'll be back in 10 minutes and we will walk down together.

Ten minutes later. Nurse returns.

Nurse: I'll walk down to O.T. with you now, Betty.
Betty: (Silence, gets up and starts walking.) Why do you make me do things I don't want to do? I wish you would leave me alone, all of you.
Nurse: You are irritated because you are going to O.T.?
Betty: No, I just don't want to go. It's not helping me. (She keeps on walking.)

Betty is severely depressed. She prefers to stay alone, responds minimally to others, and with negativism. Because Betty is depressed, the nurse speaks slowly and allows ample time for Betty to respond to her requests.

The nurse uses restating to encourage Betty to expand on her reason for not going to O.T. When this approach fails she states an observation she made of Betty in O.T. the previous day. A positive statement such as this helps to elevate Betty's self-esteem.

The nurse follows this statement with another positive one to help Betty alter her negative thinking. Because Betty's thinking is so deeply negative she screens out any positive statements about herself. The nurse is aware that Betty will probably continue to do this and is supportive and empathic at the same time, letting her know what is expected of her (to go to O.T.). She gives Betty some time to prepare herself to go and returns 10 minutes later, as she stated, with the expectation that Betty will go. She accepts Betty's expression of her annoyance with her and the staff for asking her to do what she does not want to do and continues walking with her to O.T.

It will be important for the nurse to provide some positive feedback to Betty on her return from O.T. about her behavior, such as "I know you didn't want to go, but I'm pleased that you did. I think you are trying to help yourself feel better."

Manic Behavior

THEORETICAL APPROACHES

Manic behavior is a mood disturbance found in clients diagnosed as having bipolar disorder. The manic episode is characterized by a predominantly elated mood with symptoms of hyperactivity, pressure of speech, *flight of ideas,* inflated self-esteem, decreased need for food and sleep, distractibility, irritability, and excessive involvement in activities that may have painful consequences. Episodes of manic behavior may be followed by periods of depression. The symptoms of depression and *mania* may alternate rapidly or last several weeks or months. Table 14-5 summarizes theories of manic behavior.

NURSING PROCESS
Assessment

Physical dimension. Manic behavior is the opposite of depressed behavior. Motor activity is increased; the client is hyperactive, restless, and involved in many activities, such as buying sprees, reckless driving, foolish business investments, and sexual behavior unusual for the individual. Dress is flamboyant and colorful. Women may wear excessive and inappropriate jewelry for the situation. Makeup may be excessive and poorly applied. Men may dress in exaggerated fashion with little or no attention to personal hygiene. There is a decreased need for sleep. The individual awakens several hours before the usual time full of energy and may go for days without sleep and without feeling tired. Appetite is decreased, and the client does not take time from his un-

TABLE 14-5 Summary of theories of manic behavior

Theory	Dynamics
Genetic	Behavior is transmitted in families in which one or more members have had a manic episode as well as a depressive episode.
Biological	Excesses in biogenic amines, norepinephrine, and serotonin predispose to periods of elation.
	Chromosomal abnormalities contribute to manic behavior.
	Defects in cell membranes are found in clients with bipolar disorder.
Psychoanalytical	Loss, real or imagined, may precipitate a manic episode and defend against depression. Anxiety and tension are denied, resulting in elated and uninhibited behavior.

ceasing activities to eat. Lack of sleep and failure to eat may become life threatening. He also fails to take note of minor ailments or physical complaints and becomes susceptible to infection and illness.

✳ *Emotional dimension.* During manic episodes the client's mood is euphoric. He is overly cheerful, excessively enthusiastic, and appears "high." He may exhibit a wide range of mood swings, becoming irritable and angry easily when his desires are thwarted. There is an infectious quality about his mood and an unwarranted optimism. Feelings of inadequacy and inferiority lurk beneath his euphoria.

✳ *Intellectual dimension.* Thought processes in the manic client are accelerated, and he is easily distracted. As a result of responding to various environmental stimuli (noises, movements, pictures, colors, temperature, other people, activities), his speech becomes pressured. He has flight of ideas resulting from his thoughts racing ahead of his speech. Communication may be humorous—full of jokes, puns, plays on words and amusing irrelevancies. The client may become theatrical, with singing and dramatic mannerisms. Sounds rather than meanings govern word choice (clanging). Thoughts may become grandiose and delusional, with the client thinking he is a well-known entertainer, writer, or political or religious figure. Judgment and insight are impaired. The client may give away valued possessions or very expensive belongings.

✳ *Social dimension.* Self-esteem is unrealistically inflated. Overconfidence in one's self and one's abilities is exhibited. Increased sociability may result in calling old friends and acquaintances at all hours of the day and night. The intrusive, domineering, demanding, and meddling nature of his interactions is unrecognized by the manic client. He is often involved in excessive planning and participation in multiple activities—sexual, political, religious, and occupational.

296.4x MANIC BIPOLAR DISORDER

ESSENTIAL FEATURES

The individual's predominant mood is elevated, expansive, or irritable, accompanied by hyperactivity, flight of ideas, and inflated self-esteem.

MANIFESTATIONS
Physical Dimension

Hyperactivity
Decreased need for sleep
Participation in multiple activities
Flamboyant, bizarre dress

Emotional Dimension

Elevated, euphoric mood
Irritable
Excessive enthusiasm

Intellectual Dimension

Pressure of speech
Flight of ideas
Distractability
Lack of judgement
Theatrical, dramatic speech
Puns, jokes, plays on words, amusing irrelevancies
Delusions of grandeur

Social Dimension

Inflated self-esteem
Grandiosity
Excessive involvement in activities of others
Increased sociability
Intrusive
Domineering
Demanding in relationships

Adapted from American Psychiatric Association: Diagnostic and statistical manual of mental disorders (DSM-III-R), Washington, D.C., 1987, The Association.

✳ *Spiritual dimension.* Clients with recurring episodes of manic behavior may come to value the "highs" in their lives. As a way to avoid the painful realities in their own lives, they may choose not to adhere to their medication regimen to maintain their "high." Life may become far more bearable and pleasurable when the individual is elated and euphoric than when depressed. It then becomes important to assess the meaning and value of the illness to the client.

Analysis

Nursing diagnosis. The following list provides examples of NANDA-accepted diagnoses related to manic behavior with causative statements.

1. Disturbance in self-concept related to exaggerated sense of self-importance
2. Impaired social interactions related to demanding, meddling behavior
3. Sleep pattern disturbance related to hyperactivity

4. Alterations in thought processes related to delusions of grandeur
5. Noncompliance related to thinking that medications are no longer needed

DSM-III-R diagnoses. The diagnosis of bipolar disorder is subclassified as mixed, manic, and depressed. Mixed bipolar disorder involves the client's having symptoms of both manic and depressive episodes. A diagnosis of bipolar disorder, depressed, is made when the client, in a major depressive episode, has had one or more manic episodes. With a diagnosis of bipolar disorder, manic, the client is in a manic episode.

A diagnosis of *cyclothymia* is made when the client has both manic and depressive symptoms, but not of sufficient severity or duration to be diagnosed as a major depression or a manic episode. The essential features and manifestations of the features of bipolar disorder according to the DSM-III-R are listed in the box on p. 282.

The following Case Example demonstrates manic behavior.

Case Example

Sondra Bowen, a 39-year-old opera singer, is admitted to a psychiatric hospital after keeping her family awake for several nights with prayers and a song marathon. She is flamboyantly dressed in a floor-length red skirt and peasant blouse and is adorned with heavy earrings, numerous necklaces and bracelets, and medals pinned to her bosom. She speaks rapidly and is difficult to interrupt as she talks about her intimate relationship with God. She often breaks into song, explaining that her beautiful singing voice is a special gift that God has given her to compensate for her insanity. She uses it to share the joy she feels with others who are less fortunate.

Planning

See Table 14-6 for examples of long-term and short-term goals and outcome criteria related to disturbance in self-concept. These serve as examples of the planning stage of the nursing process.

Implementation

Physical dimension. The client who exhibits manic behavior needs external controls until he is able to set limits on his own physical activity. Providing a structured, subdued environment helps to limit some of the restlessness and hyperactivity. A private room with minimal furnishings and neutral colors is helpful. The nurse selects noncompetitive, solitary activities, such as walking, swimming, gymnastics, raking leaves, writing, finger-painting, and jogging, that help the client direct energy appropriately. By providing activities or projects that can be completed in a short time, the nurse gives the client opportunities to experience success, reduce feelings of inadequacy, and develop self-control. It is important to assist the client with his grooming so that clothing is in good repair and appropriate for the season, activity, and time of day. An appropriate appearance helps the

---

TABLE 14-6 Long-term and short-term goals and outcome criteria related to disturbance in self-concept

Goals	Outcome Criteria
NURSING DIAGNOSIS: DISTURBANCE IN SELF-CONCEPT RELATED TO AN EXAGGERATED SENSE OF SELF	
Long-term goals	
To have a realistic perception of self	Makes realistic statements about self
To cope with the stress of life	Identifies situations that cause stress
	Identifies responses to stress
	Identifies consequences of responses to stress
	Explores alternative ways of coping
	Uses an adaptive method of coping
To comply with medication regimen	Takes medication as directed
	Verbalizes importance of taking medication, perhaps for the rest of his life
Short-term goals	
To express painful feelings	Verbalizes painful feelings
	Gives self permission to feel angry, sad, anxious
To strengthen relationships	Identifies problem areas in relating to others
	Initiates an activity with another person
	Listens to another person's problem
To increase self-esteem	Completes a task or project successfully
	Makes positive statements about self
	Is less anxious
	Makes appropriate decisions
	Learns a new skill
	Does something for another person

client maintain his identity and prevents ridicule from others. The nurse reduces environmental stimuli as much as possible, particularly at bedtime, to promote sleep.

Comfort measures such as a warm bath, darkness, and the administration of prescribed medications prevent fatigue and exhaustion. It is important for the nurse to closely supervise the administration of medications, because the client may "cheek" it and dispose of it later. A change to the liquid form of medication may alleviate this problem.

A high-calorie, high-vitamin diet with supplemental feedings and adequate fluids promotes an adequate dietary intake and prevents excessive weight loss. Finger foods such as sandwiches, fruits, and milkshakes, which can be eaten when the client is too restless to sit down and eat, ensures healthy nutrition.

Because the client tends to ignore physical ailments, it is important for the nurse to carefully monitor his vital signs and weight and any signs of injury or misuse.

Emotional dimension. When the client's mood is euphoric and elated, he is pleasant to be with; however, it is important that staff and others do not encourage behavior that promotes or accelerates his elation and euphoria. Helping the client to express his feelings of inadequacy and inferiority may lessen his sense of a constant state of threat and reduce psychomotor activity. The irritability and anger that erupts easily when his desires are not met can best be handled with a kind, firm, and persuasive approach that promotes external controls before the anger escalates and becomes destructive.

Intellectual dimension. Listening quietly and attentively will provide a sounding board for the verbally active client. It is helpful to attempt to interrupt the constant stream of conversation and encourage him to focus on one topic at a time, to direct his attention to real concerns and limit his flight of ideas. Laughing at or encouraging jokes, puns, and humorous anecdotes tends to escalate the behavior and has little therapeutic benefit. The nurse may ignore grandiose thinking or distract him by focusing his attention on real activities and events. Short, simple, direct requests and explanations for activities and procedures are more easily heard and may eliminate some of the arguing, belligerance, and impetuousness of the manic client. The nurse promotes opportunities for the client to see himself realistically. Such simple statements as "You are Gary Johnson" when the client claims to be the well-known singer Michael Jackson helps reorient the client to reality.

Social dimension. Realistic self-esteem is promoted by simple, matter-of-fact reality statements. It is essential to avoid arguing or being irritated by the client's persistence and repetitiveness in proclaiming his competence and achievements. Scheduling short, frequent times for interactions helps to maximize the client's short attention span. Reducing the number of contacts with others and assigning the same person to work with the client each day promotes more meaningful relationships with a consistent person and may prevent attempts to dominate, meddle, and demand from others. Setting limits on involvements in business investments and political and reli-

gious activities is crucial during a manic episode to prevent future negative consequences and embarrassment. Involving the family in setting limits in these areas is an important part of the treatment. Manic-depressive self-help groups are available in some communities for clients to receive additional support and information about the illness.

Spiritual dimension. Clients with manic behavior need to learn to value themselves realistically. Promoting self-worth reduces the underlying feelings of inadequacy and inferiority and lessens his need to inflate ideas about himself. Helping the client see himself as a unique individual with realistic positive attributes and a member of a family or larger community increases the client's valuing himself in spite of the limitations caused by his illness. It is also important to help the client discuss the meaning of his illness. Avoiding painful realities by becoming "sick" (manic) may be seen as a pleasant way to handle life stress, and he may come to enjoy the feeling rather than face life's problems. It becomes essential that the client accept his illness as one that is treatable so that he can function effectively throughout his lifetime.

Suicide

Suicide is the intentional action taken by a person to end his own life. The ultimate level of self-destruction, suicide is a perplexing problem in a culture that teaches the value of life and abhors death. The term *suicide* is used to describe a thought, a threat, gesture, attempt, or completed act. *Suicidal ideations* are thoughts a person may have about killing himself. Many people harbor ideas about suicide without ever verbally expressing the idea. A *suicidal threat* is a verbal indication that the person is considering a self-destructive act. A suicidal gesture is an act of self-harm that generally is not a threat to the person's life. The *suicidal gesture* is seen as a cry for help in many situations. A *suicidal attempt* may follow a gesture and occurs when the person believes his behavior will result in his death. Many times the attempt is unsuccessful because the person is unexpectedly rescued; for example, someone returns home and interrupts the suicide attempt or takes the person to the hospital. Suicide attempts and gestures may be used to communicate anger, frustration, and despair to significant persons in his life. Completed suicide results when a person takes his own life with conscious intent.

A recent and controversial type of suicide, rational suicide, proposes that individuals carry out their death wish in a planned manner using a method of choice and with the cooperation and participation of family members and friends at a time selected by the individual. Although not widely accepted, it is subject to much discussion today (see the following Case Example).

Case Example

John and Delores Sanders, both 81, were found dead of gunshot wounds in the front seat of their auto in a pasture 5 miles

TABLE 14-7 Summary of theories of suicide

Theory	Theorist	Dynamics
Psychoanalytical	Freud	The death drive, inherent in all persons, is in constant struggle with the instinct to live. It is this struggle that accounts for the ambivalence seen in suicidal persons.
Sociological	Durkheim	The nature of a society (for example, unstable socioeconomic conditions) influences suicide.
	Farberow	Religion, legal sanctions, and philosophical beliefs determine the meaning and pattern of suicide in a society.

from their home. On investigation, the murder-suicide was found to be a deliberately planned act by both Mr. and Mrs. Sanders. Mrs. Sander's failing vision, heart congestion, and stroke had forced her husband to place her in a nursing home earlier. He brought her home when she complained bitterly and wanted to be at home with Mr. Sanders. A note found on the floorboard of their car had typewritten funeral instructions and the telephone number of their son. The note, in part, said, "Dear Eric, we know this will be a terrible shock and embarrassment. But as we see it, it is one solution to the problem of growing old. We greatly appreciate your willingness to try to take care of us. After being married for 60 years, it only makes sense for us to leave this world together because we loved each other so much. Don't grieve for us, as we had a good life and saw you turn out to be a fine person. Love, Mother and Dad." Eric, their son, shocked and horrified, looked at the options they could have taken and sadly stated he could find none that would have been satisfactory to his parents.

Other types of self-destructive behavior exist: overeating, smoking, reckless driving, participation in hazardous sports or hobbies, and substance abuse.

THEORETICAL APPROACHES
Psychoanalytic

According to Freud,[30] an individual's two significant insticts are eros (instinct for life) and thanatos (instinct for death). The death drive, thanatos, is inherent in all persons and is engaged in a constant struggle with eros. This accounts for the ambivalence experienced by suicidal persons—they wish to live and they wish to die. Freud explained that a stressful event evokes confusion, guilt, and shame, which activate the death wish. The person kills himself instead of the object that he wants to destroy. Freud's anger-turned-inward theory is discussed on p. 264.

Sociological

Durkheim[24] discussed suicide within a sociological context. He stated that the nature of a society predisposes to suicide and that suicide can be expected when certain conditions exist. He believed any condition that interfered with a stable socioeconomic status is influential in the commission of suicide. For example, consider the high suicide rate during the Depression in 1929. His studies showed a direct relationship between social conditions and the incidence of suicide. Durkheim described four forms of suicide, as follows:

Egoistic	The individual lacks group support, resulting in extreme individualism.
Altruistic	The individual indentifies strongly with a group and is willing to die for ideas and purposes of the group.
Anomie	The individual is in a period of normlessness, as occurs when society undergoes changes and moral authority is weakened.
Fatalistic	The individual receives excessive regulation, the opposite of anomie.

Farberow[26] emphasized sociocultural conditions associated with suicide. Sociocultural influences such as religion, legal sanctions, and philosophical beliefs determine the meaning and pattern of suicide in a society. According to Farberow, suicide cannot be studied without consideration of the impact of these influences on the suicidal person. (See Table 14-7 for a summary of theories of suicide.)

NURSING PROCESS
Assessment

✦ ***Physical dimension.*** Any person in poor physical health who has chronic pain or a chronic or terminal illness is considered at risk for suicide. Many persons who successfully complete suicide have been found to have visited their physician for a variety of physical complaints within 6 months of their deaths. They described headaches, chest pain, insomnia, fatigue, gastrointestinal upsets, backaches, and anorexia. These symptoms may indicate depression, and it is imperative that the nurse be aware of the potential for suicide among these clients.

Other persons considered at high risk for suicide include those abusing alcohol and drugs, those engaged in risk-taking activities such as mountain climbing, hang-gliding, and car racing, and those who are accident prone. Age is also a factor to consider with adolescents and older white males having the highest rates of suicide.

It is important to inquire about arrests, motor vehicle accidents, and court involvements, because many persons attempt suicide after being jailed. Inquiring about previous suicide attempts is equally important. A person with a previous attempt is likely to make another attempt.

✳ ***Emotional dimension.*** Any depressed person, particularly one with feelings of hopelessness, is considered at risk for suicide (see the Research Highlight on p. 286). Not all depressed persons are suicidal, but it is important that the nurse be aware of the possibility

Research Highlight

Hopelessness and Eventual Suicide: A 10-Year Prospective Study of Patients Hospitalized With Suicide Ideation

A. Beck, R. Steer, M. Kovacs & B. Garrison

PURPOSE

This study was designed to ascertain whether hopelessness, depression, or suicide ideation would predict eventual suicide in clients hospitalized because they had suicidal ideas.

SAMPLE

The sample included 207 clients admitted to two psychiatric inpatient wards between 1970 and 1975. They were considered to be having suicidal ideas, had not made a recent attempt, and were between 17 and 65 years of age.

METHODOLOGY

A detailed clinical interview was done by a psychologist or psychiatrist within 24 to 48 hours of admission. A research assistant administered the Beck Depression Inventory (BDI), the Hopelessness Scale, and the Scale for Suicide Ideation. After each client's discharge, contact was maintained for a period of 5 years. If the client was deceased, data regarding the cause, manner, and mode of death were obtained.

FINDINGS

Fourteen of the clients completed suicide. Of these, the greatest number were diagnosed with neurotic depression (35.8%). The Hopelessness Scale differentiated significantly between the two groups of persons with suicidal ideas. Persons with suicidal ideas who completed suicide had higher mean scores than those who did not die from suicide. The pessimism rating in the BDI was also higher among those who later completed suicide.

IMPLICATIONS

There is a relationship between hopelessness and suicide; therefore the assessment of hopelessness is useful as an indicator of suicide risk. Interventions that reduce hopelessness may lower the suicidal potential. There is evidence in the literature that cognitive therapy acts faster in lowering hopelessness than does pharmacotherapy. Thus prompt cognitive interventions or a combination of cognitive therapy and pharmacotherapy may be directed at reducing hopelessness and, consequently, suicide risk.

Based on data from the American Journal of Psychiatry **142**(5):559, 1985.

with depressed persons. Persons with excessive guilt may also attempt suicide.

Intellectual dimension. The suicidal person may be preoccupied with thoughts of self-harm or self-destruction. He may actively state his wish to die, or he may give out subtle clues, such as saying "Good-bye" or "You won't have to bother with me any more."

Ambivalence may be seen in the suicidal client. It is essential to assess this behavior so that emphasis can be placed on the person's need to live.

The person with disorganized, fragmented, and distorted thinking is considered a high risk for suicide. Because of his confusion and disorientation, he may be unable to reason effectively or control his behavior, and may act impulsively. Persons with schizophrenia or psychoses have a high potential for suicide. The client may describe hallucinations with voices telling him to jump out a window or walk out in front of moving vehicles, or he may describe delusions of being Superman and attempt to fly off a roof. Because the risk is great in these persons, the nurse thoroughly assesses judgment, thought content, and impulsiveness.

Social dimension. Most people who commit suicide have experienced turmoil or losses in their interpersonal relationships. Sudden changes in life situations, such as separation, divorce, or death, may have created what is perceived by the client as insurmountable problems. The nurse assesses the nature of the client's relationships with family and friends and his perception of supportive persons. Frequently isolation and alienation from significant others is seen, and the client withdraws from others. He may reject any offers of help from supportive persons. Dependence brought on by illness or injury may generate feelings of hopelessness and helplessness, with suicide seen as the only choice, since he thinks nothing can be done about the situation and no one can help.

An assessment of the person's personal, family, school, and work history may provide significant information. Persons living alone, particularly older, single, divorced or widowed men, are prone to suicide. Persons with a family history of a committed suicide or an attempt are considered a risk for suicide. It is important to ask whether anyone in the family has ever attempted suicide. Failure at school or perceived failure at school as well as unemployment and job stress are contributing factors to suicide. The nurse needs to be aware that the anniversary date of a lost loved one may precipitate a suicide attempt as grief is reawakened.

Additional clues that may be significant in assessing suicide risk include the following behaviors: giving away possessions, arranging personal and business affairs, contacting friends and relatives, and writing a will.

The client's self-concept is assessed. Because of upheavals in relationships and loss of loved ones, the individual's esteem may be lowered. Feelings of inferiority, incompetence, inadequacy, and worthlessness are common. It is also essential that the individual's resources are assessed, including family, friends, agencies, employment, and finances, so that support systems can be strengthened.

✷ ***Spiritual dimension.*** The nurse explores the client's religious affiliation. Most studies indicate that white Protestants in the United States have the highest rate of suicide. However, this does not preclude the fact that people of other races and religions do commit suicide.

A discussion of the client's beliefs about life and death provide data on the client's potential for suicide. For some, death may be seen as a punishment for guilt or a way to punish others for inflicting guilt and pain. Others may view life as having no meaning or purpose or may believe that there is no help or hope that life will ever be better. Others see death as a relief from pain and suffering, and better for themselves, the family, and loved ones.

The nurse assesses the client's sense of value and worth as a person. Many who attempt suicide feel unimportant and insignificant, that their life or death makes little difference to anyone.

Analysis

Nursing diagnosis. The following list provides examples of NANDA-accepted nursing diagnoses with causative statements.

1. Potential for violence: self-directed, related to threats of suicide
2. Potential for violence: self-directed, related to suicidal gestures
3. Potential for violence: self-directed, related to inability to realistically evaluate the problem
4. Potential for violence: self-directed, related to inability to control behavior associated with suicide attempt

Potential for violence: self-directed is a NANDA-approved nursing diagnosis that applies to the suicidal client. The defining characteristics of this nursing diagnosis are listed in the box at right.

The following Case Example demonstrates the characteristics of the nursing diagnosis, potential for violence, self-directed.

Case Example

Terry, age 15, attempted to kill herself by taking an overdose of a combination of medications including Valium, aspirin, Sominex, and Dalmane. She had a fight with her boyfriend of 7 months and had been grounded by her father for talking on the telephone too long. She does not have a good relationship with her mother, who she said "never listens to her." On returning from school she became angry at her hopeless situation and searched the house for any medications she could find and swallowed them. Thirty minutes later her mother returned, and on learning what Terry had done, had her admitted to a psychiatric unit for adolescents.

POTENTIAL FOR VIOLENCE: SELF-DIRECTED

DEFINITION
The state in which an individual experiences behaviors that can be physically harmful to self.

DEFINING CHARACTERISTICS
Physical Dimension
Body language that indicates effort to control; clenched fists, tense, rigid posture
Current self-harm behavior
Previous self-harm attempt
Decreased self-care
Putting personal and business affairs in order
Lack of impulse control
Pain
Possession of destructive means (gun, knife)
Substance abuse/withdrawal
Emotional Dimension
Depression
Sudden mood elevation (paradoxic calm)
Increased anxiety, panic
Feelings of "I can't take it"
Intellectual Dimension
Verbal statement of intent to harm self
Self-derogatory statements
Egocentricity
Delusional thoughts
Hallucinations
Deliberate noncompliance with medical regimen
Impaired judgement
Boasting
Social Dimension
Low self-esteem
Isolated
Seclusive
Helplessness
Life crisis
Aggressiveness
*Oppressive environment
Spiritual Dimension
*Hopelessness
*Lack of future plans
*Lack of meaning and purpose in life

Adapted from North American Nursing Diagnosis Association Classification of Nursing Diagnosis: Proceedings of the seventh conference, St. Louis, 1987, The C.V. Mosby Co.
*Indicates characteristics other than those defined by NANDA.

Planning

See Table 14-8 for examples of long-term and short-term goals and outcome criteria related to potential for violence, self-directed. These serve as examples of the planning stage of the nursing process.

Implementation

✦ ***Physical dimension.*** Hospitalization is generally the treatment of choice when a client has attempted

TABLE 14-8 Long-term and short-term goals and outcome criteria related to potential for violence: self-directed

Goals	Outcome Criteria

NURSING DIAGNOSIS: POTENTIAL FOR VIOLENCE, SELF-DIRECTED RELATED TO DEPRESSED MOOD

Long-term goals

Goals	Outcome Criteria
To develop more realistic and positive concept of self so that feelings of self-esteem, self-respect, acceptance by others, and belonging are enhanced.	Makes positive statements that describe self. Makes positive statements about significant others. Participates in an activity that is pleasurable. Learns a new skill. Engages in an activity that results in success.
To establish meaningful relationships with significant members of the family or friends.	Initiates a conversation or an activity with a significant person. Makes positive statements about the significant person. Responds positively to praise or compliments person. Responds positively to praise or compliments from others. Smiles when praised or complimented.

Short-term goals

Goals	Outcome Criteria
To accept protection from self-destruction until able to assume responsibility for self.	Makes statements indicating that client knows reasons for close observation. Verbalizes acceptance of protective measures.
To make a contract not to harm self.	Signs a written contract. Verbalizes acceptance of need for contract. Talks with a member of the health care team when thinking becomes suicidal.
To express anger constructively	Talks about angry feelings. Attends exercise classes. Statements indicate anger is a normal feeling. Talks about healthy ways to deal with angry feelings.
To meet physical needs.	Dresses self attractively and appropriately each day. Eats three fourths of all food on meal trays. Sleeps all night without interruptions. Asks for medication for constipation or headaches. Walks outdoors one time each day. Experiences satisfactory sexual relations.
To participate in ward activities.	Makes bed, performs other housekeeping activities as assigned (such as cleaning bathrooms, pushing wheelchair patients to meals). Is on time for meetings with physician or team, scheduled activities and meals. Joins in a small group conversation or activity.

suicide or appears in imminent danger of harming himself. Most hospitals have written policies about the care of suicidal persons that include the following:

1. Removing potentially harmful items: belts, socks, boot strings, matches, lighters, hairpicks, sharp objects, watches, glass cosmetic containers.
2. Observing the client 24 hours a day on a one-to-one basis.
3. Having client sleep in a dimly lit area for observation purposes.
4. Having the client eat on the unit.
5. Maintaining special awareness at times when suicide attempts are known to be likely: early morning, on arising, during busy routines, while shaving, when there is a shortage of staff, change of shift, when suddenly cheerful.
6. Isolating, if progressing toward destruction, to decrease stimulation.
7. Encouraging to participate in activities.

The client is given antidepressant medications to elevate his mood and make him more amenable to treatment. Electroconvulsive therapy (ECT) is an additional treatment that has proved effective (see Chapter 23).

Because the risk of suicide is high after the diagnosis of a terminal illness, during a chronic illness, or after an arrest for a motor vehicle accident, the nurse alerts the client's significant others to the possibility of suicide when clues have been observed. Physical complaints are treated as prescribed to promote comfort and a caring attitude.

Emotional dimension. Anguish, anger, depression, and hopelessness are the most common emotions expressed by clients who are suicidal. Nursing interventions for these feeling states are discussed in the Depression section of this chapter, p. 269.

Intellectual dimension. Threats of suicide are taken seriously. Listening attentively conveys an attitude of caring so desperately needed by the suicidal person. Because of a narrowing focus on the perception of his situation, the nurse helps the client expand his thinking to consider options with more favorable consequences for himself and others. When the suicide threat is a manipulative maneuver for control of others, assisting the client to sort out the meaning underlying the suicide threat is more helpful than labelling him a "manipulative client."

No-suicide contracts are an effective treatment method. The client states in writing that he will not hurt or kill himself, and if he has these feelings he will talk with a staff member about them. The presence of threatening delusions or hallucinations requires protection from impulsive actions. Close observation and medication may be necessary. Once the risk of suicide is lessened, the client can be taught new methods of coping. Problem solving, decision making, and assertiveness are methods used to reduce the impact of stress.

Social dimension.
A vital task in working with a suicidal client is helping him improve his self-concept. It is important to involve the client in activities to prevent preoccupation with self-destructive behavior and to provide opportunities for increasing self-esteem through accomplishment of useful and worthwhile tasks. This involves him with others and lessens the isolation and alienation. Helping the client reestablish relationships with family and friends who are significant to him also reduces the isolation. Until contact with family is made, the nurse may be the significant person. Family, friends, and other supportive persons need to be involved in the treatment plans.

It is helpful to plan for a friend or family member to be with the client on the anniversary of the death of a loved one. This contact may prevent loneliness and help the client reintegrate positive relationships with others.

Providing the telephone number of hotlines and the name of a contact person at crisis intervention centers is an additional effective nursing action.

Spiritual dimension.
The perception by the suicidal client of an intolerable life situation requires the greatest nursing expertise. Feelings of hopelessness, purposelessness, and meaninglessness are diminished by warmth and a caring, confident attitude and by offering alternatives for solving problems. The relationship with the nurse may satisfy his need for relatedness such that he finds the strength to come to terms with life, gain confidence, value himself, and live an enriched life.

Evaluation

In the evaluation process the goals are points of reference against which the nurse notes what behaviors have changed, and what new behaviors have emerged. Favorable outcomes are seen in the depressed client when he has fewer physical complaints, his mood is animated, he is less preoccupied, negative thinking is decreased, he has initiated new friendships, and he derives pleasure from daily life. The nurse keeps in mind the depressed client's reluctance to acknowledge progress within himself, even though progress is evident to others.

For the manic client, evaluation is based on the client's level of activity, stability of emotions, realistic self-concept and thought processes, understanding of his illness, appropriate social behavior, and compliance with his medication regimen.

Evaluation of the suicidal client involves noting daily changes in mood and activity level. Continuous evaluation of the client's potential for suicide is imperative. A mood that is less depressed, participation in activities, social interactions with others, and a stated desire to not harm or kill himself indicate a positive evaluation. However, the nurse is cautioned to be aware that these behaviors may indicate the client has already made the decision to commit suicide. Family and significant others are included in the evaluation of depressed, manic, or suicidal clients.

NURSING PROCESS SUMMARY: DEPRESSION

ASSESSMENT

Physical Dimension
Anorexia
Insomnia/excessive sleeping
Mutism
Psychomotor retardation or
   agitation
Exhaustion
Heart pounding
Diarrhea
Constipation
Vomiting
Fainting
Impotence
Drug or alcohol abuse

Physical illnesses
Accident proneness
Inability to carry out
   activities of daily living
Somatic complaints

Emotional Dimension
Anger
Hostility
Lack of feeling
Torment
Anxiety
Suicidal feelings
Guilt
Powerlessness
Unworthiness
Emptiness
Boredom

Intellectual Dimension
Delusions
Hallucinations
Confusion/disorientation
Lack of concentration
Preoccupation with self
Ruminations over wrong
   doings (real or imagined)
Rigidity
Poor judgment
Inattentiveness
Grandiosity
Forgetfulness
Self-blame
Self-criticism
Suicidal thoughts

Social Dimension
Poor self-concept
Isolation/clinging
Alienation
Helplessness
Withdrawal from others
Dependence

Spiritual Dimension
Meaninglessness
Purposelessness
Sense of failure in life
Hopelessness
Lack of belief and value
   in self
Alienation from God or
   supreme power

NURSING PROCES SUMMARY: DEPRESSION—cont'd

ANALYSIS

See list of nursing diagnoses on p 287.

PLANNING AND IMPLEMENTATION

Physical Dimension

Provide genetic counseling.

Assist with activities of daily living with particular attention to appearance and grooming.

Provide between-meal snacks and serve attractively to stimulate appetite.

Relieve physical symptoms such as constipation and headache.

Promote sleep with comfort measures such as warm bath, wine, music, and back rub.

Schedule short, regular times with client to demonstrate interest and acceptance.

Plan regular exercise schedule.

Give physical contact to client with handshake, touch on the shoulder, or hug when appropriate.

Observe for side effects of prescribed medications.

Increase environmental stimulation with colors, pictures, and plants.

Assist with electroconvulsive therapy if ordered.

Emotional Dimension

Promote expression of sad or angry feelings.

Provide emotional support to client with empathy, warmth, and genuineness.

Plan activities that are a source of pleasure.

Use an active, friendly, confident approach to client to promote a feeling of hopefulness and worth.

Decrease feelings of powerlessness by encouraging decision making.

Help the client experience successes.

Observe for potential suicide (e.g., a lifting depression).

Intellectual Dimension

Allow the client time to think and respond when depressed.

Help the client distinguish between thoughts and feelings.

Explore with client strengths and positive attributes.

Limit negative thoughts and worrying.

Provide positive visualization and imagery when preoccupied with negative thinking about self.

Assist with decision making by limiting choices.

Encourage family members to help with business decisions.

Help client to accept personal flaws without blame.

Observe continuously when suicidal thoughts are expressed.

Social Dimension

Enhance client's self-concept.

Promote meaningful relationships with appropriate degrees of dependence and independence.

Involve family, friends, or neighbors to enlarge the social network.

Offer activities that demand interacting with others, such as card playing, puzzles, or ceramics.

Encourage the client to do things for others.

Teach assertiveness skills.

Know and recognize pertinent cultural expressions of depression.

Provide occupational activity, exercise, or music therapy.

Spiritual Dimension

Encourage expression of religious values and beliefs.

Promote creative opportunities for client to move beyond self-centeredness.

Provide a relationship that fosters a sense of hope and meaning to life.

EVALUATION

Evaluation is based on the client's ability to prevent or cope with depressive symptoms. Positive evaluation reflects a decrease in depressive episodes, including increased energy, participation in usual activities, a more animated affect, decreased negative thinking and increased self-esteem, social interactions, and feelings of hope, worth, and value. Evaluation also includes the client's ability to recognize signs and symptoms of depression and to seek help before the depression becomes severe or immobilizing.

BRIEF REVIEW

Hope, despair, manic behavior, and suicide describe behaviors along the hope-despair continuum. Hope enables a person to accomplish a goal and is related to trust and the expectation that help from another person is forthcoming. Despair, the inability to grieve, results in a pathological state (depression) following a loss. Manic behavior, an affective illness, is characterized by symptoms that are the opposite of depression; these include hyperactivity, elation, and excessive verbal activity. Suicidal behavior is the ultimate act of self-destruction and frequently accompanies depression.

Theoretical explanations for depression include displaced anger, loss of esteem as a result of failure to achieve developmental goals, heredity, chemical imbalances, negative thinking, lack of positive reinforcement, learned helplessness, losses, and a combination of variables such as chemicals, experiences, and behaviors. Explanations for manic behavior include heredity, chemical excesses, defects in cell membranes, and losses. Explanations for suicide include the individual's innate death drive, the nature of society, and religious and legal sanctions.

The nursing process is a systematic and organized method of working with clients who have lost hope, who grieve, or who are depressed and possibly suicidal. The increasing numbers of suicides, particularly among adolescents and the elderly, challenge the nurse to identify persons at risk for suicide, to intervene quickly to prevent suicide, and to strengthen the person's coping skills so that life becomes bearable and meaningful.

REFERENCES AND SUGGESTED READINGS

1. Akiskal, H., and McKinney, W.: Overview of recent research in depression, Archives of General Psychiatry **31**:285, 1975.
2. American Psychiatric Association: Diagnostic and statistical manual of mental disorders (DSM-III-R), Washington, D.C., 1987, The Association.
3. Arieti, S.: Roots of depression: the power of the dominant other, Psychology Today **13**(1):54, April 1979.
4. Baker, C., editor: Physician's desk reference, Oradell, N.J., 1980, Medical Economics Co.
5. Baldessarine, R.: Biomedical aspects of depression and its treatment, Washington, D.C., 1983, American Psychiatric Press.
6. Beck, A.: Depression: causes and treatment, Philadelphia, 1967, University of Pennsylvania Press.
7. Beck, A., and others: Hopelessness and eventual suicide: a 10-year prospective study of patients with suicidal ideation, American Journal of Psychiatry. **142**(5):559, 1985.
8. Becker, E.: The revolution in psychiatry, New York, 1964, The Free Press.
9. Belmaker, R., and van Pragg, H.: Mania: an evolving concept, Jamaica, N.Y., 1980, Spectrum Publications, Inc.
10. Berk, J.: The down comforter, New York, 1980, Avon Books.
11. Bibring, E.: The mechanism of depression. In Greenacre, P., editor: Affective disorders, New York, 1953, International Universities Press.
12. Blattner, B.: Holistic nursing, Englewood Cliffs, N.J., 1981, Prentice-Hall, Inc.
13. Blazer, D.: Depression in late life, St. Louis, 1982, The C.V. Mosby Co.
14. Bowlby, J.: Processes of mourning, International Journal of Psychoanalysts **42**:317, 1961.
15. Burns, D.: Feeling good, New York, 1981, The New American Library.
16. Cameron, N., and Rychlak, J.: Personality development and psychopathology, Boston, 1985, Houghton Mifflin Co.
16a. Campbell, L.: Hopelessness: a concept analysis, Journal of Psychosocial Nursing and Mental Health Services **25**(2):18, 1987.
17. Cappodanno, A., and Targum, S.: Assessment of suicide risk: some limitations in the prediction of infrequent events, Journal of Psychosocial Nursing and Mental Health Services **21**(5):11, 1983.
18. Carroll, B.: The blood test for depression: how to use it, Diagnosis **3**(9):71, 1981.
19. Ciaramitao, B.: Help for depressed mothers, ed. 2, Edmunds, Washington, 1982, Charles Franklin Press.
20. Clayton, P., and Barrett, J.: Treatment of depression: old controversies and new approaches, New York, 1983, Raven Press.
20a. Davis, J., and Maas, J.: The affective disorders, Washington, D.C., 1985, The American Psychiatric Association.
20b. Deakin, J.: The biology of depression, Washington, D.C., 1986, The American Psychiatric Association.
21. Depression/awareness, recognition, treatment (DART), National Institute of Mental Health, 1986, U.S. Dept. of Health and Human Services, U.S. Government Printing Office.
22. DeRosis, H., and Pellegrino, V.: The book of hope, New York, 1981, Bantam Books.
23. Dixon, D.: Manic depression: an overview, Journal of Psychosocial Nursing and Mental Health Services **19**:28, 1981.
23a. Dufault, K.: Hope: its spheres and dimensions, Nursing Clinics of North America **20**(2):379, 1985.
24. Durkheim, E.: Suicide, New York, 1951, The Free Press.
25. Erikson, E.: Childhood and society, ed. 2, New York, 1964, W.W. Norton & Co., Inc.
26. Farberow, N.: Suicide in different cultures, Baltimore, 1975, University Park Press.
27. Farberow, N.: Suicide prevention in the hospital, Hospital and Community Psychiatry **32**:99, 1981.
28. Feighner, J.: New generation antidepressants, Audio-Digest Psychiatry **10**(17):1, 1981.
29. Fieve, R.: Mood swing, the third revolution, New York, 1981, Bantam Books.
30. Freud, S.: Mourning and melancholia. In The complete psychological works of Sigmund Freud, vol. 14, London, 1957, The Hogarth Press, Ltd. (Translated from the German under the general editorship of J. Strachey and A. Tyson.)
31. Gallant, P., and Simpson, G.: Depression: behavioral, biochemical, diagnostic, and treatment concepts, New York, 1955, Spectrum Publications, Inc.
32. Gleit, C.J., and Tatro, S.: Nursing diagnoses for health individuals, Nursing and Health Care **2**:456, 1981.
33. Harris, E.: The dexamethasone suppression test, American Journal of Nursing **82**:784, 1982.
34. Hatton, E., and Valente, S.: Suicide, assessment and intervention, Norwalk, C.V., 1984, Appleton-Century-Crofts.
35. Hatton, C., and Balente, S.: Suicide, assessment and intervention, ed. 2, Norwalk, Ct., 1984, Appleton-Century-Crofts.
36. Hollister, L.: Current anti-depressant drugs: their clinical use, Palo Alto, Calif., 1981, ADIS Press Australia.
37. Jackson, E., and Cardon, A.: New drug evaluations, Drug Intelligence and Clinical Pharmacy **14**:585, 1980.
38. Jacobson, A.: Melancholy in the twentieth century: causes and prevention, Journal of Psychiatric Nursing **18**(7):11, 1980.
39. Jourard, S.: Suicide: an invitation to die, American Journal of Nursing **70**:269, 1970.
40. Kaplen, R., Kottler, D., and Francis, A.: Reliability and rationality in the prediction of suicide, Hospital and Community Psychiatry **33**:212, 1982.
41. Klerman, G.: The age of melancholy, Psychology Today **13**(11):37 April 1980.
42. Kline, N.: From sad to glad, New York, 1981, Ballantine Books.
43. Kovacs, M.: The efficacy of cognitive and behavior therapies for depression, American Journal of Psychiatry **137**:1495, 1980.
44. Kovacs, M., and Beck, A.: Maladaptive cognitive structures in depression, American Journal of Psychiatry **135**:525, 1978.
45. Kübler-Ross, E.: On death and dying, New York, 1969, The Macmillan Co.
46. Lattaye, T.: How to win over depression, New York, 1980, Bantam Books.
47. Lewinsohn, P.: A behavioral approach to depression. In Friedman, R., and Katz, M., editors: The psychology of depression: contemporary theory and research, Washington, D.C., 1974, V.H. Winston & Sons.
47a. Lewis, S., McDowell, W., and Gregory, R.: Saving the suicidal patient from himself, RN, December, 1986.
48. Menninger, K.: Hope, American Journal of Psychiatry **116**:481, 1959.
49. Merz, B.: Cell membrane defects in mental illness, Journal of the American Medical Association **248**:633, 1982.
50. Miller, J.: Inspiring hope, American Journal of Nursing **85**(1):22, 1985.
51. Motto, J., Heilbron, D., and Juster, R.: Development of a clinical instrument to estimate suicide risk, American Journal of Psychiatry **142**(6):680, 1985.
52. Murray, R.: Model for psychiatric and mental health nursing: negative self-concept. In Carlson, J., Craft, C., and McGare, A., editors: Nursing diagnosis, Philadelphia, 1982, W.B. Saunders Co.

52a. Nolen-Itoeksema, S.: Sex differences in unipolar depression: evidence and theory, Psychological Bulletin **101**(2):259, 1987.

53. Parent, C., and Whall, A.: Are physical activity, self-esteem and depression related? Journal of Gerontological Nursing **10**(3):8, Sept. 1984.

53a. Richman, J.: Family therapy for suicidal people, New York, 1986, Springer Publishing Co., Inc.

54. Rippere, V., and Williams, R.: Wounded healers: mental health workers' experiences with depression, New York, 1985, John Wiley & Sons.

55. Rogers, C., and Ulsafer-van Lanen, J.: Nursing interventions in depression, Orlando, 1985, Grune & Stratten, Inc.

56. Roose, S., and others: Depression, delusions and suicide, American Journal of Psychiatry **140**(9):1159, 1983.

57. Roy, A.: Risk factors for suicide in psychiatric patients, Archives of General Psychiatry **39**(9):1089, 1982.

58. Rush, J., and Altshuler, K.: Depression—basic mechanisms, diagnosis and treatment, New York, 1986, Guilford Press.

59. Rutter, J., Izard, C., and Read, P.: Depression in young people, developmental and clinical perspectives, New York, 1986, Guilford Press.

60. Sartorius: Depressive disorders in different cultures, Geneva, 1983, World Health Organization.

61. Schmale, A.: A genetic view of affects with special reference to the genesis of helplessness and hopelessness. In Nagera, H.: The psychoanalytic study of the child, Monograph No. 2, New York, 1964, International Universities Press, Inc.

62. Seligman, M.: Depression and learned helplessness. In Friedman, R., and Katz, M., editors: The psychology of depression: contemporary theory and research, Washington, D.C., 1974, V.H. Winson & Sons.

63. Shopsin, B.: Manic illness, New York, 1979, Raven Press.

64. Shortridge, L., and Lee E.: Introduction to nursing practice, New York, 1980, McGraw-Hill Book Co.

65. Smith, D.M.: Guided imagination as an intervention in hopelessness, Journal of Psychosocial Nursing and Mental Health Services **20**(6):29, 1982.

66. Smitherman, C.: Nursing actions for health promotion, Philadelphia, 1981, F.A. Davis Co.

67. Stutland, E.: The psychology of hope, San Francisco, 1969, Jossey-Bass, Inc., Publishers.

68. Travelbee, J.: Interpersonal aspects of nursing, ed. 2, Philadelphia, 1971, F.A. Davis Co.

69. Tuskan, J., and Thase, M.: Suicides in jails and prisons, Journal of Psychosocial Nursing and Mental Health Services **21**(5):29, 1983.

70. Weissman, M., and Paykel, E.: The depressed woman, Chicago, 1974, University of Chicago Press.

71. Willner, P.: Depression: a psychological synthesis, New York, 1985, John Wiley & Sons.

72. Zung, W.: A self-rating depression scale, Archives of General Psychiatry **12**:63, 1965.

ANNOTATED BIBLIOGRAPHY

Beck, A.: Depression: causes and treatment, Philadelphia, 1967, University of Pennsylvania Press.

This text presents theoretical frameworks for understanding depression as well as symptoms, classifications, and investigative studies. Methods of treatment, including drugs, electroconvulsive therapy, and psychotherapy, are also discussed.

Peck, M., Farberow, N., and Litman, R.: Youth suicide, New York, 1985, Springer Publishing Co.

An emphasis of this book is prevention of suicide, ranging from the need to educate young children on the meaning of death to a plea for gun control. Psychodynamic issues related to self-destructive behaviors and treatment issues are also discussed.

Rogers, C., and Ulsafer-van Lanven, J.: Nursing interventions in depression, Orlando, 1985, Grune & Stratton, Inc.

This book is an excellent guide for nursing interventions for persons with affective disorders, in a variety of treatment settings and age groups. The book also raises critical questions about the direction of psychiatric nursing practice and education.

CHAPTER 15

FLEXIBILITY–RIGIDITY

Cathleen Shultz

After studying this chapter the learner will be able to:

Discuss historical perspectives of flexibility and rigidity.

Describe the theoretical development of flexibility and rigidity.

Use the nursing process to care for clients experiencing difficulties with flexible or rigid behaviors.

Identify research findings relevant to flexibility and rigidity.

Change is inevitable in life, and adaptation is essential to healthy maturation. Central to flexibility is the capacity to respond to change easily.

Flexibility means that the person responds and can be influenced to change. The flexible person has many responses and maintains an open mind. Adjectives such as resilient, pliant, accommodating, and adaptable describe the flexible client.

Failure to adapt and alter one's behavior as conditions change characterizes "rigidity." The rigid client may not acquire new behaviors or responses different from previously established change responses. Remaining with the familiar, the rigid client seeks security by minimizing risks and avoiding the unknown. The rigid client is also characterized as being obstinate, unyielding, closed minded, or unwilling or unable to consider new information. Thought processes involving decision making, problem solving, and the quality of interpersonal relationships are profoundly affected by the client's rigidity. Typically rigidity has been linked exclusively with aging, but current research suggests this is not so.[78]

A client's response to change reveals his place on the flexibility-rigidity continuum (Figure 15-1). Cues are seen in the person's activities and interactions, which are formed by developmental stages, early experiences, culture, and personality. The environment contributes to the flexible or rigid responses. If the client perceives the environment as stressful, there is greater tendency to respond rigidly.

When unhealthy, the flexible individual resembles a chameleon, which cannot be clearly identified in its native environment. Readily adopting others' beliefs and values, the client demonstrates little consistency, predictability, separateness from others, or sense of commitment. Terms such as "wishy-washy," "wimpy," "weak" and "mimicking others" may be used to describe this client.

The rigid person needs structure, consistent expectations, specific instructions, and clear lines of authority. Excessive rigidity restricts the range of healthy behaviors. The client may have a diminished capacity to initiate and maintain interpersonal relationships.

However, rigid behaviors may actually aid an individual. Denial of feelings and predominantly rigid responses enabled prisoners of war to withstand solitary confinement and torture.[42] The rigid person may cope better in a regimented society. Denying feelings makes an indifferent and hostile environment more tolerable.[41]

Rigid behaviors are rooted in fear. Rigid or repetitious behaviors are commonly seen in compulsive personality disorders and disorders of impulse control.

Considering clients' change response patterns assists in accurately minimizing or preventing health problems re-

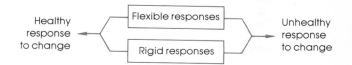

FIGURE 15-1 Flexibility-rigidity continuum.

Historical Overview

DATE	EVENT
1500s-1800s	Discussion of rigidity first appeared in the literature in the sixteenth century.
	Rigid behaviors were believed to be due to a religious melancholy or the devil's work; treatment involved a ritual of exorcism by witch doctors, mystics, or religious leaders.
1900-1920s	Rigid behaviors were first identified as a medical concern by Freud in 1915; he conceptualized symptomatology as unconscious with psychosexual roots in the libido.
1930s-1940s	A neurophysiological cause for rigid behaviors was sought; researchers discovered that the personality's socialization influenced the degree of rigidity.
1950s-1960s	Attempts were made to link the process of socialization with personality characteristics. Adorno[4] documented the authoritarian personality and thus caused a shift from a neurophysiological to a socialization basis.
	Rubenowitz confirmed the impact of socialization on the development of rigidity.[94] He revealed that both flexibility and rigidity existed in adults and influenced their thinking, attitudes, and behavior.
1960s-1980s	Behavioral therapy began with the conditioning studies of Pavlov[80] in the Soviet Union and Thorndike[108] in the United States. Until the development of behavioral treatments, the prognosis for clients with obsessive-compulsive personalities was poor and nurses were only peripherally involved in treatment.
	Phobias have emerged as the second most common mental health problem with at least one in nine Americans having some form of phobia; only alcoholism occurs more often.
	Rigid behaviors are considered the mental health problem of the 1980s, corresponding to an increasingly insecure and complex world.
Future	Nurses, especially those with counseling credentials, will be more directly involved with treatment using relaxation, imagery, and desensitization.

lated to flexibility and rigidity. Intervening during pertinent developmental stages may help those at risk individuals whose creative potential and capacity for enjoying life is already compromised by problems of rigidity or flexibility.

A broad spectrum of obsessional behavior exists that incorporates rigidity. The terms "rigidity" and "obsessions" may be used interchangeably.

Obsessive-compulsive disorders are common, rigid behaviors frequently treated on an outpatient basis. Unfortunately no studies have been undertaken to determine the inpatient or outpatient occurrence using DSM-III-R criteria.[88] Other studies have reported an incidence from 0.1% to 2.5%.[20,48,61] Preliminary data from a National Institute of Mental Health (NIMH) study suggests obsessive-compulsive disorders may be far more prevalent than is commonly believed.[95]

Seventy-six percent of obsessive-compulsive disorders in a child psychiatric population were in males.[43] No sex comparison studies exist for adults.

Treatment of these disorders challenge the nurse to find and use meaningful interventions. Clients rarely report themselves symptom free at the completion of a treatment regimen. About 20% of clients find maintaining their gains difficult. Relapse is common among those clients who are only partially improved at the end of treatment.[51] However, the nurse is reminded that successful treatment is possible, with the success rate enhanced by the nurse's encouragement.

For brevity this chapter will address only these disorders of impulse control: compulsive gambling, kleptomania, and pyromania. This chapter focuses on general information applicable to rigid personalities.

THEORETICAL APPROACHES
Biological

Increasingly, researchers have explored the relationship between rigid behaviors and biological causes and biochemical changes. Several interesting facts have emerged. One is summarized in the Research Highlight on p. 295. Positive responses occurred by treating obsessive-compulsive clients who manifested abnormal dexamethasone suppression with antidepressants and behavioral therapy.

Some theorists speculate that rigidity is associated with

Research Highlight

Abnormal Dexamethasone Suppression Test in Primary Obsessive-Compulsive Patients: A Confirmatory Report

J. Cottraux, M. Bouvard, B. Claustrat & C. Juenet

PURPOSE

Numerous studies have suggested a relationship between obsessive-compulsive disorder and an abnormal response to the dexamethasone suppression test. This study examined those relationships.

SAMPLE

Twenty subjects (10 males and 10 females with a mean age of 37 years) made up the sample. All had been referred to the psychology department of a neurological hospital. Each had met the DSM-III criteria for obsessive-compulsive disorder. Twelve also had a secondary major depressive disorder. All were treated as outpatients.

METHODOLOGY

Plasma cortisol levels were determined on diluted samples by radioimmunoassay. Dexamethasone was to have been self-administered at 11 PM the evening before the dexamethasone suppression test.

The week before the dexamethasone suppression test, all were assessed for obsessive-compulsive disorder based on DSM-III criteria. An evaluator completed the Hamilton Rating Scale for Depression. The client completed a rating scale scoring the time spent each day in internal or external rituals and the anxiety related to situations eliciting ritual behaviors.

FINDINGS

Six of the 20 patients (30%) showed an abnormal dexamethasone suppression based on levels of plasma cortisol greater than 5 μg/100 ml at 4 PM. Suppressors and nonsuppressors did not differ significantly on age, anxiety, duration of rituals per day, major depression, family history of depression, duration of obsessive-compulsive disorder, and duration of secondary depression. There was a trend toward a stronger family history of depression in suppressors ($p = 0.06$) and an excess of male subjects in nonsuppressors ($p = 0.06$).

IMPLICATIONS

The dexamethasone suppression test results were used to indicate further treatment. Five of the six dexamethasone suppression test nonsuppressors responded favorably to 2 months of antidepressant medication. Of the dexamethasone suppression test suppressors, four showed a positive response to a combination of behavior therapy and clomipramine.

The authors believe that biological markers may be used to divide obsessive-compulsive disorder into two subcategories. Some obsessive-compulsive disorder cases may be related to anxiety disorders and some to unipolar endogenous depression. Nurses can encourage clients with obsessive-compulsive disorders to have laboratory testing for dexamethasone suppression and possible favorable, further treatment.

Based on data from Psychiatry Research **13**:157, 1984.

increased autonomic arousal. At this point whether the arousal is the cause or the result of rigid behaviors is difficult to ascertain.[12] Documented cases exist verifying that obsessive-compulsive individuals who met DSM-III criteria had elevated cerebrospinal fluid cortisol levels.[110] Head injuries have also been identified as a probable contributor to the development of obsessive-compulsive neuroses.[73]

Diets of rigid clients have been studied. Hypoglycemia secondary to an inappropriate diet has been documented as causing obsessive behavior, which cleared when a high-protein diet was administered.[90]

Some studies indicate that blood type O may be associated with a decreased development of obsessive-compulsive symptomatology.[89] Reports have also been published linking obsessive-compulsive disorders to neurological illness and depression.[68] Electroencephalogram (EEG) changes have been consistent with temporal lobe epilepsy indicating that this disorder may be associated with a brain disease. Specifically a lesion in the limbic system has been theorized.[57]

Psychoanalytic

Obsessions are intrusive recurring thoughts, images, or impulses that are unacceptable to the person, cause distress, and are ego dystonic; that is, the person does not consider them voluntarily produced. Frequently the obsession is repulsive, inane, or obscene. Obsessional content usually centers around dirt and contamination, aggression, keeping things in strict order, sex, or religion. The client feels compelled to engage in these sometimes repugnant thoughts or fantasies.[65]

Continuous brooding or repetitive thinking about real situations, unpleasant possibilities, or difficult decisions is not considered obsessional thought because the individual is engaged in thinking in a meaningful way. Because the content is not ego dystonic, it is not a true obsession.[65]

Obsessional behaviors range from a normal amount without uncomfortable anxiety to those which pervade a person's life-style. If the behaviors are distressing or incapacitating, the syndrome is labeled "neurotic." Between these extremes are obsessional traits that cluster into personality patterns called the obsessional personality, seen

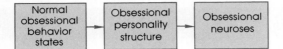

FIGURE 15-2 Obsessional behavior continuum.

in a person with obvious anxiety (Figure 15-2). Traits are fixed, long lasting, and predictable. As long as clients remain productive, they are not neurotic even though they may be using rituals extensively.[98]

In the quest for total mastery, those with rigid personalities may use intelligence or magical thinking to diminish anxiety. Although phobias are covered in Chapter 12 they are briefly discussed here because they are also one of the methods of control that may be used by the rigid personality. Phobias assist a rigid client by permitting him to avoid anything that threatens loss of control or is a potential danger.

Obsessions and compulsions can occur in the same individual simultaneously. Compulsions are repetitive acts regarded as excessive or exaggerated. Although the behaviors are voluntary, the urge to do them is so strong that the person's volition seems to be diminished.

The dynamics for compulsions are similar to those for obsessions in that compulsions are obsessive thoughts that are acted out. Some compulsions take the form of repeated urges to act; although the thought recurs, the person resists overt action.

The rigid personality has obsessive-compulsive patterns of perfection, omnipotence, and omniscience with an overriding need for certainty and absolutes. Mounting anxiety may be released in a variety of syndromes, such as alcoholism, drug addiction, compulsive overeating or undereating (anorexia nervosa), compulsive masturbation, compulsive gambling, compulsive stealing (kleptomania), or compulsive setting of fires (pyromania). In all these situations the person is driven to do the act; pleasure does not accompany the behavior; only a diminishing of anxiety is felt. Table 15-1 summarizes definitions from the psychoanalytic perspective.

As the child passes through the phases of psychosexual development, the anxiety generated from socialization is manifested through various ego defenses. Later in life, a person's anxiety may cause him to become fixated or regress to an earlier point because of conflicts that occurred during that stage. These fixations and regressions are examples of ego defenses that are part of normal development, but in the neurotic person they become rigid; even when they do not relieve anxiety, they are repeated because they at least convey the illusion of control.[65] For example, Mary does not begin important paperwork; instead, she clears the top of her desk and countertops in her office until the activity consumes the time she allotted for the paperwork.

The rigidity mechanisms are defenses against powerlessness and helplessness. When these behavioral devices fail to serve their purpose, the client may experience a total breakdown of integrative capacities resulting in responses such as depression, schizophrenia, paranoid behaviors, or grandiose states.

The defense mechanisms found in obsessive-compulsive disorders include isolation, undoing, reaction formation, and denial. Psychoanalytic theory proposes that conflicts in the anal phase are linked to obsessive symptoms. If the person unsuccessfully represses the anxiety attached to the conflicts and uses sublimation and reaction formation, obsessive and compulsive traits are likely to appear in later life but at a subclinical level.

When repression and sublimation fail, the defense mechanisms of *isolation,* undoing, reaction formation, or denial occur, in that order. With isolation the person separates feelings associated with a thought, as in the following Case Example.

Case Example

Jay had repeated thoughts that his family was dead. However, his reaction to the thoughts was unemotional. He effectively isolated the ordinary feelings that accompany such overwhelming loss. Unaware of the meaning behind such thoughts, he was annoyed with their intrusiveness and wished to be rid of them.[65] Jay will continue using isolation as long as his anxiety is minimized by its presence. When isolation fails, other defense mechanisms will replace it.

Rado elaborated on Freud's theories regarding behavioral rigidity. He considered obsessions and compulsions to be overreactive disorders. The person's emotions inflict damage rather than serving as emergency signals. Rado supported Freud's hypothesis that the cause of behavioral rigidity is the "battle of the chamber pot."

The child responds to the demands for bowel training with enraged defiance and to the mother's punishments or threats with fearful obedience. Making the child feel

TABLE 15-1 Definitions of terms from the psychoanalytic perspective

Term	Definition
Obsessions	Intrusive recurring thoughts, images, or impulses unacceptable to client
Compulsions	Repetitive acts regarded as excessive or exaggerated
Phobias	Fears that are out of proportion to the demands of the situation and cannot be explained or reasoned away
Obsessional personality	Obsessional traits in a person with obvious anxiety; not neurotic as long as person remains productive
Neuroses	Distressing or incapacitating symptoms that interfere with living
Pathological gambling	Compulsive gambling to release anxiety
Kleptomania	Compulsive stealing to release anxiety
Pyromania	Compulsive setting of fires to release anxiety

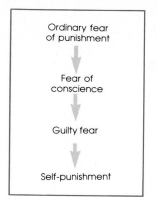

FIGURE 15-3 Steps in the development of expiratory behavior.

guilty for not obeying her becomes the mother's means of control.[65] This guilt creates a fearful conscience that demands perfection, repentance or reparations known as expiatory behaviors (Figure 15-3) (see Chapter 40).

Interpersonal

Sullivan's concept of the self-system is germane to rigid behaviors. The self-system encompasses all the energies and behaviors that an individual devotes to avoiding anxiety or increasing self-esteem and security. As the self-system forms, the person's emotional investment seems to be in maintaining the system, not in changing it. Effectively steering the individual away from anxiety-provoking situations by means of security operations, the system is difficult to change. Three security operations are closely linked to rigidity: selective inattention, false personifications, and sublimation.[65,105]

Behavioral

Behavioral therapists focus on changing the observable behavior and ignoring the inner conflicts and motivations. The emotional reaction to danger is based on the person's appraisal of his own coping efforts. When confronted with anything that they perceive as a threat, rigid individuals are more upset than are "normal" individuals. They believe that magical thinking or rituals will alter feared out-

comes. Rather than confronting their anxiety feelings directly, they prefer to use rituals. Further, loss of control or uncertainty is intolerable and therefore feared and avoided. Rigid persons are not necessarily aware of the pattern of appraisal that they are using, because the process may be preconscious and usually becomes automatic and intuitive. Figure 15-4 illustrates the rigid and normal patterns of danger appraisal and the likely outcomes.

Rigid disorders, like all other human behaviors, are responses that the individual has learned and selected, or chosen to repeat. Thus the individual who compulsively counts has learned that counting fence posts somehow helps allay anxiety. Reinforcement (any event that increases the likelihood of a response being repeated) needs to occur for behaviors to reappear. The ritualistic behavior is believed to relieve some of the anxiety and become a reinforcer, even though the relief may be momentary.

Anxiety-provoking stimuli, such as unwanted thoughts or frightening situations, become paired with other stimuli. For example, John's sexual thoughts became paired with dirty hands, which led to frequent hand washing; since the washing did not relieve all his anxiety, he had to repeat the procedure.

Cognitive

Cognitive structures (understanding, knowledge, or intelligence) designed to achieve equilibrium are organized mental activities. When a fear is perceived, the client organizes the fear response according to his past reactions to similar situations and one of three results takes place. The structure does not respond in a way different from previous experiences if the fear is congruent with past situations. If the fear has never been mentally processed, the individual does not assimilate it; usually the response is avoidance or responding without understanding. If conflict occurs between fear and the person's structure, change may result as the person strives to resolve the conflict and retain equilibrium. The change may or may not be healthy; for example, the fearful person may use compulsive rituals. Working with the fearful individual requires therapeutically enacting cognitive conflict to produce the desired changes.[84]

Cognitive processes mediate any threat that creates anxiety. The person first evaluates the degree of danger and the available resources for coping with the danger. For example, if a person perceives someone in authority

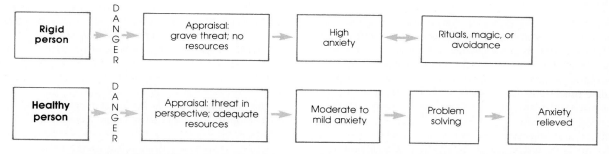

FIGURE 15-4 Paradigm of the rigid person's and the healthy person's appraisal of danger.

TABLE 15-2 Summary of theories of flexibility-rigidity

Theory	Theorist	Dynamics
Biological	Beech and Perrigault	Rigidity is associated with autonomic arousal.
	Lieberman	Obsessive-compulsive disorders have been linked to neurological illness and depression.
	Traskman	Obsessive-compulsive people have elevated cerebrospinal fluid cortisol levels.
	Rippere	Hypoglycemia secondary to an inappropriate diet causes obsessive behavior.
	Rinieris	Blood type O may hinder the development of obsessive-compulsive personality
	Jenike	A limbic system lesion has been theorized to cause obsessive-compulsive behavior. EEG changes indicate temporal lobe epilepsy in obsessive-compulsive clients.
Psychoanalytic	Freud	Rigid behaviors result when an individual is fixated at or regresses to an early stage of psychosexual development. Behavior becomes rigid to convey an illusion of control. Defense mechanisms used include isolation, undoing, reaction formation, and denial. Rigidity mechanisms are defenses against powerlessness and control. The rigid person functions effectively in most areas of living.
	Rado	Rigid behaviors are overreactive disorders that cause harm rather than convey that the individual has a problem. Behavioral rigidity begins with the "battle of the chamber pot."
Interpersonal	Sullivan	The individual's self-system uses energy and behavior to avoid anxiety or increase self-esteem or security. The rigid person's self-system seems to maintain the system, not change it. Three security operations are linked to rigidity: selective inattention, false personifications, and sublimation.
Behavioral		Focus is on changing the observable rigid behavior and ignoring inner conflicts and motivations. When confronted with anything perceived as a threat, the rigid person is more upset than "normal" individuals.
Cognitive	Piaget	Rigid disorders are viewed as responses the persons selected or chose to repeat to decrease anxiety. The rigid individual's source of threats and anxiety is unacceptable ideas and feelings close to the person's conscious awareness. Cognitive processes assist in determining the severity of anxiety and fear as well as solutions.

to be a threat, he decides how he is to behave in the presence of that person. When the individual has no idea what to do in the situation, the problem becomes frightening, whereas knowing what to do reduces the problem to a reasonable size.

Piaget[83] believes that rigid responses are selected and repeated by the client to minimize anxiety. Critics assert that cognitive theories provide a rationale for treatment that is aimed at symptom removal. They maintain that there is an oversimplification of the problem.

Table 15-2 summarizes the theories and dynamics of flexibility-rigidity.

RELATING TO THE CLIENT

Initially the nurse needs to determine the length of time she may be working with the client to change rigid behaviors. Caution is urged if the time is apt to be short because working with the rigid client usually requires long lengths of time. Change without appropriate support can cause this client's defenses to disintegrate. If the nurse does not have the time or the expertise, she needs to provide a supportive role.

Patience and tolerance are required in relating to the client who is bound by fears or rigidity. Waiting for the completion of ritualistic and compulsive behavior can be frustrating. The person's need to control everything can cause the nurse to feel manipulated into responding to irrational demands.[65]

The orientation phase can be long, even several months in duration, as the client struggles to move from an intellectual understanding to an emotional understanding of behavior. Even though repetition may be tiring, the nurse will need to repeat insights often and in different ways to assist the client therapeutically.

The client may be tempted to end therapy when some anxiety has diminished within the first few sessions. The nurse encourages the client to continue therapeutic sessions because he needs long-term counseling before permanent, beneficial changes are seen.

During the relationship, the nurse may also engage in a power struggle with the client. The nurse's own flexibility may be tested by the client's rigid demands.

Establishing a significant relationship with a constricted and inflexible person is a challenge. Personally it may not be rewarding because the client may expect perfection and voice criticism if the nurse is imperfect.

The working phase is prolonged because trust is slow to develop in someone with a rigid personality. The working phase may never reach the depth of sharing and openness that marks many therapeutic relationships because of the proclivity these clients have for intellectual discussion rather than attending to feelings.[65] The bulk of the therapeutic work involves translating the client's intellectual, often profound insight, into emotional understanding and a commitment to change.

Being aware of one's own feelings, especially anger or frustration, is essential because these can increase the client's anxiety level and exacerbate the symptoms the nurse is working to diminish. Keeping expectations realistic is important, since changing extremely rigid behaviors is a difficult and slow process that involves ongoing self-awareness.[65]

Reviewing the therapeutic session after the session closes is essential for developing insight. The nurse may provide homework material for consideration between sessions. Also the nurse needs to highlight client behaviors that are a source of pride. Interactions with the client need to contain both positive and negative statements about the client, since the balance and presence of both are important to long-term involvement with a client manifesting rigid behaviors.

When the client shows considerable insight into his behavior with manifested changes in living, the client is ready for termination. The end of therapy is approached with an organized plan including the review of the client's problem behaviors, the insights achieved, and the remaining tasks.

NURSING PROCESS
Assessment

✦ *Physical dimension.* Ordinary changes that accompany maturation and aging are readily accommodated by the flexible person. Daily routines are varied in response to schedule changes, illnesses, and the changing needs of family members or close friends. Body functions are accepted as natural phenomena and are not the object of undue concern. The flexible person is resilient in the face of adversity. Changes and some disorder are tolerable in the physical environment. A balance exists among concerns for the external world, the sensations and feelings generated within the person, and the more abstract inner thought processes of the person.[65]

The ease with which the client accomplishes ordinary daily routines indicates how much these activities are bound to rituals. Many clients have lived with their rituals and obsessions for years. Responses to certain key questions indicate whether the nurse needs to explore the responses further. For example, the nurse asks, "How long does it take you to get ready for work?" If the client responds, "Three hours," this is the cue for further data collection. Most clients do not volunteer information about their obsessions and compulsions unless distressed about them.[50]

In addition to questions, direct observation of routines or inquiry about the use of time is necessary to assess the extent of rituals or irrational fears. Rigid clients may repeat tasks such as hand washing or compulsive checking of water faucets or gas stoves.[28] Although rare, obsessive slowness can exist, such as taking 1 hour to brush one's teeth. Even when the disability becomes more public, the client often has enough successful modes of functioning to maintain a job and prevent hospitalization.

The person's health history can reveal characteristic patterns of adapting to the shifting demands of life such as illnesses associated with stress and change. Some illnesses such as ulcerative colitis have been correlated with the obsessional personality.[85] Repeated and exaggerated concerns about illness, such as cancer, AIDS, tuberculosis, or a cold, can prompt the person to seek unnecessary physical examinations and even multiple surgical treatments. Abuse of vitamins, herbal preparations, and over-the-counter medications can also be manifested.

Deficits in self-care may result from behavioral patterns that interfere with daily living. The obsessive-compulsive client is especially vulnerable to dietary deficiencies created by overeating or undereating.

Cleanliness can become a pursuit that requires hours and takes priority over all activities. For example, a strange paradox exists in some individuals who maintain scrupulous cleanliness in the bathroom while the remainder of the house is a chaotic mess with food encrusted on utensils in the kitchen and months of dust accumulated in other rooms. The person may manifest this same scrupulous behavior in his manner of dress.

The person may develop elaborate rituals around food preparation, eating, getting up, or preparing for bed. These activities, which need to be performed in a certain sequence, can consume nearly all of the client's waking hours. Any break in the routine usually means that the procedure is begun again until it is perfectly executed.[65]

The person feels inner resistance (rejects or disowns the impulse) and may even consider the act senseless but finds it necesssary to complete it. The most frequent forms of compulsions are cleaning (hand washing) and checking (making sure everything is turned off or locked). Males are more frequently checkers, and females are more frequently washers.[51]

When assessing the physical dimension of people with rigid behaviors, the nurse needs to consider the severity and type of dysfunctional behavior. Some specific physical problems arise as a consequence of stereotyped, rigid behaviors. Most frequently encountered in compulsive clients is dermatological problems. Repeated hand washing may lead to a breakdown of the skin surface. Chronic dry skin may occur from too frequent showering. Dermatitis, skin lesions, and chemical reactions to soap may be present. The client may report physical problems such as fatigue, symptoms of anxiety, anorexia, nausea, diarrhea, sweating, paresthesia, and palpitations.

The normal routines of eating and sleeping may be disrupted by phobias or premorbid obsessional thoughts.[149] The dread of dying while asleep may cause insomnia. Wanting to maintain control may cause the client to have difficulty going to sleep.[49,107]

The client's body language is eloquent. The inflexible person often has a stiff body posture with muscle tightness. The arms are frequently crossed as if to shut out everyone. The facial expression is likely to reflect few emotions.

The nurse needs to be aware that rigid clients with

problems of impulse control such as stealing, gambling, or fire setting may be a hazard to other clients during hospitalization. Precautions may be necessary to protect the rigid client and others. Assessment includes determining if the client has matches or other fire-setting paraphernalia and limiting access to items used as fuel. Agency policies on smoking, card games, and keeping personal items, such as lighters, may need to be reviewed and altered to ensure the safest possible environment for all concerned.

✳️ *Emotional dimension.* Assessing the client's response to change provides one of the major clues to flexibility. Change is a challenge that may trigger creativity and kindle enthusiasm in the flexible person, but it threatens the rigid individual, who is unable to accept it.

Similar to acceptance of change is the acceptance of differences. The flexible person accepts people with different values, skin color, language, or life-style. This acceptance carries with it a sensitivity to and appreciation of others' feelings based on trust and respect. The flexible person is comfortable with others and has a sense of self-worth and an optimistic outlook. Flexibility provides access to the entire range of human emotions that a person can experience, and this enables the person to express these feelings appropriately.[65]

Problematic, rigid behaviors are often in close association with other emotional difficulties. Therefore the nurse assesses for the presence of associated emotional problems as well as rigid behaviors. Associated problems, such as depression, need to be treated before the rigid behavior to enhance success.[51]

Anxiety at the beginning of treatment has been related to the client's response to treatment. With mild anxiety, the client is more likely to succeed. High anxiety may need reducing before treating the rigid behavior because extremely anxious clients are likely to fail.[51]

Severe fears of illness without any signs of disease and fears of dying when the person is actually in good health are also bases for psychiatric evaluation of obsessive-compulsive characteristics. Observations, examination, and laboratory tests are used to rule out the existence of any real physical problem as psychiatric treatment is initiated.

Dominated by fears and anxiety that prompt them to seek absolute control over their emotions and environment, rigid persons use only a limited range of normal human potential. Described as *pseudoplacid* (falsely calm), their emotional demeanor seems to be an unaffected, flattened emotional state unless they are confronted with one of their core concerns, as discussed in the following Case Example.

Case Example

Sharon, an efficient keypunch operator, became upset when a new employee rearranged the office supplies. Sharon "blew up" and insisted that everything be returned to its original place so that she could inventory all supplies every morning and evening. Sharon's co-workers were surprised at the anger Sharon displayed and puzzled that Sharon wanted to inventory supplies, since it was not one of her assigned tasks. Her quiet, unassuming manner changed when she perceived that she lost control of her environment.

Many of the fears and repetitious thoughts that are a part of rigidity may be known to only the sufferer or the immediate family members. Clients often feel embarrassed and disgusted about the irrational and senseless nature of their problems as indicated in the following Case Example. Disclosures of the client's distress are shared only after a trusting relationship has been established that clearly indicates unqualified acceptance of the client as a person.[65] These people typically intellectualize their feelings or do not mention them.

Case Example

Although she held an important executive position, Lois recently experienced numerous personal changes and stressors that taxed her ability to adapt. The changes included a move, her son's hospitalization for asthma, her husband's job loss, and a robbery of her jewelry. Her new job required that she hear employees' problems. After weeks of this pressure she sought counseling because her feelings frightened her.

When she was asked to describe herself and what frightened her she stated, "These people come to my office with difficult problems. After listening about 5 minutes I feel numb, like this is not real. If I touch my arm I can't feel it. The person is talking, but I can't hear all of it. I've managed to say the right thing and get them out of the office quickly. I'm frightened that someone will find that I feel like I'm falling apart and can't handle the job. I don't think anyone suspects that I feel this way. Please help me."

✳️ *Intellectual dimension.* Willingness to consider both sides of an issue and to change plans and openness to self-scrutiny demonstrate flexible thinking. How open is the person to new ideas? How able is the person to compromise or to see another's viewpoint?

Rigid people appear to have a more restricted sphere of interest and knowledge than flexible people, and they are more concrete in their thinking and less introspective. The Research Highlight on p. 301 presents another view in that rigid thinking and rigid personalities were not found to be correlated. Other studies support that concrete thinking is evident when clients focus on the present rather than working toward a future goal. The extremely rigid person is too concerned with controlling the fears and anxieties of the moment to develop any action for the future. The isolation of feelings results in a limited capacity for introspection.[26,65]

Clients with problems of extreme rigidity are often above average in intellect. However, there may be a thinking deficit specific to topics they fear.[114] Clients may also have firm beliefs that feared outcomes will definitely materialize if they do not protect themselves. They can be incapacitated by even trivial decisions. The need to always be correct and the reluctance to take any kind of risk render them ineffective at most administrative levels. If required to arrive at a decision, their solution includes finding a rule or policy to follow.

Rigid clients may appear preoccupied or have difficulty concentrating. Prioritizing is not easy for them. They may be characterized by doubt about their work and their decisions. Their thinking may be illogical. At work or school

Research Highlight

Rigid Personality and Rigid Thinking

P. Kline & C. Cooper

PURPOSE

This study explored the relationship between the rigid personality and rigid thinking. Rigid people are not generally viewed as creative. The study determined if this were so by using pen and paper tests to measure typical divergent thinking and the obsessional traits of dogmatism and authoritarianism.

SAMPLE

One hundred seventy-three undergraduate university students volunteered for 12 hours of testing. Approximately half were male, and half were female. Their mean age was 20.4 years with a standard deviation of 1.4 years. Each subject was rewarded with individual feedback about his test results.

METHODOLOGY

Tests were divided into four 3-hour sessions. Two main variables were tested: personality (using A:3Q, the Wilson-Patterson Conservatism Scale, Balanced Dogmatism and Kohn's Balanced F Scale) and thinking abilities (using the Comprehensive Ability Battery).

FINDINGS

Most of the personality variables did not correlate significantly with the creativity variables nor rigid thinking and rigid personality. The statistically significant correlations were small, thus indicating that rigid thinking and rigid personality are not closely related.

IMPLICATIONS

The findings have important implications for the training and selection of flexible thinkers. For example, authoritarian people can be taught flexible thinking. Similarly, creativity in school children appears not to depend on personality variables.

Based on data from the British Journal of Educational Psychology **55**:24, 1985.

their time may be mismanaged, especially if they have compulsive behaviors. Some have reported resisting thinking by occupying their minds with counting real or imaginary items.

Case Example

Anita typifies the intellectual problems encountered by rigid individuals with a need to be perfect and in control of their surroundings. Anita has been a senior nursing student for 3 months. As the clinical rotations become more complex, she becomes more disorganized in completing nursing care on assigned clients. She seems unsure of herself and preoccupied most of the time. Although she writes comprehensive nursing care plans she has trouble doing nursing care other than in the order written on the care plan. In conferences she can quote rationales for her nursing care almost verbatim from the book. On one occasion, when working with a client, she ran from the room when she was unable to answer a question about a new medication. A teacher found her in the restroom crying and stating, "I'll never get this all right. I'm not a good nurse."

Social dimension. A person's flexibility enables one to establish varied relationships with diverse degrees of closeness and to change the responses to these relationships over time. Success in establishing an intimate, lasting relationship suggests a certain amount of flexibility. Flexibility permits an individual to sustain a balance in dependent as well as independent relationships.

Another assessment area concerns persons' flexibility in social roles. This is important, since one's total identity can become submerged in one's primary role. For example, the general, the scientist, or the professor who responds to all situations as a professional; or the mother who responds to all situations as a mother, rather than as a person with a unique identity, is inflexible.

Rigid individuals tend to have restricted social contacts, and their relationships are characterized by aloofness and superficial involvement. Their ruminations and morbid thought often lead to compulsive avoidance of others.[24] Assessment of the individual's social network reveals few contacts, usually limited to family members and co-workers. The person whose life is circumscribed by fears and repetitious behavior may devote all energy to symptoms, leaving no time for social contacts. When asked, these individuals deny that their rituals affect social functioning, but they may express loneliness in their relationships (see Chapter 19 for further information on loneliness).[65]

Recreational activities may be entirely missing or may be pursued ritualistically, suggesting that the goal is to achieve rather than to relax and enjoy. Even in recreation the individual is driven by his belief that one "should" relax.

Assessing the family is essential for quality care of a rigid individual. Frequently the entire family is involved in maintaining the rituals because to do otherwise is to precipitate unbearable anxiety in the afflicted member and create retribution and chaos within the family. Therefore knowing how the family functions and the role that each member plays in relation to the rigid person is important. The common pattern is for the entire family to be controlled by the members' idiosyncratic needs. Some research indicates that major contributors to the development of obsessive-compulsive disorders are the parental symbiotic needs combined with perfectionistic family interaction styles.[46,52,65]

In the work setting, compulsion or overachieving may be evident. Clients may complain of chronic job dissatisfaction or may fear success and unconsciously manifest behavior such as lateness or not meeting deadlines, which ensures there will be no promotions.[118]

Although some clients with rigid behaviors may be involved with such antisocial behavior as fire setting and shoplifting, they do not readily admit their involvement. Even when caught they usually deny wrongdoing. In their minds the act makes them feel better or is done to help someone.

Cultural background needs to be assessed, since preliminary studies show ethnic groups such as the Irish are more likely to be obsessive. In addition, marital status and geographical location are influences; females living in rural areas without outside employment and bachelors are more likely to be obsessional. The common factor among all three groups (the Irish; unemployed, rural females; and bachelors) is that they are either emotionally or geographically isolated.

The avoidance patterns used by people with rigid behaviors often lead them to abandon most of their friends and compromise personal aspirations. Even though they define their behaviors as self-defeating, they rationalize what they are doing as necessary and become skillful at inventing excuses so that others will not be aware of their fears. This is illustrated in the following Case Example. Although Betty could do her job well she would probably be viewed more effectively and obtain more co-worker cooperation if she did not isolate herself from them. Her compulsions affected her social contacts as well as her overall job performance.

Case Example

Even when her anxiety was minimal, Betty, an accountant, washed her hands 10 times before and after she ate. Because she did not want others to know this she did not date, did not invite people to her apartment, and did not eat with her co-workers. She believed she was effective at work and did not need to socialize with her colleagues to be good at her job.

Spiritual dimension. A person who is flexible is able to develop a philosophy that guides conduct. The flexible person has religious or philosophical convictions that are personally satisfactory and can be used as a source of strength and self-renewal. Flexibility enables an unsatisfied person to search for a fulfilling faith.

Rigid people tend to profess faith in a supernatural power who is obeyed without thinking or questioning. This type of client seems to draw an imaginary box around his spiritual self and is intolerant if the box's lines are crossed. Religious principles tend to be accepted literally rather than searched for philosophical or historical significance. Scrupulous moral standards or religious practices are very important and rigidly followed, often resulting in an unwillingness to recognize the validity of differing faiths.[65] Similarities have been found between religious compulsions (such as compulsively attending church services or obsessively praying) and the obsessive-compulsive personality.[39]

Rigid adherence to religious and ethical beliefs creates guilt and feelings of inadequacy for many inflexible people. They set exceedingly high standards for themselves and for others; then, with failure, they are left guilty and disillusioned. Their need for perfectionism is also manifested as an inability to forgive themselves or others (see Chapter 14 for further information about guilt).

Thus in assessing the spiritual dimension the nurse needs to understand the clients' meaning and perceptions of their faith. Are their beliefs a source of comfort or primarily a rigid demand for compliance? Does their faith offer hope and tolerance for others instead of judgmental attitudes? What activities unrelated to compulsive behavior do they do for spiritual fulfillment?[65]

Measurement tools. Numerous scales exist to determine varying facets of flexibility and rigidity. Table 15-3 summarizes the more common scales.

The Maudsley Obsessional-Compulsive Inventory, introduced in 1977, is a 30-item, true-false quesionnaire (see the upper box on p. 303). It identifies four varieties of compulsive behaviors: checking, cleaning, obsessional slowness, and conscientious doubting. Although this tool is primarily used to study obsessive-compulsive behaviors, it also identifies the problematic rigid behaviors most often seen in treatment settings.[65,100]

TABLE 15-3 Instruments to measure flexibility-rigidity

Instrument	Measures
California F Scale[4]	Antisemitism and ethnocentrism
Gough-Sanford's Rigidity Scale[16]	Resistance to habit change and preference for order and detail
Rokeach[91] Dogmatism Scale	Authoritarianism, belief-disbelief, and open- and closed-mindedness; focuses on political and religious beliefs
Obsessional scales[67-69]	Self-reporting presence of obsessions
Gibb's Scale[35]	Degree of obsessive-compulsive traits
Sandler-Hazari Obsessionality Inventory[31]	Obsessional traits and symptoms in clinical and non-clinical populations
Hopkins Psychiatric Rating Scale[76]	Obsessive-compulsive judgments
Crown-Crisp Experimental Index[76]	Diagnostic information about obsessions
SCL-90-R Brief Symptom Inventory[76]	Obsessive-compulsive dimension
Leyton Obsessional Inventory[18,77]	Presence of obsessions

THE MAUDSLEY OBSESSIONAL-COMPULSIVE INVENTORY (MOC)

Instructions: Please answer each question by putting a circle around the *true* or the *false* following the question. There are no right or wrong answers and no trick questions. Work quickly and do not think too long about the exact meaning of the question.

1. I avoid using public telephones because of possible contamination.	True	False
2. I frequently get nasty thoughts and have difficulty getting rid of them.	True	False
3. I am more concerned than most people about honesty.	True	False
4. I am often late because I can't seem to get through everything on time.	True	False
5. I don't worry unduly about contamination if I touch an animal.	True	False
6. I frequently have to check things (e.g., gas or water taps, doors, etc.) several times.	True	False
7. I have a very strict conscience.	True	False
8. I find that almost every day I am upset by unpleasant thoughts that come into my mind against my will.	True	False
9. I do not worry unduly if I accidentally bump into somebody.	True	False
10. I usually have serious doubts about the simple everyday things I do.	True	False
11. Neither of my parents was very strict during my childhood.	True	False
12. I tend to get behind in my work because I repeat things over and over again.	True	False
13. I use only an average amount of soap.	True	False
14. Some numbers are extremely unlucky.	True	False
15. I do not check letters over and over again before mailing them.	True	False
16. I do not take a long time to dress in the morning.	True	False
17. I am not excessively concerned about cleanliness.	True	False
18. One of my major problems is that I pay too much attention to detail.	True	False
19. I can use well-kept toilets without any hesitation.	True	False
20. My major problem is repeated checking.	True	False
21. I am not unduly concerned about germs and diseases.	True	False
22. I do not tend to check things more than once.	True	False
23. I do not stick to a very strict routine when doing ordinary things.	True	False
24. My hands do not feel dirty after touching money.	True	False
25. I do not usually count when doing a routine task.	True	False
26. I take rather a long time to complete my washing in the morning.	True	False
27. I do not use a great deal of antiseptics.	True	False
28. I spend a lot of time every day checking things over and over again.	True	False
29. Hanging and folding my clothes at night does not take up a lot of time.	True	False
30. Even when I do something very carefully I often feel that it is not quite right.	True	False

From Rachman, S.J., and Hodgson, R.J.: Obsessions and compulsions, Englewood Cliffs, N.J., 1980, Prentice-Hall, Inc.

Analysis

Nursing diagnosis. Fear is a nursing diagnosis approved by NANDA that applies to the rigid person. The defining characteristics of this nursing diagnosis are listed in the lower box on p. 304.

The following Case Example illustrates the characteristics of the nursing diagnosis of fear.

Case Example

Evelyn is a 30-year-old married administrative assistant at a small university. She sought a nurse counselor 8 months after her father's death. Her peace of mind was devastated, and she was preoccupied with the circumstances surrounding his death from lung cancer.

She denied the reality of his death and how it had changed her life. She believed she would never be able to get the close relationship with him that she had desired all of her life. She had excessive, hostile thoughts toward him.

Although she had functioned successfully as a professional her competence and job performance were decreasing. She repeatedly told her co-workers that she believed her father was alive.

Inwardly, she became frightened by her irrationality, and she became panicky as she feared the humiliation that would come when others learned the truth. She had difficulty concentrating and recalling promises. When discussing her lack of concentration and poor recall, she appeared as if she were in control because she could identify that her problems were the result of her response to her father's death.

Evelyn also worried about her diminished activities as she forced herself to avoid reminders about him. She would not enter a room at home that contained her desk because his clothes had hung in the closet. She had a phobic reaction to a house her father had visited the day of his death. She reacted with profound anxiety as she passed the funeral home in her car.

During the initial assessment she was pale and nervous. She altered between soft, nervous laughter and tears. She was aware of her bursts of anxiety, irrational thoughts, and phobic behavior, but her intellectual insights were insufficient to alter her behavior.

The following list provides examples of additional NANDA-accepted nursing diagnoses with causative statements.

1. Ineffective coping caused by fear

FEAR

DEFINITION

Client experiences a painfully uneasy feeling related to an identifiable source perceived by the client as dangerous.

DEFINING CHARACTERISTICS

Physical Dimension
Diaphoresis
Voice tremors/voice pitch changes
Feeling of physiological disruption
*Chronic disease can become evident
*Ritualistic practices
*Stereotyped routines
*High autonomic arousal including increased pulse, respiratory rate, and blood pressure

Emotional Dimension
Feeling of emotional disruption
Feeling of loss of control (actual or perceived)
*Phobias
*Anxiety
*Low self-esteem
*Dysphonic mood
*Pseudoplacidness
*Anger

Intellectual Dimension
Increased questioning/verbalization
*Obsessions
*Ethnocentrism
*Concreteness
*Above average intellect
*Dogmatism

Social Dimension
*Withdrawal
*Isolation
*Hyperchondriacal
*Symptoms dominate interactions
*Concern about status and prestige

Spiritual Dimension
*High moral values
*Pessimism about future
*Conservatism

Adapted from North American Nursing Diagnosis Association Classification of Nursing Diagnosis: Proceedings of the seventh conference, St. Louis, 1987, The C.V. Mosby Co.
*Indicates characteristics in addition to those defined by NANDA.

---

2. Potential for exacerbation of fear leading to compulsive hand washing because of recent death of spouse
3. Potential fear of success related to job promotion
4. Fear of imaginary animals related to client's age of 5 years
5. Fear related to possible harm related to germ contamination
6. Fears related to thoughts of dying during sleep
7. Fear of performing poorly on the job related to harsh superego with obsessional thoughts
8. Fear related to anxiety associated with leaving the house

DSM-III-R CLASSIFICATIONS RELATED TO FLEXIBILITY-RIGIDITY

ANXIETY DISORDERS
300.30   Obsessive-compulsive disorder (or obsessive-compulsive neurosis)

PERSONALITY DISORDERS
301.40   Obsessive-compulsive

IMPULSE CONTROL DISORDERS NOT ELSEWHERE CLASSIFIED
312.32   Kleptomania
312.31   Pathological gambling
312.33   Pyromania
312.39   Trichotillomania
312.39   Impulse control disorder (not otherwise specified)

Adapted from American Psychiatric Association: Diagnostic and statistical manual of mental disorders (DSM-III-R), Washington, D.C., 1987, The Association.

---

9. Ineffective family coping related to accommodating client's rigid behaviors
10. Spiritual distress related to the fear of not controlling self and others
11. Potential for fearing harm to self because of recent divorce
12. Noncompliance related to anxiety
13. Noncompliance related to obsessions
14. Noncompliance related to compulsive hand washing
15. Severe fear of death related to hospitalization
16. Fear of surgery related to loss of control while under anesthesia

DSM-III-R diagnoses. The DSM-III-R classifications related to flexibility-rigidity are listed in the box above. The essential features and manifestations of the features of obsessive-compulsive anxiety disorder and obsessive-compulsive personality disorder, according to the DSM-III-R, are listed in the boxes on p. 305.

Planning

See Table 15-4 for long-term and short-term goals and outcome criteria related to fear. These serve as examples of the planning stage in the nursing process.

Implementation

Physical dimension. The nurse reduces demands on the client when there is evidence of increasing tension such as agitation or escalation of ritualistic behavior. Medications may be ordered, especially during acute periods, when the client is near panic. Interventions include administering the medications as ordered and observing for side effects. Self-management techniques for controlling anxiety are preferable when possible. (See Chapter 12 for further information about anxiety.)

Antidepressant medications have been used with some success for depressed clients with obsessions, since depression appears to accelerate or maintain obsessive symptoms. Antidepressants seem to have a primary effect of reducing the depression and a secondary effect of reducing obsessions. The nurse observes hospitalized clients for medication side effects and teaches outpatient clients to observe for side effects in their health regimens.

For the hospitalized client, the nurse allows time for the rituals that the person needs to perform. Some routine nursing activities may need to be modified to accommodate the client's needs. The extremely ritualistic person may require prompting to eat meals on time or to meet specific appointments.

Skin protection may be indicated for clients who wash their hands or shower frequently. Lotions, topical medications, or gloves can provide some protection for hand washers, and clients may need reminders to use prescribed soaps and lotions. Harsh soaps are to be eliminated so that the client will not continue to irritate the vulnerable skin surface. The client will need reminding to thoroughly dry the wet skin, expecially when irritation is present or in hot weather.

Both obsessions and phobias may be somatic. Such phobias as fear of contracting cancer or the obsession that cancer has developed are best dealt with by not focusing on them. Following examination to ensure that no pathological condition is present, diversion to activities that interest the client, or a matter-of-fact acceptance of the complaints is indicated.[65]

300.30 OBSESSIVE-COMPULSIVE ANXIETY DISORDER

ESSENTIAL FEATURES

The individual experiences recurrent obsessions or compulsions without recognizing the senselessness of the behavior and does not get pleasure from completing an activity.

MANIFESTATIONS
Physical Dimension

Repetitive, purposeful, and intentional behavior performed according to certain rules or in a stereotyped fashion.

Emotional Dimension

Marked distress.

Intellectual Dimension

Recurrent or persistent ideas, thoughts, impulses, or images experienced as intrusive, unwanted, and senseless or repugnant (at least initially).

Attempts to ignore or suppress obsessions or to neutralize them with some other thought or action.

Recognizes that the obsessions are the product of his own mind and not imposed from without.

Content of the obsession is not related to another disorder, that is, does not include thoughts about food in the presence of an eating disorder.

Compulsion is not an end in itself, but is designed to neutralize or to prevent discomfort or some dreaded event or situation.

Either the activity is not connected in a realistic way with what it is designed to neutralize or prevent, or it is clearly excessive.

Is aware that his behavior is excessive or unreasonable.

Social Dimension

Obsessions or compulsions are time consuming, or interfere with occupational functioning, social activities, or relationships with others.

Adapted from American Psychiatric Association: Diagnostic and statistical manual of mental disorders (DSM-III-R), Washington, D.C., 1987, The Association.

301.40 OBSESSIVE-COMPULSIVE PERSONALITY DISORDER

ESSENTIAL FEATURES

A pervasive pattern of perfectionism and inflexibility beginning by early adulthood and present in a variety of contexts.

MANIFESTATIONS
Emotional Dimension

Restricted expression of affection

Inability to discard worn out or worthless objects even when they have no sentimental value

Intellectual Dimension

Preoccupation with details, rules, lists, orders, organization, or schedules to the extent that the major point of the activity is lost.

Indecisiveness: decision making is either avoided, postponed, or protracted; for example, the individual cannot get assignments done on time because of ruminating about priorities.

Social Dimension

Lack of generosity in giving time, money, or gifts, when no personal gain is likely to result.

Perfectionism that interferes with task completion.

Unreasonable insistence that others submit to exactly his way of doing things.

Unreasonable reluctance to allow others to do things because of the conviction that they will not do them correctly.

Excessive devotion to work and productivity to the exclusion of leisure activities and friendships.

Spiritual Dimension

Overconscientiousness, scrupulousness and inflexibility about matters of morality, ethics, or values (not accounted for by cultural or religious identification).

Adapted from American Psychiatric Association: Diagnostic and Statistical manual of mental disorders (DSM-III-R), Washington, D.C., 1987, The Association.

TABLE 15-4 Long-term and short-term goals and outcome criteria related to fear

Goals	Outcome Criteria

NURSING DIAGNOSIS: FEAR RELATED TO RECENT CAR WRECK RESULTING IN RITUALISTIC BEHAVIOR

Long-term goals

To have a less constricted life-style	Develops a "wish list" of activities he would like to have as part of his life-style
	Identifies those aspects of his life he desires to be less constricted
	Encourages his family to assist him in altering his life-style
To develop a positive self-concept	Lists those activities and people that enable him to feel good about himself
	Participates in therapy for at least 6 months
	Says two positive things about himself each day

Short-term goals

To decrease hand washing to 30 or less times per day within 1 week of hospitalization	Counts the number of times hand washing is done each day and reports this to one nurse
	Experiences an increase in emotional comfort as hand-washing frequency diminishes
	Uses prescribed soaps and lotions within 24 hours following hospitalization
To decrease all ritualistic behavior within 1 month after beginning outpatient therapy	Begins discussing fears with nurse during second scheduled session
	Identifies poor coping responses to his fears by third scheduled session

Emotional dimension. Rigidity demands tolerance, understanding, and acceptance by the nurse and significant others. Pressures for clients to hurry or to make decisions create anxiety that results in increased rigidity. Familiar routines provide a reassuring structure. Discussing the situations and the accompanying feelings while encouraging clients to confront the problems that have compromised their ability to function are reassuring and can decrease anxiety.[65]

Since theories of causation differ, it follows that therapy sessions also differ. The psychoanalytic theory that obsessive-compulsive problems occur as a result of unresolved conflicts in the anal stage of development leads to the analysis of childhood experiences. The cognitive model focuses on the individual's evaluation or cognitive appraisal of the threatening ideas or feelings that are central to the major symptoms. Since the person's belief system can be elicited by the nurse's focusing on self-statements and beliefs about the problem area, treatment such as desensitization is of shorter duration and more direct than the psychoanalytic approach.[101]

Current treatment methods can be divided into two types: (1) exposure procedures designed to reduce the anxiety related to obsessions and (2) blocking or punishing procedures developed to decrease the frequency of either obsessive thoughts or compulsive behaviors. Exposure procedures (paradoxical intention, imaginal flooding, satiation, and aversion relief) use systematic desensitization and procedures using prolonged exposure to feared cues. Blocking or punishing procedures consist of thought stopping, aversion therapy, and covert sensitization. The latter two have proved the most successful. Table 15-5 gives definitions and examples.

Verbal support may help when the person becomes anxious, but the modeling of calmness and empathy provides a more meaningful message. Praise is helpful as the ritualistic behavior decreases. If possible, the nurse provides opportunities for the client to talk with someone who has been successful in overcoming similar problems. Often persons with fears believe that they are the only ones in the world who are so fearful.[65]

With the nurse's assistance, clients need to first learn to recognize the existence of feelings such as anger, guilt, and loneliness before discovering the presence of and expressing appropriately their own feelings. For example, the client may not initially realize anger is an appropriate response to a put-down by a friend. In an effort to avoid conflict and maintain a "nice" image the client may deny his anger and not acknowledge the put-down. The client needs to first know that anger exists and then learn how to recognize its presence within himself before therapeutically working with the anger. By being available and supportive, expecially during periods of anxiety or an escalation of behavior, the nurse can encourage the client's expression of independent feelings and reward any initiative he assumes for dealing with feelings as illustrated in the following Case Example.

Case Example

Kevin was critical of everyone because he missed an occupational activity. The nurse who was working with Kevin sat down and discussed the situation. Kevin was asked to describe his feelings. After some hesitancy he said he felt left out and that no one cared enough to tell him that he missed the activity. The nurse pointed out that Kevin's behaviors indicated anger and resentment and how these were related to feeling rejected. The nurse also mentioned the progress he had made in describing his feelings.

TABLE 15-5 Definitions and examples of treatment methods

Term	Definition	Example
Imaginal flooding	Repeatedly recalling situations in the mind that precipitate undesired behavior	A client recalls an image in his mind of a high wall as he learns to conquer his fear of heights. He repeats the image, often combined with relaxation, until anxiety is minimized.
Satiation	Designed to decrease potency of a reinforcer	The compulsive eater is placed before a large table of food and must eat until the compulsive desire is gone. The schedule is repeated until he no longer acts out his compulsive behavior with eating.
Thought stopping	Self-induced technique to stop undesired thoughts	A client actively recalls an unwanted thought and commands himself to "stop." At the same time he relaxes. The procedure is repeated until he satisfactorily stops the undesired thought.
Aversion therapy	Use of stimuli designed to create repulsion following undesired behavior	Disulfiram (Antabuse) is given to an alcoholic client to induce nausea when he drinks alcohol.
Modeling	Imitation as a method of behavior change	The nurse demonstrates the desired social skill that the client wishes to adopt.
Behavioral rehearsal	A rehearsal situation that simulates role-playing; client rehearses new responses to problem situations after learning new adaptive responses portrayed through modeling	The client rehearses the social skill (for example, answering the phone) that causes an anxiety response. The client is taught by the nurse until he can do the skill without the undesired behavior occurring.
Social reinforcement	Positive reinforcement to new behavior; both behaviors occur in a social setting important to client	The client demonstrates the changed behavior (for example, answers the phone and talks coherently without stuttering) and is complimented for his ability to do this by those who knew he had difficulty with the behavior.
In vivo exposure	Placing client in artificial situation that resembles the real situation causing problematic behavior	The client who fears bridges is shown a video that mimics going over a bridge in a car. The situation is combined with a method (for example, relaxation or thought stopping) designed to prevent the undesired behavior. The client can view this situation as safer and able to be controlled.
Flooding	Repeated exposure to a situation that causes the undesired behavior; client is not to stop the exposure scheduling	The client is repeatedly driven down a street that causes anxiety; this is done over and over until the client no longer fears the street. Usually this is combined with a relaxation method to assist the client in changing the undesired behavior.

Kevin may need many encounters like the preceding example. By conveying patience and understanding the nurse assists Kevin to verbalize his emotions. Rigid clients have spent many years unaware of their internal self. Self-awareness is the foundation for their behavioral changes.

Homework assignments are useful between counseling sessions with rigid clients. Their ruminations may be helpful because they will remember and ponder these assignments. For example, the nurse may tell the client about the topic of the next session and ask the client to think about and discuss his reaction and feelings about the topic. These clients cannot acknowledge the presence of feelings until they understand that feelings exist in every situation.

Treatment for both fire setting and stealing can be similar. A newly developed technique of line graphing has been helpful in sequentially correlating external stress, behavior, and feelings. For example, a child fire setter is requested to discuss his feelings and behavior before, dur-

ing, and after a recent fire-setting episode. Feelings and behaviors are graphed with the child present to visually represent the situation; this assists the child to see the cause-and-effect relationship between feelings and behavior. The child is then given a choice of adaptive responses other than setting fires. Graphing helps the child observe his feelings as well as provides strategies to interrupt the fire-setting act before it occurs.[15] To date, use of this treatment for adults has not appeared in the literature.

Intellectual dimension. Offering the client new ways to view the core problem and alternative responses to that problem forms the basis for developing more effective coping skills. For example, a client has obsessive thoughts that a co-worker is her enemy; the nurse helps her consider other possible ways to interpret the co-worker's behavior.

A time when the client's anxiety is low is the best opportunity for teaching new coping skills. When the person is receptive, the nurse provides only the information about emotional insights that can be assimilated.[65] If the client's anxiety escalates or the person is resistant, it is better not to press the issue.

Imagery or thinking in pictures has gained increasing popularity since the 1960s.[32] Nurses have used this with relaxation for clients with various problems to reduce phobias, anxiety, fear, pain, and sleeplessness. Systematic desensitization (see Chapter 12) has also been a helpful intervention in clients' rigid behaviors.

Argument and persuasion make one's viewpoint rigid, whereas a matter-of-fact presentation of information is more likely to be acceptable to the client. Rigid clients are more apt to portray remarkable intellectual understanding of their situation and do not benefit from intellectualization during therapeutic sessions. This only reinforces continuing the behavior that contributed to their denial of internal feelings. The nurse strives to help the client connect intellect and emotions by encouraging related homework between thearpy sessions.

A number of behavioral management techniques have been developed in recent years. For example, staff use of response prevention involves preventing the client from doing ritualistic behavior by distracting attention, redirecting activity, or cajoling.[120]

Self-help information relevaant to problems of rigidity is available to the general public. One technique that can be self-taught is thought switching, and is briefly outlined in the box below. Another useful technique, thought-stopping, is found in Chapter 14.

Self-help readings are included in the Annotated Bibliography at the end of this chapter. Reading materials are more likely to be helpful to clients who are only moderately dysfunctional. Severely impaired individuals require assistance to implement self-help measures; the family or significant others need to be involved in this treatment.

Social dimension. After the nurse establishes a trusting relationship with the client, she encourages interpersonal relationships as an important part of intervention with the rigid person, for example, by giving the client assignments such as calling a friend or meeting one new person each week. Social skills training to diminish anxiety may be needed before the client is able to increase the quality or quantity of social contacts. For example, the client may need to role-play telephone skills with a nurse before actually phoning a friend.

When the client's anxiety is low, participation in small-group activity is encouraged. Meaningful responsibilities such as committee work, volunteer efforts, or assisting with work at home help thrust the person into social participation. Membership in a self-help group composed of persons with similar problems or in a therapy group can assist the client to increase social skills.[65]

Family members often experience intense frustration because of the client's symptoms, expecially as clients have become more socially or occupationally dysfunctional. Impatient to see results, the family may need the nurse's guidance to convey patience while assisting in treating the symptoms. Also, the family may have years of dysfuncional communication patterns and years of protecting the client from anxiety-provoking situations. If the client's progress is hindered by the home situation, therapeutic intervention such as hospitalization or family therapy may be necessary.

Family members are encouraged to continue contact with the client during hospitalization. The nurse provides contact with both following the client's discharge to promote continuity in care as the family conveys the effect of the client's behavior on their interaction patterns. By sharing with the family the plans and expectations for change that have been developed, the nurse promotes the family's ongoing involvement in the client's treatment. The home will be the crucial test of the new behavioral changes and whether they will be lifelong.

Encouraging and supporting mature family relation-

THOUGHT-SWITCHING TECHNIQUE

Aim: To replace fear-inducing self-instructions with competent self-instructions.

Thought switching involves replacing negative thoughts with positive ones until the positive ones, through practice, become so strong that they replace the anxiety-provoking negative ones. A series of positive thoughts are deliberately strengthened until they override unwanted ones.

Following are steps in thought switching:

1. Recall anxiety associated with the fearful stimuli. List all self-instructions used in the situation. (For example, "As I enter the elevator, people will stare," and "As I enter the elevator, the walls will collapse.") Include small, detailed thoughts as well as overwhelming ones.
2. List an opposite set of coping self-instructions. (For example, "As I enter the elevator, I'll tell myself it doesn't matter if people stare," and "As I enter the elevator, I'll tell myself the walls will not collapse.")
3. Put each coping self-instruction on a separate card. Keep cards in a convenient place, such as in a purse, in a pocket, or by the telephone. Their sequence does not matter.
4. Identify a high-frequency activity carried out every day, such as using the telephone, combing hair, or drinking coffee. Each time before the activity is carried out, the top card is read.
5. Use the coping self-instructions in real-life situations.
6. If better self-instructions are developed, use them but do not switch too often. Practice each one enough for it to be useful.

Adapted from Fensterheim, H., and Baer, J.: Stop running scared! New York, 1977, Dell Publishing Co., Inc.

ships that provide opportunities for the client to exercise autonomy and independence are useful strategies. Family members often are locked into a pattern in which they foster and maintain the client's dependence. Both the client and the family need help to change these dependence patterns.

Various family therapies have had moderate to good success in changing problematic family patterns.[22] In a group setting, family members can explore decisions to be made, such as how money may be spent or where to go on vacation. The nurse's presence can help them feel freer to explore previously unavailable options. The nurse can interject comments or questions designed to promote thinking and diverse responses. By ignoring rigid behaviors and concentrating on healthier ones, rigid behaviors can decrease.

Because of societal stigmas associated with gamblers, kleptomaniacs, or pyromaniacs, clients with an impulse control problem may not be readily included in social activities. Developing an individualized social network plan may be necessary for these clients.

Pathological gamblers may need their economic and job status reviewed for specific interventions that will assure their return as a contributing member of society. Kleptomaniacs may have stolen items accumulated in their home; someone needs to accompany the client and inventory their possessions, returning that which can be returned to others. The nurse may directly work with store personnel to assist the client in returning stolen items or making a plan for restitution. The pyromaniac may have destroyed his living area by fire, so the nurse may be involved with finding available housing when the client is discharged or referring him to a social worker for further assistance.

Because clients with pyromania or kleptomania may have broken the law by destroying property, stealing, or harming people, the nurse may need to assist these clients when facing legal charges or being sent to jail. The client may be temporarily hospitalized for a court-ordered evaluation. The client with pyromania is never to be taken lightly, since he may be dangerous to himself or others unfortunate enough to be in the buildings he is planning to destroy by fire. Valuables need to be secured when accessible to the client with kleptomania.

Spiritual dimension. Rigid clients frequently have a constricted spiritual dimension. Typically they have unrealistic expectations for perfection and become entangled with the religious rules and not with the predominant concepts offered by the religious beliefs.

Guilt may absorb the rigid client who is unable to strictly adhere to religious beliefs. The nurse can encourage the client to discuss these superhuman ideals in a factual manner. She can also exhibit acceptance and unconditional regard as she moves the client toward self-acceptance. (See Chapter 13 for additional information about guilt.)

Referral to counselors, ministers, or religious leaders with counseling experience may be necessary to assist these clients in moving from "the letter of the law" practice to a more tolerant and kind approach toward self. Focusing the client on self-acceptance rather than on changing others' behaviors may require repeated reinforcement.

Obsessions and compulsions may be manifest with self-depreciating religious thoughts and compulsive practices. When the client is hospitalized, the nurse may need to facilitate the compulsive acts. For example, the client may use a rosary and finger the beads throughout a catheterization procedure. Removing the beads without an awareness of the compulsive need can heighten anxiety in the rigid client who requires some control in unfamiliar surroundings. Providing a quiet room away from those who may be disturbed by the religious practice will assist the rigid client in practicing his beliefs.

INTERACTION WITH A COMPULSIVE CLIENT

Nurse: (Approaching hospitalized female client who is repeatedly and rapidly washing her hands. It is time for the client's antianxiety medication.) Miss Clark, your medication is ready for you to take.

Client: Okay. (No attempt is offered to stop the activity.)

Nurse: I brought water for you to take with the pill. Here it is. (The medication and pill are handed to the client.)

Client: (The client takes the pill and hands the empty containers to the nurse.) Thanks.

Nurse: I'll be back in 5 minutes so we can talk.

The client in the preceding interaction is preoccupied with compulsive hand washing. Compulsive behavior usually temporarily releases the anxiety of the rigid client. Rather than interrupt the hand-washing activity and risk a further increase in the client's anxiety, the nurse chose to focus on administering the antianxiety medication.

This is not the time to engage the client in a discussion of her hand-washing ritual, nor does the client need censorship or berating. Usually, rigid clients are well aware of the absurdity of their behaviors; they need help in associating their feelings with their actions. The nurse wisely allows the medication some time to be effective before exploring with the client those thoughts or activities preceding the hand-washing act.

In a matter-of-fact manner, the nurse approaches the client, truly expecting the client to take the medicine. Adding the choice of when the client wanted the nurse to give the medicine might have further increased the amount of anxiety.

Evaluation

Successful treatment may lead to unscheduled time in the client's day as the rituals are diminished. Time previously devoted to the rituals becomes available for entertainment, relationships, or projects. Clients may need assistance in acquiring new skills and in planning social and occupational activities. Evaluation provides an excellent opportunity to review this aspect of the client's life to determine new needs for nursing intervention.

In working with these difficult and long-term clients,

NURSING PROCESS SUMMARY: RIGID BEHAVIOR

ASSESSMENT

Physical Dimension
Physical evidence of anxiety
Daily rituals
Illnesses such as ulcerative colitis
Compulsive acts such as excessive hand washing or "checking" behavior
Dietary deficiencies
Use of time (for example, taking an inordinate amount of time to prepare for work)
Dermatological conditions
Sleep disturbances
Inflexible body language
Pseudoplacidness
Work compulsion

Emotional Dimension
Fears (for example, illness without presence of disease)
Dysphoric mood
Depression
Anxiety
Constricted personality
Need for self-control and environmental control
Flattened emotional state
Feelings of depersonalization and derealization
Feelings of inadequacy
Inappropriate affect

Intellectual Dimension
Restricted sphere of interest and knowledge
Concrete thinking
Diminished introspection
Obsessive thoughts
Intellectualization of feelings
Difficulty concentrating
Thinking deficit with feared topics
Doubt
Ambivalence
Diminished risk taking
Need to be correct or perfect
Inflexibility
Rumination
Morbid thoughts
Overachieving
Dogmatically believes that laboratory tests and procedures are wrong
Negative thoughts about future
Inflexible attitude toward change

Social Dimension
Impaired marital status or social success with significant others
Decreased amount and frequency of social interaction (social network)
Not satisfied with the quantity and quality of relationships
Social skill deficits
Aloofness and compulsive avoidance of others
Decreased self-esteem
Lack of recreational activities
Unhealthy family relationships
Inability to work with others to accomplish work goals
Loneliness
Expectation that others will rigidly meet his demands
Antisocial acts such as kleptomania and pyromania

Spiritual Dimension
Inflexibility in beliefs
Unquestioning belief in supernatural power
Rigid religious practices
Black or white spiritual issues
Intolerance of other's belief
Difficulty accepting own behaviors

Need for religious perfectionism
Unforgiving of self
Hopelessness

ANALYSIS
Refer to the nursing diagnosis section of this chapter (p. 304).

PLANNING AND IMPLEMENTATION

Physical Dimension
Reduce demands when increased anxiety is evident.
Limit behavior when it threatens health (excessive hand washing).
Establish routine daily activities so that some anxiety is avoided.
Allow sufficient time to complete tasks.
Encourage adequate rest, nutrition, and activity.
Arrange time for hospitalized client to complete rituals.
Provide skin protection if needed.
Observe for side effects of prescribed medications.

Emotional Dimension
Promote expression of emotions.
Encourage client to verbalize when anxious or fearful.
Provide diversional activities of interest to client to promote pleasurable experiences.
Accept the client without scolding or criticizing.

Intellectual Dimension
Assist client with new ways to solve problems and thus develop more effective coping skills.
Provide information and teaching when anxiety is low.
Avoid arguing or persuasion.
Use a matter-of-fact approach.
Use systematic desensitization to help client control feelings in presence of fearful stimuli.
Use thought stopping and thought switching to help client change to more positive thinking.
Explore prejudices and stereotypes that hinder self-growth.
Demonstrate flexibility in self and explore with client his reaction to others who demonstrate flexible thinking.
Explore prejudices and stereotypes that hinder self-growth.

Social Dimension
Plan activities to enhance social skills.
Plan meaningful social activities.
Increase client's self-concept to relieve loneliness and isolation.
Provide supportive relationships.
Encourage family to participate in client's treatment.
Avoid focusing on physical symptoms when interacting with client.
Role play effective social skills.
Provide activities leading to positive accomplishments to increase self-esteem and feelings of adequacy.

Spiritual Dimension
Assist client to have realistic expectations of self and others.
Refer to clergy or other appropriate person when client is disillusioned with faith.
Promote self-acceptance despite shortcomings.

EVALUATION
Measurable goals and outcomes provide the data for evaluating the intensity of the rigid behavior, the client's growth in understanding the origins of rigidity, new ways to cope with the problems, and the diminishing or eliminating of rigid behaviors.

the nurse may easily become discouraged with her own interventions. Meaningful employment evaluations that measure achievements by what the nurse has done as well as what the client has done may help provide satisfaction for the nurse.

BRIEF REVIEW

Flexibility and rigidity are reactions to change that can be functional or dysfunctional. Inflexible behaviors alter one's capacities for developing interpersonal relationships and managing daily living. Rigidity, repetition, anxiety, fear, and a driven quality characterize rigid disorders, including obsessive-compulsive disorders, impulse control disorders, and phobias.[67]

Freud's theories on neuroses influenced psychiatrists to favor psychoanalytic treatment. Learning theories emphasizing cognitive change as a means for altering behaviors are gaining acceptance. A holistic approach to the nursing problems related to rigidity involves a comprehensive assessment of all dimensions of the client's life.[67]

As rigid behaviors have become more prevalent, nurses have become more involved in their direct treatment. Treatment of rigid clients with behavioral interventions rather than psychoanalysis has facilitated this role change for nurses. The future promises expansion of nursing practice into broader care of rigid clients as more is learned about this complex problem.

REFERENCES AND SUGGESTED READINGS

1. Adams, P.: Obsessive children: a sociopsychiatric study, New York, 1973, Brunner/Mazel, Inc.
2. Adams, P.: The obsessive child: a therapy update, American Journal of Psychotherapy 39(3):301, 1985.
3. Adler, J., and others: The fight to conquer fear, Newsweek 103(17):66, 1984.
4. Adorno, W.T., and others: The authoritarian personality, New York, 1950, Harper & Brothers.
5. American Psychiatric Association: Diagnostic and statistical manual of mental disorders, ed. 3, Washington, D.C., 1980, The Association.
6. Apter, A., and others: Severe obsessive compulsive disorder in adolescence: a report of 8 cases, Journal of Adolescence 7(4):349, 1984.
7. Badding, N.C.: Educating phobic clients about the physiology of their feelings. . . physiological bases of common physical responses to panic, Health and Social Work 10(1):23, 1985.
8. Ballenger, J.: Biology of agoraphobia, Washington, D.C., 1984, American Psychiatric Press.
9. Baralt, A.R.: Systematic desensitization and cognitive restructuring in the treatment of a self-injection phobia, Journal of Rehabilitation 51(1):35, 1985.
10. Barron, A.P., and Earls, F.: The relation of temperament and social factors to behavior problems in three-year-old children, Journal of Child Psychology and Psychiatry 25(1):23, 1984.
11. Baxter, L.: Two cases of obsessive-compulsive disorder with depression responsive to trazodone, Journal of Nervous and Mental Disease 173(7):432, 1985.
12. Beech, H.R., and Perrigualt, J.: Toward a theory of obsessional disorder. In Beech, H.R., editor: Obsessional states, London, 1974, Methuen & Co., Ltd.
13. Behar, D.: Computerized tomography and neuropsychological test measures in adolescents with OCD, American Journal of Psychiatry 141(3):363, 1984.
14. Berntson, G.C., and others: Cardiac reactivity and adaptive behavior, American Journal of Mental Deficiency 89(4):415, 1985.
15. Bumpass, E., Fagelman, F., and Brix, R.: Intervention with children who set fires, American Journal of Psychotherapy 37:328, July 1983.
16. Buros, D.K., editor: The fifth mental measurement yearbook, Highland Park, N.J., 1959, The Gryphon Press.
17. Carpenito, L.: Nursing diagnosis: application to clinical practice Philadelphia, 1983, J.B. Lippincott Co.
18. Clark, D., and Bolton, D.: Obsessive-compulsive adolescents and their parents: a psychometric study, Journal of Child Psychology and Psychiatry and Allied Disciplines 26(2):267, 1985.
19. Clifford, C., and others: Genetic and environmental influences on obsessional traits and symptoms, Psychological Medicine 14(4):791, 1984.
20. Coryell, W.: Obsessive compulsive disorder and primary unipolar depression: comparisons of background, family history, course mortality, Journal of Nervous and Mental Disorders 169:220, 1981.
21. Crossley, T., and Guzman, T.: The relationship between arson and pyromania, American Journal of Forensic Psychology 3(1):39, 1985.
22. Dalton, P.: Family treatment of an obsessive-compulsive child: a case report, Family Process 22(1):99, 1983.
23. Eisenberg, J., and Asnis, G.: Lithium as adjunct treatment in obsessive compulsive disorders, American Journal of Psychiatry 142(5):663, 1985.
24. Farkas, G., and Beck, S.: Exposure and response prevention of morbid ruminations and compulsive avoidance, Behavior Research and Therapy 19(3):257, 1981.
25. Foa, E.B.: Failure in treating obsessive-compulsives, Behavior Research Theory 17:169, 1979.
26. Foa, E.B.: Phobias; how to keep your fears under control, U.S. News and World Report 91:69, 1981.
27. Foa, E.: Success and failure in the behavioral treatment of obsessive-compulsives, Journal of Consultant and Clinical Psychology 51(2)287, 1983.
28. Foa, E. and others: Deliberate blocking and exposure of OC rituals: immediate and long term effects, Behavior Therapy 15(5):450, 1984.
29. Foa, E., and others: Imaginal and in vivo exposure: a comparison of obsessive-compulsive checkers, Behavior Therapy 16(3):292, 1985.
30. Fontana, D.; Some standardization data for the Sandler-Hazari Obsessionality Inventory, British Journal of Medical Psychology 53(3):267, 1980.
31. Freud, S.: The ego and the id, New York, 1962, W.W. Norton & Co., Inc. (J. Strachey, editor.)
32. Gagan, J.M.: Imagery: an overview with suggested application for nursing, Perspectives in Psychiatric Care 22(1):20, 1984.
33. Gatz, M., and others: older women and mental health, Issues in Mental Health Nursing 5(1/4):273, 1983.
34. Geller, J., and Bertsch, G.: Fire-setting behaviors in the histories of a state hospital population, American Journal of Psychiatry 142(4) 464, 1985.
35. Gibb, G., and others: The measurement of the obsessive-compulsive personality, Educational and Psychological Measurement 43(4):1233, 1983.
36. Goldsmith, R.E.: Some personality correlates of open processing, Journal of Psychology 116:59, 1984.

37. Goldstein, W.: Obsessive-compulsive behavior, DSM-III, and a psychodynamic classification of psychopathology, American Journal of Psychotherapy 39(3):346, 1985.

38. Green, S.: Mind and body: the psychology of physical illness, Washington, D.C., 1985, American Psychiatric Press.

39. Greenburg, D.: Are religious compulsions religious or compulsive: a phenomenological study, American Journal of Psychotherapy 38(4):524, October, 1984.

40. Heath, G., and others: Diagnosis and childhood fire setting Journal of Clinical Psychology 41(4):571, 1985.

41. Henry, P.J., and Stephens, P.M.: Stress, health, and the social environment, New York, 1977, Springer Verlag.

42. Hinkel, L.E.: The effect of exposure to cultural change, social change and changes in interpersonal relationships on health. In Dohrenwend, B.S., and Dohrenwend, B.P., editors: Stressful life event: their nature and effects, New York, 1974, John Wiley & Sons, Inc.

43. Hollingsworth, C., and others: Long-term outcome of obsessive-compulsive disorder in childhood, Journal of American Academy of Child Psychiatry 19:134, 1980.

44. Hollingsworth, C., and others, (1984). The outpatient treatment of patients with OCD, Behavior Research and Therapy 22(4):455, 1980.

45. Hoogduin, K.: The diagnosis of OCD, American Journal of Psychotherapy 40(1):36, 1986.

46. Hoover, C., and Insel, T.: Families of origin in obsessive-compulsive disorder, Journal of Nervous and Mental Disease 172(4):207, 1984.

47. Hunter, R., and MacAlpine, I.: Three Hundred Years of Psychiatry, London, 1983, Oxford University Press.

48. Ingram, I.: Obsessional illness in mental hospital patients, Journal of Medical Science 107:382, 1961.

49. Insel, T.R.: Obsessive-compulsive disorder: five clinical questions and a suggested approach, Comprehensive Psychiatry 23:241, 1982.

50. Insel, T.R.: The psychopharmacological treatment of obsessive compulsive disorder, Journal of Clinical Psychopharmacology 1:304, 1982.

51. Insel, T.R.: New findings in obsessive-compulsive disorder, Washington, D.C., 1984, American Psychiatric Press.

52. Insel, T.: Obsessive-compulsive disorder, Psychiatric Clinics of North America 8(1):105, 1985.

53. Insel, T., Hoover, C., and Murphy, D.: Parents of patients with obsessive-compulsive disorder, Psychological Medicine 13(4):807, 1983.

54. Insel, T., and others: Tricyclic response in obsessive compulsive disorder, Progress in Neuro-psychopharmacology and Biological Psychiatry 9(1):25, 1985.

55. Jacobson, R.R.: The subclassification of child firesetters, Journal of Child Psychology and Psychiatry 26(5):769, 1985.

56. Jenike, M.: The EEG in OCD, Journal of Clinical Psychiatry 45(3):122, 1984.

57. Jenike, M.: Obsessive compulsive didsorder: a question of a neurologic lesion, Comprehensive Psychiatry 25(3):298, 1984.

58. Jolley, J.M.: The relationship between self, structure, and adaptability and age, American Psychology Bulletin 6:95, 1984.

59. Junginger, J., and Diatto, B.: Multitreatment of obsessive compulsive checking in a geriatric patient, Behavior Modification 8(3):379, 1984.

60. Kline, P., and Cooper, C.: Rigid personality and rigid thinking, British Journal of Educational Psychology 55:24, 1985.

61. Kolb, L.C., and Brodie, H.K.H.: Modern clinical psychiatry, Philadelphia, 1982, W.B. Saunders Co.

62. Kolko, D.: A conceptualization of firesetting in children and adolescents, Journal of Abnormal Child Psychology 14(1):49, 1986.

62a. Kretch, D.: The elements of psychology, New York, 1982, Alfred A. Knopf, Inc.

63. Kringlen, E.: Obsessional neurotics: a long-term follow-up, British Journal of Psychiatry 10:709, 1965.

64. Lapsley, D.K., and Enright, R.D.: A cognitive developmental model of rigidity and senescence, International Journal of Aging and Human Development 16(2):81, 1983.

65. Larson, M.L.: Flexibility-rigidity. In Beck, C.M., Rawlins, R.P., and Williams, S.R. editors: Mental Health-psychiatric nursing: a holistic life-cycle approach, St. Louis, 1984, The C.V. Mosby, Co.

66. Leone, C.: Thought-induced change in phobic beliefs: sometimes it helps, sometimes it hurts, Journal of Clinical Psychology 40(1):68, 1984.

67. Lerner, P.: The development of a self-report inventory to assess obsessive compulsive behavior, Dissertation Abstracts International 43(9-B):30, 1983.

68. Lieberman, J.: Evidence for a biological hypothesis of OCD, Neuropsychobiology 11(1):14, 1981.

69. Magaro, P.: The personality of clinical types; an empirically derived taxonomy, Journal of Clinical Psychology 37(4):796, 1981.

70. Mallinger, A.: The obsessive's myth of control, Journal of the American Academy of Psychoanalysis 12(2):147, 1984.

71. Marks, I: Behavioral psychotherapy for anxiety disorders, Psychiatric Clinics of North America 8(1):25, 1985.

72. McFall, M.E., and Wollersheim, J.P.: A cognitive-behavorial formulation and approach, Cognitive Therapy and Research 3:333, 1979.

73. McKeon, J., McGuffin, P, and Robinson, P.: Obsessive-compulsive neurosis following head injury: a report of four cases, British Journal of Psychiatry 144:190, 1984.

74. McKeon, J., and others: Life events and personality traits in OC neurosis, British Journal of Psychiatry 144:185, 1984.

75. Mellman, L., and Gorman, J.: Successful treatment of OCD with ECT, American Journal of Psychiatry 141(4):596, 1984.

76. Mitchell, J., editor: The ninth mental measurement yearbook, Lincoln, Neb., 1985, University of Nebraska Press.

77. Mothersill, K., and Neufeld, R.: Probability learning and coping in dysphoria and obsessive-compulsive tendencies, Journal of Research in Personality 19(2):152, 1985.

78. Panek, P.E., and others: Behavioral rigidity in young and old adults, The Journal of Psychology 114:199, 1983.

79. Pasnau, R.: Diagnosis and treatment of anxiety disorders, Washington, D.C., 1984, American Psychiatric Press.

80. Pavlov, I.P.: Experimental psychology and other essays, New York, 1959, Philosophical Library, Inc.

81. Peplau, H.: The power of the dissociative state, Journal of Psychosocial Nursing 23:31, 1985.

82. Persons, J.: Processing of fearful and neutral information by OC's, Behavior Research and Therapy 22(3):259, 1984.

83. Persons, J., and Foa, E.: Processing of fearful and neutral information by obsessive-compulsives, Behavior Research and Therapy 22(3):259, 1984.

84. Phillips, J.: The origins of intellect; Piaget's theory, San Francisco, 1975, W.H. Freeman and Co. Publishers.

85. Rabavilas, A.: Relation of obsessional traits to anxiety in patients with ulcerative colitis, Psychotherapy and Psychosomatics, 33(3):155, 1980.

86. Rado, S.: Adaptational psychodynamics: motivation and control, New York, 1969, Science House, Inc.

87. Rachman, S., and Hodgson, R.: Obsessions and compulsions, Englewood Cliffs, NJ, 1980, Prentice-Hall, Inc.

88. Rasmussen, S.: The epidemiology of obsessive compulsive disorder, Journal of Clinical Psychiatry **45**(11):450, 1984.

89. Rinieris, P., and Stefanis, C.: Obsessional personality traits and ABO blood types, Neuropsychobiology **6**(3):128, 1980.

90. Rippere, V.: Dietary treatment of chronic obsessional ruminations, British Journal of Clinical Psychology **22**(4):314, 1983.

91. RoKeach, M.: The open and closed mind, New York, 1960, Basic Books, Inc. Publishers.

92. Rosenheim, E., and Golan, G: Patients' reactions to humorous interventions in psychotherapy, American Journal of Psychotherapy **40**(1):110, 1986.

93. Rowan, V., and others: A rapid multi-component treatment for an obsessive-compulsive disorder, Journal of Behavior Therapy and Experimental Psychiatry **15**(4):347, 1984.

94. Rubenowitz, S.: Emotional flexibility-rigidity as a comprehensive dimension of the mind. Stockholm, 1963, Almquist, Wiskell, & Forlag.

95. Runck, B.: Research is changing views on obsessive compulsive disorder, Hospital Community Psychiatry **34**(7):597, 1983.

96. Salkoviskis, P.: Obsessional-compulsive problems: a cognitive behavioral analysis, Behavior Research and Therapy **23**(5):571, 1985.

97. Salzman, L.: The value of psychotherapy over antidepressants in treating OCDs, Integrative Psychiatry **1**(1):28, 1983.

98. Salzman, L.: Psychotherapeutic management of obsessive compulsive patients, American Journal of Psychotherapy **39**(3):323, 1985.

99. Salzman, L.: Treatment of the obsessive personality, New York, 1985, Aronson.

100. Sanavio-Ezio, A., and Vidotto-Giulio, D.: The components of the Maudsley Obsessional Compulsive Questionnaire, Behavior Research and Therapy **23**(6):659, 1985.

101. Scott, A., and others: Regional differences in obsessionality and obsessional neurosis, Psychological Medicine **12**(1):131, 1982.

102. Sifneos, P.: Short-term dynamic psychotherapy of phobic and mildly obsessive compulsive patients, American Journal of Psychotherapy **39**(3):314, 1985.

103. Steketee, G., and others: Obsessive compulsive disorder; differences between washers and checkers, Behavior Research and Therapy **23**(2):197, 1985.

104. Stewin, L.: The concept of rigidity: an enigma, International Journal for the Advancement of Counseling **6**(3):227, 1983.

105. Sullivan, H.S.: The interpersonal theory of psychiatry, New York, 1953, W.W. Norton & Co., Inc.

106. Swenson, R.: Response to tranylcypromine and thought stopping in obsessional disorder, British Journal of Psychiatry **144**:425,1984.

107. Tan, T., and others: Biopsychobehavioral correlates of insomnia, American Journal of Psychiatry **141**(3):357, 1984.

108. Deleted in proofs.

109. Thyer, B., and others: Fear of criticism is not specific to OCD, Behavior Research & Therapy **22**(1):77, 1984.

110. Traskman, L., and others: Cortisol in the cerebral spinal fluid of depressed and suicidal patients, Archives of General Psychiatry **37**(7):761, 1980.

111. Travers, J.: Clarifying the issue: the issue of clarity, Psychotherapy Patient **1**(2):5, 1984.

112. Turner, R. and others: Assessing the impact of cognitive differences in the treatment of OCD, Journal of Clinical Psychology **39**(6):933, 1983.

113. Turner, S. and others: Biological factors in obsessive compulsive disorders. Psychological Bulletin **97**(3):430, 1985.

114. Turns, D.: Epidemiology of phobic and obsessive compulsive disorders among adults, American Journal of Psychotherapy **39**(3):360, 1985.

115. Volavka, J., and others: Clomipramine and imipramine in obsessive-compulsive disorder, Psychiatry Research **14**(1):85, 1985.

116. Warneke, L.: The use of intravenous chlorimipramine in the treatment of OCD, Canadian Journal of Psychiatry **29**(2):135, 1984.

117. Warneke, L.: Intravenous chlorimipramine in the treatment of obsessional disorder in adolescence: case report, Journal of Clinical Psychiatry **16**(3):100, 1985.

118. Wasylenski, D.: Psychodynamic aspects of occupational stress, California Journal of Psychiatry **29**(4):295, 1984.

119. Weeks, D.J.: Transcutaneous nerve stimulation: two cases with phobia-resolving consequences, Journal of Behavioral Therapy and Experimental Psychiatry **15**(1):37, 1984.

120. Weiner, M., and White, M.: The use of a self psychology approach in treating a compulsive 84 year old man, Clinical Gerontologist **3**(4):64, 1985.

ANNOTATED BIBLIOGRAPHY

Fensterheim, H., Baer, J.: Stop running scared! New York, 1977, Dell Publishing Company, Inc.

This paperback for anyone with distressing fears is a compendium of information on phobias and how to control them. The authors discuss fear and fear-control training. Programs for mild obsessive-compulsive symptoms are provided. Appendices include examples of relaxation exercises and hierarchies for systematic desensitization.

Kellerman, J.: Helping the fearful child, New York, 1981, Warner Books.

The author discusses how the child learns to be afraid. Common childhood fears such as darkness and new situations are covered. Those who raise children are offered methods to deal with the child's fears in the home and how adults may cope with the fears. The authors suggest finding professional help if the book's advice is ineffective or needs professional reinforcement.

Rachman, S.J., and Hodgson, R.J.: Obsessions and compulsions, Englewood Cliffs, N.J., 1980, Prentice Hall, Inc.

This book presents detailed theoretical explanations for the development of obsessions and compulsions. Research findings to support treatment methods are included. Discussions cover both conventional treatment and psychological modification.

CHAPTER 16

DEPENDENCE–INDEPENDENCE

Mary Flo Bruce

After studying this chapter the learner will be able to:

Trace the historical development of dependent, independent, and interdependent behaviors.

Identify theories of dependent, independent, and interdependent behaviors.

Use nursing process to provide care to clients with maladaptive dependent and independent behavior.

Identify current research related to dependence and independence.

Dependence on others is a fundamental human need during normal growth and development and a healthy response to crises throughout the life cycle. As individuals mature, they move toward increasing independence, with the goal of becoming interdependent. Western society values independence and views dependency generally as a weakness or inadequacy. Because of society's views, children are often prematurely pushed toward independence. Dependent behavior in adults is often regarded as maladaptive. Conflict often arises from frustration of dependent and independent needs.

Maladaptive dependence is of central significance in the psychopathology of personality disorders and in individuals who are addicted to chemical substances. Some people may manifest pseudo-independent behavior. Nurses need to understand adaptive and maladaptive dependence and independence to assist clients to meet their needs.

THEORETICAL APPROACHES

Dependent behavior is behavior in which one person relies on another individual or object for support or aid. *Independence* involves taking initiative in meeting one's own needs; the individual is self-reliant. Dependent and independent behavior may be adaptive or maladaptive.

Adaptive dependence allows an individual to be dependent when the external and internal environments preclude autonomous functioning. Development of adaptive dependence assists one to accept physical and emotional limitations. *Maladaptive dependence* is a method of cop-

ing that is inappropriate or unrealistic; an individual relies too much on others to make his decisions or take care of him. One may develop a physical or emotional illness as a result of this manner of coping.

Adaptive independence occurs when the individual is able to act according to his own judgment. *Maladaptive independence* is a behavior that interferes with an individual's ability to attain a high level of health. The person is so independent that he refuses aid from another even when it is appropriate. This mode of coping may be learned when a child receives negative reinforcement for displaying adaptive dependent behavior.

Interdependence, a balance between dependence and independence, occurs when the individual uses dependent or independent behavior as appropriate for the situation. Interdependent functioning requires use of the individual's problem-solving abilities and is not a mere patterned response to environmental stimulus.

One can use the health-illness continuum as a framework to conceptualize adaptive and maladaptive dependence and independence. The individual who maintains adaptive coping behavior is on the healthy end of the continuum (Figure 16-1) and thus able to develop interdependence that enables him to cope optimally within his abilities.

Psychoanalytic

Freud[20] dealt with the development of dependence in the oral phase, which occurs during the first 2 years of life. During this phase the infant learns to depend on the

Historical Overview

DATE	EVENT
Pre-Industrial Age	The individual was dependent on nature and became more independent when tools and material were developed.
Industrial Age	Technology made interdependent behavior essential for survival.
Post-Renaissance	The frontier woman was expected to be dependent, while cherishing the spirit of independence. This dichotomous expectation of women continues to some extent to the present.
	Western society came to view independence as a God-given right, with dependent behavior being discouraged.
	The patient was expected to assume a passive, dependent role.
1952	World Health Organization recognized the individual's dependence on alcohol in their definition of alcoholism.
1970s	Holistic medicine emphasized independence with its belief that the individual is responsible for self-care.
	Men and women were more apt to work interdependently in fulfilling family responsibility.
1980s	Alcohol continues to be the number one chemical substance abused in the United States.
	Dependence on drugs such as opiates, cocaine, and hallucinogens cause a major health problem, cutting across socioeconomic groups.
	The nurse's role in the care of substance abusers is more active than previously.

parent for both emotional and physical life support. The infant learns that dependence needs are met by the parent, and survival occurs only if minimal needs are satisfied.

According to Freud, if dependence needs are not met during the oral phase, the individual becomes fixated at this stage. This fixation results in one's attempting to meet one's dependence needs. Fixation at the oral stage can result in substance dependency, development of a dependent personality disorder or other problems related to meeting dependent needs, such as eating disorders or smoking. The dependent individual relies on significant others to make his choices. The person's superego is very inhibited by the demands and prohibitions of others. Use of chemical substances allows the release of the inhibitions of the superego. The person is able to be himself, to

talk more freely, and be more sociable. The individual's ego boundaries are loosened, and the person may even act on id impulses that are ordinarily repressed. However, adaptive dependence occurs when the infant's dependence needs are adequately met, and he progresses successfully through the oral stage to the next stage of development.

Adaptive independence is learned at a later stage than adaptive dependence. According to Freud, during the anal stage the toddler begins to learn independent behavior. At this stage the child is able to move about somewhat without assistance, and the parent begins to expect certain things of the child, such as walking. The child learns that certain actions cause certain behaviors in others. For instance, when the toddler goes to the toilet, the parent acts

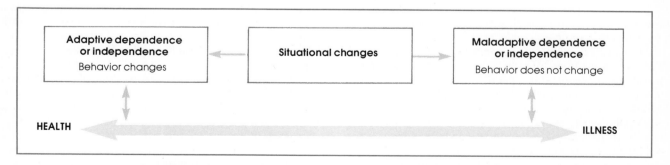

FIGURE 16-1 Dependence-independence on the health-illness continuum.

pleased; when the child wets the diaper, the parent shows disapproval. Parents start reinforcing behavior that is less dependent, and the child develops a need for achievement. This need activates internal pressure, which initiates a response from the child to relieve the pressure. Positive parental response to the child's beginning mastery over the environment rewards the child. Gradually, increasingly independent behavior is rewarded, and the toddler learns adaptive independence.

Erikson[16] called the first 18 months of life the trust versus mistrust period. The infant learns to trust himself and the environment by "asking" the parent for caring behavior. The asking behavior is repeated, and an effective response is expected. If the parent continues to deliver the necessary care, the baby learns trust and acceptance.

During the development of trust the infant begins to realize he is a separate entity from the parent. Parental behavior such as rejection or overprotection leads to dependent, attention-seeking behaviors. When rejected, the infant may hold his breath or stomp his feet to get attention. On the other hand, the overprotected child may be quiet and withdrawn so the caretaker will say, "What a good boy!" or "What a good girl!" Development of these dependent behaviors leads the infant to feel powerless and inadequate. As the dependent person gets older, he often finds the use or abuse of chemical substances allows him to feel better about himself. The person feels a false sense of control, more adequate, and more independent. While "high" one often feels one can accomplish anything.

Erikson labeled the beginning of adaptive independence as the autonomy versus shame and doubt stage. To progress successfully through this stage the toddler needs to receive positive reinforcement for doing things for himself. At the same time the parents need to exert firm outer control. The toddler must be allowed to make decisions within his ability. During the next stage, initiative versus guilt, independent behavior is expanded. Concurrently the ability to communicate is enhanced. The child demonstrates independence by saying "no" to parental demands.

The most vital stage in the development of independent behavior is the industry versus inferiority stage. At this age the child wants to do things for himself, takes initiative, and works diligently to overcome obstacles. All of these are tasks of independence, and it is important for the parent to reinforce such independent behavior. Praise from the parents and others is an excellent positive reinforcer during this stage. Positive, consistent reinforcement needs to be given for both physical and emotional acts that reflect adaptive independent behavior.

Erikson dealt with independent behavior at all stages. The last stage of life, integrity versus despair, is an important stage for maintaining adaptive independence. Erikson described ego integrity as all previous phases coming together while despair leaves the individual angry and filled with self-disgust. The aging individual with ego integrity is able to develop adaptive independence, which is the opposite side of the coin of the adaptive dependence discussed earlier. The elderly person faces many changes. Along with increasing physical dependence, emotional in-

dependence is threatened by many losses that occur during the latter part of life. While the aging individual is attempting to cope with these losses, society says, "Independence is important" and "Worthwhile people work." The aging individual needs to receive positive reinforcement for realistic independent behavior to counteract the increased physical dependence and society's negative attitude. Rewards, such as positive statements and sincere praise, can be given for both adaptive dependent and adaptive independent behavior. During this phase, because of forced dependence in some areas, the client with interdependent coping skills is able to age more successfully.

Erikson described two stages in which interdependent behavior is developed, the identity stage and the intimacy stage. The identity stage occurs in adolescence. If the youth has accomplished the previous tasks adequately, the development of interdependent behavior is facilitated. Having previously received positive reinforcement for adaptive dependent and adaptive independent behavior, the adolescent has already learned some interdependent behavior. The adolescent has a need to be psychologically independent from the family and may express this independence by renouncing the values and norms of the parents. However, the individual is extremely dependent on peers. It is because of this need for approval from peers that the adolescent may become involved with chemical substances and become chemically dependent. The parents have the task of allowing the youth to make independent decisions and judgments when possible, while assuring the adolescent of continued love and support from the family. This period is often difficult for the parents and the adolescent. Frequently it appears to the parents that their child who had excellent judgment just a couple of years earlier is incapable of making any sound judgments at all. During this time the parent allows independent decisions while setting firm and consistent rules.

During the intimacy stage, adaptive coping behavior consists of having the ability to move from a dependent to an independent position. Developing an independent coping style, the young adult then assumes a role that requires interdependence. If the individual has previously developed a realistic trust in others and is secure in his own identity, he is able to be self-disclosing and form an intimate relationship with another. This relationship fulfills affiliation needs and achieves interdependence.

Bowlby emphasized the importance of bonding between the infant and the parental figure.[8] He discussed the attachment phenomenon that begins immediately at birth. A bond occurs between mother and infant at birth, and the newborn is soon conditioned to meet his dependence needs. Klaus and Kennell[27] expanded Bowlby's theory to include the newborn and both parents. The mother and father need to see, touch, and cuddle the baby soon after birth. This time is critical in conditioning the parents to perform the role of parent. The sooner the bonding occurs, the more rapidly the parents receive positive reinforcement from the baby's touch, and the adaptive dependence needs of both the baby and parents are met.

Bowlby believed that independent behavior is fostered

by parents who provide unfailing support along with consistent encouragement that the child become independent. The parent gives unfailing support by allowing and encouraging the child to perform tasks that he can successfully accomplish. At the same time, the parent needs to assist the child with tasks that are too difficult. While developing autonomy, the child needs to feel confident that the attachment figure will be available when needed. Development of independent behavior extends throughout childhood and adolescence; however, once the behavior is developed, it persists fairly consistently through the life cycle. Having had both dependent and independent needs met, the individual may use interdependent behavior.

According to Bowlby, the self-reliant person is not as independent as Western culture stereotypes project. The self-reliant individual is able to develop adaptive interdependent behavior. The well-adapted person and his attachment figure both give and receive support and love, are available when needed, and slowly build confidence in each other's availability.

Mahler[29] considered the first few months of life as symbiotic months, which means that at this time a union between the baby and the mother is essential. During these months the baby learns to identify with the mothering half of the baby's symbiotic self and responds mainly to the internal environment.

Maladaptive dependence is developed when the infant's dependence needs are not rewarded in a manner that allows the infant to progress from one stage to another. The infant who receives sufficient care for survival but does not receive loving care from the parental figure will not have dependence needs met adequately. This infant develops maladaptive dependence. The opposite side of the coin is the parental figure who has a smothering relationship with the infant, which results in maladaptive independence. In both cases the infant is taught a maladaptive mode of coping. Either the toddler tries harder to get dependence needs met or withdraws and develops a maladaptive independence.

According to Mahler the development of independent behavior begins at 4 or 5 months, the peak of the symbiotic phase. At this time the infant begins the first subphase of "separation-individuation," which are two separate but intertwined tasks. *Separation* is the development of the physical ability to move away from the mother, along with the mental awareness of being separate. *Individuation* is a cognitive, affective development that allows the infant to cope with the separateness. The subphases of the separation-individuation process are described in Table 16-1.

Interpersonal

Sullivan[42] considered infancy the "learning to count on others" phase. He stressed interpersonal relationships and socialization and contended that if dependent needs are met in infancy, the infant learns to trust himself with others. Through the interpersonal relationship with mother, the baby's dependency needs are met and thus adaptive dependence occurs.

According to Sullivan adaptive independence begins in the latter part of the infantile stage, when the baby learns to satisfy some of his own needs independent of the

TABLE 16-1 Subphases of Mahler's separation-individuation process

Phase	Age	Description	Example
Differentiation	5-9 months	Becoming aware of being separate from mother. A powerful bond between mother and infant. Physical and psychological dependence on mother.	Smiles at sound of mother's voice and at sight of mother.
Practicing	9-14 months	Expanding independence. In latter part of phase learns to walk. Adaptive independence learned from games played with mother and other nurturing individuals. First notices inanimate objects in environment. Separation anxiety.	Plays game in which child runs away from mother and mother chases and catches child.
Rapprochement	14-24 months	Many conflicts need to be resolved. Increased awareness of external environment. Increased sense of physical separateness. Adaptive development depends on child resolving conflict related to wish to replace parent of same sex. Separation anxiety.	Shares achievements with mother.
Consolidation	24-36 months	Beginning of object constancy—the ability to hold a symbolic picture of loved object when object is absent. Child moves away from mother with less anxiety. Increased independence. Future mental health depends on the development of increased individuality and emotional object constancy.	Plays alone without physical presence of mother.

TABLE 16-2 Development of dependence, independence, and interdependence according to various theories

Theorist	Development of Dependence	Development of Independence	Development of Interdependence
Bowlby	Birth—attachment	Childhood to adolescence—unfailing support	Adolescence—assurance of availability of attachment figure
Erikson	Birth—trust	Age 2 to 3 years—autonomy Age 3 to 6 years—initiative	Age 13 to 18 years—identity Age 18 to 40 years—intimacy
Freud	Birth to 2 years—oral phase	Age 2 to 3 years—anal phase	
Mahler	Birth—symbiotic phase	Age 4 to 5 months—separation individuation Age 2 years—reapprochement Age 3 years—consolidation	
Sullivan	Birth—learning to count on others	Childhood—self-reliance	Age 6 to 9 years—looks to peers for a sense of companionship Age 9 to 12 years—forms an intense love relationship with person of same sex ("chum relationship") Age 13 to 18 years—able to establish relationships with persons of opposite sex—to be dependent, independent, and interdependent

mother. The growth of independence occurs during the second stage, childhood, which begins with articulate speech is learned. This is when the child develops a self-concept and recognizes himself as separate from others.

Sullivan's interpersonal relationship theory proposes that interdependent behavior is initiated during the juvenile stage. During this time the child learns both to cooperate and compete. The school-age child learns to work and play with other children. They work together to attain goals they have established. At the same time they compete against those who are outside of their own group. At this age children form clubs and gangs. Internal control is strengthened, and external control is lessened somewhat.

The growth of interdependent behavior continues through the next two periods, preadolescence and adolescence. During preadolescence the child learns to form relationships that require reciprocity and mutual sharing. By the end of adolescence the young adult has learned the rights and the responsibilities of living in society. The self-system is stabilized, and the individual is capable of forming indepth interpersonal relationships.

Behavioral

The learning theories propose that maladaptive dependence occurs when positive reinforcement is not sufficient to meet the infant's needs. The baby learns to search for methods to meet these needs. As an adult the individual may learn to rely on chemical substances to meet their needs. Alcohol or other chemical substances reinforce one's positive feelings about oneself. When the chemical action wears off, the good feelings are replaced by feelings of guilt, inadequacy, and dependence, so the person uses the substance again to regain the good feelings.

The psychodynamics of maladaptive independence are similar to those of maladaptive dependence. Maladaptive independence occurs at a later stage of development, dur-

ing early childhood. Maladaptive independent behavior interferes with an individual's ability to attain optimal health. This mode of coping may be learned when a child receives negative reinforcement for displaying adaptive dependent behavior. Rewarding inappropriate independent behavior can also result in maladaptive independent behavior. The individual who has developed a maladaptive independent coping style has difficulty accepting external control. When external control is necessary, the individual experiences a conflict between internal and external needs. Examples of this conflict are the elderly person who is confused at times and can no longer live alone and the alcoholic individual at a cocktail party. Both of these individuals want to pursue an independent course. The elderly person wants to live independently but is too confused to do so. An external control—living with someone else—is imposed. The alcoholic has an internal conflict. At cocktail parties the external control says, "Drink—it is the sociable thing to do." However, the alcoholic cannot drink socially.

Table 16-2 summarizes the development of dependence, independence, and interdependence according to various theories.

Table 16-3 is a summary of theories relating to independence and dependence.

RELATING TO THE CLIENT

The nurse needs to be aware of her own values and beliefs in her relationships with these clients who have problems with dependence and independence. If a block appears to be interfering with the nurse's working with the client the nurse needs to ask several questions; for example, "Is the client's dependence or independence in conflict with my values?" and "Am I making judgments that interfere with my working with the client?" Self-disclosure may help the nurse remove any blocks that she

TABLE 16-3 Summary of theories of dependence-independence

Theory	Theorist	Dynamics
Psychoanalytic Intrapsychic	Freud	Maladaptive dependence results from the fixation of adaptive dependency needs that were not met during oral phase.
		Independent behavior is learned during anal phase in response to being allowed to exert appropriate control over actions. Becomes maladaptive when this need is frustrated.
	Erikson	As the infant learns to trust his caretaker and himself, he learns adaptive dependence.
		Adaptive independence is learned during the stage of autonomy versus shame and doubt as the child receives positive reinforcement for doing things for himself. Both dependence and independence become maladaptive when the need is frustrated.
	Bowlby	Adaptive dependence is learned during bonding between mother and infant.
		The child develops independent behavior when parent encourages him to perform realistic tasks for himself.
	Mahler	The infant has a symbiotic dependent relationship with mother.
		Maladaptive dependence develops when child's dependence needs are not rewarded by mother.
Interpersonal	Sullivan	Adaptive dependence learned during infancy when child learns he can count on others to meet his needs.
		Independent behavior begins in late infancy and continues into childhood in response to being rewarded for satisfying some needs independent of mother.
Behavioral		Dependence becomes maladaptive when positive reinforcement is not sufficient to meet infant's needs.
		Maladaptive dependence occurs when the child receives negative reinforcement for displaying adaptive dependent behavior.

interjects into the relationship. Since the therapeutic relationship is based on trust between the nurse and the client, the nurse needs to resolve any negative feelings about either dependence or independence, as well as clients with these disorders, such as substance abuse and personality disorders. During the initial stage of working with the client who displays maladaptive dependent behavior, the nurse needs to meet the dependence needs of the client. It may be necessary to assist the client in activities of daily living, help him in making decisions, and offer much praise and attention.

Clients who abuse chemical substances frequently do not see a problem or seriously believe that they can quit using the substance anytime they really want. Until the client admits he has a problem, therapy may be ineffective. However, it is important to engage the person actively in the treatment program as early as possible. Often the person enters therapy because of problems related to the substance abuse. Others enter as the result of court action. Either way the nurse is challenged to rapidly develop a therapeutic relationship with the client and assist the client to develop a treatment plan. The nurse's approach is to confront the client in a nonjudgmental manner concerning the physical symptoms caused by the addiction, his responsibility in creating his own situation, and the treatment methods open to the client. Once the client has set realistic goals, the nurse may use therapy sessions to assist the client in finding ways to meet these goals. As the relationship advances the nurse needs to gradually change the role, allowing the client to become more independent. Termination of the therapy is a very important phase. The client needs ample time to work out negative feelings that arise in the termination phase. However, when the client is able to handle the problems a termination date is set and the client assisted in reaching a successful termination of therapy.

NURSING PROCESS
Assessment

Physical dimension. Assessment of the physical dimension consists of determining the client's willingness and ability to perform tasks of daily living. The person with an interdependent coping style has achieved a balance between dependent and independent behavior that is appropriate to the situation. For example, an executive who is hospitalized for a possible myocardial infarction is able to accept the forced dependence and allows others to perform his activities of daily living. He relies on health providers to bathe him, assist him in getting out of bed, and perform whatever other physical care is needed. However, as his condition improves, he performs self-care as appropriate. This client follows the regimen necessary to return to an optimal level of health.

The client who exhibits predominantly maladaptive dependent behavior is reluctant to perform tasks of daily living. Illness, for example, provides an excellent rationalization for being dependent. The nurse observes the hospitalized client for behaviors such as refusing to take his own bath, not feeding himself, and not performing other hygienic care of which he is capable. This individual may actively refuse to care for himself or may passively wait for the nurse or family to provide the care.

Since the dependent client may demonstrate signs of

poor physical health, the nurse assesses the client's total physical appearance and health status. Physical deterioration is more apparent in certain types of maladaptive dependent behavior than in others. An individual dependent on chemical substances may neglect his physical needs as he relies more and more on a chemical substance, such as alcohol or drugs. The nurse may observe inadequate hygiene, inadequate nutrition, inactivity, weight loss, poor skin turgor or muscle tone, and unkempt appearance. Obtaining the chemical substance becomes the person's overriding objective.

The nurse takes a history of the chemical substance the client abuses, and the amount and length of use to assess his degree of dependence. Whether the dependence is psychological or physical depends on the substance used. For example, marijuana produces psychological dependence, whereas alcohol causes psychological and physical dependence. Physical dependence on a substance is referred to as *addiction*. When a person is physically addicted to a substance, he experiences a *withdrawal syndrome* when usage is stopped. Alcohol withdrawal can range from mild to severe, depending on the length of time the person has been drinking and the amount he drank. A mild form of alcohol withdrawal is commonly known as a "hangover." When the individual has been drinking for several hours or longer he may experience withdrawal symptoms shortly after he had the last drink or reduced the amount he drank. When doing an assessment the nurse observes for withdrawal symptoms.

The person may develop an alcohol withdrawal delirium, delirium tremens (DTs). This is a severe syndrome that is a serious threat to the person's life. DTs generally occur within 48 to 72 hours after cessation or reduction in a heavy and consistent intake of alcohol that lasted for a period of several weeks or longer. This response confirms the individual's physical dependence on alcohol. The symptoms the nurse observes include incoherent speech, disturbance in sleep, perceptual disturbance (hallucinations and illusions), agitation, restlessness, increased or decreased psychomotor activity, disorientation, memory impairment, tachycardia, sweating, and elevated blood pressure. This syndrome most often runs its course in 2 to 3 days and typically lasts less than a week.

The client who is experiencing alcohol withdrawal is assessed for convulsions. One early warning sign of the potential for the client to have a convulsion is a tremor of the tongue. Without proper medical management, the convulsion may result in status epilepticus, a life-threatening condition of continuous seizures. Withdrawal from diazepam (Valium) is especially dangerous because of the potential for seizures. The client who is withdrawing from diazepam can, on approximately the seventh day of withdrawal, begin having seizures that can lead to status epilepticus. Withdrawal from diazepam usually involves a tapering off period of weeks.

When assessing a client for withdrawal from other drugs, the nurse will observe withdrawal symptoms similar to those for alcohol withdrawal. Withdrawal from barbiturate-like drugs or hypnotics may result in delirium. Symptoms are the same as alcohol withdrawal delirium.

The nurse assesses the client for evidence of physical abuse, because the individual with maladaptive dependent behavior may accept physical abuse from significant others. The client may have a number of bruises, small burns, or even human bites. When asked about these, the client may ignore the questions or have difficulty in trying to talk about how the marks were incurred. The dependent person may find physical abuse less threatening than the fear of having to rely on himself. (See Chapter 36).

The person with maladaptive dependent behavior has a poor self image, which leads to the firm belief that he is not capable of caring for himself. The individual also has a fear of being alone. These characteristics are often displayed by individuals with personality disorders, such as avoidant personality disorder and dependent personality disorder.

Distortion of an individual's body image may result from maladaptive dependence. A person's body image can be distorted by feelings of low self-esteem, lack of confidence, and helplessness, which are characteristics of a dependent person. Body image is also distorted by the individual who possesses a grandiose sense of self-importance and is vain and self-indulgent, such as an individual with a narcissistic personality disorder.

A characteristic of maladaptive independence is that the person needs to be in control of the external environment. One indicator of this behavior is the performance of tasks that are contraindicated by the person's physical or emotional status. For example, the individual insists on controlling his finances while he is emotionally too unstable to manage them.

Emotional dimension. The emotional dimension of an individual with a maladaptive dependent or independent coping style is characterized by deep-seated feelings of resentment and anger, although the individual may not be aware of these feelings. Anger may be manifested by loud, threatening outbursts, threats of bodily harm to oneself or another, sullen withdrawal, or questions such as "Why did this happen to me?" The client may throw things or refuse medications or other necessary treatments. The dependent client has an underlying anger at himself because of his preceived inability to act and toward others because they help him be dependent and yet they don't do enough for his dependence.

An individual who is extremely dependent may show signs of depression. Occasionally helplessness and suicidal feelings are present. The nurse needs to look for signs and symptoms of depression and suicidal ideation. These feelings are pronounced during and following the detoxification period. (See Chapter 14).

The individual who uses a maladaptive independent coping style has difficulty accepting a dependent role. The client's internal message is "Be in control," but the external message is "You are not in control." Because there is a basic mistrust that anyone else can perform the task, any attempt to compel the client to accept external control is met by angry resistance.

The person who is using chemical substances has either shallow emotions or denies that he has emotions. Often the purpose of substance abuse is to replace painful feelings with the feeling of euphoria. When doing an assessment, the nurse may observe emotional blunting and shallowness, or the client may be hostile and belligerent. Life without the chemical substance often seems impossible, since the substance has been used as a coping method.

❋ *Intellectual dimension.* The individual who functions in an interdependent manner is able to assess situations in a realistic way. Because his perception is not clouded by unmet dependence or independence needs, the person is able to objectively evaluate each situation. When ill, the well-adapted person listens to a health care provider and then decides on a course of action. The person neither blindly accepts the health care provider's word nor immediately rebels against any restrictions. This individual needs to have time to work through the emotional impact of any illness or trauma, whether emotional or physical, before being able to decide which course of action is best.

The intellectual dimension is affected by the degree of maladaptive dependent or independent behavior a person displays. The more severe the maladaptive behavior, the more rigid the client's functioning. The nurse assesses the person's ability to comprehend what is occurring, the knowledge base the person possesses, and the person's ability to analyze the relationships involved. The individual with maladaptive dependent behavior appears to accept any explanation of the problem or condition that the nurse or other authority figures offer.

Lack of appropriate decision making characterizes the intellectual functioning of the person who uses chemical substances. The person does not know how to solve problems and cannot think beyond the moment. Delayed gratification and meeting goals are foreign to the substance user, who must have immediate and complete gratification of his needs. The nurse observes limited impulse control, lack of concentration and insight, and faulty judgment, cognitive skills, and thought processes.

After a period of detoxification, the chemical substance user often still lacks decision-making skills and will show lack of insight, faulty judgment, and limited impulse control; however, not to the same degree as during the intoxication period. Some of these attributes will return commensurate with the person's abilities after the person is free of chemical substances.

Denial is the defense mechanism most frequently used by the dependent person. The dependent person accepts society's belief that one "should" be independent; therefore, the individual uses denial to prevent himself from experiencing anxiety. The person who abuses chemical substances uses denial even more frequently than other dependent people. Part of the denial occurs because society considers chemical substance abuse not only a weakness but a moral disgrace. This makes the role of the nurse extremely difficult, because it is almost impossible to work with a client to change maladaptive behavior when the client denies the existence of the behavior. An alcoholic is a prime example of a person who uses denial in a detrimental manner. Alcoholics firmly believe their drinking is no different from that of anyone else. This attitude

is exemplified by statements such as "I could quit tomorrow if I wanted to," and "Oh! I drink quite a bit, but as soon as things let up at work I'll slow down."

Projection is another frequently used defense mechanism. Projection allows the dependent person to place blame and responsibility on someone else. It demonstrates the person's lack of self-confidence and feelings of helplessness and powerlessness. The use of projection is illustrated by the following statements: "I got drunk because my wife kept pushing me," and "I stole it because my dad said I was a coward. It is his fault."

❋ *Social dimension.* In the United States young children are taught to be competitive and to value independence; children are urged to leave home when they become young adults. These values are not the same in some other cultures. Both the Japanese and Mexican cultures teach children to value interdependence. Families tend to stay close, and several generations may live together.

Awareness of individual and family developmental tasks is also important when assessing dependent and independent behavior. Is the client performing at the correct developmental level for his age and culture? It is usually considered appropriate for the 20-year-old youth to find a job and move away from home. However, this is not considered appropriate for most 14-year-olds. Is the family accomplishing its developmental tasks?

It is in the social dimension that the nurse can most easily assess interdependent coping behavior. The interdependent person is able to function in both social and occupational settings. Some characteristics of interdependent behavior include the development of meaningful relationships, the ability to provide and accept nurturing care, and the maintenance of a good work record. In the occupational setting an interdependent coping style allows the individual to accept authority when it is appropriate and to be the authority when needed. The interdependent person accepts the responsibility for his own actions.

Both maladaptive dependent and maladaptive independent coping styles have many social ramifications for the client and the family. Manipulation of others is a characteristic of both styles.

The person who used chemical substances is often seen as a manipulative and exploitative client. Within the drug culture, manipulation is a way of life. The payoff is in conning others into meeting the person's needs at their own expense. (See Chapter 21). The nurse may find such behaviors from these clients as wanting special favors, wanting to bend the rules, and disregarding rules. Other behaviors such as seduction, helplessness, or interpersonal exploitativeness may be displayed. The manipulative client acts out his feelings rather than stating them verbally.

The client who uses helplessness tells the nurse how well the nurse is able to do things with remarks such as "I wish I were as competent as you," "I don't know how you manage everything so well. I just can't seem to do it," or "I can't seem to do anything by myself. I am so dumb."

The individual with maladaptive dependent behavior

frequently has many social contacts. However, when left alone, even for a short time, this person becomes fearful and anxious. The spouse may miss work often because the dependent individual demands attention. When the client is ill and hospitalized, the family devotes full time to the client. Although there are many visitors, the social contacts do not reassure this individual, and as soon as he is alone, he becomes very demanding of the nursing staff.

The effects of maladaptive dependent behavior on interpersonal relationships depend on the type of behavior and the severity of the maladaption. The behavior can range from suspiciousness and withdrawal from social contacts to overt acting out, such as lying or stealing to get attention. Characteristics to observe include clinging, many acquaintances but no close friends, too much concern for the feelings of others and jealousy. There may be overt acting out, in which the individual engages in verbal or physical violence and aggression. In some cases the violence is self-directed.

The client may have legal problems caused by violent acts, thefts, illegal occupations, failure to honor debts, or reckless driving. These problems often occur in persons with a maladaptive coping style who use chemicals to meet their dependence needs.

Family assessment is essential because of the relatedness of the family dynamics to the emotional problems of the client. The nurse interviews the family to identify the family patterns and investigate how the individual with the identified maladaptive coping style fits in the family dynamics.

The family may reinforce pattern of maladaptive dependence by doing for the client or insisting that the nursing staff do for him what he needs to do for himself. The nurse asks all family members how they see themselves and the other family members contributing to the problem. When talking with more than one member of the family, the nurse can observe the family's interactions with each other, including how they address each other, whether any one person is excluded from the conversation, what tone of voice they use with each other, and the nonverbal messages that are sent. The nurse also needs to find out how the client views each member of the family. The client can describe what role he believes the family plays in the present problem.

Once the family dynamics are identified, the nurse can assess both the client's and the family's perception of the maladaptive dependent behaviors.

Family dynamics also play an important role in the development of the members' self-concepts. Parents who are comfortable with themselves are able to portray this to their children and are also able to accept their children as they are. Through positive acceptance and appraisal from the parent, the children develop positive self-concepts and high self-esteem. The children are then able to make decisions when appropriate and thus experience some independence. Positive interactions with parents throughout the different developmental stages enable an individual to learn adaptive interdependence.

The effects of maladaptive dependent behavior are also demonstrated in social interactions. The degree of social impairment depends on the severity of the dependence needs. The individual who believes his dependence needs cannot be met feels pain; to allay this pain, the individual may go to extreme lengths and display behavior such as whining or being very self-centered. The client tends to exclude the needs of others, and they gradually withdraw. As people withdraw from the client in response to his behavior, the behavior of the client becomes more extreme.

Many persons with personality disorders demonstrate maladaptive dependence. Individuals with avoidant and dependent personality disorders have a need for uncritical acceptance by others. This need greatly interferes with social functioning. The individual's behavior estranges him from his family and other interpersonal relationships. The person then may experience loneliness and may seek excessive attention or he may withdraw completely. The client may ask the nurse, "Why doesn't anyone like me?" or "Why am I always alone?" The client's response to this loneliness includes frequent touching, speaking loudly, asking for unneccessary help, soliciting praise for accomplishments, asking for approval of personal appearance, and other attention-seeking behavior.[7] This type of coping behavior is self-defeating. The client is attempting to meet a basic need that was not met in infancy. The attention the client receives is never enough.

Individuals with chemical dependence, especially alcohol abuse, have the potential for causing family disintegration. (See the Research Highlight on p. 323). The nurse assesses the family dynamics in terms of the effects the client's behavior has on the family as well as the family's needs that are met by his behavior. In the early stages of alcoholism the family may make excuses for the behavior of the alcoholic member. Later they may lie to relatives and friends in an attempt to conceal the problem. On the other hand, the family members may facilitate the alcoholic's drinking by buying alcohol for him or creating and promoting situations that they know lead to increased stress that results in drinking. The family may also use the alcoholic member as a scapegoat by focusing on his problem as the sole cause for the underlying family conflict. The family may become dysfunctional if the alcoholic gets well. However, the family problems increase as the alcoholic's intake increases, and sometimes the family unit dissolves, leaving the alcoholic alone. At other times the family stays together, continuing the same dynamics that perpetuate the problem.

Assessment of the occupational history of the client with maladaptive dependent or independent behavior is important, since the individual may have varying degrees of occupational impairment. The extent of occupational impairment varies with the substance used and the amount of dependence on the substance. Job-related behaviors include increased absenteeism, absence from the job on Mondays, and prolonged breaks. The client who displays maladaptive independence to the extent of disregarding social norms has difficulty in keeping a job. The behaviors that cause the individual to have legal problems also affect occupational functioning. The individual is impulsive, shows litle or no responsibility, is late or does not show up, and often just walks off the job.

Research Highlight

Stability/Instability in the Alcoholic Marriage: The Interrelationship Between the Course of Alcoholism, Family Process, and Marital Outcome

P. Steinglass, L. Tislenko & D. Reiss

PURPOSE

The study was designed to investigate the effect of alcoholism on marital stability and the relationship between family behavior and different types of alcoholism.

SAMPLE

The sample consisted of thirty-one families containing one alcoholic spouse with a 5-year drinking history (the spouse was not necessarily currently drinking) and one nonalcoholic spouse. Both spouses lived at home and were economically self-sufficient. Of the thirty-one alcoholic spouses, twenty-three were men and eight were women. The sample was white, middle-aged, into their second decade of marriage, highly educated, and middle-class or upper middle-class. Many but not all of the families contained children. The alcoholic spouses's history of alcoholism was based on two criteria sets: the Goodwin et al. criteria and the Self-Administered Alcoholism Screening Test (SAAST).

METHODOLOGY

Two sets of data were collected: the initial phase (t_1) and the second phase (t_2). During the initial 6-month phase of data collection, the researcher made observations of family behavior nine times (4-hour sessions each). The families were divided into three groups based on drinking patterns of the alcoholic spouse: stable wet subjects who were actively drinking at the start of the study and continued throughout the 6 months of data collection; stable dry subjects who were dry at the outset and remained so; and alternators who were either actively drinking at the start but were dry when the 6 months had ended or were dry when data collection began and drinking when the study ended.

The second phase of the study was 2-year follow-up and included collection of detailed data about the alcoholic spouse's current drinking and marital status as well as the drinking and treatment history for the 2-year period between t_1 and t_2. The SCL-90 Outpatient Psychiatric Rating Scale questionnaire was used. Home observations were also made.

FINDINGS

Families who converted to dry drinking patterns between t_1 and t_2 had higher levels of intrafamily engagement (physical and verbal contact with each other) than those in which active drinking continued. The stable wet families demonstrated variance in marital stability at t_2, with 50% of the spouses separating.

IMPLICATIONS

With knowledge that alcoholism adversely affects family interaction and marital stability, the nurse can provide family therapy for the family. If the alcoholic spouse denies the need for help, the nurse can begin therapy with other family members. The family members may be referred to self-help groups, Al-Anon and Alcoholics Anonymous, if they are resistant to institutional family therapy.

Based on data from Family Process 24:3, 1985.

The maladaptive dependent individual who is placed in an unstructured work situation has difficulty structuring his work. The person also has difficulty with jobs that require independent decisions. Behaviors that interfere with occupational functioning include procrastination, stubbornness, indecisiveness, impulsiveness, depression, and frequent mood swings. The effect on the individual's ability to work depends on the severity of the maladaptation.

The maladaptive independent individual usually appears to do well alone. The family dynamics are reversed from those of the dependent person's family. Often the family feels left out and not needed. In cases of extreme maladaptive independent coping behavior, the individual feels in total control of the external and internal environment. This interferes with social contacts, family, and occupational functioning.

Spiritual dimension. Interdependence allows the individual to develop spiritually and to continue to strive for his full potential. By definition, interdependence permits one to be dependent on others (including a supreme being) or to be dependent on self. Therefore the individual has the freedom to believe or not to believe in a supreme being or power. The interdependent person does not have an excessive need for *affiliation,* that is, a need to be very closely associated with an organization. Neither does the interdependent person have to feel totally in control of the internal and external environment.

Maladaptive dependent behavior makes it difficult for a person to develop a realistic, meaningful philosophy. The extremely dependent person may avow a belief in a supreme being; however, this belief is colored by the person's internal stimuli, which produces an excessive need for affiliation. These are the same stimuli that influence the person to cling to family and friends. The dependent person does not allow enough self-growth to reach his full potential. He may gravitate to cults because of a need to be told what to do.

Maladaptive independent coping behavior also interferes with needs related to the spiritual dimension. The person has difficulty forming a relatedness to a supreme being or to other people because of a basic mistrust of himself and others. In severe cases the individual may have no respect for the morals and values of others. This individual is not able to attain self-actualization.

MEASUREMENT TOOLS

Several tools have been developed to measure dependence and independence. A checklist using Bellar's 10

TABLE 16-4 Description of a behavioral checklist for dependence and independence for a hospitalized adult client*

Behavior	Example
Dependence subscales	
1. Seeks physical contact	Initates touching behavior
2. Seeks proximity	Draws a chair up close
3. Seeks attention	Speaks to everyone
4. Seeks help	
Physical	Asks for assistance that is not needed
Psychological	Asks for help in making decision
5. Seeks praise	Asks for praise in regard to personal appearance
Independence subscales	
1. Takes initiative	Initiates activity on own
2. Overcomes obstacles	Asks visitors to leave when tired
3. Is persistent	Completes activities of daily living
4. Wants to do something	Walks about unit for exercise
5. Wants to do by oneself	Does routine things without assistance

Adapted from Derdiarian, A, and Clough, D.H., Copyright © 1980. American Journal of Nursing Company. Reproduced with permission from Nursing Research 29:1, 1980.
*This checklist describes specific behaviors in each subscale. The rater lists the frequency of each observed behavior during a specific time period. The items under each component serve as operational definitions. There are a different number of items under each component.

components[6] of dependent and independent behavior was devised to measure, through direct observation, changes in both dependence and independence.[7] The nurse who cares for the client is the observer-rater. Table 16-4 describes this tool.

Another scale that measures dependence and independence is the D-1 Scale (Table 16-5) used by Derdiarian and Clough.[12] This scale is based on Bellar's 10 components[6]; however, it is not confined to a hospital situation. The scale consists of 51 examples of dependent and independent behaviors. The subject rates himself on a scale of 1 to 5. The scale has both validity and reliability.

Analysis

Nursing diagnosis. Powerlessness is a nursing diagnosis approved by NANDA that applies to dependence-independence. The defining characteristics of this nursing diagnosis are listed in the box on p. 325. The following lists provide examples of NANDA-accepted nursing diagnoses with causative statements related to maladaptive dependence and independence:

Related to substance abuse
1. Powerlessness related to dependence on chemical substance
2. Ineffective individual coping related to dependence or denial resulting in inability to manage stressors without chemical substance
3. Impaired social interactions related to behavior while under influence of chemical substance
4. Alteration in family process related to substance use
5. Anxiety related to loss of control secondary to substance use

Related to personality disorders
1. Ineffective individual coping related to maladaptive dependence on others
2. Impaired social interaction related to inability to maintain close relationships with others
3. Ineffective individual coping related to resistance to accepting responsibility for one's own actions

---

TABLE 16-5 Examples from the D-1 Scale*

Behaviors	1	2	3	4	5
1. I put my arm around my friends, pat them on the back, or hold hands while conversing.					
2. I feel comfortable when someone I am close to reaches out to hold my hand or pat me on the back when we are conversing.					
3. I ask my friends or loved ones to stay with me when I am depressed or in pain.					
4. I carry pictures of my family or friends in my wallet and look at the pictures when I am depressed or lonely.					
5. It makes me sad when my friends have to leave, and I will ask them if they can stay a little longer.					
6. I find myself describing my difficulties at length to friends.					
7. I spend time reading about topics that I am interested in.					
8. I can refuse help offered for tasks I can perform myself.					

From American Journal of Nursing Company. Reproduced with permission from Nursing Research 29:1, 1980.
*The scale consists of 51 items denoting dependent or independent behaviors. The subject rates the items on a 1-to-5 scale: *1.* not at all. *2.* occasionally. *3.* moderately; *4.* well; *5.* very well.

4. Ineffective individual coping related to lack of impulse control

For an example of a nursing diagnosis related to alcohol abuse, see the box below. The following Case Example demonstrates the nursing diagnosis powerlessness.

ALCOHOL ABUSE

Powerlessness

DEFINITION

State in which an individual perceives a lack of personal control over events.

DEFINING CHARACTERISTICS

Physical Dimension

Loss of appetite
Restlessness
Agitation
Tremors
Increased intake of chemical substances and tolerance
Lack of participation in care
Delirium
*Tachycardia
*Elevated blood pressure

Emotional Dimension

Apathy
Anger
Resentment
Guilt
Anxiety
Depression
Hostility
*Withdraws emotionally from situation

Intellectual Dimension

Verbal expression of lack of control over situations and outcomes
*Lack of motivation
Unable to seek information regarding care
*Rationalization
Lacks decision-making skills
Doubts own abilities in role performance
Resignation

Social Dimension

Withdraws from friends and co-workers
Fears alienation from co-workers
Acting out and manipulative behavior
Passivity
Violent behavior
*Social isolation
*Aggressive behavior
Lack of self-respect

Spiritual Dimension

*Hopelessness
*Devalues self
*Lack of faith in self

Adapted from North American Nursing Diagnosis Association Classification of Nursing Diagnosis: Proceedings of the seventh conference, St. Louis, 1987, The C.V. Mosby Co.

*Indicates characteristics in addition to those defined by NANDA.

Case Example

Paul, age 52, is an executive in a high-technology firm. He has been employed there for 26 years. Just recently the firm merged with an out-of-state firm. All the decisions are passed from headquarters without consulting anyone in the local office. Paul is a high achiever and had been in a control situation for over 10 years. He now has a feeling of powerlessness. His opinion is no longer important. Although he has drunk alcohol on social occasions since college, he always felt he was in control of his drinking. As his feelings of powerlessness have increased, so has his drinking. It has now reached a point where he is frequently late for work or misses work altogether.

DSM-III-R diagnoses. The DSM-III-R diagnoses related to maladaptive dependent or independent functioning are listed in the box on p. 326.

The essential features and manifestations of the features of dependent personality disorder, alcohol abuse, cocaine abuse, and alcohol withdrawal, according to the DSM-III-R, are listed in the boxes on p. 327.

Classification as a *substance use disorder* requires that there be behavioral changes, regular use of the substance, and effects of the substance on the central nervous system. Use is categorized into two groups: *substance abuse* and *substance dependence* (see the box below). Substance abuse has three characteristics: a pattern of pathological use, interference with social or occupational functioning, and duration of pathological use of 1 month or more. Use is considered pathological when there is intoxication throughout the day, inability to stop use, use of the substance even when contraindicated by serious physical disorder, daily need of the substance for functioning, and repeated medical complications from use.

Substance dependence is more severe than substance abuse. An individual who is substance dependent exhibits physiological dependence; that is, the person either develops a tolerance for the drug or has withdrawal symptoms when the drug is not taken. *Tolerance* occurs when the individual must take increasing amounts of the substance to achieve the desired effect. *Withdrawal* occurs when the individual shows specific physical symptoms when the substance intake is reduced or ceased.

Text continued on p. 330.

CHARACTERISTICS OF SUBSTANCE ABUSE AND SUBSTANCE DEPENDENCE

SUBSTANCE ABUSE

Pattern of pathological use
Interference with social or occupational functioning
Duration of pathological use of 1 month or more

SUBSTANCE DEPENDENCE

Exhibits physiological dependence
Develops tolerance (must take increasing amounts of substance to achieve desired effect)
Develops withdrawal (shows specific physical symptoms when substance intake is reduced or ceased)

DSM-III-R CLASSIFICATIONS RELATED TO DEPENDENCE AND INDEPENDENCE

PERSONALITY DISORDERS

301.50	Histrionic
301.89	Atypical, mixed or other personality disorder
301.83	Borderline
301.82	Avoidant
301.60	Dependent

SUBSTANCE USE DISORDERS

Substance Abuse

305.0x	Alcohol
305.4x	Barbiturate or similarly acting sedative or hypnotic
305.5x	Opioid
305.6x	Cocaine
305.7x	Amphetamine or similarly acting sympathomimetic
305.9x	Phencyclidine or similarly acting arylcyclohexylamine
305.3x	Hallucinogen
305.2x	Cannabis
305.9x	Other, mixed, or unspecified substance

Substance Dependence

304.9x	Alcohol
304.1x	Barbiturate or similarly acting sedative or hypnotic
304.0x	Opioid
304.4x	Amphetamine or similarly acting sympathomimetic
304.3x	Cannabis
305.1x	Tobacco
304.6x	Other specified substance
304.9x	Unspecified substance
304.7x	Combination of opioid and other nonalcoholic substances
304.8x	Combination of substances, excluding opioids and alcohol

PSYCHOACTIVE SUBSTANCE-INDUCED ORGANIC MENTAL DISORDERS (123)

Alcohol

303.00	Intoxication (127)
291.40	Idiosyncratic intoxication (128)
291.80	Uncomplicated alcohol withdrawal (129)
291.00	Withdrawal delirium (131)
291.30	Hallucinosis (131)
291.10	Amnestic disorder (133)
291.20	Dementia associated with alcoholism (133)

Amphetamine or Similarly Acting Sympathomimetic

305.70	Intoxication (134)
292.00	Withdrawal (136)
292.81	Delirium (136)
292.11	Delusional disorder (137)

Caffeine

305.90	Intoxication (138)

Cannabis

305.20	Intoxication (139)
292.11	Delusional disorder (140)

Cocaine

305.60	Intoxication (141)
292.00	Withdrawal (142)
292.81	Delirium (143)
292.11	Delusional disorder (143)

Hallucinogen

305.30	Hallucinosis (144)
292.11	Delusional disorder (146)
292.84	Mood disorder (146)
292.89	Posthallucinogen perception disorder (147)

Inhalant

305.90	Intoxication (148)

Nicotine

292.00	Withdrawal (150)

Opioid

305.50	Intoxication (151)
292.00	Withdrawal (152)

Phencyclidine (PCP) or Similarly Acting Arylcyclohexylamine

305.90	Intoxication (154)
292.81	Delirium (155)
292.11	Delusional disorder (156)
292.84	Mood disorder (156)
292.90	Organic mental disorder NOS

Sedative, Hypnotic, or Anxiolytic

305.40	Intoxication (158)
292.00	Uncomplicated sedative, hypnotic, or anxiolytic withdrawal (159)
292.00	Withdrawal delirium (160)
292.83	Amnestic disorder (161)

Other or Unspecified Psychoactive Substance (162)

305.90	Intoxication
292.00	Withdrawal
292.81	Delirium
292.82	Dementia
292.83	Amnestic disorder
292.11	Delusional disorder
292.12	Hallucinosis
292.84	Mood disorder
292.89	Anxiety disorder
292.89	Personality disorder
292.90	Organic mental disorder NOS

PSYCHOACTIVE SUBSTANCE USE DISORDERS (165)

Alcohol (173)

303.90	Dependence
305.00	Abuse

Amphetamine or Similarly Acting Sympathomimetic (175)

304.40	Dependence
305.70	Abuse

Cannabis (176)

304.30	Dependence
305.20	Abuse

Cocaine (177)

304.20	Dependence
305.60	Abuse

Hallucinogen (179)

304.50	Dependence
305.30	Abuse

Inhalant (180)

304.60	Dependence
305.90	Abuse

Nicotine (181)

305.10	Dependence

Opioid (182)

304.00	Dependence
305.50	Abuse

Phencyclidine (PCP) or Similarly Acting Arylcyclohexylamine (183)

304.50	Dependence
305.90	Abuse

Sedative, Hypnotic, or Anxiolytic (184)

304.10	Dependence
305.40	Abuse
304.90	Polysubstance dependence (185)
304.90	Psychoactive substance dependence NOS
305.90	Psychoactive substance abuse NOS

From American Psychiatric Association: Diagnostic and statistical manual of mental disorders (DSM-III-R), Washington, D.C., 1987, The Association.

301.60 DEPENDENT PERSONALITY DISORDER

ESSENTIAL FEATURES

A disorder in which the individual passively allows others to assume responsibility for major areas of his life because of lack of confidence and inability to function independently.

MANIFESTATIONS

Physical Dimension

Tolerates physical abuse

Emotional Dimension

Experiences intense discomfort when alone for more than a brief period

Intellectual Dimension

Leaves major decisions to others
Preoccupied with being abandoned

Social Dimension

Social relations limited to a few on whom dependent
Makes no demands on people they depend on
Belittles abilities and assets
Views self as stupid
Impaired occupational function in job that requires independence

Adapted from American Psychiatric Association: Diagnostic and statistical manual of mental disorders (DSM-III-R), Washington, D.C., 1987, The Association.

305.6X COCAINE ABUSE

ESSENTIAL FEATURES

A pathological pattern of use of cocaine for at least 1 month that causes impairment in social and occupational functioning.

MANIFESTATIONS

Intellectual Dimension

Paranoid ideation
Ritualistic behavior occurs late in course
Suspicion of abuse of cocaine
Inability to reduce or stop use
Hallucinations
Delusions

Emotional Dimension

Depression

Social Dimension

Fights
Loss of friends
Absence from work
Loss of job
Legal difficulties

Adapted from American Psychiatric Association: Diagnostic and statistical manual of mental disorders (DSM-III-R), Washington, D.C., 1987, The Association.

305.X ALCOHOL ABUSE

ESSENTIAL FEATURES

A pattern of pathological use of alcohol for at least a month that causes impairment in social or occupational functioning.

MANIFESTATIONS

Physical Dimension

Need for daily intake of alcohol
Continuous drinking despite serious physical disorder

Intellectual Dimension

Repeated efforts to control or reduce excessive drinking

Social Dimension

Absence from work
Loss of job
Legal difficulties: traffic accidents while intoxicated
Arguments or difficulties with family or friends because of excessive drinking

Adapted from American Psychiatric Association: Diagnostic and statistical manual of mental disorders (DSM-III-R), Washington, D.C., 1987, The Association.

291.80 ALCOHOL WITHDRAWAL

ESSENTIAL FEATURES

Cessation of or reduction in prolonged ingestion of alcohol followed within several hours by the manifestations listed below.

MANIFESTATIONS

Physical Dimension

Coarse tremors of hands, tongue, and eyelids
Nausea and vomiting
Malaise or weakness
Sweating
Tachycardia
Elevated blood pressure
Orthostatic hypotension

Emotional Dimension

Anxiety
Depressed mood
Irritability

Adapted from American Psychiatric Association: Diagnostic and statistical manual of mental disorders (DSM-III-R), Washington, D.C., 1987, The Association.

TABLE 16-6 Characteristics of commonly abused drugs

Drugs	Physical Dependence	Psychological Dependence	Tolerance	Effects	Effects of Overdose	Withdrawal Symptoms

Narcotics
Heroin
Morphine
Codeine
	High	High	Yes	Physical
				    Decreased response
				        to pain
				    Nausea
				    Constricted pupils
				    Drowsiness
				Psychological
				    Euphoria, "high"
				    Apathy
				    Detachment from
				        reality
				    Impaired judgment
				    Addiction
					Physical
					    Slow and shallow
					        breathing
					    Clammy skin
					    Convulsions
					    Coma
					    Possible death
						Physical
						    Watery eyes
						    Running nose
						    Yawning
						    Loss of appetite
						    Tremors
						    Chills and sweat-
						        ing
						    Cramps
						    Nausea
						Psychological
						    Irritability
						    Panic

Stimulants
Amphetamines
Cocaine
	High	High	Yes	Physical
				    Extra energy
				    Increased alertness
				    Increased cardiac ac-
				        tivity
				    Seizures
				    Respiratory distress
				Psychological
				    Euphoria
				    Aphrodisiacs; "sex
				        pot" drug
				    Paranoia
				    Addiction
					Physical
					    Increase in body
					        temperature
					    Convulsions
					    Possible death
					
					Psychological
					    Agitation
					    Hallucination
						Physical
						    Apathy
						    Long periods of
						        sleep
						
						Psychological
						    Irritability
						    Depression
						    Disorientation

Depressants
Barbiturates
Sedatives
	High	High	Yes	Physical
				    Slurred speech
				    Unsteady gait
				
				Psychological
				    Eurphoria then
				        depression
				    Hostility
				    Decreased inhibitions
				    Impaired judgment
				    Lack of concentra-
				        tion
				    Addiction
					Physical
					    Shallow respira-
					        tion
					    Cold and clammy
					        skin
					    Dilated pupils
					    Weak and rapid
					        pulse
					    Coma
					    Possible death
						Physical
						    Insomnia
						    Tremors
						    Convulsions
						    Possible death
						
						Psychological
						    Anxiety
						    Delirium

Hallucinogens
LSD
	None	High	Yes	Physical (LSD)
				    Self-destructive be-
				        havior
				Psychological
				    Changes in thinking,
				        perception, emo-
				        tional arousal
				    Increased sensory ex-
				        periences
					Physical (LSD)
					    Possible death
					
					Psychological
					    Longer, more in-
					        tense "trips"
					    Psychosis
						Not reported

TABLE 16-6 Characteristics of commonly abused drugs—cont'd

Drugs	Physical Dependence	Psychological Dependence	Tolerance	Effects	Effects of Overdose	Withdrawal Symptoms
Hallucinogens— cont'd				Time perception is slowed down Illusions Hallucinations Changes in self-image Flashbacks Synesthesias		
PCP				Physical (PCP) Hypertension Muscular rigidity Sweating Nystagmus Decreased pain response Nausea Vomiting Seizures Coma Self-destructive behavior Agitation Violence Antisocial behavior Psychological Precipitates a psychosis		
Marijuana	Moderate	Moderate	Yes	Physical Impairs sensory integrity (alters time perception) Decreased energy Reflexes slowed down Dry mucus membranes Red eyes Pulmonary changes Possible sterility Psychological Euphoria Reduces inhibitions Impairs cognition Learning Thinking Memory Comprehension Apathy Loss of motivation "Hang loose" lifestyle Impaired scholastic, academic activities Illusion Hallucinations Addiction	Physical Fatigue Psychological Paranoia Possible psychosis	Physical Insomnia Hyperactivity Decreased appetite occasionally reported

TABLE 16-7 Long-term and short-term goals and outcome criteria related to dependence-independence

Goals	Outcome Criteria

NURSING DIAGNOSIS: INEFFECTIVE INDIVIDUAL COPING: DEPENDENCE RELATED TO INABILITY TO CONSTRUCTIVELY MANAGE STRESSORS WITHOUT ALCOHOL

Long-term goal

To develop coping mechanisms other than alcohol to deal with daily stresses	Discusses how he uses alcohol Discusses lifestyle without alcohol Has a contact with Alcoholics Anonymous (AA) Has tried out at least one alternative coping mechanism

Short-term goals

To socialize effectively without alcohol	Structures social activities that do not include alcohol Participates in leisure activities without using alcohol
To accept the support of others	Attends AA meetings Discusses how others can help him live without alcohol Communicates with family about problem

NURSING DIAGNOSIS: IMPAIRED SOCIAL INTERACTION RELATED TO MANIPULATION OF OTHERS

Long-term goal

To form positive relationships without using manipulation	Identifies own manipulative behavior States how the behavior can be modified Discusses manipulative behavior with family Asks directly for needs to be met

Short-term goal

To accept responsibility for manipulative behavior	Verbalizes feelings concerning behavior Verbalizes awareness of other's feelings Accepts limits set on the behavior Accepts consequences of noncompliance

Five classes of substances produce both abuse and dependence: narcotics, stimulants, depressants, hallucinogens, and marijuana. Commonly abused drugs and their physical and psychological responses are listed in Table 16-6.

Planning

Table 16-7 provides long-term goals, short-terms goals, and outcome criteria for nursing diagnoses related to dependent-independent behavior. These serve as examples of the planning stage in the nursing process.

Implementation

Physical dimension. Once the nurse has ascertained the physicial abilities of the client, the nurse works with the client to develop a plan stating (1) the activities of daily living the client can execute independently, (2) the activities with which the client needs assistance, and (3) the activities that the nurse needs to perform for the client. The nurse may use positive reinforcement when the client demonstrates initiative in performing the activities of daily living as outlined. The positive reinforcement can consist of simply praising the client for doing the tasks or, for hospitalized clients, of allowing the client extra privileges, such as a walk or other types of recreation. The nurse also uses the therapeutic relationship to work with the client who has difficulty either in taking initiative in doing these activities or

in staying within the established limitations. Treatment of toxic reaction is based on detoxification. *Detoxification* is the process of withdrawal from alcohol occurring in a controlled environment. It is the first step in the process of rehabilitation. Detoxification can be a threat to the person's physical existence, so effective intervention is essential. Maintaining the client's physical needs for fluid and food is especially important during withdrawal from alcohol. Fluids need to be forced to a daily intake of at least 2500 ml., and as soon as possible, the client is encouraged to eat. The nurse can provide him with foods he prefers in small, frequent feedings. Snacks that are high in protein and calories may also be used to meet the client's nutritional needs.

Careful supervision of the client during the detoxification process is necessary to protect him from physical injury. Siderails may need to be used for the client's physical safety. Mechanical restraints are not used because of the possibility of injury.

The nurse administers the client's medication as prescribed to control symptoms. Addictive substances are not left within the client's reach, nor any medication with an alcohol base that he may use to meet his craving for alcohol, such as shaving lotion and cough syrup. The distinct and overlapping stages of alcohol withdrawal are described in Table 16-8.

The client experiencing withdrawal delirium needs constant reassurance in a firm, positive way to allay his fear. If the client "sees" spiders crawling on him, he needs to be assured that there are none. The nurse conveys her

TABLE 16-8 Stages of withdrawal syndrome

Stage I	Psychomotor agitation, tremors, hyperactivity, hypertension, tachycardia, diaphoresis, anorexia, insomnia, and illusions. This stage is usually self-limiting and lasts from a few hours to one to two days.
Stage II	Stage II consists of stage I symptoms plus hallucinations: auditory, visual, tactile and olfactory (rare), and paranoid ideation and behavior. The hallucinations may be transient and intermittent.
Stage III	This stage is called delirium tremens. Stage III consists of stage I and stage II symptoms with the addition of disorientation, delusions, and delirium. There may be seizure activity. There is an increased incidence of death at this stage.

Adpated from Knott, D.H., Fink, R.D., and Morgan, J.C.: Intoxication and the alcohol abstinence syndrome. In Schwartz, G.R., and others, editors: Principles and practice of emergency medicine, Philadelphia, 1978, W.B. Saunders Co.

understanding of the client's feelings. She clearly communicate his fears and apprehensions as well as the treatment plan to others who care for him.

Once the client has discontinued his use of a chemical substance, the nurse needs to assist him to recognize and discuss that life without the substance is a major loss. The nurse's intervention needs to be directed toward helping the client grieve the loss of a significant aspect of his lifestyle (see Chapter 14).

❋ *Emotional dimension.* Since a characteristic of dependent behavior is allowing the significant other to physically or psychologically abuse them, the nurse needs to recognize signs of abuse and implement plans to change this behavior (see Chapter 36).

Anger is often an underlying emotion of the dependent person. Once anger is identified, the nurse works with the client to express it using some of the interventions discussed in Chapter 12. One method for dealing with anger is to learn how to be assertive. *Assertiveness* is the ability to express one's needs and desires directly to the appropriate person in an appropriate manner. Assertiveness, as opposed to aggressiveness, does not rely on sarcasm or belittling of others. It involves assuming responsibility for one's self and one's emotions and not projecting these onto another individual. At the same time, the assertive person does not allow others to belittle him, nor does he accept responsibility for the other's behavior or emotions. Assertive behavior is difficult for the dependent individual to learn. An example of assertive behavior occurs when an alcoholic accuses his wife of being responsible for his drinking, and she informs him that it is he, and not she, who is responsible for his behavior. The nurse needs to work with the client to implement assertive behavior. Frequently in developing assertiveness the client displays aggression. It is important for the nurse to point out the difference in the two behaviors.

Assertiveness training is one method for reducing passive and aggressive behavior and increasing assertive behavior. Assertiveness training is communication skill train-

ing designed to promote more effective behaviors with respect to (1) firm, direct presentation of self, (2) active work orientation, (3) constructive work habits, (4) effectiveness in giving and taking criticism, (5) better control of anxiety or fear, and (6) satisfaction with performance.[9]

Assertiveness training typically involves people in a series of sessions in which various aspects of problematic situations are addressed. Such problems may include management of aggression, speaking effectively, identification of intimidating factors, and stress management. The specific arrangement of content and sessions varies considerably, but these programs consistently emphasize the development of new behaviors that express assertiveness. These programs typically limit training to a number of weeks or a few months at most. Learning assertiveness in a short-term program can create significant problems in day-to-day living.

When a client unexpectedly and abruptly becomes assertive in a situation in which he formerly was relatively passive, the new behavior often evokes anger rather than praise. Others have become comfortable with the person's lack of assertiveness, and the new behavior evokes punishment rather than reward.

A second potential consequence of assertiveness training can occur. If the client's personality pattern and organization of defenses are dependent on the use of a passive stance, the seemingly simple change to more assertive behaviors is likely to produce unexpected and intense anxiety and uncertainty.

For the healthy person, assertiveness training may be another useful method for positive changes in behavior. (See the Research Highlight on p. 332.) However, for the person with subtle serious underlying mental health difficulties, in whom passivity is an integral part of the personality, the risk is significant and the training is ideally undertaken only as a complement to ongoing counseling or psychotherapy.

❋ *Intellectual dimension.* To help the client develop an interdependent coping style, the nurse encourages the client to generate solutions for his problems. She assists the client in working out solutions by having him identify a simple problem and set easy, short-term goals to reach a solution. An example of this is a client who does not take care of his own hygiene. The nurse has the client identify the aspect of hygiene that would be easiest for him to initiate himself. The client then sets a short-term goal, such as "I will comb my hair by 9 AM daily without being reminded to do so." The nurse compliments the client when he initiates the action on his own. The nurse thus can assist the client in making decisions that are sound and setting goals that he can accomplish. A positive approach is used, involving the client without the client having the entire pressure of making a decision. The environment can be structured so that the client can succeed in establishing and reaching goals.

Since denial is a defense mechanism used by the person with dependent behavior, especially the one who abuses chemical substances, sound nursing judgment is essential. The nurse does not attempt to force the client through the denial stage. It is important to consider the importance of the denial mechanism to the client and to

Research Highlight

The Effects of Assertiveness Training on Older Adults

A. W. Franzke

PURPOSE

The purpose of this study was to determine whether assertiveness training is an effective intervention method for improving the quality of life for older adults.

SAMPLE

Eighty-four people (thirty males and fifty-four females) over 65 years of age living in the San Antonio, Texas area made up the sample. Forty-two people rated as upper class and were members of the American Association of Retired Persons (AARP). Forty-two were lower or lower middle class people from a nutrition center for the elderly. There were 21 people in each experimental and control group. The AARP people in the sample were volunteers obtained at a national meeting by the researcher's offering a free assertiveness training class. The participants from the nutrition center were a convenience sample. Participants were chosen for the experimental and control groups after rating by the researcher on the Shevy and Bell Constructs of Social Rank allowed control for socioeconomic status. The participants were rated by preretirement occupation and educational level. The occupation of the husband was used for women who had not been employed outside the home.

METHODOLOGY

The experimental group was given a 6-week course in assertiveness training by the researcher; the control group was not given the training. Both groups were given pretests and posttests. Two self-report scales were administered: the Assertiveness Inventory and the Burger Scale for Expressed Acceptance of Self. For the assertiveness training, the experimental group was divided into four groups: two groups of AARP members and two groups from the nutrition center. The researcher taught six classes for all the groups.

FINDINGS

The findings indicated that the assertiveness training had a significant effect on scores for assertiveness and self-concept. The upper class experimental and control group (AARP) reported a more significant increase in positive self-concept than the lower classes (nutrition group). The difference between the pretest and posttest was significant for both groups on the assertiveness measure. Differences resulting from sex were not significant.

IMPLICATIONS

The results of this study suggest that nurses working with older clients can assist them to achieve a more productive and satisying life by using an assertiveness training course as an intervention method. The clients can learn and apply the assertiveness skills at a significant level.

Based on data from The Gerontologist **27**:13, 1987.

explore the fears and anxieties underlying the denial. For instance, the person who abuses the substance is more apt to be receptive to dealing with the problem when in a physical or emotional crisis. During this time denial is less pronounced, and the client is more willing to accept that there is a problem and something needs to be done about it. The nurse can now help the individual verbalize his feelings and perception of his problem. With verbalization, anxiety subsides, and denial may not be necessary.

Instead of confronting the client about a drinking problem, the nurse may need to approach the situation by assisting the client to identify behaviors displayed while drinking. Once the client identifies the behaviors, the nurse can confront the client about the result of these behaviors. What is the impact on the client, the family, the client's job? While exploring these behaviors and their overall impact, the reality of drinking as a problem may come to the client's conscious attention. Once this occurs, the client is able to begin accepting the treatment regimen. The family of the alcoholic also uses denial and needs to be worked with to accept the reality of the situation and to help change it.

The individual with a maladaptive independent coping style also uses denial to a degree that is detrimental to optimal health. In some cases, such as a diabetic client or a client with a severe myocardial infarction, denial can be life threatening. Because denial is usually based on a need to be independent, the nurse assists the client in identifying dependent behaviors that are comfortable and those that are uncomfortable. She assists him to accept comfortable dependent situations. She also allows the client as much control of the external environment as possible. For example, the client can make decisions such as when he will bathe or when his appointment with the nurse will be. The nurse needs to reinforce behaviors that indicate an acceptance of the reality of dependent situations.

The nurse points out to the user of chemical substances his responsibility in creating his situation. In conversations with the nurse, clients are not allowed to place the blame elsewhere and must acknowledge their hand in creating their problems. The nurse will often encounter resistance to this process. Setting limits is another useful technique. Through the use of rules and regulations, clients learn to follow guidelines and accept consequences for their behavior. This forces the client to give up manipulative behavior and to be responsible for his actions.

The individual with a dependent life-style, whether dependent on people or chemical substances, needs to learn decision-making skills. The client is taught how to make small decisions and is supported throughout the process. First, the client is taught to specify the problem and to gather data about it. Second, the client is taught to propose alternatives. Next, the client discusses the pros and cons of the alternatives and selects one. The client then applies the alternative and evaluates the result. By practicing these steps and receiving increasingly harder decisions to make, the client can learn how to make decisions for himself unaided. Support from the nurse is essential in teaching the client how to problem-solve throughout the process.

Social dimension. As the nurse begins the relationship with the client whose dependence is maladaptive, she meets his dependency needs, and then gradually she assists him to do more for himself. The guidance to increased self-care conveys recognition of the client as a responsible person. However, from the outset of the relationship, the nurse sets limits on the amount and type of dependent behavior that will be tolerated and clearly communicates these to the client.

The nurse can help the client feel more in control of the situation and less dependent by anticipating his dependency needs. Early in the relationship this approach helps to develop a trusting relationship. Assisting the client in identifying ways he expresses his dependence as well as sources of the dependent behaviors is helpful. As he becomes aware of the dependent behavior, he needs support to move toward greater independence. In the process of moving toward the goal of interdependence, the client may demonstrate exaggerated independent behavior. The nurse accepts this behavior and discusses possible motivations of the behavior with the client.

Behavior modification may be used for intervention in the client's attention-seeking behavior. Positive reinforcement involves giving consistent, positive rewards for identified desirable behavior. The nurse clearly communicates to the client and the health team members what is desirable behavior. She may positively reinforce the client's behavior by giving him attention at times other than when he asks for something. She praises him when he does not engage in the attention-seeking behavior. Negative reinforcement is achieved by consistently ignoring behavior that is clearly identified as undesirable. To implement this approach, the nurse ignores the client's attention-seeking behavior.

When the client uses excessive attention-seeking behaviors, the nurse also confronts the client about the behaviors and assists him in identifying them. The client is encouraged to talk about the feelings evoked by the behaviors. The nurse assists the client in identifying and establishing mature types of behavior to meet his needs. For example, the nurse can explore with the client independent or interdependent behaviors that can replace the negative attention-seeking behaviors. She helps the client identify behaviors that are somewhat comfortable for him and then sets stages for initiating this behavior. The client may start doing the comfortable behavior once a day and then increase it in small increments until the behavior is spontaneous. As the client changes to more interdependent behavior, the nurse gives the client positive reinforcement by praising him for displaying more adaptive behavior.

Maladaptive dependent behavior can lead to low self-esteem, resulting in numerous problems such as loneliness and allowing oneself to be physically and psychologically abused. The nurse uses a nonjudgmental approach, accepting the client's positive and negative attributes. The nurse can work with the client to set attainable goals so that the client can achieve greater self-esteem. The nurse approaches the client in a consistent, accepting manner, thus indicating to the client that she considers him a person of value. The first step in treatment of the abused client is to find out if the client recognizes the abusive treatment as such. The nurse can ask questions such as "Who abuses you?" "When does it occur?" and "What are your feelings about the abuse?" Developing increased self-esteem and encouraging the expression of feeling allows the abused client to recognize the abuse and the feelings generated. (See Chapter 36 for further discussion of abuse.)

Many individuals with a maladaptive dependent coping style engage in manipulative behavior. Individuals with personality disorders and substance abuse disorders are especially prone to display manipulative behavior. It is of foremost importance that the nurse identify and set limits on the manipulative behavior; otherwise the behavior may be inadvertently reinforced. (See Chapter 21).

The client with maladaptive dependence frequently feels lonely and needs to develop an interdependent coping style. The nurse may assist the client by first arranging to spend time with the client. It may be necessary to just sit with him. Once a therapeutic relationship with the nurse is established, the client may talk about his feelings of loneliness. The nurse then helps the client balance his needs for dependence with his needs for independence. As the client's maladaptive dependent behavior decreases and he is able to take initiative, the nurse explores ways of increasing contact with others. The nurse works with the client to identify the behaviors that result in loneliness and to adapt these behaviors to a more socially acceptable mode (see Chapter 19).

Because the individual's maladaptive behaviors occur within the family, knowledge about how the family interacts is needed for successful treatment of the individual. Some alcoholic treatment centers use family intervention and milieu therapy, which involves the family in a family group night. Community mental health agencies are also used to work with the family. To ensure continuity of care, the community mental health nurse and the hospital-based nurse maintain open communication. It is essential that all involved personnel from different agencies work together and communicate.

Alcoholics Anonymous (AA) is the primary and most successful resource for rehabilitation of alcoholic clients.

THE TWELVE STEPS OF ALCOHOLICS ANONYMOUS

1. We admitted we were powerless over alcohol—that our lives had become unmanageable.
2. Came to believe that a Power greater than ourselves could restore us to sanity.
3. Made a decision to turn our will and our lives over to the care of God *as we understood Him.*
4. Made a searching and fearless moral inventory of ourselves.
5. Admitted to God, to ourselves, and to another human being the exact nature of our wrongs.
6. Were entirely ready to have God remove all these defects of character.
7. Humbly asked Him to remove our shortcomings.
8. Made a list of all persons we had harmed and became willing to make amends to them all.
9. Made direct amends to such people wherever possible, except when to do so would injure them or others.
10. Continued to take a personal inventory and when we were wrong promptly admitted it.
11. Sought through prayer and meditation to improve our conscious contact with God *as we understood Him,* praying only for knowledge of His will for us and the power to carry that out.
12. Having had a spiritual awakening as a result of these steps, we tried to carry this message to alcoholics and to practice these principles in all our affairs.

From Alcoholics Anonymous: The story of how many thousands of men and women have recovered from alcoholism, ed. 2, New York, 1955, Alcoholics Anonymous World Services, Inc.

The aim of AA is day-by-day sobriety through total abstinence. The person learns that he can have a satisying life free from alcohol. AA emphasizes the spiritual dependence of the individual in The Twelve Steps of Alcoholics Anonymous listed in the box above. These twelve steps ideally lead to recovery. The membership of AA is composed entirely of former alcoholics and recovering alcoholics. Membership is open to the person who admits that he is an alcoholic and wants to quit drinking. Members are expected to attend weekly meetings. Genuine fellowship, support, and encouragement exist among the members. They are available to one another for crises on a 24-hour basis.

Al-anon is a self-help group for the spouse, adult relatives, and close friends of alcoholics that is based on the principles of AA. The purposes of Al-anon are (1) to learn about alcoholism as an illness and (2) to facilitate discussion and resolution of common problems related to being closely associated with an alcoholic. Family members and friends receive insights as to the roles they play in relation to the behavior of the client, emotional support, and understanding.

Alateen is an organization for individuals 12 to 20 years of age in the family of a person with alcoholism. This organization provides a group in which the participants can (1) discuss stressors in the family that affect them, (2) learn coping skills, and (3) gain support and encouragement from peers.

Synanon and *Narcotics Anonymous* (NA), organizations similiar to AA, are for drug-dependent individuals. Synanon is an encounter group run by ex-addicts. NA is similiar to Synanon, but its confrontation is less severe. Various other groups have been organized using the AA format. Some of the groups also include family members.

The nurse is not usually involved with client legal problems that may result from chemical abuse. However, the nurse can explore the client's perception of the legal problem. What does the client see as the cause of the problem? The nurse can point out behaviors that have resulted in the legal problem and then explore with the client his responsiblity for his problem.

Occupational impairment frequently occurs as a result of maladaptive dependent or independent coping behavior. The nurse assists the client in realistically assessing personal capabilities and limitations by having the client list both strengths and weaknesses. The nurse can point out strengths and weaknesses that the client overlooks. The nurse can also refer the client for job or educational counseling.

Spiritual dimension. To help the client meet his spiritual needs, the nurse needs to encourage the client to discuss his beliefs and values, to explore his own philosophy of life, and to identify whether his maladaptive dependent or independent coping has led him to develop values that are interfering with treatment. The nurse may need to encourage the client to seek spiritual guidance of his own choice.

INTERACTION WITH A CLIENT WHO ABUSES ALCOHOL

Client: Well, I have been drinking again. It was John's fault. He made me so mad yesterday that I got more and more anxious. I had to drink. (Tone angry and hostile. Leaning toward nurse.)

Nurse: Sit down, Jim, and tell me what happened.

Client: (Sitting down, relates what occurred and concludes by saying,) See, I was so anxious I had to drink. (Sounding more relaxed.)

Nurse: I can understand your anger at John. (Leaning toward client.) Jim, do you remember the last time you got drunk? Tell me about it.

Client: (Relates that the last time he got drunk was when he got a ticket for speeding, and the police officer treated him like a child.) And I got real mad then. I wasn't breaking any laws. He had no reason to pick me up.

Nurse: Jim, do you see any similiarity between the two occasions? It seems that you allow your anger to get out of control. As you become more anxious you drink to relieve the anxiety. However, the result seems to lead you further into trouble and more anxiety. You may get angry at other people's behavior, but you cannot change their behavior. However, you can assume responsibility for your behavior.

Client: Yes, we have discussed my responsibility before. I can talk about it now, but when someone makes me angry I forget.

Nurse: Tell the person that you are angry and your reason. Confront him before your anger gets out of control and before your anxiety builds up.

Client: OK. Let's role play again, and maybe next time I'll remember.

Nurse: Let's make that, "I will remember."

The client arrives in a hostile state so the nurse has him relate what happened and his feelings. As he calms down the nurse has him recall a previous occasion of drinking and how it was similiar to the present event.

While the nurse needs to listen to the client and encourage expression of feeling, it is also important to confront an alcoholic with his behavior and teach methods such as assertiveness for dealing with anger and anxiety. This client has previously been taught assertiveness, and the nurse reiterates the need for him to own his responsibility and confront others appropriately.

Evaluation

Treatment is considered successful when the client recognizes the maladaptive ways he expresses his dependency needs and comfortably alternates between being dependent, independent, and interdependent. The individual who abuses substances shows success as he begins attending the appropriate self-help group, admits his dependence on the chemical substance, and has developed new behaviors for meeting his needs.

NURSING PROCESS SUMMARY: DEPENDENT BEHAVIOR

ASSESSMENT

Physical Dimension

Refusal to perform self-care
Substance abuse
Physical abuse
Poor general health
Poor body image

Emotional Dimension

Mistrust
Anger
Resentment
Helplessness
Lack of confidence

Intellectual Dimension

Rigid thinking
Inability to make decision
Acceptance of explanations from anyone
Denial
Rationalization

Social Dimension

Attention seeking behavior
Low self-esteem
Mistrust
Loneliness
Negative self-concept
Many social contacts, few close friends
Manipulation
Demanding behavior
Exploitation
Absenteeism from work
Family patterns and coping styles that reinforce dependent behavior

Legal problems
Excessive need for affiliation with others

Spiritual Dimension

Limited inner freedom and creativity
Limited self-growth
Abdication of responsibility for future to God

ANALYSIS

Refer to nursing diagnosis section, pp. 324-325.

PLANNING AND IMPLEMENTATION

Physical Dimension

Do only what client cannot do for himself to foster independence.
Encourage self-care by determining what client can do for himself, what he needs assistance with, and what needs to be done for him.
Teach relaxation.
Attend to physical health with prescribed treatments, nutrition, and exercise.
Encourage discussion of misconceptions of body image.

Emotional Dimension

Develop a trusting relationship, one-to-one initially, then help to establish one with others.
Encourage expression of feelings of anger, depression, resentment, loneliness, and helplessness.

Intellectual Dimension

Teach problem-solving skills.
Encourage decision making.
Reinforce client's attempts to solve problems or make decisions.
Assist client to face reality by looking at the consequences of his behavior.

Continued.

NURSING PROCESS SUMMARY: DEPENDENT BEHAVIOR—cont'd

Help client identify the source of anxiety that motivated his use of denial and rationalization.

Social Dimension
Enhance client's self-concept.
Set limits to avoid manipulative behaviors.
Give attention when client is not demanding or seeking attention.
Know client's cultural orientation and how this relates to the dependence.
Confront attention-seeking behavior.
Include family when explaining client's need to be more independent.

Spiritual Dimension
Use values clarification exercises to help client clarify beliefs and learn to value himself.
Help client become more fully functioning by increasing independence and self-confidence.

EVALUATION
The nursing plans have been effective when the client verbalizes understanding of the dependence and new ways to deal with it. The client can explain the differences between dependence, independence, and interdependence. He is capable of comfortably relying on himself or seeking assistance when the situation dictates the need to do so.

BRIEF REVIEW

The human infant begins life totally dependent on others for nurturing of all facets of his person. If the infant's needs are adequately met in the dependent phase, the infant is able to move on to the independent phase. Once the independent needs are met to a satisfactory degree, the toddler is able to begin learning interdependent behavior.

The interdependent individual is capable of using dependent and independent coping styles as appropriate. Interdependent coping is the most adaptive mode of coping. However, everyone at times has difficulty accepting forced dependence or independence. This difficulty does not indicate an overall maladaptive coping style as does that which occurs when the individual predominatly uses one style to handle all situations. Such a rigid pattern is detrimental to attaining an optimal level of health.

Maladaptive behaviors include (1) doing more or less than one's physical capabilities allow, (2) seeking approval, praise, and proximity in a manipulative manner, (3) low self-esteem, (4) basic mistrust, (5) anger, (6) denial, (7) rationalization, (8) social isolation, (9) occupational impairment, (10) a rigid pattern of coping, and (11) a poorly defined philosophy of life, values, and mores. These behaviors are displayed by individuals with personality disorders and those who engage in substance abuse.

The nurse's role is to assess the client for interdependent coping behaviors, discussing any maladaptive behaviors with the client, and working with him to change them.

REFERENCES AND SUGGESTED READINGS

1. Aguilera, D., and Messick, J.: Crisis intervention: theory and methodology, ed. 5, St. Louis, 1986, The C.V. Mosby Co.
2. Alcoholic Anonymous: the story of how many thousands of men and women have recovered from alcoholism, ed. 2, New York, 1955, Alcoholic Anonymous World Services, Inc.
3. American Psychiatric Association: Diagnostic and statistical manual of mental disorders (DSM-III-R), Washington, D.C., 1987, The Association.
4. Arakelian, M.: An assessment and nursing application of the concept of locus of control, Advances in Nursing Science **3**:25, 1980.
5. Astbury, C.: Recording patient dependency, Nursing Times **82**:40, 1986.
6. Bellar, E.: Dependency and independence in your children, Journal of Genetic Psychology **87**:25, 1955.
7. Booth, T.: Institutional regimes and induced dependency in homes for the aged, The Gerontologist **26**:418, 1986.
8. Bowlby, J.: Attachment and loss, vol. 1, New York, 1980, Basic Books, Inc., Publishers.
9. Clark, C.: Assertiveness skills for nurses, Wakefield, Mass., 1978, Nursing Resources, Inc.
10. Clough, D.H., and Derdiarian, A.: A behavioral checklist to measure dependence and independence, Nursing Research **29**:55, 1980.
11. Davis, R.A.: Testing Kohn's self-reliance hypothesis among high school adolescents, Adolescence **21**(82):443, 1986.
12. Derdiarian, A., and Clough, D.H.: Patient's dependence and independence levels on the prehospital-postdischarge continuum, Nursing Research **25**:47, 1976.
13. Dowling, C.: The Cindrella complex: women's hidden fear of independence, New York, 1981, Summit Books.
14. Evans, R.G.: MMPI dependency scale norms for alcoholics and psychiatric inpatients, Journal of Clinical Psychology **40**:345, 1984.
15. Estes, N.J., and Heinemann, M.E.: Alcoholism: development, consequences, intervention, St. Louis, 1986, The C.V. Mosby Company.
16. Erikson, E.: Childhood and society, ed. 2, New York, 1964, W.W. Norton & Co., Inc.
17. Evers, H.: Old women's self-perceptions of dependency and some implications for service provision, Journal of Epidemiological and Community Health **38**:306, 1984.
18. Faugier, J.: The changing concept of dependence—in the drug and alcohol field, Nurse Practitioner **1**:253, 1986.
19. Franzke, A.W.: The effects of assertiveness training on older adults, The Gerontologist **27**:13, 1987.
20. Freud, S.: An outline of psycho-analysis, New York, 1969, W.W. Norton & Co., Inc.
21. Gibson, S., and others: Measuring patient dependency, Nursing Times **82**:36, 1986.
22. Green, P.: Impaired nurse: the chemical dependency, Focus on Critical Care, **11**:42, 1984.

23. Higley, R.: Independence vs. dependence: whose decision?, ANNA Journal 13:286, 1986.
24. Homer, M., Leonard, A., and Taylor, P.: The burden of dependency, Sociological Review (Monograph) 31:77, 1985.
25. Hutchinsen, S.: Chemically dependent nurses: trajectory toward self-annihilation, Nursing Research 35(4):196, 1986.
26. Kim, M., McFarland, G., and McLane, A.: Classification of nursing diagnosis: proceedings of the fifth national conferences, St. Louis: Mosby, 1984.
27. Klaus, M.H., and Kennell, J.H.: Parent-infant bonding ed. 2, St. Louis, 1982, The C.V. Mosby Co.
27a. Knott, D.H., Fink, R.D., and Morgan, J.C.: Intoxication and the alcohol abstinence syndrome. In Schwartz, G.R., and others: Principles and practice of emergency medicine, Philadelphia, 1978, W.B. Saunders Co.
28. Lion, J.: Personality disorders, Baltimore, 1981, The William & Wilkins Co.
29. Mahler, M.: On human symbiosis and the vicissitudes of individuation, New York, 1976, International Universities Press, Inc.
30. Milan, J., and Ketcham, K.: Under the influence: a guide to the myths and realization of alcoholism, New York, 1983, Bantam Books.
31. Miller, A.: Nurse/patient dependency—a review of different approaches with particular reference to studies of the dependency of elderly patients, Advances in Nursing Science, 9:479, 1984.
32. Miller, A.: Nurse/patient dependency—is it iatrogenic?, Advances in Nursing Science, 10:63, 1985.
33. Miller, A.: A study of the dependency of elderly patients in wards using different methods of nursing care, Age and Ageing 14:132, 1985.
34. Miller, A.: Does the process help the patient?, Nursing Times 81:24, 1985.
35. Murphy, R.E.: Patient's advocate: when independence is good medicine, RN 47:15, 1984.
36. Murray, J.B.: Marijuana's effects on human cognitive functions, psychomotor functions, and personality, Journal of General Psychology 113:23, 1986.
37. Neal, M.C., and others: Nursing care planning guides for psychiatric and mental health care, Pacific Palisades, Calif., 1981, Nurseco, Inc.
38. Pasquali, E., and others: Mental health nursing: a biosychocultural approach, St. Louis, 1981, The C.V. Mosby Co.
39. Peplau, H.E.: Interpersonal relations in nursing, New York, 1952, G.P. Putnam's Sons.
40. Schuster, C.S., and Ashburn, S.: The process of human development: a holistic approach, Boston, ed. 2, 1986, Little, Brown, & Co., Inc.
41. Shives, L.: Basic concepts of psychiatric–mental health nursing, Philadelphia, 1986, J.B. Lippincott Co.
42. Sullivan, H.S.: The interpersonal theory of psychiatry, New York, 1953, W.W. Norton & Co., Inc.
43. Willis, J.: Simple scale for assessing level of dependency of patients in general practice, British Medical Journal (Clinical Research, Ed.) 292:1639, 1986.
44. Zimberg, S.: The clinical management of alcohol, New York, 1982, Brunner/Mazel, Publishers.

ANNOTATED BIBLIOGRAPHY

Estes, N.J., and Heinemann, M.E., editors: Alcoholism: development, consequences, and interventions, ed. 3, St. Louis, 1986, The C.V. Mosby Co.

The third edition of this book is highly recommended as a resource that provides a broad spectrum of topics related to alcoholism. Timely content on substance abuse in nurses and the elderly is included in this edition.

Kurose, K., and others: A standard care plan for alcoholism, American Journal of Nursing, 81:1001, 1981.

A standard care plan for acute and chronic alcoholism is described. The care plan has four categories: usual problems, expected outcomes, outcome deadline, and initial nursing orders. The care plan was a minimal guideline for nursing care. The nursing staff completed care plans in less time by using the standard care plan and focused in more depth on unusual problems of the individual. The article also includes the observations and conclusions that have been drawn from the use of this care plan.

Shramski, T., and Harvey, D.: Paradox of independence, American Mental Health Counselors Association Journal 3:4, 1981.

Independence emphasizing total self-reliance is an ideal often projected by mental health workers. However, to function in the community, an individual must adapt to interdependence. This paradox often leads to frustration for mental health counselors and their clients. To resolve the frustration, the goal of independence must be incorporated with the development of mutual support systems and group interactions. Goals need to assist the client in developing an interdependent coping style.

Waterman, A.: Individualism and interdependence, American Psychologist 36:762, 1981.

Waterman contends that to develop a truly synergistic society built on voluntary participation, individualism must be supported. Research indicates that individuals who are able to express personal beliefs are more able to develop identity, self-actualization, and moral reasoning. These characteristics enable one to function interdependently in society.

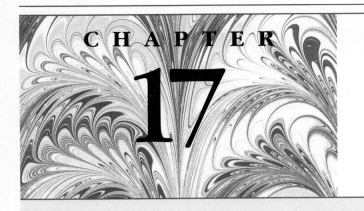

CHAPTER 17

TRUST–MISTRUST

Sharon Holmberg

After studying this chapter the learner will be able to:

Define trust and mistrust.

Trace the historical perspectives of trust and mistrust.

Describe theories of trust and mistrust.

Use the nursing process in caring for clients who mistrust.

Identify current research findings related to mistrust.

A mixture of trust and mistrust in one's basic social attitudes is crucial in the development of a healthy personality. At certain times interactions clearly require caution. Naiveté or too little caution in adult life can lead to the individual's feeling vulnerable. On the other hand, too much caution can lead the individual to interact with an immense degree of wariness. An extreme position of watchfulness puts the individual at risk for disturbed interactions and may lead to questions about one's value, raise one's level of anxiety, and may lead to behaviors that others find difficult to understand.

A sense of the trustworthiness of others usually sets the tone for positive interactions. Doubts about trusting arise normally under certain circumstances, such as when promises go unfulfilled. These doubts for most individuals are temporary and circumscribed. Inability to establish and maintain trusting relationships is a potential problem to be explored. When such circumstances prevail, pronounced distortions can occur in one's ability to relate to others, including serious distortions in perception, reality testing, and behavior.

THEORETICAL APPROACHES

The development of the individual's ability to trust, in general, cannot be considered separately from the development of mistrust. Trust and mistrust can be viewed as a continuum (Figure 17-1). This section of the chapter focuses on normal aspects of trust and mistrust, followed by the evolution of pathological states in which mistrust appears to predominate.

Trust is basic to one's ability to interact successfully with others. It requires that the individual have an idea of what meaning to attribute to the words and behavior of another person. The trusting person accepts the fact that others can be relied on and that trust is related to ideas of consistency. Consistency and reliability allow the individual to develop a trust that similar actions when repeated produce a similar outcome each time. Thus trust is reinforced.

When an expected outcome does not happen, the trusting person feels disappointed but is able to cope and can examine the situation carefully. The trusting person is capable of evaluating his own verbal exchanges and behaviors as well as the other person's. He may seek help from others to review a particular puzzling or disappointing situation. In doing so, the individual's purpose is most likely to test the reality of his perceptions and to more fully understand that which was misunderstood. Trust, then, is related not only to the expectation of similar outcomes in similar circumstances but also to the willingness and ability to objectively analyze deviations from expected outcomes to realistically understand and explain the outcome.

People who are able to trust others are able to depend on others. The trusting person relates to others with the expectation that help from others will be forthcoming in time of need and that it will be offered in a reasonably straightforward way. Trusting persons are able to outline what they need, with the expectation that negotiating takes place in an atmosphere of mutual respect.

Trust is related to faith in the goodwill of the human

Historical Overview

DATE	EVENT
Primitive Times	Efforts were made to comprehend the environment, rendering it more manageable and trustworthy by ascribing magical qualities to natural forces such as the sun.
	Trust or mistrust was stongly influenced by and reflected in dominant cultural values. People thanked the "good gods" when economic conditions were good and harvests plentiful.
1950	Advances in treatment approaches, such as the introduction of the phenothiazines, allowed for significant improvement in the mistrusting behavior of clients.
1960	With deinstitutionalization and the emphasis on shorter hospital stays followed by outpatient treatment and rehabilitation the nurse needed to be prepared to work with clients who were mistrusting both in the hospital and in the community.
1980	Contemporary society demonstrates its vulnerability and lack of trust by the use of fences, walls, and security systems.
	Increases in crime, particularly in inner cities, result in elderly and disabled persons reacting as prisoners in their own homes.
Future	Research on the effectiveness of the therapeutic nurse-client relationship may provide additional understanding of the mistrusting client and lead to new approaches for nursing intervention.

race. This philosophical approach assumes that people are basically kind and considerate.

Too much trust can have devastating impact on an individual. Blind trust may evolve from an individual's fantasy that "all of my needs will be fulfilled." Blind trust can lead to easy and repeated psychological injury and result in a reluctance to trust at all.

Mistrust is a mental state in which basic assumptions are fraught with suspicions regarding the likelihood of being able to understand and predict potential outcomes. When an individual perceives a response from others to be incompatible with factual data, it is difficult to understand the response. Interactions also become increasingly difficult when the outcome of an exchange cannot be anticipated or validated. Individuals who lack trust approach others with an assumption that they will not be accepted, understood, or valued. Consequently, productive interaction is not possible. A certain amount of judicious mistrust is normal in relationships and is desirable in certain situations. When individuals develop the ability to make judgments and discriminations about factual data, then mistrust is based on sound reasoning. When judgment is impaired, as in mental illness, mistrust and suspiciousness may dominate interactions.

Pathological mistrust arises when feelings of mistrust are generalized indiscriminately, without sufficient regard to the nature of the relationship and the context in which the relationship takes place. This pathological mistrust leads to a number of psychological responses. Fear of the unknown and the unpredictable, as when similar situations repeatedly result in dissimilar responses, can gen-

erate mistrust. Feelings of having little control combined with the fear of the unknown often lead to suspiciousness and withdrawal. The environment seems threatening and unpredictable. Withdrawal can reflect the individual's sense of helplessness, or it may reflect the fear that any action will have catastrophic consequences. The person may feel very alienated. Alienation, withdrawal, and perhaps even an individual sense of nonexistence are means of coping with extreme mistrust.

Certain individuals are wary of others' motivations throughout life. The ability to exchange ideas and expressions of feelings or to fully articulate one's own wishes is considered fruitless. Paranoia is an extreme form of this suspiciousness. Paranoid thinking is based on the suspicion that others have devious, if not evil, intentions. A sense of the world as basically good is lost. The world is viewed as evil and motivations of others are viewed as attempts to thwart individual survival needs.

Genetic and Biological

Pathological mistrust can be seen in numerous clinical syndromes but is a predominant characteristic in schizophrenia and paranoia. Several theories have been developed to explain these pathological syndromes in which mistrusting behaviors predominate (Table 17-1).

Genetic potential for the development of schizophrenic syndromes is strongly supported by research. Twin and family studies indicate that schizophrenia occurs more frequently in the children of schizophrenic parents than those with nonschizophrenic parents.

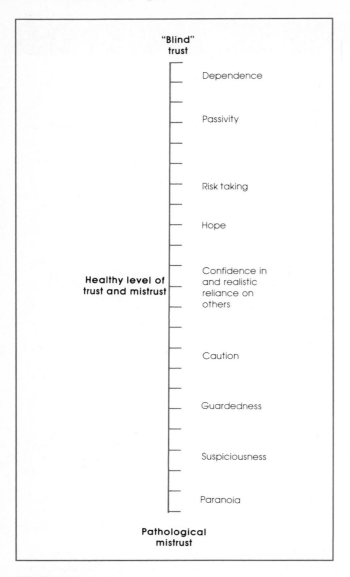

"Blind"
trust

Dependence

Passivity

Risk taking

Hope

Healthy level of
trust and mistrust

Confidence in
and realistic
reliance on
others

Caution

Guardedness

Suspiciousness

Paranoia

Pathological
mistrust

FIGURE 17-1 Trust-mistrust continuum.

The major groups of biochemical theories related to schizophrenia have been developed from attempting to understand the mechanisms of action of psychotropic drugs. By studying the cause of *extrapyramidal symptoms, tardive dyskinesia,* and the nervous system the mechanisms of action of psychoactive drugs have been better understood. These studies suggest the likelihood of imbalances in dopamine, serotonin, and norepinephrine in the neurotransmission process. The antipsychotic action of neuroleptic drugs is thought to result from the blockage of dopamine receptors.

Related studies have focused on the possible dysfunction of the endocrine glands. In particular the focus has been on the study of prolactin and growth hormone secretion from the pituitary gland, since the secretion of both may be controlled by the same neurotransmitters

thought to be relevant to the cause of schizophrenia. It is well established that drugs which decrease dopaminergic activity, as do neuroleptics, increase serum prolactin levels.

Another focus of biochemical research is the study of monoamine oxidase (MAO) activity.[18] MAO is an enzyme crucial to the metabolism of biogenic amines, and its activity is largely genetically determined. Generally MAO activity has been found to be lower in persons diagnosed as having chronic schizophrenia. When persons diagnosed as having acute schizophrenia are studied, there seems to be little, if any, variation from normal MAO activity.

The search for physiological factors in schizophrenic illness is being pursued in a number of other areas as well. The development of computed tomography and pneumoencephalography has allowed study of structural deviations of the brain. Recent evidence suggests that persons diagnosed as having schizophrenia may be likely to have structural abnormalities.[38,47]

The prominence of cognitive and language difficulties in schizophrenia may suggest abnormalities in brain hemisphere functioning, especially the left hemisphere, which is specialized for language and analytic processing. Tests for eye dominance, handedness, and lateral eye movements are associated with hemispheric dominance and have been used to evaluate the possible existence of left hemispheric dysfunction. Some studies support the theory of specific left hemispheric dysfunction in schizophrenia (see the Research Highlight on p. 341).

Psychoanalytic

Freud[14] suggested that mistrusting behaviors are a consequence of the failure of the ego as a mediator between drives and reality. The ego functions that maintain contact with reality may be incompletely developed, weakened or impaired; primitive modes of thinking and feeling predominate. Communication with others becomes distorted. The individual cannot comprehend his experiences and becomes more suspicious as the level of anxiety increases.

Erikson[12] described the first emotional developmental stage as basic trust versus basic mistrust. He stated specifically that the way in which body needs are met has a direct bearing on the establishment of emotional trust. Consistency and the mother's ability to accept the baby's biological needs and functions are factors that influence the degree of self-acceptance and social trust an infant ultimately develops.

Interpersonal

Sullivan[41] suggested that feedback from significant others influences the development of trust. The child gradually incorporates experiences with others into images of "good me," "bad me," and "not me." "Good me" concepts develop from positive and rewarding experiences with significant others, usually parenting figures. The child views himself in a positive way and the environment as caring and responsive. Most children develop parts of the self that are "good me" and parts that are "bad me." These

TABLE 17-1 Summary of theories of mistrust

Theory	Theorist	Dynamics
Biological		
Genetic		Genetic tendencies are linked with pathological mistrust.
Biochemical		Imbalances in chemistry of nervous system related to pathological mistrust, decreased prolactin secretions, and lowered MAO activity. Brain structure abnormalities and left hemisphere dysfunction may also contribute to pathological mistrust.
Psychoanalytic	Freud	The incompletely developed, weakened or impaired ego contributes to distorted communication. The individual has difficulty comprehending his experiences and becomes increasingly suspicious as his anxiety increases.
	Erikson	Inconsistency or failure to meet infant's basic needs results in infant developing mistrust.
Interpersonal	Sullivan	The "not me" aspect of personality accompanied with anxiety and confusion contributes to lack of trust.
Psychoanalytic and Interpersonal	Mahler	When child's separation tasks are not fully accomplished, person lacks a strong sense of self and is threatened, insecure, and mistrustful when interacting with others.
Cognitive	Piaget	Cognitive development during months 4 to 9 results in infant's recognition that his actions initiate reactions that may contribute to development of a sense of trust or mistrust.
Family Interaction	Lidz	Overt marital conflict and parental characteristics of overprotective mother and passive father may lead to mistrust of others. Lack of respect for infant's individual traits contributes to feelings of insecurity and suspiciousness.
Communication	Bateson	Double-bind communication promotes insecurity and mistrust.

Research Highlight

Brain Function in Psychiatric Disorders: Regional Cerebral Blood Flow in Unmedicated Schizophrenics

R.E. Gur, R.C. Gur, B.E. Skolnick, S. Caroff, W. Obrist, S. Resnick & M. Reivich

PURPOSE

The intent of this study was to further examine previous research which suggests that there may be regional brain dysfunction in schizophrenia. Behavioral evidence suggests left hemispheric dysfunction and left hemispheric overactivation. It is hypothesized that there will be an increase in left hemispheric blood flow for schizophrenics when compared to matched controls.

SAMPLE

Eleven male and eight female subjects, all right handed, with no history of drug abuse, alcoholism, neurological disease or medical disease were selected from two inpatient psychiatric hospitals to participate in the study. Subjects were free of neuroleptic medication for at least 1 week before the study. Nineteen control subjects were matched with subjects for sex, age, and education.

METHODOLOGY

Trace amounts of xenon XC 133 were inhaled through a face mask by subjects while the uptake and clearance of the isotope were measured by 16 collimated sodium iodine crystal detectors placed over the scalp. Subjects were tested under three conditions: (1) resting baseline, (2) verbal analogies, and (3) spatial line orientation test.

FINDINGS

There were significant differences between the schizophrenic subjects and the control subjects under all conditions tested in this study. Regional cerebral blood flow was equal in the two hemispheres for control subjects and higher in the left than the right hemisphere for schizophrenic subjects during the resting baseline test. When activation procedures were used, schizophrenic subjects continued to demonstrate different blood flow changes in anterior and posterior regions. When there was a difference in lateralization of flows, it was always in the direction of increased left hemispheric flows in schizophrenic subjects.

IMPLICATIONS

The results support the hypothesis of left hemispheric overaction. Greater numbers of subjects need to be studied, and repeated measures of the same individuals will permit better specificity in identifying brain regions that are implicated in schizophrenic psychopathology.

Based on data from Archives of General Psychiatry **42**:329, 1985.

patterns of self-understanding become somewhat stable during the first 3 years of life.

Mahler and Sullivan also developed concepts that apply to understanding mistrusting behaviors. Mahler[28] described the development of emotional object constancy and individuality. When these separation tasks are not fully accomplished, the person lacks a strong sense of self and feels more vulnerable and threatened when interacting with others, thereby decreasing the level of trust in both himself and others. Sullivan described a similar process in the development of self-concept. In his terminology the "not me" is that aspect of personality accompanied by anxiety, confusion, and lack of trust.

Cognitive

Piaget and Inhelder,[33] conceptualizing the cognitive development of the child, state that it is between the fourth and ninth months that the child first begins to recognize that his actions result in reactions; then slowly he realizes that *he* is an integral part of the sequence of events. From this understanding a beginning sense of self-trust is established. In this phase, between 4 and 9 months of age, the infant begins to give up spontaneous smiling to demonstrate more selective responses. When seeing strangers the child has a reaction that appears to be fear or anxiety.[40] Recent research seems to indicate that this change in response is a result of cognitive development. The earlier egocentrism of the infant gives way to a more objective perception of reality. The infant has the cognitive ability to realize that "things" can act on their own and may be unpredictable or even alarming.

As the child recognizes the existence of causes that are independent of his own action, he can establish the fact of his own separateness and experience a sense of trust and confidence in others. Cognitive development is a necessary prerequisite and a preparation for physical separation from the mother, requiring the child to "trust" that his mother will not disappear during the separation.

Throughout the remainder of life, the foundations of trust are tested with each developmental phase. These foundations can be reestablished and renewed or modified with each crisis and conflict. At any time during the remaining developmental phases, the individual may confront situations that seriously challenge his ability to trust. When basic trust cannot be restored through a series of interactions with the environment, the individual may experience a serious undermining of his previous concept of self and may develop distorted modes of relating to others.

Information processing as a cognitive dysfunction is seen in persons with pathological mistrust. It has been suggested that persons in a psychotic state such as schizophrenia have difficulty making correct associations. Ideas and perceptions seem to develop without the logical thought process and are reflected in cognitive, linguistic, and perceptual deviations. Reasons for these association disorders are poorly understood but may be a consequence of the individual's difficulty with attention. Zubin[50] has conceptualized three dimensions of attention:

(1) selecting a focus, (2) maintaining a focus, and (3) shifting a focus. Most people can select relevant stimuli in the environment toward which they direct their attention and at the same time become almost totally unaware of other stimuli. For example, a person wishing to read a book will focus on the book and disregard the radio playing, the fluorescent lamp's buzz, other people's talking, flashing headlights through the window, and any other environmental noise. Persons who are unable to maintain a focus or who constantly shift their focus soon become confused, distracted, and unable to decipher relevant stimuli requiring a response. It has been suggested that such responses may be a result of impairment of the cognitive-perceptual filtering mechanism and result in a mistrust of others.

Family Interaction

Initially, theorists took their views of the family from what the client said about his family in the therapeutic process. The mother was viewed as problematic and as "causing" schizophrenia. The label "schizophrenogenic mother" was applied. Essentially this means that the client viewed the mother as hostile, overtly or subtly rejecting, aloof, cold, overanxious, and overprotective. The outwardly harmonious families, termed "skewed" by Lidz, Fleck, and Cornelison,[27] are characterized by a mother who is exceedingly intrusive into her child's life and overprotective, feeling that the child cannot exist without her supervision. The child realizes, over time, that his mother opposes any movements toward autonomy from her and becomes fearful of engulfment or incorporation, yet on some level believes that neither can he get along without his mother nor she without him. The father in such a family structure is generally passive, in deference to the wife, and may feel excluded from the family, based on the intensity of the relationship between mother and child. In extreme form, the father may be psychotic or alcoholic and unable to provide support or satisfaction to the wife. A second family interactional dynamic of schizophrenia described by Lidz and associates is that of the "schismatic" family. In these families overt conflict predominates between the spouses, who compete for the loyalty of the children. The child may feel caught in a bind, trying to please both parents, and ultimately accepts the role of family *scapegoat* and behaves in ways that seem to cause parental conflicts.

In both family structures, the communication patterns become confusing, distorted, and even irrational. The ability of various members to separate self from others and to recognize differences in feelings and reactions is impaired. The overprotection undermines the child's ability to develop basic trust in his world and abilities. The child represses his feelings and needs in an effort to fit into the parents' requirements.

Communication

Distorted patterns of communication with inconsistent verbal and nonverbal messages can severely undermine trusting relationships. This pattern of *double-bind* communication does not allow for clarification. This repetitive pattern of interaction prevents a clear understanding or resolution of the inconsistencies in levels of communication and leaves all participants feeling confused (see Case Example).

Case Example

A nurse was attempting to establish a therapeutic alliance with Jerome, whose history indicated that he was paranoid, trusted no one, and usually stopped therapy after one or two sessions. After several therapy sessions, Jerome telephoned the nurse and said to her, "Let's run off to Paris and get married." The verbal communication was accompanied by Jerome's laughter, and a radio was playing very loud disco music in the background. Jerome's message was unclear. The situation was resolved by communicating *about* the communications. She responded to him by saying, "You know, I am your nurse, not your girlfriend. It's not clear what you mean when you're laughing and at the same time suggesting something serious." This communication allowed for clarification of the meaning of the message and the relationship between the nurse and Jerome.

Double-bind interactions occur rather commonly in normal human interactions both within and outside the family. When caught in a double bind, a healthy individual usually responds defensively. The individual experiences discomfort, but corrective interactions and the nonrepetitive nature of the exchange prevent a pathological state.

Table 17-1 summarizes the major theories.

RELATING TO THE CLIENT

Relating to the pathologically mistrusting client can be difficult. The nurse may be puzzled by the actions she sees or may respond with fear. She may have a strong personal reaction to some of the client's bizarre behaviors. The client who mistrusts is particularly sensitive to the insincerity of another's behavior, even at times when the other person is unaware of not having made a full commitment. It is essential that the nurse is aware of having strong reactions or negative thoughts and feelings about the client within herself before interacting with the client.

To facilitate the interaction the nurse needs to be accepting and genuine, not offering a conditional relationship contingent on the client's offering expressions of gratitude. The client quickly recognizes conditional behaviors on the part of the nurse. Trusting relationships are based on the nurse's emotional accessibility.

The client is unlikely to relay information about the meaning he attributes to the relationship. He may present a multitude of indifferent behaviors, resistances, or efforts to test the interaction between himself and the nurse. The nurse may experience frustration, disappointment, and perhaps even anger and feelings of rejection when progress is slow or nonexistent.

During the introductory stage of the relationship, behaviors of the nurse intended to create a positive environment may be readily misinterpreted by the client. For instance, a smile from the nurse, in an effort to be friendly, may be interpreted as a threat. Demonstrating an understanding of the client's mistrust without responding with mistrust and rejection will help establish a basis for trusting relationships. The client is likely to be unable to look directly at the nurse for a prolonged period. Initially the nurse responds to these messages by also avoiding the intensity implied by prolonged, direct eye contact. The nurse who is able to nonverbally express a willingness to listen to the client, to demonstrate empathy and is nonjudgmental without seeming to be a threat, is likely to receive a better response. At times it will be necessary to set limits on the client's behavior, which can produce strong emotional reactions in the nurse. She may fear for her own safety and yet feel guilt, anger, frustration, or even sympathy and regret for the client who needs to be physically restrained. The nurse may have strong ethical and moral reactions to measures for behavior control that may have to be initiated.

Occasionally mistrusting clients admitted to a psychiatric inpatient unit have become sufficiently withdrawn to require total physical care. Nursing care to meet these basic needs is provided in the context of repeated efforts to establish a means of communication with the client. The nurse may feel frustrated in her efforts to communicate with a client whom she knows to be physically able but psychologically unable to interact. Patience and perseverance are required. Gradually the client will become increasingly capable of responding to the nurse and the supportive environment and will find it possible to give up some of the regressive needs.

The working phase of the relationship with an excessively mistrusting client requires the nurse to be verbally and emotionally consistent. Establishing a trusting relationship with a person who misinterprets signals requires creative thinking; translation skills can be developed to facilitate the client's correct understanding of environmental cues. For example, a frightened client told the nurse that an alarm bell rang very often. When the nurse realized that the client's response was to the ring of the ward telephone, she was able to reassure the client.

An initial task of the working phase is to ensure physical well-being and reestablish regular life patterns. In reestablishing regular life patterns the nurse is required to be persistent with small and tedious details without receiving much response from the client. As the nurse's understanding of the client and his life experiences begins to expand, it may be possible for the nurse to begin to decode delusions and *hallucinations*. It is not helpful to confront the client with the unreality of delusions or hallucinations directly. A more productive approach is to ask questions in a manner that facilitates understanding of how reality has been distorted. This nonconfrontational approach is more likely to facilitate the relationship and allow the client to broach alternate explanations.

Just as the client has difficulty trusting the nurse, the nurse may not trust the client. Behaviors from clients that seem inconsistent or ambivalent may draw out countertransference reactions in the nurse related to times when she felt insecure, frightened, and unsure of herself or how to react. Clients may articulate uncanny insights and be able to present the nurse with an aspect of her personality that she dislikes and has considered well hidden from most people. When hearing comments about this aspect of her personality, the nurse may feel uncomfortable and exposed, vulnerable to the client's ability to understand her. Recognizing and accepting herself assist the nurse in developing the ability to acknowledge that the client may be right but that does not mean that she is bad.

The client who has been able to establish some trust may demonstrate an increase in regressive and dependent behaviors as termination approaches. The nurse needs to help the client realize that he can cope with the stress of returning to a less protective setting. She can point out to the client the new behaviors or means of coping that have been developed. Recognizing and discussing feelings of sadness at the time of termination continue the established process of testing and confirming reality.

NURSING PROCESS
Assessment

Physical dimension. A pathologically suspicious individual may appear strikingly different from the "ordinary" person. It may be that there is something that is "just not quite right" about the person, such as makeup slightly off, eyebrows arched too much, or lipstick too bright and too thick. Or it may be that the plaid jacket of blue, green, and brown seems strange when combined with plaid pants, three sizes too large, of bold red and purple. The client may appear disheveled, unkempt, or even dirty and have a body odor. Sometimes the usual manner of dress reflects the individual's distorted body image. Distortions in body image may be evident. The client who considers his body physically changed will report, for example, that a body part is no longer in proportion, or that his skull has become flat, or that he is falling apart at the joints. Distortions in body image can be severe enough for some individuals that they cannot recognize photographs of themselves or even identify their own body parts. Distortions may involve confusion of sexual identity and a feeling of having some body parts that are of the opposite sex or a feeling of lacking body parts that should be there. Homosexual or promiscuous behavior may be efforts to clarify sexual identity.

Preoccupation with somatic complaints is common for the person with a distorted body image. The body feels strange. The client who has become exceedingly self-focused may also be much more aware of normal body functions (for example, breathing, heartbeat, and peristaltic movements of the bowel) and consider them abnormal. Physical assessment needs to include attention to these physical complaints to separate realistic physical problems from hypochondriacal complaints. Equally important to assess are the client's diet and sleep patterns. Some clients may neglect necessary health care such as eating, dressing properly, elimination, and sleeping. Because of their fears of being poisoned or harmed these can become a serious threat to survival.

The suspicious client may be unable to look directly at others. Often the person who is suspicious wears sunglasses as a way to protect himself from eye contact. Persons who cannot maintain eye contact may stare out the window, keep their eyes down toward the floor, or wander about the room.

Motor activity for clients who are schizophrenic may be within the normal range or may be on either of two extremes: too little or too much. Those with too little motor activity, *catatonic* clients, show marked withdrawal, sometimes to the point of being totally immobilized and unable to respond to commands. They may move themselves into unusual, seemingly uncomfortable positions and remain there for hours. *Waxy flexibility* is the term applied when it is possible to place a client's limbs in a given position that the individual makes no effort to change, sometimes for hours. At times movements will be repetitive and stereotyped, such as plucking at the skin or pulling out hair. Other unusual or bizarre movements may also be seen, such as facial grimacing or sucking movements of the mouth. Some bizarre movements can result from psychotropic medications. Chapter 22 further discusses drug-related movements.

An increased rate of motor activity in suspicious clients is usually demonstrated by agitation, pacing, inability to sleep, loss of appetite, and weight loss. Increased motor activity may be accompanied by emotional lability, flight of ideas, and impulsiveness. When an individual is unable to exert the usual, socially expected controls, impulsive behavior may result. This behavior appears to be sudden, unpredictable, unmotivated, and illogical. The client may become verbally destructive, aggressive, or even violent. Persons who have been withdrawn and quiet for considerable periods may also demonstrate impulsive behavior. It is particularly important to recognize that such impulsive behavior can include suicidal attempts that are likely to be serious.

Obtaining a thorough history as part of the assessment has two purposes. The first is to establish if any other family members have been treated for serious psychiatric disturbances, since some research supports a genetic predisposition to schizophrenia. The second purpose is to clarify where and how the client's symptoms began. Acute drug intoxication, especially amphetamines, hallucinogenic drugs of various types, and sometimes alcoholic hallucinosis may produce symptoms similar to the behavior of schizophrenia. Laboratory studies of blood and urine may show toxic levels of some of these substances. Neurological conditions such as Huntington's chorea, Gilles de la Tourette's disease, tertiary syphilis, some forms of epilepsy (especially temporal lobe epilepsy), and brain tumors may manifest themselves with extreme suspiciousness in addition to psychotic components. A thorough medical examination is essential to rule out physical causes of the behavior.

Emotional dimension. The person who demonstrates trust is able to express his own feelings relatively freely, in an honest and forthright manner, and expects the same from others. Emotions can be shown in an acceptable manner, accurately reflecting how the individual may feel in a given situation. Facial expressions are a key to how one feels. Other behaviors such as body movements and posture are consistent with the person's facial expressions.

For the suspicious individual, feelings may not be easily interpreted. Since the individual experiences the world as threatening and unsafe in many respects, feeling comfortable, relaxed, and free to express himself is almost impossible. The person himself may be uncertain of his own feelings or may not realize what is being communicated by his behavior. The client can appear angry and threatening or withdrawn and suspicious, or it may be difficult to interpret his mood at all. Characteristic feelings are negativism, helplessness, decreased self-esteem, anxiety, fear, anger, guilt, depression, and ambivalence. These feelings may not always coincide with what seems to be the dominant mood of the client.

Distortions in feelings may make it exceedingly difficult to interpret what is being communicated. The client usually is unaware of the distortions, since he may find nothing unusual in his expression of feelings. Emotional lability is a common characteristic. For example, a client may laugh hysterically while describing an experience. A few moments later, the same individual may burst into tears, with little having occurred to precipitate such an extreme change. When questioned, the client is not always able to explain this shift in expressed mood and may or may not be aware of its having occurred. Generally the shift in mood is extreme, with the expression of feeling being an *overreaction* to what would normally be expected to accompany the content of the discussion. The client may explain the shift in mood as being a response to other stimuli, such as hallucinations; thus the change, from the client's perspective, seems perfectly comprehensible.

The opposite of overreaction is emotional blunting. This refers to a decreased intensity of emotion from that which one would normally expect from the specific situation. Such clients frequently seem to be apathetic, minimally responsive, or indifferent to the environment or events that happen to them. Another somewhat similar but more severe emotional response, known as *flat affect,* is demonstrated when a client does not communicate any feelings in his verbal and nonverbal responses. It is impossible to interpret any emotional tone. For instance, a client, in describing having been raped a few days ago, may talk of the event as if she had read it in a newspaper, showing no personal feelings or reactions. With such clients, it is extremely difficult to understand their emotional reactions.

Equally difficult to interpret are affects that are clearly inappropriate to the situation. An inappropriate expression of emotion is seen when the content of a thought or an idea is very different from the emotional tone being expressed. For example, a client may be describing having threatened his wife with a knife during an argument and be laughing as he describes the event.

Feelings experienced by the suspicious person can be potent despite the possible difficulties in interpreting them. The individual who has become uncertain of his identity has difficulty understanding his environment. One likely outcome of this is a sense of overwhelming anxiety accompanied by feelings of impending doom. For exam-

ple, a young woman was brought into the emergency room almost in shock after having collapsed in exhaustion. She had been running for 4 hours in an effort to escape unknown "pursuers" wishing to kill her. The client may be unrealistically convinced that death is almost certain but chooses to struggle against it. Such a reaction to overwhelming anxiety yields expression of fear or anger that may be difficult to differentiate from each other. The client who reacts in this manner to overwhelming anxiety can be volatile, threatening, aggressive, and often suspicious or paranoid. This person is particularly sensitive to feeling trapped or closed in. Small rooms, limited access to exits, close physical proximity, and emotional intensity may cause the client to express his fear by fleeing or by explosive behavior. The client is generally more able to express anger than to acknowledge anxiety and fear. Clients may express their fear through paranoid ideas as in the preceding example. Emotionally, the individual may experience *depersonalization,* a feeling of strangeness or unreality concerning the self. The client may feel a loss of identity, different, changed, or empty. Clients who experience depersonalization are likely to make statements such as the following:

"My body is like a pillar of salt. Chips fall when I move."

"I can't look in a mirror because it isn't me anymore. Who is it?"

A closely related experience, *derealization,* addresses the feeling of strangeness or unreality with respect to the environment, as if the environment has changed. Following are examples of statements that reflect this experience:

"I've been walking around in a dream for days."

"Something has happened to the world. It's become evil and red."

A second means of expressing confusion in self-identity and response to overwhelming anxiety may be withdrawal from the environment. The client becomes passive, may be unresponsive and withdrawn, and may feel and act helpless. Severe withdrawn behavior, as in catatonia, can occur, but a more common response is the client's gradual or partial withdrawal from relationships. The client feels depressed, lonely, and guilty. Feelings of guilt may arise from a sense of having failed himself and others. The experience of being unable to cope with self and others adequately (a low self-esteem) accompanied by the discomfort (mistrust) felt in relating to others can further reinforce the passivity.

Ambivalence (the coexistence of contradictory emotions, attitudes, ideas, or desires with respect to a particular person, object, or situation) may be a temporary feeling for most people. The healthy individual recognizes the contradictory feelings but can choose the one option expected to be most satisfactory. When excessively ambivalent feelings are experienced, the choice of alternatives cannot be made. The highly suspicious individual may continually alternate between choices, feeling and expressing a wish to do one and then the other. For example, a client may repeatedly state that he wants to call his mother on the telephone but is constantly sidetracked by other activities on the way to the telephone. Ambivalent

TABLE 17-2 Some behavioral manifestations of ambivalence

Behavior	Description	Example
Compulsive rituals	Attempts to solve conflicting feelings by constant, repetitive activity that may be stereotyped or seem meaningless	John has difficulty leaving his room. He gets up from the chair, takes three steps forward and then three steps backward, sits again, touches the bed, stands up, taps the window, sits down, taps his knee three times, and then gets up and begins to walk forward again.
Negativism	Attempts to avoid opposing feelings by refusing, either verbally or nonverbally, to participate	Elizabeth's response to any request is always no. She refuses to get out of bed in the morning or participate in any ward activities. Once engaged in a given activity, the effort to have her change the activity is equally problematic.
Overcompliance	Attempts to deny responsibility for any action by doing only what another exactly instructs should be done	Harold agrees to play checkers but will not move the pieces unless someone sits beside him to tell him exactly which way to move them and where to place them.

feelings can seriously disrupt the individual's ability to function and may produce any of the following behaviors: (1) compulsive rituals, (2) negativism, or (3) overcompliance (Table 17-2). The constant indecision of the ambivalent person most likely indicates that motivation to accomplish a task is missing. Independent positive volition is lacking, perhaps because the individual believes that whatever action he chooses will be wrong; he will feel guilty, hurt someone, or increase the seriousness of his own predicament. Commitment to a specific action or feeling means that the individual may be held accountable for the choice, producing an intolerable situation for the person already feeling vulnerable.

✳ ***Intellectual dimension.*** One of the major characteristics of pathological mistrust is multiple difficulties in the process and character of thought. It is hypothesized that, as a person becomes increasingly anxious and experiences multiple stressors or fears, the ability to think clearly and logically is impaired and the person regresses to a more primitive level. Each individual is susceptible to some degree of impairment in thinking when under extreme stress. Persons who have extreme difficulty in trusting relationships are more likely than others to develop problems with thinking clearly or with their ability to abstract, communicate, and accurately perceive the environment. The cognitive mechanisms employed to arrive at conclusions do not follow the rules of ordinary logic employed by adults but follow some other process so that the conclusions reached are different from those ordinarily considered acceptable. This process of arriving at conclusions may be experienced normally in dreams, when the connection between two events seems logical and obvious. This "dreaming" thought process in the awake adult is called *primary process thinking* (regressed thinking) and can be considered a less mature form of cognition. Primary process thinking may be employed in an effort to allay anxiety, at least temporarily. As the level

of anxiety increases, there is a likelihood of increasingly distorted thinking. So that these interrelated cognitive distortions can be more clearly explored, they will be described in the following categories: (1) disturbances in thought processes, (2) perceptual difficulties, (3) disturbances in language usage and communication, and (4) other intellectual disturbances.

Disturbances in thought processes. Three major disturbances in thought processes that commonly occur in highly suspicious clients are fragmented thinking, autistic thinking, and delusional thinking. *Fragmentation* of the thought process occurs either by thoughts becoming split off so the individual will "lose track of" thoughts or by the individual's blocking of thoughts. Thought blocking can be observed when an individual in the midst of a discussion suddenly stops or abruptly changes the topic. When fragmented thinking predominates, thoughts usually do not seem to occur logically. Consequently the listener experiences the ideas being expressed as only slightly related to each other, or the transition between topics cannot be deciphered. The listener may find the interaction to be confusing or impossible to follow. For example, a client asked about his bus ride to the clinic responded, "The bus was late and warm; my bed was warm and comfortable; comfort for tears and sadness like my mother, when she was home yesterday."

Autistic thinking in the adult can be viewed as similar to the typical, normal childhood thought processes that occur before the child has sufficient intellectual and emotional maturity to perceive the environment in other than a self-centered way. This thought process requires a minimal distinction between self and others and an inability to distinguish internal stimuli from external stimuli. For instance, the client may think "I want a glass of water," and then believe that others know his wish. An understanding of reality may be based on fantasy or wishes rather than on objective observations. Events or interactions may take on special, personal meanings for anxious and suspicious individuals, meanings not understood or universally accepted by others.

Magical thinking is a form of autistic thinking whereby the individual equates thinking with doing. The logical link missing is that the client does not grasp the realistic relationship between cause and effect but believes he has secret powers or influences that "cause" other things to happen. For example, a client who lived near an air force base believed he controlled the taking off and landing of airplanes because the planes would fly in search of him when he was having "bad thoughts."

Concrete thinking is another type of autistic thinking. Concrete thinking reflects an inability to conceptualize meaning in words or thoughts. Therefore the ability to process information accurately may be lost. Understanding based on the context of words and nuances of meaning is lost. For example, *pare, pair,* and *pear* may seem to be the same, confusing the client because the client does not grasp the context of use and is therefore unable to determine which word is meant. The ability to classify in logical categories or abstract common qualities may fail; for example, when asked to explain the similarity between a car and a truck, the client may respond "They are both big," emphasizing a concrete quality. The client may be unable to associate other, more abstract qualities, such as that both are means of transportation. Concrete thinking does not allow the client to organize facts in a manner that makes sense. Misinterpretations of casual remarks or jokes are common. The individual may not understand the subtleties in a joke and cannot interpret proverbs in other than a concrete way. For example, the proverb "People who live in glass houses should not throw stones" will be understood to mean that if a person in a glass house throws a stone, it will break a window.

The third major disturbance in thought processes is the *delusion,* or belief system that is not validated or tested against reality. It is firmly maintained, even in the face of contradictory information or obvious proof to the contrary. Delusions usually reflect the client's denial of certain physical traits or feelings that he initially acknowledges but considers unacceptable. The delusional thought process begins to develop when the individual feels threatened by others or experiences anxiety related to a real or imagined trait of his own. As a protective measure, the individual projects outward these assumed negative qualities and may ascribe them to other persons, which can be accomplished by misinterpreting impressions of events and things. Thus, for the individual, unacceptable thoughts, feelings, actions, and wishes come from outside rather than inside himself. For example, a person who considers himself lazy may develop the idea that others are talking about his laziness. Each time he sees people talking, he is certain they are talking about him.

The individual may also attribute to others his own traits that he considers unacceptable. Delusions develop essentially by reversing the usual deductive reasoning process. Usual logical thought processes move from description to conclusion. For the person with delusional thoughts the conclusion is already clear; then evidence is mobilized, and events are interpreted to support the conclusion. As the individual continues to use this false reasoning system, it can take on more organization, meaning, and complexity. Delusions may become systematized. That is, the delusional beliefs become more organized and are worked out in such a way as to seem logical, and they become integrated into the rest of the individual's life. When the person becomes utterly convinced of his false belief and all evidence to the contrary is ignored, a fixed delusion has developed. See Table 17-3 for definitions of the more common delusions.

Perceptual difficulties. The five senses facilitate one's accurate perception of the environment. Normal perceptions are those that can be consensually validated by other

TABLE 17-3 Types of delusions

Term	Definition	Example
Ideas of reference	Belief that certain occurrences are directly related to oneself	An elderly woman, convinced she had a bad body odor, believed she caused others around her to rub their noses or sneeze.
Delusions of grandeur	An exaggerated sense of self-importance	A young woman who delivered a baby a few weeks before was brought to a psychiatric hospital because she was convinced she had given birth to the baby Jesus.
Somatic delusions	Belief that the body is changing or responding in an unusual way	A 22-year-old woman refused to wash her face, apply makeup, or look in a mirror because she believed that she had "turned into an old woman" as a result of being unfaithful to her husband.
Delusions of persecution	Belief that one is in danger, under investigation, persecuted, or at the mercy of some powerful force	A 52-year-old policeman under a great deal of job-related stress began to think his coworkers were against him. He was convinced they would harm him and refused to socialize with them.

individuals in the environment. For example, if a school cafeteria is serving fish on a particular day, most persons who walk by the cafeteria will receive some olfactory stimulation, and there will most likely be general agreement that the smell is one of fish cooking. As this example shows, perception involves a two-step process: recognition of the stimulus and an understanding or interpretation of the stimulus. Difficulties with perception may occur at either of these steps. The client may inaccurately perceive the nature of the stimulus or misinterpret it. Interpretation of and reaction to the stimulus are based on emotional associations with the stimulus. However, regardless of previous experiences of the same or similar stimuli, the suspicious client may misinterpret or produce seemingly dissonant reactions to the current stimulus situation.

Perceptual distortions are common but usually transitory. Almost every person has experienced a situation such as waking up suddenly to misperceive an object in the room as an unknown person or catching a glimpse of an object out of the corner of the eye, such as a ball, and interpreting it as an airplane. These distortions, known as *illusions,* are misrepresentations or misinterpretations of reality. They are usually brief, transitory experiences that may be accompanied by an equally temporary emotional reaction such as surprise or fear. Illusions are most often visual or auditory, but they can also be olfactory, tactile, or gustatory. Much more profound perceptual difficulties occur commonly in conjunction with distortions in body image. Depersonalization and identity confusion are examples of distortions in body image.

Other profound distortions in perception are *hallucinations* (Table 17-4). Hallucinations are perceptions of objects, sensations, or images that have no basis in reality. No stimulus exists; yet the individual perceives a stimulus and acts on it.

Hallucinations are frequently experienced as real sensations by the individual, or they may have an uncanny quality whereby the individual acknowledges their nonexistence in reality but claims "they are real to me." For example, the client may be able to engage in a conversation about the voices in his head. Most likely, hallucinations are a response to severe anxiety. As anxiety increases, dissociated components of the self-system begin to seem real and can meet needs such as improving self-esteem, control, or communication that are not being supplied in reality.

Four phases in the development of hallucinations have been described. At first, in response to anxiety, stress, or loneliness, daydreaming increases and focuses on comforting thoughts to relieve the discomfort. The client remains reality based and can still identify the thoughts as part of himself. However, as anxiety continues to increase, perceptual awareness becomes more intense, and the client develops a "listening state" to hear the sensations, which are now becoming dissociated with the self and are only vague, muffled sounds or whispers. The client, with ever increasing anxiety, wishes to put distance between himself and the developing hallucination by projecting the experience outward; thus it may seem to be coming from some place other than the self. In the third phase, the hallucination develops more prominence. The client adjusts to the experience and may find that the hallucination provides a sense of temporary security or comfort. Finally, the hallucination may lose its quality of comfort and become commanding, threatening, or disparaging. The client may feel controlled by the hallucination and become so involved with the experience that the possibility of outside interaction diminishes significantly. In this phase, hallucinations can powerfully influence the client's behavior. Command hallucinations that tell the individual to hurt himself or others are likely to be acted on.

TABLE 17-4 Types of hallucinations

Sense	Definition	Example
Auditory	Voices or sounds that have no basis in reality are heard. Voices may be a projection of inner thoughts, which can be comforting, derogatory, threatening, or commanding.	A young woman, very frightened of interaction with other people, hears a voice telling her what to do and how to act each time she leaves home.
Visual	Visual images of figures, objects, or events are experienced in the absence of external stimuli.	A middle-aged woman repeatedly sees glimpses of herself handcuffed and tied in a chair.
Gustatory	Tastes are experienced as distorted, or the client may experience taste without a stimulus.	A client who is concerned that some unknown person wants him dead experiences a bitter taste when he eats food in a restaurant.
Olfactory	Nonexistent odors that may arise from a specific or unknown place are smelled.	An adolescent girl, shortly after beginning menstruation, says her body smells bad. Repeated washing does not remove the odor.
Tactile	Strange body sensations are felt. Tactile hallucinations may be associated with distortions in body image. This hallucination frequently occurs with alcohol toxicity.	A young psychotic man repeatedly reports that he is unable to sleep because his penis is being massaged throughout the night by an unknown force.

TABLE 17-5 Language disorders

Language Change	Definition	Example
Asyndetic expression	A language disorder manifested by a juxtaposition of elements or meanings without adequate linkage	A client, when asked the name of the president, responds, "White House."
Metonymic speech	The use of imprecise terms or words with approximate meaning	"I have eaten three meals" becomes "I have had three menus."
Echolalia	The purposeless repetition of a word or phrase just stated by another individual	The nurse says, "Turn on the lights," and the client responds, "The lights, the lights, the lights, the lights."
Neologisms	A private word or phrase coined by the speaker that has special meaning to the speaker and cannot be understood by others	A client responds to a question by saying, "Ethuel, tanigram."
Clang associations	The repetition of words or phrases that have a similar sound but no other relationship	The nurse says, "What would you like to eat?" The client's response is "Eat, feet, meet, beat."
Word salad	The linking of ordinary words and phrases in a meaningless, illogical, disconnected manner	A client, pacing the hallway, says, "Vanilla reason lopsided can go left and right he is."

The most common hallucinatory experiences are auditory or visual. Olfactory, tactile, and gustatory hallucinations are occasionally experienced by the psychotic individual but occur more commonly with persons who have an organic condition or are in alcohol or drug toxicity.

Disturbances in language usage and communication. Satisfactory interaction with others is based on the ability to adequately exchange ideas and thoughts, to share perceptions, and to express feelings. Disorders in language usage prevent this exchange from occurring. The resulting effect is a serious constriction or even total failure to establish a relationship.

When the individual experiences serious disruption in abstract thought patterns, speech patterns are likely to reflect the degree of chaos and fragmentation that the client experiences. Communication disorders can occur either because the individual is unable to organize his language properly or because a private language has developed. Inability to organize language properly can result from an association disorder or the loss of logical thought processes that occurs as autistic thinking develops. For example, a client who had begun to experience more symptoms told the nurse that he had begun to read normal words, like "China," as "C-hina." He wished to pronounce words in this manner, but doing so had a special meaning. He could not explain further. The individual fails to use conceptually based language patterns and may break speech into segments or fragments. As the breakdown of ideas and their expression continues, a single word or phrase may come to represent a whole meaning to the person. The person may feel he has communicated adequately but fails to be understood by the listener. Table 17-5 describes the most common language disorders.

Other intellectual disturbances. In addition to the assessment of thought processes, perceptual difficulties, and communication disorders in the suspicious client, it is important to evaluate other parameters of intellectual functioning. Clients with a low level of intellectual ability may never have developed intellectually beyond primitive thinking characterized by concreteness and magical thinking. Such thought processes in a mentally retarded individual may be normal. Disorders of orientation can have an organic or psychological basis. Orientation to person, place, and time is the normal state but is influenced by multiple factors. For example, a client who is suspicious and withdrawn, socially isolated, and preoccupied with hallucinatory experiences may know who he is and where he is but have no clear idea about the month or year.

A disturbance in the client's level of consciousness and ability to remember, particularly an abrupt change in these functions, may indicate a primary organic disease process rather than a schizophrenic delusional disorder. Further neurological evaluation may be indicated.

When clients demonstrate severe impairment in attention span or ability to concentrate, they are experiencing severe anxiety and may be delusional, experiencing hallucinations or other disturbances in the thinking process.

❊ *Social dimension.* Persons who trust readily show a willingness to meet others, feel relaxed and comfortable in making approaches, know that they have something of value to offer, and demonstrate some enthusiasm for doing so by displaying expressions of interest in another's feelings and reactions.

Social adjustment needs to be assessed by exploring specific details of the individual's life. For example, clients who have very few social contacts may respond to questions with "Oh, I don't do anything," or ultimately by admitting, "Oh, I watch the afternoon 'soaps.'" These comments can be explored further by assessing the level of involvement the client can maintain. Assessment includes evaluating both the client's current and premorbid adjustment. Previous levels of adjustment can predict, to some

IMPAIRED VERBAL COMMUNICATION

DEFINITION

State in which an individual experiences a decreased or absent ability to use or understand language in human interaction.

DEFINING CHARACTERISTICS

Physical Dimension
  Stuttering
  Slurring
  Whispering
  Fragmented sentences
  Deafness
  Dyspnea
Emotional Dimension
  *Angry and hostile
  Suspicious
  *Ambivalent
  *Facial expression incongruent with verbal content
Intellectual Dimension
  Illogical ideas (loose associations)
  Autistic thinking
  Distractable
  Disoriented
  Confused
  Loss of memory
  *Hallucinations
  *Delusions
  Inability to speak dominant language
  Speaks or verbalizes with difficulty
  Does not or cannot speak
  Difficulty forming words or sentences
  Difficulty expressing thoughts verbally
  Inappropriate verbalizations
Social Dimension
  *Isolates self from others
  *Minimal feedback from others
Spiritual Dimension
  Despair

Adapted from North American Nursing Diagnosis Association Classification of Nursing Diagnosis: Proceedings of the seventh conference, St. Louis, 1987, The C.V. Mosby Co.
*Indicates characteristics in addition to those defined by NANDA.

degree, the client's potential. A positive change in social adjustment skills may indicate that the client is able to cope with the expansion of his social network. He may be receptive to socialization or job training programs that he previously refused. A client's refusal to participate or withdrawal may be viewed as one means of coping with an environment that seems overwhelming. Assessing the client's apparent "readiness" for rehabilitation programs is essential to successfully engaging the client at the appropriate time. Equally important is that the nurse recognize the value social and work programs can have in the overall improvement of the client's health.

Interpersonal trust plays a significant role in the successful establishment and maintenance of a social network. The nurse assesses the client's social network, his contacts with relatives, friends, and neighbors, through which he maintains a social identity and receives emotional support, material aid, services, and information and develops new social contacts.[29] The establishment and maintenance of a social network is closely related to one's ability to trust. For individuals who experience pathological mistrust, a successful interaction as superficial as purchasing gasoline may be impossible.

One's concept of self is defined in part by responses from others. When early childhood relationships create much anxiety, the socialization process is disrupted, leading to inadequate social development. Socially inadequate development resulting in the person's being unable to maintain communication with others can lead to private thinking, unique ways of experiencing the world, and a loss of the emotional meaning of social experiences. Socially accepted attitudes and roles may never be learned or can become distorted and are experienced by the client as loneliness, social isolation, withdrawal, and dependence. The disordered interpersonal and object relations of the client do not result in a total rejection of social relatedness but are often characterized by an intense wish for, and an equally intense fear of, close relationships with other people, a need-fear dilemma.

Spiritual dimension. The healthy, trusting individual may recognize a sense of spirituality as a natural part of his existence, providing a sense of meaning to life. For the trusting individual, reaffirmation of relatedness to a higher being is facilitated by interaction and communication with others. Through relationships, the individual is able to maintain the sense of identity and inner strength necessary to cope with the stressors of normal development and the demands of human existence. When stresses become most severe, it is not unusual for a healthy person to seek spiritual connectedness as a source of support and guidance. Crises may produce opportunities for spiritual growth.

Individuals experiencing pathological mistrust are, in a major way, cut off from opportunities to reestablish a sense of being connected to a larger universe. The individual has lost a feeling of connectedness with significant others in his environment. Therefore he no longer has access to resources critical for maintaining trust. When mistrust is severe, the individual experiences a loss of the meaning to life. This experience can lead to despair, hopelessness, and withdrawal to the point of "feeling dead" while living.

The individual who begins to experience disintegration of self-image and with it a loss of the personal meaning to life will usually struggle against the powerful feelings of potential doom and despair. The person may not be clearly aware of the subtle changes that occur in thinking processes, emotional experiences, and changing modes of interaction. Some individuals may begin to seek religious groups and organizations as a means to "shore up" the self-concept, to cope with a sense of impending doom, and to remain connected with a purpose to life. The effort to maintain self-identity often occurs in the prepsychotic phase of illness. Experiences directly related to losing touch with reality, such as uncanny feelings or *déjà vu* experiences need to be explored. A rational explanation to the mistrusting client is to place these experiences in a religious context. The individual may suddenly begin to express increased interest in spiritual, religious, and philosophical questions, hoping to relieve the intense discomfort. It is not unusual for the client to change his religious affiliation, disclaim former beliefs, and insist that finally he has "found the truth"; no other approach is right, and he has been misled, fooled, or deceived by significant others.

The first task of the nurse is directed toward gaining some understanding of a client's long-standing religious beliefs and values, as contrasted with beliefs that have developed as a consequence of personality disintegration. The client may have developed a complex system of beliefs, well supported by Biblical teaching, or may have adopted philosophical positions that have been taken out of context.

The nurse needs to also be aware of the potential for suicide in clients who suffer a profound sense of isolation and meaninglessness in life. Suicidal behaviors in such clients are likely to be successful, since motivation for suicide is rarely directed toward efforts to reestablish a connectedness to others but more toward acknowledging the feelings of "being dead." Suicidal behavior may be impulsive; it may be difficult to recognize the danger signs.

Measurement tools. The Interpersonal Trust Scale[35a] based on social learning theory, is directed toward measuring general trust expectancies rather than more specific behavioral manifestations of trust. Another scale of general interest is the Trust Scale for Nurses.[46] This scale consists of ten items, six of which are a subscale directed toward measuring the nurse's trust of clients and four of which are a subscale directed toward measuring the nurse's trust of other nurses.

Analysis

Nursing diagnosis. The following list provides examples of NANDA-accepted nursing diagnoses with causative statements.

1. Noncompliance with prescribed medication regimen related to thinking the medication is poisoned
2. Disturbance in self-concept related to distorted body image
3. Potential for violence related to hallucinatory voices
4. Noncompliance related to impotence associated with antipsychotic medications
5. Sleep pattern disturbance related to fears associated with delusions
6. Alteration in thought processes related to delusions
7. Sensory-perceptual alteration: hallucinations related to anxiety associated with multiple stressors
8. Impaired verbal communication related to loose associations
9. Ineffective coping: hostile behavior related to fear of others
10. Social isolation related to extreme suspiciousness

Impaired verbal communication, sensory perceptual alterations, and alterations in thought processes are three nursing diagnoses approved by NANDA that apply to a person who mistrusts. The defining characteristics of the nursing diagnoses are listed in the boxes on the opposite page, at right, and p. 352.

The following Case Example illustrates characteristics of the nursing diagnosis of impaired verbal communication.

Case Example

Alan was brought to the hospital by the police. He had been found in a restricted area near the airport hiding in the underbrush. Alan was dirty and unshaven and wore torn clothing. In the hospital admitting office Alan sat rigidly in one corner watching everyone in the room, his eyes reflecting sometimes fear and sometimes sadness. When asked questions, Alan made some mumbling sounds, from which no words could be understood. It was later discovered that Alan had been missing from home for 2 days. Before abruptly leaving home, Alan had spent the previous 3 weeks sitting alone in his room. He had refused food and would talk to no one.

SENSORY PERCEPTUAL ALTERATIONS

DEFINITION

State in which an individual experiences a change in the amount, pattern, or interpretation of incoming stimuli accompanied by a diminished, exaggerated, distorted, or impaired response to such stimuli.

DEFINING CHARACTERISTICS

Physical Dimension
Apathy
Hypervigilance
Body image changes
Body posture alterations
Sleep pattern disturbances
*Muscle tension
Altered sensory activity
Restlessness
Change in usual response to stimuli

Emotional Dimension
Emotional lability
Anxiety, fear
Apathy
Irritability
*Feeling expressed incongruent with reality

Intellectual Dimension
*Distractable
Disorientation to time, place, or person
*Non-reality-based thinking
Hallucinations
Altered conceptual or abstraction ability
Altered ability to problem solve
Altered communication

Social Dimension
Inappropriate social interaction
Change in behavior pattern

Spiritual Dimension
*Alteration in previously held religious ideas

Adapted from North American Nursing Diagnosis Association Classification of Nursing Diagnosis: Proceedings of the seventh conference, St. Louis, 1987, The C.V. Mosby Co.
*Indicates characteristics in addition to those defined by NANDA.

The following Case Example illustrates characteristics of the nursing diagnosis of sensory-perceptual alterations.

Case Example

Peter, a 29-year-old computer programmer, has worked alone in an office in the basement of a large manufacturing firm for the past 7 years. When the firm was bought by another company, Peter was told he could move to Baltimore, the new company headquarters, or he would be given compensatory pay for 6 months, allowing him time to find another job. Having to make such a difficult decision so disturbed Peter that he became unable to concentrate at work and believed the new company president was talking to him through the ventilators and sometimes followed him home. Peter became very tense on the walk home and would turn around to look for the new president and believed he saw a glimpse of a shirt sleeve or hat disappearing around the corner. One evening Peter believed he saw the company president sitting at the kitchen table talking. Peter yelled and screamed in anger and could not be calmed down.

The following Case Example illustrates characteristics of the nursing diagnosis of alteration in thought processes.

Case Example

Ellen, a 20-year-old unemployed woman, lives with her mother. She has been unable to finish high school and has never worked. In the first session with her nurse she says to the nurse, "Can you give me feelings? I have no feelings. I am empty." She goes on to describe in a very disorganized manner that she is more than one Ellen. One Ellen is a famous movie actress, the other is a bad evil person, maybe the devil, and the third is the Ellen sitting in the room. She insists that she knows this because it was reported in a national magazine and furthermore demands that the nurse arrange a television appearance for her so that "The whole world will know."

DSM-III-R diagnoses. The DSM-III-R diagnoses related to schizophrenic and delusional disorders are listed in the box below.

ALTERATION IN THOUGHT PROCESSES

DEFINITION

State in which an individual experiences a disruption in such mental activities as thinking, reality orientation, problem solving, judgment, and comprehension.

DEFINING CHARACTERISTICS

Physical Dimension
*Hypervigilance or hypovigilance
*Catatonic
*Compulsive rituals
 Regression

Emotional Dimension
*Flat facial expression
*Ambivalence
*Inappropriate, unusual, or bizarre emotional expression
 Irritability

Intellectual Dimension
*Does not distinguish between cause and effect
*Loss of ability to categorize logically
 Will not talk
 Delusions
 Distractability
 Disorientation to time, place, or person
 Memory deficits
 Inaccurate interpretation of environment
 Egocentricity
 Inappropriate, nonreality based thinking

Social Dimension
 Inappropriate verbal responses to others
 Behavior of others misunderstood

Spiritual Dimension
*Misinterprets religious teachings
*Religiosity (may believe self to be God or the devil)

Adapted from North American Nursing Diagnosis Association Classification of Nursing Diagnosis: Proceedings of the seventh conference, St. Louis, 1987, The C.V. Mosby Co.
*Indicates characteristics in addition to those defined by NANDA.

DSM-III-R CLASSIFICATIONS RELATED TO SCHIZOPHRENIA AND DELUSIONAL (PARANOID) DISORDERS

SCHIZOPHRENIC DISORDERS

295.1x	Disorganized type
295.2x	Catatonic type
295.3x	Paranoid type
295.9x	Undifferentiated type
295.6x	Residual type

DELUSIONAL (PARANOID) DISORDERS

297.10	Delusional (paranoid) disorder
	Persecutory
	Jealous
	Erotomanic
	Somatic
	Grandiose
	Other

PSYCHOTIC DISORDER
NOT ELSEWHERE CLASSIFIED

295.40	Schizophreniform disorder
295.70	Schizoaffective disorder
298.80	Brief reactive psychosis
297.30	Induced psychotic disorder
298.90	Psychotic disorder not otherwise specified

PERSONALITY DISORDERS

301.00	Paranoid
301.20	Schizoid
301.22	Schizotypal

Adapted from American Psychiatric Association: Diagnostic and statistical manual of mental disorders (DSM-III-R), Washington, D.C., 1987, The Association.

The essential features and manifestations of the features of the disorganized type and paranoid type of schizophrenia and delusional (paranoid) disorder according to the DSM-III-R classification are listed in the following boxes.

Planning

See Table 17-6 for examples of long-term and short-term goals and outcome criteria related to mistrust. These serve as examples of the planning stage in the nursing process.

Implementation

✦ ***Physical dimension.*** Attention is first directed toward meeting the clients physical and safety needs. Clients who have experienced severe symptoms for a long time without care may be suffering from malnutrition, dehydration, infections, and other physical disorders. Facilitating treatment for these physical problems is the first priority. Physical illnesses in conjunction with a psychiatric disorder can produce a synergistic effect of increasing the symptoms of either illness. For example, a mistrusting client who is also diabetic may refuse to eat because she believes her intestines have turned to stone. The resulting physiological imbalances created by refusal to eat may further stimulate other distortions in body image as specific symptoms of hypoglycemia begin to occur. Prompt inter-

---

295.3X SCHIZOPHRENIA, PARANOID TYPE

ESSENTIAL FEATURES

The individual shows a disturbance in thinking characterized by persecutory or grandiose delusions or hallucinations with a persecutory or grandiose content.

MANIFESTATIONS
Physical Dimension

Doubts about gender identity
Violence

Emotional Dimension

Unfocused anxiety
Anger
Argumentativeness
Fear of being thought of as homosexual

Intellectual Dimension

Persecutory delusions
Grandiose delusions
Delusional jealousy
Hallucinations

Social Dimension

Stilted, formal social relations

Adapted from American Psychiatric Association: Diagnostic and statistical manual of mental disorders (DSM-III-R), Washington, D.C., 1987, The Association.

295.1X SCHIZOPHRENIA, DISORGANIZED TYPE

ESSENTIAL FEATURES

The individual shows a disturbance in thinking characterized by incoherence, flat, silly, or inappropriate affect, delusions (nonsystematized), and hallucinations.

MANIFESTATIONS
Physical Dimension

Oddities of behavior (poor or eccentric grooming)
Grimaces
Mannerisms

Emotional Dimension

Flat facial expression
Facial expression incongruous with verbal expression
Silly

Intellectual Dimension

Hypochondriacal complaints
Fragmentary delusions
Hallucinations
Incoherence

Social Dimension

Extreme social withdrawal

Adapted from American Psychiatric Association: Diagnostic and statistical manual of mental disorders (DSM-III-R), Washington, D.C., 1987, The Association.

297.10 DELUSIONAL (PARANOID) DISORDER

ESSENTIAL FEATURES

The individual exhibits delusional system related to themes of jealousy, persecution, body changes, or grandiosity.

MANIFESTATIONS
Physical Dimension

Eccentricities of behavior (for example, wears towel around neck or sunglasses inside, staring)

Emotional Dimension

Appropriate expression based on content of delusion
Resentment and anger
Suspiciousness

Intellectual Dimension

Persistant persecutory delusions
Delusions of jealousy
Grandiosity
Ideas of reference

Social Dimension

Social isolation or seclusiveness
Litigious activities

Adapted from American Psychiatric Association: Diagnostic and statistical manual of mental disorders (DSM-III-R), Washington, D.C., 1987, The Association.

TABLE 17-6 Long-term and short-term goals and outcome criteria related to mistrust

Goals	Outcome Criteria
NURSING DIAGNOSIS: SENSORY-PERCEPTUAL ALTERATIONS: AUDITORY HALLUCINATIONS RELATED TO ANXIETY ASSOCIATED WITH MULTIPLE STRESSORS	
Long-term goals	
To extinguish auditory hallucinations	Recognizes that the voices are not real
	States that he no longer hears voices talking to him
	Recognizes that auditory hallucinations occurred in relationship to high anxiety
To improve ability to concentrate	Stays involved with a task for at least 20 minutes
	Does not describe interruptions in thought processes
To continue taking antipsychotic medications	Expresses recognition that medications alleviate hallucinations
	Asks questions about use of medications
Short-term goals	
To decrease anxiety	Understands hospital routine
	Feels comfortable in a "protected" environment
	Describes "feeling better" in response to antipsychotic medications
	Expresses verbally a feeling of confusion about the reality of voices heard
	Uses effective methods to decrease anxiety
To discuss hallucinations and accompanying feelings	Describes content of auditory hallucinations
	Describes feelings when hearing voices
	Accepts support from other people to ignore instructions from hallucinations
	Controls impulsive behaviors
To participate in ward meetings	Attends group therapy three times per week
	Responds in ways that demonstrate attention maintenance
	Avoids talking to hallucinatory voices in group meetings
NURSING DIAGNOSIS: IMPAIRED VERBAL COMMUNICATION RELATED TO LOOSE ASSOCIATIONS AND FRAGMENTED SPEECH	
Long-term goals	
To discuss premorbid functioning	Discusses habits, interests, activities, previous medical treatment
To develop ability to express some thoughts and ideas	Articualtes words clearly
	Talks in sentences
	Makes requests for basic needs
To demonstrate consistent verbal and nonverbal behavior	Articulates feelings clearly, accompanied by appropriate expression of affect
	Expresses both positive and negative feelings
Short-term goals	
To feel less fearful in new environment	Responds to brief, explanatory statements
	Appears more relaxed, with less rigid posture
To interact with others	Accepts information about medical tests ordered
	Asks questions about hospital routine
	Tolerates activity group three times per week
	Spends at least 2 hours daily in dayroom
	Holds brief conversations with other clients or staff
To communicate with logical associations	Speaks without loose associations or fragmentation

ventions to ensure adequate nutritional intake are necessary for maintenance of physical balance. Psychological interventions can be initiated after the life-threatening physical illness is controlled.

Occasionally the nurse meets clients who have developed bizarre or socially unacceptable means of meeting basic needs, for example, eating with fingers when a fork is indicated. These behaviors are sometimes a result of desocialization, which can happen in the hospital or at home, especially when the individual has little contact with or feedback from others about his behavior. The nurse may wish to implement a program to change these behaviors, which can be as simple as reminding the client of alternatives. The change may require more intensive behavior modification programs, with a reinforcement system to encourage systematic behavioral change.

In the hospital, several measures are taken to prevent self-destructive behavior, including checking the client's personal belongings for any instruments that can be used to inflict physical harm, such as razors, matches and cigarettes, and even forks and knives, as well as ensuring that the length of electrical cords on lamps is as short as possible, using unbreakable glass in the windows or mirrors, and maintaining furniture in excellent repair so that sharp or broken edges do not exist. If the client is treated in an outpatient setting, continual awareness of the client's ability to meet self-care needs is relevant to maintaining the living situation. Self-destructive behaviors in an outpatient setting may be more subtle and nonspecific but require an equal amount of attention. For instance, a client who repeatedly exposes himself to harsh weather without proper clothing or who walks alone for hours at night may be passively self-destructive rather than actively suicidal. Attention to these behaviors and appropriate intervention, such as facilitating a change in the treatment setting, may be necessary.

A common difficulty for suspicious clients is the ability to maintain proper sleeping and eating patterns. For the acutely psychotic individual, sleep may be disrupted by nightmares or severe anxiety, so that the individual cannot fall asleep, or it may be that the person feels more comfortable in a less stimulating environment. Reversals of the sleep-wake pattern may be seen. Sleeping too much may be a way for the individual to manage difficulties relating to others. Of primary importance is to understand in a more precise way the cause of difficulties experienced by the client. It is usually advisable not to encourage the use of medication for sleep but to provide whatever intervention is necessary in response to the cause of the sleeping problem. An active program during the day that keeps the client involved and prevents retreats to bed for daytime naps can also facilitate normal sleep patterns, as can vigorous physical exercise. In a hospital or day treatment program, these activities can be part of the overall treatment program. Referral to rehabilitation programs, job training programs, sheltered workshops, or volunteer activities may be necessary for persons out of the hospital to maintain a daily life structure that enables more normal sleeping habits.

Body image distortions and identity confusion are best managed by helping the client describe his perception as concretely as possible. Once the distortions are understood, the nurse can facilitate correction by suggesting alternate ways to understand the client's experience. For instance, the nurse observed a 20-year-old client's acne but had not discussed it with her. When the client explains that her face is rotting away the nurse can express doubt about her perception or present reality. Helping the client maintain a separate sense of self can be facilitated by using proper pronouns to clarify a given situation. For instance, "I am Jean Johnson, your nurse, and I have come to help you, George, prepare for breakfast" encourages a recognition and reinforcement of separateness. It may be important to continually remind the client who is around him and what activities are in progress. Specific information, given in anticipation of activities or changes at the time of the event can be helpful in maintaining a sense of control and a sense of self-identity for the client. Orientation to surroundings is helpful for clients who have a sense of identity confusion, for example, "You and I are

going to walk down this long hallway to the very end to my office." Anticipatory guidance, as in this example, can facilitate the client's ability to cope with events that seem distorted and unreal. Realizing the degree of body image distortion may require the nurse to make inferences from observed behaviors, since the client may not realize or be able to articulate his difficulty. Seeing the client in inappropriate clothing may precipitate a discussion of how the client views himself. Sexual identity problems are often not addressed openly or directly by clients. The client may express a fear of being homosexual as one way to relay concerns about sexuality. Providing information about normal sexual functions and behavior or discussions with the client about normal body and sexual functions can be exceedingly important.

Psychotropic medications are a common intervention for coping with distortions. Chapter 22 provides more specific information about the use of medications.

Emotional dimension. The mistrusting individual may be totally out of touch with any feelings and thus cannot express them accurately or is so fearful of his own or the other's reactions that he relies on a number of mechanisms to hide, distort, or miscommunicate feelings. Interventions in the emotional dimension are directed toward understanding the client's emotional reactions and facilitating his interpretation of them, by recognizing and acknowledging them and ultimately supporting the client's ability to accurately communicate them in a culturally acceptable manner. To do this, the nurse needs to attend to a number of factors that inhibit full expression of feelings, such as poor social skills, lack of self-confidence, a fear of rejection or punishment, the client's need to protect himself from emotional hurt, and memories of past unpleasant emotional experiences.

Nonverbal communication takes on a profound meaning: body postures, amount of eye contact, physical proximity, and the degree of apparent tension in the nonverbal exchange are all measures of how the relationship is progressing. The nurse maintains an emotional posture of accessibility, respect, and interest. She directs her efforts toward stimulating interest in the client and not filling in silences with chatter or talking about herself as a means to manage her own feelings of discomfort in the silence. The client easily recognizes these ploys and may respond with increased withdrawal. The nurse may be able to facilitate the relationship by using a number of nonverbal methods of relating to the client, such as looking at magazines, playing games, or going for a walk. The manner in which questions are phrased is important. Open-ended questions or comments, such as "Tell me about your day's activities," and then a pause to communicate interest and expectation of an answer are usually more productive than direct questions. The client plays a key role in the pace of closeness that develops. The nurse may need to help facilitate the expression of feelings by noticing subtle changes in expression.

As the client is able to more comfortably relate to the nurse in an individual setting, the behavior can be generalized to other interactions. The client may be more accepting of the perspective of others and can gradually learn to more accurately identify his own feelings and express them to others. Self-identity is then strengthened, which initiates a cycle of increasingly healthy expression of feelings. As the client begins to gain confidence in being able to accurately reflect his own feelings, he is rewarded by accurate responses from others.

Clients who express emotional reactions with ambivalence, flat affect, or inappropriate affect are using these means to keep their emotional reactions hidden, distorted, unclear, vague, or diffused. Behaviors such as compulsive rituals, negativism, and overcompliance can create serious restrictions on the client's ability to perform activities of daily living. When this occurs, active intervention by the nurse may be required to ensure task accomplishment. Firm limit setting, with a focus on reality and recognition that certain tasks need to be done, can be adequate intervention. At times, the nurse may be required to provide specific, detailed, step-by-step directions or to actually do the task for the client. When a client's feelings and thoughts are exceedingly disorganized, the ability to make decisions is severely impaired. It is impossible for the client to decide which of the massive number of inputs requires a response. When such circumstances prevail, the nurse needs to limit choices. As the client becomes increasingly organized, the choices can be expanded. Gradually, as increasing integration of feelings and thoughts occurs, the client becomes more capable of self-care activities and will be able to choose for himself.

Principles to keep in mind when interacting with clients who have difficulty with expression of affect are the following:

1. The angry client is rarely angry at the nurse personally but may be projecting feelings from another relationship. It may be safest for the client to express anger at the nurse rather than the individual who actually generated the anger. If the nurse becomes angry with the client, she tells him so in a matter-of-fact way without making him feel guilty or depriving him of care.

2. The nurse does not encourage the client to express feelings unless she is comfortable with the client's expression of feeling and can be available to listen.

3. Expression of feelings may not always be therapeutic. Catharsis may be good in certain situations, but expression of the same feelings over and over can serve as a constant forcus on the feeling and become merely ruminations.

4. Too much focus on negative feeling may reinforce them or bring them into focus to the point that the client feels a need to destructively act out rather than to cope with intense feelings over a period of time.

5. Emotional expression and the experience of intense feelings can be painful, even for the client who seems out of contact with reality.

6. Clients may experience shame or be embarrassed by expressing feelings. The nurse needs to be aware of these reactions and provide appropriate interventions, such as privacy to discuss significant feelings in a quiet and comfortable atmosphere and offering emotional support and sensitivity.

✳ *Intellectual dimension.* Sometimes clarification is difficult, since the client's ability to communicate is severely limited. The nurse needs to express clearly that she does not understand, which she can do gently, without emotionally rejecting the client as an individual. Both the client and the nurse will need to continue trying to communicate. Sometimes the communication is similar to understanding a foreign language—a portion is comprehensible, but the whole does not fall together into a sensible meaning. The nurse needs to listen carefully and then share what is understood. The accuracy of understanding is checked with the client. If the content of the communication remains unclear, the feelings relayed may be more obvious than the verbal message. Recognizing and acknowledging the feelings the client is expressing can facilitate the understanding of meaning of the message.

Hallucinations are a particularly disturbing experience for the client. Such experiences are often frightening and can frequently lead to increased anxiety and further distortions of reality. Hallucinations may be a means of expressing feelings that are otherwise unacceptable to the client. If, when clients describe hallucinations, the nurse is judgmental or attempts to argue with the client, the result may be a further decrease in trust and confidence. On the other hand, if the nurse encourages the client to share his perceptions, the client can begin to build a trusting relationship with the nurse. The nurse can aid reality testing for the client by acknowledging that, although the perceptions are real to the client, they are not shared by others. With sufficient observation and interaction, the nurse may be able to recognize the precipitants of the client's increased anxiety resulting in hallucinations. Once a pattern is identified, the nurse can discuss the precipitants and encourage the client to express whatever feelings were being experienced. Eventually the client may be able to realize the relationship between the hallucination and particular strong feelings. The nurse can cast doubt on the hallucination without directly challenging the client's experience. Some clients readily recognize hallucinations as "out of reality" and will describe this experience. Even so, the client may feel out of control. Severe hallucinations, such as command auditory hallucinations, can cause the client to lose control of his behavior. Usually the nurse can recognize this and intervene before the client loses control by setting firm limits or moving the client to a quieter place. Setting up competing stimuli such as whistling or humming can interrupt the hallucination. Engaging in conversation, a game, or going for a walk can help divert the client's attention to something else.

Delusional thoughts, from the client's perspective, are real and seem absolutely true, regardless of how far-fetched the ideas. Arguing with the client about the reality of the delusional content will only reinforce his wish to convince others of the belief and can facilitate a solidification of the delusional system. A delusional system develops as a defense that serves to protect the client from formidable feelings. With time the nurse can learn what symbolic meaning the delusion probably contains for the client and may be able to respond to the underlying theme. For example, a client who had become convinced that out-of-state cars followed him and were after him may actually have been expressing the wish for his family, who lived out of state, to pay more attention to him and not reject him. When this client began to discuss the idea that cars were following him, the nurse, understanding the meaning, can refocus the discussion of his feelings of loneliness and rejection. It is very important to let the client know that, although his interpretation of reality seems right, others have arrived at a different conclusion. The nurse shares her idea that she interprets information in a different way and may make suggestions that cast doubt on the validity of the delusional thought process without directly challenging it.

Clients with paranoid delusions are generally suspicious and will promptly reject any questioning of their thought processes. They may consider anyone who challenges them to be dangerous. Communication with the very suspicious and delusional person needs to be direct, clear, and concrete. Providing accurate data as straightforwardly as possible is essential, as is being clear about boundaries. The nurse's use of "I" and "you" helps such clients differentiate themselves from the surroundings that seem so dangerous. The extremely paranoid client also needs to maintain a sense of being in control. Clear messages about what is expected, what are "rules," and what the individual has a choice about let the paranoid person know exactly what he can and cannot do. This is beneficial to prevent the client's feeling that he has somehow been wronged by the staff or the nurse. For example, a paranoid client, upset that his primary nurse had been ill, asked her if he could be transferred to another unit. He, of course, knew that this was possible. The nurse responded to the situation by agreeing that, if he wished, he could be transferred, but she did not think it would be a good idea, since he had got to know people on this unit and she felt that they had been working well together, despite her having been sick and taken 2 days off. The nurse suggested to the client that he think about it for a while and they could talk more about it later. Later in the day the nurse approached the client, who said to her, "Oh, you are right. I guess I had better stay here."

Misinterpretation of reality as a consequence of disorders in thought processes can result in impulsive or autistic behaviors. It is not always possible for the client to stop autistic behavior, even at the request of the nurse. Clients rarely refuse to comply not because of obstinacy but because they cannot as a result of their own perceptions of reality. If the behavior is not harmful to the client or others nearby, it may not be helpful to persist in attempting to have the client stop. A person will not do something he absolutely does not want to unless physical force is used. The nurse can be prepared to make a decision about whether the behavior is destructive enough to require physical force. If the nurse decides that the client is not harming himself or others, she will not pressure the client to the point where he responds by lashing out. The nurse attends to the behavioral cues that indicate the client is unwilling to cooperate and tries again later. As a last resort, it may occasionally be necessary to restrain a client for his own or others' protection.

As the client's thought disorder begins to disappear, it is important for the nurse to adopt a plan of care that further builds on the changes in behavior. More opportunities for task mastery can be provided. Gradually the client becomes able to accomplish increasingly complex tasks and can build positive feelings about himself from experiences such as occupational therapy or tasks such as keeping his own room in order. The use of these interventions can rebuild self-esteem and help the client obtain personal satisfaction. Another purpose for these therapeutic interventions is to provide the nurse with opportunities to observe the strengths and weaknesses of the client in areas such as manual skill, concentration and attention, and ability to follow directions. Information of this nature is exceedingly valuable in making realistic plans for rehabilitation and can provide data to determine the client's readiness for alternative opportunities to develop skills. Sometimes previously unknown organic deficits may be recognized, a special talent noticed, or a specific limitation in ability to relate to others noted. Observations can be discussed with the client, to further understand what has been noticed. Knowing a client's limitations is important to ensure that the client is not frustrated by being asked to perform tasks he cannot do.

✤ *Social dimension.* Initial efforts are directed toward reestablishing interpersonal contact on a one-to-one basis. This may require consistent, repeated, brief approaches to initiate social participation and facilitate communication. Gradually the client's relationships with others can be expanded.

When it is clear that there is a pathological family pattern of interaction and communication, treatment of the whole family may be indicated, with efforts directed toward repatterning the communication and role relationships. (See Chapter 29 for a discussion of family therapy.) It is not unusual for the family to experience guilt, self-blame, anger, frustration, and disappointment with the ill member. These feelings need to be recognized, acknowledged, and explored by the nurse. Families who blame themselves for the client's difficulty are particularly sensitive to comments that may implicate them as responsible for the behaviors of the client. The nurse needs to be aware of this possibility and approach the family with sensitivity to the difficulties they have experienced in their relationships with the mistrusting client. Krauss and Slavinsky[25] point out the importance of establishing a working alliance with the family, especially the family of the client with a long-term disorder, to exchange information, provide guidance and support, relieve the family of guilt and responsibility, and prevent further deterioration of the family unit. Families of the mistrusting client often are isolated and do not have an adequate system of support, as a result of having to cope with the client's unusual behaviors. The financial burdens of providing treatment can become overwhelming for the family as well as decreasing the resources available for social interaction with others. Interventions may need to be directed toward helping the family of the client to reestablish previous network ties or to develop new ones. Families may profit from referral to self-help groups or family support groups. Providing families with information about the illness and helping them develop skills in regard to management of daily activities is beneficial.

Clients may need help establishing themselves in the community after discharge from the hospital. Planning for community living includes attention to the basic minimal requirements: some form of economic support including sufficient resources for food, a safe place to live, and referral to some form of follow-up treatment including a means of obtaining medications. The nurse can be involved in any of these aspects of implementation. Ideally the client is also taught about the use of his medication and a number of other self-care skills that may be lacking. The nurse's referral to other nurses and other professionals who will be providing further treatment includes the assessment of the client's daily living skills and any special techniques that have been found helpful in facilitating accomplishment of self-care tasks. Nurses who work with clients in the community focus their attention on helping the client build a social network. Often the client's social network is very small, including perhaps a visit to the therapist in an outpatient clinic and occasionally interacting with a family member. Expanding the client's social network can be a slow process but proceeds gradually and consistently. It is generally recommended that clients who have demonstrated vulnerability to the stress of change need to be encouraged to make no more than one major life change at any given time. Abrupt changes may actually precipitate an exacerbation of symptoms. Careful monitoring and timing are relevant to the interventions. Some clients need firm expectations and specific goals set for expansion of their social network.

Often the client and frequently the nurse fail to recognize the importance of integration into and support from the community to enhance coping mechanisms. The importance of a structured daily life has been recognized as a way to prevent regression. The nurse who monitors the status of clients living in the community needs to place an emphasis on the monitoring of activities of daily living. Support for establishing a social network is often maintained in a concrete and specific way in the group or individual therapy provided in outpatient settings.

An individual's work is a central theme in his definition of self. Even persons who have retired or are not currently employed think of themselves as "a retired shoemaker" or say, "I was a steel worker before the plant closed." Work not only provides a source of income but also can be a major source of social interaction, a means of self-satisfaction, and a way to feel one has contributed to society. Many clients who experience symptoms such as hallucinations or some other thought disorder can, despite these difficulties, maintain productive employment. Those who cannot retain a job may need referral to rehabilitation programs or sheltered work environments. An important task for the nurse is not only to facilitate appropriate referral but also to support communication between the various service providers and aspects of treatment.

✿ *Spiritual dimension.* Work with the mistrusting client in the spiritual dimension is directed toward facilitating a sense of relatedness and meaning to life. Often this begins by establishing a sense of connectedness in a relationship of trust. Facilitating the client's indirect expression of feelings through creative arts, poetry, or music is a positive way for the nurse to make contact with a deeply disturbed client.

The nurse, in her effort to differentiate between the client's psychotic processes and long-standing religious beliefs, needs to have some general knowledge of the major emphasis in various religious denominations. She may find her own philosophy of life and religious beliefs challenged by the client. The nurse recognizes that maintaining a personal connection with the client is more therapeutic than is a debate over specific beliefs. The nurse may openly acknowledge differences in religious teachings without presenting this as a barrier to a therapeutic relationship with the client.

Interpersonal relationships the client has had may be lost or change dramatically as a consequence of pathological mistrust. Once having regained a reality base, clients may be ashamed or embarrassed by the behaviors they demonstrated and may need help understanding the impact of these behaviors on others. The client may also experience feelings of loss and grief when more realistically able to articulate his own strengths and limitations. The nurse will need to facilitate the client's grieving process while helping the client establish realistic life goals for himself.

INTERACTION WITH A MISTRUSTING CLIENT

Nurse: (In medication room, about to give fluphenazine hydrochloride [Prolixin decanoate] injection) Mr. Evans, this is your usual medication. The amount you will get is what you have had before.

Client: I've been wondering, is there a way that someone can be killed with no trace of what caused it afterward?

Nurse: What are you referring to, Mr. Evans—this medication?

Client: Well. . . .(pause) I was just wondering about, you know, my father died . . . .

Nurse: I don't know of any way to kill someone without there being evidence of what caused the person's death. I am giving you the medicine to help you, not to hurt you. What about your father?

Client: Well, he was a good man and yet he died at such a young age. The Mafia must know something. He was such a good man, God would not punish him.

Nurse: As we've talked about before, Mr. Evans, your father died from a heart attack. . .is it 20 years ago now?

Client: Yes.

Nurse: The anniversary of his death is next week, isn't it?

Client: Yes, I always dedicate that day to him. I go to his grave and say a prayer.

Nurse: I guess you must feel it was unfair that he died so young. Do you feel very sad at this time of year?

Client: Yes, I do. Can I call you if I want to talk some more?

This client demonstrates his lack of trust and severe paranoia by indicating indirectly that he does not feel very safe with the nurse who has been giving him the same medication for several months. His delusion soon becomes quite apparent.

The nurse approaches the situation through clear, direct questions that facilitate a better understanding of what the client is thinking. The client's concerns are responded to specifically and directly. It is important to assure him of his safety and to emphasize the present reality. By stating facts in a nonargumentative tone and focusing on obtaining more information from the client, the nurse is better able to give accurate feedback. Sometimes the client's delusional thoughts confuse past memories, present activity, and thoughts about future plans. Here, the nurse has helped the client put each in proper perspective.

Ultimately the nurse helps the client identify some of the feelings that are associated with the discussion and may have contributed to the expression of delusional ideas. Over time, the client can better understand the relationship between his feeling state and thought process and he may eventually draw conclusions that include both the real facts and the real feelings.

Evaluation

In acute treatment settings, the mistrusting client may demonstrate dramatic behavioral changes, among which are significant increase in reality orientation, increased ability to articulate feelings with appropriate affect, improved decision-making ability, and increased ability to tolerate interpersonal relationships. The client may be unable to acknowledge or directly articulate changes in a specific manner but will clearly demonstrate more healthy behaviors.

NURSING PROCESS SUMMARY: MISTRUST

ASSESSMENT

Physical Dimension
Failure to make eye contact
Quick, darting eye movements
Furtive glances over shoulder or behind self
Body image distortions
Failure to eat and take medicine
Inability to sleep
Sitting on edge of chair

Emotional Dimension
Anger   Ambivalent feelings
Feeling threatened   Feeling of rejection
Helplessness   Feeling that people
Anxiety   cannot be trusted
Insecurity   Feeling of aloneness
Guilt   Aloofness
Fear of loss of control   Secretiveness

Intellectual Dimension
Irrational thinking   Belittling
Perceptual disturbances—   Accusations
   illusions, delusions,   Impaired memory
   or hallucinations   Disorientation
Inability to think abstractly Inflexible thinking
Negativism   Difficulty learning
Criticism   Preoccupation with
Blaming   physical symptoms

Social Dimension
Poor self-concept
Role conflicts and distortions
Lack of involvement with others
Lack of involvement in activities
Limited social network
Decreased mutual interaction
Increased dependence
Inadequate social skills
Isolation
Social withdrawal

Spiritual Dimension
Loss of connectedness with significant others
Loss of meaning to life with feelings of despair and withdrawal

ANALYSIS
See the nursing diagnosis section on p. 351.

PLANNING AND IMPLEMENTATION

Physical Dimension
Meet physical and safety needs.
Manage hypochondriacal symptoms.
Provide behavior modification to promote self-care.
Prevent self-destructive behavior.
Promote adequate eating and sleeping patterns.
Encourage physical exercise.
Refer to job training and rehabilitation programs.
Provide information about normal sexual functioning.
Monitor psychotropic medications.
Respect privacy and distance.
Avoid touching
Restrain client for protection of client or others when
   out of control.

Emotional Dimension
Recognize and acknowledge emotional reactions.
Support client's ability to accurately communicate
   feelings of anxiety, mistrust.
Attend to factors that inhibit expression of feelings of
   anxiety, mistrust.
Provide privacy for expression of feelings.
Encourage expression of feelings such as anxiety and
   fears.

Intellectual Dimension
Orient client to surroundings.
Use clear, direct, concrete communication.
Ask for clarification to understand meaning of private
   language.
Recognize precipitants of hallucinations (anxiety).
Distract client from hallucinations by conversation, a
   game, or other diversion.
Decode meaning of delusions.
Focus on reality.
Accept resistances in the relationship.
Set limits on negativism.
Avoid confrontation.
Teach relaxation techniques.

Continued.

NURSING PROCESS SUMMARY: MISTRUST—cont'd

Social Dimension

Develop a one-to-one relationship to establish a basis for trust.

Reestablish interpersonal contact with consistent, brief approaches.

Include family in treatment regimen, for example, family therapy.

Plan for community living.

Promote social activities.

Provide work that is self-satisfying to enhance self-concept.

Prevent withdrawal and isolation.

Spiritual Dimension

Facilitate a sense of relatedness to others.

Promote indirect expression of feelings through creative arts.

Help client cope with feelings of loss and despair by promoting realistic hope to enhance life goals.

EVALUATION

Evaluation is based on the degree, intensity, and appropriateness of mistrust demonstrated in the client's behavior. Progress is reflected when the client identifies situations where he feels mistrust, when he has learned to validate his perceptions with a trusted person, and when he interacts socially with others.

BRIEF REVIEW

Trust and mistrust are influencing factors in personality structure and in relationships. The ability to trust is strongly influenced by early parent-child relationships, family relationships, and inherited traits. Trust develops from consistent, reliable interpersonal exchanges in which the individual feels accepted, understood, and valued. Trusting relationships are maintained by a willingness to evaluate one's own behavior, the behavior of others, and the circumstances of the interaction in an objective and realistic manner. The individual's ability to trust may change or be modified in response to significant or traumatic events in adulthood. Healthy individuals establish relationships, assuming others are basically trustworthy, but are able to rationally discriminate and evaluate this during the process of interaction.

Mistrust can develop into a pathological state whereby interaction with others is characterized by suspiciousness of others, withdrawal, and difficulty in interpersonal relationships. Mistrust is seen in doubts about one's ability to communicate accurately, to understand others, and to predict the potential outcome of interactions. Multiple theoretical approaches have been applied to understanding the pathological states, such as schizophrenia and paranoid disorders, in which mistrust is a predominant characteristic. No single theoretical approach has been accepted as fully explaining the multiple clinical syndromes in which a defective interpretation or loss of contact with reality is one of the significant aspects of the clinical picture.

The nurse approaches work with mistrusting clients in a systematic, goal-oriented manner, facilitating the client's movement toward increasing healthy behaviors. As the nurse makes an assessment and begins to plan and implement treatment, she can relate her knowledge of the client to theories of behavior. Evaluation of care includes reviewing the client's movement toward health and planning for further treatment, if indicated.

REFERENCES AND SUGGESTED READINGS

1. American Psychiatric Association: Diagnostic and statistical manual of mental disorders, ed. 3, Washington, D.C., 1987, The association.
2. Andreasen, N.: The broken brain: the biological revolution in psychiatry, New York, 1984, Harper & Row, Publishers.
3. Andreasen, N.C., and others: Hemispheric asymmetries and schizophrenia, American Journal of Psychiatry **139**:427, 1982.
4. Baxter, C., and Melnechuk, T.: Perspectives in schizophrenia research, New York, 1980, Raven Press.
5. Beard, M.T.: Trust, life events, and risk factors among adults, Advances in Nursing Science **4**(4):26, 1982.
6. Bellack, A.: Schizophrenia: treatment, management and rehabilitation, Orlando, Fla., 1984, Grune & Stratton, Inc.
7. Callaway, E., and Naghdi, S.: An information processing model for schizophrenia, Archives of General Psychiatry **39**:339, 1982.
8. Carpenter, W.T., Murphy, D., and Wyatt, R.J.: Platelet monoamine oxidase activity in acute schizophrenia, American Journal of Psychiatry **132**:438, 1975.
9. Caton, C.: Management of chronic schizophrenia, New York, 1984, Oxford University Press.
10. Colliton, M.A.: The spiritual dimension of nursing. In Beland, I., and Passos, J.: Clinical nursing, ed. 4, New York, 1981, Macmillan Publishing Co., Inc.
11. D'Arcy, C., and Siddique, C.M.: Social support and mental health among mothers of preschool and school aged children, Social Psychiatry **19**:155, 1984.
12. Erikson, E.H.: Childhood and society, ed. 2, New York, 1964, W.W. Norton & Co., Inc.
13. Erikson, E.H.: Identity and the life cycle: selected papers, New York, 1959, International Universities Press, Inc.
14. Freud, S.: Analysis: terminable and interminable. In Freud, S.: Collected papers, vol. 5, London, 1950, The Hogarth Press, Ltd.
15. Fromm-Reichmann, F.: Psychotherapy of schizophrenia, American Journal of Psychiatry **111**:410, 1954.
16. Glazer, W., and others: Chronic schizophrenics in the community: are they able to report their social adjustment? American Journal of Orthopsychiatry **52**:116, 1982.
17. Gordon, M.: Nursing diagnosis: process and application, New York, 1982, McGraw-Hill Book Co.

18. Gruen, R., and others: Platelet MAO activity and schizophrenic prognosis, American Journal of Psychiatry **139**:240, 1982.

19. Gur, R.E., and others: Brain function in psychiatric disorders. III. Regional cerebral blood flow in unmedicated schizophrenics, Archives of General Psychiatry **42**:329, 1985.

20. Hemmings, G.: Biochemistry of schizophrenia and addiction: in search of common ground, Baltimore, 1980, Univesity Park Press.

21. Kim, M.J., and Moritz, D.A., editors: Classification of nursing diagnoses: proceedings of the third and fourth national conferences, New York, 1982, McGraw-Hill Book Co.

22. Klein, M.: Love, guilt and reparation, New York, 1975, The Melanie Klein Trust.

23. Koontz, E.: Schizophrenia: current diagnostic concepts and implications for nursing care, Journal of Psychosocial Nursing and Mental Health Services **20**(9):44, 1982.

24. Korner, A., and others: The relation between neonatal and later activity and temperament, Child Development **56**:38, 1985.

25. Krauss, J.B., and Slavinsky, A.T.: The chronic psychiatric patient and the community, Oxford, England, 1982, Blackwell Scientific Publications, Ltd.

26. Leff, J.: Expressed emotion in families, New York, 1985, Guilford Press.

27. Lidz, T., Fleck, S., and Cornelison, A.: Schizophrenia and the family, New York, 1965, International Universities Press, Inc.

28. Mahler, M.S.: A study of the separation-individuation process, Psychoanalytic Study of the Child **26**:403, 1971.

29. McKinlay, J.B.: Social network influences on morbid episodes and the career of help seeking. In Eisenberg, L., and Kleinman, A., editors: The relevance of social science for medicine, New York, 1980, D. Reidel Publishing Co.

30. Millen, T.: Disorders of personality, New York, 1981, John Wiley & Sons, Inc.

31. Northouse, P.G.: Interpersonal trust and empathy in nurse-nurse relationships, Nursing Research **28**:365, 1979.

32. Pai, S., and Kapar, R.L.: The burden on the family of a psychiatric patient: development of an interview schedule, British Journal of Psychiatry **138**:332, 1981.

33. Piaget, J., and Inhelder, B.: The psychology of the child, New York, 1969, Basic Books, Inc., Publishers.

34. Platt, S.: Social adjustment as a criterion of treatment success: just what are we measuring? Psychiatry **44**(5):95, 1981.

35. Ritzler, B.A.: Paranoia—prognosis and treatment: a review, Schizophrenia Bulletin **7**:710, 1981.

35a. Rotter, J.B.: A new scale for the measurement of interpersonal trust, Journal of Personality **35**:651, 1967.

36. Rosenthal, T., and McGuiness, T.: Dealing with delusional patients: discovering the distorted truth, Issues in Mental Health Nursing **8**:143, 1986.

37. Ruditis, S.E.: Developing trust in nursing interpersonal relationships, Journal of Psychiatric Nursing and Mental Health Services **17**(4):20, 1979.

38. Schweitzer, L., Becker, E., and Welsh, H.: Abnormalities of cerebral lateralization in schizophrenic patients, Archives of General Psychiatry **35**:982, 1978.

39. Seiver, L.L., and others: Smooth pursuit eye tracking impairment, Archives of General Psychiatry **39**:1001, 1982.

40. Spitz, R.A., and Wolf, K.M.: The smiling response and contribution to the ontogenesis of social relations, Genetic Psychology Monographs **34**:59, 1946.

41. Strauss, J., and Carpenter, W.: Schizophrenia, New York, 1981, Plenum Medical Books.

42. Sullivan, H.S.: The interpersonal theory of psychiatry, New York, 1953, W.W. Norton & Co., Inc.

43. Szasz, T.: The myth of mental illness, New York, 1974, Harper & Row, Publishers.

44. Tudor, G.E.: A sociopsychiatric nursing approach to intervention in a problem of mutual withdrawal on a mental hospital ward, Perspectives in Psychiatric Care **8**(1):11, 1970.

45. Ulin, P.: Measuring adjustment in chronically ill clients in community mental health care, Nursing Research **30**:229, 1981.

46. Wallston, K.A., Wallston, B.S., and Gore, S.: Development of a scale to measure nurse's trust of patients, Nursing Research **22**:232, 1973.

47. Wasow, M.: Coping with schizophrenia, Palo Alto, Calif., 1982, Science and Behavior Books.

48. Weinberger, D., and others: Poor premorbid adjustment and CT scan abnormalities in chronic schizophrenia, American Journal of Psychiatry **137**:1410, 1980.

49. Wright, T.L., and Palmer, M.L.: An unobtrusive study of interpersonal trust, Journal of Personality and Social Psychology **32**:446, 1975.

50. Zubin, J.: Problems of attention in schizophrenics. In Kietzman, J.L., Sutton, S., and Zubin, J., editors: Experimental approaches to psychopathology, New York, 1975, Academic Press, Inc.

ANNOTATED BIBLIOGRAPHY

Falloon, I.: Family management of schizophrenia, a study of clinical, social, family and economic benefits, Baltimore, 1985, The Johns Hopkins University Press.

The author recognizes the family as a major contributor to a positive outcome for persons with schizophrenia. Empirical evidence for the effectiveness of family therapy is presented, and methods of family management are discussed.

Krauss, J.B., and Slavinsky, A.: The chronic psychiatric patient and the community, Oxford, England, 1982, Blackwell Scientific Publication, Ltd.

This book focuses on the management of chronically ill psychiatric clients in the community. The multiple aspects of assessment and approaches to nursing management in a community setting are described.

Strauss, J., and Carpenter, W.: Schizophrenia, New York, 1981, Plenum Medical Book Co.

The authors approach schizophrenia with an interactive developmental systems approach. This model emphasizes the impact of the bio-social-psychological components of schizophrenia. Guidelines for treatment and current research are also discussed.

PAIN

Sharon Holmberg

After studying this chapter the learner will be able to:

Define and describe the differences between acute and chronic pain.

Discuss the historical development of pain and pain management.

Describe theories of pain.

Use the nursing process to care for clients with pain.

Identify current research findings related to the pain syndrome.

Pain is a universal human experience. The broadest definition of pain is that it is a personal, private sensation of hurt. This definition describes pain in the subjective realm, implying that the individual experiencing pain is the true expert on the sensation. Other definitions of pain suggest its usefulness to the human organism. For example, pain has been defined as a harmful stimuli that warns of current or impending tissue damage and as a pattern of responses used to protect the person from harm. Pain is the most common symptom of disease or injury that precipitates entry into the health care system. Acute pain usually serves to trigger self-protective behaviors that prevent the person from further harm, such as withdrawing one's hand from a hot stove, or supporting behaviors that encourage healing, such as immobilizing a twisted ankle. Acute pain is usually time limited and likely to disappear once the precipitating cause has been resolved and healing has taken place. On the other hand, chronic pain may or may not be associated with pathological findings, can lose its specific meaning in relationship to disease processes, and may actually be a hindrance to the individual's health and well-being. Such pain may be experienced by some persons without demonstrated pathological findings. Persistent pain either with or without pathological findings may become a health problem in its own right, affecting all aspects of the individual's life.

Chronic pain is the most frequent cause of disability in the United States. In one survey[38] internists estimated that

approximately 13% of their clients could be classified as chronic pain sufferers. Estimates of the economic cost of this syndrome through the loss of work productivity, the cost of workers' compensation payments, health care costs, and related expenses are as high as 60 billion dollars annually. These numbers relate to economic expenditures and do not begin to address the emotional cost to the individual experiencing pain, who comes to view the suffering as endless, purposeless, and unavoidable.

Nurses, as the professionals with the most direct contact with clients experiencing pain, are in positions that require knowledge of pain assessment and management. This proximity allows the nurse to assess the degree of pain experienced by the client and by intervening appropriately, to significantly minimize both the pain experience and the effect of pain on the client's life.

Many clients in psychiatric settings complain of pain. Whether the pain is real or imagined (psychogenic) the nurse needs to know ways to help the client manage. This chapter focuses on the problem of pain with emphasis on chronic pain syndromes.

THEORETICAL APPROACHES

Pain taxonomies have been developed based on two factors: the duration of pain and various aspects of the causes and pathological factors. Pain of less than 6 months' duration is considered acute, whereas chronic

Historical Overview

DATE	EVENT
3000 BC	Early Hindu culture considered pain a life energy imbalance and a punishment for sinful living. Pain was once thought to emanate from the heart since the heart was considered the center of human feelings.
1800s	Theories about the causes of pain changed following Pasteur's (1822-1895) discovery of germs. Pain came to be viewed as something inflicted by a pathological condition rather than a wrongdoing.
1850	Nightingale, in her book *Notes on Nursing,* pointed out that the suffering (pain) experienced by an individual may be caused by many other factors than the disease process.
1920s and 1930s	Medical efforts attempted to cure pain with surgery or chemicals that interrupted pain pathways or destroyed parts of the neurological system. Although unsuccessful, this approach to the cure of pain served to point out the complex neurological, endocrinological, social, and emotional factors related to pain.
1980s	Contemporary theories now recognize pain as a holistic experience influenced by both pathological and individual factors. Nurses are challenged to use the technological knowledge available and integrate it with the more traditional methods for relief of pain. Today pain management is defined as a priority for clinical nursing research.
Future	The current emphasis on the biological aspects of mental illness may promote a clearer understanding of pain mechanisms. Individuals may assume responsibility for their own pain management through self-help groups and hypnosis. An increasing number of pain clinics will be established.

pain lasts for more than 6 months. Pain is also described as limited, intermittent, or persistent. Limited pain relates directly to the presence of some physical condition in the healing process and ends once the healing process is complete. Both intermittent and persistent pain may or may not be caused by a pathological condition. Persistent pain is often considered resistant to treatment and may cause individuals to seek many different treatments in an effort to find relief. It is usually this pain that is described as a pain syndrome.

Agnew, Crue, and Pinsky[1] classified pain as follows:

1. Acute pain, with a duration of a few days, can be mild to severe. As a symptom of an underlying physical problem, it will abate once the pathological condition is treated. An example is postoperative pain.
2. Subacute pain, which has a somewhat longer duration, can be either mild or severe, is caused by a known pathological conditions, and involves a prolonged period of healing. An example is the pain experienced by someone with a bone fracture.
3. Chronic, malignant pain is defined as pain caused by uncontrolled neoplastic disease. Metastatic cancers can cause severe pain in various parts of the body, depending on the disease process and what organ systems are involved.
4. Chronic, benign pain is pain that has persisted for more than 6 months. It may have an unknown or a known cause other than neoplastic disease. The client demonstrates an adequate ability to cope. A client with rheumatoid arthritis may experience this type of pain.
5. Chronic intractable benign pain is the same as chronic benign pain except that the client demonstrates inadequate coping mechanisms. Pain then becomes a primary diagnosis.

The experience of chronic pain can arise from many different circumstances. It may begin with an acute episode of painful physical illness. In other situations the curative treatments produce residual damage that causes pain or the client has developed an illness with a slow insidious progression of symptoms and perhaps progressive deterioration. An additional group of clients have made multiple, unsuccessful efforts to find a physical cause for their pain and have been seen by many specialists without obtaining a specific medical diagnosis. In all cases, each physiological explanation of pain includes an emotional component. The experience of pain is a combination of the stimulation of neural receptors with a substrate of past experience, anxiety, cultural learning, and meaning of the illness. The term "somatogenic" is often used to refer to pain produced by a physiological process, and "psychogenic" is applied to pain that originates in the mind. *Psychogenic pain* is not necessarily experienced any differently than pain with an obvious physical cause. Qualities of psychogenic pain, such as severity, intensity, and location, may be exactly the same as with somatogenic pain. Psychogenic pain implies that adequate physical explanations for the experience of pain cannot be given but that psychological explanations better clarify the cause.

Certain psychiatric disorders may be expressed through pain syndromes. *Hysterical pain* may be brought on by a specific, highly charged emotional event that is related to earlier unconscious emotional conflicts. Known as a conversion disorder it is similar to other hysterical physiological symptoms, such as blindness (see Chapter 34). A related term, *hypochondriacal pain,* describes per-

sons who have a constant preoccupation with their bodies, fear disease or body malfunction, and also experience pain. A hallucination of pain is relatively rare but may be experienced by the psychotic individual who usually has body delusions also such as the body changing size. *Munchausen's syndrome* is the term applied to persons who repeatedly come to acute care settings with convincing but false symptoms of almost any illness or injury, at times accompanied by falsified documents that support evidence of the disease. This is a relatively rare disorder. The most common pain experiences related to emotional stress and occasionally experienced by most people are headaches, muscle aches, or low back pain.

Biological

At present, the most widely accepted, comprehensive theory of pain is the "gate control theory," which suggests that pain is modulated by a gating mechanism located in the spinal cord, as well as by activities in the higher cen-

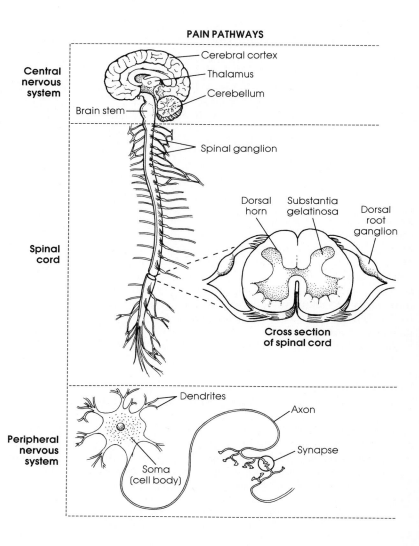

FIGURE 18-1 Pain pathways. The peripheral nervous system, made up of millions of neurons, transmits pain and other sensations by chemical exchange at the synapse into the dorsal horn of the spinal cord and then up through the substantia gelatinosa into the central nervous system. Pain perception is the outcome of multiple chemical exchanges in this complex pathway.

PAIN PATHWAYS

Central nervous system
Cerebral cortex
Thalamus
Cerebellum
Brain stem

Spinal cord
Spinal ganglion
Dorsal horn
Substantia gelatinosa
Dorsal root ganglion
Cross section of spinal cord

Peripheral nervous system
Dendrites
Axon
Synapse
Soma (cell body)

tral nervous system structures. Therefore other central nervous system activities such as memories and emotions can influence the perception of pain. Sensations are transmitted from nerve receptors into the spinal cord and eventually to the brain, but these impulses can be modulated or altered in the spinal cord, brain stem, or cerebral cortex.

The nerve fibers transmit impulses to the spinal cord. At the dorsal horn of the spinal cord the impulses encounter a "gate," which may be open, partially open, or closed. The "gate" is thought to be the substantia gelatinosa, consisting of highly specialized cells throughout the length of the spinal cord that can modulate the transmission of nerve impulses.

If this gate is open or partially open, the pain impulses stimulate T cells (transmission or trigger cells) allowing the pain sensation to proceed through the spinal cord to the brain. If the gate is closed, pain impulses are blocked. As the pain impulses ascend to the brain, activity in the brain stem, thalamus, or cerebral cortex, all of which influence or control emotions, memory, and attention, influence the individual's perception of pain. (Figure 18-1)

Cerebral processes descending from the brain may also have an impact on the gating mechanism. Melzak and Wall,[44] who originally developed this theory, have proposed three types of cerebral processes: (1) sensory-discriminative, which relays information about time, space, location, and intensity; (2) motivational-affective, which provides information about the presence of unpleasantness or discomfort, resulting in action that decreases noxious stimuli, and (3) central control processing, the cognitive aspect of the brain, which analyzes the meaning of pain as well as past experiences and probable outcomes. Together this cerebral processing defines the pain experiences, determines motivation for alternative responses, and projects possible outcomes, thus interacting to influence the perception of and response to pain. In this way cerebral processing influences the physiological processes of the gating mechanism.

Psychological

Pain may occur primarily in conjunction with psychological factors. Persistent somatogenic pain may lead to psychological distress, expressed as depression, anxiety, anger, and feelings of loss of control. In these cases the psychiatric disorder is a secondary consequence of pain but may take on primary importance in the treatment.

Psychoanalytic

Early psychoanalytic theoretical writings discuss pain primarily in the context of the pleasure-pain principle (see Chapter 3), but little is written about physical pain. In describing her observation of infants during the first year of life, Anna Freud[21] believed that "any tension, need or frustration is probably felt as 'pain' because the infant is not yet mature enough to separate bodily events from emotional events."

Szasz[60a] formulated a general psychoanalytic theory of pain by articulating some basic assumptions. First, the ego system relates to the body as an object, just as the ego system relates to other persons as objects. Second, anxiety is an emotional state that occurs as a signal of danger to the ego. For an adult, danger could be the threat of losing a needed object, for example, another person who is important. Third, according to Szasz, pain is an emotional state (affect) that has to do with the relationship of the ego to the body. As such, pain serves to warn the ego of the potential loss (or damage) of a part (or the whole) of the body.

Szasz noted that the terms "organic" and "psychogenic" as applied to pain serve only to locate it in an area of the body, rather than to differentiate the experience. A parallel is drawn between these terms and the psychoanalytic application of "objective fear" and "neurotic anxiety." Just as the source of objective fear can be validated by others (for example, being stopped by police with drugs in the car) so can the source of organic pain be validated (for example, a fractured leg). In this case, pain is a symptom. The source of neurotic anxiety is not validated by others because it is not "objectively" dangerous (for example, fear of cats) but represents something specific to the individual. Similarly, psychogenic pain cannot be validated by objective tests (for example, most headaches) but is nonetheless experienced by the individual as pain. In this case, pain becomes a form of communication, a means of soliciting help.

Pain or at least discomfort is experienced by every small child. This signals to the child that something is wrong, a message that is likely to be communicated to others in a variety of ways. The response depends on a multitude of factors from the child, the situation, and significant others. The cause of the pain, either physical or emotional, the perceived seriousness of the cause, and whether these perceptions are mutually shared influence the response. Also important to determining the response are factors in significant others such as how the child's message is interpreted, what the expectations of the child are, and cultural expectations, values, and attitudes of the significant others. Through a series of experiences beginning in earliest life, each person develops a set of assumptions about expressing pain and what the "correct" response should be. Certain response patterns can be established that may be repeated later in life (see the following Case Example).

Case Example

As an infant, Sara had a particularly sensitive gastrointestinal tract. She frequently developed colicky symptoms an hour or so after being fed. These symptoms usually coincided with her mother leaving for work. Sara's mother, anxious to arrive at work on time, was frequently impatient with her irritable, crying child and rushed to dress Sara and drop her off at a babysitter. Sara, now 10 years old, sometimes gets a "stomachache" before school in the morning and was unable to attend a 3-day sleep-over camp last summer because she developed abdominal pain, nausea, and vomiting the day before camp was to start.

The experience of acute pain is usually accompanied by fear or anxiety or both: fear related to the loss or injury of a body part and anxiety about the response of the significant others. A small child's response to acute pain includes looking to others for relief. If the wished-for response is not soon forthcoming, anxiety may increase as the child becomes concerned about a real or threatened separation or loss of love from an important person. This is one of the psychological processes by which anxiety can become associated with pain in the emotional life of an individual. Another is an injury or hurt induced by significant others, as in receiving punishment. Pain is directly linked to the withdrawal of love. Not only is the physical pain accompanied by anxiety but also anxiety and fear can recur if the individual believes that punishment is anticipated or deserved.

Anticipatory anxiety has a role in explaining the psychological mechanisms related to chronic pain. When what is feared (that is, loss of something important) actually does or seems to have come to pass, the individual's response may be to feel grief and anger or disappointment, to feel punished, or to expect punishment. These dynamic psychological processes are very similar to those that occur in depression. Instead of depression, however, experiencing pain becomes the predominant manner used to express the sense of loss, inwardly turned anger, hostility, and feelings of being responsible and guilty. This theory of anger turned inward and repressed hostility has been used to describe the *pain prone person*. A history of physical abuse as a child, with pain used as a means of discipline, and parents who are attentive only when the child is sick or hurt are thought to be common experiences of the pain-prone person.

Given certain circumstances, individuals with certain character traits, such as being somewhat demanding and complaining, are more likely to develop chronic pain. It has also been suggested that having a limited formal education, a manual or routine job, and a lack of environmental supports may contribute to the development of chronic pain. Many clients may express emotional distress through physical language because they do not have a vocabulary that is adequate for explaining the emotional concepts that lead to pain. Somatic symptoms may be used as a defense against intolerable feelings. For example, a person who has learned that the expression of anger is unacceptable may experience and describe his feeling of anger as physical pain. It is thought that some persons with chronic pain use that symptom as an emotional de-

---

Research Highlight

Chronic Pain: Lifetime Psychiatric Diagnoses and Family History

W. Katon, K. Eagan & D. Miller

PURPOSE

This study was conducted to develop more information about the relationship between chronic pain and psychiatric disorders. Specifically the lifetime psychiatric diagnoses and family history of both psychiatric illness and chronic pain were examined in a group of people with chronic pain.

SAMPLE

From a pool of all persons admitted to an inpatient chronic pain treatment program over 8 months, 37 persons (two of every three) agreed to participate in the study. There were 20 women and 17 men. They ranged from 24 to 70 years of age. Subjects had experienced chronic pain severe enough to cause substantial impairment for at least 1 year, and a medical cause had been ruled out. Those excluded were persons with a history of severe abuse of or dependence on narcotic analgesics and those with an extensive psychiatric treatment history.

METHODOLOGY

Subjects were interviewed using the NIMH Diagnostic Interview Schedule. A family history of mental illness and chronic pain was obtained in the interview. Subjects also filled out an extensive packet of psychological tests. Among those scales used for this report were the Beck Depression Inventory, the Sarason Social Support Questionnaire, and the Beck Hopelessness Scale.

FINDINGS

The most common psychiatric diagnoses were either current or past depressive episodes or both (56.8%) and current or past alcohol abuse (40.5%). Twenty-four subjects (64.9%) had a past diagnosis of either alcohol abuse or major depression or both. Nineteen (51.4%) had an onset of these problems before developing chronic pain. A total of 56.4% of subjects had family histories of alcoholism, depression, or both.

IMPLICATIONS

This study demonstrates the association of chronic pain symptoms with either a past or present diagnosis of depression, alcohol abuse, or both. A strong association between a past history of alcohol abuse and the future development of chronic pain is shown. Since more than half the subjects experienced depressive episodes or alcohol abuse before the onset of chronic pain, the pain may be an expression of chronic psychiatric illness. Another group may be exhibiting a distinct sick role response, modeled in their families, which was brought on by common medical disorders such as back strain.

Based on data from The American Journal of Psychiatry **142**:1156, 1985.

fense against a core conflict or a psychotic process. Without the symptoms of chronic pain such individuals may become acutely psychotic.

The individual who develops chronic pain related to physical illness or injury may experience both psychological losses and real losses, among which may be loss of mobility, loss of job, loss of independence, or significant changes in appearance. These losses can then lead to depression. The depression and pain, accompanied by feelings of being punished (perhaps unfairly), perpetuate and complicate the problem. According to Sternbach[59] chronic pain and depression seem almost interchangeable; chronic pain usually leads to reactive depression, and a reactive depression is frequently accompanied by complaints of pain. Recent research supports the interrelationship of depression and chronic pain (see the Research Highlight on p. 366).

RELATING TO THE CLIENT

When relating to the client with pain, the nurse keeps in mind that no pain, from the slightest to the most severe, is purely physical or purely emotional. Seeing the client as a whole person can facilitate the development of an effective supportive relationship. In the orientation phase of the relationship with the client, pain assessment and establishing a positive alliance are essential. An initial, positive relationship with a client can be established by conveying to the client that you know "it hurts." Frequently, the client's behavior does not invite an empathic or positive response. The client is likely to be angry and resentful, or depressed, sullen, and withdrawn. Referral to a psychiatric treatment setting may be viewed as just another way for others to communicate that the pain is not "real" and this recommendation viewed as just another treatment attempt doomed to failure. The nurse takes into account the impact that previous negative reactions have had on the client and works toward building trust. The client needs to trust the nurse to believe in his pain.[39]

Equally important is for the nurse to respect the client's response to pain. The client and the nurse may have very different attitudes about what is considered appropriate behavior with regard to the reporting of pain and the verbal and nonverbal expressions of pain. Because of the differences in cultural expectations, values, beliefs, and previous experiences (memories) of pain, there may be significant communication gaps between the nurse and the client. Sometimes it may be difficult for the nurse to

---

Research Highlight

Assessment of the Pain Experienced in Relation to Selected Nurse Characteristics

S.R. Dudley & K. Holm

PURPOSE

The impact of some nurse characteristics, including years in practice, age, job satisfaction, educational preparation, clinical practice area, cultural background, and shift assignment, was investigated to determine if these characteristics were relevant to the assessment of clients' pain and emotional distress.

SAMPLE

From a pool of 114 full-time nurses, employed on general surgical, general medical, and a combined intensive care/coronary care unit, 50 nurses were randomly selected and asked to participate in the study. The study was conducted in a large university medical center. The nurses had been educated in associate degree, diploma, or baccalaureate programs, ranged in age from 21 to 61 years, and included 45 women and 5 men.

METHODOLOGY

The subjects were administered a sociodemographic questionnaire, and the Standard Measure of Inferences of Suffering Scale, which consists of brief vignettes describing clients and situations encountered in nursing practice. A 7-point rating scale is used for the subject to rate each vignette on the degree of pain and psychological distress. A third instrument was the Job Descriptive Index, which was used to investigate the degree of the subject's job satisfaction, based on type of work, pay, supervision, coworkers, and promotional opportunities.

FINDINGS

When the subjects' responses were divided into separate categories for pain and emotional distress, subjects inferred significantly more emotional distress than pain. This finding was unrelated to any of the nurse characteristics such as educational preparation, years in practice, age, clinical practice area, job satisfaction, or shift assignment. When looking at the client characteristics of age, sex, and illness/injury, only the category of illness/injury influenced the subject's inference of suffering. Emotional distress was ranked significantly higher than pain, regardless of client characteristics.

IMPLICATIONS

The perception that a client is not experiencing pain but rather considerable emotional distress when, in fact, the client may be experiencing both can lead to mismanagement of care. Relief of pain is a major concern. More understanding of how personal characteristics and personality variables enter into the process of assessing clients' pain needs to be developed. Not only does the degree of emotional distress associated with illness vary, but also the degree of pain varies.

Based on data from Pain **18:**179, 1984.

acknowledge patients' pain (see the Research Highlight on p. 367).

There are a number of misconceptions and prejudices held by members of the health care team that can interfere with adequate and accurate treatment. Chief among them are personal notions that prevent the nurse from accurately interpreting behavior. The nurse needs to understand her own attitudes and feelings related to pain behaviors. This allows her to more objectively analyze discrepancies between her own expectations of behavior and the real behaviors of the client. Clients sometimes feel that their responses to pain are negatively judged, that they cannot measure up to the expectations of others, or that they are ashamed of their behavior. Comparing one client's pain response to another's or comparing a client's response to what the nurse considers ideal is an injustice to the individual. Discussions with clients can serve both to facilitate the acceptance of behavioral responses and to arrive at mutually agreeable acceptable, and appropriate behavioral expressions of pain.

Relief of pain is a joint venture of the client and the treatment team. The evolution of consistent, mutually shared definitions of the pain experience is essential to the establishment of treatment goals. A determination of the type and degree of pain relief that is both achievable and acceptable to the client is negotiated. Although total relief from pain may not be possible, the nurse's behavior reflects confidence and enthusiasm, without including false or impossible promises.

In the termination phase, it is important to review, with the client, accomplishments toward the established treatment plan as well as to review those areas of minimal improvement. Positive changes are reinforced, and discussion of these contributes to the client's positive sense of self. Anxiety about maintaining the improvement is a common concern of the client that will need to be addressed. More difficult, but necessary, is a realistic discussion of treatment goals not completed and an evaluation of what else may be possible.

NURSING PROCESS
Assessment

Physical dimension. The physical expressions of pain vary depending on the conditions causing pain. Therefore it is important to begin the physical assessment of the client with an understanding of the client's medical history and to be aware of any documented medical conditions. The nurse then familiarizes herself with the pain patterns usually associated with that condition. This knowledge helps the nurse develop precise and clear questions for discussion with the client.

The following list provides questions and topics for discussion relevant to physical assessment:

1. Where is the pain? Have the client point to specific painful areas of his body or ask the client to draw painful areas on a diagram of the front and back of the human body (Figure 18-2).

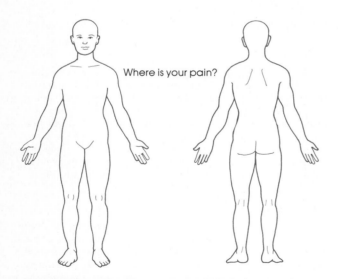

FIGURE 18-2 Identification of pain sites. Instruct the client as follows: please mark, on the drawings, the areas where you feel pain. Put *E* if external, or *I* if internal, near the areas which you mark. Put *EI* if both external and internal. (From Jacox, A.: Pain: a source book for nurses and other health professionals, Boston, 1977, Little, Brown & Co.)

WHAT DOES YOUR PAIN FEEL LIKE?

Some of the words below describe your *present* pain. Circle *ONLY* those words that best describe it. Leave out any category that is not suitable. Use only a single word in each appropriate category—the one that applies best.

1	2	3	4	5
Flickering	Jumping	Pricking	Sharp	Pinching
Quivering	Flashing	Boring	Cutting	Pressing
Pulsing	Shooting	Drilling	Lacerating	Gnawing
Throbbing		Stabbing		Cramping
Beating		Lancinating		Crushing

6	7	8	9	10
Tugging	Hot	Tingling	Dull	Tender
Pulling	Burning	Itchy	Sore	Taut
Wrenching	Scalding	Smarting	Hurting	Rasping
	Searing	Stinging	Aching	Splitting
			Heavy	

11	12	13	14	15
Tiring	Sickening	Fearful	Punishing	Wretched
Exhausting	Suffocating	Frightful	Grueling	Blinding
		Terrifying	Cruel	
			Vicious	
			Killing	

16	17	18	19	20
Annoying	Spreading	Tight	Cool	Nagging
Troublesome	Radiating	Numb	Cold	Nauseating
Miserable	Penetrating	Drawing	Freezing	Agonizing
Intense	Piercing	Squeezing		Dreadful
Unbearable		Tearing		Torturing

Adapted from Jacox, A.: Pain: a source book for nurses and other health professionals, Boston, 1977, Little, Brown & Co.

HOW INTENSE IS YOUR PAIN?

People agree that the following five words represent pain of increasing intensity. They are:

1	2	3	4	5
Mild	Discomforting	Distressing	Horrible	Excruciating

To answer each question below, write the number of the most appropriate word in the space beside the question.

1. Which word describes your pain right now? ____
2. Which word describes it at its worst? ____
3. Which word describes it when it is the least? ____
4. Which word describes the worst toothache you ever had? ____
5. Which word describes the worst headache you ever had? ____
6. Which word describes the worst stomachache you ever had? ____

Adapted from Jacox, A.: Pain: a source book for nurses and other health professionals, Boston, 1977, Little, Brown & Co.

HOW DOES YOUR PAIN CHANGE WITH TIME?

1. Which word or words would you use to describe the *pattern* of your pain?

1	2	3
Continuous	Rhythmic	Brief
Steady	Periodic	Momentary
Constant	Intermittent	Transient

2. What kind of things *relieve* your pain?

_____
_____
_____
_____

3. What kind of things increase your pain?

_____
_____
_____
_____

Adapted from Jacox, A.: Pain: a source book for nurses and other health professionals, Boston, 1977, Little, Brown & Co.

2. When did the pain start? Details of the client's first experience of this pain and its cause can be significant to the treatment.
3. Is the pain continuous or episodic?
4. Do you recognize patterns of occurrences associated with time of day, mood, emotional stress, or work demands?
5. How would you describe the quality of the pain? Is it well-localized or dull, diffuse pain? (See the box on p. 368).
6. How intense is the pain? The use of rating scales helps to objectify intensity and provides a standard measure for the client and the nurse to measure changes. (See the left box above).
7. Does the description of pain change over time? Such changes may reflect an actual change in the physical status of the client.
8. Discuss physical and environmental factors that influence the severity of pain. (See the right box above.) Body functions such as eating, coughing, or defecation may influence pain experiences, as does body posture, the weather, room temperature, and noise.

The physiological processes that change as a consequence of pain are related to the autonomic nervous system and are common with experiences of acute pain but may be totally absent in clients with chronic pain. The nurse observes for elevated blood pressure, elevated pulse and respirations, pupil dilation, skin color changes (pallor or flushing), and diaphoresis. Acute pain may also lead to nausea, vomiting, or diarrhea. Because clients with chronic pain may have few if any observable physiological changes, these are not necessarily reliable indicators of the presence of pain. Chronic pain may affect other physiological processes, for example, decreased appetite, sleep disturbances, and the lack of sexual desire.

Most clients with pain do not describe significant changes in perception of the body's shape, size, or appearance except when these changes are based on reality. For example, an individual with chronic pain as a result of severe arthritis or a person who had lost a limb in an accident will have significant, obvious changes. Such changes will influence the person's perception of his body and require significant emotional adjustment. Other individuals who experience pain as one aspect of another psychiatric disorder, especially psychotic disorders, may believe that the body has actually changed dimensions or is distorted.

Other physical signs of pain include body posture and facial expression. The body part with pain may be held stiffly or immobile. Limps or paralysis can also occur. The person with acute pain sometimes moans or shows pain by facial grimaces. The facial expression of chronic pain sufferers reflects tension or anxiety.

Emotional dimension. Emotions associated with chronic pain are complex. Over time the pain experience may have taken on a variety of meanings and be attached to emotional experiences that have little to do with the original causes of the pain. Pain begins to develop a symbolic meaning. Living with chronic pain produces significant real and emotional changes in the person's life and may mean adopting a totally new life-style. Once the person has accepted the notion that the pain cannot be cured, loss is the most common feature of the emotional experience. Anger, frustration, and resentment may be the first expressions of loss. These feelings can be directed outward toward others who are blamed for the situation. The health care team is especially vulnerable to receive the blame and anger, since the client's expectation is that it is their job to cure the problem. When anger is directed inward, the client may feel both guilt and the wish for or expectation of punishment. Self-destructive behaviors in the form of noncompliance or not caring for self are expressions of guilt and punishment. Guilt is also associated with self-blame. The individual may express this by stating "I have brought this on myself" and also relates feeling responsible for disrupting the lives of others. Anhedonia is a prevalent emotional tone. The client feels there is little opportunity to experience joy and happiness.

When discussing the client's pain, it is necessary not only to listen to the content of what the person says about the location of, intensity of, changes in, and type of pain, but also to listen for the emotions expressed at the same time. There are three phases to the emotional experience of pain: anticipation, the sensation itself, and the aftermath. These phases occur in sequence, especially with acute pain, but vary in length and intensity depending on the nature of the pain. For example, in acute pain, anticipation may be short, whereas for the person with intermittent pain, it may be a common emotional state. The individual with continuous pain usually experiences all three phases.

Persons with acute pain are most likely to feel anxiety related to causes and consequences. Anticipating pain accompanying diagnostic procedures or surgery raises the individual's anxiety. When the onset of pain is sudden, unanticipated, and unexplained, anxiety is related to a lack of understanding. This anxiety is expressed by agitation, restlessness, irritability, and demanding behavior. The client may seem pressured and may demand time, attention, and explanations. As the individual obtains more information about the cause of the acute pain and its meaning relative to body injury or illness, the anxiety may change to fear or relief. Fear about the meaning of the illness or injury and worry about long-term consequences may lead to further anxiety.

Depending on the location of the pain, clients may feel embarrassed to discuss it. This is particularly true when pain is located in the groin, genitals, or rectum. Shame is another common emotion associated with pain, particularly for those individuals referred to psychiatric treatment or specialty clinics for the treatment of chronic pain. The person may have had repeated experiences of others not believing that the pain is "real" or may have been told "it's all in your head" with the implicit message being that the individual is simply complaining, has control over the pain, and should "make it go away." Discussion of pain has become associated with humiliation. Persons reluctant to describe their pain are asked how others have responded to them in the past.

Grief and depression over the significant losses that accompany major physical illness or injury are appropriate and necessary for the individual's emotional adaptation to chronic pain and adjustment to a changed life. These emotional responses are expected as one aspect of the recovery process and require the nurse's attention.

On the other hand, pain may be a symptom of intolerable stress. In these cases, pain is a secondary consequence and a means of coping with "pain" in other aspects of life. Depression, anger, guilt, or frustration may be expressed as physical pain. The experience of physical pain may mask serious emotional disturbances. Clients are likely to be less resentful of the physical sensation of pain and more willing to talk about the pain than about any other emotions or feelings. Assessment and understanding of the emotions of such clients are done slowly and carefully in order to avoid precipitating severe depression or a psychotic state.

Intellectual dimension. A state of hyperresponsiveness to sensations may accompany pain. The client is more sensitive to noxious stimuli and may negatively interpret interactions with others in the environment. Irritability that accompanies discomfort can lead to a negative interpretation of verbal exchanges. The client can easily misinterpret the meaning of comments and may take offense or view comments meant as neutral in a negative light. For example, in responding to a request for assistance, the nurse may say, "Can I help you?" only to receive an angry or sarcastic reply from the client such as, "I didn't mean to interrupt your busy day." Perception may also be heightened. The weight of a blanket or the smell of a cigarette, for example, may be interpreted as an exceedingly noxious stimulus by the client, whereas these same sensations experienced without pain are not troublesome. A diminished response to sensations and lack of perception occurs frequently when the individual is both depressed and in pain. Then there may be minimal reaction to others and the environment.

The client's ability to maintain attention and concentration are likely to be disturbed by acute pain. The pain and attempts to manage the pain may so absorb thinking and cognition that he cannot attend to other matters, which seem trivial to him. Clients with intermittent or chronic pain may ruminate about previous pain experiences, relating them to the current sensations.

Social dimension. The impact of pain on the individual has significance for all aspects of social role functioning. Not only does the perception of self change but also close relationships with family and close friends may change. The ability to function adequately in previously established work roles can be severely curtailed, thus significantly influencing one's income, social status, and life-style and ultimately reinforcing a negative view of self.

A person's perception of self (self-esteem, self-worth) may change in a negative direction in association with the meaning of pain for the person and the real physical damage to the body as a result of illness or injury. Persons who suffer extreme physical changes may alter their emotional concept of self to include these real changes. Those persons who are adaptable and flexible with a secure sense of self are likely to require a period of adjustment to accommodate the change but then continue to think of themselves in a changed but positive way. As previously stated, chronic pain is frequently associated with depression, one aspect of which is low self-regard. This low self-regard may have been a personality trait before the experience of pain or may develop as a consequence of the meaning given to chronic pain, as well as the stress of coping with it. In order to assess a person's change in self-perception, self-reports as well as data from significant others need to be obtained.

A positive sense of self is related to feelings of independence and the ability to maintain control of one's body and feelings and to having some influence on the environment. These abilities are sometimes lost or relinquished. For example, in most health care facilities, the client is required to give over control of medications to the nursing staff, resulting in the need to rely on others for pain control. This situation leads to dependence, similar to childhood, and will bring up memories or emotional conflicts about child-parent interactions. Although comforting for some persons and threatening for others, the fact of dependence produces more regressive behaviors. The client may begin to make equally as many complaints about what seem to be trivial matters as about important matters. Other clients will express nothing, on the assumption that others do not care about their problems or discomforts, including pain. Assessment of dependence or independence includes the environmental expectation of dependent behavior as well as the client's reaction to increased dependence. Clients who develop pain syndromes as an unconscious wish to withdraw from social and environmental demands may actually receive some "secondary gain" from the dependent position.

Coping with pain can take considerable emotional energy. Clients feel too exhausted or depressed to maintain social contacts and slowly withdraw from their social networks, which leads eventually to loneliness and isolation. The person loses interest in others, including the desire for intimacy and sexual relations with their significant other. Friends and family members are likely to withdraw from the person in pain, not wishing to face their own emotional trauma caused by seeing suffering in someone close to them. These significant others both identify with the suffering and feel helpless to intervene. Family members, in an effort to protect the person in pain, sometimes decide to withhold certain information or do not express their concerns to the client. Rather than discuss stresses of daily living, the family members attempt to project a happy, if superficial, image, further isolating the individual through emotional distance, lack of knowledge, and lack of mutually shared experiences. Family dynamics change. Other family members attempt to pick up the tasks of the person in pain, changing the expectation of who is to fulfill any given family role.

Loss of employment is common for the individual with chronic pain. Physical disability with or without chronic pain may make return to a previous job impossible. Job retraining may be possible but is accompanied by lost earning time and the cost related to retraining. Beyond the real expenses entailed, however, is the question of whether the person with chronic pain is able to and desires to either return to a former job or be retrained. According to Unikel[61] people who display symptoms of pain and sickness learn, either through their own experience or from observations, that there are three consequences to pain: attention, avoidance of stressful situations, and economic advantage. Assessment of how these three factors influence the individual's pain experience is impor-

tant. The relationship between chronic pain and economic supports is significant to treatment planning. Factors to consider in the assessment process are success or failure at the job, ability to cope with work-related stress, positive or negative feedback from others, a sense of control or powerlessness, and general job satisfaction. Some persons receive disability payments or workers' compensation payments roughly equivalent to their previously earned income. This may serve as an unconscious incentive for continued uncontrolled symptoms, especially if the job was stressful and the person finds relief in avoiding stressful situations. Only rarely does the individual consciously and deliberately avoid employment by developing symptomatic behavior. The individual experiences a real illness or injury and discovers that his needs continue to be met, and perhaps with less "effort" on his part. He may feel more gratification from the role of sick person than he receives in his job. These emotional factors then serve as reinforcers to maintain the illness.

The client's present experience and expression of pain are strongly influenced by early experiences with pain and associated memories. Cultural factors, especially the means of reacting to and expressing pain within the family culture, influence present behavior. These subtle but strong influences are usually difficult for the client to verbalize directly because they are based on early, preverbal, learned behaviors. For example, in general, women have been found to have a lower maximum tolerance for pain than men although individual variations are great.[47] This is thought to be culturally determined since men are not supposed to cry out in pain as quickly as women, especially in Western cultures.

Spiritual dimension. An important aspect of the assessment process is to understand what meaning the client gives to the experience of pain. The following are questions the person may or may not express but probably often thinks about: "Is pain associated with death? Will it be permanent? Do I deserve to suffer? Am I devalued as an individual because of pain and infirmity?"

Feelings of decreased value and worthlessness develop with persistent pain, especially when accompanied by physical incapacitation. Life may not seem worth living because the pain is sometimes unbearable. The individual feels that the pain represents punishment for being bad or unworthy or that life with physical incapacitation and pain is too difficult. Persons may also feel they are a burden for the family. The risk of suicide can be great at these times and needs to be carefully assessed.

The client's philosophy of life, religious beliefs, and spiritual ideas may be seriously challenged by living with pain. The values, beliefs, morals, and ethics that have held meaning for the individual in the past, such as "God is good," may seem to be a mockery given present experiences. The client who attempts to think through questions related to the "why" of pain will at least confront, if not need to accommodate, his philosophy to fit the present situation. The person with no meaningful philosophy of life may be overwhelmed by the experience of pain and lack a belief system that can provide some solace and aid with coping.

The nurse inquires about the client's religious beliefs and explores with the client how his belief system fits the present experience. For example, the client who believes pain is a punishment for wrongdoing may spend considerable time and energy mentally searching for those things that may be deemed "bad enough" to deserve the level of pain being experienced. Such persons are also likely to be consumed with feelings of guilt. Clients may express this belief by wishing to "do over" some aspect of their life, continually regretting having failed, and becoming preoccupied with the extent of their "punishment." Doubts about either the existence of or the fairness of a deity may be expressed. Assessment of the strength of the client's belief system is important to understanding the client's perspective.

Another common reaction to pain is for the client to view the experience as a test of commitment to his religious beliefs. The client with this perspective can be reticent to complain of discomfort or ask for medication to relieve the pain. Pain becomes something that is to be endured as a means of proving worthiness. Proving that one can meet these religious challenges can mean unnecessary suffering and ultimately the client will probably express anger and frustration or even question whether the effort to endure has any benefit. Hopelessness may be clearly expressed by the individual. When the nurse notices that a client seems to be in pain but says nothing, an exploration of his belief system may provide some understanding of how the client hopes to cope with pain or whether he has abandoned all hope.

The assessment includes an understanding of how the client views prayer and meditation. Some questions to consider include the following:

1. Has the use of prayer or mediatation been useful in the past?
2. Does the client receive help or satisfaction from these activities?
3. Under what circumstances do these activities help?
4. Do they produce relaxation, improve self-control, or facilitate a more positive sense of self?
5. Is the client knowledgeable about any of the relax-

ation or meditation techniques that may help, such as transcendental meditation or self-hypnosis?

Measurement tools. Measurement tools are useful to assist the nurse in systematically assessing the client's subjective experience of pain. One of the most common measurement tools is a simple descriptive scale, sometimes called a "pain ruler," that asks the client to select a place on the scale which most accurately reflects the level of pain experienced. One end of the scale indicates pain while the other end indicates severe pain (Figure 18-3).

The McGill-Melzack pain Questionnaire includes both an effort to measure the strength (severity) of pain and attempts to delineate pain location. In addition, the client is asked to choose from lists of word descriptors that specify different aspects of the pain experience. The words are categorized into three major classes:

1. Words that describe the sensory qualities of the experience
2. Words that describe the affective qualities of the experience
3. Evaluative words that describe the intensity of the pain experience

The advantage of this measurement tool is its sensitivity to the subtle changes in aspects of the pain sensation that would not be reflected by other measurement tools.

Analysis

Nursing diagnosis. The following list provides examples of NANDA-accepted diagnoses, with causative statements related to pain.

1. Impaired physical mobility related to pain secondary to paraplegia
2. Sleep pattern disturbance related to pain
3. Self-care deficit related to low back pain secondary to need for assistance with dressing and grooming
4. Powerlessness related to intolerable pain

Altered comfort: chronic pain is a nursing diagnosis approved by NANDA that applies to the person in pain. The defining characteristics of this nursing diagnosis are listed in the left box on p. 373.

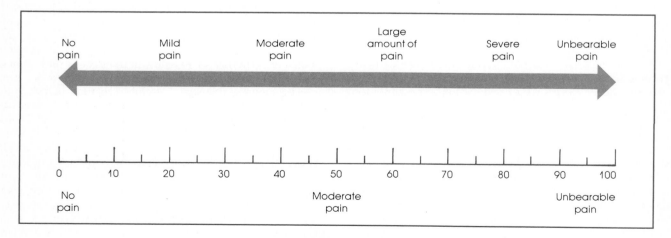

FIGURE 18-3 Pain rulers.

ALTERED COMFORT: CHRONIC PAIN

DEFINITION
State in which the individual experiences pain that continues for more than six months.

DEFINING CHARACTERISTICS
Physical Dimension
Altered muscle tone
Protective guarded behaviors
*Sleep disturbance
Restlessness
Observed evidence of pain
Facial expression of tension, anxiety
Autonomic nervous system changes (acute pain): increased blood pressure, pulse, respirations, diaphoresis, dilated pupils
Altered ability to continue previous activities
Anorexia
Weight fluctuations
Emotional Dimension
*Anxiety
Fear of another injury
*Irritability
*Anger
*Anhedonia
Intellectual Dimension
Verbal report of pain for more than 6 months
*Rumination about pain experiences
*Inattentiveness
Social Dimension
*Withdrawal from significant others
*Changes in family roles
*Changes in work roles
*Loss of libido
*Low self-esteem
Spiritual Dimension
*Questions philosophy of life
*May doubt existence of a diety
*Hopelessness
*Concern with meaning of pain

Adapted from North American Nursing Diagnosis Association Classification of Nursing Diagnosis: Proceedings of the seventh conference, St. Louis, 1987, The C.V. Mosby Co.
*Indicates characteristics in addition to those defined by NANDA.

The following Case Example demonstrates the characteristics of altered comfort: chronic pain.

Case Example

Frank, a 47-year-old former employee of a public works department, received an on-the-job injury to his arm 8 months ago. He had been in a manhole attempting to repair a leaking water main. As the work progressed, water accumulated to about 4 inches in the bottom of the manhole. Frank began to panic and asked the boss if he could go out to "get some air." The boss said "no" and became angry. Frank, increasingly anxious, attempted to climb the ladder anyway but slipped. The ladder fell, hit Frank, and knocked him into the water. He developed difficulty breathing and paralysis and pain in the arm where the ladder struck him. He has seen four physicians who can find no

307.80 IDIOPATHIC PAIN DISORDER

ESSENTIAL FEATURES
The individual with idiopathic pain disorder complains of pain in the absence of adequate physical findings.

MANIFESTATIONS
Physical Dimension
Excessive, severe, or prolonged pain
Indeterminate or absent organic findings

Intellectual Dimension
Complaints of pain in excess of what would be expected from the physical findings
Preoccupation with pain

Social Dimension
Impaired social activities
Impaired work role

Adapted from American Psychiatric Association: Diagnostic and statistical manual of mental disorders (DSM-III-R), Washington, D.C., 1987, The Association.

physical damage. Frank, now at home and unemployed, needs assistance with dressing because the arm remains painful and paralyzed. He has filed for workers' compensation and feels very angry that no one has been able to find out what is wrong with his arm and tell him how to cure it.

DSM-III-R diagnoses. The DSM-III-R diagnoses related to pain include idiopathic pain disorder. The essential features and manifestations of the features according to the DSM-III-R are listed in the box above.

Planning

The Case Example below gives an example of the nursing diagnosis idiopathic pain disorder. Table 18-1 provides some examples of long-term and short-term goals and outcome criteria related to pain. These serve as examples of the planning stage in the nursing process.

Case Example

Paula, 37 years old, was referred to a pain treatment program after all physical and neurological studies failed to show organic cause for her severe headaches, tingling on the scalp, and the sensation of her head swelling up at night, symptoms that have increased in frequency and severity for the past several months. Paula quit her job 4 years ago due to persistent headaches brought on by conflict with her boss. She has been living with her parents, providing company for her mother who experiences chronic leg pain secondary to diabetic neuropathy. Six months ago, Paula's father retired and is now home every day caring for his wife. With a reduced family income, there are financial pressures. Paula resents her father's presence, admits that she sometimes feels "in the way" now, and says she should consider finding a job to help the financial situation but cannot do so because of her medical problems. After coping with the pain that keeps her awake all night, Paula has no energy left for a job.

TABLE 18-1 Long-term and short-term goals and outcome criteria related to pain

Goals	Outcome Criteria
NURSING DIAGNOSIS: ALTERED COMFORT RELATED TO HEADACHE	
Long-term goals	
To describe positive feelings about self	Accepts compliments from others
	Describes accomplishments in occupational therapy program
	Shows interest in appearance and dress
To understand that increased emotional stress makes headache worse	Describes stressors that increase headaches
	Considers ways to avoid stressors
	Explores alternate behaviors to cope with stress
Short-term goals	
To reestablish regular sleep pattern	Stays in bed at night, even if not asleep
	Stays out of bed all day in spite of symptoms or tiredness
	Negotiates with treatment team about use of sleep medications
To monitor the frequency of symptom occurrence	Records an hourly account of symptoms over a 24-hour period for 3 consecutive days
	Reviews symptom frequency chart with treatment team
To discuss the pattern of symptom occurrence	Records activities and feelings on hourly basis over a 24-hour period for 3 consecutive days
	Reviews activities chart with treatment team
	Attempts to determine relationships between symptoms, activities, and feelings
To participate in family meetings with parents	Attends family meetings three times per week
	Can express verbally, positive and negative feelings toward parents
	Is able to accept criticism from parents

Implementation

★ Physical dimension. Implementation of treatment for pain may be done in a variety of settings. Clients with pain syndromes are usually first seen in medical clinics or hospitals because the client believes the cause to be physiological. When determination has been made that there are no definable physiological causes or that the pain experience has become further complicated by emotional factors, the client is likely to be referred to a psychiatric treatment setting or a specialty clinic for chronic pain sufferers. Clients with pain from emotional causes rarely seek psychiatric treatment initially and may be unwilling to acknowledge an emotional component. Therefore implementation of treatment for pain involves a combination of approaches.

Specific interventions for pain include the use of medications, nerve blocks, and occasionally surgical interventions. Other possible interventions more frequently used in physical care settings and less often in psychiatric settings include massage and application of heat or cold. The use of *transcutaneous electrical nerve stimulation (TENS)* or acupuncture has become more common in recent years.

Medications used in the treatment of chronic pain range from analgesics to antidepressants and also include placebos. A placebo is any medical or nursing measure that works because of its implicit or explicit therapeutic intent instead of its specific chemical or physical properties. It may be a pill containing lactose, an injection of saline, or even a surgical procedure. Contrary to popular belief, the use of placebos does not differentiate "real" pain from psychogenic pain. Placebos can and do relieve pain, both psychogenic and that caused from obvious physical stimuli. They may work by reducing anxiety or by the classical conditioning response. That is, the association of taking a pill or receiving an injection is expected to relieve pain so it does. There may also be a biochemical response. It has been theorized by some researchers that the cognitive expectation of a response actually stimulates a physiological response of producing more of the body's natural pain-relieving substances, endorphins.

The use of sedatives and narcotic analgesics in the treatment of acute pain is a standard practice. However, in the treatment of chronic pain, these drugs may be more problematic. The possibility for development of tolerance, dependence, or addiction is always present when these drugs are used. In general, physical tolerance (but not necessarily addiction) develops after continuous use of narcotics for 2 weeks or longer but can be quickly reversed when the drug is no longer needed for pain relief.

Neurosurgical techniques are sometimes employed for the treatment of intractable pain. All neurosurgical techniques cause permanent lesions of the nervous system and thus are used cautiously. In general, these techniques are not highly successful in the long-term treatment of pain.

Nerve blocks are one form of neurological technique and are intended to interrupt pain pathways in the peripheral nervous system. Nerve blocks may be temporary, of the type dentists use to block pain or the spinal blocks used in labor and delivery. A temporary block is used for diagnostic purposes to investigate the anatomical pain pathways. It can also be used prognostically so that the client can experience the probable effect before a permanent procedure is done. The nurse needs to be aware of possible complications, such as severe systemic reactions to the anesthetics that could require emergency interventions such as intubation and cardiopulmonary resuscitation during the procedure.

Transcutaneous electrical nerve stimulation (TENS)

consists of electrodes powered by a battery-operated generator that send a mild electrical current into the body at or near the pain site and can be used to control both acute and chronic pain. TENS are the most common peripheral stimulation technique but others, such as vibratory stimulation and acupuncture, have come into use over the past 10 years and have been shown effective for some clients and some types of pain. Just why TENS and other stimulation techniques are effective is unknown, but theories are (1) blood flow is increased near the electrodes, increasing muscle relaxation and healing; (2) the body may be stimulated to release endorphins, increasing natural pain relief; or (3) electrical stimulation closes the neurological "gate" to pain impulse transmission. Some clients who benefit from TENS will use these units continuously and need to be taught correct application of electrodes and other important aspects of how the unit functions so they can use it at home. The nurse observes for possible complications, such as skin irritation or electrical burns from the electrodes. Therapeutic controversies about acupuncture, another form of peripheral stimulation, are far from resolved, but research shows possible benefit in 60% to 75% of patients with chronic pain,[35] at least for short periods of time.

Two of the most traditional, effective, and universal nursing measures for pain control are the use of massage and the application of heat and cold. Not only does massage facilitate relaxation and help to relieve anxiety, but also the action of massage stimulates large-fiber nerve impulses, according to the gate control theory, and thus closes off the reception of pain impulses. Massage can be done lightly or deeply. Back massage can be used to reduce pain regardless of the site, although the specific pain site can sometimes be massaged.

The application of heat increases blood flow to injured tissues and thereby reduces inflammation. It is especially useful for bruises, muscle spasms and arthritis. Heat also has a stimulating effect on large nerve fibers similar to that of massage, thus reducing the small fiber pain sensations. Application of heat will not relieve some types of pain, such as that caused by pressure on a nerve. Superficial dry heat is applied by use of heating pads or heat lamps. Moist heat is applied by the use of hot-water bottles or hot baths. The nurse needs to be particularly cautious of and alert to avoid the possibility of burns. Occasionally deep heat from an ultrasound device may be administered for specific types of pain, such as back pain. Cold therapy is more effective for acute pain than for chronic pain and is especially useful for burns or sprains.

Emotional dimension. For the client with acute pain, the most common emotional experience is anxiety and fear. Interventions from the nurse are directed toward the reduction of anxiety. The nurse needs to respond to the demands of the client, provide accurate, clear, and simple explanations of procedures and treatments, and respond to the client's questions. Verbal interaction and the presence of others help to reduce the client's anxiety. It's important for the nurse to control her own responses to situations such as severe injury or uncomfortable procedures. The nurse realizes that the client may be able to see her face but not the site of the injury or procedure, and thus his emotional response may be guided by what is reflected on the nurse's face.

Clients with chronic pain present complicated emotional features. Some of the most common psychotherapeutic interventions are individual psychotherapy (see Chapter 8), group therapy (see Chapter 28), and marital therapy (see Chapter 30). Since the phenomenon of pain arises from physiological, emotional, and social factors, multimodel therapy is likely to be more effective than any single approach.

The major goals of psychotherapy are to help the client with chronic pain reduce helpless and hopeless attitudes by gaining control of the symptoms. This can be done by identifying and reducing anxiety states, identifying irrational cognitions;, thinking, and personal beliefs, and then helping the client to make modifications.

Intellectual dimension. The theories related to pain mechanisms show that the individual can influence experiences of pain by thought processes. Clients can be taught to block pain sensations at the cortical level by a number of cognitive strategies, including distraction, relaxation, guided imagery, biofeedback, and hypnosis. Major advantages of these approaches are that the client is given a participatory role in pain relief and can develop a sense of control over the problem. Effective teaching from the nurse allows the client to use several of the cognitive approaches without assistance and on an as-needed basis. Most treatments have the added advantage of requiring little technical equipment. The most important elements in these techniques are that the nurse is confident of their helpfulness, can project this attitude to the client, and has been able to establish an alliance that facilitates the teaching process.

Reality testing and teaching the client to identify patterns of response that cause pain and to develop new response patterns are interventions that have been found to be helpful. Many clients with chronic pain need assistance to identify and express their emotional responses rather than respond with an expression of physical pain. On the inpatient unit the nurse is responsible for designing and implementing a carefully conceived milieu. This includes developing relationships with clients: encouraging them to problem solve, to develop better communication skills, and to understand the relationship between emotional stress and pain. A therapeutic milieu is an ideal environment for clients to develop an understanding of their emotional responses to daily life stresses.

Distraction is a simple technique employed by nurses often without awareness of its being a treatment approach. Pain is relieved by focusing one's attention on something other than pain. When concentrating on a book, a television program, or a conversation with another person, pain is no longer at the client's center of attention and will be felt less intensively. This is a short-term relief technique that may be especially helpful for managing periods of more acute pain but does not generally provide a long-term solution to the pain problem. Effective distracters are those involving the client's sense of hearing, sight, or touch. If the nurse knows of the client's hobbies or interests, this information helps in the selection of an appropriate distraction. Rhythm and repetition facilitate these techniques so the use of music, rhythmic breathing exercises, frequent repetition of a word or phrase, poetry, singing, or tapping of the foot or hand is encouraged. Other examples are to give the client a picture and ask him to describe it in detail or ask him questions about it. On an inpatient unit, encouraging visitors or the client's interaction with others can also serve as an effective distraction. The client needs to be taught these techniques, which can then be employed at will once the benefits are experienced.

Guided imagery and relaxation exercises are related techniques for pain control. Guided imagery utilizes the client's ability to create images in the mind of pleasant places or experiences based on previous life experiences. It resembles a form of self-hypnosis. A comfortable environment with minimal noise and interruptions facilitates the exercise. Relaxation exercises may be used before guided imagery exercises to help induce a relaxed state. Initially, guided imagery involves an interaction with the nurse who helps the client create a relaxed, comfortable mental image by encouraging and asking questions that stimulate the client to create the imagined scene. Once the client has learned techniques of relaxation or imagery, client-specific cassette tapes can be made. The tape can then be used by the client to re-create the imagery and induce a relaxed state. A period of 15 to 20 minutes is usually long enough to be helpful (see the Research Highlight below). Imagery uses the mind's ability to create physiological responses. Just as watching a frightening scene in a movie can increase an individual's pulse rate, so can imagery facilitate the body's ability to relax. Clients often experience drowsiness after using this technique.

When used properly, hypnosis can alleviate severe pain. *Hypnosis* is an altered state of consciousness whereby distraction is minimized and concentration is heightened. Pain signals may be processed by the brain at

---

Research Highlight

Imagery Coping Strategies in the Treatment of Migraine

J.M. Brown

PURPOSE

It has been suggested that for imagery to be effective, the subjects must be able not only to imagine the scene, but also to respond emotionally as if present in the image. This investigation explores the effects of response versus stimulus strategies on tolerance and reported magnitude of pain associated with hand immersion in cold water.

SAMPLE

Forty-five persons who suffer from migraine headache were recruited through media advertising to participate in this study. Of these, six dropped out due to time constraints or because they did not have at least four headaches in the baseline period. Thirty-five of the 39 subjects were women, mean age was 38 years, and nearly all had experienced migraine headaches for at least 5 years. Most had used medication, and some had used other treatments such as acupuncture, relaxation exercises, biofeedback, or chiropractic. Subjects were randomly assigned to three groups.

METHODOLOGY

All subjects kept diaries throughout the 8-week experiment that rated headache duration, frequency, and type and amount of medication taken. Subjects were given a pretest and posttest involving putting one arm in cold water to measure the subject's report of pain magnitude and pain tolerance. Subjects were randomly assigned to three groups as follows. (1) The response group was taught to imagine a scene that included descriptors of mood response (for example, relaxed, tension drained away, calm). (2) The stimulus group was taught to imagine the same scene but in greater detail and without mood descriptors. (3) The control group was shown unfocused vacation slides in rapid sequence, accompanied by a somewhat plausible explanation that this treatment was subconscious reconditioning. Each subject was given a pretest for tolerance and magnitude of pain response and then seen in five weekly sessions for treatment. A posttest was then administered.

FINDINGS

Both the response and stimulus imagery groups did not differ from each other and were superior to the placebo group, gaining increased control over both the magnitude and tolerance of pain. The imagery treatment groups gained control in both experimental pain (placing the arm in cold water) and clinical pain (headaches). This difference in groups could not be explained by other possible variables such as attitude about the treatment or amount of medication used.

IMPLICATIONS

That the imagery treatments were superior to a credible placebo indicates that the improvement can be attributed to the imagery treatments. This improvement was maintained through a 2-month follow-up. It would seem that the content of coping imagery does not make a difference but that the frequency of the subject's use of the strategy at home did improve its effect.

Based on data from Pain **18**:157, 1984.

an unconscious level but are not felt consciously. In responsive subjects all pain can be removed for controlled periods of time by the use of hypnotic suggestion. It can be used selectively to block pain in certain regions of the body or to only partially block pain. It has been suggested that blocking all pain by hynotic suggestion is not to be done, especially with some organic conditions since a change in the course of a clinical condition needs to be detectable by the clinical signs and symptoms of pain. Important diagnostic clues can be missed with a total block of pain sensation. The length of time that hypnotic analgesia is effective varies from a few hours to several days or weeks. With repeated hypnotic suggestion, pain relief can be reinforced and the effective time extended. Clients can be taught self-hypnosis, effectively gaining control over their pain.

Biofeedback is a means of providing the client with information about specific body functions such as skin temperature, pulse rate, blood pressure, or muscle tension by using equipment that measures these functions and provides feedback information to the client by means of visual or auditory signals. Its major use in chronic pain is to help the client control muscle tension, anxiety, and some autonomic nervous system functions, thereby influencing the physiology of the body and aiding in pain control.

Social dimension. It is important to stress that certain pain behaviors can be learned and unlearned. Once pain behaviors begin to occur, they can be influenced by factors outside the person and may be controlled by various environmental factors. It has been found that reported intensity of pain by clients is systematically influenced by social reinforcers. Treatment is an effort to manage excess disability from pain by focusing on the actions of clients and their families to determine what pain behaviors are reinforced and how they are reinforced. The theoretical approach is based on learning theory. A behavior is learned by being reinforced from others' responses, but the behavior can be unlearned or modified by changing those factors that reinforce it (see Chapter 3).

Family and social roles can be significantly changed when the individual develops a serious medical condition accompanied by pain. Most often these changes are initially protective, intended to allow the individual time and opportunity for recovery. Any individual in the process of recovery from an extended illness will be faced with giving up a "sick role" and again take on a more functional, productive role. This task is more difficult when symptoms of the illness, such as pain, persist. Identifying variables that serve to reinforce and maintain sick role behavior is important in implementing behavior modification techniques. Clear limit setting and consistency of responses are necessary for a positive outcome.

Clients who have been unemployed for long periods and especially those who receive monetary compensation, such as workers' compensation, are particularly difficult to rehabilitate. The longer an individual stays away from work, the less likely he is to eventually return to work. Behavioral techniques that address the client's low level of motivation and stimulate emotional insight have been

successful. Behavioral therapy focuses on increasing the client's physical abilities, such as increasing activity levels, reducing the amount of pain medications used, and a specific program designed to reinforce nonpain behaviors. Behavioral therapy is almost always combined with several other therapeutic approaches.

Spiritual dimension. Some clients need or ask for spiritual guidance that can be provided by clergy. This may be especially helpful for those who feel unfairly punished by their God and find their religious beliefs challenged. Some beliefs and religious ideas may interfere with treatments, such as the case when a client has lost hope and the will to live. Discussions with the client concerning these beliefs are necessary in order to help the client reestablish the will to participate in treatment programs.

Some specific treatments use the client's belief system in the treatment process. The aim is for the client to gain existential knowledge about himself through introspection and meditation. Especially relevant are yoga and transcendental meditation (see Chapter 38). A passive attitude, relaxation, and focused concentration are particularly helpful aspects of meditation for the person in pain.

INTERACTION WITH A CLIENT IN PAIN

Client: (Partially sitting in bed with eyes downcast.) Don't trouble me this morning with breakfast or anything else. This has been the worst night.

Nurse: What has made it the worst night?

Client: Oh, the pain in my back was just awful. I couldn't sleep.

Nurse: What was it like?

Client: It went down my leg and then . . . . oh, never mind.

Nurse: Mr. B., I am interested in hearing how you describe the pain. It will help us work together on this problem.

Client: I don't think it can be solved.

Nurse: Are you feeling more hopeless after the bad night you had?

Client: I don't see how being in this hospital is going to help.

Nurse: Right now you sound discouraged. First, I'd like to help you get into a more comfortable position, then we can talk to get a better understanding of what the pain is like.

This client and nurse are in the process of establishing a working alliance. Many people would look to the nurse for assistance, but the client with chronic pain may have learned that others do not wish to hear about his pain, depression, and hopelessness. Such expectations can produce initial rejection of the nurse.

The nurse responds with a direct question that indicates her interest in the client's experience. The tone of voice is nonjudgmental, reflecting concern and interest. She does not become frustrated by his initial hesitance to explain but rather indicates the essential need for a shared understanding of the problem. The nurse has begun the process of involving the client in the process of finding

NURSING PROCESS SUMMARY: PAIN

ASSESSMENT

Physical Dimension
  Elevated blood pressure, pulse, respirations
  Dilated pupils
  Flushed or pallid appearance
  Diaphoresis
  Nausea
  Vomiting
  Diarrhea
  Sleep disturbances
  Decreased appetite
  Decreased sexual functioning
  Pained facial expression
  Moaning, groaning
  Exhaustion

Emotional Dimension
  Anxiety
  Fear
  Embarrassment
  Humiliation
  Anger
  Frustration
  Resentment
  Guilt
  Grief
  Depression

Intellectual Dimension
  Hyperresponsiveness
  Irritability
  Negativism
  Increased or decreased perception
  Decreased concentration
  Rumination

Social Dimension
  Disturbed relationships
  Negative self-concept
  Increased dependence
  Increased demands on others
  Withdrawal from social networks
  Isolation
  Loss of employment
  Loss of income
  Secondary gains
  Cultural factors (women have a lower tolerance for pain than men, stoicism)

Spiritual Dimension
  Meaning of pain (associated with punishment, death)
  Decreased value as a person
  Suicide risk
  Religious beliefs (pain as punishment for sins or to be endured)
  Views of prayer, meditation

ANALYSIS

See the nursing diagnosis section on p. 372.

PLANNING AND IMPLEMENTATION

Physical Dimension
  Refer for nerve blocks, TENS
  Explain use of massage.
  Explain use of heat and cold.
  Give medications.

Emotional Dimension
  Reduce anxiety.
  Facilitate expression of negative feelings: fear, anger, frustration, resentment, guilt, embarrassment, humiliation, grief, depression.
  Provide psychotherapy.

Intellectual Dimension
  Teach distraction for pain (for example, music).
  Teach relaxation, guided imagery.
  Refer for biofeedback, hypnosis.
  Assist to identify patterns of response that cause or relieve pain.

Social Dimension
  Promote giving up sick role.
  Use behavioral therapy.
  Encourage client to return to work.
  Refer for vocational counseling.
  Increase independence.
  Assist to improve social networks.
  Increase self-concept.

Spiritual Dimension
  Refer to clergy for spiritual guidance when client feels punished, sinful, abandoned by God or other power.
  Promote will to live.
  Assist to learn to live with pain.
  Encourage introspection and meditation.
  Provide accurate information concerning permanence of pain, possibility of death.

EVALUATION

The following behaviors indicate a positive evaluation: shows awareness of events or situations that trigger pain, manages pain with appropriate reduction techniques, accepts the fact that he will have some pain, and knows community resources available for treatment and counseling.

solutions to his pain and has conveyed a willingness to further engage the client in the pain assessment.

The nurse has also introduced the idea that the client's mood is relevant to the experience of pain and includes it in a discussion of pain. She does not pursue further discussion of mood at this time because the client, in this phase of the alliance, has defined the problem as pain and is unlikely to understand the interrelationship. There is a general acknowledgement and acceptance of the client's feeling state.

Ultimately the intervention suggested by the nurse implies that she does not believe the situation is hopeless. The client's expectation of rejection has been derailed by the nurse's offer to further explore the situation with him.

Evaluation

Evaluation of the nursing interactions for the client with pain is based on both what the client says about the level of pain and behavioral cues. In general, successful outcome is indicated when the client is able to describe a decrease in the severity or frequency of pain. For those clients with chronic pain it is important to consider what techniques for pain management have been learned successfully and to ensure that the client understands them. When used successfully, the client may describe feeling more in control of himself, may be better able to function in daily activities, and will demonstrate improved self-confidence. Family interventions may result in changed family dynamics that encourage the client to perform in expected roles. Some clients with chronic pain can have sufficient return of functioning so that they return to work or consider participation in retraining programs. Evaluation also considers which treatment programs are most successful.

BRIEF REVIEW

Pain is an abstract concept whose presence is indicated by the client's expression of the feeling and by his behaviors. As a syndrome, pain continues to be an economically and emotionally costly problem for both the individual and society. In part because of the economic and emotional burden, the problem of pain in health care has received much more attention during the past 20 years. New theoretical constructs have facilitated interest and research related to pain management.

Pain involves not only physiological mechanisms, but also emotional, intellectual, social, and spiritual components. The interaction of all factors determines the client's experience and expression of pain. There are several classifications of pain. Classification is based on cause and time factors. Persistent pain with no known physiological cause is known as psychogenic pain. The most commonly accepted theory of pain is the gate control theory described first by Melzack and Wall in 1965.

The nurse has a significant responsibility in working with clients experiencing pain. Chronic pain can be severely disabling. In addition to the discomfort of the client, social role functions are lost and the individual loses productivity and a positive sense of self. Together with the client the nurse assesses severity, location, intensity, and duration of pain, as well as contributing emotional, social, cultural, and spiritual factors. From the assessment a plan of care is developed and implemented. The first intervention is to establish a working relationship with the client, and then goals can be developed. In addition to medications, there are several other effective interventions. The nurse becomes involved with teaching clients both about their pain and about the techniques, such as guided imagery, that alleviate pain. Evaluation of progress is based on criteria established for the client to achieve.

REFERENCES AND SUGGESTED READINGS

1. Agnew, D., Crue, B., and Pinsky, J.: A taxonomy for diagnosis and information storage for patients with chronic pain, Bulletin of the Los Angeles Neurological Societies **44**:84, 1979.
2. American Psychiatric Association: Diagnostic and statistical manual of mental disorders (DSM-III-R), Washington, D.C., 1987, The Association.
3. Barber, J., and Adrian, C.: Psychological approaches to management of pain, New York, 1982, Brunner/Mazel.
4. Beckman, C.E., and others: Self-concept: an outcome of a program for spinal pain, Pain **22**:59, 1985.
5. Blazer, D.G.: Narcissism and the development of chronic pain, International Journal of Psychiatry in Medicine **10**(1):69, 1980.
6. Blessing, D.: Free yourself from pain, New York, 1981, Simon & Schuster.
7. Bonica, J.J.: The management of intractable pain in general practice, General Practitioner **33**:107, 1966.
8. Brena, S.F., editor: Chronic pain: America's hidden epidemic, New York, 1978, Atheneum/SMI.
9. Brena, S.F., and Chapman, S.L.: Management of patients with chronic pain, New York, 1983, Spectrum Medical and Scientific Books.
10. Bromm, B., editor: Pain measurement in man: neurophysiological correlates of pain, New York, 1984, Elsevier Press.
11. Brown, J.M.: Imagery coping strategies in the treatment of migraine, Pain **18**:157, 1984.
12. Catchlove, R., and Cohen, K.: Effects of a directive to work approach in the treatment of workmen's compensation patients with chronic pain, Pain **14**:181, 1982.
13. Crook, J., Rideout, E., and Brown, G.: The prevalence of pain complaints in a general population, Pain **18**:299, 1984.
14. Davitz, J.R., and Davitz, L.L.: Inferences of patient's pain and psychological distress: studies of nursing behaviors, New York, 1981, Springer Publishing Co.
15. Davitz, L.J., and others: Nurses' inferences of suffering, Nursing Research **18**:2, 1969.
16. Dudley, S.R., and Holm, K.: Assessment of the pain experience in relation to selected nurse charcteristics, Pain **18**:179, 1984.
17. Fordyce, W.E., and others: Pain measurement and pain behavior, Pain **18**:53, 1984.
18. Fordyce, W.E., Roberts, A.H., and Sternbach, R.A.: The behavioral management of chronic pain: a response to critics, Pain **22**:113, 1985.
19. France, R.D., and Houpt, J.L.: Chronic pain: update from Duke Medical Center, General Hospital Psychiatry **6**:37, 1984.

20. France, R.D., Houpt, J.L., and Ellinwood, E.H.: Therapeutic effects of antidepressants in chronic pain, General Hospital Psychiatry **6**:55, 1984.

21. Freud, A.: The role of bodily illness in the mental life of children. In Frend, A. The psychoanalytic study of the child. New York, 1952, International Universities Press, Inc.

21a. Geach, B.: Pain and coping, Image **19**(1):12, 1987.

22. Gorsky, B.H.: Pain: origin and treatment, Garden City, N.J., 1981, Medical Exam Publishing Co.

23. Hendler, N.: Diagnosis and nonsurgical management of chronic pain, New York, 1981, Raven Press.

24. Hendler, N.H., Long, D.M., and Wise, T.N.: Diagnosis and treatment of chronic pain, Boston, 1982, John Wright, P.S.G., Inc.

25. Houpt, J.L., Keefe, F.J., and Snipes, M.T.: the clinical specialty unit: the use of the psychiatric inpatient unit to treat chronic pain syndromes, General Hospital Psychiatry **6**:65, 1984.

26. Jacox, A.: Pain: A source book for nurses and other health professionals, Boston, 1977, Little, Brown & Co.

27. Jacox, A., and Stewart, M.: Psychosocial contingencies of the pain experience, Ames, Iowa, 1973, University of Iowa Press.

28. Katon, W., Eugan, K., and Miller, D.: Chronic pain: lifetime psychiatric diagnoses and family history, American Journal of Psychiatry **142**:10, 1985.

29. Keefe, F.J., and Bradley, L.A.: Behavioral and psychological approaches to the assessment and treatment of chronic pain, General Hospital Psychiatry **6**:49, 1984.

30. Kerr, F.W.L.: The pain book, Englewood Cliffs, N.J., 1981, Prentice-Hall, Inc.

31. Khatami, M., and Rush, J.A.: A one year follow-up of the multi-model treatment for chronic pain, Pain **14**:45, 1982.

32. Kim, M., McFarland, G., and McLane, A.: Classification of nursing diagnoses, St. Louis, 1984, The C.V. Mosby Co.

33. Kramlinger, K.G., Swanson, D.W., and Maruta, T.: Are patients with chronic pain depressed? American Journal of Psychiatry **140**:6, 1983.

34. Lester, M.C., editor: Pain control: practical aspects of patient care, New York, 1981, Masson Publishing U.S.A.

34a. Levitan, S., and Berkowitz, H.: New developments in pain research and treatment, Washington, D.C., 1985, American Psychiatric Association.

35. Lewith, G.T., and Machin, D.: On the evaluation of the clinical effects of acupuncture, Pain **16**:111, 1983.

36. Lipton, S.: Persistent pain: modern methods of treatment, New York, 1983, Grune & Stratton, Inc.

37. Lipton, S., and Miles, J., editors: Persistent pain: modern methods of treatment, vol. 5, New York, 1985, Grune & Stratton, Inc.

38. Margolis, R.B., and others: Internists and the chronic pain patient, Pain **20**:151, 1984.

39. McCaffry, M.: Nursing management of the patient with pain, ed. 2, Philadelphia, 1979, J.B. Lippincott Co.

40. Meinhart, N.T., and McCaffery, M.: Pain: a nursing approach to assessment and analysis, Norwalk, Ct., 1983, Appleton-Century-Crofts.

41. Melzack, R., editor: Pain measurement and assessment, New York, 1983, Raven Press.

42. Melzack, R., and Wall, P.: The challenge of pain, New York, 1983, Basic Books, Inc., Publishers.

43. Melzack, R., and Wall, P.D.: Pain mechanisms: a new theory, Science **150**:971, 1965.

44. Melzack, R., and Wall, P.D.: Psychophysiology of pain. In Jacox, A., editor: Pain: a source book for nurses and other health professionals, Boston, 1977, Little, Brown & Co.

45. Nightingale, F.: Notes on nursing, London, 1970, Brandon Systems Press, Inc.

46. Nigl, A.J.: Biofeedback and behavioral strategies in pain treatment, New York, 1984, Spectrum Medical and Scientific Books.

46a. North American Nursing Diagnosis Association Classification of Nursing Diagnosis: Proceedings of the seventh conference, St. Louis, 1987, The C.V. Mosby Co.

47. Notermans, S.L.H., and Tophoff, M.M.W.A.: Sex differences in pain tolerance and pain appreciation. In Weisenberg, M., editor: Pain: clinical and experimental perspectives, St. Louis, 1975, The C.V. Mosby Co.

48. Nursing Now: Pain: nurse 85 books, Springerhouse, Pennsylvania, 1985, Springerhouse Corporation.

49. Paul, R.P.: Chronic pain primer, Chicago, 1979, Year Book Medical Publishers, Inc.

50. Reich, J., Tupin, J.P., and Abramowitz, S.I.: Psychiatric diagnosis of chronic pain patients, American Journal of Psychiatry **140**:11, 1983.

51. Roy R., and Tunks, E., editors: Chronic pain: psychosocial factors in rehabilitation, Baltimore, 1982, Williams & Wilkins Co.

52. Schaffer, C.B., Donlon, P.T., and Bittle, R.M.: Chronic pain and depression: a clinical and family history survey, American Journal of Psychiatry **137**:1, 1980.

53. Schiffer, R.B., and others: Depressive episodes in patients with multiple sclerosis, American Journal of Psychiatry **140**:11, 1983.

54. Schwartz, D.P., and others: A chronic emergency room visitor with chest pain: successful treatment by stress management training and biofeedback, Pain **18**:315, 1984.

55. Shacham, S., Dar, R., and Cleeland, C.S.: The relationships of mood state to the severity of clinical pain, Pain **18**:187, 1984.

56. Skevington, S.M.: Chronic pain and depression: universal or personal helplessness? Pain **15**:309, 1983.

57. Steger, J.C., and Fordyce, W.E.: Behavioral health care in the management of chronic pain. In Millon, T., Green, C., and Meagher, R., editors: Handbook of clinical health psychology, New York, 1982, Plenum Press.

58. Sternbach, R.A.: Pain: a psychophysiological analysis, New York, 1968, Academic Press, Inc.

59. Sternbach, R.A.: Pain patients: traits and treatment, New York, 1974, Academic Press, Inc.

60. Swerdlow, M., editor: Relief of intractable pain, ed. 3, New York, 1983, Elsevier Science Publishers, B.V.

60a. Szasz, T.: Pain and pleasure: a study of bodily feelings, ed. 2, New York, 1975, Basic Books, Inc., Publishers.

61. Unikel, I.P.: How we learn chronic pain and sickness. In Brena, S.F., editor: Chronic pain: America's hidden epidemic, New York, 1978, Atheneum/SMI.

62. Urban, B.J.: Treatment of chronic pain with nerve blocks and stimulation, General Hospital Psychiatry **6**:43, 1984.

63. Urban, B.J., Keefe, F.J., and France, R.D.: A study of psychophysical scaling in chronic pain patients, Pain **20**:157, 1984.

64. von Knorring, L., and others: Pain as a symptom in depressive disorder. II. Relationship to personality traits as assessed by means of K.S.P., Pain **17**:377, 1983.

65. Wain, H.J., and Devaris, D.P., editors: The treatment of pain, New York, 1982, Jason Aronson, Inc.

66. Weh-Hsein, W., editor: Pain management, assessment, and treatment of chronic and acute syndromes, New York, 1987, Human Sciences Press.

ANNOTATED BIBLIOGRAPHY

Jacox, A.J.: Pain: a source book for nurses and other health professionals, Boston, 1977, Little, Brown & Co.

This book contains an overview of pain and pain assessment including excellent detailed descriptions of the physiological mechanisms, pathology, and social and psychological aspects of pain. An overview of pain treatment describes the majority of currently used pain treatment methods. Alleviations of pain associated with specific conditions focus primarily on physical conditions. Psychosomatic pain is not specifically discussed.

Meinhart, N.T., and McCaffery, M.: Pain: a nursing approach to assessment and analysis, Norwalk, Ct., 1983, Appleton-Century-Crofts.

This book gives an excellent description of current research, theory, and facts related to pain and its effects on clients. Included are helpful methods and tools that can be used when working with clients in pain.

CHAPTER 19

LONELINESS

Cathleen Shultz

After studying this chapter the learner will be able to:

Define loneliness.

Discuss historical perspectives of loneliness.

Describe theories of loneliness.

Apply the nursing process to care for clients experiencing loneliness.

Identify current research findings relevant to loneliness and client care.

Usually loneliness is defined as the absence of expected relationships. Thus the individual's perceptions, learned behavior, social skills, and social network have considerable effect on whether he acknowledges loneliness. Nurses usually describe loneliness negatively, especially regarding its chronicity and potential harm to the individual's health.

Loneliness is caused by the lack of certain kinds of social contact. In the everyday world, clients may not share the same description of loneliness, but they can easily report its presence or absence. Usually the person feels deprived or that something is missing because certain expected relationships are absent or deficient.

Loneliness is a dynamic, cyclical process that can create, as well as be part of, numerous health problems. In other words, loneliness can precipitate illness and illness can precipitate loneliness. Scholars agree on three important points: loneliness results from deficiencies in a person's social relationships; it is subjective and often not directly related to social isolation; and it causes unpleasant feelings.

The best estimates of incidence indicate that between 50 and 60 million Americans, or one fourth of the population, are lonely at some time during any given month.[45] Loneliness appears to be age related. Data from many studies suggest that loneliness is a major social problem among adolescents with as many as 10% to 15% labeled as seriously lonely.[5] Peaking at adolescence, the incidence of loneliness declines with increasing age until it reaches a rather constant incidence at about age 70.[62]

Adaptive loneliness is healthy because it helps the client turn inward and gather strength from internal resources. At these times loneliness is not a problem needing nursing intervention, but a normal reaction to life's circumstances. Ending a friendship, beginning a new job, moving, and changing marital status are common occurrences that may have a loneliness component. Loneliness does not automatically cause damage; it can provide time to develop potential and generate creative endeavors such as poetry, art, and music.

Beyond the effect on the individual, loneliness affects a society's health and human relationships. When people are lonely they are not benefiting from personal contacts.

THEORETICAL APPROACHES
Psychoanalytic

Those psychoanalytic theorists who wrote about loneliness obtained their data in clinical situations with emotionally troubled individuals. This influenced their view that loneliness is harmful and negative.

Zilboorg[76] distinguished between lonesome and lonely. Lonesome is transient and normal; loneliness is a consuming, negative experience with underlying hostility and narcissism. The lonely person has infantile, omnipotent feelings and is egocentric. Loneliness has roots in infancy when the child learns the pleasure of being cared for and loved and the dismay associated with temporarily unmet needs.

Sullivan[69] claimed that loneliness appears first in childhood with a need for human intimacy. From the infant's initial desire for human contact to the preadolescent's de-

🌿 *Historical Overview* 🌿

DATE	EVENT
Ancient Times	Historical accounts of the Jews and Christians acknowledged man's loneliness as the impetus for Eve's creation. Strong leaders such as David and Solomon sought people and God to reduce their lonely states.
	Numerous religions and other social groups urged frequent contacts between members to continue the groups' beliefs and maintain a social network.
Before 1960	In 1955 Hildegard E. Peplau, a nurse, was among the first to write about loneliness as a concept.[56]
	Only 12 publications about loneliness existed in English, including works by Sullivan[69] and Fromm-Reichmann.[19]
1970-1975	Written material on loneliness, including research, grew rapidly during this time.
	Weiss, the father of loneliness, wrote his classic book entitled *Loneliness: The Experience of Emotional and Social Isolation.*[71]
1975-Present	Loneliness has obtained major attention by those involved in health care.
	In the nursing literature loneliness is interwoven with commonly occurring events such as hospitalization, institutionalization of elderly individuals, bereavement, and suicide.
	Published information evolves from descriptions of loneliness and the behavior of lonely people to loneliness intervention programs.
	A loneliness prevention industry emerges and is thriving via self-help books, support groups, video dating clubs, and video and cassette tapes.
Future	With the development of an increasingly high technological-low touch society, it is probable that the incidence of loneliness will become greater.
	Public awareness of loneliness will increase, and nurses will be challenged to include loneliness prevention and treatment interventions in all health care settings.

sire for a friend, persons need relationships. Failing to gain social skills because of faulty parent or peer interactions can later lead to adult loneliness.

Fromm-Reichmann,[19] agreeing with Sullivan, also believed loneliness to be unpleasant and originating in childhood. In the extreme, loneliness could lead to a psychosis.

Cognitive

Cognitive theorists suggest that loneliness results from discrepancies between actual and perceived levels of social contact.[58] Causes are multifaceted, including character and situational factors as well as past and present influences.

Loneliness is one endpoint of the social interaction continuum (Figure 19-1). Everyone has an optimal level of social interaction: too little and loneliness results, too much and crowding or feeling that one's privacy is invaded occurs.

Sociocultural

For sociologists the cause of loneliness is outside the individual and shaped by society. Social learning theorists believe lonely behavior originates in childhood, is reinforced, and continues in adult life. In modern society three sociological forces create increased loneliness: (1) a decrease in meaningful group relationships, (2) an increase in geographical mobility, and (3) an increase in social mobility.

Three kinds of loneliness have been described: transient, situational, and chronic. Transient loneliness is not recognized as needing professional intervention. Clients either relieve their own loneliness by seeking the companionship of others, or the unpleasant feeling subsides with time.

Situational loneliness is precipitated by a specific life event. Loneliness may then be a companion to or cause of other emotional manifestations such as bereavement and depression. Common events causing situational loneliness include moving, entering college away from home, divorce, death of a family member or friend, obtaining a new job, or a changing social network because of others moving or removing themselves as the client's friends. The client's reactions are beyond just the feeling of being lonely; those additional reactions include headaches, depression, sleep disturbances, anxiety, and somatic complaints. Clients with situational loneliness are more likely

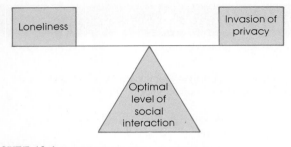

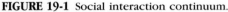

FIGURE 19-1 Social interaction continuum.

TABLE 19-1 Types of loneliness

Types	Characteristics
Transient	Duration: few minutes or hours; loneliness relieved by client
Situational	Precipitated by a life event of significance to the client; severe reactions, possibly lasting up to 1 year
Chronic	Extends beyond temporary circumstances to become a way of life; faulty interaction patterns; minimal or nonexistent intimacy

to seek professional assistance than those experiencing transient loneliness.

For some, loneliness is likely to extend beyond temporary circumstances. Loneliness becomes chronic and a way of life. Patterns of interaction are faulty even when environmental circumstances are optimal. These people have difficulty establishing a social network and becoming involved with others beyond superficial interactions. Intimacy is minimal or nonexistent. When loneliness exists longer than 2 years with no apparent traumatic event, it is considered chronic. The three types of loneliness are described in Table 19-1.

Like so many emotions, maladaptive loneliness creates other cyclic problems. Inwardly, those with chronic loneliness blame themselves and feel hopeless in changing their circumstances. Because these persons perceive themselves as lacking in power to alter their life and expect others to shun their company, loneliness becomes their predominant feeling state. They may also experience the previously mentioned symptoms and have poorer health.

Others view the lonely client's main deficiency as a lack of social reinforcement. Social relations are believed to be a method of reinforcement. Each person has a number and type of relationships with others that are uniquely satisfying. Clients may have different levels of optimal social reinforcement. For example, some need many very close friends while others need only one close confidant. If the perceived optimal level is removed, loneliness results.

Two sociological positions predominate: the other-directed position[60] and the individualism position.[65] When people become other directed and desire to please, they become conformists, alienated from their inner beings, including their feelings and goals. These traits are shaped by significant others and the mass media. Consequently, diffuse anxiety results because the need to please others motivates behavior and is rarely completely satisfied. The members of the other-directed society form what Reisman[60] calls "the lonely crowd."

Slater believes individualism is the problem in America. People desire community and other people. The American pursuit of individualism (need to control one's behavior and to be self-directed) contradicts the basic nature of humans, which is to be with others. The result is loneliness.

In either sociological position, loneliness is normal, is commonly experienced in society and frequently changed by sociological forces, and is shaped by both the past and the present.

Not all people who are alone are lonely. Although frequently used interchangeably, aloneness, solitude, and boredom are not synonymous with loneliness (Table 19-2). People can be by themselves and not be lonely because they still perceive themselves with friends, neighbors, or a higher being to whom they can turn for comfort and company. Being bored is not being lonely; people can have a strong social network at the same time that they are bored or they lack something to do.

Humanistic

In his theory of personality, Rogers proposed that there is a discrepancy between one's inner self and the self seen by others. He believed that clients are pressured by society to behave in certain ways and that loneliness becomes a natural outcome of performing one's roles. As the individual performs various roles, an empty existence emerges.

People remain "locked in their loneliness" because they believe their real inner selves are unlovable. Fearing rejection prevents them from truly exposing their real selves. People continue their social roles with their accompanying feelings of emptiness; consequently, they can expect to experience loneliness. The cause lies within the client and is more shaped by current experiences than by childhood experiences.

TABLE 19-2 Definitions of loneliness and related terms

Term	Definition
Loneliness	A negative experience caused by lack of contact; feeling that something is missing
Aloneness	An observable deficiency in social contacts; may or may not lead to loneliness
Solitude	Voluntary withdrawal from interpersonal relationships
Boredom	Lack of something to do

TABLE 19-3 Summary of theories of loneliness

Theory	Theorist	Dynamics
Psychoanalytic	Zilboorg	Loneliness has roots in infancy. The lonely person has infantile, omnipotent feelings. Lonesome is transient and normal; loneliness is a consuming, negative experience.
	Sullivan	Loneliness first appears in childhood with a need for human intimacy. Failing to gain social skills can lead to adult loneliness.
Cognitive	Fromm-Reichman	Loneliness originates in childhood, can be unpleasant, and can lead to psychoses.
	Perlman and Peplau	Loneliness results from discrepancies between actual and perceived levels of social contact. Loneliness is one endpoint of a social interaction continuum.
Sociocultural	Reisman, Glazer, and Denney	Loneliness is shaped by society, originates in childhood, and is reinforced in adulthood.
	Slater	Loneliness results from a pursuit of individualism that contradicts human nature which is to be with others. Loneliness is normal and commonly experienced.
Humanistic	Rogers	Loneliness is a natural outcome of performing one's societal roles. People are "locked in their loneliness" because they believe their inner selves to be unlovable. The cause of loneliness is within and is more shaped by current experiences than by childhood experiences.
Existential	Moustakas	Loneliness is viewed as a positive. Real loneliness and loneliness anxiety are different entities.
Interactionist	Weiss	Loneliness is caused by the interaction of personality factors and situational factors. Two types of loneliness exist: social loneliness and emotional loneliness.

Existential

Moustakas[49,50] differentiates between "loneliness anxiety" and "real loneliness." Loneliness anxiety results from a discrepancy between what one is and what one pretends to be; the results include defense mechanisms that prevent people from examining themselves and frequently seeking activity with others. Facing genuine life experiences and realizing one's aloneness cause real or existential loneliness. Almost exclusively, Moustakas regards loneliness as a positive experience.

Interactionist

Weiss[71] regards the cause of loneliness as the interaction of personality factors and situational factors. Based on his clinical work, he has described two types of loneliness. Emotional loneliness occurs when a close intimacy is lacking; social loneliness happens when meaningful friendships or a sense of community is lacking. Emotionally lonely individuals feel restless and empty, whereas socially lonely people are bored and feel socially inadequate. Interactionists also view loneliness as normal.

Table 19-3 summarizes the theoretical approaches.

RELATING TO THE CLIENT

The meaning of loneliness varies from person to person. Consequently, when an individual admits to feeling lonely, no clear, precise, single description emerges to guide the nurse.

The nurse searches her feelings and beliefs about loneliness in the preinteraction phase. Many people believe the common myth that nothing can be done to alter lonely people's behaviors. This myth has prevented lonely persons from seeking help. The nurse cannot convince the lonely client to change unless she believes changes can occur. Without hope and encouragement from the nurse, the relationship may not progress beyond the initial interaction.

In the orientation phase the nurse demonstrates caring and understanding to further explore the nature and extent of the client's lonely feelings. Trust is crucial as the nurse attempts to determine the degree and type of the client's loneliness.

During the relationship the client may become overly dependent on the nurse as he finds acceptance and understanding, perhaps for the first time. The client needs continual encouragement to explore other relationships, test newfound social skills, or incorporate an animal in the home. The nurse may find sessions trying, especially ones the client spends rehashing minute details of interactions. Clients need frequent reminders that relationships are subject to human error as they build confidence in their social abilities. Pain and hurt are inevitable in the client's relationships, and the nurse needs to be sensitive to the negative aspects of trying new social behaviors.

The working phase involves teaching social skills to the client or altering the client's life-style to meet relationship needs. Time in the working phase depends on how quickly clients learn new behaviors and the number and quality of relationships needed to alleviate their loneliness.

As with other deeply rooted behaviors, the lonely client may feel hopeless; this can affect the nurse negatively. Maintaining a healthy personal life, including a support system outside the work setting, assists the nurse in functioning at maximum capacity. By actively working on her life-style, she can have the energy to resist long-term personal reactions such as depression, frustration, rejection, and failure. Being sensitive to her past experiences as well as successes and failures in lonely situations can minimize countertransference.

During termination the nurse's needs for human relationships may cause her to consider becoming part of the lonely client's social network. The nurse is encouraged to determine her own lonely feelings throughout interactions so the therapeutic relationship can be terminated in a healthy manner and not prolonged to meet the nurse's needs. The nurse decreases the lonely client's dependence slowly while ensuring that there are adequate resources to assist the client when needed.

Loneliness has developed over a lifetime so setbacks may occur. If the client seeks the nurse's assistance following termination, the nurse needs to be accepting of the setback, willing to resume the relationship, and pursue new goals or the same goals with a hopeful attitude.

NURSING PROCESS
Assessment

✦ Physical dimension. Loneliness can cause physical health problems by placing the client at risk for serious health problems, and physical health problems can cause loneliness. A comprehensive life-style assessment provides clues to identify not only potential physical problems but also risks for future loneliness development.[64] The box on p. 387 lists possible health problems with a loneliness component. Some physical problems necessarily lead to loneliness because human contact is minimized. Diseases and physical problems throughout history have carried a social stigma, causing others to avoid people with those medical diagnoses. Despite increased knowledge and awareness, the stigmas still exist in some parts of the world.

Loneliness can develop in clients who have various physical disorders affecting not only the individual but also the client's family or support system. Generally any physical problem that carries a social stigma affects the client's capacity to relate to others or creates an altered life-style; that is, decreasing intimacy or quality and quantity of relationships can cause loneliness. Assessment considers clients and their family members' physical health status because a client's loneliness can be caused by a family member's health problem. For example, the child with an alcoholic parent may have limited social contacts because of the family's denial of the alcohol problem.

Hospitalization requiring isolation and limited visitors can create temporary loneliness as can recovering from an acute illness that leaves the client too weak for socializing. In situations such as these, temporary loneliness is inevitable. Both social isolation and feelings of loneliness among hospitalized and dying clients have been found, especially those in acute-care, cure-focused settings.[16,37] Consider the lonely state of Mary Beth in the following Case Example.

Case Example

Mary Beth is a 25-year-old artist with a traumatic injury to her right arm that resulted in a below-elbow amputation. She was right handed. She has been hospitalized 8 days and has been out of the intensive care unit for 2 days.

Because of his job, her husband's visits are brief and infrequent; she has not seen her children, 4 months old and 5 years old, since her hospitalization on the day of the accident. She cries frequently, snaps at hospital personnel when answering their questions, has been unable to sleep easily at night, and claims she is useless to anybody.

She will not look at staff when they try to engage her in conversation; she tells them she wants to be alone. She has asked to see her parents and children; neither has been possible at this time because of distance from the hospital, lack of funds, and her parents' lack of desire to visit. She has no interest in television or reading.

During her hospitalization the staff learned that Mary Beth operated her own craft business from a building near her home. Mary Beth has been selling her oil paintings and giving art lessons at her business establishment. A friend has agreed to operate the business while she recuperates.

Medications can contribute to the development of loneliness. Drugs such as antipsychotics and strong sedatives alter the client's thinking. Medications can cause communication disorders or neurological dysfunctions. Long-term cortisone therapy alters the client's physical appearance and activity level. These can alter the client's ability to relate to others and the desire of others to be with the client.

Loneliness can cause sleep disturbances, and sleep disturbances can cause loneliness. Lonely clients often manifest sleep disturbances similar to those of depressed clients.

Esthetic problems can diminish the desire for others to be with the client. Offensive odors, incontinence of stool or urine, and mutilating surgery need to be addressed as possible impediments to socialization and intimacy.

Poor nutrition among elderly persons is often due to loneliness rather than to food or money. Women who have cooked for family or friends and who ate with them are especially vulnerable to loneliness at mealtimes when these significant others are gone. Meals are avoided to prevent the feelings of loneliness.

Chronic diseases requiring numerous treatments, such as renal dialysis, and chronic pain limit the client's quantity and quality of social activities. Social activities often become secondary to treatment of the client's health problem.

Lonely people have reported lower pain tolerance levels. Also, for those clients who present somatic complaints or require higher doses of pain relief medication, the nurse may need to explore the client's needs for the presence of other persons to relieve loneliness. The astute nurse will assess the loneliness needs of clients who request frequent pain relief or higher doses of pain relief medication.

❋ Emotional dimension. There is not one simple way to describe how lonely clients feel. They may express themselves similar to these clients who were asked to describe what it was like to be lonely:

HEALTH PROBLEMS CREATED BY PROLONGED LONELINESS OR WITH A POSSIBLE LONELINESS COMPONENT

CARDIOVASCULAR CONDITIONS

Myocardial infarction
Congestive heart failure
Coronary thrombosis
Ventricular fibrillation
Hypertension
Sudden death
Alcoholism in self or family member

BODY IMAGE CONDITIONS

Overweight or underweight
Limb amputation
Scars
Facial deformities
Mastectomy
Colostomy

CONDITIONS WITH A SOCIAL STIGMA

Cancer
Tuberculosis
Alcoholism in self or family member
Acquired immune deficiency syndrome (AIDS)

COMMUNICATION DISORDERS

Dyslexia
Stuttering

SLEEP DISTURBANCES

Hypersomnolence
Hyperactivity

CONDITIONS ALTERING SOCIAL RELATIONSHIPS

Chronic disease
Malnutrition
Chronic pain
Somatic illnesses

CONGENITAL MALFORMATIONS

Achondroplasia
Craniofacial defects
Amelia or hypomelia

DERMATOLOGICAL CONDITIONS

Port-wine stains
Acne
Ichthyosis
Scleroderma
Visible skin cancers

CONDITIONS USUALLY REQUIRING LIMITED PEOPLE CONTACT

Hemophilia
Osteogenesis imperfecta
Immunodeficiencies
Leukemia

ILLNESS-RELATED CONDITIONS LIMITING PEOPLE CONTACT

Isolation
Limited visitors
Acute-care settings

ALTERED ACTIVITY LEVELS

Cushing's disease
Paraplegia
Quadriplegia
Gait disturbances

CONDITIONS ALTERING SEXUAL ACTIVITY

Impotence
Premature ejaculation
Frigidity
Sexual deviance
Genitourinary surgery
Herpes zoster or shingles
Surgeries
Colostomy
Hysterectomy
Foul body odors

"I felt so empty inside."

"I was totally unlikeable."

"I did not know what to do with myself. Nothing I did was satisfying, and I felt so aimless."

"I was depressed and felt unwanted. I was leprous and unclean."

"Nothing meant anything to me. I had no one to share my life with . . . everyone was gone."

"I feared being with people."

These statements indicate the complexity of the client's lonely feelings. They express a variety of reactions from depression and hopelessness to phobic behavior. The nurse needs to explore the intensity of the client's loneliness, the reasons behind the loneliness, the times or days when loneliness is present, and measures used to relieve loneliness to obtain a total perspective.

A client can feel afraid to express feelings toward others when faced with difficult circumstances. Unless his feelings are expressed he can feel alienated. Promoting his expression of feelings in a safe environment and conveying acceptance of his feelings clarifies his perspective on the situation.

Loneliness can be masked by the presence of overriding emotional states such as hopelessness, depression, and anger. The nurse explores loneliness as a component of other emotional states; it is seldom seen in isolation.

✳ ***Intellectual dimension.*** When an individual's need for relationships is met, he can be more creative, rational, and logical. Problem solving is easier. Extreme loneliness can lead to altered perceptions and ultimately suicidal thoughts and actions.

Sensory stimulation provides data for the client's thoughts. If the senses are malfunctioning, the client can be prevented from receiving accurate cues. His logical thinking may be altered, creating loneliness. Consider the following Case Example.

Case Example

Auda, 75 years old, has numerous lifelong friends. She is widowed and lives alone in a rural community where friendships are the essence of living. She has diminished hearing that began 2 years ago; she refuses to get a hearing aid.

Several friends came by to wish her a happy birthday. She has more difficulty hearing when there is considerable background noise. The kitchen is humming with activity. Two of her friends, Exie and Darlene, are laughing and talking to each other; Darlene says, "That Auda is such a darling." Auda barely catches the conversation. She heard "That Auda is such a . . ." and completes the sentence with the word ". . . bother."

Moments later Auda is found crying in her bedroom. She is inconsolable. The party atmosphere comes to a halt.

In the Case Example the client's diminished hearing caused her to hear only part of the conversation. Her perceptions were based on inaccurate information. She may find herself increasingly lonely as her friends tire of her inability to relate to them as before.

Situations similar to this are common among persons with impaired hearing. If family or friends cannot cope with the person's behavior changes or if the hearing loss is not corrected, the hearing impaired individuals can soon find themselves with a smaller social network.

Loneliness has been associated with cynicism and rejection toward life and others and pessimistic beliefs, including being unable to control one's destiny. Researchers have found that lonely people have a more pessimistic view of marriage and either see themselves as never marrying or report the likelihood of a marriage ending in divorce.[29,48,67] If clients actually believe that others are not worth knowing and there is little that can be done to change one's relationships, then clients probably have little motivation to change and will continue their behavior of isolating themselves from others.

✳ *Social dimension.* Assessment of the social dimension of loneliness includes determining the client's numbers and types of social contacts, recent moves, status of pets, desire for human contact, relationship satisfaction, self-concept, times when loneliness occurs, marital status, income level, recent life or role changes, recent losses such as divorce or death, culture, economic factors, social skills, and the concept of trust. This information contributes to knowing if clients are at risk for loneliness development and their coping strategies for relieving and preventing loneliness. (See the Research Highlight below.)

Social skills are necessary to form relationships and meet the human's need for companionship. Lonely people

seem to have problems relating to others; thus they experience a social skill deficiency.

A lonely client may describe feeling awkward in social situations, may suffer from a self-esteem problem, or may feel alienated from family members or friends. Thus the meaning of loneliness to the client is important to know because in differing circumstances, lonely clients need interventions specific to the type of loneliness felt by these clients.

Typically lonely people take fewer social risks such as purposely meeting new friends, include fewer people in their social network, express less affection for others, and have minimal self-disclosure. They have difficulty being close to others and letting others be close to them. Lonely people often report being shy, introverted, and self-conscious.

Some lonely people have increased self-focused attention that prevents them from being empathic and respon-

---

Research Highlight

Loneliness Among the Elderly: A Causal Approach

R. Creecy, W. Berg and R. Wright, Jr.

PURPOSE

This study attempted to specify and test a causal model of loneliness among elderly adults. Their loneliness was viewed as a product of a cumulative deficit caused by social isolation. The tested model has three major concepts: (1) social activity, or the amount of time spent in formal and informal social activities; (2) social fulfillment, or the quality of involvement in social activities or other interactions; and (3) loneliness, or the degree of felt loss, separation, or isolation and the recognition that these feelings are problematic.

SAMPLE

Data were obtained from a national survey of 4,254 non-institutionalized adults from 18 to 99 years. Participants were selected using a multistage cluster sampling design, stratified by region, city size, and age. This study used data from the 65 years and older group (n = 2,797).

METHODOLOGY

Participants answered demographic questions to obtain the background variables of sex, age, income, marital status, and health. Each variable had previously been related to lonely feelings.

Social activity was measured by a 4-item index obtaining the amount of time the respondent spent participating in select activities (recreation and hobbies; clubs, fraternal or community organizations; socializing with friends; doing volunteer work). Social fulfillment was measured by a 3-item index rating the degree the respondent faced problems with not enough friends, not enough to do to keep busy, and not feeling needed. The dependent variable was measured via a question about whether loneliness was (1) not a problem, (2)

a somewhat serious problem, or (3) a very serious problem to the respondent.

Data were analyzed using multiple regression within the framework of path analysis.

FINDINGS

Five of the seven explanatory variables (marital status, self-perceived health status, income, social activity, and social fulfillment) directly predicted feelings of loneliness. Age and sex did not meet the criterion of explained variance. Three of the five background variables (marital status, income, and self-perceived health status) had significant direct effects on loneliness. Namely, those without a spouse, with limited incomes, or with poor health tended to experience loneliness.

Social fulfillment was the most important predictor of loneliness in the causal model. A sense of social fulfillment debases feelings of loneliness. Social activity, through its relationship with social fulfillment, had a significant indirect causal effect on loneliness. Therefore the higher one's social activity level, the greater the sense of social fulfillment and the lower the loneliness level.

IMPLICATIONS

The model represents one method to assess loneliness as an end product of various social and psychological interrelationships. Sufficient variation in the loneliness felt by elderly persons was found to support the hypothesis that loneliness is not inherent in the aging process. Loneliness was found to be directly related to limiting factors such as marital status, health, and income. The loss of spouse, health, or income tends to isolate aged persons from contacts necessary to prevent loneliness.

Based on data from The Journal of Gerontology **40**:487, 1985.

sive to others' needs and feelings. Others are inhibited socially and do not enjoy parties or the company of others. Lonely people are more likely to coerce others to meet their goals, which may prevent relationships from developing.

Loneliness has been found to be age related in that its intensity is more prevalent among adolescents and older adults. Among older people, loneliness is more related to socioeconomic status than to age or health. Elderly persons may be unable to form new friendships since their social circle decreases because of death and disability. Fixed incomes alter their life-styles and ability to maintain friendships; for example, if they can no longer drive they may not be able to as readily visit family and friends. Loneliness is acutely painful and widespread among adolescents, particularly those who live in divorced families. Adolescent loneliness is more frequent on Fridays and Saturdays. Adolescents also are more likely to feel isolated from parents, teachers, and peers. Adolescents of the lowest social classes, regardless of culture, are more likely to be lonely in their search to belong. Social skill deficits have been found in adolescents who describe themselves as unpopular, shy, and passive. The most vulnerable group seems to be 13-year-old females.[42] Williams[73] has linked delinquent behavior with loneliness as seen in the Research Highlight below.

An association has been found between loneliness and various personal relationships, that is, friends, dating partners, and mates. Adults without mates have greater loneliness than those with mates. For college students the absence of dating partners and friends is closely related to loneliness development. Students who have never had steady dating partners have more loneliness than students who have had steady dating partners.

Economic factors may also relate to loneliness, especially as they affect the client's self-esteem. Particularly important is the link between low socioeconomic status and loneliness. Poor persons may view their status as minimal and consequently not relate to others because they may be embarrassed about their clothing or housing.

Surprisingly, loneliness is not related to the total number of friends.[52] One friendship can meet the client's needs for relationships. Loneliness, then, is in the eye of the beholder. Consider the following Case Example.

Research Highlight

Adolescent Loneliness

E.G. Williams

PURPOSE

Previous studies indicated that one way adolescents express lonely feelings is by delinquent behavior. This study sought to answer questions about whether delinquent adolescents expressed high amounts of general loneliness and whether that loneliness correlated with their need for inclusion, control, and affection as well as demographic characteristics and the offenses committed.

SAMPLE

Participants consisted of 98 volunteers from three detention centers in metropolitan areas. The subjects were between 10 and 18 years of age and were housed in the detention facilities because of delinquent or antisocial acts.

METHODOLOGY

Subjects completed three instruments to obtain self-reported expressions of loneliness. One was the Loneliness Questionnaire (LQ) consisting of 14 items with a Likert-type response scale; the higher the score, the higher the amount of loneliness. Another elicited demographic information and the reason the participant was in detention. The last was the Fundamental Interpersonal Relations Orientation–Behavior (FIRO–B) Questionnaire used to measure need for inclusion, control, and affection.

Independent variables were divided into subgroups on sex, family rank, family structure, income, offense, age, race, religion, locale, wanted inclusion, wanted control, wanted affection, expressed inclusion, expressed control, and expressed affection. Subjects were assigned to these groups based on their delinquency offenses, demographic characteristics, and FIRO-B scores. The dependent variable was measured by the LQ score.

Analysis of variance was the statistical technique used to assess the effects of the independent variables on the amount of loneliness. Multiple comparison tests were done.

FINDINGS

The results revealed no significant correlation between the amount of loneliness and types of delinquent offenses committed or any specific demographic variable. No significant correlations were found between the amount of loneliness and needs for inclusion and control. However, a significant correlation was found between the amount of loneliness and the need for expressed and wanted control ($p \leq 0.05$).

IMPLICATIONS

From a social learning perspective, the delinquent acts of adolescents may have been an attempt to control others or force others in authority to control them to satisfy their needs for control. Those working with delinquent adolescents may see acting-out behavior as a symptom of loneliness.

Based on data from Adolescence **18**:51, 1983.

Case Example

Michelle, 35 years old, was widowed 3 years ago. She had had a close relationship with her husband, and all social activities had involved them as a couple. As a career woman she made the decision to remain near her friends rather than move close to her family, who was over 2,000 miles away.

Grieving was intense as was the loneliness she felt over the next 2 years. She attended many social functions, dated often, and visited friends frequently. Despite these social activities and numerous friends, loneliness was prolonged and a severe depression occurred. Michelle felt hopeless and entertained suicidal thoughts. Her loneliness was unrelieved by social activity and professional involvement.

Knowing that experiencing a death, divorce, or loss of a lover places clients at risk, the nurse assesses Michelle's social dimension beyond the number of persons in her social network. Obviously the one close relationship had provided satisfaction; remove that relationship, and the client becomes vulnerable.

Satisfaction with relationships is more important than frequency or length of interactions. Many lonely people have reported frequent interactions with strangers and acquaintances and fewer interactions with family and friends. In other words, lonely people meet many individuals, but they remain lonely because these individuals are not as important as family, friends, or work.

Not to be overlooked is the client's physical environment relative to whether he is housebound or lacking mobility. The nurse needs to assess the location of the home or apartment relative to meaningful social activities, resources to seek social activities (that is, car, money, or phone), the size of the home, the number of people in the home and rooms for privacy, the home's appearance and cleanliness, the presence of pets, and safety factors. Persons who live in urban areas and in high-crime communities are more vulnerable to loneliness because they fear venturing out or cannot afford transportation for social activities.

Employment factors may contribute to loneliness. Workers who are primarily technical and perform repetitive tasks that require minimal thinking may feel of no value to the work setting and isolated from even their co-workers. On the other hand, the higher one rises in the organization and the more power one attains, the more likely one may develop loneliness.

Time of day may affect the client's loneliness and needs to be considered in the assessment of a hospitalized client. O'Dell's research[54] summarizes specific hours clients feel most lonely when hospitalized; one of these is late in the evening after visitors have left and before bedtime. The nearness of meaningful holidays or anniversary dates heightens loneliness feelings. Adolescents are typically vulnerable to loneliness on the weekends.

Various cultures experience social relationships and thus loneliness differently. Even expressions of friendship differ among groups of people. Some minority groups value extended families more than friends. Some Europeans, such as the English, may not value exploring feelings as do Americans; consequently, they relate differently and these cultural differences need to be addressed through accurate assessment.

Other relationship barriers with implications for developing loneliness are cultural or related to upward mobility, such as moving to different geographical regions or changing one's socioeconomic status. Cultural exclusion occurs when one cultural group does not accept another.[7] With the frequency of upward mobility and moves from one area of the country to another, people require time to learn a new group's values. Until that occurs, loneliness may be experienced. If for any reason a person does not attain full group membership, the lonely feelings increase in intensity.

Typically, lonely people not only dislike themselves, but also dislike others. Lonely people express less interest in sustaining contact with people, perhaps to avoid the pain of rejection or possibly because of lack of positive social reinforcement. They can avoid or distance others by projecting their own inadequacies and expecting perfection in acquaintances and friends.

Reasons for being lonely are as diverse as the expressions of loneliness. Rubenstein and Shaver[84] placed reasons for being lonely into the five categories summarized in the box below.

✿ *Spiritual dimension.* Feeling alone and without others can be a painful experience. Determining the client's meaning of and attitude toward life and desire for relationships provides an indicator of the extent of loneliness. Lonely clients may not have much hope to be liked or even tolerated by others. Without a faith in themselves, others, or God, they are unlikely to explore new relationships or take risks with current relationships.

For those who believe in a higher power, that being encourages companionship among believers. Most reli-

---

CLIENT-REPORTED REASONS OF LONELINESS

CATEGORY 1: BEING UNATTACHED

Having no spouse
Having no sexual partner
Breaking up with spouse or lover

CATEGORY 2: ALIENATION

Feeling different
Being misunderstood
Not being needed
Having no close friends

CATEGORY 3: BEING ALONE

Coming home to an empty house
Being alone

CATEGORY 4: FORCED ISOLATION

Being housebound
Being hospitalized
Having no transportation

CATEGORY 5: DISLOCATION

Being far from home
Being in a new job or school
Moving too often
Traveling often

CLIENT FEELINGS WHEN LONELY

CATEGORY 1: DESPERATION

Desperate
Panicked
Helpless
Afraid
Without hope
Abandoned
Vulnerable

CATEGORY 2: DEPRESSION

Sad
Depressed
Empty
Isolated
Sorry for self
Melancholy
Alienated
Longing to be with one special person

CATEGORY 3: IMPATIENT BOREDOM

Impatient
Bored
Desirous to be elsewhere
Uneasy
Angry
Unable to concentrate

CATEGORY 4: SELF-DEPRECATION

Unattractive
Down on self
Stupid
Ashamed
Insecure

NYU LONELINESS SCALE

1. When I am completely alone, I feel lonely. (almost never . . . most of the time)
2. How often do you feel lonely? (all the time . . . never)
3. When you feel lonely, how lonely do you feel? (extremely lonely . . . I never feel lonely)
4. Compared to people your own age, how lonely do you think you are? (much lonelier . . . much less lonely)

How much do you agree with each of the following?

5. I am a lonely person.
6. I always was a lonely person.
7. I always will be a lonely person.
8. Other people think of me as a lonely person.

From Peplau, L., and Perlman, D.: Loneliness: a sourcebook of current theory, research and therapy, New York, 1982, John Wiley & Sons, Inc. Reprinted by permission.

gious groups foster this. In Western culture a continuing relationship between individuals and God and among individuals is at the center of beliefs and practices. Assessment includes the focus of the clients' worship, their concept of a higher being, and the degree of support clients perceive they need from the higher being.

General principles of conduct permeate religious teachings. People are reminded to love self and others and to actively express love to a higher being and fellow humans. Assessment can include determining the beliefs the client actively practices in relating to his fellow human beings.

These questions may guide the nurse in assessing the client's spiritual dimension:

How frequently are you in the company of others? alone?

Do you view others as friendly or hostile?

What does your religion believe about solitude?

When have you felt alone from a higher being? from family and friends?

What religious practices do you use to relieve loneliness?

What are your creative abilities? Do you do these alone or with others?

Measurement tools. Several tools using two different approaches to measure loneliness are available. One approach is unidimensional and describes loneliness as a single experience with common themes. Another approach is multifaceted.

The most widely used unidimensional measure of loneliness is the UCLA Loneliness Scale consisting of 20 items.[57] The scale can be used to determine the presence and degree of loneliness in clients so that appropriate interventions can be developed.

Another popular scale is the NYU Loneliness Scale (see the box above). It measures long-term loneliness from a multifaceted perspective. It is useful when one needs to know the extent of loneliness since interventions may differ between situational and chronic loneliness.

In one of the earliest attempts to describe feelings associated with loneliness, Rubenstein and Shaver[62] used the NYU Loneliness Scale, which lists feeling adjectives as possible descriptions of loneliness. Factor analysis identified clusters of responses that could be used to isolate dimensions or factors of loneliness. The responses were intercorrelated and factor analyzed to form four main categories summarized in the left box above.

Category 1 received the largest number of responses and was observed in those experiencing emotional isolation. These people were distressed and most often had severed their most intimate social ties through divorce, death, or abandonment. Cateogy 3 was viewed as similar to the social isolation that occurs when clients move or enter new jobs. Impatient boredom was seen more as an indicator of loneliness in young persons than among old persons. Categories 2 and 4 were conceptualized as reactions to loneliness. If loneliness was encountered long enough, self-blame and depression would probably result.

Analysis

Nursing diagnosis. The NANDA nursing diagnoses related to loneliness are impaired social interaction and social isolation. The defining characteristics of these two diagnoses are summarized in the boxes on p. 392.

The following Case Example illustrates characteristics of the nursing diagnosis of impaired social interaction.

Case Example

Jason is a 15-year-old who has recently moved with his parents from a rural area of Arkansas to Atlanta, Georgia. The move occurred several months before his graduation from the junior high school he has attended for the last 3 years.

His parents have become concerned because after 3 months

IMPAIRED SOCIAL INTERACTION

DEFINITION
State in which an individual participates in an insufficient or excessive quantity or ineffective quality of social exchange.

DEFINING CHARACTERISTICS
Emotional Dimension
*Fears about interacting with others
Intellectual Dimension
Verbalized or observed inability to receive or communicate a satisfying sense of belonging, caring, interest, or shared history
Social Dimension
Verbalized or observed discomfort in social situations
Observed use of unsuccessful social interaction behaviors
Dysfunctional interaction with peers, family, and/or others
Family report of change of style or pattern of interaction

Adapted from North American Nursing Diagnosis Association Classification of Nursing Diagnosis: Proceedings of the seventh conference, St. Louis, 1987, The C.V. Mosby Co.
*Indicates characteristic in addition to those defined by NANDA.

in his new school he continues to verbalize his inability to meet new friends. He complains every weekend about being bored and not having anything to do. When his parents suggest that he call someone, he gets very angry and says that "the kids here don't like to do the same things I like."

The following Case Example illustrates characteristics of the nursing diagnosis of social isolation.

Case Example

James, a 59-year-old Korean War veteran, is single and has been chemically dependent since spending several years of his military service in the Aleutian Islands. As a child, he was indulged by parents who rarely punished him, met his every need, and required no accountability from him. He had developed no intimate friendships and never learned how to relate to his classmates. He had no household chores and seldom stayed with one activity for long.

Today he leads a lonely existence in an unkept trailer. Receiving disability benefits, he holds no job and has no social ties other than occasionally visiting two close aunts. His parents died years ago.

Last week one of his aunts suddenly died. As he had done so often in the past, James reacted to the crisis by turning to diazepam (Valium), neperidine (Demerol), and beer. His chemically altered consciousness prevented his experiencing the loss and subsequent loneliness. He did not attend the funeral.

Emotional pain is intolerable to him so he escaped via drugs and avoided the experience. Chemicals prevented feeling the pain by altering his awareness and thinking. He is a very lonely individual because of his past behavior and experiences.

SOCIAL ISOLATION

DEFINITION
Person needs or desires contact with others but is unable to make that contact.

DEFINING CHARACTERISTICS
Physical Dimension
Increased irritability
Restlessness
Change in previously good health state to illness state
Sleep disturbances (too much sleep or insomnia)
Change in eating habits (overeating or anorexia)
*Sighing
Emotional Dimension
Unexplained dread
Abandoned feeling
Useless feeling
Depression, anxiety, or anger
*Fears about interacting with others
Intellectual Dimension
Inability to concentrate and make decisions
Postponement of important decisions
Belief that time passes slowly
Doubts about ability to survive
*Boredom
Social Dimension
Desire for more family or nurse contact
Failure to interact with others who are nearby
*Unsatisfactory social network (self-reported)
*Desire for more friend contact
*Feeling of social inadequacy
Spiritual Dimension
*Inability to relieve loneliness by religious practices that previously had assisted client to cope

Adapted from North America Nursing Diagnosis Association Classification of Nursing Diagnosis: Proceedings of the seventh conference, St. Louis, 1987, The C.V. Mosby Co.
*Indicates characteristic in addition to those defined by NANDA.

The following list provides examples of additional NANDA-accepted diagnoses with causative statements.
1. Social isolation related to chronic illness
2. Impaired social interaction related to negative self-concept
3. Dysfunctional grieving related to child moving from the home
4. Social isolation related to absence of significant others
5. Hopelessness related to feelings of loneliness
6. Social isolation related to move to a new community
7. Social isolation related to recent diagnosis of Acquired Immune Deficiency Syndrome (AIDS)
8. Potential social isolation related to initiation of reverse isolation
9. Impaired social interaction related to admission to a nursing home

DSM-III-R diagnoses. Loneliness can lead to and be masked by psychopathological conditions. Among those conditions most often seen with a loneliness component are depression, withdrawal, hostility, despair, and anger. The reader is referred to Chapters 12, 14, and 17 for further information on these topics.

Planning

Table 19-4 provides some long-term and short-term goals and outcome criteria related to loneliness. These serve as examples of the planning stage of the nursing process.

Implementation

·ːᐧ· ***Physical dimension.*** Loneliness has been linked *·✦·* with alcoholism, suicide, and physical illness. Because loneliness has life-threatening consequences, the nurse uses the loneliness health-illness continuum model as a reference for client care (Figure 19-2). The nurse strives to prevent or minimize the detrimental effects of loneliness on health.

The nurse arranges programs where clients eat together in restaurants or eat meals in each other's homes. Groups can be formed for at-risk people. Churches and senior citizen groups have regular meetings that include meals; Sunday dinners for widowed individuals provide companionship at a vulnerable time of the week.

Regular physical exercise (for example, using a stationary bike, weight lifting, walking, golfing, and swimming) not only improves physical health but also contributes to general emotional health because endorphins are produced, promoting a sense of well-being.

Relieving lonely feelings may require the client's acceptance of an unalterable physical problem such as a congenital syndrome or changing an alterable problem such as obesity. Changing the client's perceptions or the

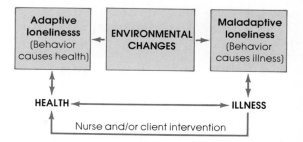

FIGURE 19-2 The client's response to loneliness on a health-illness continuum.

body image problem is paramount to developing relationships.

Correcting disfigurements that can be changed by cosmetic surgery is possible. As a result the client may be more likely to desire being with others. Persons with missing or nonfunctioning body parts can be referred to organizations that provide support and guidance for obtaining and using prostheses. These organizations can assist the client to locate stores that sell clothing for persons who have had disfiguring surgeries.

When the problem is decreased mobility as a result of a fractured hip or paralysis, physical supports such as canes, walkers, and wheelchairs are available. These supports increase mobility, which can increase social interaction.

If the client is homebound, visiting nurses from the private or public health sector are incorporated into discharge planning. The community nurse facilitates continuity of care into the home and work with clients to keep social isolation to a minimum. In some states social services provide transportation to buy groceries, keep

---

TABLE 19-4 Long-term and short-term goals and outcome criteria related to loneliness

Goals	Outcome Criteria
NURSING DIAGNOSIS: SOCIAL ISOLATION RELATED TO RELOCATION	
Long-term goals	
To use effective coping strategies to relieve feelings of loneliness	Shares coping strategies used to resolve previous times of loneliness
	Participates in support groups of adults who have experienced losses
To establish meaningful relationships	Attends one activity per week with a person he perceives to be positive
	Maintains relationships that relieve lonely feelings
Short-term goals	
To engage in a constructive life-style to meet loneliness needs	Uses thought-stopping techniques to prevent dwelling on lonely feelings
	Lists activities and people he enjoys by fifth visit
	Participates in one activity with a significant other within 2 weeks after counseling began
To maintain social network relationships he perceives as positive	Lists people in his social network that he views as positive
	Develops a plan to maintain contact with these people

health-related appointments, or to ensure social outings.

Odors can contribute to isolation. Simply improving personal hygiene may also eliminate the problem. In managing these esthetic problems, professionals such as enterostomal therapists are available for consultation. Bowel and bladder training regimens as well as odor eliminators are identified in the nursing literature if specific instructions are needed.

Urban clients who live in unsafe neighborhoods are especially likely to be lonely. Moving may be impossible and may create more problems than it solves. Interventions are designed considering the client's habits and habitat. For example, a lonely client living in a ghetto can use community-supported transportation to receive health care in free neighborhood clinics; the client may only need assistance in identifying transportation and the clinic location. Another challenge is presented by the client who lives in a high-income area distant from neighbors. Neighborhood support groups, law enforcement officials, and community organizations may be used to develop an informal social network to check these individuals periodically.

Emotional dimension. The nurse can help lonely clients by acknowledging their loneliness. Encouraging clients to describe what they feel may prevent avoidance or denial of loneliness. They may need assistance in expressing loss of power, diminished prestige, anger, and dependence.

The client's predominant feeling state, such as depression and anger, will initially direct the nursing interventions. The nurse's communication portrays hopefulness, concern, acceptance, and a willingness to spend time with the client. If the client is in an acute care setting, sometimes the nurse's being available and willing to talk are all that is needed. The nurse can become an alternate support system during hospitalization. Hospitalized clients with few visitors or with long spans of time between visitors have found visits by the nurse to be helpful. Using short, frequent visits and expressing interest and concern have proved to minimize loneliness.[54]

Rubenstein and Shaver[62] found several activities that individuals do when they feel lonely to relieve the uncomfortable feelings. These include crying, sleeping, thinking, doing nothing, overeating, taking tranquilizers, watching television, drinking or getting "stoned," studying or working, writing, listening to music, exercising, walking, working on a hobby, going to a movie, reading, playing music, spending money, calling a friend, and visiting someone. Some are therapeutic; others are not. The most commonly used activities were reading, listening to music, and calling a friend. At first glance they appear simplistic, but clients have documented that these kinds of activities work and nurses can incorporate them to relieve client loneliness.

Because loneliness is so prevalent and accompanies numerous disorders and situations, the expert psychiatric nurse may be a consultant for lonely clients. Helping staff to develop interventions or providing direct care through counseling in nonpsychiatric settings has become increasingly needed.

Intellectual dimension. If the client has negative thoughts about himself and others, the nurse directs him in using thought-stopping techniques. Converting negative thoughts to positive thoughts can break the self-deprecation cycle and prepare the client for better relationships.

Scheduling diversional activities for evenings or weekends when loneliness is most likely to occur prevents the client from having time to think about how lonely he is. Elderly people who can participate in activities have found these sorts of activities to be extremely helpful[26,39]: hobbies; sports; reading; playing cards; watching television; praying; meditating; work such as housework, cooking, and gardening; and completing jigsaw or crossword puzzles.

Identifying tasks the client can do during high-risk times can prevent lonely feelings. Relatives and friends can be included in activities if the client desires. Holiday and anniversary activities are more meaningful if planned according to the way the client once celebrated them.

If sensory perceptions are altered and the problem is correctable, the nurse can explore ways to obtain items such as glasses and hearing devices. Community organizations such as the Lions Club and Kiwanis Club assist in purchasing these items for low-income individuals. Support groups exist for hearing and visually impaired persons. The client may need to learn a new method of communication such as the Braille alphabet or sign language. Tutors and volunteers are available in most large communities. Attachments to amplify voices may be placed on the client's telephone.

Therapeutic reminiscing has proved helpful for older clients who can share interesting events about their past. Previous successes and coping mechanisms can prove to the client he is worthwhile and his life has meaning. By reflecting on skills used previously to solve socially related problems, clients can gain hope to face present problems leading to loneliness.

Social dimension. Interventions to enhance social skills and the number and quality of relationships are firmly established on what the client values. The client's need for autonomy affects the success of the intervention. For example, clients who value their independence will benefit the greatest from interventions that allow them to maintain control. For the lonely client who is able, this means helping him develop his own plan to minimize loneliness.

With a motivated client, the nurse encourages learning new coping behaviors or assists the client to retain successful coping behaviors to obtain an optimal health state. The client then adapts in a healthy way to the frequent encounters with situations producing loneliness. For example, the client who has moved to a new city with no acquaintances may exhibit disturbed sleep patterns, such as waking in the early morning hours. Over time, exhaustion interferes with work productivity and health, even further reducing the client's ability to develop new friendships. The client needs assistance to alter this cycle and regain optimal health before the maladaptive behavior leads to permanent or destructive results.

Developing a social network plan to "repeople" the client's world can be a challenging task. A social network plan involves evaluating the scope of a client's social contacts and enacting a plan to increase the quantity or quality of those contacts. Budget, geographical location, resources, transportation, likes and dislikes, availability of significant others, and health state are considerations in implementing a social network. Willing family members or friends can be included in the treatment. The plan belongs to the client; the nurse is the facilitator. For those persons who have lost their major source of human intimacy, the nurse can give support while assessing and determining the need to "repeople" their world.

Day care centers, garden clubs, foster grandparent programs, senior citizen groups, community coffee klatches, church groups, mixers, summer Elderhostel programs, and college classes open to handicapped or senior citizens are methods for various age groups to make new social contacts. The nurse gathers pertinent information about these activities to assist the client's decision making. Informing, discussing advantages and disadvantages, prioritizing, and periodically checking the client's progress toward becoming part of these groups are important nursing interventions. The nurse may assist in forming these activities if none exist within the community.

If the client has a diminished self-esteem, some situational changes can be considered. For example, a retired client may have recently moved to a retirement village. Esteem is lessened because the person no longer views himself as contributing meaningfully to life. Usually a niche can be found for the client's talents and abilities. Organizing parties, participating in community political campaigns, volunteering for hospital work, and visiting others in the same area who are temporarily housebound are activities involving the client's ability to relate to others.

Sharing past experiences as a volunteer consultant to those who may benefit from them is a method to develop work-related contacts. Retirement communities with planned activities provide additional options to "repeople" one's life.

Sharing housing with someone who is compatible can also prevent loneliness. Some individuals have successfully attempted communal living to provide companionship, share expenses, achieve safety, and give meaning to life.

Nursing of clients in long-term care settings such as nursing homes or mental hospitals requires that nurses teach unskilled workers how to meet companionship needs during routine care. Talking while ambulating clients, touching clients when entering their rooms, and allowing clients to talk during mealtimes offer opportunities to enhance the quality of institutional living while encouraging the client's reality orientation. Workers can be taught this information and need to see nurses modeling expected caring behavior.

Companion animals serving as people substitutes, have been especially helpful to young and old individuals, and are particularly helpful to persons with illnesses that leave them housebound or in nursing homes. As a source of comfort they can offer meaning to clients who view the world as hopeless. If the client's life-style, resources, and desires permit, a pet can offer companionship and occupy the client's time. Usually a veterinary medical association has guidelines for placing animals in private dwellings as well as nursing homes. When hospitalized, the client needs contact with the pet, if only through the caregiver telling the client that his pet is being fed and cared for or the caregiver arranging a "visit" by the pet.[15]

Social skills can be developed by methods such as role-playing. Imagery assists the client to view himself as successful in social situations. Big Brother, Big Sister, Adopt-a-Grandparent, and Adopt-a-Grandchild groups offer meaningful social outlets and also promote role development.

Spiritual dimension. Interventions will depend on past practices the client has used to relate to the Higher Being acknowledged by his beliefs. To a client who values and practices his beliefs, the inability to do so can create an all-consuming loneliness. Encouraging prayer and meditation can bridge the feelings of alienation. Visits to the hospital or nursing home chapel can offer an atmosphere conducive to interacting more meaningfully with God.

When a client is doubting, suffering, lonely, or hurting, prayer can bring relief. When an individual feels alone, reaching out to others can become a means to forget one's aloneness while fulfilling scriptural intent.

A client can be in conflict with his beliefs and thus feel alienated from his known world. Verbalizing this conflict without fear of censure may relieve the tension and enable the client to solve the problem. Also, reading favorite passages of the Bible or other inspirational books may provide comfort when loneliness is imminent.

The nurse fosters the client's own spiritual resources in coping with loneliness rather than imposing new, unfamiliar practices. If the nurse feels inadequate about discussing spiritual matters or cannot support the client's beliefs or practices, obtaining a chaplain, minister, or rabbi would be the logical step.

Some churches have members or ministers who regularly check the religious status of persons admitted to hospitals. These groups schedule frequent visitation and offer services specific to the client's beliefs. Paid or voluntary hospital chaplains may provide the same services. For example, communion can be brought to the client's bedside and served.

Depending on the religious group's outreach services, a member may expect numerous cards, assistance with caring for his family or home, regular visitation, and home care after discharge. Clients may spend years developing relationships with their church groups; the nurse would do well to foster and incorporate this support system into the client's needed interventions.

INTERACTION WITH A LONELY CLIENT

Nurse: (Making afternoon rounds, entering the room of a hospitalized adult male client who is several hundred miles from home; he is sitting in a chair, the television is on, and he is staring out a window.) Good afternoon, Mr. Graddy; how are you?

Client: (He offers no eye contact and continues staring out the window.) Okay.

Nurse: You're all alone.

Client: (Turning to face her.) Well, yes I am.

Nurse: (Indicating an empty chair near him and maintaining eye contact.) May I sit with you?

Client: (Nods affirmatively and pulls the chair closer to him so they are sitting across from each other.) Sure. I need some company.

Nurse: (Sitting down and placing her paperwork on the dresser nearby.) What can I help with?

Client: (Speaking slowly and with hesitation.) Nothing . . . not really. I was just thinking about my kids and how much I miss them. My boy is coming home from the service this weekend and my wife and I were. . .

The preceding conversation continued for about 5 minutes, and the nurse agreed to come by his room again later in the evening.

Mr. Graddy was lonely, and the nurse encouraged him to acknowledge how he felt. Her conversation prevented him from denying the presence of loneliness. By conveying acceptance and spending some time with Mr. Graddy she provided a caring human contact. She can become an alternate support system to him during this hospitalization by making short, frequent visits part of her nursing interventions with him.

The nurse used verbal and nonverbal communication skills to convey interest, concern, acceptance, and caring to Mr. Graddy. She was not discouraged by his initial lack of interest in her presence. She did not remain standing in an authority position, and she put down her "professional equipment" to indicate this time was his. He easily responded to her cues, and this visit may become the basis for future positive nurse-client interactions.

Evaluation

Evaluation centers on the client's expression of loneliness, reduction or elimination of health problems caused by loneliness, and the client's awareness of changes. Generally people cope with loneliness in one of three ways: 1) changing their relationships, 2) changing their social desires or needs, and 3) decreasing the importance of their relationships. When changes do not occur, new goals are developed and more pertinent strategies are incorporated into the nursing process. Positive evaluation indicates that maladaptive loneliness behavior has changed or been modified and new social skills have emerged.

Evaluation includes an assessment of the nurse's behaviors. Identifying and modifying behaviors that create problems in relating to lonely clients are essential to effective nursing care. For example, being less authoritarian when talking with a lonely client who is expressing his feelings may allow him to more freely discuss his perceptions. Supportive work environments can provide the ingredients to enhance self-evaluation and lead to personal and professional growth that ultimately promotes more effective nursing care of the lonely client.

NURSING PROCESS SUMMARY: LONELINESS

ASSESSMENT

Physical Dimension
- Chronic illness
- Altered body image
- Socially unacceptable disease
- Chemical dependence
- Sleep disturbances
- Congenital defects
- Sensory impairment
- Headaches
- Nausea
- Overeating
- Tears

Emotional Dimension
- Aimlessness
- Uneasiness
- Empty feeling
- Melancholy
- Isolation
- Feeling of being unattractive
- Hopelessness
- Vulnerability
- Depression
- Insecurity
- Anger
- Sadness
- Aloneness
- Boredom
- Self-pity
- Self-deprecation
- Self-consciousness
- Despair
- Isolation
- Alienation
- Impatience
- Stupidity
- Shame

Intellectual Dimension
- Altered perceptions
- Suicidal thoughts
- Rationalization
- Intellectualization
- Difficulty making decisions
- Impaired judgments
- Pessimistic beliefs
- Doubting

NURSING PROCESS SUMMARY: LONELINESS—cont'd

Social Dimension
Decreased intimacy
Recent death or divorce
Role change
Social skill deficits
Decreased social network
Unsatisfying relationships
Living alone
Change in living quarters
Recent relocation
Upward or downward social status mobility
Shyness
Helplessness

Spiritual Dimension
No meaningful relationship with God or supreme being
Feeling of alienation
Altered beliefs and practices

ANALYSIS

Refer to the nursing diagnosis section on pp. 391-393.

PLANNING AND IMPLEMENTATION

Physical Dimension
Arrange programs for clients to eat together.
Assist client to accept unalterable physical problems.
Encourage corrective surgery.
Refer those with missing or nonfunctioning body parts to organizations for support and guidance.
Obtain physical supports such as canes or walkers to increase mobility.
Plan a regular exercise schedule.
Relieve physical symptoms such as sleeplessness.
Arrange transportation needs.
Manage esthetic problems such as odors and foul drainage.

Emotional Dimension
Acknowledge client's lonely feelings.
Promote expression of lonely feelings.

Plan meaningful activities.
Portray hopefulness, concern, and acceptance.
Provide short, frequent visits with friends.
Acknowledge client's need for autonomy in **interventions**.

Intellectual Dimension
Assist client to use thought-stopping techniques to decrease negative thoughts.
Schedule diversional activities.
Provide aids to correct sensory perception problems.
Encourage therapeutic reminiscing for older clients.
Assist client in distinguishing between thoughts and feelings.
Provide positive visualization and imagery when client is preoccupied with lonely feelings.
Observe continuously if client expresses suicidal thoughts.
Encourage client to attend therapy sessions.

Social Dimension
Design activities to enhance social skills.
Develop a social network with the client.
Minimize social isolation through discharge planning services.
Plan meaningful social activities.
Assist the client to change relationships as needed.
Encourage family and friends to visit client.
Obtain a companion animal.
Alter the client's social skills through role-playing.
Use imagery to assist the client in viewing himself as successful in social situations.
Encourage the client to do activities with others.

Spiritual Dimension
Encourage expression and practice of religious values and beliefs.
Promote creative endeavors.

EVALUATION

Refer to the evaluation section of this chapter on p. 396.

BRIEF REVIEW

Loneliness is a universal phenomenon often viewed as negative and unpleasant. Caused by the inadequacy or lack of certain kinds of important contacts, loneliness has been linked to numerous health problems.

The study of loneliness has only recently developed, and nurses such as Hildegard Peplau have contributed to loneliness information and treatment. Heightened public awareness of the problem provides an excellent opportunity for nurses to assist lonely clients.

Loneliness theories emerged from the psychological and sociological sciences. Most theorists believe loneliness is unpleasant and linked to current situational factors.

Among the at-risk groups for loneliness are adolescents, dying persons, those with chronic or socially unacceptable illnesses, those with body image problems, those who have lost significant relationships, and those who have relocated geographically.

Loneliness and health problems are cyclic; each can cause the other. Health problems related to loneliness occur in all dimensions and are associated with cardiovascular diseases, body image problems, chronic diseases, emotional illnesses, impaired hearing, divorce, moves, role changes, transportation problems, employment factors, and spiritual difficulties.

Nursing diagnoses for the lonely client center on social isolation and impaired social interaction. Interventions designed by the nurse and client assist the client to cope by changing the client's relationships or social desires and needs or by decreasing the importance of relationships. Strategies such as obtaining companion animals, determining transportation needs, altering social skills, and encouraging spiritual beliefs work to prevent or minimize lonely feelings.

The nurse is unable to meet all the loneliness needs of her clients in their various developmental stages. However, she can offer a climate conducive for preventing or minimizing loneliness. This climate contains recognition, regard, respect, understanding, caring, and encouragement to enter relationships with others. In such a climate the client can express himself without fear, test new ways to handle his relationships, reevaluate his behavior, change negative attitudes toward himself and others, and grow toward becoming a more integrated and less lonely human being.

REFERENCES AND SUGGESTED READINGS

1. Anderson, C., Horowitz, L., and French, R.: Attributional style of lonely and depressed people, Journal of Personality and Social Psychology 45(1):127, 1983.
2. Bernikow, L.: Alone: yearning for companionship in America, New York Times Magazine, p. 24, August 15, 1982.
3. Booth, R.: Toward an understanding of loneliness, Social Work 28:116, March-April 1983.
4. Brennan, T.: Loneliness at adolescence. In Peplau, L., and Perlman, D.: Editors: Loneliness: a sourcebook of current theory, research, and therapy, New York, 1982, John Wiley & Sons, Inc.
5. Brennan, T., and Auslander, N.: Adolescent loneliness: an exploratory study of social and psychological pre-dispositions and theory, vol. 1. National Institute of Mental Health, Juvenile Problems Div., Grant no. R01-MH 289 12-01, Behavioral Research Institute, Washington, D.C., 1979.
6. Brickel, C.M.: A review of the roles of pet animals in psychotherapy and with the elderly, International Journal of Aging and Human Development 12(2):119, 1980.
7. Brody, E.B.: Cultural exclusion, character and illness, American Journal of Psychiatry 8:852, 1966.
8. Carpenito, L.: Nursing diagnosis: application to clinical practice, Philadelphia, 1983, J.B. Lippincott Co.
9. Carter, A.: A nurse's Christmas carol, RN, p. 36, 1984.
10. Cochrane, N.: An explanatory study of social withdrawal experiences of adults, Nursing Papers 15:22, Summer 1983.
11. Cohen, N.: On loneliness and the aging process, International Journal of Psychoanalysis 63:149, 1982.
12. Creecy, R., Berg, W., and Wright, R.: Loneliness among the elderly: a causal approach, Journal of Gerontology 40(4):487, 1985.
13. Davis, J.H.: Children and pets: a therapeutic connection, Pediatric Nursing 11:377, September-October 1985.
14. Ellison, E.S.: Social networks and the mental health caregiving system: implications for psychiatric nursing practice, Journal of Psychosocial Nursing and Mental Health Services 21:21, March 1983.
15. Erickson, R.: Companion animals and the elderly, Geriatric Nursing, p. 92, March-April 1985.
16. Feifel, H.: The meaning of dying in American society. In Davis, R.H., editor: Dealing with death, San Diego, 1973, University of Southern California, Ethel Percy Andrus Gerontology Center.
17. Francis, G.: Loneliness: measuring the abstract, International Journal of Nursing Studies 17(2):127, 1980.
18. Francis, G.M.: Loneliness: the syndrome, Issues in Mental Health Nursing 3:1, January-June 1981.
19. Fromm-Reichmann, R.: Loneliness, Psychiatry 22:1, 1959.
20. Gatz, M., Pearson, C., and Fuentes, M.: Older women and mental health, Issues in Mental Health Nursing 5:273, 1983.
21. Hamilton, J.: Development of interest and enjoyment in adolescence. II. Boredom and psychopathology, Journal of Youth and Adolescence 12(5):363, 1983.
22. Hartog, J., Audy, J.R., and Cohen, Y.A., editors.: The anatomy of loneliness, New York, 1980, International Universities Press, Inc.
23. Hillestad, E.A.: Is it lonely at the top? Nursing Administration Quarterly 8:1, Spring 1984.
24. Hogstel, M.O.: Old, alone, and in need. . . a right radical mastectomy (case study), Journal of Gerontological Nursing 8:337, June 1982.
25. Hojat, M.: Loneliness as a function of parent-child and peer relations, The Journal of Psychology 112:129, 1982.
26. Hood, P.H.: Perceived loneliness among the aged and associated factors, unpublished master's thesis, Seattle, 1974, University of Washington.
27. Horowitz, L., French, R., and Anderson, C.: The prototype of a lonely person. In Peplau, L., and Perlman, D., editors: Loneliness: a sourcebook of current theory, research and therapy, New York, 1982, John Wiley & Sons, Inc.
28. Hoskins, L.M., and others: Nursing diagnosis in the chronically ill: methodology for clinical validation, Advances in Nursing Science 8(3):80, 1986.
29. Jones, W., Hobbs, S., and Hockenberry, D.: Loneliness and social skill deficits, Personality Processes and Individual Differences, p. 682, 1983.
30. Jones, W.H.: Loneliness and social contact, Journal of Social Psychology 113:295, 1981.
31. Jones, W.H., Freemon, J.A., and Goswick, R.A.: The persistence of loneliness: self and other determinants, Journal of Personality 49:27, 1981.
32. Kahn, R.: Aging and social support. In Riley, M., editor: Aging from birth to death, vol. 30, Boulder, Col., 1979, Westview Press, Publishers.
33. Kaplan, B.H., Cassel, J.C., and Gore, S.: Social support and health, Medical Care 15(suppl.)47, May 1977.
34. Kayser-Jones, J.S., and Abu-Saad, H.: Loneliness: its relationship to the educational experience of international nursing students in the United States, Western Journal of Nursing Research 4:301, 1982.
35. Kim, M.J., McFarland, G.K., and McLane, A.M., editors: Pocket guide to nursing diagnoses, ed. 2, St. Louis, 1987, The C.V. Mosby Co.
36. King, K.: Three strikes against her: female, old, and . . . drunk, Journal of Gerontological Nursing 10(7):30, 1983.
37. Kubler-Ross, E.: On death and dying, New York, 1969, Macmillan Publishing Co., Inc.
38. Leiderman, P.H.: Loneliness: a psychodynamic interpretation. In Hartog, J., Audy, J.R., and Cohen, A., editors: The anatomy of loneliness, New York, 1980, International Universities Press, Inc.
39. Lopata, H.Z.: Loneliness: forms and components, Family 35:2, 1971.
40. Lund, D.A., and others: Can pets help the bereaved? Journal of Gerontological Nursing 10:8, June 1984.
41. Madrid, M.: Nurses can turn the tide. Journal of Gerontological Nursing 10(5):8, 1981.
42. Mahon, N.E.: The relationship of self-disclosure, interpersonal dependency, and life changes to loneliness in young adults, Nursing Research 31:343, 1982.
43. Mahon, N.E.: Developmental changes and loneliness during adolescence, Topics in Clinical Nursing 5:66, April 1983.
44. Martocchio, B.: Living while dying, Bowie, Md., 1982, Robert J. Brady Co.
45. Meer, J.: Loneliness, Psychology Today 7:28, July 1985.
46. Meis, M.: Loneliness in the elderly, Orthopaedic Nursing 4:63, May-June 1985.
47. Michela, J., Peplau, L., and Weeks, D.: Perceived dimensions of attributions for loneliness, Journal of Personality and Social Psychology 43:929, 1982.

48. Miller, J.: Assessment of loneliness and spiritual well-being in chronically ill and healthy adults, Journal of Professional Nursing, p. 79, March-April 1985.

49. Moore, J.A., and Sermat, V.: Relationship between self-actualization and self-reported loneliness, Canadian Counsellor 8(3):84, 1974.

50. Moustakas, C.: Loneliness, Englewood Cliffs, N.J., 1961, Prentice-Hall, Inc.

51. Moustakas, C.: Loneliness and love, Englewood Cliffs, N.J., 1972, Prentice-Hall, Inc.

52. Norbeck, J.S.: Social support: a model for clinical research and application, Advances in Nursing Science 3:48, July 1981.

53. North American Nursing Diagnosis Association Classification of Nursing Diagnosis: Proceedings of the seventh conference, St. Louis, 1987, The C.V. Mosby Co.

54. O'Dell, S.H.: Someone is lonely, Issues in Mental Health Nursing 3:7, January-June 1981.

55. O'Hanlon, J.: Boredom: practical consequences and a theory, Acta Psychologica 49:53, 1981.

56. Peplau, H.: Loneliness, The American Journal of Nursing 55(12):244, 1955.

57. Peplau, L., and Perlman, D., editors: Loneliness: a sourcebook of current theory, research and therapy, New York, 1982, John Wiley & Sons, Inc.

58. Perlman, D, and Peplau, L.: Theoretical approaches to loneliness. In Peplau, L., and Perlman, D.: loneliness: a sourcebook of current theory, research and therapy, New York, 1982, John Wiley and Sons.

59. Rainwater, A.J.: Elderly loneliness: its relation to residential care, Journal of Gerontological Nursing 6:593, June 1980.

60. Reisman, D., Glazer, N., and Denney, R.: The lonely crowd: a study of the changing American character, New Haven, Conn. 1961, Yale University Press.

61. Robb, S.S., and others: A wine bottle, plant and puppy: catalysts for social behavior, Journal of Gerontological Nursing 6:721, December 1980.

62. Rubenstein, C., and Shaver, P.: The experience of loneliness. In Peplau, L., and Perlman, D., editors: Loneliness: a sourcebook of current theory, research and therapy, New York, 1982, John Wiley & Sons, Inc.

63. Russell, D., Peplau, L.A., and Cutrona, C.E.: The revised UCLA loneliness scale: concurrent and discriminant validity evidence, Journal of Personality and Social Psychology 39:472, 1980.

64. Shultz, C.: Lifestyle assessment: a tool for practice, Nursing Clinics of North America 19:271, 1984.

65. Slater, P.: The pursuit of loneliness, Boston, 1976, Beacon Press.

66. Smith, R.: Boredom: a review, Human Factors 23:329, June 1981.

67. Solano, C.: Two measures of loneliness: a comparison, Psychological Reports 46:23, 1980.

68. Solano, C., Balten, P., and Parish, E.: Loneliness and patterns of self-disclosure, Journal of Personality and Social Psychology 43(3):524, 1982.

69. Sullivan, H.S.: The interpersonal theory of psychiatry, New York, 1953, W.W. Norton & Co.

70. Weeks, D.G., and others: The relation between loneliness and depression: a structural equation analysis, Journal of Personality and Social Psychology 39:1238, 1980.

71. Weiss, R.S.: Loneliness: the experience of emotional and social isolation, Cambridge, Mass., 1973, MIT Press.

72. Welt, S.R.: The developmental roots of loneliness, Archives of Psychiatric Nursing 1:1, 1987.

73. Williams, E.: Adolescent loneliness, Adolescence 18:51, 1983.

74. Wright, M.: This silence we could break, RN 44:62, December 1981.

75. Zack, M.: Loneliness: a concept relevant to the care of dying persons, Nursing Clinics of North America 20:403, June 1985.

76. Zilboorg, G.: Loneliness, Atlantic Monthly 1:45, 1938.

ANNOTATED BIBLIOGRAPHY

Peplau, H.: Loneliness, American Journal of Nursing 55:244, December 1955.

In this classic article by a renowned nurse, the author shares insights about loneliness that remain helpful to contemporary nurses.

Peplau, L., and Perlman, D., editors: Loneliness: a sourcebook of current theory, research and therapy, New York, 1982, John Wiley & Sons, Inc.

In this comprehensive overview of loneliness, knowledge and summaries of relevant research are combined into a practical sourcebook. Historical and current concepts are explored including self-help practices of lonely people.

Welt, S.W.: The developmental roots of loneliness, Archives of Psychiatric Nursing 1:1, 1987.

This article addresses the phenomenon of loneleness. Loneliness is defined as emotional isolation that develops in an interpersonal context and as a manifestation of the need for human intimacy. The article explains the interpersonal antecedents of loneliness and healthy loneliness. Clinical case data are used to illustrate the theoretical constructs of loneliness, premature aloneness, defensive aloneness, and healthy aloneness.

BOREDOM

Cathleen Shultz

After studying this chapter the learner will be able to:

Discuss historical perspectives of boredom.

Describe theories of boredom.

Apply the nursing process to care for clients experiencing boredom.

Identify current research findings relevant to the care of clients experiencing boredom.

Boredom is an affective mental state primarily caused by prolonged exposure to dull, uninteresting, or monotonus stimulation. Boredom, a common phenomenon, can result in harmful stress capable of leading to disease and accidents. Those who are particularly vulnerable to experiencing the negative results of boredom include those who do repetitive tasks over a long period of time, those who are institutionalized or recuperating from a lengthy illness, those in prolonged isolation or solitary confinement, the retired, the socially withdrawn, adolescents, and those with handicaps creating sensory deprivation.

Boredom is frequently confused with monotony, tedium, or apathy. They are related to boredom and have common features as summarized in Table 20-1. Those who work in isolation or view their work as monotonous are less efficient and alert following only short times with the tasks. Accidents causing injury and death are inevitable without intervention.

Monotony alone, however, is not sufficient to cause boredom. Other factors include emotional lability, age, and satisfaction with personal life.[26,59,65,67] In addition, others believe that boredom results when the activity lacks meaning to the person or he perceives it as boring.[16,38]

People with monotonous jobs tend to be more neurotic and less mentally healthy than those in other jobs.[27,48] Also, boredom characterizes the narcissistic and borderline personality disorders and is found within the DSM-III-R descriptions of these problems. Clearly the phenomenon needs a nursing perspective since nurses are challenged to incorporate known interventions to minimize the effects of boredom and to produce empirical investigations pertinent for enhancing care of the bored client. Table 20-2 lists types of boredom and their causes.

THEORETICAL APPROACHES
Biological

Biological theories view boredom as a consequence of inattention. Biological theorists have linked cortical maturation to the development of the capacity to be attentive.[56] Myelination of certain nerve fibers may not be completed until 12 years of age, and measures such as EEG and reaction time reflect the ability to be attentive.[21]

Conflicting reports link boredom with a decreased heart rate[41] and an increased heart rate variability.[3,73,74] Perkins[53] found a significant decrease of both during boring tasks. Hill and Perkins[27] believe this discrepancy to be caused by the attitude of the worker to the task rather than whether the task is identified as boring. Further study is needed before cardiac difficulties are definitely associated with boredom. Work continues on biological causes and results of boredom as it is studied in individuals' personal lives and occupations.

Psychoanalytic

Information about boredom has emerged in bits and pieces through numerous psychoanalytic theories. In general, boredom is perceived as a complicated, internal, af-

Historical Overview

DATE	EVENT
1860	Florence Nightingale wrote that sick patients are adversely affected by seeing the same walls and ceiling while confined.
1913	Munsterberg recognized boredom in actual working situations.
1920s-1940s	A series of papers was published in England describing an ongoing concern with boredom and monotony affecting work.
1927	McDowall and Wells published an account of the genesis of boredom.
1930-1937	Earliest systematic psychoanalytic discussions of boredom were written by Fenichel,[15] Spitz, and Winterstein.
1953	Greenson[18] distinguished between an apathetic and an agitated boredom.
1972	First nursing article addressing boredom was published; the topic has since appeared in 10 publications with nurse authors.
1975	Berstein[5] integrated psychoanalytic and sociological constructs to describe the recent increase in boredom. He proposed a dual taxonomy by differentiating between responsive and chronic boredom created by internal causes. Wangh[75] viewed boredom as an outcome of intrapsychic struggle.
1981	The first research on boredom conducted by nurses was published by Savitz and Friedman.[61] Smith's work[65] indicated that only about 40 papers have been published on boredom since 1926. Boredom is associated with narcissistic and borderline personality disorders.
Future	Nurses are challenged to incorporate knowledge about boredom into practice as they learn to recognize boredom, distinguish it from related states of confusion and adaptation, and develop and use interventions to change the bored state.

fective experience that results in the client's disinterest in the environment. This disinterest prevents a clash between desires and constraints. For example, the school-aged child with a desire to fulfill a fantasy to play outdoors is unable to do so because he is confined to his desk. The chief cause of boredom is prevention of intrapsychic conflict. Thus the cause is internal and self-created.[75,76]

Fenichel's classic work[15] related boredom to depression, neurotic states, narcissistic needs, oral-sadistic needs, and diminished self-esteem. Narcissistic clients express vague complaints including feelings of emptiness and lack of initiative.[32-34] The symptoms are linked to chronic boredom, and Fenichel believed that they relate to a lack of empathetic mothering. He noted that people frequently

TABLE 20-1 Definitions of boredom and related terms

Term	Definition
Boredom	An affective mental state primarily caused by prolonged exposure to monotonous stimulation
Monotony	Tedious uniformity or lack of variety
Apathy	Lack of interest or concern
Emptiness	Lack of feeling
Sensory deprivation	Removal or minimization of sensory stimulation
Tedium	Disgust or weariness
Ennui	Feeling of mental weariness produced by lack of interest in surroundings

TABLE 20-2 Types of boredom

Type of Boredom	Cause
Apathetic	Repression of forbidden instincts and a decreased imagination
Agitated	Secondary state caused by failure of available activities to gratify wishes and fantasies
Responsive	Inevitable reaction to a monotonous task or life situation
Chronic	Unresolved inner struggle causing boredom to persist
Existential	Extraneous, multiple factors
Interpersonal	Other people

relieved bored feelings by oral activities such as eating, drinking, and smoking.

Although Fenichel primarily focused on internally caused boredom, he believed that boredom can be externally caused. The best example is the assembly-line worker whose many impulses conflict with his work; he resists acting out his impulses to briefly stop the work flow because he will be unemployed.

Hartocollis[23,24] studied boredom in certain mental health problems and believed boredom to be particularly characteristic of borderline personality disorders. He concluded that borderline and narcissistic clients are chronicly bored.

Behavioral

Behaviorists believe that boredom is caused by the client's environment. As the first to study boredom, McGill University researchers placed individuals on a bed with planned decreased stimulation, called "perceptual isolation." Their eyes were covered, they heard a constant buzzing noise through earphones, and their arms and hands were covered with cardboard cuffs. The experience became unpleasant within a few days, and diverse effects were found, including mood lability, visual and auditory hallucinations, electroencephalogram (EEG) alterations, and an increase in persuasability.[25]

Building on the early studies,[16,54,56] more studies expanded and included the McGill findings. Behaviorists then renamed the concept "sensory deprivation."

Boredom is recognized as a unique psychophysiological state that is best explained as an unusual emotional response to predictability (Frank, 1961). When individuals experience too much predictability, boredom exists; too little predictability causes confusion.

When the client is bored, task performance becomes impaired and perceptions altered. The ideal aim then is an adaptive response with optimal predictability (Figure 20-1).

Not to be ignored is the fact that for some bored clients, reward is inherent in the boredom. When bored they concentrate on the past and the familiar. By choosing the known over the unknown, they avoid undesired emotions.

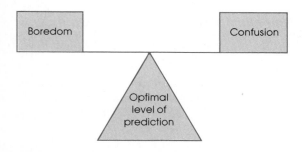

FIGURE 20-1 Continuum of human predictability.

Cognitive

Cognitive theorists generally believe attention is a factor in the development of boredom. Attention is viewed as essential to learning and creative problem solving.[19]

Perkins and Hill[54] found that a person can subjectively develop boredom in response to lack of interest in a task. They found that a person could initially be interested in the task only to later be bored because of his own perceptions.

Sociocultural

Generally the sociological viewpoint holds that both individuals and society may become bored and that boredom is less caused by personality traits than by the various situations in which people find themselves. This is best illustrated by sociologist Robert Nisbet's warning in 1969 that society's authority was being undermined. During this time of social upheaval, he believed that authority was greatly diminished and gradually boredom and apathy were becoming apparent. Sociologists link boredom with physical disease, cruelty, and nihilism. Harlow Shapley even placed boredom as third in a list of five possible causes of world destruction.[31]

Orcutt[51] believes there are two forms of boredom. Existential boredom occurs without people present, whereas interpersonal boredom occurs when others are present. Studies reveal that younger and lower income people are more likely than the older and more wealthy respondents to experience existential boredom; the older and more wealthy group reports more interpersonal boredom.[52]

Table 20-3 summarizes the theoretical approaches.

RELATING TO THE CLIENT

In the preinteraction phase, the nurse explores boredom as it affects both her and the client. Countertransference occurs particularly with bored clients.[36,44,71] Especially in therapy sessions is the nurse likely to become bored, lack energy, and have a decreased motivation to interact with the boring client. Maintaining an awareness that one can become bored with a chronically bored client is the first step in preventing one's own boredom.

During the orientation phase, the nurse who is attuned to both negative and beneficial aspects of boredom will more likely convey hope and develop a broader range of nursing interventions. The results of boredom are discussed later in this chapter.

The nurse works with the client to differentiate and clarify his boredom. Throughout the working phase the nurse encourages increased motivation by the client. Support is necessary to assist the client in reversing his attitude toward his professional and personal life.

The nurse strives to teach the client that his worth is separate from his behavior and that alleviating boredom is a worthwhile goal. Warmth is conveyed by the nurse through active attempts to assist the client in resolving difficulties caused by boredom. Attention to detail becomes necessary as the nurse asks the client for specific examples and assists him to comprehensively explore these difficult situations.

TABLE 20-3 Summary of theories of boredom

Theory	Theorist	Dynamics
Biologic	Pribram	Altered EEGs and decreased reaction time are among the physiological variables indicative of the presence of and reaction to boredom.
Psychoanalytic	Wangh	Boredom results from conflicting internal forces.
	Greenson	Boredom is due to repressing forbidden instincts causing conflict.
	Fenichel and Harticollis	Boredom is associated with persons experiencing neuroses; it involves narcissistic needs, oral-sadistic needs, and diminished self-esteem.
Behavioral	Herron	Boredom results from sensory deprivation caused by the environment.
Cognitive	Piaget	Formal operational thinking occurs in adolescence, enabling the client to counteract boredom.
	Hamilton	Boredom occurs with inattention.
Sociocultural	Shapley and Orcutt	A society may experience boredom because of a perceived loss of authority; societal boredom is viewed as destructive.

The working phase involves assisting the client to risk greater unpredictability, which may be accompanied by fear. The client needs support to change his behavior.

When terminating the therapeutic relationship, the nurse focuses on behavioral change, goal attainment, and the client's ability to grasp situations. Ensured that support exists, the client assumes more responsibility for his actions as he moves to decrease boredom. The client is encouraged to practice new learned behaviors daily.

NURSING PROCESS
Assessment

Physical dimension. The negative effects of boredom, especially in the work environment, have been found to adversely affect job performance, morale, and eventually the actual work quality. Table 20-4 summarizes susceptible occupations and activities that place clients at risk for accidents and personal injury caused by boredom. Especially vulnerable are those whose jobs are characterized by fast, machine-paced work requiring heightened attention to avoid serious personal injury. These people include forklift drivers and assemblers who both do and do not use machine pacing. The machine-paced assemblers reported somatic complaints, anxiety, depression, and fre-

TABLE 20-4 Occupations and activities that place clients at risk for accidents and personal injury caused by boredom

Sample Activity	Sample Occupation
Industrial inspection	Lathe operator
Radar target detection	Punch press operator
Radar navigation	Drill operator
Television surveillance	Air traffic controller
(night watch person	Train controller
or security guard	Airplane pilot
watching monitors)	Truck driver
Prolonged driving	Assembly workers

quent visits to the company's health clinic. The first survey of the physical consequences of occupation-related, severe boredom revealed a high incidence of psychosomatic diseases such as gastritis and peptic ulcers.[60] As one gets older while in the same job, occupational boredom seems to diminish.[26,46,67] It is not known if this is due to adaptation to the work setting or the fact that bored, younger workers leave the setting.

Boredom may also be present in seeing or hearing impaired persons, the physically restrained, clients in lengthy isolation, those in protected environments such as the laminar airflow rooms in which the client has little people contact, those recovering from drug or alcohol abuse, the alert but physically limited terminally ill, and those individuals institutionalized in rehabilitative facilities, mental health centers, and nursing homes.

The physical environment can contribute to boredom. For example, when in drab hospital rooms or workrooms, while eating visually unappealing food, and while using broken, dysfunctional, or inappropriate hearing aids or glasses, clients can experience boredom. Dim or flickering lights, uncomfortable room temperatures, and annoying or humming noise may alter attentiveness, thus increasing the client's susceptibility to boredom.

A myth prevails that obese people eat more when bored. In actual studies obese persons ate significantly more food than normal persons but boredom markedly increased food consumption for both obese and non-obese persons.[1]

The nurse assesses the severity and meaningfulness of the problem by determining the intensity of boredom, the presence of related feeling states, the client's need and desire to reduce the effects of boredom on his life, and the possibility of developing successful coping mechanisms that can be incorporated into the client's life-style. When these bored feelings capitulate into chronic resignation, frustration, fear, resentment, apathy, depression, and hostility the problem further challenges the client's coping abilities.

The nurse and client determine if boredom is related to fatigue, anger, grief, fear, avoidance, conflict, or loss of purpose. Changing the client's life-style depends on the client's motivation, his resources, the length of boredom, and how quickly he can make necessary changes.[63]

Occasionally bored clients actively seek stimuli to remove the feeling or prevent its occurrence. These are the excessively action-oriented, self-destructive thrill seekers, including those who abuse stimulant and depressant drugs. On psychological tests they will favorably respond to items such as "I would like to hunt lions in Africa" and "I would like to race motorcycles."

Adolescents are at risk for boredom. If boredom is present, then further assessment involves eliciting information about alcohol and drug consumption. In other words, the nurse also determines what clients do to relieve feelings associated with boredom.

The chronically bored client with borderline personality disorder also actively relieves boredom by oscillating moods or expressing intense anger. Splitting and projective identification are two defense mechanisms that are frequently used to mask boredom. Splitting enables the client to view the world as all bad with no positive attributes, or as all good. Projective identification allows the client to displace their self-hatred and anger. Both defense mechanisms may mask the presence of boredom, but the nurse assesses the borderline client's boredom intensity.

Boring activities are associated with a high level of frustration and monotony (see the Research Highlight below).[54] Keen[30] believed the bored person has lost momentum and has a limp will. Nothing appears exciting to these people.

❋ *Intellectual dimension.* Boredom can affect one's intellectual dimension both positively and negatively. When a person is bored, creativity comes to a halt. However, following boring experiences some persons have produced creative endeavors such as painting and writing.

❋ *Emotional dimension.* Initially boredom seems to be simple inertia. The bored client has lost momentum, motivation, and nothing appears exciting. For some, boredom is a temporary result of a lack of adequate stimuli or a retreat from overstimulation. Clients' statements such as "I feel trapped," "I'm bored to death," "It's a blah day," "I've nothing to do," and "I just do not want to do that" reveal the uniqueness of the boredom experience.

Sensory deprivation can also resemble a stimulant that can lead to a heightened awareness and readiness to act. The relationship is U-shaped; as arousal increases, performance first improves and then diminishes to the beginning performance level.[42] Particularly affected is the person's heightened ability to memorize lists and to recall previously learned material following sensory deprivation.

Research Highlight

Cognitive and Affective Aspects of Boredom

R.E. Perkins & A.B. Hill

PURPOSE

This study's purpose was to investigate whether boredom is associated with subjective monotony, boredom is associated with a high degree of frustration, and whether boredom occurs when the stimuli lack personal meaning.

SAMPLE

Twenty-four undergraduates were chosen after responding to a set of eight questions about motorcycles. Their mean age was 21.6 years. Two groups were developed; each had six men and six women. One group would likely find the study task interesting (I); the other group would likely find it boring (B).

METHODOLOGY

Seven 6 × 8 inch color pictures of motorcycles were shown to each subject individually. The subject was given a list of constructs related to the quality and use of motorcycles and was asked to rate these constructs on a seven-point scale. At the end of the task, the subjects were asked to rate their degree of interest or boredom on a six-point scale (slightly, reasonably, very interesting/boring).

Total discrepancy scores (TDSs) were obtained for each elicited construct (TDSE) and for supplied constructs (TDSS). The higher the TDS, the more meaningful the stimuli or picture was to the subject.

FINDINGS

Using a t test of the TDS, means of the I group and B group indicated a significant difference. No evidence supported that boredom was associated with a lack of meaningful stimulation.

In the second experiment, boredom was found to be associated with subjective monotony, and the third experiment provided strong support for previous speculations that boredom is associated with frustration.

IMPLICATIONS

The study presented more data to describe the cognitive and affective activity associated with monotony and boredom. Questions remain about the origins of boredom. The authors believe that subjective monotony may induce or represent boredom and that boredom occurs as a result of unknown processes. The field remains open for further investigation.

Based on data from British Journal of Psychology **76**:221, 1985.

Short periods of decreased stimuli with no people contact, no radio or television, minimal sound, closed eyelids, and lying down would then be helpful for those studying for tests requiring memorization.[69,70]

The bored person may have more difficulty with long-term projects and situations requiring creative problem solving. When bored with a task, some persons may leave it incomplete or mechanically complete it without giving attention to detail or quality. Also the long-term project in itself may be boring.

Chronic physical problems such as posttraumatic head injury or cardiovascular accident and emotional problems such as autism, psychoses, drug abuse, or drug treatment that alters the mind's ability to function normally may contribute to boredom.

Determining the school progress of the student may be a clue to a decreased attention span and the presence of boredom. Learning is intense during primary and secondary school years, yet the young child or adolescent may not be able to attend to learning that accompanies minimal stimulation or requires long periods of intense attention. Generally educators agree that boredom inhibits learning.[17] For information about the Boredom Confusion Adaptation Scale (BCAS), an instrument designed to diagnose boredom in school children, see the Research Highlight below. Because boredom is inversely related to crea-

---

Research Highlight

Diagnosing Boredom, Confusion, and Adaptation in Schoolchildren

S.B. Frick

PURPOSE

Using Friedman's rational theory as a framework, this study was designed to develop and test an instrument that could diagnose middle-school children's bored (B), confused (C), or adapted (A) states of mind.

SAMPLE

Subjects were from two middle schools in central South Carolina. One hundred fifty-four students in the seventh grade participated with the median age being 11.9 years (range was 11 to 15). Ninety were male, and sixty-four were female; 30 did not identify their race, 28 were black, and 96 were white.

METHODOLOGY

Middle-school counselors, using definitions of B, C, and A, identified school situations specific to each construct. From the situations, declarative statements pertinent to B, C, and A were developed for the BCAS instrument, which then was independently reviewed and rated by five experts including Friedman. Only statements agreed on by all five experts remained. Sixty items, twenty for each construct, were retained and randomly arranged in the final instrument. Each statement was followed by two blanks that students could respond to with "like me" or "unlike me."

The BCAS was read aloud to each student who then checked his own responses. The researcher was not involved in this phase of data collection. Other information was obtained from school records including the Comprehensive Test of Basic Skills (CTBS) subscale and total skills scores; year-end grades received by students in mathematics, social studies, language arts, and reading; and total number of times tardy and absent. All data related to the school year in which the BCAS was given were collected.

Kuder Richardson 20 reliability estimates were obtained for each subscale (confusion = .77, and adaptation = .71). Other statistical correlations and factor analyses revealed 33 significant items (14 confusion, 12 boredom, and 7 adaptation), which were included in the final form of the BCAS.

Pearson product moment correlation coefficients were calculated to obtain relationships between the BCAS subscales and the other data.

FINDINGS

The results revealed several significant findings, including support of assumed instrument reliability and validity. Generally scores and grades compared as follows:

Scale Scores	CTBS Scores	Teacher Grades
Increase on the confusion score	Decreased	Decreased
Increase on the boredom score	Decreased	Decreased
Increase on the adaptation score	Increased	Increased

IMPLICATIONS

The BCAS score may be used diagnostically by school health professionals to determine boredom, confusion, or adaptation states. Interventions specific to the confused or bored state may be individually determined to achieve a more adaptive state in the learning environment. Bored students would need varied assignments and teaching methodologies to enhance learning. Confused students could benefit from simplification of assignments, increased structure such as an assignment calendar, more regulation at school, and a decreased amount and variety of classroom stimuli. These states are challenges for the teacher, especially when both types are in the same classroom.

Boredom and confusion are considered situation specific so the measurement tool may differ in other settings. The development and determination of the effects of interventions to change the confused or bored state remain areas to be explored.

Based on data from Journal of School Health **55**:7, 1985.

tivity,[62] the nurse assesses the client's creativity by asking about hobbies and work.

Case Example

Virgil, a 68-year-old retired businessman, moved to a retirement community in Arkansas. Following 50 years of work, he anticipated a life of fishing and small farming. Instead he does not keep busy and becomes increasingly bored and depressed. His wife, at a loss for what to do and feeling overwhelmed by his need for attention, wishes they could return home to New York. Clearly, preparation would have helped; now they need assistance to solve a difficult situation.

✿ ***Social dimension.*** Assessment of the social dimension includes determining if the client is an introvert or an extrovert. Extroverts are more likely to be bored, especially in a socially isolated situation.[59]

Boredom has often been called the culprit in "problem drinking." Numerous respondents to public surveys report that their deviant drinking was due to trying to kill time because there was nothing to do.[58]

While assessing occupational status including unemployment, the nurse may also determine the client's attitude toward the job or position. For the unemployed person, obtaining sample schedules of their daily activities may provide information about how they occupy their time. Busy and creative people seldom complain of boredom, especially over a prolonged period of time.

Case Example

Greg is a 16-year-old who dropped out of high school because he was bored. His days are now occupied with watching television and smoking marijuana. He lacks the social and occupational skills to get a job, and his friends are in school all day. His own efforts to fill the void are ineffective, and he looks to the outside world for needed stimulation. Stealing cars, racing, and speeding occupy his time until he is finally arrested. Boredom has resulted in serious consequences for Greg.

A client may perceive himself as bored from being in a job, friendship, or marriage too long. Another example occurs when a person is transferred to a new job, especially when the activity level decreases from that of his previous position.

Boredom can be especially devastating to a person planning to retire. The nurse assesses persons of retirement age for their preparedness. Questions such as "When does your retirement occur?"; "What do you and your family plan to do following your retirement?"; and "What activities do you do regularly other than work?" will provide the nurse with helpful information to guide her actions.

The home-bound, nursing home, or hospitalized client may experience boredom without sufficient diversional activities. The assessment will include questions about the presence of a phone, television, or radio; the frequency and length of television or phone use; and the frequency and purpose of visitors.

When bored in social situations, the client may with-

draw. Bored clients do not draw people to themselves. Consequently clients with few contacts with people may have more opportunity to experience boredom.

✳ ***Spiritual dimension.*** The chronically bored, withdrawn client has difficulty relating to his world. Aimless and lacking purpose, this person is alienated from a higher being during boredom. Assessing his attitude toward goals and his desire to relate to himself and others provides information about the extent of his boredom. Whether or not the client participates in creative activities can give the nurse information about the client's bored state relative to his spiritual dimension.

Measurement tools. Tools to measure the presence and severity of boredom have primarily emerged from industry and studies of vigilance, attention, and sensory deprivation. Nurses can use these tools in a variety of settings to determine boredom susceptibility, the presence of the types of boredom, and the client's ability to cope with boredom.

Zuckerman's Sensation Seeking Scale (SSS) was revised to the Sensation Seeking Scale, Form V (SSS-V), a 72-item, forced-choice scale exploring the need for stimulation and boredom susceptibility.[38] It focuses on whether one is bored or not and whether the subject is averse to repetitive experiences, routine work, or dull or predictable people. Males score higher on this scale.[77]

Another scale, the Boredom Coping Scale (BCS), reflects the individual's ability to alter perceptions of and ability to participate in potentially boring activities. The BCS is a brief, self-reported measure using nine statements with forced-choice responses assigned points from zero to 9.[22] Its aim is to decrease boredom.

Orcutt[50] devised two scales to differentiate between interpersonal and existential boredom. Combined with an altered version of the BCS each scale had less than 10 statements with four Likert-type options ranging from

---

TABLE 20-5 Tools to measure boredom

Measurement Tool	Purpose
Sensation Seeking Scale, Form V (SSS-V)	Determines number and diversity of stimuli desired by individual; explores boredom susceptibility and need for stimulation
Boredom Coping Scale (BCS)	Reflects how the person copes with boredom; measures person's ability to alter his perceptions of and ability to participate in boring activities
Orcutt's Scale	Differentiates between interpersonal and existential boredom
Boredom Confusion Adaptation Scale (BCAS)	Diagnoses the presence of boredom, confusion, or adaptation to predictable circumstances

DIVERSIONAL ACTIVITY DEFICIT

DEFINITION

A feeling state experienced by the person in an environment with minimal stimulation or in which the person holds minimal interest.

DEFINING CHARACTERISTICS

Physical Dimension
Yawning
Body language indicative of disinterest
Fidgeting
Immobility
Weight gain or loss
*Diminished sensory stimulation
*Accident proclivity, especially in work setting
*Oral activities such as frequent eating, drinking, or smoking
*Sleepiness
*Confinement to a room or building

Emotional Dimension
Flat affect
Unpleasant thoughts or feelings
Restlessness
Hostility
*Fatigue
*Depression
*Frustration
*Lethargy
*Emptiness
*Powerlessness
*Thrill-seeking activities
*Bored

Intellectual Dimension
Inattentiveness
*Lack of motivation
*Decreased attention span
*Learning difficulties
*Disinterest in activities

Social Dimension
*Withdrawal
*Lack of significant support system
*Ineffective social skills
*Diminished social activity
*Retirement
*Occupation that has repetitive paced tasks
*Children or significant others leaving home
*Career changes, including termination of a job

Spiritual Dimension
*Decreased creativity
*Aimlessness
*Lacking of purpose
*Alienation

Adapted from North American Nursing Diagnosis Association Classification of Nursing Diagnosis: Proceedings of the seventh conference, St. Louis, 1987, The C.V. Mosby Co.
*Indicates characteristics in addition to those defined by NANDA.

"agree" to "disagree." Following are samples of these items:

1. I get bored seeing the same old faces.
2. I'm always too busy to be bored.
3. It bores me to engage in small talk with people.
4. I feel my life has clear direction and purpose.

A fourth scale, the Boredom-Confusion-Adaptation Scale (BCAS), is discussed in the preceding Research Highlight.

A summary of the tools to measure boredom is presented in Table 20-5.

Analysis

Nursing diagnosis. Boredom logically is associated with the diagnoses of sensory-perceptual alteration, social isolation, and ineffective individual coping (see Chapters 17, 19, and 34). The defining characteristics of the NANDA-accepted nursing diagnosis of diversional activity deficit are presented in the box at left. Other possible nursing diagnoses with causative statements for the client with boredom include the following:

1. Social isolation: boredom related to hospital isolation procedures
2. Sensory-perceptual alteration: boredom related to need to immobilize hip joint for recent hip replacement surgery
3. Ineffective individual coping: boredom related to recent occupational retirement
4. Diversional activity deficit related to boredom during retirement
5. Potential diversional activity deficit related to monotonous environment in hospital isolation room

The following Case Example illustrates characteristics of the nursing diagnosis of diversional activity deficit.

Case Example

Raymond worked for 45 years as an engineer, always arriving at least an hour before the scheduled workday. He worked hard and received a good income, but his job was boring and he felt trapped. When he realized he would never attain the level in the company that he desired, he lost interest in his work and resigned himself to tolerate it until retirement. He did.

Although Raymond was educated and bright, he had no outside interests other than his lawn. He and his wife had few friends and spent most of their time at home. With his work interest removed, he felt lonely and bored.

He quickly lost interest in anything new he attempted. Nothing needed the old skills he had used for decades. He wanted to help his wife, but he felt in the way. She had her own schedule and had not retired from those activities. Gradually he lost his appetite and interest in anything. He began waking at 4 AM. When his movements and speech slowed down, and he joked about ending it all, his wife arranged for him to see a counselor. Raymond's situation was serious and required intervention. Boredom specifically required attention as it was inherent in his depression and suicidal thoughts.

DSM-III-R diagnoses. Boredom has been linked with the DSM-III-R categories of narcissistic and borderline personality disorders. The boxes on p. 408 give essential features and manifestations of the features of these two diagnoses.

301.81 NARCISSISTIC PERSONALITY DISORDER

ESSENTIAL FEATURES

A disorder in which there is a pervasive grandiose sense of self-importance, achievements, talents, or uniqueness. Begins in early adulthood and is present in a variety of situations.

MANIFESTATIONS
Emotional Dimension

Preoccupied with feelings of envy

Lack of empathy

Cool indifference or marked feelings of rage, inferiority, shame, humiliation, or emptiness in response to criticism, defeat, or disappointment

Aware but indifferent to feelings of others

Intellectual Dimension

Preoccupation with fantasies of unlimited success, power, brilliance, beauty, or ideal love; when fantasies are pursued, it may be with a driven, pleasureless quality and an insatiable ambition

Unrealistic overestimation of abilities and achievements

Sense of self-importance possibly alternating with feelings of special unworthiness

Preoccupation with how well one is doing or how well one is regarded by others

Greater concern with appearances than with substance

Expects to be noticed without appropriate achievement

Believes problems are unique and understood only by special people

Social Dimension

Exhibitionistic need for constant attention and admiration

Relationships that alternate between the extreme of overidealization and devaluation

Extreme self-centeredness

Fragile self-esteem

Constant seeking of admiration and attention

Expectation of special favors without assuming reciprocal responsibilities (entitlement)

Advantage taken of others to indulge one's own desires or for self-aggrandizement (interpersonal exploitation)

Spiritual Dimension

Disregard for personal integrity and rights of others

Adapted from American Psychiatric Association: Diagnostic and statistical manual of mental disorders (DSM-III-R), Washington, D.C., 1987, The Association.

Planning

Table 20-6 provides long-term and short-term goals and outcome criteria related to boredom. These serve as examples of the planning phase of the nursing process.

Implementation

✴ *Physical dimension.* Everyone experiences fleeting boredom that is easily relieved by changing

301.83 BORDERLINE PERSONALITY DISORDER

ESSENTIAL FEATURES

A disorder in which there is instability in a variety of areas, including interpersonal behavior, mood, and self-image. Begins in early adulthood and is present in a variety of situations.

MANIFESTATIONS
Physical Dimension

Gender identity disturbance

Emotional Dimension

Chronic feeling of emptiness and boredom

Unstable mood: shifts from normal to dysphoric

Anxiety lasting from a few hours to a few days

Depression

Suicidal gestures

Inappropriate intense anger or lack of control of anger

Self-mutilation

Intellectual Dimension

Impulsive or unpredictable behavior in at least 2 self-damaging areas consisting of spending, substance abuse, overeating, sex, shoplifting, reckless driving, and alternating between extremes of over-idealization and devaluation

Pessimistic outlook

Uncertainty about career goals

Extreme stress; transient psychotic disorder

Social Dimension

Intense and unstable interpersonal relationships

Intolerance of being alone

Manipulative behavior

Uncertainty about friendship patterns

Alteration between dependency and self-assertion

Frantic efforts to avoid real or impaired abandonment

Spiritual Dimension

Idealization of people

Devaluation of people

Adapted from American Psychiatric Association: Diagnostic and statistical manual of mental disorders (DSM-III-R), Washington, D.C., 1987, The Association.

one's thoughts, engaging in an activity, or varying activities. The type of boredom that can create potential harm such as accidents or depression is usually subtle and complex, and the client is unable to use his usual coping strategies. Environmental constraints such as office rules may prevent an individual from using his previously successful coping mechanisms. Effective coping generally incorporates changing one's habits to minimize what causes the boredom and changing one's attitude toward the activity associated with boredom.

The bored client needs a balance between routine activities, novel activities, and change to alter the predictability of his situation. Placing readable calendars, clocks, newspapers, and televisions in client's rooms or lounge

TABLE 20-6 Long-term and short-term goals and outcome criteria related to boredom

Goals	Outcome Criteria
INEFFECTIVE INDIVIDUAL COPING: BOREDOM RELATED TO RECENT OCCUPATIONAL RETIREMENT	
Long-term goals	
To use effective coping strategies during retirement from engineering position	Lists interests and sets priorities
	Chooses two interests and obtains information to implement at least one of them
	Invests time and resources into developing at least one new interest area before scheduled retirement date
To maintain positive social network following retirement	Lists those people valued by him and his spouse
	Develops a plan with his spouse to continue contact with these people after retirement
Short-term goals	
To alter home environment to minimize the amount of boredom experienced	Discusses with his wife the need to decrease his boredom
	Schedules frequent planned breaks doing enjoyable activities
To minimize anxiety felt when bored at home	Learns relaxation methods and uses at home as needed

areas is a simple but significant strategy to prevent confusion and also boredom. In addition, altering the environment by moving furniture can change the quantity and content of conversation between staff and clients. A sensitively designed environment reinforced with caring personnel can positively influence client behaviors and feelings.[50] The nurse teaches those clients with impaired hearing and vision to periodically assess their hearing aids or glasses.

Touch becomes essential for some isolated, institutionalized, or dying clients who are bored. The back rub may be a welcome contact to clients with decreased sensory stimulation.

Although boredom is most often linked with negative consequences, there are reports of its therapeutic uses. For example, if a person with a history of deviant sexual arousal does not respond to aversion therapy, then creating conditions to produce boredom while the client engages in sexual activities and fantasies to the saturation level has been found sufficient to alter the behavior.[43]

Sensory deprivation, long linked with boredom, has value in treating clients with conditions such as stuttering, esophoria, infantile colic, snake phobia, narcotic addiction, compulsive overeating, smoking, alcoholism, hypertension, autism, and retardation. In addition, increased short-term memory, enhanced visual concentration, in-

creased daydreams, and increased persuasibility may follow periods of decreased stimulation.[70]

The boring work setting may or may not be alterable to diminish the causes of boredom. Explore with the client what may be changed such as the type of work, the location of office equipment or lounges, pictures on the wall, and varying the type of tasks. Reassigning personnel may be needed to maintain productivity as well as enhance creativity. The client may consider instituting small frequent breaks and varying activity. If these are not possible the client may need to consider other employment, especially when safety or health is a concern.

Thrill seekers may need interventions to specifically prevent physical harm to themselves and others. Because their bored behavior may accompany drug abuse, both the drug abuse and the boredom may simultaneously need the nurse's attention.

Emotional dimension. Clients may need assistance in acknowledging their boredom. Encouraging them to express their feelings may be a new experience, especially for the chronically bored who believe boredom is a way of life. Verbalization can occur directly with the nurse or during group therapy with those who have similar problems. Music therapy may offer soothing sensory stimulation and may be scheduled before a group session to promote communication and relax the group members.

The predominant feeling states of frustration, restlessness, and apathy best respond to strategies used with the depressed or lonely client. (See Chapters 14 and 19 for additional information.)

Intellectual dimension. Preventing boredom using intellectual processes may involve altering both the client's activity level and his attitude. Dividing a complex task into attainable steps may help the client to see it as achievable. As each step is successfully completed, positive rewards that are meaningful to the client can be offered. For example, the client may have a large report due as part of his work. Since the topic is boring, he has a hard time initiating and continuing production of the document. By breaking the report into smaller sections that take one day each to prepare, the task is perceived as more manageable. At the end of each day in which one section is finished he treats himself to some time reading a book he had long wanted to finish. The success keeps his momentum, and he interspaces a boring task with a pleasurable activity.

Other choices may be presented such as taking small frequent breaks or decreasing the total amount of time spent on the task during any one workday. Intellectual stimulation, especially strategies to develop original responses, encourage creativity. For example, during therapy the nurse may give scenarios that urge the client to use his imagination while problem solving. The idea is to produce a response that shows the client understood the scenario and generated relevant solutions.

Breaking goals into measurable steps creates a sense of progress in these clients who are emotionally removed from thoughts of the future. With each step, congratulations and encouragement are warranted.

Alleviating classroom boredom that inhibits learning

requires teacher cooperation. The nurse may facilitate meetings between student, parents, teachers, and guidance counselors so that a team approach to problem solving is used.

※ **Social dimension.** If the client is hospitalized for short-term, acute illnesses, the nurse may facilitate socialization opportunities. Providing client lounge areas, ensuring that client rooms have adequate space and furniture for visitors, and promoting visiting hours that consider the schedules of visitors are strategies the nurse may use to alleviate boredom.

When clients do not have visitors, especially while in isolation, staff members need to periodically visit the client at times not requiring medication administration or treatment. The personal touch and attention become meaningful for the client. Those clients who are institutionalized either permanently or for a lengthy rehabilitation may benefit from planned as well as unplanned diversionary activities. The goal is to reach the client's optimum level of activity whether through singing, games of checkers, or walking field trips. Dining rooms for group eating are excellent places not only to enjoy meals but also to break up the long hours of the day. Clients need encouragement to maintain communication by telephone calls, writing letters, or sending cards. It is essential to increase their social options wherever possible. The client's social skills may also need altering to produce more satisfying relationships with people and to prevent boredom.

Boredom can result from external pressures to conform.[62] When the client does not feel free to respond differently from his peer group and he chooses to remain with his peer group, then boredom may become a coping method. The client would rather be bored than become alienated from his peers.

Preventatively all people need to prepare for their retirement to decrease the likelihood of boredom. Joint decision making with significant others is needed to determine future goals so that the retirement period can indeed be meaningful.

※ **Spiritual dimension.** A client may decrease his boredom by concentrating on his relationship with himself, others, or a higher being, which may require the nurse's support as the client changes his behavior. Encouraging prayer, meditation, and the development of meaningful goals may also help the client decrease boredom.

Each client has his unique cadre of spiritual resources that can be incorporated into the nursing care plan. Whether that be organized church groups, time alone, use of a religious group's practices, or seeking a more meaningful existence, the nurse can incorporate what the client values to help him alleviate boredom.

INTERACTION WITH THE CLIENT EXPERIENCING BOREDOM

(Nurse enters room of hospitalized male client who is staring at walls as he sits in the lounge chair. His morning care is completed; no visitors are expected since his spouse and friends work during the day. He is 45 years old and has been admitted because of depression secondary to an adjustment to disability. He has not worked in 3 months. The nurse has been in the room twice this morning. She has interacted with him daily since his admission.)

Nurse: Mr. Sayers, I see you glanced at the magazines your wife left. What did you find that was interesting?

Client: (Talking slowly and softly.) Oh, one article on cars but I finished it.

Nurse: What are your plans for this morning? (The unit's activity schedule has already been discussed with him; a printed schedule is in his room and in the hall and lounge area.)

Client: None really. Time sure drags in here. I'm bored.

Nurse: (Sitting beside him and extending the printed schedule.) This morning some recreational activities are planned in the lounge. You mentioned yesterday that you liked classical music. Today a group is getting together to listen to Chopin. Afterward they talk about the artist and his music. It may interest you.

Client: (Indicates a little interest as he leans forward in his chair and gives her eye contact for the first time.) Well, yeah, it might . . . . (Hesitates and pauses.)

Nurse: I would be glad to go with you to the area and introduce you to the people. (He nods affirmatively.) I've got to finish giving these medications; then I'll come back for you in about 20 minutes.

Client: (Smiles slightly.) Sure, I would like to.

Even though Mr. Sayers's primary problem was depression, boredom was an integral component of his problem, his hospitalization, and his coping with a changed work status. The nurse entered the room with an awareness of all three and attempted to focus on the first two.

Her visit provided stimuli in the form of a forced but friendly interruption. The visit prevented him from dwelling on his own thoughts and encouraged him to do some constructive planning of his time. Without the interaction and attention to the unit's resources, Mr. Sayers may have spent the morning alone more bored than ever.

The nurse focused him on unit activities. She encouraged him by blending the unit activities with knowledge she had gained during a previous nursing assessment. She supported him by offering to take him to the setting where the activity was scheduled and introducing him to unfamiliar people. By doing both she increased the likelihood that this could be a successful intervention and one that the client would incorporate into his hospital routine.

Although this was a brief interaction, the nurse used a number of strategies to alleviate situational boredom. These included maintaining trust, offering a suggestion, respecting the client's individuality, varying his hospital routine, using diversional activities, offering hope, providing support and encouragement, considering the client's interests, and promoting his independence. She does not let his lack of energy, insight, initiative, or attention to surroundings such as the posted schedule interfere with the possibility of relating to others through a meaningful activity.

Nursing interventions in similar situations require a sensitive, creative nurse who is aware of the client as an individual and the practice setting's resources and capabilities. This nurse also plans to address the chronic boredom that contributed to the client's depression as she strengthens her relationship with him.

Evaluation

Evaluation of the nursing process includes an examination of the concrete data and the client's self-reporting about his progress in changing his activities, environment, and attitude.

Logically one would expect boredom and its accompanying feelings to decrease or be alleviated. If neither occurs, new goals and more relevant strategies are implemented until new behaviors are evident.

NURSING PROCESS SUMMARY: BOREDOM

ASSESSMENT

Physical Dimension
Yawning (relationship is unknown)
Vocation characterized by fast, machine-paced work, by viewing monitors, or by monotonous activities
Frequent clinic visits at work or school
Somatic illnesses such as gastritis and peptic ulcers
Change in job's activity level
Vision or hearing impairment
Isolated physical environment
Physical restraints
Protected environment such as a laminar airflow room
Hospital isolation procedures
Terminal illness
Living in long-term care or rehabilitation facility
Increased food consumption
Chewing fingertips and nails
Occupation-related accidents and injuries

Emotional Dimension
Anxiety
Depression
Drug or alcohol abuse
Trapped or bored feeling
Chronic resignation
Frustration
Fear
Resentment
Apathy
Hostility
Thrill seeking to occupy time

Intellectual Dimension
Decreased creativity
Diminished readiness to act
Inattentiveness
Decreased attention span
Misses details
Decreased task quality
Diminished ability to learn
Lack of educational achievement

Social Dimension
Social isolation
Introvert or extrovert personality
Diminished daily activities
Unemployed
Home-bound
Decreased access to transportation, television, or radio
Lack of or ineffective social skills
Difficulty relating to self and others

Spiritual Dimension
Aimlessness
Lack of purpose
No or minimal future orientation
Alienation from self, others, and higher being

ANALYSIS
Refer to the Nursing Diagnosis section on p. 407.

PLANNING AND IMPLEMENTATION

Physical Dimension
Balance schedules between routine and novel activities
Alter predictability of situations
Remove or minimize sameness
Orient to reality
Alter environment such as furniture and wall colors
Encourage participation in recreational activities
Frequently touch those with sensory deprivation
Keep prostheses such as hearing aids and glasses functioning properly
Encourage small, frequent breaks during boring tasks
Vary activities where possible

Emotional Dimension
Encourage use of music therapy and group therapy
Reward successful completion of boring tasks
Break boring projects into manageable steps
Eliminate or minimize thrill-seeking activities especially if potentially harmful to clients or others
Reduce predominant feeling states of restlessness, frustration, and apathy
Promote activities at which clients can succeed

Intellectual Dimension
Decrease the complexity of the task
Encourage client to develop meaningful rewards
Encourage creative responses to problems and boring tasks
Assist client to develop an individualized retirement plan that includes attention to activities and desires
Facilitate meetings with student, teachers, parents, and guidance counselors to confront problems associated with boredom in the classroom
Minimize or eliminate conformity
Develop time to think or do unplanned activities in a client's busy schedule
Encourage altering busy, tight schedules at work or in the client's personal life

NURSING PROCESS SUMMARY: BOREDOM—cont'd.

Social Dimension
  Facilitate socialization opportunities
  Encourage development of social skills
  Provide an environment that prevents boredom
  Visit clients in isolation or protected environments
  For those who are home bound or institutionalized,
    develop a schedule of planned activities and the
    opportunity for unplanned activities
  Encourage the client's optimum level of activity
  Encourage clients to maintain communication with
    others via telephone calls, letters, or cards
Spiritual Dimension
  Encourage a more optimistic attitude
  Assist clients to develop future plans
  Encourage the development of more meaningful
    relationships and behaviors
  Encourage clients to know themselves better
  Assist clients to use previously successful spiritual
    resources

EVALUATION

Evaluation includes examining the concrete data and the client's self-reporting on the success of the nursing process. Goals and outcomes concentrate on decreasing or alleviating boredom. Interventions are evaluated in terms of the intensity of boredom, the presence of related feeling states, the client's need and desire to reduce the effects of boredom on his life, and the development of successful coping mechanisms that the client can eventually incorporate into his life-style.

BRIEF REVIEW

Boredom is a common experience that has received little attention by health professionals until recently. Since boredom is linked with predictability, researchers found that subjects functioned best when their stimulation level was moderate. If the subjects were overstimulated, they became confused; if they were understimulated, they became bored.

Boredom has been addressed by numerous theorists. All acknowledge boredom as a feeling state with diverse causes that can be generally categorized as internal, external, or a combination of internal and external. Initially believed to only have unpleasant consequences, boredom is now known to have numerous benefits for different population groups. Among them are clients with stuttering, autism, mental retardation, alcoholism, hypertension, and compulsive overeating.

Adolescents, retired persons, those with monotonous occupations, the hearing and vision impaired, and those experiencing social isolation, confinement, and restriction of movement are among the at-risk groups for developing boredom. Most in these groups experience some form of sensory deprivation creating too little stimulation with too much predictability.

The negative effects of boredom include altered job performance and work quality, missed work time, somatic complaints, anxiety, depression, and accidents that could possibly lead to death. In the work setting, the results have been costly in lost working hours, injuries, and even death. Boredom is associated with decreased attention, gastritis, peptic ulcer, chronic resignation, frustration, apathy, hostility, thrill seeking, decreased creativity, altered learning, and alienation from self and others.

Nursing diagnoses for the bored client involve sensory-perceptual alteration, social isolation, ineffective individual coping, and diversional activity deficit. Joint planning by the nurse and client promotes such strategies as increasing or varying sensory stimulation, creating opportunities for success, completing tasks with minimal interruptions, decreasing task complexity, increasing socialization opportunities and skills, decreasing repetition, preparing for retirement, minimizing conformity, and altering the physical work environment to alleviate or minimize boredom and its accompanying feelings.

REFERENCES AND SUGGESTED READINGS

1. Abramson, E.E., and Stinson, S.G.: Boredom and eating in obese and non-obese individuals, Addictive Behaviors **2**:181, 1977.
2. Azima, H., Vispo, R., and Azima, F.J.: Observations on anaclitic therapy during sensory deprivation. In Solomon, P., and others, editors: Sensory deprivation, Cambridge, Mass. 1961, Harvard University Press.
3. Bailey, J.P., and others: Boredom and arousal: comparison of tasks differing in visual complexity, Perceptual and Motor Skills **43**:141, 1976.
4. Bell, L.: Boredom and the yawn, Review of Existential Psychology and Psychiatry **17**(1):91, 1980.
5. Bernstein, H.E.: Boredom and the ready-made life, Social Research **42**:512, 1975.
6. Braverman, B.G., and Shook, J.: Spotting the borderline personality disorder, American Journal of Nursing **87**(2):200, 1987.
7. Bressler, B., and others: Research in human subjects and the artificial traumatic neurosis: where does our responsibility lie? American Journal of Psychiatry **116**:552, 1959.
8. Caplan, R.D., and others: Job demands and worker health,

Washington, D.C., 1975, U.S. Department of Health, Education, and Welfare.

9. Chang, G.S., and Lorenzi, P.: The effects of participative versus assigned goal setting on intrinsic motivation, Journal of Management 9(1):55, 1983.

10. Cleland, C., and others: Creativity of faculty as influenced by body typology and boredom, Academic Psychology Bulletin 3:191, June 1981.

11. DiMattia, D.J., and Huber, C.H.: A new clinical conceptualization: prediction therapy, American Mental Health Counselors Association Journal 5:123, July 1983.

12. Dong, H.K.: Method of complete triads: an investigation of unreliability in multidimensional perception of notions, Multivariate Behavioral Research 18:85, January 1983.

13. Drory, A.: Individual differences in boredom proneness and task effectiveness at work, Personnel Psychology 35:141, 1982.

14. Fahmy, N.R.M., and Noble, J.: Digital osteomyelitis due to boredom, The Hand 13(3):285, 1981.

15. Fenichel, O.: On the psychology of boredom. In Fenichel, H., and Rapaport, D., editors: The collected papers of Otto Fenichel: first series, New York, 1953, W.W. Norton and Co.

16. Fiske, D.W.: Effects of monotonous and restricted stimulation. In Fiske, D.W., and Maddi, S., editors: Functions of varied experience, Homewood, Ill., 1961, Dorsey.

17. Frick, S.R.: Diagnosing boredom, confusion, and adaptation in school children, Journal of School Health 55:254, September 1985.

18. Greenson, R.R.: On boredom, Journal of the American Psychoanalytic Association 1:7, 1953.

19. Hamilton, J.A.: Attention, personality and the self-regulation of mood. In Maher, B.A., editor: Progress in experimental personality research, vol. 10, New York, 1981, Academic Press.

20. Hamilton, J.A.: Development of interest and enjoyment in adolescence. Attentional capacities, Journal of Youth and Adolescence 12(5):355, 1983.

21. Hamilton, J.A.: Development of interest and enjoyment in adolescence. II. Boredom and psychopathology, Journal of Youth and Adolescence 12(5):363, 1983.

22. Hamilton, J.A., Haier, R.H., and Buchsbaum, M.S.: Intrinsic enjoyment and boredom coping scales: validation with personality, evoked potential and attention measures, Personality and Individual Differences 5(2):183,, 1984.

23. Hartocollis, P.: Affects in borderline disorders. In Hartocollis, P., editor: Borderline personality disorders: the concept, the syndrome, the patient, New York, 1977, International Universities Press.

24. Hartocollis, P.: Affective disturbance in borderline and narcissistic patients, Bulletin of the Menninger Clinic 44:135, 1980.

25. Herron, W.: The pathology of boredom, Scientific American, p. 52, January 1957.

26. Hill, A.B.: Work variety and individual differences in occupational boredom, Journal of Applied Psychology 60:128, 1975.

27. Hill, A.B., and Perkins, R.E.: Towards a model of boredom, British Journal of Psychology 76:235, 1985.

28. Inhelder, B., and Piaget, J.: The growth of logical thinking from childhood through adolescence, New York, 1958, Basic Books.

29. Kail, R., and Bisanz, J.: Information processing and cognitive development, Advances in Child Development and Behavior 17:54, 1982.

30. Keen, S.: Chasing the blahs away: boredom and how to beat it, Psychology Today, p. 78, May 1977.

31. Kelly, G.A.: The psychology of personal constructs, vol. 1, New York, 1975, W.W. Norton & Co.

32. Kohut, H.: The analysis of self: a systematic approach to the psychoanalytic treatment of narcissistic personality disorders (Psychoanalytic study of the child, monograph no. 4), New York, 1971, International Universities Press.

33. Kohut, H.: The restoration of the self, New York, 1977, International Universities Press.

34. Kohut, H., and Wolf, E.S.: The disorders of the self and their treatment: an outline, International Journal of Psychoanalysis 59:413, 1978.

35. Kopp, T.: Designing boredom out of instruction, Performance and Instructions: The Journal of the National Society for Performance and Instruction 21:23, May 1982.

36. Kulick, E.M.: On countertransference boredom, Bulletin of the Menninger Clinic 49:95, March 1985.

37. Kurtz, J.P., and Zuckerman, M.: Race and sex differences on the sensation seeking scales, Psychological Reports 43:529, 1978.

38. Landon, P.B., and Suedfeld, P.: Complex cognitive performance and sensory deprivation: completing the U-curve, Perceptual and Motor Skills 34:601, 1972.

39. LaRocco, J.M., House, J., and French, J.: Social support, occupational stress, and health, Journal of Health and Social Behavior 21:202, September 1980.

40. Levy, S.T.: Psychoanalytic perspectives on emptiness, Journal of the American Psychoanalytic Association 32(2):387, 1984.

41. London, H., Schubert, D.S., and Washburn, D.: Increase of autonomic arousal by boredom, Journal of Abnormal Psychology 80(1):29, 1972.

42. Marsh, J.: The boredom of study: a study of boredom, Management Education and Development 14(2):120, 1983.

43. Marshall, W.L., and Lippens, K.: The clinical value of boredom: a procedure for reducing inappropriate sexual interests, The Journal of Nervous and Mental Disease 165(4):283, 1977.

44. Morrant, J.C.: Boredom in psychiatric practice, Canadian Journal of Psychiatry 29:431, August 1984.

45. Munsterberg, H.: Psychology and industrial efficiency, Boston, 1913, Houghton-Mifflin.

46. Nachreiner, F.: Experiments on the validity of vigilance experiments. In Mackie, R.R., editor: Vigilance: theory, operational performance, and physiological correlates, New York, 1977, Plenum Press.

47. Nachreiner, F., and Ernst, G.: Monotony and satiation as a person-situation interaction. Paper presented at the XIXth International Congress of Applied Psychology, Munich, Germany, 1978.

48. O'Connell, S.R.: Recreation therapy: reducing the effects of isolation for the patient in a protected environment, Children's Health Care 12(3):118, 1984.

49. O'Hanlon, J.F.: Boredom: practical consequences and a theory, Acta psychologica 49:53, 1981.

50. Olsen, R.V.: The effect of the hospital environment: patient reactions to traditional versus progressive care settings, Journal of Architectural and Planning Research 1(2):121, 1984.

51. Orcutt, J.D.: Some social dimensions of boredom. Paper presented at the Annual Meeting of the American Sociological Association, Detroit, 1983.

52. Orcutt, J.D.: Contrasting effects of two kinds of boredom on alcohol use, Journal of Drug Issues 14:161, Winter 1984.

53. Perkins, R.E.: The nature and origins of boredom, PhD thesis, Staffordshire, United Kingdom, 1981, University of Keele.

54. Perkins, R.E., and Hill, A.B.: Cognitive and affective aspects of boredom, British Journal of Psychology **76**:221, 1985.

55. Poulton, E.C.: Stresses and hazards. In Elliot, E., editor: Human factors for designers of naval equipment, London, 1975, Medical Research Council.

56. Pribram, K.H.: Languages of the brain, Englewood Cliffs, N.J., 1971, Prentice-Hall, Inc.

57. Reisser, P.C., Reisser, T.K., and Weldon, J.: What holistic healers believe, Journal of Christian Nursing **3**(1):16, 1986.

58. Robinson, W.P.: Boredom at school, The British Journal of Educational Psychology **45**:141, 1975.

59. Rosseel, E.: Fatigue and boredom resulting from reduced task motivation, Psychologica Belgica **14**:67, 1974.

60. Samoilova, A.J.: Morbidity with temporary loss of working capacity of female workers engaged in monotonous work (Russian), Sovetska Zdravookhranenie **30**:41, 1971.

61. Savitz, J., and Friedman, M.I.: Diagnosing boredom and confusion, Nursing Research **30**:16, January-February 1981.

62. Schubert, D.S.: Creativity and coping with boredom, Psychiatric Annals **8**:46, March 1978.

63. Shultz, C.M.: Lifestyle assessment: a tool for practice, Nursing Clinics of North America **19**(2):271, 1984.

64. Slater, V.: A behavioural programme for Billy, Nursing Times, p. 1267, July 28, 1982.

65. Smith, R.P.: Boredom: a review, Human Factors **23**:329, June 1981.

66. Solomon, P., and others, editors: Sensory deprivation, Cambridge, Mass., 1961, Harvard University Press.

67. Stagner, R.: Boredom on the assembly line: age and personality variables, Industrial Gerontology **2**:22, Winter 1975.

68. Strahan, C.: The retired patient: boredom, fears, and suicide, Delaware Medical Journal **52**:497, September 1980.

69. Suedfeld, P.: Changes in intellectual performance and in susceptibility to influence. In Zubek, J.P., editor: Sensory deprivation: fifteen years of research, New York, 1969, Appleton-Century-Crofts, Inc.

70. Suedfeld, P.: The benefits of boredom: sensory deprivation reconsidered, American Scientist **63**:60, January-February 1975.

71. Taylor, G.J.: Psychotherapy with the boring patient, Canadian Journal of Psychiatry **29**:217, April 1984.

72. Thackray, R.I.: The stress of boredom and monotony: a consideration of the evidence, Psychosomatic Medicine **43**:165, April 1981.

73. Thackray, R.I., Bailey, J.P., and Touchstone, R.M.: Physiological, subjective and performance correlates of reported boredom and monotony while performing a simulated radar control task, FAA Office of Aviation Medicine Reports **75-8**:9, 1975.

74. Thackray, R.I., Jones, K.N., and Touchstone, R.M.: Personality and physiological correlates of performance decrement on a monotonous task requiring sustained attention, British Journal of Psychology **65**:351, 1974.

75. Wangh, M.: Boredom in psychoanalytic perspective, Social Research **42**:538, 1975.

76. Wangh, M.: Some psychoanalytic observations on boredom, International Journal of Psychoanalysis **60**:515, 1979.

77. Wasson, A.S.: Susceptibility to boredom and deviant behavior at school, Psychological Reports **48**:901, June 1981.

ANNOTATED BIBLIOGRAPHY

Braverman, B.G., and Shook, J.: Spotting the borderline personality, American Journal of Nursing **87**(2):200, 1987.

A case example of team management of the borderline client who appears in the emergency room is offered. Presenting symptoms and behaviors including boredom as a component of the DSM-III characteristics are presented. Specific nursing interventions such as limit setting, family involvement, safety measures, and need for psychiatric consultation are discussed.

Levy, S.: Psychoanalytic perspectives on emptiness, Journal of the American Psychoanalytic Association **32**(2):387, 1984.

The author considers emptiness as a component of boredom. The article reviews emptiness from a psychoanalytic perspective and its treatment modalities. Suggestions are offered in the management of the complaint of emptiness.

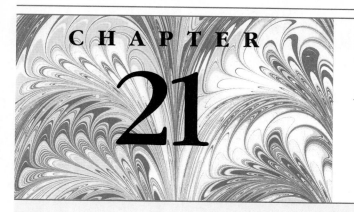

CHAPTER 21

MANIPULATION

Nancy Kowal Ellis

After studying this chapter the learner will be able to:

Discuss manipulation within a historical perspective.

Define manipulation.

Discuss theories of manipulation.

Use the nursing process to provide care for a manipulative client.

Manipulation is a method of interacting in which an individual attempts to gain control over others to fulfill his immediate needs and desires. The manipulative person often feels satisfaction when he achieves his goal of controlling others. The labels "manipulative client" or "manipulator" usually evoke a negative emotional response, because the recipient of the manipulation often feels victimized or violated.

Although manipulation is commonly perceived as negative and destructive, virtually all interpersonal interactions involve some degree of conscious or unconscious manipulation. The term manipulative has been misused to refer to any individual or client who attempts to gain control or to become assertive.

In a therapeutic relationship the nurse strives to meet the needs of a client and to encourage growth and independence. This is a broad and often difficult goal when the client is manipulative. It requires the nurse to deal with the process as well as the content of the interaction. Unfortunately, when a client manipulates as a part of his pattern of interacting, strong emotional responses are evoked, and the process of the interaction may be neglected. An understanding of the dynamics of a client's manipulative behavior can assist the nurse in dealing with her emotional response and in accomplishing the therapeutic goal of facilitating the client's growth and independence. The degree to which manipulative behavior is used will also influence the nurse's and client's range of possible long-term and short-term goals. Extreme destructive manipulation in a patterned response is a common characteristic of clients diagnosed with an antisocial personal-

ity disorder. How this disorder relates to the use of destructive manipulation will be discussed.

THEORETICAL APPROACHES
Psychoanalytic

Manipulation is defined by Webster's as skillful handling or operation, or artful management and control with the use of shrewd influence, especially in an unfair or fraudulent manner.

Psychoanalytic theory views the use of manipulation to be associated with the development of the superego. The superego emerges in an infant in response to external rewards and punishments from significant others, most often parents. For this development to begin, the infant needs to have the capacity to identify and internalize various parental responses, demands, and prohibitions.

The infant's developing superego is reinforced as he experiences an increased sense of self-esteem and fulfillment as he lives up to the standards and demands of the superego. Failure to meet these standards results in feelings of guilt and shame. The development of primary morality can therefore be directly linked to the morality of the significant others to which the infant is exposed.

The maturing child is also exposed to the standards and demands of his peer groups. As this peer group becomes a primary source of identification for the child, he begins to become socialized according to the morality of this group. As an individual continues to develop, the internalized morals of early significant others and the modifying impact of the peer socialization process contribute

Historical Overview

DATE	EVENT
1500s	Machiavelli published *The Prince*, which described manipulative strategies to succeed in politics. Power, not ethics, was stressed.
Early 1800s	The labels "morally deficient" and "morally insane due to genetic impairments" were introduced. They included individuals who demonstrated obvious destructive manipulation.
Early 1900s	The label "psychodynamically impaired" replaced the moral labels. Destructive manipulative behavior was included in this category. The term "psychopath" was commonly used to describe individuals who functioned without regard to others' rights and outside of social rules and laws.
1930	Cleckley[3] replaced the term "psychopath" with "sociopath," explaining that these individuals' destructive behaviors were directed toward society.
1952	The first DSM offered the diagnostic category sociopathic personality, which included manipulative behavior.
1963	Kumler,[13] a nurse, published an article on manipulation that recognized the impact of manipulation on the nurse-client relationship.
1968	DSM-III placed the diagnostic category *sociopath* under the general heading *personality disorders.* Wiley, a nurse, published her conceptualization of manipulation.[29]
1970s	Christie and Geis, researchers in Machiavellian behaviors, extensively studied manipulative individuals' abilities to exploit others, remain emotionally detached, and be continually opportunistic. They predicted that manipulative behaviors would increase in society, because these behaviors were reinforced by role models.
1970s	Several popular books on how to succeed through manipulation began to appear (for example, *How to Win Friends and Influence People*).
1980	DSM-III altered the previous diagnostic category to *antisocial personality disorder.*
1986	An article written by Chitty and Maynard[4] reflected renewed interest in managing manipulation.
Future	The nurse's understanding of manipulation will increase and she will become a key professional in coordinating the care of individuals with manipulative behavior.

to the developing conscience. An individual's moral stance and experience of guilt when using manipulative behavior is influenced by both the developed conscience and the individual's perception of the values of his current peer group or society.

The development of the superego and the conscience is influenced by various factors of early infancy and childhood. An infant who has very strong aggressive feelings and who fears retaliation from his parents may turn his aggressive feelings inward. The result may be an overly severe superego and conscience. Such an individual would probably manipulate very little, if at all.

An infant may develop a weak superego as a result of his inability to internalize social expectations or demands. The morality or demands of the parents may be inconsistent, with parents reinforcing a false impression to society as opposed to what they did or how they did it. The re-

sultant weakly formed superego would offer the child a decreased sense of guilt or remorse (or a lack of these), and a weakly formed conscience.

A child who experiences a particularly strong identification with his peer group may experience guilt in situations in which he, as an individual, manipulates. However, manipulation in collaboration with his peers or colleagues may free this individual from experiencing guilt.

An individual with a manipulative personality often uses the manipulative act as his primary goal. Punishment or reward has no effect on this individual, as the gain is experienced from the act itself. Psychoanalytic theorists view the individual with a manipulative personality to be a fragile form of a *narcissistic personality*. The narcissistic individual manipulates as a response to experiencing a narcissistic wound that causes shame and anxiety. The need to restore a sense of balance becomes primarily important to the individual. This involves restoring a lost sense of pride and decreasing the contempt experienced from the feelings of shame that are overriding. Such an individual manipulates and experiences a sense of relief and exhilaration at having pulled something over on someone and setting the balance right.

The narcissist views others as an extension of himself and uses them to mirror his own grandiose self-image. Any imperfection in others cannot be tolerated, and therefore the narcissistic manipulator avoids all genuine intimate relationships. The individual with a manipulative personality places his appearance as a priority over all other aspects of himself. Any threat to his appearance results in manipulative attempts to redeem his image, regardless of the impact on others or the violation of rights or rules. If the manipulative act is exposed, the manipulator often insincerely displays contrition to fulfill the image that society expects. Guilt or remorse are only acted out, because the individual with a manipulative personality has not developed a strong enough superego to truly experience these reactions.

Bursten,[2] in his psychoanalytic study of manipulation, emphasized the conscious nature of manipulation. The individual does not necessarily know the unconscious motivator of his behavior; however, he is aware or can become readily conscious that he is controlling another person by some fradulent or crafty means to his own advantage. Bursten identifies four essential components of manipulation[2]:

1. Conflict of goal—the manipulator must perceive accurately or inaccurately a conflict of goals between himself and the other person. The manipulator must want something from the other person that the person doesn't want him to have.
2. Intentionality—the manipulator must have a conscious intent to influence the other person. This component requires anticipatory planning by the manipulator with an intent that is conscious or readily accessible to consciousness.
3. Deception—the manipulator's reality testing is such that he knows his plan is to deceive the person.
4. Sense of satisfaction—the manipulator must experience exhilaration (a sense of satisfaction) in having deceived the other person.

The four components are interrelated; in some instances one may be more easily recognized, and in other situations another component may be more obvious. Bursten emphasized that all components must be observed or reasonably inferred for the behavior to be identified as manipulation.

Bursten[2] described three groupings of manipulative situations. A person in group I does not ordinarily use manipulation. The person may occasionally use manipulation to achieve a goal or attain satisfaction and pleasure. For example, this person may manipulate to gain a special privilege or to draw attention to himself.

The second group consists of people who may use manipulation to avoid perceived danger and discomfort. Examples of this type of manipulation are an attempt to avoid situations that increase anxiety or to avoid anticipated punishment, as when a child does a special favor for a parent when he thinks punishment is forthcoming. People in this group and the first one do not manipulate repeatedly or chronically. Their reason for manipulation usually becomes obvious during the interaction, and the advantages are at a conscious level.

People in the third group seem to manipulate for the sake of manipulating. Manipulation is the person's lifestyle; he has a manipulative personality. The manipulative behavior may be silly, involving pranks that may lead to repeated punishment. The basis for the manipulation is primarily a need to "pull something over" on another person. People in this group may be classified as having an antisocial personality disorder.

Interpersonal

Wiley[29] described two types of manipulation that occur in interpersonal relationships: constructive and destructive.

Constructive manipulation is using one's strengths and abilities in interpersonal situations to promote successful relationships. The constructive manipulator knows he is using manipulation and accepts responsibility for it.[29] Communication continues consciously and maturely. Both parties in the interaction know what is occurring and can make a conscious choice whether to participate in the interaction based on their own needs.

Destructive manipulation is using or playing others for one's own purposes. This manipulator promotes difficulties in or destroys interpersonal relationships, and personal growth does not result. Communication is often at an unconscious level, with the victim unaware of the dynamics. The victim, however, experiences negative feelings and often responds with anger and withdrawal. The manipulator may feel rejected after this exchange, resulting in further anxiety and an increased need to manipulate.

Shostrom[26] proposes that manipulative behavior is never totally eliminated; rather, all individuals use some degree of manipulation throughout their lives. These behaviors can be viewed on a continuum of manipulative behavior to actualized behavior. The manipulative range of the continuum includes individuals who conceal sincere emotions in a variety of behaviors to serve their needs and desires, with disregard for others. The actualized range of the continuum includes individuals who trust their own emotions and openly communicate their needs and desires. Shostrom characterizes the manipulator as deceiving by playing roles to create calculated impressions. Finally, he has a constant need to control others. The actualizer is characterized by honesty and genuineness of emotion. The actualizer is aware and trusts himself and others. He is free and spontaneous in interactions. Most individuals fall somewhere between these two extremes. An individual in the actualized range may engage in manipulation but is aware of the behavior and accepts responsibility for it.

Kumler[13] used the term *adaptive maneuvering* to describe the manipulative responses of newborns. She defines it as an automatic behavioral pattern to which a person adapts to decrease anxiety without learning or experiencing interpersonal growth. Newborns learn several adaptive maneuvers to fulfill basic needs. They influence or manipulate without regard for others' needs and without responsibility. Although this is necessary and acceptable for newborns, it is usually viewed as unacceptable in adults and has negative consequences.

A developing child tests a variety of adaptive maneuvers to manipulate the environment to meet his needs. Significant others begin to respond to these behaviors by setting limits. However, the child is allowed to experiment and test his limits and to occasionally fail. If the child's experimentation is met with consistent, clear limits and unconditional love and acceptance, he begins to develop a sense of self-control, self-worth, and self-esteem and to form a healthy identification with his parents. Gradually the child replaces the adaptive maneuvers with more independence and self-regulation. He learns to clearly express his needs and to trust that they will be fulfilled.

A child may remain at the manipulative end of the continuum if the ideal responses to his adaptive maneuvers do not occur. This child's experimentations are met with inconsistent limits or no limits, conditional love, and nonacceptance. The child does not learn how to fulfill his needs or gain acceptance and love from others, resulting in increased anxiety and fear. He becomes insecure and submissive to external controls, lacking self-esteem and self-worth.

As this individual grows, he becomes trapped in a vicious cycle of relating to the environment: he has needs to be met, but he has learned that inconsistency and lack of fulfillment are to be expected. He therefore becomes anxious when faced with his needs or fears and begins to disregard the needs and rights of others. Adaptive maneuvers learned in infancy—in this case manipulation—are repeated to gain fulfillment. If the individual receives a positive response and his needs are met, his anxiety temporarily decreases. However, his use of manipulation will be reinforced, and this pattern of relating continues. If he is met with a negative response and his needs remain unfulfilled, his fears, insecurities, and anxiety greatly increases, and he becomes angry and frustrated. His self-esteem and self-worth diminishes, while feelings of helplessness and insecurity thrive. In an attempt to fulfill his needs and control his anxiety, he again tries to manipulate. Learned adaptive maneuvers will be attempted for self-protection. The inability to trust others to respond to his needs and frustrations with the external world are reinforced, and the individual's sense of worthlessness and helplessness increases.

This individual has learned that he cannot risk losing control or feeling vulnerable. His inability to take a risk makes a sincere relationship impossible. Lacking basic trust, he is trapped in an attempt to gain and maintain control.

Table 21-1 summarizes the theoretical approaches.

RELATING TO THE CLIENT

In the orientation phase of a nurse-client relationship the nurse is aware of the potential for destructive manipulation on both sides. Health care providers typically use constructive manipulation in giving care. They expect to be in control and to have clients conform to certain rules and regulations. However, the degree to which clients comply depends on their personality, the personality of

TABLE 21-1 Summary of theoretical approaches

Theory	Theorist	Dynamics
Psychoanalytic		Manipulation develops in response to a weak superego.
		The individual with a manipulative personality uses manipulation as a primary goal.
	Bursten	Manipulation operates on a conscious level.
		There are four essential, interrelated components of manipulation: conflict of goal, intentionality, deception, and sense of satisfaction.
		There are three groupings of persons who manipulates—those who (1) manipulate occasionally to achieve a goal or satisfaction, (2) sometimes manipulate to avoid danger and discomfort, (3) manipulate as a life-style—manipulate for the sake of manipulation.
Interpersonal	Wiley	Constructive manipulation occurs on a conscious level.
		The person uses assets to promote successful interpersonal relationships.
		Destructive manipulation is unconscious and destroys relationships.
	Shostrom	All people use manipulation throughout their lives.
		The behavior can be placed on a continuum of manipulative behavior (conceals emotion and serves own needs) to actualized behavior (trusts own emotions and openly communicates needs).
	Kumler	Manipulative behavior of the newborn is adaptive maneuvering to meet his needs.
		Positive responses to adaptive maneuvering leads to the development of independence and self-regulation.
		When adaptive maneuvering is not successful for getting needs met, the person remains manipulative.

those offering care, the interactions between these two parties, and the nature of the goals and plan of care.[12] The nurse's position can foster destructive manipulation if she has strong, unconscious needs that she attempts to satisfy in her work setting. A nurse who uses destructive manipulation has a need to appear powerful and may therefore force the client to depend excessively on her.

A client engages in constructive manipulation when he enters the health care system and assesses the role he is expected to assume. He often becomes dependent to fit into the system and avoid confrontations to ensure that his needs are met. The potential for destructive manipulation exists also; the client may exploit the situation to meet unconscious needs. By understanding the dynamics underlying manipulative behaviors, the nurse can respond effectively to the client and avoid inappropriate, nontherapeutic labeling.

When destructive manipulation is identified, the nurse questions the context in which it is occurring. Is the client open to change and growth at this time, or does the client's increased anxiety prevent this? A client whose anxiety level is high because of physical illness or the stress of a life change often clings to old coping behaviors. The nurse cannot expect this client to change patterns of interacting and coping. However, the nurse can be a role model of mature interaction patterns, regardless of the client's anxiety.

To be a role model of mature communication, the nurse needs to be aware of her reactions to the client throughout their relationship. As the recipient of manipulative behavior, the nurse may feel victimized and respond with anger and frustration. Frustration is common if the nurse, consciously or unconsciously, expects some change in the client and expends a great deal of energy toward this goal. Anger may result if the manipulative client tries to play staff members against each other. The skillful manipulator may choose certain nurses as protectors or friends, telling them they can assist him in a special way. The client also chooses certain nurses to be enemies, disrupting the health care team. Nursing reactions, if not openly discussed, can lead to punitive responses that may foster further manipulation and anger.

The nurse's conscious and unconscious reactions to the client affects how various manipulative behaviors are viewed and labeled. For example, one client may buy a nurse gifts in exchange for "good service," while another client threatens to notify the hospital administration if "service is not good." Both clients fear that their needs will not be met because of their vulnerable positions; both are manipulating. However, the way their behavior is labeled may vary based on the nurse's personal reaction to the client. The nurse's own needs may also influence her perception of the client's behaviors. For example, the nurse who is insecure in her role may encourage the client to offer compliments and to continue to manipulate.

Assessing whether a manipulative client has engaged in the working phase of a relationship can be extremely difficult. Focusing on this issue may only foster more frustration and anger among the staff. Regardless of the client's commitment to the relationship, the goal of role modeling healthy communication patterns and avoiding reinforcement of the destructive manipulation remains the same. The nurse need not try to change the client; this will surely result in power struggles, frustration and anger, or alienation for both. Such a goal may also result in the nurse's using manipulation to force compliance. In the working phase of a relationship the client is also likely to test limits and trust. It is therefore important for the nursing staff to communicate openly as often as possible.

Focusing on the sincerity of the client's reaction to termination can also result in negative nursing reactions. Regardless of the client's expressed reaction, he is experiencing the ending of a relationship, and the opportunity for constructive role modeling exists. If the relationship has been short term, expecting real engagement of the client can be unrealistic because of his inability to form a trusting relationship. A client may attempt to deceive the nurse to avoid sharing any sincere reactions to termination. He might enact a role he thinks the nurse expects of him (for example, he may give excessive gifts to the whole staff). The termination process may also cause the client to feel increased anxiety and to regress to maladaptive communication patterns and coping behaviors. The role change required in terminating a relationship that has been protective and nurturing may even cause the highly actualized client to feel anxiety and regress to a more manipulative coping pattern. By viewing these reactions as part of the termination process, the nurse can avoid feeling like a failure because of the client's regression.

NURSING PROCESS
Assessment

✦ ***Physical dimension.*** The nurse first assesses the client's perception of the threat to his physical security. Any threat may prompt increased anxiety and a regression to maladaptive coping mechanisms. Physical illness often results in a sense of loss of control and a fear of becoming helpless and dependent. Further, the health care system often strips a client of control. In the health care system a client often feels extremely vulnerable and anxious and attempts to manipulate the environment to increase his security. He may rely on manipulative maneuvers to fulfill the physical needs that he has been able to independently meet in the past. The nurse assesses the client's stress level and past coping responses. Verbal and nonverbal behaviors cue the nurse that the client is feeling a threat or increased stress.

The client's physical dimension becomes difficult to assess when his manipulations interfere with his ability to accurately express his physical needs. This occurs because depending on the nurse to meet physical needs makes the client vulnerable. The client may react by offering exaggerated or false expressions of a physical condition or need or by withholding important information. For example, the client who exaggerates his pain to get extra medication ensures that his need (pain relief) will always be fulfilled and under his control. A client desiring discharge or special visiting privileges may also withhold essential information. To validate these clients' physical condition or needs, the nurse objectively observes both verbal and nonverbal signals. An accurate pain assessment, for example, includes both the client's perceptions of pain and observation of his appetite, sleeping pattern, ability to concentrate, and level of activity.

✳ *Emotional dimension.* The nurse attempts to determine whether the client's manipulative behavior is a response to anxiety or an established, destructive pattern of interaction. A client who temporarily regresses may be aware of his behavior and disturbed by it. This client may be able to discuss the fears or anxieties that triggered the behavior. Further exploration may reveal that manipulative behavior occurs only in response to very high stress.

A client who manipulates destructively as a pattern of relating may appear pleased when his manipulations are successful; sincere remorse or embarrassment are not seen. When the behavior is explored with this client, he may respond with self-pity, anger, or frustration instead of accepting responsibility for it.

The nurse differentiates among assertive, aggressive, and manipulative behaviors. Many clients are encouraged to become assertively involved in their care and to question the health care providers, yet the system often remains rigid, and these attempts may be met with anger or power struggles. Clients may be negatively labeled because they have confronted the health care team or changed a routine. An objective awareness of the differences between these behaviors assists the nurse in identifying whether the behavior is a constructive coping response or a destructive pattern of relating and coping.(See Chapter 16)

The destructive manipulator often displays emotional superficiality; the expression of sincere anxiety, guilt, or fear makes the client vulnerable. The nurse may observe that the client can only express hostility and anger when he is anxious or fearful and frustration when he feels guilty.

✳ *Intellectual dimension.* Manipulative behaviors are often learned as survival skills in childhood; therefore a client who is cognitively impaired may still be a skillful manipulator. The manipulator often expresses seemingly rational reasons for his behaviors and may present a sound defense when threatened by feedback. The client may continually express a conflict between his perceived needs and the needs of others. The nurse is likely to observe difficulties with roommates, conflicts with hospital routines and rules, and a resistance to limits set by the hospital staff. As the client's anxiety builds, complaints may escalate to involve several levels of hospital administration.

The client may use compliments and excessive flattery to get people "on his side." He may express and expect special privileges because of his perceived "special circumstances." When staff does not respond positively to his manipulative behavior, the client may get angry and frustrated. He believes that staff members are resistant because, as in his other relationships, they are "against him."

The client who has been in the health care system for a long time may have learned several effective maneuvers to gain control. He may use medical jargon, drop board members' names, or refer to physicians and nurses as personal friends. These behaviors often elicit a threatened, withdrawn, or placating reaction from the health care team.

The nurse assesses the client's motivation to alter his behavior. She ascertains how the client perceives his behavior and whether his behavior has caused difficulties in the past. The nurse can ask him directly if he is willing to change his behavior and if he is committed to working toward this goal now.

✳ *Social dimension.* Wiley[29] categorized a client's destructive manipulative behavior into three groups: (1) *aggressive maneuvering,* exemplified by multiple demands, threats, requests for special considerations, and playing members of the health care team against each other, (2) *distracting maneuvering,* exemplified by changes of subject, flattery, expressions of helplessness, tearfulness, dawdling, and last minute stalling, and (3) *disparaging maneuvers,* exemplified by reprimands or self-pity.

The destructively manipulative client is often severely impaired in the social dimension of his life. This dimension can be assessed by observing the client's present interactions and exploring past social interactions. A social history may reveal no sincere relationships. The client may also transfer frustrations and anger onto any significant social support that does remain involved. If family members are present, the nurse may assess ambivalence in their reactions to the client.

Exploration of the client's job history may reveal an inconsistent work pattern, possibly resulting in financial instability. The client often speaks of a troubled past, in which he has been victimized by external circumstances. A manipulative pattern of relating may be evident since early childhood. A review of the client's childhood and adolescence may reveal periods of aggressiveness and early sexual behaviors. The abuse of drugs or alcohol may also be discovered. These behaviors may have continued into adulthood, possibly resulting in poor work performance and poor parenting skills. A lack of respect for social norms, values, and laws may be seen.

What may initially appear to be manipulative behavior may actually be the client's cultural pattern of relating. For example, many cultures view women as submissive and allow men to make demands and to dominate. Objectivity is essential in such a case; an angry reaction from the nurse can interfere with an accurate assessment. At times it becomes necessary for the nurse to use the responses of the staff to assist in assessing a client's behaviors.

When a health care team is involved with a destructively manipulative client, the team often becomes unable to work together harmoniously. The treatment plan is often a widely debated issue, because each team member perceives the client differently. It is common for the nurse to expend a great deal of energy on the client, while the client appears to be uninterested and uninvolved. As the nurse is manipulated, she may begin to give special privileges. According to Wiley,[23] the nurse commonly responds to destructive manipulation by feeling threatened or alienated or by reinforcing the behavior by pitying or mothering the client. These reactions, objectively identified, suggest that the client is manipulating.

Spiritual dimension. Shostrom[26] identified that a client's behavior can be influenced by religions that are manipulative as opposed to actualized. *Manipulative religions* stress the inability of individuals to trust their own nature and encourage helplessness. The nurse may observe overdependence on the religious community. The client may refuse to think through situations, because he has learned to respond only as the religion demands. Such a client may also resist helping himself, assuring the nurse that his religion will take care of him. Difficult events may be avoided or rationalized as God's will. *Actualized religions* stress trust in one's own nature and encourage self-direction and growth. A client of this style of religion may rely on his religious community for support, guidance, and strength but attempts to accept responsibility for his behavior and the direction of his future. The client's past religious involvements, then, may influence his present behavior.

The nurse remains objective by assessing the client's perception of the meaning of religion in his life. The client may blame God or his religion for his situation or his dissatisfaction with life. Such a client may also attempt to use religion in a manipulative pattern. The client's level of self-actualization and life satisfaction are typically low because of his chronic inability to fulfill his basic needs and his lack of success in forming relationships. He may also have been involved in activities that are illegal, unethical, or outside social norms and values and may express pride in past violations of others' rights.

MANIPULATIVE COPING MODE*

DEFINITION

An enduring pattern of use of behavior aimed at immediately satisfying one's needs while disregarding the rights and needs of others.

DEFINING CHARACTERISTICS

Physical Dimension

- Sense of helplessness or loss of control related to the stress of a physical disease or physical vulnerability
- Threat to physical security
- Past periods of aggressiveness

Emotional Dimension

- Emotional superficiality
- Hostility, anger, or frustration expressed when feeling anxiety, guilt, or fear
- Insincerity
- Exhilaration at successfully manipulating others
- Self-pity
- Anger and hostility expressed toward past or remaining social supports

Intellectual Dimension

- Deceptive
- Persistent requests for special privileges
- Avoidance through change of subject or flattery
- Mental status usually intact
- IQ usually in normal range
- Conflicts between perceived needs and needs of others

Social Dimension

- Lowered self-esteem
- No identifiable sincere relationships and lack of support network
- Inconsistent work history
- Perception of self as victimized
- Engagement in early sexual behaviors
- Poor parenting and work performance
- Lowered self-worth
- Lack of respect for others

Spiritual Dimension

- Lack of respect for social values, norms, and laws
- Chronic inability to feel fulfilled
- Blames God or religion for situation
- Lack of personal growth from experiences

*This diagnosis has been proposed but is not yet approved by NANDA.

Analysis

Nursing diagnosis. Manipulative coping mode is an example of a nursing diagnosis that applies to clients with manipulative behavior. This nursing diagnosis was proposed but has not been accepted by NANDA. The box at left lists defining characteristics of this nursing diagnosis.

Other nursing diagnoses with causative statements appropriate for clients with manipulative behavior include:

1. Powerlessness related to altered ability to meet social responsibilities
2. Impaired social interaction related to inability to maintain enduring relationships
3. Ineffective individual coping related to disregard for social norms
4. Ineffective individual coping related to lack of impulse control

The following Case Example illustrates the characteristics of the nursing diagnosis of manipulative coping mode.

Case Example

John, age 26 years, has lost his third job as a salesman. He blames his boss for "being against him" and his co-workers for "setting him up." He expresses a great deal of anger at all his former co-workers for being jealous of him. John relates that his whole life has been this way. External circumstances consistently stand in the way of his fulfillment. At present John is hospitalized for elective surgery. He demands that his visiting hours be extended because he is expecting contacts for future employment. He is aware of his roommate's condition and need for sleep but sees this as just another obstacle in his way. John continues to enlist the assistance of other patients in violating the visiting hours and appears to enjoy deceiving the staff. When confronted, John immediately appears very sorrowful and states that he only breaks rules because his life has been so difficult.

DSM-III-R diagnoses. Although manipulative behaviors are not solely related to personality disorders, the use of destructive manipulation is a common characteristic of

301.70 ANTISOCIAL PERSONALITY DISORDER

ESSENTIAL FEATURES

A personality disorder in which there is a history of continuous and chronic antisocial behavior which violates the rights of others, occurs in a persistent pattern beginning before age 15 and continues into adult life wherein the adult fails to sustain good job performance over a period of several years. (This may not be evident in persons who are self-employed and those who have not been gainfully employed, such as students and housewives).

MANIFESTATIONS
Physical Dimension

Diagnosis made at age 18 years or later
Not due to mental retardation, schizophrenia, or mania
Repeated drunkenness or substance abuse

Emotional Dimension

Irritability and aggressiveness
Impulsivity, failure to plan ahead
Recklessness

Social Dimension

Truancy
Expulsion or suspension from school
Delinquency
History of running away from home at least twice
Repeated sexual involvement in casual relationships
Thefts
Vandalism
Chronic violation of rules at home
Initiation of fights
Patterned violation of the rights of others
Inability to sustain work
Inability to function as adequate parent
Disregard for social laws and norms
Inability to sustain sincere sexual relationship
Failure to honor financial obligations

Intellectual Dimension

Persistent lying
Low grades in school inconsistent with IQ

Spiritual Dimension

Disregard for truth

Adapted from American Psychiatric Association: Diagnostic and statistical manual of mental disorders (DSM-III-R), Washington, D.C., 1987, The Association.

TABLE 21-2 Long-term and short-term goals and outcome criteria related to manipulation

Goals	Outcome Criteria
NURSING DIAGNOSIS: MANIPULATIVE COPING MODE RELATED TO NO SINCERE RELATIONSHIPS	
Long-term goal	
To replace manipulative behaviors with more actualized, mature patterns of relating	Demonstrates mature behaviors role modeled by the health care team. Engages in long-term therapy as an outpatient to continue to gain support for new behaviors and patterns of relating.
Short-term goals	
To become aware of the use of manipulation and its affect on the ability to gain true fulfillment of one's needs and desires	Begins to identify own manipulative behavior. Explores what it feels like to be manipulated. Explores past uses of manipulation and assesses outcomes of those experiences.
To recognize the stimuli that prompts the use of manipulative behaviors	Explores past situations that prompted the use of manipulation and identifies feelings experienced. Understands the process of manipulative communication that occurs during hospitalization after the situational anxiety has decreased.
To experiment with alternative, more actualized methods of identifying and meeting needs	Begins to maturely express emotions and needs without manipulating. Substitutes new methods of relating while hospitalized. Accepts feedback on new behaviors.
To self-evaluate behaviors and identify when support is needed to avoid relying on old patterns of communication	Identifies when old, manipulative patterns of relating are used and begins to accept responsibility for them. Expands the use of new behaviors to any support systems or significant others. Begins to request support when anxiety or stresses are high to avoid reliance on old patterns of relating.

these disorders. The essential features and manifestations of the features of antisocial personality disorder according to DSM-III-R are listed in the box on p. 422.

Planning

Table 21-2 gives examples of long-term and short-term goals and outcome criteria related to manipulation. These serve as examples of the planning stage in the nursing process.

Implementation

✦ *Physical dimension.* The nurse providing physical care for the manipulative client ensures that basic physical safety is maintained while holding the client responsible for his own behavior. The client may have a variety of basic physical needs. A client who manipulates and reacts with a sense of helplessness, making him dependent, is encouraged to assume responsibility for self-care. After assessing the client's perception of the threat to his physical well-being, the nurse can intervene to decrease that threat by allowing the client to assume as much control as possible. For example, a manipulative client may not ask for an explanation of a procedure for fear of exposing his vulnerability and losing control. Anticipating the client's need and carefully explaining the procedure without a request may lower the client's perceived threat and anxiety.

✳ *Emotional dimension.* Anxiety often stimulates a regression to maladaptive communication or destructive manipulation patterns. A manipulative client feeling a high level of anxiety may defend himself by camouflaging his emotions and attempting to gain external control. The nurse looks beyond these defensive maneuvers, discusses the client's perceptions of his current anxiety level, and explores his past patterns of coping with anxiety. Stripping such a client of all of his defenses is not a useful intervention.

A priority intervention is to establish expectations, set the appropriate and necessary limits, and clearly communicate these to the client and the health care team. Limits are only effective if communicated consistently and firmly and are routinely reviewed to ensure they do not become punitive. Client requests are objectively considered and not automatically opposed. The box at right gives an approach to setting limits. Inappropriate limit setting may result when the nurse becomes angry or exerts excessive control. Limits need to be reasonable and easily applied, since the manipulative client has probably been exposed to inconsistent, idle threats throughout his life. For example, the threat of not providing care if he does not cooperate cannot be enacted; it only perpetuates the cycle of maladaptive communication. The client's ability to set his own limits is assessed and encouraged. Encouraging self-control not only deters power struggles but also provides for role modeling mature relating.

Power struggles may result if the nurse phrases limits in a personal manner, beginning with "I want" or "you must." This sets up a situation conducive for struggling over control. Limit setting is done in an impersonal manner (for example, "Part of your treatment plan is that you attend one group today.") so that the nurse does not become the focus of the client's anger.

The client will test limits and expectations. Consistent responses from the entire health care team are essential. As the client learns that the limits and expectations are firm and constant, he may begin to substitute one maladaptive behavior for another. Again, clear communication and consistency are integral in responding.

LIMIT SETTING

EXPECTATIONS

Make expectations clear to client and other staff members.

CLIENT-CENTERED LIMITS

Be sure that limits are in the best interest of the client and not punitive.

COMMUNICATION

Avoid using personal statements, such as "I don't want you to drink alcohol while I'm on duty." Offer the true rationale: "Alcohol is not allowed in the hospital."

CONSEQUENCES

When consequences are needed, avoid those that are absurd or cannot be enforced, such as "Put the alcohol away or I won't come into your room." Offer only enforceable consequences, such as "If you don't dispose of the alcohol, I will call security to dispose of it."

TESTING

Remain firm and consistent as the client tests the limits that have been set.

VENTING

Allow the client to vent feelings about limits, but do not become engaged in power struggles or attempt to rationalize (for example, "The hospital policy was written because things would get out of control if all clients could drink alcohol . . ."). Instead, verify the client's feelings and repeat the limit as necessary: "I hear that you are angry about this, but alcohol is not allowed."

POSITIVE REINFORCEMENT

Return to the client's room when the affect has subsided to demonstrate that you are not angry and have not withdrawn from the client. Offer positive reinforcement for strengths.

CLARIFICATIONS FOR STAFF

Explain the expectations, limits, and consequences discussed with the client to all staff members to provide consistency and avoid confusion.

Although the entire health care team remains aware of expectations and limits, to the extent that is possible, one primary nurse handles the client's requests. This approach lessens the possibility of confusion and inconsistency, which a manipulative client can readily take advantage of. The primary care nursing system is ideal in this situation; requests for special privileges or changes in treatment are referred to one nurse, who knows all aspects of the client's treatment.

Power struggles may be avoided if the nurse clearly explains to the client that confidentiality is maintained in the health care system. If the client requests that a nurse keep a special secret or not share certain information, the nurse is clear in her response and consistently avoids becoming engaged in any special relationship with the client.

When manipulative behavior occurs, the nurse responds to the process or meaning of the behavior to avoid unnecessary power struggles over content. This allows the nurse to respond to the client's affect objectively. For example, if a client wants to slip out of the hospital for an hour, the nurse acknowledges that it must be difficult to be hospitalized and unable to continue with normal routines. This allows the nurse and client to explore the client's actual need, instead of struggling over the content of the client's request. A manipulative client often responds to limit setting with anger. The nurse may respond to this anger by acknowledging that the client is angry and that his situation is difficult and frustrating. Such a response avoids punitive reactions or power struggles with the client. If possible, the nurse discusses the process when the client's anxiety has decreased. The client's needs at the time of the reaction to limit setting and his ineffective communication can be explored. More constructive patterns of coping and communicating are discussed if the client is receptive.

It is difficult to avoid reinforcing the cycle of manipulative behavior. For example, a client may angrily demand that his medications be given 30 minutes later than usual, and a busy nurse may comply to save time and avoid a conflict. But this response reinforces the manipulative behavior, and learning does not occur. If a client's request is possible, he may be allowed the control he is seeking. However, the nurse provides constructive role modeling and encourages learning by later exploring the client's angry reaction and indirect request for control with him. Gratifying a client's manipulative requests without encouraging learning or growth only reinforces the manipulative behavior. Ignoring or neglecting the client also reinforces the behavior, since the client expects his needs to not be met.

Finally, the entire health care team's responses to the client need to be continually explored. Conscious and unconscious anger, frustrations, and judgments are common. Remembering to respond to the client's behaviors from a dynamic perspective is helpful. The nurse reminds the team that the client's behavior is a result of a life-long pattern of relating and is unrelated to any particular team member. For example, a client may be compliant and complimentary with the day nurse and noncompliant with the evening nurse, blaming her for his noncompliance. These nurses objectively assess their treatment of this client, but remember that his reactions to them are most likely not personal or sincere. Rather, they are part of a pattern of relating that somehow meets the client's perceived needs.

Intellectual dimension. If manipulative behavior has been consistently reinforced and supported, the client's motivation for change may be minimal, especially if stress is high and he is relying on previously successful coping mechanisms to control anxiety. Attempts to change the behavior of an unmotivated client may be unsuccessful. However, the nurse continues to offer constructive role modeling and avoids reinforcing manipulative behaviors by not responding emotionally. Again, responding to the process of the interaction assists the nurse in controlling her own possibly affect-laden response. For example, the nurse may simply tell a client that a particular subject (such as another nurse's personal life) is not appropriate. She may then offer a more appropriate subject in its place.

The most effective intervention for an extremely skillful manipulator is to explore the meaning of the behavior with him and the health care team. A client who appears very intelligent does not necessarily have the ability to change a behavioral pattern without some form of therapy. Such a client may be able to identify and discuss his own maladaptive behavior. However, he may not be able or willing to work at changing the behavior. The nurse may first explore with the client past ineffective interactions that prevented him from attaining his desires and meeting his needs. The client can then be encouraged to review past events to identify how his behavior was destructive. With this information the client can be encouraged to plan new methods for meeting his needs and positively reinforced when these new methods are attempted.

Social dimension. The nurse offers the client the opportunity to identify the destructive nature of past relating patterns and role models constructive alternative patterns. She encourages the client to explore his reactions to being manipulated by others as a first step in realizing how his manipulative behavior affects others. The client is encouraged to identify the use of manipulation in the past and to try out new communication techniques. The nurse encourages these new techniques only when the client's anxiety is low. Attempting a behavioral change when anxiety is high sets up the client for frustration and failure. The nurse discusses past and present behaviors nonjudgmentally; the client and nurse explore the consequences of these behaviors, such as his failure to learn from past events. The nurse demonstrates to the family or significant others techniques that do not reinforce manipulative communication. These persons can also benefit from observing constructive communication and effective limit setting.

The client's strengths are supported to increase self-esteem. He needs encouragement and room to test new techniques; periods of temporary regression are common.

A structured setting is ideal for this testing period, since it provides consistency, opportunities for learning, and safety. In a structured milieu the nurse can encourage the client's strengths and interactions with others, while the client remains independent. A structured environment can also support the nurse in holding the client responsible for his behaviors.

In a group setting the manipulative client often emerges as a leader because of his need for control, and power struggles with the staff may ensue. Although this can be difficult for the health care team, the positive aspects of the client's behavior can be emphasized; leadership ability is a strength.

Any change in the client's long-term pattern of relating needs consistent and continued reinforcement after he leaves the health care system. Long-term psychotherapy can provide this reinforcement and an opportunity to learn to gain true fulfillment of needs. Family therapy can help the entire family learn constructive communication patterns.

✄ *Spiritual dimension.* The nurse remains constantly aware of her own values and judgments and of how they affect her perceptions of the client. Even if the client is involved in activities that are illegal or outside social norms and values, objectivity remains necessary.

Some clients may ask to include clergy in their care just to have another person to manipulate. However, some clients may appear insincere in requesting religious support to cover their vulnerability and maintain control. Regardless of the perceived rationale, the client's requests for religious assistance are supported. If the client involves a consistent religious representative, such as a hospital chaplain, in his case, this person is to be regarded as a part of the treatment team. The plan of care can be shared to keep channels of communication open and to maintain consistency in limits and expectations.

INTERACTION WITH A MANIPULATIVE CLIENT

Client: I want my medication at 9:30 AM. Any earlier than that is inhumane! You nurses are all worthless idiots anyway. Call my doctor. I'm leaving right now!

Nurse: John, it sounds like it has really been difficult for you to be in the hospital and on a hospital routine. I can discuss changing your medication time with your primary nurse and doctor.

Client: What's the matter? Can't you make a decision on your own? Or are you too new?

Nurse: A decision like this involves all of us. It is important that we make it together and then stick to it.

Client: Well, that could take time. When you're here, you can accommodate me. You're the nicest one, you know. You seem to understand more than those others.

Nurse: It sounds like its difficult for you to work with a team of people. But we will meet and try to work it out.

Client: Please, do it for me just this one time. I promise I won't tell.

Nurse: The unit policy is that medications are given within 30 minutes of when they are ordered. But we will discuss it as a team with your doctor.

John attempted to manipulate the nurse several times. First, he attempts to change her behavior through his anger. The nurse avoids responding to the affect (anger) and the personal insults by responding to the process of the interaction (John's difficulty with being on a hospital schedule). She also avoids a power struggle and remains objective by offering to discuss the client's request with the appropriate team members. John again attempts to manipulate by first trying to make her feel insecure, then special. The nurse avoids manipulation by responding to his difficulty with the hospital routine (a control issue) and consistently offering the same solution. The nurse reinforces the limit in an impersonal manner in her last statement. The unit policy sets the limits, not herself; she therefore avoids being the focus of John's anger and power issues. The nurse also reinforces her proposed solution consistently. The consistent and depersonalized limits set by the nurse will reinforce a mature communication pattern and maintain the necessary consistency among the health care team. If this pattern is reinforced, John can learn that his needs are met when appropriate, without the use of manipulative techniques.

Evaluation

The evaluation of a change in a client's manipulative behaviors is based on the client's actions, not on his verbalizations. Promises and plans to change are respected; however, they are not true indicators of change in the manipulative client. Regression to former behaviors can be expected and is not evaluated as a failure.

The nurse can base an evaluation on small changes in a client's behaviors; more obvious, long-term changes will most likely only result from long-term therapy. The nurse also evaluates her own expectations of the client and the reality and dynamics of these expectations. The prognosis for the client diagnosed with an antisocial personality disorder is often poor, and little change is expected. In such a case constructive role modeling of mature interacting by the staff can be considered a success. All evaluations are based on the long-term goal of promoting learning through role modeling constructive, mature behavior. With this the client is given the opportunity to learn and grow; change is supported as it occurs.

The evaluation of the manipulative client's care can be divided into four areas to ensure a thorough and objective review.

Adequacy

Was the client's behavior assessed objectively, or was he labeled negatively?

Did the behavior meet the criteria for destructive manipulation, or was it a regression because of stress?

Was a distinction made among aggressive, assertive, and manipulative behavior?

Did the treatment plan encourage client learning?

Was communication and limit setting clear and consistent, or was the cycle of manipulative behavior reinforced through inconsistency and staff anger?

Appropriateness

Were consistent limits and plans established early and communicated to the entire health care team?

Were interventions objective and punitive responses avoided?

Were the client's needs considered and met when possible?

Was the process of the client's interactions, not just content, addressed?

Effectiveness

Did the client demonstrate any behavioral change?

Was the client able to identify a need for continued learning and support?

Was the client able to identify manipulative communication patterns when his anxiety was low?

Were basic needs fulfilled by a supportive staff?

Efficiency

Did the health care team experience open, clear communication?

Did they support each other during the client's manipulative attempts?

Was the health care team able to identify the dynamics involved in interactions with the client and with each other?

Were limits and expectations consistently maintained by the entire team?

Was the manipulative behavior identified early?

Was information shared with all persons involved with the client?

Has the health care team learned and grown from working with this client?

NURSING PROCESS SUMMARY: MANIPULATION

ASSESSMENT

Physical Dimension
  Manipulates to meet physical needs
  False expression of physical needs
Emotional Dimension
  Constructive manipulation
  Increased anxiety
  Regression to maladaptive coping patterns
  Inaccurate (exaggerated or hidden) expressions of physical needs
  Destructive manipulation
  Exhilaration at successful manipulation
  Emotional insincerity
  Anger and frustration
Intellectual Dimension
  Awareness of behavior
  Denial of behavior
    Deception
  Externalizes blame
  Conflict between perceived needs and others' needs
  Resistance to rules and limits
  Excessive flattery or complaining
  Excessive name dropping
  Excessive use of medical jargon
  Perceives threat to security
Social Dimension
  Multiple demands
  Threatens
  Requests special considerations
  Plays members of health care team against each other
  Stalls
  Helplessness
  Tearfulness
  Self-pity
  Lack of social support network

Lack of sincere relationship with significant other(s)
Inconsistent job history
Repeated perception of himself as a victim
Staff disruption
Involves several persons in case (administrators, representatives, lawyers)
Spiritual Dimension
  Overdependence on religion
  Use of religion as an excuse
  Low life satisfaction
  Low self-fulfillment

ANALYSIS
See the nursing diagnoses on p. 421.

PLANNING AND IMPLEMENTATION
Physical Dimension
  Ensure basic needs are met while holding client responsible for his behavior.
Emotional Dimension
  Discuss client's perception of his anxiety.
  Explore patterns of coping with anxiety.
  Set appropriate, client-centered limits.
  Respond to the process of the behavior.
Intellectual Dimension
  Allow client to assume as much control as possible.
  Channel all requests to primary nurse.
  Maintain confidentiality in the health care system.
  Role model constructive communication.
  Explore the meaning of behaviors with client.
  Explore past ineffective interaction and failure to learn.
Social Dimension
  Respond consistently to testing of behaviors.
  Explore client's reactions to being manipulated.

NURSING PROCESS SUMMARY: MANIPULATION—cont'd

Explore past patterns of interaction.
Encourage client to try out new communication techniques.
Support client's strengths.
Reinforce new constructive behaviors.
Encourage client to seek long-term psychotherapy.

Spiritual Dimension

Support client's requests for religious assistance.
Involve clergy in the treatment team.

EVALUATION

The client's progress toward achieving the nursing care goals is evident when he demonstrates awareness of ways his manipulative behavior is expressed and situations that motivate him to use manipulation. There is improvement in his behavior when he assumes responsibility for asking directly for his needs to be met, verbalizes positive ideas about himself, and develops interpersonal relationships without using manipulation.

BRIEF REVIEW

An infant learns manipulative behavior to ensure that basic needs are met. Usually, as a child grows, manipulative behaviors are replaced with actualized behaviors. To some extent, all individuals continue to use some degree of constructive or destructive manipulation. A child who receives inconsistent and conditional love often learns maladaptive relating and coping patterns and continues to manipulate to fulfill his needs. An individual falls into a manipulative cycle when needs are not met and anxiety increases because of negative past experiences. He disregards the needs of others and begins to manipulate to fulfill his needs. When the individual's attempts are successful, the behavior is reinforced. When the attempt is unsuccessful, he feels increased anxiety and frustration, often manifested as anger and hostility toward the persons who are perceived as failing him. This reaction leads to further attempts to manipulate to decrease the anxiety.

Destructive manipulative behaviors are often associated with the DSM-III-R diagnostic category of antisocial personality disorder. A client with this diagnosis may come into contact with the health care system for a number of related reasons. The long-term goal of the nurse is to role model constructive, actualized patterns of interpersonal behavior to help the client change his behavior. This may result in an initial behavioral change, and the client is encouraged to pursue long-term change through long-term therapy.

Anger and frustration are common health care team reactions to manipulative behaviors. Open communication and consistency are essential for the staff to continue working together toward the therapeutic goal of offering constructive role modeling. The early identification of manipulative behavior is integral. The nurse is often the key individual in identifying this behavior and mobilizing the health care team and extended resources to coordinate the client's plan of care. The nurse also plays a key role in helping the client become aware of the available long-term therapeutic modalities. Major changes are rarely seen during short-term contact; however, success can be evaluated on the basis of the health care team's ability to consistently offer constructive role modeling and opportunity for growth.

REFERENCES AND SUGGESTED READINGS

1. American Psychiatric Association: Diagnostic and statistical manual of mental disorders (DSM-III-R), Washington D.C., 1987, The Association.
2. Bursten, B.: The manipulator: a psychoanalytic view, New Haven, Conn., 1973, Yale University Press.
3. Cleckley, H.: The mask of sanity, St. Louis, 1982, The C.V. Mosby Co.
4. Chitty, K.K., and Maynard, C.K.: Managing manipulation, Journal of Psychosocial Nursing and Mental Health Services 24(6):8, 1986.
5. Davidson, G.C., and Neale, J.M.: Abnormal psychology: an experimental clinical approach, ed. 3, New York, 1982, John Wiley & Sons, Inc.
6. Finch, J.: Nurse and mental health law: psychopaths—who are they?, Nursing Mirror 119(4):24, 1984.
7. Groves, J.E.: Taking care of the hateful patient, New England Journal of Medicine 298(16):883, 1978.
8. Hare, R.D.: Psychopathy: theory and research, New York, 1970, John Wiley & Sons, Inc.
9. Hare, R.D., and Schalling, D.: Psychopathic behavior: approaches to research, New York, 1978, John Wiley & Sons, Inc.
10. Hood, M.: New horizons: special units, the psychopathic patient, Nursing Times 81:(12):53, 1985.
11. Holderby, R.A., and McNulty, E.G.: Feelings: how to make a rational response to emotional behavior, Nursing 79 9:39, 1979.
12. Hughes, J.: Manipulation: a negative element in care, Journal of Advanced Nursing 5:21, 1980.
13. Kumler, F.R.: The interpersonal interpretation of manipulation. In Burd, S.F., and Marshall, M.S., editors: Some clinical approaches to psychiatric nursing, New York, 1963, The Macmillan Co.
14. Luetje, V., and Murray R.: The person whose behavior is abusive. In Murray, R., and Huelskoether, M.: Psychiatric mental health nursing: giving emotional care, Englewood Cliffs, N.J., 1983, Prentice-Hall, Inc.
15. Lyon, G.G.: Limit setting as a therapeutic tool. In Backer, B., Dubber, P., Eiseman, E., editors: Psychiatric mental health nursing: contemporary readings, New York, 1978, Van Nostrand Reinhold Co., Inc.
16. MacMillan, J., and Kofued, L.: Sociobiology and antisocial personality: an alternative perspective, Journal of Nervous and Mental Disease 172:701, 1984.
17. McMorrow, M.E.: The manipulative patient, American Journal of Nursing 81:1188, 1981.

18. Murphy, G.E., and Guze, S.B.: Setting limits: the management of the manipulative patient, American Journal of Psychotherapy **14**:30, 1960.

19. Pasquali, E., and others: Mental health nursing: a holistic approach, St. Louis, 1985, The C.V. Mosby Co.

20. Reid, W.H.: The psychopath: a comprehensive study of antisocial disorders and behaviors, New York, 1978, Brunner/Mazel, Inc.

21. Reid, W.H.: The treatment of antisocial syndromes, New York, 1981, Van Nostrand Reinhold Co., Inc.

22. Reid, W.H.: The antisocial personality: a review, Hospital and Community Psychiatry **36**:831, 1985.

23. Richardson, J.I.: The manipulative patient spells trouble, Nursing **11**:48, 1981.

24. Ruesch, J.: Disturbed communication, New York, 1972, W.W. Norton & Co.

25. Schultz, J.M., and Dark, S.L.: Manual of psychiatric nursing care plans, Boston, 1982, Little, Brown & Co.

26. Shostrom, E.: Man the manipulator, Nashville, 1967, Abingdon Press.

27. Smith R.J.: Personality and psychopathy: a series of monographs, texts, and treatises, New York, 1978, Academic Press.

28. Widiger, T.A., and Frances A.: Axis II personality disorders: diagnostic and treatment issues, Hospital and Community Psychiatry **36**:619, 1985.

29. Wiley, P.L.: Manipulation. In Zderad, L.T., and Belchen, H.C., editors: Developing behavioral concepts in nursing, Atlanta, 1968, Southern Regional Education Board.

30. Zamora, L.C.: Anger. In Haber, J., Leach, A.M., Schudy, S.M., and Sideleau, B.F., editors: Comprehensive psychiatric nursing, New York, 1982, McGraw-Hill, Inc.

ANNOTATED BIBLIOGRAPHY

Cleckley, H.: The mask of sanity, St. Louis, 1982, The C.V. Mosby Co.

This book gives a classic description of the sociopath and highlights 16 specific personality traits. Several case examples illustrate these traits. The author discusses the use of the descriptive label *sociopathy* instead of the term *antisocial personality disorder.*

Reid, W.H.: The antisocial personality: a review, Hospital and Community Psychiatry **36**:831, 1985.

This article reviews antisocial personality disorder and discusses the difficulty of identifying and understanding this disorder. Various theories of the pathology of the antisocial personality disorder, from classic theories to the most recent theories, are presented. Epidemiology and treatment are also thoroughly discussed.

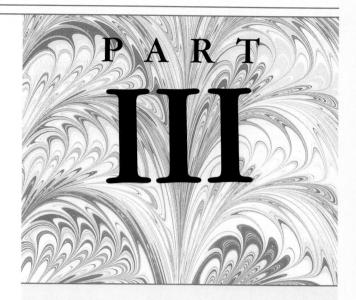

PART III

Therapeutic Modalities

Mental health–psychiatric difficulties may respond to a single treatment modality or a combined regimen. Part III addresses the most frequently used of these treatment modalities. Each chapter lays a foundation for the nurse to develop strategies for maintaining mental health as well as for intervening in psychiatric illnesses. Following a general introduction, selected theoretical approaches are discussed for each treatment modality. Specific characteristics of each type of therapy are presented. In addition, the psychiatric nurse's role, goals for therapy, and qualifications for practice are described. Each chapter concludes with an application of the five-step nursing process.

Part III begins with a discussion of psychotropic drugs (Chapter 22) and other types of somatic therapies (Chapter 23) that are vital aspects of the psychiatric nurse's responsibilities. Milieu therapy is presented in Chapter 24. Chapter 25, Community Mental Health, applies the nursing process to the community and to major community mental health problems. Chapters 26 and 27 cover the use of therapy identifiable by its length: crisis intervention and short-term psychotherapy. The focus of Chapter 28 is group therapy, one of the predominant types of therapy for clients of all age groups. Building on the foundations established in group therapy, the treatment modalities of family therapy, marital therapy, and sex therapy are described in Chapters 29, 30, and 31. Therapy directed toward the mental health–psychiatric nurse's role in chronic psychiatric illnesses, organic mental syndromes, psychophysiological illnesses, eating disorders, abuse situations, and dying are explored in Chapters 32 to 37. Chapter 38 considers nontraditional treatment approaches for maintaining a state of health.

C H A P T E R

22

PSYCHOTROPIC MEDICATIONS

Virginia Burke Karb   Richard E. Stull

Charlene Uthoff Bradham   Michael Roark

After studying this chapter the learner will be able to:

Define the five major classifications of psychotropic medications.

Trace the historical development of the use of psychotropic medications.

Discuss indications, usual dosage, common side effects, and nursing implications of psychotropic medications.

Describe psychotropic medication interactions with foods and other drugs.

Discuss tolerance and physical dependence.

Discuss the medication compliance problem.

A *psychotropic medication* is any medication that alters the mind. The major categories of psychotropic medications are the *antipsychotic agents, antianxiety agents, antidepressant agents* and *antimanic agents. Antiparkinson* medications are also discussed here because they lessen the side effects of many of the antipsychotics. Although these medications calm agitated, excited, and hyperactive clients, they are more than sedatives or tranquilizers; the term *tranquilizer* is a misnomer and is not used today.

Medications are used with other therapies to treat psychiatric problems. Medications can control violent, dangerous, or destructive behavior, improve the client's subjective feelings, shorten inpatient treatment times, and hasten the recovery of some clients. With medications, many clients who once required inpatient treatment can be treated at home, in the physician's office, or at the community mental health center.

As the use of psychotropic medications grows, so does the awareness that many of the agents can be abused, attract those using illegal drugs, and be addictive. Research continues to search for the ideal psychotropic medications: those that alleviate symptoms, produce no side effects, have low abuse potential, do not cause dependence or addiction, are inexpensive, and do not interact with other medications.

NURSING PROCESS
Assessment and Analysis

When psychotropic medications are prescribed, the nurse returns to the database to make sure that necessary baseline data have not been omitted from the assessment. For example, certain laboratory tests not needed for all clients may be needed for clients receiving specific medications. The nurse also obtains information on previous use of the prescribed agent and the client's response to it; known allergies; and other medications used by the client, especially over-the-counter prescriptions, birth control pills, and illegal drugs. The client's reliability may be an important factor when considering self-medication.

Planning

The nurse works with the client and family to establish realistic therapeutic goals based on knowledge of the client and the medications. For example, the nurse may determine the times of day that the client takes the medication after considering his usual schedule, mealtimes, and use of other medications. The nurse also plans how to monitor for desired effects and side effects. If a prescribed drug is known to contribute to weight gain, for example, the plan may include regular weighing and exercising.

🌿 *Historical Overview* 🌿

DATE	EVENT
Pre-1800	Before the development of psychotropic medications, psychiatric care was limited to custodial care. Clients were committed to asylums where restraint or seclusion were the only methods to control behavior.
	In India natural products such as powdered root of Rauwolfia serpentina, a component of reserpine, were found effective in changing behavior.
1800s	The bromide salt of lithium was used to treat gout and as a sedative and anticonvulsant. Its toxic effects prevented its use as a treatment for mania in the United States until early 1970.
1950s	Chlorpromazine was synthesized as an antihistamine in France by Charpentier and later was used to treat psychomotor excitement and mania.
	Clinical studies of antitubercular agents led to the discovery that isoniazid and iproniazid were effective in diminishing depression and associated symptoms in psychotic clients.
1959	Librium was introduced in the United States.
1980s	Today there is a changing awareness among physicians of the role of medications in psychiatric care, with emphasis on research rather than anecdotal notes. It is no longer assumed that clients must tolerate uncomfortable side effects; within limits, medications, dosages, and schedules can be altered based on the client's response. Clients are encouraged to be knowledgeable about their medications.
Future	Because *noncompliance* with medication is commonly associated with psychiatric clients, nurses are challenged to identify factors that contribute to noncompliance, to predict those at risk for noncompliance and to initiate interventions that foster compliance.

Implementation

The nurse teaches the client in detail about the medications, desired effects, side effects, and symptoms that should prompt the client or family to contact the health care team. Unfortunately, many clients still get much of their information on medications from other clients or the media (see the Research Highlight).

Evaluation

In most cases one goal of therapy is to enable the client to return to the community, responsible for self-medication. The nurse needs to determine the following:

1. Are the medications having the desired effects? What data support this?
2. Are side effects occurring? If so, are they tolerable?
3. Is the plan complete and appropriate for the client?
4. How does the client feel about the effects of the medications? Are the client's expectations about the results being met?
5. How do family members feel? Are their expectations being met?
6. If side effects cannot be eliminated, can they be controlled or treated, or can the client learn to live with them? Which ones can (or cannot) the client live with?
7. If the medications are not effective or produce side

effects requiring discontinuance of the agent(s), how does the client feel about it?
8. Is the client reliable and informed enough to be discharged for self-medication? If not, what alternative plans can be made?
9. Does the client have the finances to purchase the medication when going from inpatient to outpatient care?

General guidelines for teaching clients about psychotropic medications are found in the box on p. 434.

Special Nursing Considerations

The effects of psychotropic medications. The client's age can affect his response to psychotropic medications. In the elderly, medications that cause dry mouth (antidepressants and antipsychotics) can be particularly troublesome, because saliva production decreases with age. Constipation may alter medication excretion and contribute to use and sometimes abuse of laxatives and enemas, which in turn contributes to dehydration and electrolyte imbalances. As body fat increases, the action of medications stored there is lessened in intensity but prolonged.[18] Reduced renal function can contribute to medication toxicity at lower doses. Reduced vision and hearing may contribute to misunderstandings about medications and doses.

Research Highlight

Client Perception of Role in Psychotropic Drug Management

S.H. Durel & B.A. Munjas

PURPOSE

This study was designed to investigate whether community mental health center (CMHC) clients perceived their role as medication consumer as active or passive and whether they had enough knowledge to assume an active role. The literature suggested that medication efficacy and client safety are contingent on the client's ability to be an active participant in the health care plan.

SAMPLE

Forty-six clients were chosen randomly from a CMHC. Data were collected using a cross-sectional exploratory survey. All subjects had received psychotropic medications for at least 6 months.

METHODOLOGY

Data were collected through individual interviews using two investigator-developed instruments. The Medication Consumer Scale (MCS), a 28-item scale, measured congruency of clients' perception with prescribed role. The Medication Questionnaire (MED Q), a structured interview, assessed clients' knowledge of their medications.

FINDINGS

Findings indicated that clients did not understand the general effects of their medications and that they were passive medication consumers. There was evidence of client readiness to assume a more active role. Three factors contributed to the client's difficulties: inadequate knowledge of drug effects, perceived powerlessness in making decisions about their health care, and lack of understanding about the relationship between medication treatment of the psyche and general physical health.

Analysis of the MED Q indicated that relying on memory alone, 80% of the clients would be unable to give the name, dosages, and frequency of prescribed drugs. Clients also reported that most of what they knew about their medications came from other clients during hospitalization or the media.

IMPLICATIONS

This research suggests that health care providers need to examine current teaching efforts. Also, health care providers need to lessen the sense of powerlessness that clients feel about their health care management. Finally, the apparent readiness of clients to assume a more active role can be used by nurses to improve client understanding of psychotropic medications.

Based on data from Issues in Mental Health Nursing 4:65, 1982.

The physiological differences and smaller body size of children also affect reactions to psychotropic medications. Cardiac output and blood flow, related to body surface area, result in faster distribution of medications. For these reasons doses for pediatric clients are often determined by ratios of milligram per kilogram of body weight or by the body surface area method.[1] Fortunately, psychotropic medications are usually not needed for young children.

Tolerance, dependence, and withdrawal. *Tolerance* is a state of decreased responsiveness to a medication resulting from prior exposure and usually requires an increased dosage of the medication. When the continuously increased dosage results in a need for the medication for the client to maintain normal functioning, and when abrupt cessation results in the characteristic *withdrawal syndrome,* the condition is called *physical dependence.* Tolerance can occur without physical dependence, but physical dependence without initial tolerance is uncommon. Terms such as *need* and *craving* describe *psychological dependence.* Information on tolerance, dependence, and withdrawal is included in the discussion of each category of medications.

ANTIPSYCHOTIC MEDICATIONS
Uses

The antipsychotic medications often called *neuroleptics,* are used to treat psychoses such as schizophrenia, paranoia, major depressions, and mania. Antipsychotic medications also have antianxiety properties and frequently are prescribed for treatment of severe anxiety. Other conditions treated with antipsychotic medications are intractable hiccups, Huntington's chorea, and Tourette's syndrome (Table 22-1).

Action and Side Effects

Neuroscientists hypothesize that excessive activity of the neurotransmitter dopamine in certain areas of the CNS leads to psychosis. The antipsychotic agents are thought to block dopamine receptors. The action of antipsychotics is believed to occur in the brainstem reticular formation, which may be a site of dopamine receptor blockade. The brainstem reticular formation controls the inflow, integration, and outflow of information through the brain. For example, schizophrenic clients are extremely aware of pe-

PSYCHOTROPIC MEDICATIONS

Guidelines for teaching client use

1. Caution client not to "share" medications.
2. Caution client to keep all health care providers—physicians, nurses, dentists, therapists, pharmacists, chiropractors, and midwives—informed of all medications being taken.
3. Caution client that the dosage of any medication is not to be decreased, increased, or discontinued without the advice of the health care provider.
4. Remind client that unless specifically instructed to do so, he is not to double up or catch up with missed doses. He is to wait until the next dose is due and take only that dose. If in doubt, the client needs to contact a member of the health care team.
5. Remind client to keep all medications out of the reach of children. Child-proof caps need to be used.
6. Emphasize that the client is not to drink alcohol. Most medications discussed in this chapter are central nervous system (CNS) depressants and *cannot* be combined with another CNS depressant.
7. It is often impossible for clients to remember all possible medication interactions; therefore, instruct client to avoid over-the-counter drugs unless permitted by the physician. This includes cold and cough remedies, allergy medication, aspirin, acetaminophen or other pain relievers, antacids, laxatives, and vitamins.
8. Psychotropic medications are usually contraindicated during pregnancy and lactation. Counsel female clients to use birth control while taking any of these medications. If a client suspects she is pregnant, instruct her to consult her physician immediately. If a client wishes to become pregnant while using one or more of these medications, advise her to see her physician first.
9. Discuss common side effects. Because everyone may respond differently to a medication, encourage client to report any unusual sign, symptom, or subjective feeling.
10. Caution outpatients not to keep medicine bottles on the nightstand or in other places where there is a greater likelihood of accidental overdose or repeating a dose in the night. Instruct clients to keep medications in the labeled containers and never to mix different medications in a single container.

Reminders for the administering nurse

1. Question client carefully about history of medication allergy before therapy is begun.
2. Many psychotropic medications are toxic, have high abuse potential, or are frequently used in suicide attempts. Medications are often prescribed in small quantities, requiring the client to return often to have the prescription refilled.
3. Any client may refuse or pretend to take a medication, but this can be a serious problem with psychiatric clients. Missed doses may cause the health care team to increase a dosage or use another medication unnecessarily. A client may be storing doses for a later suicide attempt. Carefully supervise all clients to ascertain that doses have actually been taken.
4. When preparing medications for more than one client at a time, never leave the prepared doses unattended.
5. In an outpatient setting, be alert for clients who are returning with increasing frequency for prescription refills; this may indicate that the medication is being abused or used inappropriately. Carefully assess the client who seems depressed or severely anxious for possible suicidal tendencies.

---

ripheral stimuli but have difficulty sorting out their meanings. Many researchers believe that an important action of antipsychotics is the impairment of the schizophrenic client's ability to respond to peripheral stimuli, while allowing him to respond to direct stimuli.

Alteration of neurotransmission in other areas of the CNS may account for other effects of antipsychotic agents. Dopamine receptor blockade probably leads to endocrine and extrapyramidal side effects. Components of the extrapyramidal system degenerate in Parkinson's disease, and a clinical picture resembling this disease often occurs in clients treated with antipsychotic agents, presumably as a result of dopamine receptors blockade in this area of the CNS. There appears to be a balance of inhibition and excitation in the *extrapyramidal system.* Dopamine is the transmitter for inhibition, acetylcholine for excitation. The blockade of dopamine receptors leads to an excita-tion that may be therapeutically diminished with agents that block acetylcholine receptors (anticholinergic agents). Alteration of this balance may lead to motor dysfunction. Chronic use of antipsychotics may produce such an alteration, perhaps leading to *tardive dyskinesia* or other extrapyramidal side effects (Table 22-2).

The various antipsychotic agents differ primarily in potency and side effects (see Table 22-1). The effectiveness of antipsychotic agents is similar; for ease of comparison, doses of the medications are based on the *chlorpromazine equivalent*—an approximation of the quantity needed to equal the therapeutic effect of 100 mg of chlorpromazine. It does not imply equivalence of adverse effects. Adverse effects of antipsychotic agents are the following:

Anticholinergic effects (blurred vision, constipation, dry mouth, tachycardia)

Increased lactation in women
Gynecomastia in men
Sedation
Orthostatic hypotension
Cholestatic jaundice
Allergic reactions (rashes, dermatitis)
Photosensitivity
Extrapyramidal side effects (described in Table 22-2)

Absorption, Distribution, and Fate

Chlorpromazine (the prototype of the aliphatics) is only partially absorbed from the gastrointestinal tract after oral administration. Peak plasma levels are usually reached in 2 to 4 hours. (Plasma levels are four to 10 times higher after intramuscular injection and are usually reached in 2 to 3 hours.) A significant proportion of the drug is degraded in the intestine, which may account for the diminished absorption when taken orally. Differences in strength, the presence of food in the gastrointestinal tract, and concomitant therapy with drugs such as antacids and antiparkinsonian agents may significantly alter its absorption.

The piperidine group of phenothiazines includes mesoridazine and thioridazine. Side effects within the group are similar (see Table 22-1). Mesoridazine is the only piperidine available in a parenteral (intramuscular) form. Six medications form the piperazine class (see Table 22-1). In addition to their antipsychotic activity, the piperazines have potent antiemetic properties. Blood dyscrasias and jaundice are less likely to occur with this group of drugs.

Fluphenazine is available in two depot forms, fluphenazine decanoate and fluphenazine enanthate. The duration of action is approximately 2 weeks, although in some clients 4 weeks between doses may suffice for maintenance therapy. Depot forms, useful for noncomplying clients, are given by deep intramuscular injection in a large muscle mass, avoiding the deltoid muscle.

Haloperidol, butyrophenone, is readily absorbed when taken orally, reaching peak plasma levels in 3 hours. Peak plasma levels are reached in 1 hour after intramuscular injection. The half-life varies with the route of administration. Haloperidol decanoate is given once a month in a dose approximately 20 times the daily oral maintenance dose.

TABLE 22-1 Antipsychotic medications, dosages, and side effects

Generic and Trade Name	Usual Oral Dosage Range for Adults (mg)	Sedation	Orthostatic Hypotension	Anticholinergic	Extrapyramidal†
PHENOTHIAZINES					
Aliphatic					
Chlorpromazine (Thorazine)	200-1000	+++	++	++/+++	++
Triflupromazine (Vesprin)	50-150	+++	++	++/+++	++/+++
Piperidine					
Mesoridazine (Serentil)	100-400	+++	++	++	+
Thioridazine (Mellaril)	150-800	+++	++	++/+++	+
Piperazine					
Acetophenazine (Tindal)	60-120	++	+	+	+++
Carphenazine (Proketazine)	75-400	++	+	+	+++
Fluphenazine (Prolixin)	1-10	+/++	+	+	+++
Perphenazine (Trilafon)	6-64	+/++	+	+	+++
Prochlorperazine (Compazine)	15-150	++	+	+	+++
Trifluoperazine (Stelazine)	2-10	++	+	+	+++
BUTYROPHENONES					
Haloperidol (Haldol)	2-100	+	+	+	+++
THIOXANTHENES					
Chlorprothixene (Taractan)	75-600	+++	++/+++	++/+++	+/++
Thiothixene (Navane)	6-60	+	+/++	+	++/+++
OTHERS					
Loxapine (Loxitane)	20-250	++	+/++	+/++	++/+++
Molindone (Moban)	15-225	++	+/++	++	++/+++

*Relative potency in producing side effects: +, low; +++, high.
†Excludes tardive dyskinesia, which can be produced to the same degree by all antipsychotic agents.

TABLE 22-2 Extrapyramidal side effects of antipsychotic medications

Side Effect	Signs and Symptoms	Difficulties in Assessment	Comments and Treatment
Acute dystonia	Buccolingual reactions (tongue protrusion, grimacing, trismus), opisthotonos, neck twisting, spastic torticollis, abdominal wall spasm, gait abnormalities, scoliosis, lordosis, kyphosis, abnormal eye movements, *oculogyric crisis* (paroxysm of the eyes, eyes held in a fixed position for minutes to hours); may be accompanied by anxiety, tachycardia, respiratory distress, cyanosis, fever; mentation unchanged	Reactions often acute in onset; have been mistaken for tetanus, hysteria, convulsions, meningitis, stroke, strychnine poisoning	Symptoms are most common after parenteral administration in clients under 25 years of age. Symptoms rarely persist but are distressing to client and onlookers. Acute dystonia may be severe enough in children to cause death.[13] Treatment consists of discontinuing the antipsychotic medication and administering a centrally acting anticholinergic (such as benztropine) or antihistamine (such as diphenhydramine)
Akathisia	Restlessness, difficulty sitting still, agitation, uncontrolled pacing	May mimic dyskinesia; may be mistaken for psychotic agitation, resulting in inappropriate increase in dose of antipsychotic medication	Treatment consists of reducing dose of antipsychotic medication and/or administering anticholinergics and/or a sedative such as diazepam until symptoms are controlled. If adaptation occurs antipsychotics can be administered.
Tardive dyskinesia	Protrusion of the tongue, puffing of cheeks, chewing movements, involuntary movements of the extremities and trunk, choreiform movements manifested as a single muscle jerk or tic; worsens under stress	Client may attempt to mask movements by developing semipurposeful movements in response to jerks; poorly fitting dentures in the elderly may result in facial movements resembling tardive dyskinsia; dyskinesia disappears during sleep; tremors have a to-and-fro component, while dyskinesia does not; postures are sustained in dystonia but not in dyskinesia; in severe cases may resemble Huntington's disease	Symptoms are more common with long-term use (more than 1 year) and in women and the elderly. They may be unmasked by suddenly discontinuing medication. Medication treatment is not satisfactory for most clients. This condition may not be as relentless as once thought. Health care team, with client and family, weigh the potential risks of tardive dyskinesia with psychosis.
Parkinsonism	Tremors, rigidity, motor retardation, excessive salivation, shuffling gait, loss of postural reflexes, masklike expression	May be difficult to differentiate between motor retardation, masklike expression, and apathy of parkinsonism and the affect of a major depression	Treatment consists of anticholinergics or amantadine. Routine prophylactic use of these medications is not recommended.

Medication Interactions

The antipsychotics are used cautiously with other medications that also depress the CNS, such as antianxiety agents and hypnotics, alcohol, narcotics, analgesics, preanesthetic sedatives, and general anesthesia. If possible antipsychotics are discontinued temporarily if the client has spinal or epidural anesthesia. Heavy smokers may require a larger dose of an antipsychotic. If antipsychotics are used with a tricyclic or tetracyclic antidepressant or an anticholinergic, there may be additional *anticholinergic* activity and CNS depression. Antipsychotics may interfere with the action of guanethidine by inhibiting antihypertensive effects.

Overdoses of antipsychotics are seldom fatal in adults.

Children may experience more serious reactions and are treated with immediate gastric lavage.

Dosage

Table 22-1 gives the usual oral dosage ranges of the commonly used phenothiazines.

Contraindications

Antipsychotics are contraindicated in children under 3 years of age, comatose clients, and clients with severe CNS depression, severe hypertensive or hypotensive heart disease, and preexisting bone marrow depression. Clients reporting hypersensitivity to a particular agent do not receive it again. Antipsychotics may alter the seizure threshold and are used cautiously in clients with a history of seizures.

Tolerance, Dependence, and Withdrawal

Some tolerance develops to the sedative, anticholinergic, and hypotensive effects, usually in weeks to months. Little or no tolerance to the antipsychotic action develops. Medication dependence does not occur, but some physiological adaptation occurs. Abrupt withdrawal after prolonged therapy often results in nausea, vomiting, diaphoresis, headache, restlessness, and insomnia. Withdrawal symptoms begin in 2 to 3 days and may persist for up to 2 weeks. Slowly withdrawing the antipsychotic may help.

Nursing Implications

When the psychotic client is hospitalized, the treatment focus is generally on attaining an effective dosage level. The expected results are decreased aggressive, hyperactive behavior and disorganized thought. Possible side effects require close observation, especially when medication is begun.

Weeks or months of treatment may be needed before optimal behavioral changes are seen. The client and family are reassured that early side effects or lack of desired effect is normal. Drowsiness is usually temporary and often diminishes in days to weeks. The client takes regular naps if possible and avoids driving and using hazardous equipment. Side rails and a nightlight are used.

Dry mouth may be alleviated by rinsing frequently with water, practicing good oral hygiene (brushing and flossing), sucking on hard candy (sugar free), and chewing gum. Commercially available saliva substitutes can be used. Lemon and glycerin swabs are drying and irritating and are not used. Dry mouth may contribute to denture irritation of the gums. The nurse questions the client about dry mouth or inspects the mouth regularly. Dry mouth may diminish with time.

Blurred vision is annoying and potentially dangerous. The nurse cautions the client to report this side effect if it occurs and to avoid potentially hazardous activities until it clears.

The client needs to report any difficulty with urination. This problem is more common in those confined to bed and in males with an enlarged prostate gland. The nurse monitors intake and output and encourages an adequate fluid intake (at least 2500 ml per day).

Orthostatic hypotension can be serious. Clients may merely be slightly dizzy when sitting or standing up or may actually faint. The nurse monitors blood pressure regularly when therapy is begun and when the dose is increased. The nurse instructs clients to sit at the edge of the bed with their feet on the floor for a minute before trying to stand, ensures that side rails are used at night, and supervises ambulation. She cautions clients to avoid hot showers and may instruct them to wear elastic support stockings. Orthostatic hypotension usually diminishes in time, but until it does, the potential for injury from falls is serious.

Weight gain can become a problem. The client is weighed before medication therapy begins and regularly during the treatment course. Dietary intake is supervised, and calories may be restricted for some clients. The nurse encourages the client to be active and plans regular exercise.

Extrapyramidal reactions (Table 22-3) can often be diminished by dosage adjustments or changing drugs, but it may be necessary to treat the side effects with additional medications.

Tardive dyskinesia is characterized by irregular movements of the lower facial muscles, jaw, tongue, and extremities, which may disappear during sleep, and vary in severity. As many as 10% to 20% of clients receiving antipsychotics for more than 1 year will have appreciable tardive dyskinesia. It may be aggravated or unmasked by suddenly discontinuing antipsychotics and persist after the medication is stopped. Most clients improve after several months, but some require years.

Tachycardia and electrocardiographic changes can occur. The nurse monitors vital signs regularly and may obtain a baseline electrocardiogram. Clients with preexisting heart disease are at greater risk for cardiovascular effects.

Photosensitivity has been reported with many antipsychotic agents. The nurse cautions clients to limit direct exposure to the sun and to wear a broad-brimmed hat and sunglasses and use non-PABA sunscreen when in the sun. Occasionally in long-term therapy the skin may become yellowish brown, changing later to a grayish purple. Clients and families need to report skin or allergic reactions.

Additional side effects of antipsychotic agents include signs and symptoms of cholestatic jaundice: fever, upper abdominal pain, nausea, jaundiced sclera, and diarrhea. Clients are to report these symptoms. If jaundice is suspected, the nurse withholds the dose and notifies the physician. Agranulocytosis is a rare side effect, with symptoms

TABLE 22-3 Medications for the treatment of extrapyramidal side effects

Generic and Trade Name	Usual Daily Oral Dosage Range for Adults (mg)
Anticholinergics	
Benztropine (Cogentin)	1-8
Biperiden (Akineton)	2-6
Procyclidine (Kemadrin)	6-20
Trihexyphenidyl (Artane)	1-15
Antihistamines	
Diphenhydramine (Benadryl)	75-100
Dopamine-Releasing Agent	
Amantadine (Symmetrel)	100-200

of sore throat, fever, and generalized weakness. Clients report these signs also. The nurse observes clients for blurred vision, increased intraocular pressure, opacities, and photophobia. The physician may obtain baseline ophthalmic examinations before therapy and regularly during therapy. The nurse tactfully and sensitively questions clients about menstrual irregularities, breast engorgement, changes in libido, and impotence.

Many of the oral concentrates will precipitate when mixed with coffee or tea. It helps to mix these forms with juices, soups, puddings, or other diluents suggested by the manufacturer to improve the taste.

Medications for Extrapyramidal Side Effects

Uses. Many antipsychotic agents have extrapyramidal side effects (see Table 22-2), which resemble symptoms of Parkinson's disease. *Drug-induced parkinsonism,* or *pseudoparkinsonism,* is characterized by rigidity, akathisia, tremor, *akinesia,* changes in voice tone, drooling, masklike facial expression, and loss of posture control.

Anticholinergics, antihistamines, and amantadine are used to treat these side effects (see Table 22-3). When medication side effects are treated with another medication, client response is difficult to evaluate. The nurse working with such cases thoughtfully considers the appearance of any new sign or symptom to determine its cause and possible treatment.

Anticholinergics. Anticholinergics are the medications of choice to treat *akathisia,* acute *dystonia,* and parkinsonism. They are not effective against tardive dyskinesia.

Classically, the anticholinergics block secretions, depress the tone of the gastrointestinal tract, dilate pupils, paralyze the eye's ability to accommodate, increase the heart rate, and counteract the toxicity of cholinergic agents. These actions result in dry mouth; blurred vision; photophobia; flushed, dry skin; increased heart rate; constipation; urinary retention; mental confusion and excitement. The mental confusion and excitement can manifest as agitation, disorientation, delirium, paranoid reactions, or hallucinations. Clients with a history of closed angle glaucoma, urinary or intestinal obstruction, or tachycardia are not considered for this treatment.

Anticholinergics are not used prophylactically; they are given only when treatment of extrapyramidal side effects is indicated. Benztropine, intramuscularly or intravenously, is particularly effective in reversing an acute dystonic reaction.

Antihistamines. Some antihistamines are used to treat extrapyramidal side effects because of their anticholinergic-type actions. Antihistamines' side effects are milder than but similar to the anticholinergics. Antihistamines are more likely to produce sedation. Side effects are drowsiness, dizziness, anorexia, nausea, vomiting, euphoria, hypotension, headache, weakness, and tingling of the hands. Like anticholinergics, antihistamines have no effect on tardive dyskinesia.

Antihistamines are well absorbed orally, their action lasts 4 to 6 hours. They are metabolized to inactive compounds by the liver and kidneys. Diphenhydramine, given orally, intramuscularly, or intravenously, can be used to treat acute dystonic reactions. Antihistamines are used only when treatment of extrapyramidal side effects is needed.

Dopamine-releasing agent. Amantadine, an antiviral drug that promotes the release of dopamine from central neurons, is used infrequently to treat extrapyramidal side effects. Studies show that it may be effective in some clients with tardive dyskinesia.[1,4]

Amantadine is absorbed well orally. Because the *half-life* is about 12 hours, it can be given in a single daily dose. Most of the medication is excreted unchanged in the kidneys, so it is given with caution to clients with renal impairment.

Side effects are mood changes, dizziness, nervousness, inability to concentrate, ataxia, slurred speech, insomnia, lethargy, blurred vision, dry mouth, gastrointestinal upset, and rash. Livedo reticularis (a red-blue, netlike discoloration of the skin, which worsens in cold weather) is fairly common, especially in women. It may subside or continue through therapy and will disappear gradually in 2 to 12 weeks after the medication is stopped. Edema of the ankles has also been noted.

Nursing implications. Monitoring the client receiving an antipsychotic and additional medication to treat the side effects can be challenging. It is often difficult to determine if a particular behavior is related to the initial diagnosis or a side effect. Furthermore, some side effects can be caused by two or more medications simultaneously.

ANTIDEPRESSANT MEDICATIONS

There are three major groups of medications used to treat depression—the tricyclic and tetracyclic antidepressants (TCAs), the monoamine oxidases (MAO) inhibitors, and a drug chemically unrelated to the others, trazodone hydrochloride (Table 22-4).

Tricyclic and Tetracyclic Antidepressants

Action and side effects. Most of the TCAs' effects can be attributed to one of three classic pharmacological actions. The agents inhibit the reuptake of norepinephrine, serotonin, or both from the synapse from which they are released after stimulus, thus increasing available monoamine neurotransmitters. TCAs are potent antagonists of certain acetylcholine effects, both in the CNS and the periphery. Furthermore, the tricyclic drugs antagonize certain central effects of histamine. The side effects of TCAs follow:

Anticholinergic effects (flushing, diaphoresis, dry mouth, blurred vision, constipation)

Hemodynamic effects (orthostatic hypotension, tachycardia, electrocardiographic changes)

Increased potential for seizures

In the elderly:

  Aggravation of angle-closure glaucoma

  Urinary retention

  Adynamic ileus

  Confusion

Allergic skin reactions
Photosensitivity
Hematological disorders
Ejaculation problems
Sedation
Tremors
Speech blockage
Anxiety
Insomnia
Increased appetite
Parkinsonism
Tardive dyskinesia

TABLE 22-4 Medications for mood disorders: antidepressants and antimanics

Generic and Trade Names	Adult Outpatient Daily Dose Range During Initial Treatment (mg)	Sedation*	Anticholinergic Symptoms*
TRICYCLICS			
Amitriptyline (Elavil)	75-300	+ + +	+ + +
Amoxapine (Asendin)	75-300	+	+
Desipramine (Pertofrane)	75-200	+	+
Doxepin (Sinequan)	75-300	+ + +	+ + +
Imipramine (Tofranil)	75-300	+ +	+ +
Nortriptyline (Aventyl)	20-100	+ +	+
Protriptyline (Vivactil)	15-60	+	+ +
Trimipramine (Surmontil)	75-300	+ + +	+ +
TETRACYCLIC			
Maprotiline (Ludiomil)	75-300	+ +	+ +
MAO INHIBITORS			
Isocarboxazid (Marplan)	20-30		
Phenelzine (Nardil)	45-90		
Tranylcypromine (Parnate)	20-30		
OTHERS			
Trazodone (Desyrel)	75-600	+ +	+
ANTIMANICS			
Carbamazepine (Tegretol)	600-1600		
Lithium (Eskalith)	600-2100		

*Relative potency in producing side effects: +, low; + + +, high.

Although depression is the main indication for TCAs, other uses exist, such as childhood enuresis and chronic pain management. Less well-documented uses are for the treatment of obsessive-compulsive phobic states, minimal brain damage and hyperactivity in children, and attacks of catalepsy in narcolepsy.

Absorption, distribution, and fate. As a class the TCAs are well absorbed after oral administration. High doses of the compounds, however, may delay their own absorption as a result of a potent anticholinergic effect, which slows gastric motility and therefore absorption from the gastrointestinal tract. TCAs are metabolized by the intestine and liver and slowly eliminated. The plasma half-lives vary from 8 hours for amoxapine to 30 to 60 hours for maprotiline. Because of their long half-lives, any of the currently used TCAs can be administered once a day.

Acute toxicity. TCAs are not addictive and seem to have low abuse potential. Acute toxicity can occur, however, especially when used by depressed clients in suicide attempts. The potentially fatal toxicity is essentially an anticholinergic (atropine-like) poisoning and is alleviated by physostigmine. The symptoms of toxicity follow:

Confusion
Inability to concentrate
Visual hallucinations
Body temperature initially high, then low
Dilated pupils
Hyperactive reflexes
Cardiac effects (tachycardia, bradycardia, dysrhythmias)
Delirium
Seizures
Coma

Medication interactions. TCAs have numerous medication interactions. When TCAs are administered with barbiturates, benzodiazepines, or alcohol, CNS depression is potentiated. They also block the antihypertensive effect of guanethidine or clonidine. TCA effectiveness may be diminished if the client is a heavy smoker or barbiturates are given concurrently. When combined with MAO inhibitors, TCAs can contribute to *hypertensive crisis,* high fever, or both. TCAs with anticholinergics can potentiate anticholinergic effects; with sympathomimetics, they can potentiate sympathomimetic effects.

Dosage. Therapy generally starts with a low dosage (50 to 75 mg of amitriptyline per day), which is increased every 2 to 3 days by 25 mg until the usual adult dosage of 150 mg (amitriptyline equivalent) is reached. Unresponsive clients may require up to 300 mg per day or more; however, dose-limiting side effects, such as sedation and orthostatic hypotension, may halt dosage increase at relatively low levels (75 mg per day).

Response to TCAs usually occurs in 7 to 10 days, beginning with improved sleep, appetite, and occasionally elevated mood. However, full therapeutic response may require 3 to 4 weeks or longer. The *initial treatment period* is defined as the 4 to 8 weeks of therapy needed until the client becomes nearly symptom free. Most clients require therapy for at least 4 to 6 months. Gradual tapering of dosage is recommended at the end of therapy, allowing the physician as much as a month to slowly reduce the dosage to 25 to 50 mg per day before discontinuing the drug entirely. Abrupt cessation may produce withdrawal symptoms of headache, malaise, anorexia, and fatigue.

Monoamine Oxidase Inhibitors

Action and side effects. The exact mechanism of MAO inhibitors' antidepressant effect is unknown. MAO is an enzyme involved in the metabolism of seratonin and catecholamine neurotransmitters such as epinephrine, norepinephrine, and dopamine. Reduced MAO activity increases concentration of these neurotransmitters in the CNS, which is thought to be the antidepressant mechanism.

Although MAO inhibitors have been used to treat depression longer than TCAs, they are used only in a small percentage of clients. Side effects and interactions with food have limited their usefulness more than lack of effectiveness.

The major side effect is the hypertensive crisis caused by eating foods that contain a high concentration of *tyramine.* Symptoms generally are high blood pressure, headache, nausea, vomiting, stiff neck, muscle twitching, chills, and diaphoresis with pallor. Cerebral hemorrhage and death may result. The nurse instructs the client and family not to eat foods that contain tyramine (see the box below).

MAO inhibitors lower blood pressure and have been used as antihypertensives. Like TCAs, MAO inhibitors can cause dry mouth, constipation, urinary retention, skin

---

EXAMPLE OF A TYRAMINE-RESTRICTED DIET

GENERAL DIRECTIONS

1. Designed for clients on monoamine oxidase (MAO) inhibitors, medications reported to cause hypertensive crises when used with tyramine-rich foods include foods in which aging, protein breakdown, and putrefaction are used to increase flavor. Studies indicate that as little as 5 to 6 mg tyramine can produce a response, and 25 mg is a danger dose.

2. Food sources of other pressor amines such as histamine, dihydroxyphenylalanine, and hydroxytyramine are also avoided.
3. Avoid all foods listed. Limited amounts of foods with a lower tyramine amount such as yeast bread may be included in a specific diet.
4. Avoid over-the-counter medications such as decongestants, cold remedies, and antihistamines.

FOODS TO AVOID (REPRESENTATIVE TYRAMINE VALUES IN μG/G OR ML)

Cheeses
N.Y. State Cheddar	1416
Gruyère	516
Stilton	466
Emmentaler	225
Brie	180
Camembert	86
Processed American	50

Wines
Chianti	25.4
Sherry	3.6
Riesling	0.6
Sauterne	0.4

Beer, ale
Varies with brand
Highest	4.4
Average	2.3
Least	1.8

ADDITIONAL FOODS TO AVOID

Other aged cheeses
  Blue
  Boursault
  Brick
  Cheddars (other)
  Gouda
  Mozzarella
  Parmesan
  Provolone
  Romano
  Roquefort
Yeast and products made with yeast
  Homemade bread
  Yeast extracts such as soup cubes, canned meats, and marmite
Italian broad beans with pod (fava beans)
Meat
  Aged game
  Liver
  Canned meats with yeast extracts
Fish (salted dried)
  Herring, cod, capelin
  Pickled herring
Other
  Cream, especially sour
  Yogurt
  Soy sauce, vanilla, chocolate
  Salad dressings

From Williams, S.R.: Essentials of nutrition and diet therapy, ed. 4, St. Louis, 1986, The C.V. Mosby Co.

rashes, hypotension and tachycardia, and increased intra-ocular pressure.

Medication interactions. MAO inhibitors are not combined with TCAs; sympathomimetics, including over-the-counter cough and cold preparations; alcohol; amphetamines; narcotic analgesics; barbiturates; or anesthetics. During a medication change or before surgery, MAO inhibitors are withheld for 7 days.

Other Antidepressants

Trazodone (Desyrel) is chemically unrelated to TCAs and has no MAO-inhibiting properties. Onset of action is 3 to 7 days, with optimal effect noted in about 6 weeks. Readily absorbed orally, the time to peak effect is about 2½ hours in nonfasting individuals; the manufacturer recommends it be taken with food to decrease side effects of dizziness and lightheadedness. It is metabolized in the liver; two thirds is excreted in the urine, one third in the feces. The mean half-life is about 5 hours.

Trazodone is well tolerated. The most common side effect is drowsiness; anticholinergic effects and cardiac effects (tachycardia, hypotension, and palpitations) are rare.

Nursing Implications

The nurse needs to work closely with the client and family when antidepressants are prescribed. Many side effects encountered early in treatment diminish in days to weeks. As the client begins to improve, the nurse observes for suicidal tendencies. The client who feels better may develop the emotional energy to plan suicide.

Drowsiness is usually temporary and often diminishes as the client develops tolerance to the medication. The client is cautioned against driving or operating hazardous equipment. Daily naps may be appropriate. It may also be possible to change the time of medication administration to bedtime. Side rails are kept up at night, and a nightlight is provided. The nurse cautions the client to avoid other medications that also produce drowsiness, such as cold remedies, alcohol, sleep medications, and other prescription drugs. Blurred vision may also occur; the client needs to report this symptom when it appears.

Anticholinergic side effects are treated symptomatically. Constipation can be alleviated by increasing daily fluid intake to at least 2500 ml and dietary intake of high-fiver and other foods known to stimulate defecation and regularly exercising. Clients need to avoid excessive caffeine. Occasionally, especially in the elderly, adynamic ileus has been reported. The client who complains of constipation and abdominal pain is assessed for bowel sounds.

Weight gain may result from an actual medication effect or a general improved sense of well-being and increased appetite. A calorie-restricted diet may be needed. Clients are taught about well-balanced diets, with a focus on decreasing unnecessary high-calorie food items. Daily exercise may also help.

Orthostatic hypotension can be serious because of the potential for injury. The nurse monitors blood pressure regularly during medication therapy.

Tachycardia and other cardiovascular effects can occur, especially in the elderly and those with a history of cardiovascular disease. The nurse monitors clients for changes in heart rate or rhythm.

Confusion, urinary retention, and aggravation of angle-closure glaucoma can also occur, especially in the elderly. Before therapy begins the nurse obtains a careful history of glaucoma. Antidepressants are used cautiously. The nurse monitors urinary intake and output and instructs the client to report any difficulty urinating. If urinary retention occurs, it may be necessary to catheterize the client.

The nurse also carefully assesses confusion, especially in the elderly, and never automatically attributes it to the natural aging process. Nursing measures for the confused client include reorienting him to the environment, keeping staff assignments consistent and the environment well-lit, and accompanying him when ambulating.

Sexual dysfunction commonly occurs with use of antidepressants, resulting in delayed, inhibited or retrograde ejaculation and impotence. The nurse is particularly sensitive in assessing sexual problems, as clients are often reluctant to discuss them, and is aware that clients may stop taking their medication because of this adverse effect. In some cases sexual problems are due to the specific medication or dose prescribed, and a change in either or both may alleviate the problem. However, it may be necessary to help others accept this side effect. Nurses who are comfortable with sex counseling may be able to suggest alternative ways for the client to achieve sexual gratification. Selected clients may be referred to qualified sex therapists for additional help.

The nurse informs clients receiving MAO inhibitors of the hazards of food with a high tyramine content. Symptoms of tyramine-induced hypertensive crisis are headache, hypertension, tachycardia, palpitations, nausea, and vomiting. Since this can be life threatening, clients need to seek medical help immediately. Phentolamine, propranolol, or parenteral chlorpromazine are given to counteract the hypertensive crisis.

Changes in blood glucose have been reported. The nurse cautions diabetic clients to monitor their urine sugar carefully. The nurse also monitors the client's blood glucose. A change in diet or dose of insulin may be necessary.

A variety of other side effects are rare. Unexplained bleeding or excessive bruising may be symptoms of thrombocytopenia. Jaundice, abdominal pain, or change in stool color may indicate liver dysfunction. Photosensitivity may occur. Fever, chills, malaise, and a sore throat may be symptoms of agranulocytosis and need to be reported.

Antidepressants can lower the seizure threshold; clients with a history of seizures are cautioned. Fine tremor and ataxia, if they persist, may necessitate a change in medication or dosage. A variety of other side effects may also occur, including anxiety, restlessness, hypomania, and psychotic behavior. If any unexpected behavior appears, the nurse notifies the physician, who may change the medication or dosage.

ANTIMANIC MEDICATIONS
Uses

Lithium is the medication of choice to treat mania and bipolar disorders. Approximately 80% of clients treated with lithium respond. When lithium is ineffective, carbamazepine may be used (see Table 22-4).

Lithium

Action and side effects. Lithium abolishes the excitement, euphoria, and insomnia of mania without causing sedation. It produces many neurochemiocal changes in the CNS, which may be related to its interaction with the distribution of sodium and potassium across the cell membrane. Unlike other psychotropic medications, side effects are closely associated with serum levels. The nurse monitors serum levels frequently at first, monthly once the maintenance dose is reached, and finally quarterly. Table 22-5 lists the side effects commonly seen at various serum concentrations of lithium. In prolonged treatment the following side effects may occur:

Thyroid enlargement or hypothyroidism
Polyuria
Polydipsia
Transient hyperglycemia
Headache
Peripheral edema
Weight gain
Hair loss
Metallic taste
Rashes, skin reactions
Increases in white blood cell count
Electrocardiographic changes

Lithium is excreted in the kidney and may produce irreversible renal changes. Therefore it is used cautiously in clients with compromised kidney function, in those requiring fluid restrictions, and in the elderly. Clients with sodium deficiency or receiving diuretics may be predisposed to renal toxicity to lithium. It is therefore used cautiously in clients with cardiovascular or renal disease, the dehydrated, or those receiving diuretics.

Absorption, distribution, and fate. Lithium is readily absorbed from the entire gastrointestinal tract, with plasma levels reaching a maximum in 1 to 3 hours. The compound is excreted by the kidneys and has a half-life of 17 to 36 hours in normal sodium concentrations. When plasma sodium levels are low, lithium is much less effectively cleared from the body, and toxicity can result. Therapeutically effective plasma levels of lithium lie between 0.9 and 1.4 mEq/L of plasma. Serious toxicity can result from plasma levels above 2 mEq/L.

Tremor and nausea have been associated with the rapid absorption of lithium. Absorption can be slowed by using a sustained-release formula, which produces peak plasma levels in 4 to 6 hours, compared with 1 to 2 hours for the regular formula.

Medication interactions. Concurrent use of lithium and iodine is avoided. The nurse cautions clients to avoid preparations containing iodides (such as cough medicines and multivitamins). Indomethacin and phenylbutazone elevate serum lithium levels. It is important to observe for changes in serum lithium levels when these or other nonsteroidal antiinflammatory medications are given with lithium.

Acute toxicity. There is no specific antidote for lithium poisoning. When frank toxicity occurs or plasma levels exceed 2 mEq/L, the medication is discontinued and fluid and electrolyte replacement initiated.

Dosage. Lithium dosage is guided by plasma levels. During initiation of lithium therapy in an acute manic episode, dosage is usually aimed at a plasma level near 1.2 mEq/L, which generally requires 600 to 2100 mg of lithium carbonate per day. Maintenance dosage is usually lowered to 900 to 1200 mg per day to obtain plasma levels of 0.6 to 1 mEq/L 8 to 12 hours after the last dose of lithium. Clients occasionally cannot tolerate this amount and are maintained on lower dosages (see Table 22-4). Not all clients are candidates for lithium therapy because of coexisting illnesses. A "prelithium workup" establishes normal parameters to monitor during therapy (Table 22-6).

Lithium is used with caution in pregnant or lactating women. Congenital abnormalities can result from the use of lithium; it is generally avoided at least during the first trimester. Lithium is excreted in breast milk, so women are not encouraged to breast feed.

TABLE 22-5 Serum lithium levels and side effects

Blood Level (mEq/L)	Symptoms
Below 1	Nausea
	Diarrhea
	Malaise
	Fine hand tremor
1-2	Drowsiness
	Vomiting
	Abdominal pain
	Lethargy
	Dizziness
	Slurred speech
	Nystagmus
	Confusion
	Ataxia
2-2.5	Anorexia
	Persistent nausea and vomiting
	Blurred vision
	Fasciculations
	Clonic, choreiform, and athetoid movements
	Seizures and electroencephalographic changes
	Syncope
	Acute circulatory failure
	Stupor
	Coma
Above 2.5	Generalized convulsion
	Oliguria
	Death

Nursing implications. Ten days to several weeks may be needed to obtain a serum level between 0.9 and 1.4 mEq/L. Adverse reactions of gastrointestinal irritation, tremors, muscle weakness, tinnitus, vertigo, weight gain, thirst, and polyuria may occur. Many clients develop tolerance and may be symptom free within a week. The nurse stresses to client and family the importance of returning to have serum levels measured and explains the signs of lithium toxicity (see Table 22-5). Clients also need to learn that it is the persistent blood level of the lithium that produces the desired result and that they are not to discontinue it when they feel better or take it only "as needed."

Clients are weighed before therapy. Excessive weight gain or edematous swelling of wrists and ankles can occur. A weekly weight record kept by the client is helpful. The nurse watches for edema and if necessary measures the client's wrists and ankles regularly. She also monitors blood pressure regularly. If weight gain is excessive or troublesome to the client, and it is not due to fluid retention, the nurse may consider a calorie-restricted diet and daily exercise. She may also discuss the health risks of weight gain.

Lithium is not contraindicated in diabetic clients, but it may increase the serum insulin level. The drug may also cause polydipsia and polyuria. Monitoring the serum and urine glucose levels and serum electrolyte levels may help to avoid additional problems.

Because lithium may accumulate to toxic levels in the kidney in the presence of dehydration or electrolyte depletion, the nurse emphasizes to the client the need to seek medical attention for prolonged diarrhea or vomiting and to avoid activities that cause excessive sweating. The importance of an adequate fluid intake (approximately 2500 ml per day) is stressed. Any signs of alteration in kidney function—fluid retention, unexplained weight gain, new signs of lithium toxicity, polyuria, or nocturia—are noted. Monitoring weight, intake and output, serum electrolytes, urinalysis, blood urea nitrogen, creatinine clearance, and blood pressure helps avoid problems.

Some clients find persistent hand tremors embarrassing. The client may need to decrease caffeine consumption or, on physician's approval, take most of the daily dose at bedtime or slightly reduce the dose.

Metallic taste may be a nuisance but is not serious. Taking lithium with meals may lessen nausea (ideally clients take their dose(s) at approximately the same time each day).

Lithium is available from several manufacturers and has several similar-sounding brand names. Some forms, however, are sustained-release forms, and cannot be substituted for more rapidly absorbed forms without the physician's approval. Clients are taught to take only the lithium preparation prescribed.

ANTIANXIETY MEDICATIONS

Currently antianxiety medications are widely used to reduce anxiety. The major category of antianxiety agents is the *benzodiazepines.* Two nonbenzodiazepines, hydroxyzine and meprobamate, are used also.

Uses

Antianxiety, or *anxiolytic,* medications are used primarily to diminish anxiety. Benzodiazepines are also used in acute alcohol withdrawal and impending delirium tremens. In larger doses benzodiazepines produce sedation and are potent anticonvulsant agents. One benzodiazepine, flurazepam, is used to induce sleep and not to treat anxiety. Intravenous diazepam is the drug of choice to treat *status epilepticus.* Benzodiazepines also decrease muscle tone.

Benzodiazepines

Action and side effects. In general benzodiazepines act as CNS depressants. They are believed to enhance or facilitate the inhibitory neurotransmitter action of gamma-aminobutyric acid (GABA), which mediates both pre- and postsynaptic inhibition in all areas of the CNS. Since GABA is inhibitory, receptor stimulation increases inhibition and blocks both cortical and limbic arousal.

The most common side effects are listed below:

Sedation	Tremor
Hangover	Urinary incontinence
Ataxia	Constipation
Dizziness	Fatigue
Blurred vision	Dysarthria
Diplopia	Muscle weakness
Hypotension	Dry mouth
Amnesia	Nausea
Slurred speech	Vomiting

Respiratory distress, apnea, and cardiac arrest have been reported, but usually only after intravenous admin-

TABLE 22-6 Prelithium workup

Sample	Specific Test
Blood	Hemoglobin
	White cell count
	Sodium
	Potassium
	Urea
	Creatinine (24-hour clearance preferred)
	Thyroid function (T_4, T_3, free thyroxin index, thyroid-stimulating hormone)
Urine	Complete qualitative urinalysis
Other	Electrocardiogram
	Weight
	Blood pressure
	Pregnancy (when in doubt)

Modified from Johnson, F.N., editor: Handbook of lithium therapy, Baltimore, 1980, University Park Press.

istration. Only three benzodiazepines have parenteral forms: chlordiazepoxide, diazepam, and lorazepam.

Absorption, distribution, and fate. All benzodiazepines except prazepam and oxazepam are absorbed rapidly after given orally, reaching peak plasma concentration in 1 to 3 hours. Prazepam and oxazepam are slower in reaching peak plasma concentration; prazepam, the slowest, requires up to 6 hours. Most benzodiazepines have prolonged duration of effects and are slowly eliminated.

Benzodiazepines are transformed in the liver; rates and patterns vary considerably among healthy and sick clients. Some benzodiazepines are broken down to two or more active metabolites. When metabolites are active, biotransformation extends the half-life (Table 22-7). Benzodiazepines accumulate until a steady state is reached in days to weeks. Clients on long-term therapy are evaluated carefully for weeks after therapy is begun, because medications with long half-lives may accumulate excessively.

Medication interactions. Additive sedation may occur when benzodiazepines are given with other CNS depressants, including other antianxiety or hypnotic medications, alcohol, TCAs, narcotic analgesics, antipsychotics, antihistamines, and over-the-counter sleep and cold medications. Benzodiazepines with *active* metabolites (see Table 22-7) are given carefully with cimetidine, which reduces benzodiazepine clearance and therefore prolongs half-lives.

Changes in diazepam half-life have occurred when it is administered with isoniazid, rifampin, low-dose estrogen-containing oral contraceptives, or valproic acid.

Acute toxicity. Pure benzodiazepine overdosage is nonlethal in most clients. However, clients who combine benzodiazepines with other CNS depressants, particularly alcohol, often produce hazardous CNS depression.

Dosage. Because anxiety symptoms are episodic and fluctuating, dosage is often titrated to the severity of symptoms. Benzodiazepine dosage, tailored to the individual, rarely exceeds 30 mg per day of diazepam or its equivalent. Treatment is usually begun at a low level and carefully titrated upward until the desired effect (client's ability to cope and reduction of avoidance behavior) is obtained.

Tolerance, dependence, and withdrawal. Tolerance may develop during long-term therapy, manifested as decreased side effects or a need to increase the dose to induce sleep or maintain clinical benefits.

Minor withdrawal symptoms are anxiety, apprehension, insomnia, dizziness, and anorexia. Because these are also the common symptoms of anxiety, it is impossible to decide clinically whether they are signs of withdrawal or a

TABLE 22-7 Antianxiety medications, dosages, and half-lives

Generic and Trade Name	Usual Daily Oral Dosage Range for Adults		Average or Range of Half-life in Hours	
	Antianxiety	Hypnotic	Parent Compound	Major Metabolite
BENZODIAZEPINES				
Compounds with active metabolites				
Chlordiazepoxide (Librium)	10-100	—	10	24-96
Clorazepate (Tranxene)	7.5-60	—	—	50-100
Diazepam (Valium)	2-30	—	20-50	50-100
Flurazepam (Dalmane)	—	15-30	—	74-160
Halazepam (Paxipam)	20-120	—	14	50-100
Prazepam (Centrax)	10-60	—	—	50-100
Compounds with weak or inactive metabolites				
Alprazolam (Xanax)	0.5-4	—	12	
Lorazepam (Ativan)	0.5-9	1-4	15	
Oxazepam (Serax)	30-120	—	5-15	
Temazepam (Restoril)	—	15-30	15	
Triazolam (Halcion)	—	0.25-0.5	3	
NONBENZODIAZEPINES AND NONBARBITURATES				
Hydroxyzine (Atarax)	75-400	—	3	
Meprobamate (Equanil)	1200-1600	—	10-24	
BARBITURATES				
Amobarbital (Amytal)	—	50-300	25	
Butabarbital (Butisol)	50-120	50-100	100	
Pentobarbital (Nembutal)	—	50-100	15-50	
Phenobarbital (Luminal)	30-120	60-300	79	
Secobarbital (Seconal)	—	50-100	28	

recurrence of the previous disorder as a result of premature termination of therapy. If therapy has lasted less than 1 month at the traditional therapeutic dosage, physical dependence is unlikely. If higher doses have been given for longer periods, the benzodiazepine is gradually withdrawn over 1 to 2 weeks to eliminate the possibility of a withdrawal syndrome.

Signs of a more severe physical dependence are those already described plus (in order of severity) nausea, vomiting, muscle weakness, tremor, postural hypotension, hyperthermia, muscle twitches, convulsions, and confusion or psychoses.

The antianxiety medications in general serve as strong reinforcing agents, and many anxious clients become psychologically dependent on them. This dependence ranges from enjoying the effects to centering their life-style on the use of the medication. It becomes difficult for the physician to distinguish between psychological dependence and the need for extended therapy. As psychological dependence intensifies, the drive to obtain the medication increases, and tolerance is therefore likely.

Meprobamate

Meprobamate is less potent than the benzodiazepines, and long-term use of large doses produces dependence. Its usefulness is therefore limited. It does not break down in the liver to significant major metabolites.

Following are common side effects:

Drowsiness	Anaphylactic reactions
Thrombocytopenia	Hypotension
Leukopenia	Syncope
Agranulocytosis	Blurred vision
Aplastic anemia	Paradoxical euphoria
Dermatitis	Anger
Urticaria	

Hydroxyzine

Hydroxyzine, an antihistamine with sedative and antiemetic properties, is less effective than benzodiazepines in treating anxiety. Since it is not a controlled substance, however, it is suitable for selected clients. Side effects are not common; drowsiness is transient. Fatal overdose is rare. Withdrawal reactions have not been reported.

Barbiturates

The barbiturates, a group of sedative-hypnotics, are used infrequently. They are, however, still often encountered in cases of medication abuse and suicide attempts. A small dose used to calm an anxious client is called a *sedative.* A larger dose to induce sleep is called a *hypnotic.*

Action and side effects. The barbiturates are general CNS depressants, producing sedation in small doses, anesthesia in higher doses, and death in still higher doses. These compounds, which include agents such as phenobarbital, pentobarbital, and secobarbital (see Table 22-7), depress REM sleep when given as hypnotics and induce

tolerance. Therefore they are not effective in sleep disorders beyond 5 to 7 days.

Absorption, distribution, and fate. The barbiturates are absorbed well orally, with onset of action in 15 to 30 minutes. They are metabolized in the liver and excreted in the urine.

Acute toxicity. The barbiturates, widely abused, are one of the leading causes of fatal medication poisoning, usually from suicide attempts. Overdose can cause tachycardia, hypotension, shock, ventilatory depression, coma, and death. Treatment is symptomatic, and intensive care is required.

Medication interactions. The dose is reduced in the presence of other CNS depressants, including alcohol, hypnotics, antianxiety agents, TCAs, narcotic analgesics, antipsychotics, and antihistamines. MAO inhibitors may potentiate the depressant effects of the barbiturates. Administration with rifampin may decrease the barbiturate level.

Dosage. Sedative-hypnotic medications are prescribed primarily for insomnia and are not given for more than 2 to 3 weeks. The usual dosages are listed in Table 22-7.

Tolerance, dependence, and withdrawal. Tolerance and dependence occur at doses slightly larger than therapeutic levels. Withdrawal syndromes are often severe. Little justification can be found for their use as antianxiety agents.

Nursing implications. The side effects of drowsiness and ataxia are related to dosage. When tolerance is achieved, the side effects subside. If drowsiness occurs, the nurse cautions clients to avoid driving and operating dangerous equipment. Daily naps may be appropriate for several days. The client with ataxia is alerted to the danger of potential injury.

Other side effects occur less often. Urticaria (itchy rash) may appear in the groin. Gastric irritation may be decreased by giving the dose with meals or a light snack.

Fever, malaise, sore throat, persistent or unexplained bleeding, jaundice, abdominal pain, or lingering infection in clients on long-term therapy may indicate hematopoietic or liver dysfunction and need to be reported (Table 22-8). Excessive smoking may alter the effectiveness of the medications.

NONCOMPLIANCE

Noncompliance is the failure of a client to carry out a prescribed health care plan. NANDA's defining characteristics are listed in the box on p 447. A corresponding diagnosis in the DMS-III-R is noncompliance with medical treatment. The diagnosis is made, according to the DSM-III-R, when a client fails to follow a prescribed diet because of religious beliefs or to make decisions based on personal value judgments about the advantages and disadvantages of the proposed treatment or denial of illness.

Readmissions are commonly precipitated by medication noncompliance, particularly for schizophrenic clients who do not understand that they are sick and who cease taking medication when it is needed most. Blackwell[7] stated that this neglect results in a *revolving door* syn-

TABLE 22-8 Summary of common side effects and suggested nursing interventions for psychotropic medications

Side Effect	Group of Drugs*	Nursing Interventions
ANTICHOLINERGIC		
Dry mouth	AP TCA MAOI APARK	Offer or give the client frequent sips of water or other beverages; because weight gain is often also a problem, low-calorie beverages are preferred. Suggest that the client suck on hard candy or mints or chew gum; again, low-calorie or sugarless forms are preferred. Frequent toothbrushing or rinsing the mouth with a pleasant mouthwash or other solution may help eliminate a bad taste in the mouth. Commercially prepared saliva substitutes are available.
Constipation	AP TCA MAOI APARK	Record the frequency of bowel movements. Encourage the client to increase the dietary intake of bran, fresh fruits, prunes, or other foods known by the client to stimulate defecation. Have the client increase fluid intake to 2500 to 3000 ml per day if not contraindicated by other medical conditions. Have the client increase his level of activity by walking or other forms of exercise. Stool softeners or bulk-forming agents may be necessary for some clients.
Blurred vision	AP TCA MAOI APARK	Caution the client to avoid driving or other dangerous activities until the blurring clears. The client occasionally may indicate a need to reduce the drug dosage because of side effects. If blurring persists or suddenly appears when not present before, the condition may require referral of the client to an ophthalmologist.
Urinary retention	AP TCA	Although this side effect is possible at any age, it is usually more of a problem in the elderly, in immobilized clients, and in men with enlarged prostate glands. Measure intake and output. Notify the physician; catheterization may be necessary. Teach the client to notify the health care provider if retention is suspected.
Diaphoresis	TCA	Maintain adequate fluid intake (usually over 2500 to 3000 ml per day). Observe for electrolyte imbalance; monitor serum electrolytes.
ENDOCRINE AND METABOLIC		
Weight gain	AP TCA MAOI	Weigh the client weekly; instruct the client to monitor his weight at home weekly. Provide dietary instruction about nutritious but low-calorie meal planning. Assist in the development of a regular exercise program.
Hyperglycemia and hypoglycemia	TCA AP	Monitor blood sugar carefully and frequently in diabetic clients. Modification of prescribed diet, insulin, or oral diabetic agent may be necessary.
Increased or decreased libido; changes in ability to ejaculate or maintain erection	AP TCA LI	It may not be possible to eliminate these side effects if they occur. Client and spouse support may be necessary. These side effects may contribute to poor medication compliance if the client views them as severe problems. Altering the drug dose or switching medications may be helpful.
Menstrual irregularities	AP	Refer for gynecological exam if appropriate. Advise the use of birth control measures to avoid unwanted pregnancy.
Gastric irritation	TCA LI	Alter the prescribed times for taking doses to coincide with meals. Decrease the size of the dose and administer more frequently. Change the medication form (for example, switch to liquid from tablets).
NEUROLOGICAL		
Drowsiness and sedation	AP TCA MAOI APARK	Caution the client to avoid driving or other dangerous activities requiring mental alertness until the degree of drowsiness can be evaluated. With some medications or with some clients drowsiness may be a desirable effect. Daytime drowsiness, especially with antidepressants, may indicate the need to increase the nighttime dose or give the entire day's dosage at bedtime. Persistent drowsiness may indicate the need to change the medication or dose; this requires careful clinical judgment. Drowsiness may lessen with time. Encourage client to continue the medication for at least several weeks.

*AP, Antipsychotic agents; *TCA*, tricyclic and tetracyclic agents; *MAOI*, monamine oxidase inhibitors; *APARK*, antiparkinsonian agents; *LI*, lithium.

TABLE 22-8 Summary of common side effects and suggested nursing interventions for psychotropic medications—cont'd

Side Effect	Group of Drugs*	Nursing Interventions
CARDIOVASCULAR		
Orthostatic hypotension	AP	Instruct the client to rise slowly from lying to sitting or to standing from sitting.
	TCA	Keep the side rails of the bed up for hospitalized clients; suggest that they call for assis-
	MAOI	tance when getting up until they have learned to manage the problem.
	APARK	Elastic stockings may be helpful.
		Instruct the client to avoid hot showers or baths, since they may cause vasodilation and aggravate the problem.
		Monitor the blood pressure if the hypotension is severe or frequent.
Tachycardia	TCA	Monitor the pulse two to four times daily until stable.
	APARK	Withhold the dose if the resting pulse before a dose is 120 or greater (or follow the insti-
	LI	tutional policy regarding this).
		If appropriate, teach the client to record the pulse regularly at home.
		The client is to avoid excessive caffeine intake.

NONCOMPLIANCE

DEFINITION

Failure of client to take medications as prescribed in a health care plan.

DEFINING CHARACTERISTICS

Physical Dimension
*Agitation
 Persistence of signs and symptoms for which therapy was originally prescribed
 Missed appointments with health care team
*Unexpected high or low serum medication levels
*Appearance of exaggerated or unexpected side effects or disappearance of previous side effects without explanation
 Too much or too little medication remaining at the time of visit (documented by pill count or other objective data)
 Lack of finances
 Progression of disease process

Emotional Dimension
*Guilt
*Anxiety
*Anger
*Embarrassment
*Hostility
*Persistence of emotional affect present when therapy was begun

Intellectual Dimension
*Rationalization
 Statement of lack of compliance
*Negativism about prescribed therapy
*Identification of preference for therapies not prescribed by health care team
 Lack of knowledge

Social Dimension
*Social isolation
*Avoidance of associations formed while following prescribed regime
*Return to associations that existed before therapy
 Unsupportive family
 Nontherapeutic relationship between client and nurse

Spiritual Dimension
 Adherence to religious belief or doctrine prohibiting the use of specific kinds of therapy
*Feeling that dependence on therapies implies weakness and inability to cope
*Feeling that emotional difficulties are God's will

Adapted from North American Nursing Diagnosis Association Classification of Nursing Diagnosis: Proceedings of the seventh conference, St. Louis, 1987, The C.V. Mosby Co.
*Indicates characteristics in addition to those defined by NANDA.

drome—repeated admissions to and discharges from the hospital. Blackwell categorized errors in medication adherence into the following five groups:

1. Errors of omission
2. Errors of purpose (taking medication for the wrong reasons)
3. Errors of dosage
4. Errors in timing or sequence
5. Taking additional medications not prescribed by physician

The following Case Example illustrates the characteristics of the nursing diagnosis of noncompliance.

Case Example

Donald, a physician, was diagnosed at age 46 with bipolar disorder. Over the years his increasingly prolonged and pronounced periods of mania caused his family to urge him to seek psychiatric care. He was hospitalized, and therapy included lithium titrated to the desired serum level. The lithium produced a pronounced change in behavior, which Donald stated was subjectively more pleasant. He was discharged. When he returned for an appointment in 3 weeks, serum lithium levels were significantly lower than expected. He said that the fine hand tremor caused by the lithium made him appear old; he felt people would not have confidence in a physician "whose hands tremble all the time." He also felt that as a physician he should be "strong enough to handle this illness without medications," and that "people shouldn't come to rely on drugs for well-being."

The following factors may be used to predict with minimal reliability whether a client will default on medication regimes:

1. Chronic illness
2. Symptom suppression (as opposed to curative action) by the medication
3. Delayed relapse with cessation of the medication
4. Ambivalent feelings toward dependence issues
5. Need for multiple medications
6. Social isolation

Nursing Implications

Many clients treated with psychotropic medications are ambivalent about medication. The association of these medications with illegal drug use plus prevailing suspiciousness about taking any prescribed medication leads to hesitancy to comply with treatment. Following are other reasons why clients do not comply:

1. Lack of understanding of diagnosis and treatment
2. Denial of illness

Research Highlight

Compliance with Therapeutic Regimens: a Follow-up Study for Patients with Affective Disorders

F. A. Youssef

PURPOSE

This study was designed to determine the impact of client education on client compliance to psychotropic medication regimens after discharge from the hospital.

SAMPLE

The sample was 36 adults diagnosed with affective disorders, discharged from an inpatient facility, and who were to take an oral psychotropic medication. Subjects also had to have a follow-up appointment in 2 weeks and be able to read and write. They were randomly assigned to a control group and an experimental group.

METHODOLOGY

The control group received the usual agency instruction on medications: on the day of discharge, a nurse instructed the client individually about medications. The experimental group was asked to attend twice-weekly group sessions conducted by the investigator and one other nurse. Topics included medication action, minor side effects, and reasons why clients stop taking their medications.

Data were collected twice. At discharge all subjects completed a form requesting information on discharge medications: name, prescription number, time of last dose, number of pills in the bottle at discharge, and when and with whom the first return visit was scheduled. One to 2 days before the return visit, compliance data were collected by a staff member unaware of whether clients were in the control or experimental group. Data included name of drug, number of pills remaining, and prescription number. All subjects were followed for 6 months.

FINDINGS

In the control group five clients were defined as compliant, and 13 were not. In the experimental group, 11 were defined as compliant, and seven were not. Chi square was used to determine that the difference was statistically significant.

IMPLICATIONS

For clients with affective disorders a directive client-education group approach to teaching about medications seems to result in better client compliance than one-time, day-of-discharge instructions.

Based on data from Journal of Advanced Nursing **8:**513, 1983.

3. Side effects of medication
4. Fear of dependence on medication
5. Desire to remain ill to receive secondary gains
6. Feeling a loss of control over body
7. Negative relationship with health care team
8. Lack of family support
9. Cost

The nurse asks the following questions to prepare the client for discharge and self-management[8]:

1. What physiological dysfunction does the client appear to have that may interfere with carrying out the prescribed treatment regimen?
2. What beliefs does the client have about the illness or effectiveness of treatment?
3. Does the client have medication-induced side effects that make compliance difficult?
4. Is the client on a regimen that makes compliance difficult?
5. Does the client have the necessary knowledge to carry out the regimen?
6. Does the client have the necessary skills to carry out the regimen?
7. Does the client's social support system or daily routine interfere with compliance?

One criterion for discharge is the client's ability to deal with activities of daily living. The client needs to be able and willing to adhere to his medication regimen. Medication cards (see box below) are helpful, and group teach-ing sessions may also be appropriate (see the Research Highlight on p. 448).

BRIEF REVIEW

The four major categories of psychotropic medications are the *antipsychotic agents,* the *antianxiety agents,* the *antidepressant agents,* and the *antimanic agents.* The *antiparkinson agents* are also discussed because of their effectiveness in lessening the side effects of psychotropic medications.

The antipsychotics are most effective for clients with schizophrenic and paranoid disorders, major depressions, and mania. The antiparkinsons are given to clients with extrapyramidal symptoms resulting from their antipsychotic medications. The tricyclic and tetracyclic antidepressants (TCAs) and the monoamine oxidase (MAO) inhibitors are the most commonly used antidepressants. MAO inhibitors are prescribed less often than TCAs because of the danger of hypertensive crisis that may occur when the client on MAO inhibitors eats food containing tyramine. For clients with bipolar disorder, lithium is effective in treating manic episodes. Serum levels of clients taking lithium are frequently monitored to avoid toxicity. Antianxiety medications are widely used for reducing anxiety. They are also commonly misused and abused. Because of their long half-life, these medication may accumulate excessively in the body and remain for weeks after therapy is begun. The combination of antianxiety medications and other CNS depressants, such as alcohol, can be fatal. Tolerance and dependence with long-term use may develop.

Noncompliance with a medication regimen is a problem with psychiatric clients, particularly the schizophrenic client. Noncompliance results in frequent readmissions to the hospital. Medication cards and group teaching sessions may help clients to comply.

SAMPLE MEDICATION CARD

Your medication is ___Elavil___. Your dosage is 75 mg three times each day with meals.

ACTION

This medication will increase your energy level and decrease your depressed feeling.

EFFECTS AND PRECAUTIONS

1. You may experience drowsiness, blurred vision, dry mouth, and constipation while taking this medication.
2. It may take 2 to 3 weeks before you begin to feel less depressed. It is essential that you continue taking the medicine even though you do not feel any benefits.
3. Do not use alcohol while taking this medicine because of possible serious interaction of your medication with the alcohol.
4. Do not use any over-the-counter medications without informing your physician.
5. Do not drive a car until you are sure the medicine does not make you drowsy.
6. Notify your physician if you are constipated or have difficulty passing urine. Use a stool softener (Colace) and eat a diet high in fiber.
7. Do not change the dosage of your medicine without informing your physician, and do not give the medicine to anyone else.

REFERENCES AND SUGGESTED READINGS

1. American Medical Association: A.M.A. drug evaluations, ed. 5, Chicago, 1983, American Medical Association.
2. American Psychiatric Association: Diagnostic and statistical manual of mental disorders, ed. 3, Washington, D.C., 1987, The Association.
3. Anderson, G.D.: Benzodiazepines, Nurse Practitioner 5:47, 1980.
4. Bernstein, J.G.: Handbook of drug therapy in psychiatry, Littleton, Mass., 1983, PSG/Wright Publishing Co., Inc.
5. Birkhimer, L.J., and DeVane, C.L.: The neuroleptic malignant syndrome: presentation and treatment, Drug Intelligence and Clinical Pharmacy 18:462, 1984.
6. Boettcher, E.G., and Anderson, S.F.: Psychotropic medications and the nursing process, Journal of Psychosocial Nursing and Mental Health Services 20(11):12, 1982.
7. Blackwell, B.: Adverse effects of antidepressant drugs. II. "Second generation" antidepressants and rational decision making in antidepressant therapy, Drugs 21:273, 1981.
8. Brief, D.J., and Dorman, J.E.: Noncompliance: understanding and intervening when clients fail to follow the treatment plan. In Backer, B.A., Dubbert, P.M., and Eisenman, E.J.P., editors: Psychiatric mental health nursing, ed. 2, Monterey, Calif., 1985, Wadsworth Health Sciences Division.

9. Carpenito, L.J.: Nursing diagnosis: application to clinical practice, Philadelphia, 1983, J.B. Lippincott Co.

10. Ciraulo, D.A.: Psychotropic drug therapy in the emergency department, Topics in Emergency Medicine 4(4):17, 1983.

11. Clark, J.B., Queener, S.F., and Karb, V.B.: Pharmacological basis of nursing practice, ed. 2, St. Louis, 1986, The C.V. Mosby Co.

12. Cohen, M., and Amdur, M.: Medication group for psychiatric patients, American Journal of Nursing 81:343, 1981.

13. Corre, K.A., Niemann, J.T., and Bessen, H.A.: Extended therapy for acute dystonic reactions, Annals of Emergency Medicine 13:194, 1984.

14. Csernansky, J.G., and Hollister, L.E.: Carbamazepine in the treatment of lithium-resistant manic-depressive illness, Hospital Formulary 18:410, 1983.

15. Fuentes, R.J., Rosenberg, J.M., and Marks, R.G.: Sexual side effects: what to tell your patients, what not to say, R.N. 46(2):34, 1983.

16. Gold, D.D.: Pharmacotherapy of schizophrenia, Hospital Formulary 19(2):153, 1984.

17. Hahn, K.: Management of Parkinson's disease, Nurse Practitioner 7:13, 1982.

18. Hayes J.E.: Normal changes in aging and nursing implications of drug therapy, Nursing Clinics of North America 17(2):253, 1982.

19. Hayes, P.E.: Rational prescribing guidelines for antipsychotic drugs, Family and Community Health 6(3):1, 1983.

20. Hunn, S., and others: Nursing care of patients on lithium, Perspectives in Psychiatric Care 18(5):214, 1980.

21. Jann, M.W., Garrelts, J.C., Ereshefsky, L., and Saklad, S.R.: Alternative drug therapies for mania: a literature review, Drug Intelligence and Clinical Pharmacy 18:577, 1984.

22. Jeste, D.V., and Wyatt, R.J.: Therapeutic strategies against tardive dyskinesia, Archieves of General Psychiatry 39:803, 1982.

23. Lasater, M.G.: Nursing care of the patient with a tricyclic antidepressant overdose, Critical Care Nurse 4(4):28, 1984.

24. Lickey, M.E., and Gordon, B.: Drugs for mental illness, New York, 1983, W.H. Freeman & Co., Publishers.

24a. Masters, J., and Spitler, R.: Neuroleptic malignant syndrome, Journal of Psychosocial Nursing and Mental Health Services 24(9):10, 1986.

25. Moran, M.G., and Thompson, T.L.: Increased psychotropic side effects in geriatric patients, Hospital Formulary 17(11):1513, 1982.

26. Oles, K.S.: Pharmacokinetics in the aged. III. Drug use in the elderly, Hospital Formulary 19:817, 1984.

26b. McGinnis, J., and Foote, K.: Rapid neuroleptization, Journal of Psychosocial Nursing and Mental Health Services 24(10):17, 1986.

27. Oppeneer, J.E., and Vervoren, T.M.: Gerontological pharmacology: a resource for health practitioners, St. Louis, 1983, The C.V. Mosby Co.

28. Pagliaro, L.A., and Pagliaro, A.M., editors: Pharmacologic aspects of aging, St. Louis, 1983, The C.V. Mosby Co.

29. Portnoi, V.A., and Johnson, J.E.: Tardive dyskinesia, Geriatric Nursing 3:39, 1982.

30. Salem, R.B.: Recommendations for monitoring lithium therapy, Drug Intelligence and Clinical Pharmacy 17:346, 1983.

30a. Scrak, B. and Greenstein, R.: Tardive diskinesia: evaluation in a nurse managed prolixin program, Journal of Psychosocial Nursing and Mental Health Services 22(5):10, 1986.

31. Stewart, R.M.: Update on managing parkinsonism and tardive dyskinesia, Consultant 23(6):51, 1983.

32. Swonger, A.K., and Constantine, L.L.: Drugs and therapy, ed. 2, Boston, 1983, Little, Brown & Co.

33. Todd, B.: Drugs and the elderly: why are some drugs withdrawn slowly? Geriatric Nursing 4(6):393, 1983.

34. Turnquist, A.C.: The issue of informed consent and the use of neuroleptic medications, International Journal of Nursing Studies 21(3):181, 1983.

35. Vogel, P.: Lithium and the thyroid, Journal of Psychosocial Nursing and Mental Health Services 24(2):8, 1986.

ANNOTATED BIBLIOGRAPHY

DeGennaro, M., and others: Psychotropic drug therapy: antidepressants, lithium, antipsychotics, extrapyramidal side effects, sedatives-hypnotics, American Journal of Nursing 81:1303, 1981.

A separate article is devoted to each of the topics listed in the title and focuses on nursing care of clients receiving these psychotropic medications.

Symposium on drugs and the older adult, Nursing Clinics of North America 17:251, 1982.

Articles for this symposium constitute half of the June issue. Of particular interest are articles on psychotropic medications and the elderly, normal changes from the aging process and their effects on nursing implications of medication therapy, and ways to assist the elderly in managing medication therapy at home.

CHAPTER 23

SOMATIC THERAPIES

Judith Eberle Seidenschnur

After studying this chapter the learner will be able to:

Describe electroconvulsive therapy, psychosurgery, insulin coma therapy, hydrotherapy, narcotherapy, Indoklon therapy, restraints, and seclusion as modes of treatment.

Trace the historical development of somatic therapies

Identify indications, contraindications, and complications of somatic therapies

Discuss the legal and ethical aspects of somatic therapies.

Explore the role of the nurse in somatic therapies.

Somatic therapies are treatment methods using physiological agents to produce desired behavioral changes, generally in conjunction with other types of psychotherapy. Psychopharmacological agents, the most common, are discussed in Chapter 22. *Somatic therapies* examined here are electroconvulsive therapy (ECT), *psychosurgery, insulin coma therapy, hydrotherapy, narcotherapy,* and *Indoklon therapy.* Restraints and seclusion are also discussed. Some therapies are no longer used (insulin coma therapy), some are being revived as a result of new research findings (psychosurgery), and some continue to be controversial in effectiveness and safety (ECT).

ELECTROCONVULSIVE THERAPY

Electroconvulsive therapy involves the passage of an electrical stimulus of 70 to 150 volts to the brain for 0.1 to 1 second to produce a grand mal seizure. The amount of voltage and the length of application vary with each client. The dosage is adjusted to the minimal amount of electrical current necessary to produce a seizure. Individual seizure thresholds vary and are generally found to be higher in females and older people.

Seizure induction is needed to achieve the therapeutic effect, which is thought to be the result of an alteration in the postsynaptic response to the neurotransmitters in the central nervous system (CNS). Because ECT stimulates synaptic remodeling, the number of vesicles that contain synaptic protein increases, producing an enhanced behavioral response and relief of depressive symptoms.[7]

The client receives atropine sulfate subcutaneously before the procedure to decrease oropharyngeal secretions. At the beginning of the treatment an intravenous dose of Sodium Pentothal or methohexital sodium (Brevital) is given as a sedative. Electrode jelly is applied bilaterally to the temples or unilaterally to the nondominant hemisphere, and padded electrodes are applied. An airway or soft mouth gag is put in the client's mouth. Succinylcholine chloride (Anectine) is given as a muscle relaxant.

During early use of ECT fractures commonly resulted from the intense contractions. The use of a muscle relaxant prevents this and permits CNS features of a seizure while keeping muscle spasms minimal. The resulting grand mal seizure closely resembles that of spontaneous origin, with a *tonic* phase (tightening of muscles) for approximately 10 seconds and a *clonic* phase (rhythmic movement of muscles) for 30 seconds. The movements are slight and often limited to plantar flexion of the feet, followed by rhythmic twitching of the toes.

During the seizure a central vagus discharge leads to a period of bradycardia with a drop in blood pressure, followed by tachycardia and a rise in blood pressure. This also produces a rise in cerebrospinal fluid. The pituitary gland is stimulated, and there is evidence of an increase in autonomic activity. Adrenocorticotropic hormone (ACTH), epinephrine, and norepinephrine levels rise im-

🍇 *Historical Overview* 🍇

DATE	EVENT
Ancient times	The Greek and Roman practice of boring holes in the skull (trephination) to allow evil spirits to escape was a primitive form of psychosurgery.
	The use of cold water (hydrotherapy) has been a form of treatment since Galens' (120 BC) and Hippocrates' (460 BC) days.
1933	Insulin coma therapy was developed by a Viennese physician as a treatment for clients with thinking disorders.
1936	Lobotomy was introduced in the United States. The procedure, a surgical intervention that interrupts the emotional circuit in the limbic system, is infrequently used today because of the availability of psychotropic medications and other forms of treatment.
1937	ECT was introduced in Rome by two physicians who observed that there was no evidence of schizophrenia in epileptic clients. Thinking that seizures prevented schizophrenia, they promoted the use of artificially induced seizures to treat schizophrenia.
1940s	Before the discovery of psychotropic medications in the 1950s, physical restraints, seclusion, and ECT were the primary treatments for all types of mental disorders.
1980s	ECT continues to be controversial although its use has become more widespread.
	Today it is essential that the nurse be knowledgeable of the actions, indications, and contraindications of currently used somatic therapies for the safety of the client and her own legal protection.
Future	Nurses are challenged to contribute to the expanding knowledge of the biological aspects of mental illness by collaborative research with other disciplines.
	The need to explore ethical questions regarding the intrusive and unscientific use of somatic therapies is a priority as decisions that affect clients become increasingly complex.

mediately after the treatment, but return to normal several minutes later.

The seizure is accompanied by a short period of apnea and then stertorous (snoringlike) respiration. Because the muscle relaxant paralyzes the respiratory muscles, an anesthetist is present to administer oxygen to the client and assist respiration by mechanical means if necessary. Usually the client sleeps for 5 to 10 minutes after the seizure, slowly awakens, and does not remember the treatment.

The number of treatments given varies according to the severity of the disorder and therapeutic response and is not predetermined. Response varies widely, and sometimes only three treatments are needed. A risk of manic reaction or short-term confusion exists if a client is treated excessively.[9] Clients benefiting most from ECT generally show mild improvement after the first several treatments.

Treatments are usually given two or three times a week, with 48-hour intervals most desirable. Clients over 65 years of age given ECT more often than twice a week experience a significantly longer period of posttreatment confusion.[10]

Indications

ECT has a distinct advantage over some medications, which generally require several days to weeks before symptoms are relieved. When risk of suicide is high, prompt, effective ECT may reduce the risk more quickly than medication.

Clinical indications for ECT are major mood disorders with pronounced physical deterioration and risk of suicide, severe mania uncontrolled by neuroleptics or lithium, and some forms of schizophrenia (such as acute, catatonic, and paranoid) that have not responded to medication. Clients more likely to receive therapeutic benefits from ECT are those who have no psychogenic basis for their depression (see the Research Highlight on p. 453), display somatic and paranoid delusions accompanied by feelings of guilt, and have a history of depressive episodes.

ECT is preferred to antidepressant therapy in some cases, such as for clients with heart conditions, for whom tricyclics are contraindicated because of the potential for dysrythmia and congestive heart failure, and for pregnant clients, in whom antidepressants place the fetus at risk for congenital defects. ECT has not been found effective in

Research Highlight

Reevaluation of ECT in Depression

V. Bagadia, R. Abhyankan, M. Doshi, P. Pradhan & L. Shah

PURPOSE

This study was designed to evaluate the effectiveness of ECT for clients diagnosed with depression.

SAMPLE

The sample was 40 depressed clients of both sexes from 18 to 65 years of age. Two consulting psychiatrists agreed on the diagnosis of each client in independent evaluations.

METHODOLOGY

Psychiatric history, mental status, and physical examination data were obtained. A double-blind randomized technique was used in two parallel groups of clients. The clients were given either six ECT treatments and a placebo or six simulated ECT treatments and Imipramine, 150 mg per day. Psychiatric evaluations included the Hamilton Psychiatric Rating Scale for Depression, the Beck Self-Inventory Scale for Depression, and the Clinical Global Impression Scale. Clinical

and subjective evaluation of side effects were done at baseline and after 20 days. The test battery was given before ECT and 48 hours after the final treatment.

FINDINGS

When the two groups' scores on the Hamilton Rating Scale were compared, clients who received ECT and the placebo had significantly more improvement ($p \le .05$) after 7 days and after 20 days ($p \le .01$) than clients receiving simulated ECT and Imipramine. There was no significant difference in the cognitive status at the pretreatment or the posttreatment evaluation between the two groups.

IMPLICATIONS

The results confirm that ECT produces significant improvement in depressed clients compared with antidepressant medication therapy. This information is helpful to the nurse giving reassurance to clients considering ECT.

Based on data from Psychopharmacology 19(3):550, 1983.

altering the primary symptoms of thought disorder, and little evidence exists to indicate that it is effective in neurotic clients and those diagnosed with a personality disorder or grief reactions.

Contraindications

ECT is not recommended for clients with histories of cardiovascular disease, because elevated hormone levels contribute to transient hypertension and tachycardia that may increase the risk of stroke or coronary thrombosis. It is also contraindicated for clients with a brain tumor, acute myocardial infarction, congestive heart failure, pneumonia, or aortic aneurysm. Therefore it is essential that clients have a complete system review and physical examination before treatment.

The mortality for clients receiving ECT is approximately 1 in 10,000 treatments—lower than that for clients having surgery with anesthesia. An American Psychiatric Association (APA) task force found a 36% death rate by suicide in untreated or more conservatively treated severely depressed clients.[4]

Complications

Life-threatening complications of ECT are rare.[19] Back pain occasionally results and may persist for a few days or weeks. Fractures are not uncommon in elderly clients with osteoporosis. The aged with a history of coronary

disease also may develop cardiac dysrhythmia. The self-neglect and suicide potential of the depressed elderly client is far more hazardous than the possible side effects. Respiratory arrest, if it occurs, is the result of the anesthesia or muscle relaxant.

Memory loss is a common but transient side effect. As clients awaken, they are confused but become fully oriented in 2 hours. Memory for events immediately before and during the treatment remains impaired, but memory for events up to 2 years before treatment and remote memory generally return to normal.

Nursing Roles

ECT treatments can be administered in a hospital, clinic, or physician's office. Following are the nursing roles and responsibilities, which are similar to those preceding a surgical procedure:

Before treatment

1. Check the record for recent physical examination and routine laboratory work (blood count, blood chemistries, and urinalysis). Results of pre-ECT psychological evaluations of memory capability are helpful.
2. Check for a signed consent form. It is best to have a relative read the informed consent also. If the client's ability to comprehend the information is questionable, additional medical and legal opinions may be needed.

3. Involve the family as much as possible to inform them and relieve their fears and anxieties.
4. Communicate positive feelings about the procedure to the family and client.
5. Discourage cigarrette smoking just before procedure to avoid increased difficulty in managing pulmonary secretions during treatment.
6. Omit liquids 6 hours and solids 8 hours before treatment.
7. Remove dentures, glasses, and jewelry (rings may be taped) and dress the client in loose clothing.
8. Have the client evacuate bladder and bowels.
9. Monitor vital signs before, during, and after treatment.
10. Give atropine as ordered before treatment. It may also be given intravenously just before the treatment.
11. Make sure that oxygen, suction, and endotracheal intubation is accessible and functional in case of a cardiorespiratory emergency.
12. Display a warm, supportive attitude to reduce apprehension. Clients receiving ECT are somewhat anxious (especially about the first treatment), and although the procedure is painless, some feel a sense of dread. The idea of shock and subsequent seizure can be frightening.

During treatment
1. Maintain the airway and remove pharyngeal secretions with suction as necessary.
2. Observe the client continuously until he is fully recovered. He is allowed up when awake, alert, and able to ambulate.
3. Give the client a mild sedative for restlessness if prescribed.

After treatment
1. Touch the client as he awakens to demonstrate care, establish your presence, and allay fear.
2. Orient the client to time, place, and events as he awakens.
3. Give medications for minor discomforts, such as headache or nausea.
4. Provide opportunities for the client to express his feelings about the treatment.
5. Promote normal activity after the treatment to discourage incapacity.
6. Document client responses during and after treatment.

The following Case Example describes a client and her response to ECT.

Case Example

A 73-year-old, widowed woman with severe recurrent affective illness since age 38 was admitted because of a progressive 3-month deterioration demonstrated by social withdrawal, poor hygeine, agitation, feelings of hopelessness, extreme fatigue, sleeplessness, poor concentration and memory, and anorexia. She was diagnosed as having a major mood disorder with delusional features. She was unresponsive to tricyclic antidepressants, lithium, and monoamine oxidase inhibitors; ECT was indicated.

She was informed and signed the consent form. The procedure and its common side effects were explained, and she was encouraged to ask questions and express her fears and feelings. Her daughter was included in the discussion for her information and emotional support. After five treatments in 12 days her depressive symptoms improved markedly. After ten treatments her depressive symptoms disappeared, and she returned to her usual level of functioning.

Ethical and Legal Considerations

Strong public objections that ECT is inhumane are pervasive, and legal action to control its prescription has been attempted in some states. This is highly unfavorable; a legislative body is hardly qualified to rule on the appropriateness of psychiatric treatment. Excessive regulation has infringed on medical practice. Often the cost of malpractice suits is so high that doctors avoid using ECT. As a result, a pro-ECT group was formed in 1975 to promote the use of ECT to medical professionals and the public. The group hoped to counteract the effects of court actions restricting ECT and to improve its reputation.

The use of ECT provoked criticisms about informed consent and the determination of competence (see Chapter 46). An APA task force addressed these issues and recommended that the consent form include the following:
1. Information on the nature and degree of seriousness of the disorder
2. Probable course without ECT
3. Description of the procedure
4. Risks and side effects
5. Possibility of alternative treatments
6. Why ECT is recommended
7. Statement of the individual's or guardian's right to refuse or revoke consent
8. Statement that a new consent form will be obtained for additional treatment series

The task force also suggested documentation be made in the clinical record specifying that the information was given to the client and that the consent giver is competent, able to comprehend the information, and able to act responsibly. It also stated that a competent client who refuses ECT cannot be forced to receive it. It suggested that when competence is in question, an evaluation be done by a group including the client's attorney and psychiatrist. A treatment committee of one (preferably two) psychiatrist, neurologist, internist, and attorney can also review the case if any of the initial evaluators find the client to be incompetent. The treatment committee interviews each client and determines competence.

INDOKLON THERAPY

Indoklon (hexafluorodiethyl ether) is a colorless, volatile liquid given with oxygen inhalation to induce convulsions to treat depression.

Indoklon therapy is a substitute for ECT and has been an effective complement to drug therapy for clients unwilling to consent to ECT. The resulting seizure is similar to that produced with ECT; however, the onset is more gradual. Eight to 14 treatments are given at intervals determined by the client's response and the physician's preference. Atropine is given intramuscularly before treatment to decrease secretions and the possibility of vagal stimulation.

Because of the wide variability in the metabolism and effect of Indoklon, it is no longer used. ECT is seen as the safest and the most reliable method of seizure induction.

PSYCHOSURGERY

Psychosurgery is the selective surgical removal or destruction of nerve pathways or normal brain tissue to influence behavior.[51a] Psychosurgery is also a legal term defined as the practice of destroying brain tissue of psychiatric clients.

The prefrontal lobotomy, rarely done today, severs the fibers connecting the frontal lobe with the hypothalamus. It was initially considered to separate thought from emotion. The original purpose of the prefrontal lobotomy was remedial treatment for deteriorated clients placed on psychiatric unit back wards because they had not responded to any other form of therapy. It was also developed in a desperate attempt to treat schizophrenia. Potentially serious side effects are related to this procedure, including intellectual and emotional impairment, personality changes demonstrated by flattened affect and emotional withdrawal, incontinence, and some metabolic disorders.[12]

Current psychosurgery, sometimes referred to as psychiatric surgery, is the neurosurgical treatment of an extremely severe mental disorder and is indicated only after all other treatment alternatives have been exhausted. Procedures today are more localized, refined, elaborate, and less destructive and have more precise results.

Because of inadequate understanding of neurological processes and the absence of scientific evidence of the effectiveness or long-term side effects of psychosurgery, it is subject to the strictest legal and ethical scrutiny.[13] Informed consent is a problem in general surgery, and this problem of understanding is compounded when the affected organ is responsible for the cognitive process in an informed consent. It is not uncommon for the next of kin to be asked to give their permission for surgery. Activist groups advocate strong controls for elimination of psychosurgery, because without discretion it can be used to control the behavior of social dissidents. They believe this technique can lead to medical abuses under the label of "therapy," and alternative behavioral intervention strategies may never be attempted. This is a legitimate concern for everyone, because with the capacity to control behavior there is an inherent potential to misuse it. Psychosurgery will remain a controversial subject.

INSULIN COMA THERAPY

Insulin coma therapy was used originally for clients with eating and weight problems, severe agitation, and some neurological disorders. Later, observers noted that many psychotic clients, particularly newly diagnosed schizophrenic clients, improved following the comotose state produced by the insulin. Insulin therapy produces

sedative effects and rebuilds physical health. Clients responding positively felt a sense of freedom and expression; others became quiet and withdrawn. This treatment is no longer used because of the careful monitoring required and lack of evidence of its effectiveness.

HYDROTHERAPY

There are various forms of *hydrotherapy*—the use of water to achieve a therapeutic and tranquilizing effect. These techniques are used infrequently today, but two of the most common types—the wet sheet pack and the continuous tub bath—are discussed here.

A cold, wet sheet pack is applied to treat tension, agitation, and insomnia. It is indicated for drugless tranquilization. When the body is abruptly cooled, its immediate reaction is to contract cutaneous blood vessels. It is thought that the energy expended leaves the client with a feeling of lethargy, substantially decreasing restlessness and agitation and producing an overall feeling of drowsiness.

The continuous tub bath is also used to treat an agitated, hyperactive client. This treatment is 2 to 10 hours long, during which the client is continuously observed. The client is suspended in a hammock, head supported by a pillow, while he is submerged from shoulders down in continuously running water. The bath temperature ranges from 92° to 96° F. A canvas cover with an opening for the head and neck is applied over the tub to help maintain a constant temperature and to increase the overall therapeutic effectiveness.

NARCOTHERAPY

Narcotherapy is the intravenous administration of sedatives or stimulants to produce a physiological state conducive to therapeutic change. The very slow intravenous injection of Sodium Pentothal, amobarbital (Amytal), or in some cases methylphenidate (Ritalin) relaxes or stimulates the client to become more amenable to psychotherapeutic intervention.

An intravenous infusion of a 5% dextrose solution in water is started to make a vein accessible for injection. A physician administers the drug in the amount required to facilitate the client's responsiveness to the interview. During the procedure traumatic events are reexperienced, and the unconscious emotions associated with the events are expressed. Interpretation of information about traumatic or repressed experiences assists the treatment team as they formulate appropriate intervention strategies.

Narcotherapy is frequently used only once, although it may be used in a series. Sedatives are generally most effective with psychotic individuals; clients with repressed trauma or amnesia respond best to stimulants.

PHYSICAL RESTRAINTS

Physical restraints, usually leather straps, immobilize the client who cannot control aggressive impulses and who is potentially dangerous to himself or others. Restraints are applied only when there is sufficient risk of harm and when alternative means have been unsuccessful. Restraint apparatus is applied only under the supervision of a registered nurse and with a physician's order.

Behaviors considered clinical justification for restraints are the following:

1. Accelerated motor activity

2. Physical assault to self, others, and environment
3. Physical and verbal threats
4. Hyperresponsiveness to environmental stimuli

Clients demonstrating these behaviors are considered potentially suicidal or homicidal and are psychiatric emergencies. Immediate intervention is needed to prevent harm to themselves or others. Restraints are not for pun-

---

REPORT ON SECLUSION OR RESTRAINTS

Date

Care and observation code:

1 Order written/received	11 Range-of-motion exercises	21 Singing
2 In 4-point restraints	12 Medication given	22 Mumbling incoherently
3 Out of 4-point restraints	13 Meal served	23 Quiet
4 In seclusion	14 Fluids offered	24 Sleeping
5 Out of seclusion	15 Toilet offered	25 Disrobing
6 Dangerous objects removed	16 Yelling/screaming	26 Quarreling
7 1 to 1 observation	17 Crying	27 Beating door
8 Restraints removed	18 Cursing	28 Walking
9 Massage to extremities	19 Threatening	29 Standing still
10 Circulation check	20 Laughing	30 Lying or sitting

Checks made on client—code and initial

12:01 AM	6:00 AM	12:00 PM	6:00 PM
12:15 AM	6:15 AM	12:15 PM	6:15 PM
12:30 AM	6:30 AM	12:30 PM	6:30 PM
12:45 AM	6:45 AM	12:45 PM	6:45 PM
1:00 AM	7:00 AM	1:00 PM	7:00 PM
1:15 AM	7:15 AM	1:15 PM	7:15 PM
1:30 AM	7:30 AM	1:30 PM	7:30 PM
1:45 AM	7:45 AM	1:45 PM	7:45 PM
2:00 AM	8:00 AM	2:00 PM	8:00 PM
2:15 AM	8:15 AM	2:15 PM	8:15 PM
2:30 AM	8:30 AM	2:30 PM	8:30 PM
2:45 AM	8:45 AM	2:45 PM	8:45 PM
3:00 AM	9:00 AM	3:00 PM	9:00 PM
3:15 AM	9:15 AM	3:15 PM	9:15 PM
3:30 AM	9:30 AM	3:30 PM	9:30 PM
3:45 AM	9:45 AM	3:45 PM	9:45 PM
4:00 AM	10:00 AM	4:00 PM	10:00 PM
4:15 AM	10:15 AM	4:15 PM	10:15 PM
4:30 AM	10:30 AM	4:30 PM	10:30 PM
4:45 AM	10:45 AM	4:45 PM	10:45 PM
5:00 AM	11:00 AM	5:00 PM	11:00 PM
5:15 AM	11:15 AM	5:15 PM	11:15 PM
5:30 AM	11:30 AM	5:30 PM	11:30 PM
5:45 AM	11:45 AM	5:45 PM	11:45 PM

Name	Initial	Name	Initial	Name	Initial

FIGURE 23-1 General observations are coded from 1 to 30 at the top of the flow sheet. The nurse documents her observations by number in the appropriate time period.

ishment or retaliation or to free staff members from having to observe a client.

Continuous supervision is necessary during restraint to prevent untoward effects, such as suffocation or injury to an extremity. Restraints are applied only in a horizontal line—that is, to both hands and both feet. Cross-restraints (one arm and the opposite leg or one arm and leg on the same side) are extremely dangerous and unacceptable.

Because the use of restraints is an emotionally charged subject, its justification needs to be clearly documented in the progress and nursing notes. Documentation includes the type of device and length of time the restraint was in place. Many facilities have restraint flow sheets to ensure adequate documentation (Figure 23-1). A physician's written order is needed for this treatment.

To be effective, restraint is done quickly and efficiently. An adequate number of staff members are needed to restrain a client in a professional manner so that his dignity is maintained and he is managed without injury to himself or staff members. Each member of the team needs to have specific responsibilities. Restraints need to always be readily accessible and in working order. The method of restraint is practiced in advance to ensure that it can be done with ease. It is never assumed that the client understands the reason for restraint. The nurse informs him that restraints are applied because he is unable to control his behavior; he is supported and reassured that the restraints will be removed as soon as he is able to regain control of his behavior. Restraints are padded to prevent skin breakdown and restriction of circulation. The client is positioned in anatomical alignment. Medication is often administered and the client informed that it is to help him feel better. Privacy is maintained, but the client is not left alone; he is talked to to avoid the impression that he is being punished or abused. Vital signs are checked and extremities observed for any circulatory impairment. Restraints are removed for 5 minutes at least every 2 hours, the extremity is massaged, and range-of-motion exercises are permitted. Fluids are offered, and the client is fed if restrained during mealtime. The client is permitted to use the bathroom.

SECLUSION

Seclusion confines a client to a single room. The door may be locked or unlocked. There may be minimal furnishings and a limited opportunity for communication with others. Seclusion promotes therapeutic limit setting by providing security, ego boundaries, and external controls for behavior until the client regains self-control. Containment, structure, and support are the essential functions of seclusion. It is an appropriate method for controlling behavior, especially when a client has been destructive to the physical environment, is hyperactive, or has been increasingly agitated by environmental stimuli (Figure 23-2).

Seclusion is not indicated for those who are actively suicidal and require one-to-one intervention. Potentially suicidal clients; when left secluded, may harm themselves. It also is not indicated for clients who attempt to gain recognition and attention for misbehavior and view seclu-

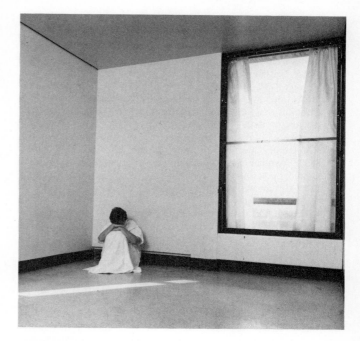

FIGURE 23-2 A seclusion room.

sion as a reward. Secluded clients may regress or become confused because of the lack of sensory stimulation.

When a client is put in seclusion, the procedure is carried out as that for the restrained client. Secluding an individual is done quickly and efficiently, with a concern for the client's dignity and value as a person. The room is prepared in advance and the purpose of seclusion explained. Potentially dangerous clothing or possessions are removed, and the client is observed continually. Food and fluids are provided, and bathroom use is permitted. Medication also is given if the seclusion is to calm the client. The nurse suggests socially acceptable behavior in a supportive, nurturing manner and helps him regain internal control of thoughts, feelings, and behavior.

The nurse documents the incident precipitating a client's seclusion and records the client's response, length of seclusion, and all nursing care given during seclusion.

BRIEF REVIEW

Somatic therapies gained widespread recognition in the 1930s with the introduction of ECT. Other somatic therapies, such as Indoklon therapy, insulin coma therapy, psychosurgery, hydrotherapy, and narcotherapy, gradually became available for treatment of psychiatric illnesses. ECT continues to be an effective treatment for depressed clients. Indoklon therapy and insulin coma therapy are no longer used. As knowledge of the brain expands and research continues, psychosurgery may be revived as a treatment modality for psychiatric disorders. Hydrotherapy and narcotherapy continue to be effective modalities, helping clients to relax and deal with emotional trauma. Restraints and seclusion are useful when clients lose control and are potentially dangerous to themselves or others.

REFERENCES AND SUGGESTED READINGS

1. Baradell, J.G.: Humanistic care of the patient in seclusion, Journal of Psychosocial Nursing 25(2):8, 1985.

2. Bartlett, J.R., and Bridges, P.K.: Psychosurgery: yesterday and today, British Journal of Psychiatry 131:249, 1977.

3. Benson, D.F., and others: The long-term effects of prefrontal leukotomy, Archives of Neurology 38:165, 1981.

4. Cochran, C.C.: Change of mind about ECT, American Journal of Nursing 84(8):1004, 1984.

5. Corkin, S.A.: Prospective study of cingulotomy. In Valenstein, E.S., editor: The psychosurgery debate, San Francisco, 1980, W.H. Freeman & Co., Publishers.

6. Cowley, P.N.: An investigation of patients' attitudes toward ECT by means of a Q analysis, Psychological Medicine 15(1):131, 1985.

7. Crowe, R.R.: Current concepts of electroconvulsive therapy: a current perspective, New England Journal of Medicine 311(3):163, 1984.

8. Evans, B.M., Bridges, P.K., and Bartlett, J.R.: Electroencephalographic changes as prognostic indicators after psychosurgery, Journal of Neurology, Neurosurgery and Psychiatry 44:444, 1981.

9. Fraser, R.M.: ECT: a clinical guide, New York, 1982, John Wiley & Sons, Inc.

10. Fraser, R.M., and Glass, I.B.: Recovery from ECT in elderly patients, British Journal of Psychiatry 133:524, 1978.

11. Fraser, R.M., and Glass, I.B.: Unilateral and bilateral ECT in elderly patients: a comparative study, Acta Psychiatrica Scandinavica 62:13, 1980.

12. Gorman, W.F.: Psychosurgery: government regulating medicine, Arizona Medicine 38:275, 1981.

13. Gostin, L.O.: Ethical consideration of psychosurgery: the unhappy legacy of the prefrontal lobotomy, Journal of Medical Ethics 6(3):149, 1980.

14. Grahame-Smith, D.G.: The neuropharmacological effects of electroconvulsive therapy in depression, Advances in Biochemical Psychopharmacology 39:327, 1984.

15. Hoffman, B.F.: Electroconvulsive therapy: a current view (editorial), 130(9):1123, 1984.

16. Holcomb, H.H., and others: Effects of electroconvulsive therapy on mood, Parkinsonism and tardive dyskinesia in a depressed patient: ECT and dopamine systems, Biological Psychiatry 18(8):865, 1983.

17. Janicak, P.G., and others: Efficacy of ECT: a meta-analysis, American Journal of Psychiatry 142(3):297, 1985.

18. Kalayam, B., and others: A survey of attitudes on the use of electroconvulsive therapy, Hospital and Community Psychiatry 32(3):185, 1981.

19. Kalinowsky, L.B.: The convulsive therapies. In Freedman, A.M., and Kaplan, H.I., editors: Comprehensive textbook of psychiatry, vol. 2, ed. 2, Baltimore, 1975, The Williams & Wilkins Co.

20. Karlinsky, H., and others: The clinical use of electroconvulsive therapy in old age, Journal of the American Geriatrics Society 32(3):183, 1984.

21. Keefe, D.: Development of care for the mentally ill, Physiotherapy 66:407, 1980.

22. Kendell, R.E.: The contribution of ECT to the treatment of affective disorders. In Palmer, R.L., editor: ECT: an appraisal, Oxford, 1981, Oxford University Press.

22a. Kendrick, D., and Wilber, G.: Seclusion: organizing safe and effective care, Journal of Psychosocial Nursing and Mental Health 24(11):26, 1986.

23. Kilok, L.G., and Aust, N.Z.: Non-pharmocological biological treatments of psychiatric patients, Journal of Psychiatry 17(3):215, 1983.

24. Kramer, P.M., and others: The Clarke Institute experience with electroconvulsive therapy. I. Development of a clinical audit procedure, Canadian Journal of Psychiatry 29(8):648, 1984.

25. Lambourn, J.: Is cognitive impairment one of the therapeutic ingredients of ECT? In Palmer, R.L., editor: ECT: an appraisal, Oxford, 1981, Oxford University Press.

26. Lepage, D., and others: Procedure for ECT: toward a more rational use of ECT, Union Medicale d   Canada 109(9):1262, 1980.

27. Lerer, B.: Electroconvulsive shock and neurotransmitter receptors: implications for mechanisms of action and adverse effects of electroconvulsive therapy, Biological Psychiatry 19(3):361, 1984.

28. Lerer, B., and others: Receptors and the mechanism of action of ECT, Biological Psychiatry 17(4):497, 1982.

29. Lerer, B., and others: Effect of vasopressin on memory following ECT, Biological Psychiatry 18(7):821, 1983.

30. Lesser, H.J.: Consent competency and ECT: a philosopher's comment, Journal of Medical Ethics 9(3):144, 1983.

31. Major, L.G.: Electroconvulsive therapy in the 1980's, Psychiatric Clinics of North America 7(3):613, 1984.

32. Maletzky, B.: Multiple monitored electroconvulsive therapy, Boca Raton, Fla, 1981, CRC Press, Inc.

33. Malitz, S., Sackheim, H.A., and Decina, P.: ECT in the treatment of major affective disorders: clinical and basic research issues, Psychiatric Journal of the University of Ottawa 7:126, 1982.

34. Martin, B.A., and others: The Clarke Institute experience with ECT. II. Treatment evaluation and standards of practice, Canadian Journal of Psychiatry 29(8):652, 1984.

35. Mauk, S.: Surprising truths about shock treatment, Cosmopolitan, November, p. 230, 1981.

36. Mielke, D.H., and others: Multiple monitored ECT safety and efficacy in elderly depressed patients, Journal of the American Geriatrics Society 32(3):180, 1984.

37. Misik, I.: About using restraints—with restraint, Nursing '81 11(8):50, 1981.

38. Parry, B.L.: The tragedy of legal impediments involved in obtaining ECT for patients unable to give informed consent (letter), American Journal of Psychiatry 138(8);1128, 1981.

39. Pettinati, H.M., and others: Cognitive functioning in depressed geriatric patients with a history of ECT, American Journal of Psychiatry 141(1):49, 1984.

39a. Phillips, P., and Nasr, S.: Seclusion and restraint and prediction of violence, American Journal of Psychiatry 140(2): 229, 1983.

40. Pisarcik, G.: Facing the violent patient, Nursing '81 11:61, 1981.

41. Price, R.: Hydrotherapy in England 1840-70, Medical History 25:269, 1981.

42. Roper, J.M., and others: Restraints and seclusion, Journal of Psychosocial Nursing 23(6):18, 1985.

43. Runck, B.: ECT: assuring benefits and minimizing risks, Hospital and Community Psychiatry 34(5):409, 1983.

44. Schmidt, D., and Schorsch, E.: Psychosurgery of sexually deviant patients: review and analysis of new empirical findings, Archives of Sexual Behavior 10:301, 1981.

45. Scovern, A.W., and others: Status of ECT: review of the outcome literature, Psychological Bulletin 87(2):260, 1980.

46. Soloff, P., and others: Seclusion and restraint in 1985: a review and update, Hospital and Community Psychiatry, 36(6):652, 1985.

46a. Swinton, W.E.: The hydrotherapy and infamy of Dr. James Gully, Canadian Medical Association Journal 123:1262, 1980.

47. Task Force on Psychiatric Uses of Seclusion and Restraint, Task Force Report no. 22, Washington, D.C., American Psychiatric Association, 1985.

47a. Talbot, K.: ECT: exploring myths, examining attitudes, Journal of Psychosocial Nursing and Mental Health Services **24**(3):6, 1986.

47b. Taylor, P.: ECT: the preliminary report of a trial in schizophrenic patients. In Palmer, R.L., editor: ECT: an appraisal, Oxford, 1981, Oxford University Press.

48. Taylor, P.G.: Consent competency and ECT: a psychiatrist's view, Journal of Medical Ethics **9**(3):146, 1983.

49. Weeks, D., Freeman, C.P.L. and Kendell, R.E.: Does ECT produce enduring cognitive deficits? In Palmer, R.L., editor: ECT: an appraisal, Oxford, 1981, Oxford University Press.

50. Weiner, R.D., and Power, D.G.: The use of ECT within the Veterans Administration hospital system, Comprehensive Psychiatry **21**:23, 1980.

51. Wexler, D.: Seclusion and restraint: lessons from law, psychiatry, and psychology, International Journal of Law and Psychiatry, **5**:285, 1982.

51a. W.H.O. Collaborative Center for Psychopharmacology in India: I. Reevaluation of ECT in schizophrenia. II. Reevaluation of ECT in depression, Psychopharmacology Bulletin **19**(3):550, 1983.

ANNOTATED BIBLIOGRAPHY

Fraser, M.: ECT: a clinical guide, New York, 1982, John Wiley & Sons

The efficacy of ECT is presented, and the indications are outlined. Legal guidelines and issues are also discussed.

Talbot, K.: ECT: exploring myths, examining attitudes, Journal of Psychosocial Nursing **24**(3):6 1986.

Myths about ECT perpetuated by clients and health care professionals are addressed. The article also discusses current concepts and treatment approaches.

CHAPTER 24

MILIEU THERAPY

Judith A. Saifnia

After studying this chapter the learner will be able to:

Define milieu therapy.

Describe the historical background of milieu therapy.

Discuss productive and nonproductive characteristics of nurses working in a therapeutic milieu.

Utilize the nursing process to provide a therapeutic milieu for care.

Identify methods for evaluating therapeutic milieu.

Two major approaches to establishing a therapeutic treatment environment have been developed: the therapeutic community and milieu therapy. Although many of the treatment strategies used in these two approaches are the same, some distinction can be made based on the specificity and philosophy of these two frameworks.

The *therapeutic community* is a structured environment with a specific philosophy of care. The focus is on health rather than illness. The client is regarded as a responsible member of a social group. The treatment setting is viewed as a community of both staff and clients. All members interact democratically to achieve therapeutic outcomes. The goal of this approach is the development of insight into behavior through feedback received from the whole population of clients and staff.[16]

A more comprehensive term, *milieu therapy,* refers to the scientific planning of an environment for therapeutic purposes. The key is planned use of the environment. Specific milieu factors and social interactions are structured to form a total treatment approach. The goal of this approach is the development of social and emotional skills that will be beneficial in everyday life.[16]

The difference between these two approaches is one of emphasis. Although the goal of the therapeutic community is insight, the desired end result is improvement in behavior. Likewise, to achieve the behavioral changes desired in the milieu therapy setting, evaluation of thoughts and feelings is often incorporated. Because of this overlap and the resulting confusion, Herz[25] suggested that the broader term of *therapeutic milieu* be used to describe all milieu treatment approaches. *Milieu* is a French word meaning environment or setting. Therapeutic milieu refers to the general setting where treatment occurs, regardless of the philosophy of treatment. The specific goals and treatment strategies for each treatment environment are specified to serve as criteria for evaluation of effectiveness.

In this chapter the terms milieu therapy and therapeutic milieu are used interchangeably. Therapeutic community is used to refer to the classical approach developed by Jones.[31]

To examine the multifaceted dimensions of a psychiatric treatment environment, a holistic approach that synthesizes information from various fields is necessary. Such an approach is based on the view that personal and environmental factors interact to determine behavior, that individual behavior cannot be predicted based on personal factors alone, and that environmental factors need to be considered as well.

Historically, the domestic service pattern and the medical intervention pattern have been the theoretical models used in providing a therapeutic milieu. The approach currently in use in psychiatric settings is the *social interaction pattern.*

Contributions were made to this chapter by Becky Lancaster, R.N., M.S.N.

Historical Overview

DATE	EVENT
Late 1700s	Pinel coined the term "moral treatment" to describe his new approach to psychiatric care, which included removing chains, using accepting attitudes, and setting examples of appropriate behavior and humanitarianism.
Early 1800s	Tuke established the York Retreat based on an atmosphere of kindness, meaningful employment of time, regular exercise, a family environment, and treatment of clients as guests.
Late 1800s	The predominant service pattern in psychiatric institutions was the domestic service pattern in which care was custodial and the staff performed essentially housekeeping tasks.
Early 1900s	Attention to hospital atmosphere declined, resulting in the development of environments that were benignly custodial or more destructively controlling, much like a prison.
1930	Sullivan[56] began to experiment again with varying the treatment milieu by selecting staff members who were sympathetic and interacted well with psychotic clients.
1939	Menninger[43] developed "prescribed" attitudes based on psychoanalytic principles that determined staff interaction patterns.
1940s	The predominant service pattern was the medical intervention pattern in which staff, including nurses, served as the physician's agents in providing care.
1946	Main[39] coined the term "therapeutic community" to describe the approach of resocialization of neurotic individuals through social interactions.
1948	Bettleheim[5] coined the term "milieu therapy" to describe his use of the total environment for treatment of disturbed children.
1953	Jones[31] used the therapeutic community approach in two experimental units for the treatment of antisocial personality disorders in which the social environment was seen as the primary treatment modality.
1960s	All nursing personnel had an active role in maintaining a therapeutic social milieu.
1970s	Treatment environments were tailored to meet the needs of the particular population they served.
Future	The future development of milieu therapy needs to be based on research to identify the milieu structure most effective for specific treatment groups.

In the social interaction pattern, the physician, client, and staff are viewed as team members, all of whom have information valuable to the client's care. All nursing personnel, including technicians, have an active role in maintaining a therapeutic social milieu, since every interaction with the client is seen as having potentially beneficial outcomes.

The principles of the interaction pattern have been identified as follows[55]:

1. The health of each individual is to be realized and encouraged to grow.
2. Every interaction is an opportunity for therapeutic intervention.
3. The client's environment is a significant component of his treatment.
4. Each client owns his behavior.
5. Peer pressure is a useful and powerful tool.
6. Inappropriate behaviors are dealt with as they occur.
7. Restriction and punishment are avoided.

The underlying expectations of this view include an emphasis on the healthy personality, individual responsibility, positive reinforcement, and the use of the whole group for behavior control. This can be accomplished only through democratic participation.

The *democratic style* of leadership emphasizes use of resources within the group. The intent is to create a climate in which members can openly express themselves, share their diversity without fear of rejection or excessive conflict, and employ their individual skills and talents to accomplish mutual tasks.[53] The democratic leader facilitates member participation. The importance of this role in

Treatment Characteristics of Effective Psychiatric Programs

J.F. Collins, R.B. Ellsworth, N.A. Casey, R.B. Hickey & L. Hyer

PURPOSE

This study was part of a large cooperative study undertaken to identify ward characteristics that positively affect posthospital adjustment.

SAMPLE

The treatment characteristics of 79 psychiatric wards in 18 Veterans Administration hospitals were evaluated in this study. To be included each ward had to be administered by a single treatment team and admit, treat, and discharge a wide variety of clients.

METHODOLOGY

Program effectiveness was evaluated by comparing 123 treatment characteristics with four measures of posthospital adjustment. The treatment characteristics were obtained using multiple measures including data from medical and ward records, client ratings of the ward, observation of the physical environment, and client and staff responses to structured scales. Posthospital adjustment was determined from responses to the Veterans Adjustment Scale, completed by each client, and the Personal Adjustment and Role Skills Scale, completed by a cooperative significant other. The scales were administered at admission (pretreatment) and by mail 3 months after discharge (posttreatment). The follow-up forms

were returned by 41% of the clients and 30% of the significant others.

FINDINGS

The results were organized into four categories: client activities, medication practices, order and organization, and staffing patterns. More effective programs had a lower percentage of socially passive clients and a higher percentage of clients off the ward. Prescribing antipsychotic medications for neurotic clients at discharge and prescribing antianxiety medications in larger than average dosages were negatively related to program effectiveness. Higher than average scores of order and organization were negatively related to program outcome. Frequent rotation of nursing staff to different shifts characterized the least effective programs.

IMPLICATIONS

This study indicates that programs that deliberately involve clients in a more active role are more effective. This includes promoting activity and interaction even though it may result in less order and organization, giving lower doses of medication so that clients can be more alert, and providing a stable staff who can play a more responsible role in monitoring clients' social and therapeutic activities.

Based on data from Hospital and Community Psychiatry 35(6):601, 1984.

---

promoting positive client outcomes was demonstrated in the study by Collins and others cited in the Research Highlight above.

Devine[18] asserted that as milieu therapy becomes more popular as a significant aspect of client care, nurses have even more opportunity to "take initiative in organizing effective therapies." Holmes and Werner[28] described this role as follows:

. . .an exciting adventure, marked by loss of traditional nursing roles, blurring of roles of all disciplines, increased responsibility for therapy on the part of both patients and staff, more intense staff-patient relationships, and a whole complex of problems for nursing that we are just beginning to explore.

This new adventure is not without anxiety and uncertainty; however, the nurse is able as never before to contribute to efficient social milieu functioning and therapeutic effectiveness.

CHARACTERISTICS OF MILIEU THERAPY

The concept of milieu therapy developed from a desire to counteract the negative, regressive effects of institu-

tionalization: reduced ability to think and act independently, an adoption of institutional values and attitudes, and loss of commitments in the outside world.[56]

Several strategies have been developed to counter the negative effects of institutionalization. These strategies include distribution of power, open communication, structured interactions, work-related activities, community and family involvement in the treatment process, and adaptation of the environment to meet developmental needs.

Distribution of Power

The milieu therapy approach involves "flattening" the control hierarchy so that all participants have a voice in decision making. Decisions are made according to the democratic process in client government meetings. The decision-making process may include the whole population of the treatment unit, or a governing council may make the final decisions based on input from various smaller groups of clients and staff members.

There is much discussion in the literature about how "flat" the hierarchy of decision making needs to be. On one hand it can be argued that a unilateral decision, no matter how wise, is contrary to the therapeutic community philosophy. On the other hand, some clients have regressed too much to participate in decision making. Staff in many treatment settings subscribe to the belief that clients are capable of decision making but act as if clients are not, creating an antitherapeutic double-bind situation.[52] Bell and Ryan,[3] in a study conducted on three different psychiatric settings in a Veterans Administration Medical Center, found that staff values may conflict with therapeutic community ideals. For example, staff felt responsible for controlling client behavior and intervening in decision-making processes while the values of the milieu were directed more at staff supporting independent decision making by clients. It appears that the best way to resolve this dilemma is through identifying a program's treatment goals and relating autonomous decision making to these goals. In any social structure, decisions need to be made at the places in which they can most effectively achieve the goals of that structure. For example, if the goal of a unit is short-term intensive treatment of severely disturbed individuals, many decisions involve medical intervention. The physician logically makes these decisions. On the other end of the continuum, if the goal of the treatment setting is to provide service to clients who remain in the community in productive social roles, the clients may make most of the treatment decisions.

The ultimate goal of any treatment program is client autonomy. This may be achieved through a stepwise progression from one treatment program to the next or by gradually increasing independence within a given program. Consciously incorporating a plan for increasing independence is a means of achieving the goal of client autonomy.

Open Communication

Although the importance of open communication has been widely recognized in the literature, it is still not a reality in many settings. Some of the reasons for this lie in the insecurity of persons in authority. Open communication requires risk taking. Questioning and criticism of a message may be threatening, whereas there is little to risk if no feedback is allowed.

In the traditional medical model of intervention, all information is directed up the hierarchy to the physician, who makes the decisions. These decisions are then passed down in the form of edicts. Information about a client's background and problems are considered "confidential," meaning that only the physician has the right to that information.

In the therapeutic milieu, treatment decisions are often made by the clients themselves, thus it is necessary for them to have information to make effective decisions. Although it is not necessary to communicate personal information, clients and staff need to have knowledge of individual treatment goals to ensure that everyone is working toward the same goals. In this atmosphere, more exclusive confidentiality is replaced by mutual trust, honesty, and open communication.

The development of open communication is difficult at times. Cultural norms, personal defenses, and established communication patterns all serve to block communications, so that opening communication channels requires taking risks and learning new patterns of expression. All members of the health care team need to work together to provide a safe atmosphere for this to occur.

Structured Interactions

K.A. Menninger[42] pioneered the concept of structured interaction patterns in the form of attitude therapy. The attitudes he prescribed are described in Table 24-1.

An advantage of structured interaction approach is that all staff members approach the client in a consistent manner that acknowledges specific diagnostic areas, thereby shortening treatment time. The difficulty with this approach is that once a diagnosis is made and an attitude prescribed there is little flexibility in the interaction pattern. Day-to-day fluctuations in the client's condition may not be accounted for, and staff members sometimes seem stilted in their responses to clients.

Currently, a behavioral intervention technique is used in many settings. Problem behaviors rather than a global interaction pattern are identified, and individual approaches are specified. For example, a client with a bipolar disorder may display several problem behaviors. In the manic phase of illness he may talk excessively, interrupt

TABLE 24-1 Approaches used in attitude therapy

Attitude	Description
Indulgence	Extremely flexible; all reasonable requests are granted and divergence from expected behavior is accepted
Active friendliness	Staff take the initiative in interactions and show special interest in the client
Passive friendliness	Staff allow the client to take the initiative in interactions; staff convey the message that they are available, but they wait for the client to approach before responding
Matter-of-factness	Suggests an element of casualness in interactions, especially regarding requests, pleas, or manipulative maneuvers; emotional responses and reassurance are avoided
Watchfulness	Observation is continuous either openly or unobtrusively, as the situation indicates.
Kind firmness	Approach is direct, clear, confident; rules and regulations are calmly cited in response to infractions and requests; directions are specific and concise with the expectation that they will be followed

the activity of others, and constantly move about. These behaviors are best managed with a kind, firm approach that sets limits and directs the client's energy into productive activity. On the other hand, during the depressive phase he may be withdrawn and passive. By using an active friendly approach, staff members make contact with him and encourage interaction and activity.

The behavioral intervention technique has several advantages over traditional attitude therapy. Specific behaviors can be targeted for change, and plans can accommodate fluctuations in the client's condition by indicating specific approaches for each behavior. Also, staff members can be more spontaneous in their interactions, basing their responses on current conditions. It may be useful to write a contract that further defines client and staff responsibility in reaching goals.

Work-Related Activities

Milieu treatment programs include work-related activities as a part of the treatment process, but the current focus of these activities is on benefits to the client rather than to the agency. Work under realistic circumstances and for appropriate rewards is probably the best central activity for all clients. Sheltered workshops and martial arts therapy provide opportunities for this type of work.

Several factors contribute to effective work therapy programs. First, clients need to choose the type of work that they wish to perform. Second, work activities are more meaningful when they are geared toward developing skills that will be useful in actual job situations. Also, a variety of activities provides the opportunity to try out different work-related areas to determine future job interests.[22]

Community and Family Involvement

The concept of the community mental health center emerged with the advent of more effective medications for behavioral control and more humane treatment philosophies. Hospitalization is only considered desirable for extreme disorders. For easy accessibility, mental health centers are placed conveniently within the surrounding neighborhood.

According to the milieu treatment approach, clients are kept in their usual environment and continue most of their routine activities while receiving treatment. An attempt is made to involve all family members in the treatment process; if one member is hospitalized, an attempt is made to continue family involvement. Visits to the hospital, home passes for the client, and family therapy sessions offer increased opportunity for all involved to practice newly acquired interaction patterns while staff members are available for support. Discharge is also coordinated with the family. Some treatment units have extended the concept of family involvement to admitting the entire family to the hospital for treatment (for example, families in which there is child abuse). This may be considered radical; however, it is effective in improving family interaction and minimizing the isolation that results from hospitalizing one family member.

Adaptation of the Environment to Meet Developmental Needs

For an individual to develop his full potential, he must have an environment adapted to his current needs. The extension of the concept of milieu therapy to all age groups and the inclusion of entire families with individuals of varying ages within the treatment milieu present a challenge to adapt the environment to meet these multiple needs.

Children. The most apparent environmental change necessary to accommodate children is a change in size of furnishings. Beds, chairs, tables, dressers, and play equipment that are designed for changing sizes facilitate a positive relationship with the environment and encourage activity and exploration.

Initially infants appear to respond better to black-and-white designs and patterns than to colors.[2] As they mature, they recognize brighter colors first, with contrasting colors being more easily comprehended.

Meaningful sound is important, even to a newborn. The most valuable sound is that of human voices directed to the child.[2] Excessive sound is harmful to concentration, whereas total acoustic dampening results in sensory deprivation.

Play equipment is important for children because toys can counteract sensory deprivation, relieve tension and feelings of hostility and aggression, and provide an avenue to "work through" problems and conflicts.[7] Blocks, puzzles, and games, as well as crayons, paint, chalk, clay, scissors, and paper encourage skill development and creative self-expression. Chapters 39 and 40 give useful suggestions for enhancing the milieu of infants and children.

Adolescents. One of the major needs of the adolescent population is a communal area for interaction with peers. Sound dampening in this area is important but should not be so great as to diminish sensory input. Soft surfaces and malleable furnishings, such as beanbag chairs, accommodate adolescents who often sit on the floor or in odd positions on furniture. Other accommodations include stereo systems, advanced creative materials such as oil paint and canvas, games and cards appropriate to their level, and sports equipment to encourage expenditure of excess energy. Individual bulletin boards encourage the display of personal items; soft drinks and simple foods promote social interaction; and participation in food preparation encourages responsibility.

Adults. Differences in the amount of responsibility that need to be granted to various types of psychiatric clients have been identified. Thus an individualized treatment approach is necessary. Clients (adults or children) who have regressed more or who are overwhelmed need more structure and support; other clients benefit from a program that promotes autonomy and responsibility. A program that provides a stepwise progression with gradual increases in responsibility would be an effective solution.

One approach divides clients into small groups according to their developmental needs. More regressed clients are placed in a group focusing on physical and safety needs, and more advanced individuals concentrate on social, esteem, and self-actualizing needs. Individuals progress to more advanced levels as their needs indicate.

While more research is needed in this area, these approaches suggest several possibilities for varying the treatment program to meet changing needs.

Aged persons. Environmental alterations that promote safety and orientation are of primary importance for the aged. Adequate lighting, nonskid surfaces, color coding of doorways, and curved mirrors at junctions can greatly assist the elderly to safely maintain orientation and mobility. Yellow-green color vision is retained the longest; therefore steps and protrusions such as doorknobs can be marked with stripes of these colors to promote safety.[2]

Diminished visual ability requires the use of brighter colors and 25% more illumination.[2] This can be provided by natural light, additional reading lights, and indirect nonglare artificial lighting. The aged have less ability to accommodate sudden increases in light; therefore windows need to be well shaded and artificial lighting placed on a rheostat system so that gradual brightening and dimming are possible.

Older individuals have a decreased ability to distinguish meaningful sound. The hum of heating, ventilating, air-conditioning systems, refrigerator units, toilets, and other appliances can be modified to dampen this background sound. Rather than increasing the volume on televisions, radios, and sound systems, earphones may be used to improve hearing without increasing environmental noise.

Often contact with the outside world is limited; therefore special attempts are made to improve input. Windows are valuable in maintaining visual contact with the outside world, and the weather provides a common topic of conversation. For those who are bedridden the ceiling can be treated as a fifth wall and designed to enhance sensory input. Entrance hallways and other hubs of activity such as nurses' stations provide needed social contact. Furniture arrangements that provide face-to-face contact or round table discussions promote social interaction.

The location of the facility used by the elderly is especially important. It is most desirable for the elderly to remain in familiar neighborhoods so that they feel safer and have an established support system. However, a once-supportive neighborhood may deteriorate. Friends and family relocate or die, crime may increase, and neighborhood shops may change hands. These factors, as well as deteriorating health, can force relocation. New surroundings need to provide opportunities to replace the social network that was left behind, and transportation needs to be provided to maintain old ties.[54]

Settin[54] contended that perceived control over the impinging environment is the most important factor in maintaining the physical and emotional status of the elderly. Freedom of choice, appropriate sensory stimulation, physical activity, social interaction, meaningful activity, and social status contribute to a sense of control and environmental mastery.

CHARACTERISTICS OF THE MILIEU THERAPIST

In the interaction pattern of milieu therapy a great deal of role blurring occurs, because any individual, including the client, can assume a leadership position. Some people work well in this environment while others are threatened by the lack of structure (see Table 24-2).

NURSING PROCESS

The physical, intellectual, and social aspects of the environment interact in contributing to the emotional atmosphere. Therefore the order of the dimensions has been changed in this chapter to provide a more logical flow of information.

Assessment

Physical dimension. The physical aspects of the treatment environment include all concrete features of the external world. These features, which set the stage on which human behavior is acted out, include the organization, structure, and interaction of many spatial features. The study of this interrelationship is called proxemics and is subdivided into three aspects: fixed feature space, semifixed feature space, and informal space.[22] (See Chapter 5.)

Fixed feature space. The internal and external design of a building and its relationship to other buildings and environmental factors constitute the "fixed" or permanent elements in space. The arrangement of these elements strongly affects interactions that influence therapeutic outcomes. The importance of locating the treatment facility close to the community it serves has already been mentioned. Another aspect of fixed feature space is the internal structure and dimensions of a treatment facility. To provide a humanizing environment newer hospitals provide greater privacy with smaller wards, each with bathrooms and showers, and personalized space for individual belongings (Figure 24-1).

Semifixed feature space. Objects within an environment that have some degree of mobility are regarded as semifixed. These are the "props" that promote a certain degree of freedom within the limits of the stable aspects of the setting such as furniture, partitions, folding doors, and planters.

Certain furniture arrangements (such as long benches found in railway stations) tend to decrease social interaction, while others (such as tables at a sidewalk cafe) tend to pull people together. Those who sit at the corners of a table at right angles to each other tend to speak more than those sitting next to each other and more than those sitting across the table from each other.

Informal space. The category of informal space, or personal distances maintained in interpersonal encounters, is probably the most significant aspect of the use of space

TABLE 24-2 Characteristics of the milieu therapist

Productive	Nonproductive
Shares problems within a context that will benefit others	Talks about personal problems without regard to the impact on others
Recognizes the risks involved in honest communication and works to minimize these risks	Interprets openness and honesty as a license to be hurtful or vindictive
Communicates an empathic understanding of others' problems	See others' problems only in terms of own difficulties
Is warm and supportive without excessive attachment	Is rejecting or becomes overly involved with others
Accepts responsibility for own actions and admits mistakes	Blames others for mistakes and failures
Works to solve problems independently; asks for assistance when problems exceed own scope or resources	Demands attention and assistance from others for any difficulty
Is self-directed in selecting activities that contribute to organizational goals	Avoids work and responsibility and relies on others for direction
Believes that others enjoy work and responsibility when given the opportunity to participate in goal setting	Believes that others need to be coerced and controlled to complete tasks
Sees their contribution in terms of the "whole"	Focuses only on own task
Works with others to achieve consensus in decision making	Makes unilateral decisions
Shares information at the appropriate time and with the appropriate people	Selectively communicates information for manipulative purposes
Acknowledges anxiety and uses resources to cope effectively	Becomes defensive in the face of anxiety
Seeks feedback about abilities and performance	Interprets feedback as criticism to be avoided
Has a sense of self-worth and self-respect	Is either egotistical or self-deprecating
Readily adapts to change	Resists change and works to maintain the status quo
Functions comfortably in various roles; acts as either a leader or a follower as the situation dictates	Strongly prefers one role assignment; adheres to a position of leader or follower regardless of the situation
Accepts conflicts and confrontation as normal aspects of life and handles them effectively	Avoids conflict and confrontation or becomes agitated when they occur
Believes that all people can change, grow, and function more effectively	Believes that the individual has little control over mental illness and that it is a permanent, recurring condition

for the individual (see Chapter 5). Humans, like animals, have territorial needs. They claim a certain space and defend it against intrusion. However, unlike animals' territorial needs, those of people vary and are flexible. The proper distance between persons in a group varies by culture. For example, a German may consider an entire room his private space and be offended if someone enters it.

Intellectual dimension.

Sensory features. The intellectual aspects of the environment are an extension of the physical properties; they include color, light, sound, texture, temperature, odor, and taste. The quality of the intellectual environment is determined by the amount and clarity of sensory stimulation. The number of stimuli becomes a problem at either end of the continuum—excessive stimuli (sensory overload) or lack of stimulation (sensory deprivation).

The intellectual quality of a psychiatric treatment setting is important because perceptual distortion may be part of the process of mental illness. Shapes, color, lighting, and textures need to be distinct and corridors and spaces clearly defined.

The major impact of color appears to be on arousal. For the normal individual, warm colors (red, pink, orange, yellow) tend to produce arousal, whereas cooler colors (green, aqua, blue) tend to induce relaxation and self-reflection. Based on this information it is logical to assume that blue will tranquilize an agitated client and red will stimulate a withdrawn one. However, the reverse has been shown. A manic client is often calmed by a hot color, not a cool color.[61] One explanation is that an individual prefers to be in the type of atmosphere that suits his mood. A color scheme that parallels a mood may be comforting. Therefore an agitated client may feel more at ease in a bright atmosphere, provided that there is not also overstimulating noise and activity to distract him.

In addition, variation in color is important. Rooms with different-colored walls are more interesting than a room painted all one color.[6] Variation in the intensity of color can also add interest, for example, one wall dark yellow and the other three pale yellow.

Closely related to color is lighting. Natural lighting is most beneficial. When natural light is not possible, the ar-

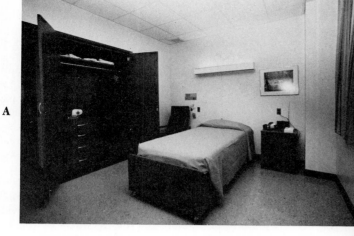
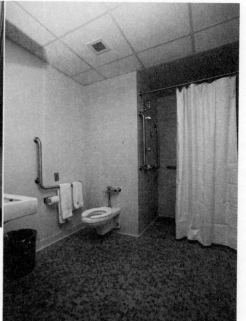

FIGURE 24-1 Personal privacy at the new John L. McClellan Memorial Hospital, North Little Rock. **A,** Private room with individual storage space. **B,** Private bathroom. (Courtesy Brian House.)

tificial lighting needs to simulate the effects of natural light, such as soft, indirect light that avoids spotlight effects. Artificial light should be balanced to contain the full spectrum of daylight color to avoid harmful effects.

Not only is the type of light important but also the duration of exposure to light. Constant light throughout the day and night can alter circadian rhythms, affecting various biological functions and emotional adjustment. Difficulty with sensory integration and orientation has been demonstrated in intensive care units with uncycled lighting.

Noise in the treatment setting is defined as unpleasant, unwanted, or intolerable sound. The sensory impact of noise is hearing loss. Besides hearing loss, high-intensity sound has social and emotional consequences. Workers continually exposed to very high–intensity noise have an increased incidence of nervous complaints, argumentativeness, sexual impotence, mood changes, and anxiety. They may also show decreased ability to perform complex tasks, reduced willingness to be neighborly, and failure to inhibit aggression. Annoyance has been found to increase as noise levels increase. Background sounds of up to 50 decibels (the level of an air conditioner) annoy only a few people. A level of 70 decibels (a vacuum cleaner) irritates a high percentage of hearers, and noise of 110 decibels (a riveting machine) is likely to bother almost everyone. While negative effects of noise were found in apparently normal individuals, respondents with psychiatric problems at the time they were surveyed were even more likely to report noise annoyance than individuals without psychiatric difficulties.[12]

Hard surfaces frequently used in hospitals reflect sound, and highly reverberant spaces add to the client's difficulty in face-to-face social relationships. Such surfaces may distort human voices or heighten the irritating qualities of sounds, making it difficult for clients to determine where a voice is coming from. A client who is facing away from a person to whom he is speaking may be merely speaking toward what he perceives as the source of the other person's voice. On the other hand, institutional spaces should not be acoustically softened so much that they eliminate all echoes.

A noisy environment has been found to increase the motor and verbal performance of withdrawn clients. Perceptual organization and sleep patterns are also improved, allowing for medication reduction.[50] The reverse is true for active clients. Therapeutically, one is again faced with the challenge of providing a balance of enough noise to stimulate withdrawn, depressed clients without overstimulating agitated, active clients.

Temperature control is basic to well-being. The comfort zone for greatest productivity varies from 64° to 74° Fahrenheit. There are individual differences in this preference, and the aged adult seems to tolerate cold and heat less well than do younger individuals.

Extremes in external temperature continue to affect hospital admissions. Besides increases in physical illness related to excessive heat and cold, mental illness also is affected by these extremes. Psychiatric admissions increase at the peaks of summer and winter.

Increases in schizophrenia, hypotension, depression, fatigue, confusion, headaches, hypoglycemic spells, and ataxia are related to combinations of heat and high humidity or heat and wind.[37] As knowledge of the impact of weather on body functions and mental health increases, it can be used to promote well-being.

Texture, the quality of roughness or smoothness of a material, has visual, acoustic, and tactile impacts. Visually, variations in roughness and smoothness contribute to orientation by making existing objects and surfaces distinct. Acoustically, more highly textured surfaces such as carpeting and textiles dampen noise, while smooth, hard surfaces reflect noise and cause it to reverberate. Tactilely, soft, nubby surfaces are comforting and warm, whereas hard, smooth surfaces are not.

Although soft textures have more therapeutic benefit, psychiatric treatment settings have most frequently used vinyl upholstery, metal, tile, plastic, and similar smooth materials because of their easy maintenance and durability.

Odor affects individuals both consciously and unconsciously. A strong odor may actually cause pain, whereas a pleasant odor is comforting. Long-term memory is closely connected with smell. For example, the smell of a rose can trigger memories of romantic occasions. Sexual arousal has also been linked with the partner's smell.

In the treatment setting, as elsewhere, both people and materials emit odors. The smell can be pleasant or distasteful, depending on cleanliness, disease, and other factors such as cigarette smoke. Room deodorizers used to mask these smells often have a biting, synthetic odor that can contribute to the problem rather than alleviate it. There is no substitute for cleanliness and fresh air in eliminating unpleasant odors. Heightened awareness and perceptual distortions such as olfactory hallucinations in the mentally ill make it especially important to be aware of the impact of odor in treatment settings.

Although the discussion of taste is more related to the subject of nutrition, a few points can be made in relation to the treatment setting. The mentally confused may experience perceptual distortions such as the tasting of color (*synthesia*). Although these behaviors cannot be totally controlled, an awareness of them is necessary.

Design features. Several design features can be used to promote orientation. Patterns in floor coverings and furnishings may be used to identify personal space and can serve as orientation supports to assist confused individuals in identifying their spatial relationship to others. Furniture size and arrangement can also contribute to defining personal space.

Differences in distances between visual planes need to be emphasized. For example, the distance between a balcony and the wall behind it can be made obvious by using contrasting colors, varying textures, or different lighting levels. Perceptual clarity is especially important for stairways to prevent accidents resulting from confusion.

Social dimension. One of the most significant environmental aspects to consider in relation to therapeutic milieu is the social aspect. The social system of a treatment milieu includes the roles of individual members, the organization of these roles into a social system based on leadership style, communication patterns that develop, and staff-client ratio.

The function of the caregiver is to respond to the needs of the client who is seeking assistance. Within psychiatric treatment settings the following professional caregiving roles have evolved.

A *psychiatrist* is a physician who specializes in the treatment of mental disorders. Training and certification prepare the psychiatrist for diagnosis of mental disorders and prescription of treatment, especially medications. Depending on their background and interest, some psychiatrists participate in various modes of psychotherapy such as individual, family, and group therapy. In most settings the psychiatrist is considered the leader of the treatment team.

The unique contribution of the *psychoanalyst* is the ability to perform analysis, the goal of which is complete understanding of the client's background and motivation for behavior, leading to changes in current behavior. Because both the training and the treatment by this method are very time consuming, there is less psychoanalysis practiced today than in the past.

The *clinical psychologist* contributes to the team through selection, administration, and interpretation of psychological tests. Clinical psychologists are prepared to conduct and guide research in the field of mental health, to design behavior management programs, and to conduct psychotherapy.

Psychiatric social workers deal with the social problems of the clients including family relationships, housing, financial support, and placement with community agencies. The needs of the client are determined after obtaining a detailed social history. Interventions include participation in individual, family, and group psychotherapy.

The *mental health–psychiatric nurse* performs many traditional functions such as assessment and intervention in medical problems, distribution of medications, and supervision of treatments. However, the role has been expanded to include many other functions as well. The psychiatric nurse is in charge of milieu management 24 hours a day. Every aspect of daily living is an opportunity for therapeutic intervention. Personal hygiene, meals, bedtime, social interactions, and therapy activities all provide opportunities for remedial approaches. The psychiatric nurse plans for these activities and supervises psychiatric technicians and practical nurses in delivering this care.

As an active member of the psychiatric team, the nurse contributes observations and suggestions for the planning of individual treatment, and participates in program planning. Much of the responsibility for coordination of team activity rests on the nurse.

The background and preparation of psychiatric nurses vary. The master's degree prepares the nurse for the most autonomous role, that of *clinical specialist.* The clinical specialist is trained for directing individual, group, and family therapy, as well as providing consultation and educational support to other nurses.

The role of the *practical nurse* in the psychiatric setting has not been clearly defined. In some settings it may be closely related to that of the registered nurse. In others it has more similarity to the psychiatric technician. In all cases it is directly under the supervision of the psychiatric nurse, who helps determine the practical nurse's role.

The *psychiatric technician,* also known as psychiatric assistant or aide, performs much of the direct care in many settings but has the least preparation. Psychiatric technicians function under the supervision of the nurse and assist in providing for the basic needs of clients. In addition, they often supervise leisure activities, have responsibility for maintaining a therapeutic environment, and may participate in individual and group therapy activities.

The *dietician* is concerned with the nutritional needs of the client. Besides providing attractive, nutritious meals, dieticians participate in education programs to improve eating habits and meal preparation. They also contribute to planning therapeutic intervention in food-related illnesses such as anorexia nervosa, bulimia, pica, rumination, and obesity.

The *occupational therapist* contributes significantly to remedial learning activities such as activities of daily living, the development of work tolerance, development of muscle strength and skills, resocialization, and prevocational assessment. The occupational therapist contributes much to the overall sense of well-being by assisting clients to be productive and creative.

There are many other specifically trained activity therapists in areas such as art, dance, poetry, and music who contribute to the well-being of the client by providing recreational and expressive outlets.

Housekeepers, secretaries, clerks, dietary aides, and canteen personnel contribute to the functioning of any setting and influence interactions that set the tone of the treatment milieu. The varied backgrounds and personalities of this group can add much to the richness of the environment.

Although each of the caregiver roles described has separate functions, many of them overlap. One area in which there is much overlap is in individual, family, and group therapy where many members of the team participate. The delegation of specific functions is largely determined by the social structure and leadership style of the treatment setting.

Communication patterns. Communication patterns are closely related to the social structure of the treatment setting. Several patterns have been identified: fan, chain, ring, wheel, and all-channel (Figure 24-2). In the *fan pattern,* messages originate at one source and are directed downward to several receivers who do not interact with each other. They may only respond to the central message sender. In the *chain pattern,* messages are initiated at one point and are passed from one receiver to the next until the message reaches the end of the chain. Feedback must return through the reverse sequence of receiving. The *ring pattern* is similar to the chain except that the last receiver reports to the sender. Messages and feedback follow a cyclical pattern. In the *wheel pattern,* messages originate at a central position. Interaction may occur between the message sender and any one of the receivers as well as between the receivers positioned next to each other. In the *all-channel pattern,* messages may originate at any point and all members may interact. The fan network is most likely to develop in groups with autocratic

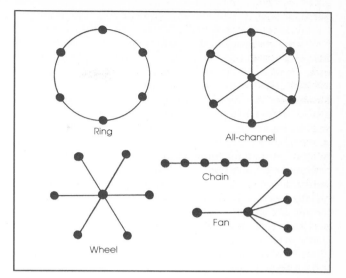

FIGURE 24-2 Communication patterns.

leadership; chain and ring networks are common with laissez-faire leadership, and wheel and all-channel communications are most common in democratic groups.

The type of communication network determines the number and nature of messages sent by members in various positions, the speed of organization, and problem-solving skill. Groups make fewer errors and organize more rapidly in the all-channel and wheel patterns and make progressively more errors and organize less rapidly in the fan, chain, and ring networks.

Besides speed and accuracy of information processing, the network of communication affects the roles within a group. The person who occupies the position nearest the center of the network is the one most likely to be recognized as leader. This implies that centrality is more important than position within the formal hierarchy of leadership.[41] While observing communication patterns on a psychiatric ward, McKeighen[41] found that the actual leader was the ward clerk, rather than the psychiatrist or head nurse, who were the official leaders. The recognition of informal leaders helps identify sources of information and clarify confusion when problems in communication arise.

Group morale is affected by communication networks. The individual in the central position will have the greatest understanding of the overall plan of action and will be most satisfied with his job. The person furthest from the center will have the least knowledge and the lowest morale.[41] Therefore the more equality in communication of information, the greater the morale of the whole group.

As part of the communication process, it is important to distinguish between constructive and destructive conflicts and to intervene to promote constructive conflict resolution. Destructive conflict occurs when it directs energy from more important activities, destroys the morale of the group, disrupts group cohesion by polarizing members, deepens differences in values, and produces negative behavior such as name calling and fighting.[23] Constructive conflict opens up and clarifies issues, results in solution of problems, increases individual involvement, enhances authentic communication, releases pent-up emotions, builds cohesiveness, and promotes individual growth.

Staff-client ratio. A concrete factor that affects social interaction in a treatment setting is the staff-client ratio. Moos[45] found that the greater the number of clients per staff member on a psychiatric ward, the more emphasis was placed on staff control and the less support and spontaneous communication. Moos also related negative factors to large numbers of clients regardless of ratio. He concludes that a decreased number of staff members and an increased number of clients have several negative effects:

1. There is greater pressure to develop a more rigid structure.
2. Staff members' need to control and manage is increased.
3. The degree of client independence and responsibility, the amount of support given, and the involvement of staff members with clients are decreased.
4. There are fewer spontaneous interactions between clients and staff.
5. There is decreased understanding of clients' personal problems and less open handling of angry feelings. Thus the staff-client ratio is extremely significant in developing positive social interactions.

Emotional dimension. The emotional atmosphere can be sensed almost immediately when one enters a treatment setting. Descriptive phrases are often used for this emotional sense: "I feel comfortable here," "Everyone is so relaxed," "Everyone works well together," and "Everything is taken care of." Bradford[9] developed a more systematic list of adjectives to describe the emotional atmosphere of a group. These have been adapted to apply to a treatment setting (Table 24-3).

Moos[45] identifies spontaneity, support, and involvement as qualities that are most beneficial for treatment. Spontaneity describes the extent to which the environment encourages clients to act openly and to freely express their feelings. Support indicates the amount of helpfulness and understanding of client needs that the staff and other clients show. Involvement describes how active and energetic clients are in the social functions of the treatment setting.

Moos states that in treatment settings with an involved, supportive, spontaneous atmosphere, clients are more satisfied, like one another and staff members more, believe that their experiences are relevant to personal development, are more self-revealing, more openly express anger, and are less submissive.

Spiritual dimension. Although providing a specific place for worship is important, the entire treatment environment can provide the background for meeting spiritual needs. Important in this assessment is the provision of quiet spaces, and opportunities for relating to nature and to other people. The importance of relatedness to nature has been recognized in different cultures throughout history as a healing force and is discussed throughout this chapter as a major therapeutic component.

TABLE 24-3 Types and characteristics of emotional atmospheres

Type	Characteristic
Rewarding	When members have worked together well on the task they set for themselves, they feel that they have gained from the experience. The members may feel rewarded if they have accomplished something, even though the task is still incomplete.
Sluggish	Often members try hard to deal with the tasks at hand but "just can't get going."
Cooperative	Members work together harmoniously. Members seem to share goals and support one another in attaining goals.
Competitive	Several members seem out to win their own points, with the result that action can only proceed out of a "win-lose" approach.
Play	Play is the opposite of being task oriented. It exists when the members avoid tasks and cannot seem to shake off a light-hearted, nonserious attitude long enough to get anything done.
Work	When the members devote themselves to tasks in a purposeful manner, the atmosphere is one of work. This may be true regardless of what other impressions result as well; for example, it is possible to fight or not accomplish the task and still "work" hard.
Fight	Often members find themselves in complete disagreement regarding the topic to be discussed, decisions to be made, or action to be taken.
Flight	Members pursue inappropriate or outside topics, horseplay, or a bull session as a means of avoiding the real task at hand (which may be threatening or unpleasant).
Tense	Members feel pressures from limited time, conflict between members, or personally threatening topics.
Relaxed	Members work together in a harmonious manner with little tension or conflict.
Cold	Insensitivity to emotional needs is apparent. Defense mechanisms are used to avoid contact. Clichés substitute for support.
Warm	An emotionally supportive climate that promotes appropriate expression of feelings and the development of mutual trust.

Adapted from Bradford, L.: Class syllabus, Searcy, Ark., 1978, Harding University School of Nursing.

NURSING ASSESSMENT TOOL: MILIEU THERAPY

PHYSICAL DIMENSION

Where is the treatment facility located in relation to the community it serves?

Are there planned interactions, such as outings, sports events, entertainment, and discussion groups, that involve both members of the treatment unit and community members?

Is transportation provided to facilitate interaction?

What is the floor plan of the building?

Does the physical layout provide areas of privacy?

Are there areas that promote interaction?

Is the furniture arranged to promote interaction?

Is there enough space to provide for individualized contact needs?

INTELLECTUAL DIMENSION

What colors are used in the environment?

Are the colors varied according to the activity of the area?

Are contrasting colors used to distinguish different visual planes?

Is the color balanced to reproduce the spectrum of daylight?

Does the lighting glare or have spotlight effects?

Is there natural lighting from windows, doors, or skylights?

What time are the lights turned on and off? Does this follow the natural circadian rhythms of the body?

What is the noise level of the environment?

Are areas provided for quiet and noisy activities?

Is the temperature of the area within the comfort zone?

Are provisions made for individual temperature control such as thermostats in bedrooms, offices, and treatment rooms?

How is the indoor temperature modified in relationship to external weather changes?

Is the humidity controlled?

Do the textures used reflect or absorb light and noise?

Are the surfaces cold or warm in appearance and touch?

Are the surfaces durable?

What odors are noticeable?

Is there a provision for circulation of fresh air?

Is the environment kept clean and waste disposed in closed areas?

Are there plants that absorb odor and give off oxygen?

Are synthetic materials used extensively?

Does the design of the building promote orientation, or is it easy to get lost?

Are there aids such as direction signs, clocks, calendars, and posted schedules to promote orientation?

What are the ward rules? Are they rigid or flexible?

What information is given to a new client arriving in the area?

Do clients have the opportunity to choose areas that are most comfortable to them?

Are clients and staff members of all levels involved in decision making?

SOCIAL DIMENSION

What are the formal roles of the members?

What are the functions (job descriptions) of the various members of the team?

Are the roles clearly distinct, or are there overlapping functions?

What is the formal administrative hierarchy?

What style of leadership is used?

What is the primary pattern of communication (who talks to whom and how frequently)?

Is the informal communication pattern the same as the formal hierarchy of communication?

Is the established pattern of communication efficient in speed, accuracy, and problem-solving capability?

What is the effect of the communication pattern on group morale?

Is there an attempt to assist clients to maintain community and family commitments?

Are family members involved in the treatment process?

What is the staff-client ratio?

What type of interaction pattern does the staff-client ratio promote?

EMOTIONAL DIMENSION

What is the emotional climate of the treatment environment? (How do you feel in the setting?)

What factors influence the emotional climate?

What blocks and facilitates the group interaction?

Does the climate allow for spontaneous expression of feelings?

What are the limits set on expression?

How is behavior that goes beyond the set limits handled?

Is support given for working through personal problems?

Is a sense of pride, camaraderie, and enthusiasm apparent?

SPIRITUAL DIMENSION

Is a place provided for meditation and religious activities?

Is a time allotted for quiet meditation and participation in religious activities if desired?

Is the staff willing to listen to explorations of the meaning of life and illness?

Do the architectural lines of the setting inspire transcendence?

Do the space and the arrangement of the furnishings promote meaningful relationships?

Is the staff available for interactions?

What is the relationship of the facility to the natural setting?

Have natural items been included in the decor?

Are opportunities provided for creative expression?

Is there a sense of peace, harmony, and balance in the setting?

Do interactions promote self-fulfillment?

The factors identified in this section form the basis for assessment of the characteristics that promote positive outcomes in milieu therapy. They also serve as a guideline for evaluation of actions. A summary of these factors for assessment is presented in the box on p. 471.

Analysis

Many factors interact to create an impression of the treatment milieu impact. Examples of such patterns that could also be seen as nursing diagnoses for a milieu treatment are presented here:
1. Overcrowded and overconcentrated hospital ward
2. Failure to provide individual privacy in bathrooms
3. Assignment of clients to bedrooms (clients not allowed to choose roommates)
4. Stark white walls, resulting in glare
5. Smooth and hard textures
6. Lack of orientation supports
7. Authoritarian power structure that prevents client involvement in decision making
8. Blocking of interaction by formal communication channels
9. Low group morale
10. Cold and competitive emotional climate
11. Blocking of emotional expression by staff members' use of cliches
12. Punishmnent of aggressive acting out rather than management to promote emotional growth
13. Locking of bedroom doors in the daytime to prevent withdrawal, resulting in lack of a quiet place for meditation
14. Lack of recognition, display, or development of creative abilities of clients
15. Lack of provision for contact with nature
16. Lack of participation in goal setting and limited knowledge of overall treatment objectives

Planning

Table 24-4 provides examples of long-term and short-term goals and outcome criteria related to the therapeutic milieu. These serve as examples of the planning stage in the nursing process.

Implementation

Physical dimension. The role that has the most impact in achieving a therapeutic physical environment is participation in the design or renovation of the setting. The nurse translates human needs into dimensional terms. For example, the size of the dayroom is especially important in both outpatient and inpatient facilities since this is the hub of activity. Design of this space needs to accommodate a variety of activities. A nurse's input concerning the number of activities and interactions that occur can determine if the design is functional.

Although not all nurses will have the opportunity to participate in designing or renovating a treatment area, much can be accomplished by arranging semifixed features to promote interaction and provide privacy. Shower curtains, lockers for personal items, bulletin boards to display personal artwork and pictures, or bedside lamps can be added at little cost.

Intellectual dimension. The nurse may interpret the needs of the client population for design experts who have knowledge about color, texture, and lighting. Some client needs that are important to consider include the level of mental confusion, common behavioral problems such as withdrawal or acting out, the developmental level of clients, the type of activity that will occur in the setting, and the type of graphics, maps, and color coding necessary to provide orientation.

Maps of the area, color coding of specific areas, name plates on doors, and wall graphics can be designed to contribute to perceptual clarity. Clocks and calendars need to be clearly visible in each area, and bulletin boards for posting treatment schedules, mealtimes, visiting hours, recreational events, and other routines need to be readily available. All of these factors combine to promote perceptual clarity and orientation.

Such decisions as when the television and lights are turned off, what activities are planned, and who can come and go in the treatment setting also have great impact on the milieu.

Several special forms of therapy have been developed to take advantage of sensory stimuli. High light levels that extend daylight time have been beneficial in treating winter depressions.[24] Sound has been used to stimulate withdrawn individuals. Both perceptual organization and sleep patterns have improved after exposure to a noisy environment.[50] Music therapy provides sensory and expressive benefits. Occupational, art, recreational, and sensory integration therapy have tactile inputs. The nurse is often responsible for making referrals, encouraging client participation, and coordinating the team members involved.

Social dimension. Social interventions are primarily directed toward increasing interaction, improving communication, and promoting involvement in decision making. Conflict resolution and confrontation are sometimes necessary to overcome barriers that prevent these interventions.

Intervention in closed communication is most effective if it begins at the top of the chain of command. The style of communication one chooses depends most on the style chosen by the person next highest in the organizational chain.[34] If the top person does not allow feedback, this blocks feedback along all other channels, and may result in frustration and a deterioration in morale.

When it is not possible to alter communication patterns at the top levels, informal patterns of communication develop in the form of rebellion and lack of productivity. However, an effective informal leader may be able to relieve some of the tension by allowing venting of frustration and promoting group interaction outside the sanctions of formal control. Unfortunately, if an authoritarian interaction pattern is firmly entrenched, it may be the only option.

In any communication system, conflicts emerge. Constructive conflict resolution requires use of confrontation

TABLE 24-4 Long-term and short-term goals and outcome criteria related to nursing diagnoses for therapeutic milieu

Goals	Outcome Criteria

NURSING DIAGNOSIS: LACK OF INTELLECTUAL CLARITY RELATED TO FAILURE TO PROVIDE ORIENTATION GUIDES

Long-term goal

To provide the necessary orientation guides from the environment	Bulletin boards in convenient places display planned daily activities. Clocks and calendars are in all client areas. Individual treatment areas are color coded. Graphics identify the function of the area. Maps are posted to indicate directions. Staff and clients participate in orienting new members and supporting the mentally confused.

Short-term goals

To have clients and staff select and develop orientation guides To have experts, such as interior designers, participate in the planning process	Areas for and placement of bulletin boards, clocks, and calendars are identified. A system for color coding functional areas is developed. Graphics and maps are designed with expert assistance. Orientation materials for new members including rules and regulations, available services, a general map, and routine schedules are developed.

NURSING DIAGNOSIS: LOW GROUP MORALE RELATED TO LACK OF PARTICIPATION IN GOAL SETTING AND LIMITED KNOWLEDGE OF OVERALL TREATMENT OBJECTIVES

Long-term goal

To have positive commitment and enthusiasm for both personal and institutional objectives	Clients list overall treatment objectives. Clients write personal goals related to overall objectives. There is verbalization of positive feelings regarding goals, personal contribution, and contributions of other clients and team members.

Short-term goals

To have all members participate in identification of overall treatment objectives To develop personal goals in relationship to overall objectives	Discussion groups are held weekly to develop goals. Each member of the team provides input. Differences of opinion are openly discussed. Decisions are made through group consensus. Personal goals in relationship to overall objectives are discussed.

NURSING DIAGNOSIS: FAILURE TO DEVELOP CREATIVE ABILITIES RELATED TO LACK OF RECOGNITION OF CLIENT'S INTERESTS OR DISPLAY OF WORKS

Long-term goal

To develop the creative ability of clients	All clients are involved in creative activities according to their ability level. Awards are given for progress in creative expression.

Short-term goals

To recognize creative ability of clients To provide opportunity for display of creative works and talents	Clients list their creative interests, hobbies, and vocational activities as they join the group. An area is selected and furnished for display of creative works. A time for creative performance such as music, dancing, singing, or theatrics is designated.

to bring the issues into the open where mutual goal setting can be achieved. Several principles enhance the effectiveness of confrontation:[32]

1. Face-to-face interaction involving all of the major participants is necessary to clarify communications.
2. Confrontation needs to occur as soon as possible after the conflict has developed. Delays in confrontation allow for polarization and the development of defenses.
3. A skilled neutral leader is necessary to analyze the factors contributing to the conflict and to plan the circumstances and timing for the confrontation to occur.
4. A setting that allows the expression of feeling without fear or reprisals is important.
5. The confrontation needs to be timed so that feelings are not too strong and overwhelming but sufficient to motivate change if growth is to occur.

The major participants need to be willing to look at themselves, examine their roles, express themselves openly, listen to other points of view, and change for conflict resolutions to result in growth. These principles provide the ideal conditions for conflict resolution. Sometimes it is necessary to diffuse strong emotions and wait for a more favorable climate. The circumstances may not always be the most desirable, and individuals may not always be willing to change. The most important factors in conflict resolution are an acceptance of conflict as a natural occurrence and a willingness to face the emotional turmoil that results.

Emotional dimension. To achieve the climate of support, involvement, and spontaneity necessary for therapeutic outcomes, it is important to develop a sense of harmony, cooperation, and group cohesiveness. Group cohesiveness holds a group together, helps it over the rough spots, allows it to fend off outside threats, and helps group members change and grow.[38] The two factors consistently identified in the literature as promoting group cohesiveness are acceptance and liking among group members and the pursuit of common goals.

People tend to like people who are similar to themselves. Similarity of group members may be enhanced by selection of a homogeneous group and by providing an opportunity to explore common interests and backgrounds through group interaction. Homogeneity may be promoted through screening criteria that select members with common goals or problems. When this is not possible, or when there is a large group in which diversity is inevitable, smaller subgroups with similar membership may be created.

For people to like each other they must know each other. This means that there must be an opportunity to spend time together. One way to achieve this is through working on a mutual project.

Another major factor affecting group cohesiveness is the development of common goals. In the treatment setting it seems logical that all group members work toward the common goal of improved mental health. However, individual clients may be pursuing their own development at the expense of others. A common error in the mental health field is to promote emotional expression at all costs. Many techniques have been developed to encourage emotional expression. Yet in society indiscriminate emotional expression can lead to ostracism from the group or to dissolution of the social network. For emotional expression to be productive, it needs to enhance not only individual well-being but also that of the social group.

Community meetings and group therapy sessions can be used to identify group goals and promote adherence to

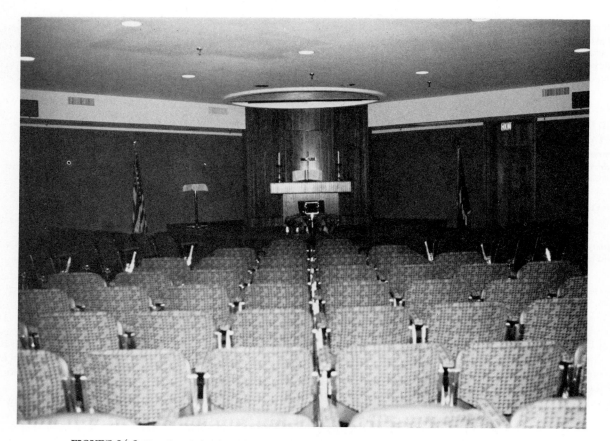

FIGURE 24-3 Focal point enhances meditation at the new John L. McClellan Memorial Hospital, North Little Rock. (Courtesy Brian House.)

the group task. For an individual to adhere to group goals, the goals need to be explicitly formulated, the path for attainment needs to be clear, and there needs to be a likelihood that they can be successfully attained.[38] The process of mutual goal setting, as well as the interaction necessary for goal achievement, can do much to enhance group cohesiveness and promote a positive emotional climate.

✤ *Spiritual dimension.* Interventions that enhance the spiritual qualities of the environment are directed toward maximizing the meaningfulness of the treatment experience, developing a sense of transcendence, increasing relatedness to other people and nature, and promoting freedom and creativity of expression.

Meaningfulness is determined by the relevance of the program to the individual. When a client's goals cannot be met in a program, he needs to be transferred to a more appropriate treatment group. This has the twofold effect of enhancing individual meaningfulness and preserving group cohesiveness, because a person who is unhappy in a group can create disharmony.

The need for both transcendence and relatedness involves creating a balance between aloneness and interaction. The physical environment can be structured to provide both private places for contemplation and reflection and larger areas for group interaction.

It is important to provide a quiet space and time to contemplate the meaning of life and to renew hope for the future. An enclosed space that blocks an external view creates a womblike effect, which promotes inward focusing of attention. Lighting may be dimmed by the use of colored glass, and low levels of interior lighting may be used in this area. A single focal point such as a brighter source of light may be used to capture attention. In a chapel the altar makes a natural focal point[40] (Figure 24-3).

The need for transcendence can be supported through vertical lines in the architectural design. McClinton[40] stated that the vertical line is inspiring, uplifting, emotional, and mystical. Strong design elements such as beams or windows focus attention upward, create a sense of transcendence and relatedness to the universe beyond (Figure 24-4).

Relatedness to God may be enhanced through worship and communion in a chapel setting. Providing an individualized religious experience is most frequently seen as a duty of the chaplain service; however, nurses can work with this service to assist clients in meeting spiritual needs.

Factors that promote relatedness to others range from furniture groupings that promote interaction to developing open channels of communication. Planned activities can encourage interaction of withdrawn and isolated members, and enforced quiet time can encourage contemplation for those who are always with a group.

Contact with nature can be provided by choosing a naturally beautiful setting, using landscaping to enhance the setting, using large windows that provide a view of the natural environment, and "bringing nature indoors" by using plants, flowers, and pictures of natural scenes (Figure 24-5).

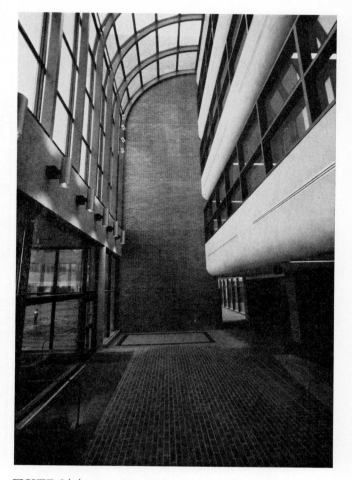

FIGURE 24-4 Upward focusing creates a sense of transcendence at the new John L. McClellan Memorial Hospital, North Little Rock. (Courtesy Brian House.)

The development of relatedness to humanity is a self-actualizing process that includes the desire for order, harmony, truth, and beauty. The creativity needed for this process is best nurtured in an environment that provides daily freedom of expression and choice. Whitehead and others[60] saw exercise of choice as a major factor in prevention of the negative effects of institutionalization. Opportunities to chose are important in sustaining autonomy and self-worth and can be facilitated in the environment.

Creativity results when all of the environmental aspects combine to promote individual growth and expression. The creativity of a treatment group reflects the capacity of the group to balance the opposing needs of the members, develop cohesive interactions, resolve conflicts productively, and effectively use the members' intellectual and physical resources to accomplish goals.

Evaluation

Evaluation of a therapeutic milieu is based on observation of desired outcomes. Several scales have been devel-

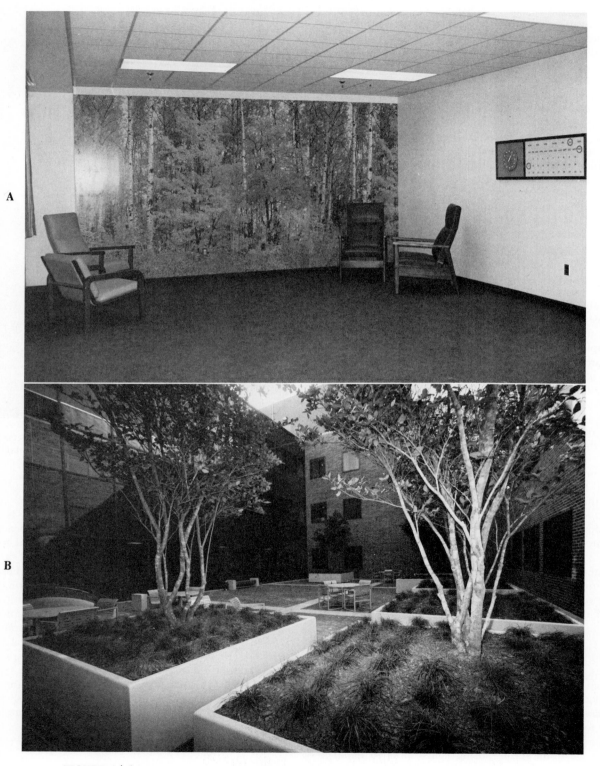

FIGURE 24-5 Bringing nature indoors at the new John L. McClellan Memorial Hospital, North Little Rock. **A,** Mural of natural scene in dayroom. **B,** Enclosed patio with plants and trees. (Courtesy Brian House.)

TABLE 24-5 Scales for objective evaluation of environmental interventions

Scale	Author	Environmental Factors Measured
Behavioral Mapping	Ittelson, Rivlin, and Proshansky	Eighteen categories of observable behavior
Ward Atmosphere Scale	Moos	Order and organization, clarity of expectations, staff control; autonomy, practical orientation, personal problem orientation; involvement, support, spontaneity, anger, aggression
Opinion about Mental Illness	Cohen and Struening	Authoritarianism, benevolence, mental hygiene ideology, social restrictiveness, interpersonal causes of mental illness
Ward Information Form	Kellam, Schmelza, and Berman	Disturbed behavior, adult status, patient-staff ratio, social contact, ward census
Group Climate Questionnaire	Johnson	Genuineness, understanding, valuing, accepting
Ward Value Scale	Almond, Keniston, and Boltax	Openness, involvement, responsibility, faith in ward

oped to objectify observations (Table 24-5). These can be effective tools in both assessment and evaluation.

Evaluation of environmental interventions, like all other steps in the nursing process, is most effective when all members of the group participate in the process. By looking at behavior and its consequences, the group can develop new awareness of effective action and interaction. This awareness can form the basis for personal growth.

BRIEF REVIEW

Milieu therapy originated in the eighteenth century with the concept of "moral treatment" developed by Dr. Philippe Pinel. This approach replaced the custodial, often punitive method of treatment employed at that time. Menninger, Main, Jones, and Bettelheim extended milieu therapy to every age group, diagnostic category, and treatment setting.

Nursing intervention in the therapeutic milieu requires knowledge of the factors that affect therapeutic outcomes. The significant physical aspects include the external and internal design of the treatment setting as well as furniture and other movable objects that are most effective when they promote constructive relationships between the members of the treatment community and the surrounding neighborhood.

The intellectual aspects of color, lighting, sound, temperature, texture, odor, and taste can be integrated to form a coherent environment that promotes stability and comfort and avoids ambiguity, complication, and sensory overload.

The social aspects of the therapeutic milieu include the organization of roles of individual members into a social system based on leadership style, the communication patterns within the system, and the staff-client ratio.

The emotional aspects include development of a positive emotional climate with elements of spontaneous expression and support of others.

The spiritual aspects provide relatedness to God, others, and nature by arranging the environment to encourage interaction and using a natural setting with natural scenes and materials.

Assessment of the factors mentioned is followed by the development of nursing diagnoses and establishment of goals and outcome criteria. Interventions focus on identified problems in each aspect of the treatment milieu and on stated goals. Examples of interventions include the following: designing a treatment setting, interpreting sensory stimuli for clients, promoting healthy conflict resolution, sharing common activities and development of goals, and promoting relatedness.

Evaluation of interventions rests on objective evaluation of multiple interacting environmental factors. This includes recognition of the role of the intervener within the total process of change.

REFERENCES AND SUGGESTED READINGS

1. Almond, R., Keniston, K., and Boltax, S.: The value system of a milieu therapy unit, Archives of General Psychiatry **19**:547, 1968.
2. Beck, W.C., and Meyer, R.H.: The health care environment: the user's viewpoint, Boca Raton, Fla., 1982, CRC Press, Inc.
3. Bell, M.D., and Ryan, E.R.: Where can therapeutic community ideals be realized? An examination of three treatment environments, Hospital and Community Psychiatry **12**:1290, 1985.
4. Benfer, B.A., and Schroder, P.J.: Nursing in the therapeutic milieu, Bulletin of the Menninger Clinic **49**(5):451, 1985.
5. Bettelheim, B., and Sylvester, E.: The therapeutic milieu, American Journal of Orthopsychiatry **18**:191, 1948.
6. Birren, F.: Human responses to color and light, Hospitals **53**:93, July 1979.
7. Blake, F.E., Wright, F.H., and Waechter, E.H.: Nursing care of children, Philadelphia, 1970, J.B. Lippincott Co.
8. Bonier, R.J.: Staff countertransference in an adolescent milieu treatment setting, Adolescent Psychiatry **10**:382, 1982.
9. Bradford, L.: Class syllabus, Searcy, Ark., 1978, Harding University School of Nursing.
10. Brown, L.J.: The therapeutic milieu in the treatment of patients with borderline personality disorders, Bulletin of the Menninger Clinic **45**(5):377, 1981.

11. Cohen, J., and Struening, E.: Opinions about mental illness, Journal of Consulting Psychology **28**:291, 1964.

12. Cohen, S.: Sound effects on behavior, Psychology Today **15**(10):38, 1981.

13. Collins, J.F., and others: Treatment characteristics of effective psychiatric programs, Hospital and Community Psychiatry **35**(6):601, 1984.

14. Cotton, N.S., and Geraty, R.G.: Therapeutic space design: planning an inpatient children's unit, American Journal of Orthopsychiatry **54**(4):624, 1984.

15. Cox, K.G.: Alzheimer's disease: milieu therapy, Geriatric Nursing **G**(3):152, 1985.

16. Cumming, E.: Therapeutic community and milieu therapy strategies can be distinguished, International Journal of Psychiatry **7**:204, 1969.

17. Davis, C., Glick, I.D., and Rosow, L.: The architectural design of a psychotherapeutic milieu, Hospital and Community Psychiatry **30**:453, 1979.

18. Devine, B.A.: Therapeutic milieu/milieu therapy: an overview, Journal of Psychiatric Nursing **3**:24, 1981.

19. Gillis, D.A.: Nursing management: a systems approach, Philadelphia, 1982, W.B. Saunders Co.

20. Golan, N.: Passing through transitions: a guide for practitioners, New York, 1981, The Free Press.

21. Good, L.R., and Hurtig, W.E.: Evaluation: a mental health facility, its use and context, American Institute of Architects Journal **59**:38, February 1978.

22. Hall, E.T.: The anthropology of space: an organizing model. In Proshansky, H.M., Ittelson, W.H., and Rivlin, L.G., editors: Environmental psychology: man and his physical setting, New York, 1970, Holt, Rinehart & Winston.

23. Hart, L.B.: Learning from conflict: a handbook for trainers and group leaders, Reading, Mass., 1981, Addison-Wesley Publishing Co., Inc.

24. Hellman, H.: Guiding light, Psychology Today **16**(4):22, 1982.

25. Herz, M.I.: The therapeutic milieu: a necessity, International Journal of Psychiatry **7**:209, 1969.

26. Herz, M.I.: The therapeutic community re-examined, Hospital and Community Psychiatry **32**(2):81, 1981.

27. Hiatt, L.G.: The color and use of color in environments for older people, Nursing Homes, p. 18, May-June 1981.

28. Holmes, M., and Werner, J.: Psychiatric nursing in a therapeutic community, New York, 1966, The Macmillan Co.

29. Ittelson, W.H., Rivlin, L.G., and Proshansky, H.M.: The use of behavioral maps in environmental psychology. In Proshansky, H.M., Ittelson, W.H., and Rivlin, L.G., editors: Environmental psychology: man and his physical setting, New York, 1970, Holt, Rinehart & Winston.

30. Johnson, D.W.: Reaching out: interpersonal effectiveness and self-actualization, Englewood Cliffs, N.J., 1972, Prentice-Hall, Inc.

31. Jones, M.: The therapeutic community, New York, 1953, Basic Books, Inc., Publishers.

32. Jones, M.: Beyond the therapeutic community, New Haven, Conn., 1968, Yale University Press.

33. Kellam, G., Schmelza, J., and Berman, A.: Variations in the atmosphere of psychiatric wards, Archives of General Psychiatry **14**:561, 1966.

34. Kepler, T.L.: Mastering the people skills, Journal of Nursing Administration **10**(11):15, 1980.

35. Kernberg, O., and Haran, C.: Interview: milieu treatment with borderline patients: the nurse's role, Journal of Psychosocial Nursing and Mental Health Services **22**(4):29, 1984.

36. Kirshner, L.A., and Johnston, L.: Current status of milieu psychiatry, General Hospital Psychiatry **4**(1):75, 1982.

37. Klosterman, V.J.: The psychological effects of weather, Journal of Psychiatric Nursing and Mental Health Services **17**(1):25, 1979.

38. Loomis, M.E.: Group process for nurses, St. Louis, 1979, The C.V. Mosby Co.

39. Main, T.F.: The hospital as a therapeutic institution, Bulletin of the Menninger Clinic **10**:66, 1946.

40. McClinton, K.M.: The changing church: its architecture, art, and decoration, New York, 1957, Morehouse-Gorham Co.

41. McKeighen, R.J.: Communication patterns and leadership roles in a psychiatric setting, Perspectives in Psychiatric Care **6**(2):80, 1968.

42. Menninger, K.A., and others: A manual for psychiatric case study, ed. 2, New York, 1962, Grune & Stratton, Inc.

43. Menninger, W.C.: Psychoanalytic principles in psychiatric hospital therapy, Southern Medical Journal **32**:348, 1939.

44. Molina, J.A.: Psychobiosocial "maps": a useful tool in milieu therapy and psychiatric education, Journal of Clinical Psychiatry **43**(5):182, 1982.

45. Moos, R.H.: Evaluating treatment environments: a social ecological approach, New York, 1974, John Wiley & Sons, Inc.

46. Mosher, L.R., and others: Milieu therapy in the 1980's: a comparison of two residential alternatives to hospitalization, Bulletin of the Menninger Clinic **50**(3):257, 1986.

47. Mulvihill, D.L.: Milieu therapy in a children's unit, Canadian Journal of Psychiatric Nursing **24**(4):17, 1983.

48. Olds, J.: The inpatient treatment of adolescents in a milieu including younger children, Adolescent Psychiatry **10**:373, 1982.

49. Osmond, H.: Function as the basis of psychiatric ward design, Mental Hospitals (Architectural Suppl.) **8**:23, 1957.

50. Ozerengin, M.F., and Cowen, M.A.: Environmental noise level as a factor in the treatment of hospitalized schizophrenics, Diseases of the Nervous System **35**:241, 1974.

51. Perry, B.A.: Getting the message across, Nursing Mirror **152**:22, March 5, 1981.

52. Sacks, R.H., and Carpenter, W.T.: The pseudotherapeutic community: an examination of antitherapeutic forces on psychiatric units, Hospital and Community Psychiatry **25**:315, 1974.

53. Sampson, E.E., and Marthas, M.: Group process for the health professionals, ed. 2, New York, 1981, John Wiley & Sons, Inc.

54. Settin, J.M.: Gerontologic human resources: the role of the paraprofessional, New York, 1982, Human Sciences Press, Inc.

55. Skinner, K.: The therapeutic milieu: making it work, Journal of Psychiatric Nursing and Mental Health Services **17**(8):38, 1979.

56. Sommer, R., and Osmond, H.: Symptoms of institutional care, Social Problems **8**:345, 1960.

57. Sullivan, H.S.: Sociopsychiatric research: its implications for the schizophrenic problem and for mental hygiene, American Journal of Psychiatry **10**:977, 1931.

58. Szekais, B.: Using the milieu: treatment-environment consistency, Gerontologist **60**(4):7, 1985.

59. van Bilsen, H.P., and van Emst, A.J.: Heroin addiction and motivational milieu therapy, International Journal of the Addictions **21**(G):707, 1986.

60. Webb, P., and Safnia, J.: Positive alternative community therapy (PACT) program, Little Rock, Ark., 1980, Little Rock Veterans Administration Medical Center, North Little Rock Division.

61. Whitehead, C., and others: The aging psychiatric hospital: an approach to humanistic redesign, Hospital and Community Psychiatry **27**:781, 1976.

ANNOTATED BIBLIOGRAPHY

Devine, B.A.: Therapeutic milieu/milieu therapy: an overview, Journal of Psychosocial Nursing and Mental Health Services 3:24, 1981.

Following a historical overview of milieu therapy, the author defines the concepts of milieu therapy and therapeutic community. Principles of milieu therapy are discussed, and the nurse's role in designing and implementing a therapeutic milieu is presented. The author also reviews research findings related to milieu therapy.

Kirshner, L.A., and Johnston, L.: Current status of milieu psychiatry, General Hospital Psychiatry 4(1):75, 1982.

Historical trends in the use of environment in treatment of mental illness are integrated with social science and empirical research studies of milieu. Research is reviewed that documents the significant effects of milieu on treatment outcomes. Also discussed in the importance of the direction of future research efforts toward more specific parameters of milieu in interaction with different diagnoses or client populations.

COMMUNITY MENTAL HEALTH NURSING

Sophronia R. Williams   Jeanette Lancaster

After studying the chapter the learner will be able to:

Identify significant events in the evolution of community mental health nursing.

Discuss theoretical approaches to community mental health nursing.

Discuss characteristics of the community mental health–psychiatric nurse.

Use the nursing process to provide nursing care to clients in community-based settings.

Community mental health nursing is the application of specialized knowledge to populations and communities to promote and maintain mental health and to rehabilitate target groups that continue to have residual effects of mental illness. The target groups include those former clients with mental illness who were discharged from state hospitals into the community. The focus of the practice of community health nursing is on change for the benefit of the whole community rather than only clients presently receiving mental health care. Thus community mental health nursing emphasizes preventive intervention.

With short-term inpatient treatment and the fact that Diagnostic Related Groups (DRGs) will limit the time a psychiatric client remains in the hospital, the number of clients needing mental health nursing care in a community-based setting will increase. The homeless chronically mentally ill and the evolving group of chronically mentally ill young adults will need the services of the community mental health–psychiatric nurse.

THEORETICAL APPROACHES
Systems

A systems theory view of the community emphasizes the community as a city, county, or state. Likewise each community is composed of numerous subsystems such as the family, groups, and the environment. The community is in constant interaction with the other subsystems. A change in one part of the community has direct and sig-

nificant influence on another part of the community. As one aspect of the community changes, other components compensate and accommodate to the changes. Changes in community functioning can be achieved by indirect or direct interventions that may be directed toward various subsystems.

Community stability, problems, tension, or conflict in one subsystem can produce ripple effects throughout the system. For example, during employee layoffs or strikes, robberies caused by financial need, boredom, depression, or outbursts of anger and hostility might increase.

Ecological

The ecological approach builds on the systems theory approach to the study of human behavior. The term *ecology* was first proposed in 1869 by a German biologist, Ernest Haeckel, to mean study of the relationship between an organism and its environment. Through the years the ecological concept has gained wide acceptance in both the biological and the behavioral sciences as a way to study the total environmental effect on organisms. An ecologic model for community mental health is a useful alternative to the model that emphasizes mental illness. Ecology emphasizes a holistic view of people and their total environment by noting the often interactive nature of the many influences on community functioning.

Human ecology, which refers to the study of people and their interdependence with the environment, is com-

🌿 *Historical Overview* 🌿

DATE	EVENT
1200	Community care for the mentally ill was evident in Gheel, Belgium, when people were placed in families for mental health care.[22]
Late 1940s	Community-based mental health care projects were developed at Menninger and Yale clinics.
1954	The community mental health–psychiatric nurse first began work at Warlingham Park Hospital.
1957	Community mental health–psychiatric nursing was provided in the hospital and community.
1963	Community Mental Health Centers Act was passed. A community-based system of mental health care was established with community mental health centers as the locus of services.
1969	The number of community psychiatric nursing services increased.
1975	Nurses working in community mental health centers were largely generalists.
Late 1970s	The number of psychiatric nursing specialists working in community mental health centers increased.
1980s	The role of the psychiatric clinical specialist in community mental health nursing will continue to expand, with emphasis on consultation and liaison roles and prevention of and early intervention in mental health problems.
Future	The nurse will increase her participation in and care of high-risk groups in an effort to assist these clients to obtain maximum functioning.

posed of essentially three parts: a philosophy, a set of principles, and an attitude. The human ecological philosophy values the study of people as holistic organisms continually affecting and being affected by their environment. From an ecological view, environment includes the external and the internal environment of a person. Thus a change in either environment influences a person's equilibrium. Within this framework, mental health and mental illness can be judged only in relation to the context in which they occur. Essentially all problems of people are specific to the individual and his particular situation.

Principles of ecology, derived from systems theory, explain how people live together within the confines of their environment. Three principles of ecology—adaptation, cycling of resources, and *succession*—elaborate on the philosophy and further explain the interaction between people and their multiple environments. People strive to adapt favorably to environmental stimuli to maintain system stability. The ways in which people behave depend on their relationship between their system stressors and their adaptive abilities. Favorable ecological conditions (adaptors) motivate a person toward a state of health or positive adaptation, whereas unfavorable influences or stressors direct the person toward illness or maladaptation. However, each person has a finite supply of adaptive responses; the rate and variability of stressors influence the quality of adaptive response. Too much change too fast can disrupt system stability.

All systems have a finite supply of physical and psychosocial resources. These resources may be tangible, such as shelter, or intangible, such as a positive, nurturing emotional climate. Because people do not have unlimited reserves of coping capacity or resources, communities need to provide mechanisms to replenish supplies before they are depleted.

The principle of succession holds that living systems are never stable or static but rather are in a constant state of change. Succession means that a state of openness and receptivity exists in the environment; this diminishes predictability and also increases the need for reserves of adaptive energy.

The focus of an ecological approach is on the essential holism of human problems. Both an ecological view and a holistic view imply that the health of a person is more than the sum of a person's body parts. Likewise the health of the community is more than the total of all residents. The community serves as a potential source of strength when an individual faces assaults against maintaining equilibrium. The community is the support system for human existence and ultimately the basis for all survival.

The theoretical approaches are summarized in Table 25-1.

CHARACTERISTICS OF THE COMMUNITY MENTAL HEALTH NURSE
Qualifications

The nurse prepared to work in a community mental setting is a registered nurse, preferably with master's level preparation as a psychiatric clinical nurse specialist. Reg-

TABLE 25-1 Summary of theoretical approaches

Theory	Dynamics
Systems	The community is composed of numerous subsystems that are in constant interaction, with compensatory changes occurring as the various components interact with each other.
Ecological	The people in the community and their environment are interdependent. A change in the internal or external environment influences the person's equilibrium.

TABLE 25-2 Direct and indirect roles with related functions

Role	Function
Direct	
Clinician	Provides direct technical nursing care (for example, giving injections and ensuring compliance with medication regimen)
Therapist	Provides various types of psychotherapy, such as family and group therapy, and crisis intervention
Educator	Teaches residents of the community about the treatment and prevention of mental illness
Indirect	
Consultant	Provides a service to other professionals in the community about the type of psychiatric nursing care the residents need
Manager	Manages the overall delivery of mental health services
Researcher	Engages in research related to clinical practice in the community develop and test theories
Educator	Provides continuing education programs and workshops for other professionals

Adapted from Carr, P.J., Butterworth, C.A., and Hodges, B.E.: Community psychiatric nursing: caring for the mentally ill and handicapped in the community, London, 1980, Churchill Livingstone.

istered nurses who have a generalist education and who have acquired increased specialized knowledge and skills in mental health–psychiatric nursing through continuing education programs, workshops, and practical experience are also qualified to provide community mental health nursing services. The nurse has internalized the ideology of community mental health and possesses an understanding of social, psychological, and interpersonal dynamics of behavior. She has a broad knowledge base of psychopathological conditions and methods for intervention in social problems. The nurse who is qualified to work in community mental health nursing services is able to work with the health team at the community mental health centers as well as with professionals and residents in the community.

Roles

The nurse who works in a community-based setting functions in various *direct* or *indirect practice roles* that are determined to some extent by her academic preparation and professional work experience. She implements her role in the community most often with a team of health care professionals, other professionals (for example, teachers), community organizers, and lay people.

Direct practice roles are those in which the nurse meets the mental health needs of the community through various treatment modalities. The nurse works directly with the client to restore his functioning to an optimal level.

An indirect practice role is one in which the nurse participates in care by providing clinical expertise and knowledge to other health care providers, who use that knowledge to meet the mental health care needs of the community. For example, the nurse may provide an indirect service to health care providers in other health care settings or in the school systems and to policy and program planners. The focus of indirect service is prevention of mental illness. The direct and indirect roles in which the nurse functions are presented in Table 25-2. The Research Highlight on p. 483 focuses on an indirect role of the community mental health nurse.

Goals

The goals of community mental health nursing are derived from the needs of clients and from knowledge and research about the prevention of emotional and mental disorders. The goals of community mental health nursing are diverse and include, but are not limited to, the following:

1. To provide prevention activities to populations and communities for the purposes of promoting mental health and securing participation in self-help activities (primary prevention)
2. To provide opportunities for interventions as early as possible when families, special interest groups, and communities experience a level of stress, tension, and lack of organization that impacts on their abilities to handle affairs of daily living and to work in satisfying and effective ways (secondary intervention)
3. To provide corrective learning experiences for client groups who have deficits and disabilities in the basic competencies needed to cope in contemporary society, and to help individuals develop a sense of self-worth and independence (tertiary intervention)
4. To anticipate when populations become at risk for particular emotional problems and to participate in

Research Highlight

Effect of a Mental Health Educational Program on Police Officers

S.M. Godschalx

PURPOSE

This study was designed to determine whether a mental health education program for police officers would increase their knowledge and change their attitudes about emotionally disturbed people in public crisis situations.

SAMPLE

Sixty police officers were randomly assigned to control and experimental groups. Experimental group members received the mental health education program.

METHODOLOGY

A pretest and posttest design was used to measure knowledge and attitudes. The experimental group received an 8-hour program on crisis management and information about emotionally disturbed people. Both groups were retested, and these scores were compared.

FINDINGS

The experimental group showed an increase in knowledge but no change in attitudes about emotionally disturbed people in public crisis situations.

IMPLICATIONS

In mental health education the goals have to be clearly specified and interventions and preventions designed to address desired changes. An increase in knowledge does not necessarily mean that other aspects of mental and social functioning will be altered.

Data from Research in Nursing and Health 7:111, 1984.

identifying and changing social and psychological factors that adversely affect people's interaction with their environments.

5. To develop innovative approaches to primary prevention activities
6. To assist in providing mental health education to populations at large to demystify stereotypes about mental health and illness and to teach people how to judge their mental health
7. To provide leadership in the field of community mental health and in the role and practice of nursing in this special area in response to the increasing emergence of different kinds of problems as care of the mentally ill becomes almost entirely a community-based endeavor

NURSING PROCESS
Assessment

Physical dimension. The physical features of the community's environment directly and indirectly influence the residents' behavior. The residents have a need to grow and develop in a clean, safe and uncrowded environment that is free of excessive noise. The nurse attends to the noise level with the understanding that noise is essential to stimulate and maintain community functioning; however, excessive amounts can detrimentally affect mental health. For example, excessive noise disrupts the performance of tasks that require concentration, increases errors in completing tasks, and causes decreased reading levels in children. Unpredictable noise can lead to increased aggression.[48] Sudden noises in the community excites an individual's autonomic nervous system and temporarily disrupts his balance.

Workers continuously exposed to high-intensity noise show an increased incidence of nervous complaints, nausea, headaches, instability, argumentativeness, sexual impotence, mood changes, and anxiety.[11] Industrial facilities in the community that have a high noise level may disrupt the residents' sleep patterns.

The nurse determines the availability and accessibility of mental health services in the community. For example, how accessible, by public transportation, are the community health centers and other aftercare facilities? Is a personal car or taxi required to reach these facilities? Highway systems that contribute to the deterioration of public transportation in the central city reduce the means residents use to get around, especially the elderly, poor and youth. These residents are less likely to use mental health services if they cannot be reached by public transportation.

When doing an assessment of the community the nurse attends to the number of persons with physical illness and disability and the type of illness. The rate of physical illness may cause emotional distress for the ill person and the person caring for him. The nurse also determines the residents who are at risk for developing physical disorders and disabilities that have the potential for affecting their mental functioning.

Emotional dimension. When assessing the emotional climate of the community, the nurse may observe fear as a predominant emotion when residents do not feel safe. The nurse collects data about the law enforcement services and patterns of patrolling the community. Such services need to be sufficient and allocated in ways that protect the safety and lives of the residents as well as their property. Break-ins, robberies, and rapes increase the fear and anxiety of community residents. High crime rates and a general feeling that their community is unsafe may also lead residents to feel despair and anger.

The nurse can gain a sense of the emotional climate by observing the freedom with which the residents use the streets and how they secure their homes. For example, if many of the homes have bars on the windows and doors, the residents feel unsafe. When walking in a community, is there a feeling that streets are safe or a feeling of impending assault?

The nurse assesses outlets the community provides for the expression of anger. For example, is there a gymnasium or recreation center equipped with a punching bag or basketball court that allows for indirect expression of anger? The nurse notes if there are discussion groups that allow for verbal expression of anger and if residents are permitted to disagree during discussion of community issues. Generally residents in a community are encouraged to control their anger. The community may even deny that anger exists among its residents. Anger in the community is evident when spouse and child abuse are prevalent (see Chapter 36). When observing behavior in a school setting the nurse will note anger expressed in various ways, such as acting out behavior and angry interactions with teachers. Most often children in schools are punished for expressing anger. Men in the community who feel powerless because they are unemployed may respond with anger and strike out verbally or physically at others.

Improvements in the community in response to needs identified by its residents may give rise to feelings of hope. However, new community programs or urban development programs that involve relocation of residents may leave them with feelings of anger and hopelessness.

The total community may express grief in response to losses that result from natural disasters such as floods, earthquakes, and tornadoes. During such experiences, the residents of the community may be unable to support one another and need assistance from the nurse. However, following a natural disaster, the nurse may observe that the residents express a kindred or fellow survivor feeling as they work together to rebuild the community. Conversely, the community residents as a whole may experience guilt when a number of rapes occur in the community. The residents may think that they could have prevented the crime.

✸ *Intellectual dimension.* The nurse assesses the residents' response to changes in the community. Some communities may be resistant to change to the extent that their mental health is adversely affected. In general, change that improves the image of the community is viewed as positive, whereas change to a lesser status tends to have a negative influence. Some communities welcome innovations, whereas others are committed to the way they have always done things. When people and organizations introduce new ideas into the community that do not involve the thinking of the residents, they are likely to encounter resistance and may be ostracized by the mainstream of the community.

Assessment of the educational services in the community is important. Educational services are needed for all residents: preschool children, school-aged children, college-aged young adults, and adults returning to school and continuing education courses, including those that meet the needs of retirees. The nurse learns about the availability of technical and vocational opportunities. She determines whether job retraining programs are available for the unemployed.

The nurse finds out how education is valued and what efforts are made by parents and community members to help young residents complete high school and attend college or acquire skills through other means that prepare them for employment. If education is devalued, some young adults may leave the community for education and employment. This action greatly affects the stability of the community.

The nurse assesses the community's coping behavior in relation to information seeking, direct action, inhibition of action, intrapsychic processes, and turning to others.[10] In appropriate information seeking, the residents are assertive in trying to find out what problems exist and what, if anything, can be done to solve the problems. The residents engage in direct action when they do anything about the problem, whether or not the action is effective. Rather than engage in action impulsively or ill advisedly, the residents, using skillful coping resources, postpone action until they have sufficient information. Denial, avoidance, and intellectualization are intrapsychic processes the residents use when they are limited in what they can do about the problems. Realizing they cannot solve the problems in isolation, residents turn to one another for supportive relationships as a form of coping.

✾ *Social dimension.* The structure of buildings in the physical environment affects health. Architectural variables affect social formation and friendship patterns according to the actual distance between houses. Neighbors meet and form friendships more readily if their dwellings face a common courtyard or if they use the same communal areas, such as a swimming pool or laundry room, at the same time.[19] The nurse attends to the size of buildings in the community. In taller buildings there seems to be a higher crime rate and lower levels of overall tenant satisfaction. This may be caused by a reduced potential to see or identify intruders, the impersonal image of the tall structures, and a lack of a feeling of territory in such buildings. The size of the community also needs to be assessed. Residents of a small community may have a stronger support system because they are likely to know other people in the community. In a large community the residents are less familiar with neighbors and may feel isolated.

The formal and informal communication system within the community is assessed. First, it is necessary to determine what media are available and their general rate of use. Next, it is useful to determine the quality and tone of the communication system. Questions may be raised about whether newspapers, radio, and television promote community harmony and competence or address the needs of predominantly one or selected groups in the community. The news covered may provide information about the community's attitude toward mental health and illness. In some communities, news reports receiving priority deal with crime, danger, and scandal. When residents are primarily exposed to negative messages, they are more likely to experience stress than if the media blend negative and positive factors. Informal channels of communication provide vital information about the community. Often people learn more about the community at the beauty shop, barber shop, or a bridge party than through multiple formal sources.

Population density can affect mental health, depending on the extent of crowding or isolation. In general, the more people living in a room, the greater the stimulation, demands on one another, and general level of frustration. Areas of high density have been related to increases in mortality, level of juvenile delinquency, and admission to a psychiatric hospital.[52] Culture influences whether crowding is perceived negatively or positively; some groups are able to tolerate closer physical proximity to family and friends. The opposite of overcrowding—isolation—may cause people to feel bored and alienated.

�֎ ***Spiritual dimension.*** The community is assessed as to the number, availability, accessibility, and variety of religious institutions. The spiritual needs of all residents of the community may not be met when a limited number of religious institutions are present in the community. Religious preferences and religious practices, regardless of denomination, have been associated with lower rates of mental disorders.[39] Nonreligious groups may be considered populations at risk because of a lack of social support, participation, and control that being a member of a religious group might contribute. Communities vary as to their beauty and provision of peace and solitude for residents. Some have beautiful parks, lakes, or walkways where residents can rest, meditate, or commune with God or another power.

The nurse attends to subtle cues that provide information about a community's spirituality. For example, are there signs advertising open forums, speakers, and musical presentations of a spiritual nature? Are gatherings with a spiritual orientation appreciated and well attended?

Analysis

Nursing diagnosis. The following list provides examples of NANDA-accepted nursing diagnoses with causative statements.

1. Potential for violence to others related to inadequate police patrol
2. Diversional activity deficit related to lack of recreational facilities
3. Social isolation related to a climate of mistrust
4. Knowledge deficit related to inadequate educational institutions
5. Spiritual distress related to lack of religious affiliation

TABLE 25-3 Long-term and short-term goals and outcome criteria related to community mental health nursing

Goals	Outcome Criteria
NURSING DIAGNOSIS: FEAR RELATED TO LACK OF SAFETY FOR RESIDENTS	
Long-term goal	
To provide a safe community	Initiates safety measures
	Accepts and adapts to changes in the community
	Demonstrates awareness of changes in safety
	Demonstrates comfort in the community
Short-term goal	
To monitor the safety of the community	Recognizes need for safety measures
	Verbalizes understanding of problem
	Reports strange activity in community
	Acquires watchdog
	Participates in crime watch program
	Enlists support of community members

Planning

Table 25-3 provides long-term and short-term goals and outcome criteria related to community mental health nursing. These serve as examples of the planning stage of the nursing process.

Implementation

∴∴ ***Physical dimension.*** The nurse may participate in encouraging the improvement and availability of mental health facilities and services by presenting statistics on mental health needs in the community and the lack of current resources. She can work with community organizations, such as local agencies on aging, to arrange for transportation to the community mental health centers and other aftercare services.

The nurse may intervene in poor reading skills among children through treatment or referral of individuals. Determining ways to restrict uncontrollable noises near schools and residential areas might prevent the problem. Nurses can join forces with other mental and environmental health workers to build a strong case for adequately insulating schools and residences and for establishing and enforcing appropriate building and zoning codes.[48]

Special implementations within the physical dimension include aiding communities to recognize the need for, seeking funding for, and providing safe playgrounds, parks, museums, and zoos where children can explore their world as well as learn and practice age-appropriate physical activities in a safe and carefully monitored setting. Since accidents are a major cause of injury and death, mental health–psychiatric nurses need to work with communities to provide safety in streets, prevent crime, regulate the use of guns, and decrease personal violence.

The nurse can assist the residents in developing a crime watch program in an effort to increase safety in the community. She can write a column or an article in the neighborhood newspaper that focuses on safety needs in the community. To ensure that all residents will have access to the material, the newspaper should be distributed free of charge. She can also solicit participation from the police, who are knowledgeable about approaches to increasing safety in the community. The police can provide or refer residents to seminars on home security and personal defense. Police can assist residents in developing a neighborhood watch program and can also provide information about gun control.

Initially the nurse intervenes in family violence by arranging for the abused spouse and children to go to a protected environment such as a domestic violence shelter. Then intervention focuses on providing emotional support while the spouse considers options such as family therapy or leaving the abused situation (see Chapter 36).

Attention to the workplace, where major hazards include chemicals, dusts, fumes, noise, heat, radiation, and vibration, is particularly important. In some factories workers are expected to complete their assigned activities in crowded, overheated, and poorly ventilated areas. A nurse can document the detrimental effects to employers of such working conditions, and lead or participate in planning a healthier work environment. She can also develop educational programs to increase workers' awareness of the hazards.

Emotional dimension. Intervention in the emotional dimension is directed at making the community a place in which residents can experience feelings of joy, hope, compassion, and responsibility for self and others, and in which they can deal effectively with such feelings as fear, anger, guilt, anxiety, hopelessness, and despair. Institutions greatly influence the emotional tone of the community. Mental health–psychiatric nurses can play a vital role in helping agencies and institutions such as day care centers, schools, hospitals, and social service agencies to recognize a need for emotional expression among residents and an environment free of undue stress, ambiguity, and feelings of alienation or rejection.

A particularly useful way to meet emotional needs is through self-help or mutual-help groups. Essentially, self-help means supporting and encouraging people to take control of and responsibility for their own lives and health. The recipients of self help also give assistance: participants help others as well as themselves.

Also, self-help groups are voluntary and involve face-to-face interactions in which participants have equal amounts of power and serve as a point of reference and support for one another. Their most useful functions are to provide social support to members through the establishment of a warm and caring group and to increase members' coping skills by providing information and by sharing their own experiences in similar situations.[22]

Support groups that can prove beneficial in most American communities are those for isolated or disrupted families, new mothers, widows, teenagers (especially teenage mothers), people who want to learn more effective ways of handling stress, and discharged psychiatric clients.

Active participation in self-help groups provides members an opportunity to experiment with and use their personal strengths to exert greater control over their health. Active participation in such groups gives members an opportunity to feel valued, in control, capable, and successful, frequently for the first time in a long time. The use of self-help groups by professionals often necessitates learning a new role. Traditionally mental health professionals have led groups. However, the key to effective self-help is for the professional members to aid in establishing the group and then decrease involvement so participants can assume responsibility. The value of such groups will increase, since they are inexpensive, available, and responsive to members' unique needs; professionals can facilitate recognition of the need for such groups, aiding in their implementation and evaluating their effectiveness.

Intellectual dimension. Health education is a common type of nursing intervention in the intellectual dimension. In many instances the goal of community-oriented health education is to increase the degree of self-responsibility among the residents of the community. Many opportunities for intellectual enrichment can be identified in the community. For example, in many communities parenting classes can enrich the health of infants and young children. Many adults have had limited experience in caring for children. Opportunities can be developed within the community both to teach parenting skills and to provide parents an opportunity to discuss their feelings and fears about their new role.

When working with mothers, the nurse can have group discussions that focus on child development and its importance for later mental health. She can distribute pamphlets that cover principles of child rearing; this information can serve as a focus for group discussions. The nurse can also show films or use television programs on effective parenting and lead a discussion of the topic afterward.

Mental health–psychiatric nurses can play key roles in supporting and developing community programs, self-help groups, and groups led by professionals designed to help residents reappraise their situation, examine potential alternatives, and learn new and more effective coping behaviors.

Social dimension. The development of organizations that provide opportunities for people to learn and practice interaction with one another is a useful approach to implementing plans in the social dimension. For example, in one college town of about 50,000 residents all youths in the junior high grades were involved in "rap groups" led by mental health volunteers. Over several years the nurse consultant with the city's mental health center had been able to develop a network in which all seventh, eighth, and ninth graders, in groups of 10 to 12 each, had a chance to informally discuss with an interested adult any topic of interest for 1 hour a week. Volunteers also met regularly with a mental health center counselor for supervision and encouragement. This program was the result of one nurse's dream and goals for enriching the mental health of young people in her community. This same type of rap group approach was also used in many of the city's elementary schools. In these schools the leaders often used a variety of methods to facilitate communication.

Mental health–psychiatric nurses participate in the implementation of a variety of community groups based on a thorough assessment of community characteristics, needs, and resources. Groups not only serve to enrich coping abilities but also can work toward improving the overall health and competence of the community. Specifically, nurses can participate with other mental health professionals and community groups in planning any of the following types of projects[58]:

1. Building projects including schools, homes, airports, shopping centers, and recreational and health care facilities
2. Programs for special populations such as children, the elderly, the handicapped, minorities, migrant workers, immigrants, chronically emotionally disturbed people, and the homeless who are emotionally ill
3. Legislation affecting social practices including substance abuse, retirement, deinstitutionalization, unemployment, and job training
4. Regulatory bodies responsible for building codes, safety procedures, professional practices and policies, and investigation of accidents and disasters
5. Contingency groups formed to plan for epidemics, influx of migrants, and terrorism

Other community efforts to meet social needs include the development of neighborhood or lay networks in which residents turn to members of their own community for support and encouragement. Mental health–psychiatric nurses can serve as catalysts in helping organize and encourage residents to form such networks.

In addition, nurses can work with or serve as consultants to a variety of social groups and institutions to help them recognize their full potential for meeting the social needs of participants. Groups such as Boy Scouts and Girl Scouts can be encouraged to recruit members not only from those eager to join but also from children who are isolated and feel alienated from their peers because of their social status, handicaps, or other factors that may differentiate them from the general population of their age-mates.

Spiritual dimension. Churches and synagogues, social groups, and other institutions influence the philosophy and orientation toward life of residents of the community. Mental health–psychiatric nurses can serve as catalysts or consultants to assist religious and other groups to recognize their role and value in helping people cope creatively and effectively with life stressors. Religious leaders provide face-to-face counseling to people dealing with stressors. These leaders are often skilled in dealing with the whole range of needs of members of their congregations. However, some clergy may profit from the support and consultation provided by a mental health–psychiatric nurse.

Religious institutions possess rich opportunities to strengthen the spirituality of members. Not only the professional staff but also lay members of these institutions can provide care and support to community groups. For example, churches and synagogues can develop helping groups for newcomers, widows, members of divorcing families, parents of handicapped children, released prisoners, or discharged psychiatric clients.

Evaluation

Community program evaluation is often completed over an extended time and at intervals. For example, if a community goal was to decrease the effects of noise on children living near an airport, evaluation may occur at intervals of 6 months or 1 year. Changing building codes and increasing insulation in homes and schools are lengthy processes; therefore accurate evaluation of the goal takes time and repeated measures. Such repeated measures provide information about how long people and communities "feel better" and how resistant they remain to stressors.

Evaluation of community programs answers questions such as the following: How well did the project work? How many people (communities) benefitted? Specifically, what gains were noted? In addition, evaluations are often most effective when they represent the thinking of the whole planning group. This does not mean that all participants are expected to have the opportunity to provide information and ideas to the person or people responsible for evaluation.

Evaluation of community-oriented efforts can seek to measure either the effectiveness of the process or the outcome derived from the program or project. Process evaluation examines the roles and activities of the participants and determines to what extent their efforts have been positive or negative. In contrast, outcome appraisal methods look at the results of the project and raise questions, for example, about the degree to which noise levels were decreased or how many parks were developed.

BRIEF REVIEW

Community mental health nursing is directed toward the mental health needs of the total community. Special attention is given to high-risk populations that include clients who were formerly institutionalized for long periods of time. Systems theory and ecological theory can be effectively applied to mental health nursing in the community. The community is viewed as a subsystem in interaction with other subsystems. Change and adaptation are ongoing processes in the community.

The nurse assumes direct and indirect practice roles in the community. She brings about changes in the community through her use of various treatment modalities, such as self-help groups. She also makes a contribution to the mental health of the community by sharing her knowledge and clinical expertise with other health care providers. The goals of the community mental health–psychiatric nurse are based on the needs of the community and are directed toward intervention and prevention.

REFERENCES AND SUGGESTED READINGS

1. Bachrach, L.L.: The challenge of service planning for chronic mental patients, Community Mental Health Journal 22(32):170, 1986.
2. Bellack, A.S., and others: A comprehensive treatment program for schizophrenia and chronic mental illness, Community Mental Health Journal 22(3):175, 1986.
3. Bloom, B.L.: Community mental health: a general introduction, ed. 2, Monterey, Calif., 1984, Brooks/Cole Publishing Co.
4. Broadley, K.: Shelter or suffering? Long-term psychiatric patients . . . from hospital, Nursing Mirror 161(18):40, 1985.
5. Bune, J.: Preventive role, Nursing Mirror 161(7):29, 1985.
6. Carling, P.J., and others: Psychosocial rehabilitation program as a challenge and an opportunity for community mental health centers, Journal of Psychosocial Rehabilitation 10(1):39, 1986.
7. Carr, P.J., Butterworth, C.A., and Hodges, B.E.: Community psychiatric nursing: caring for the mentally ill and handicapped in the community, London, 1980, Churchill Livingstone.
8. Church, O.M.: From custody to community in psychiatric nursing, Nursing Research 36(1):48, 1987.
9. Clist, L., and others: A new direction for CPNS, Nursing Times 82(1):25, 1986.
10. Cohen, F., and Lazarus, R.S.: Coping with the stresses of illness. In Stone, G.C., and Adler, N.E., editors: Health psychology—a handbook, San Francisco, Calif., 1979, Jossey-Bass, Inc., Publishers.
11. Cohen, S.: Sound effects on behavior, Psychology Today 15:38, 1981.
12. Collins, J., and others: Treatment characteristics of psychiatric programs that correlate with patient community adjustment, Journal of Clinical Psychology 41(3):299, 1985.
13. Cottrell, L.S.: The competent community. In Leighton, A.H., Kaplan, B., and Wilson, R.: New explorations in social psychiatry, New York, 1974, Basic Books, Inc., Publishers.
14. Crosby, R.L.: Community care of the chronically mentally ill: a theory for practice, Journal of Psychosocial Nursing and Mental Health Services 25(1):33, 1987.
15. Culter, D.L.: Community residential options for the chronically mentally ill, Community Mental Health Journal 22(1):61, 1986.
16. Dato, C., and others: The homeless mentally ill, International Nursing Review 32(6/264):170, 1985.
17. Echternacht, M.: Day treatment transition groups: helping outpatients stay out, Journal of Psychosocial Nursing and Mental Health Services 22(10:11, 1984.
18. Faugier, J., and others: Taking time to talk, Part I, Nursing Times: Nursing Practice 82(18):52, 1986.
19. Festinger, L., Schacter, S., and Back, K.: Social pressures in informal groups, Stanford, Calif., 1950, Stanford University Press.
20. Flaskerud, J.H., and van Servellen, G.W.: Community mental health nursing: theories and methods, Norwalk, Connecticut, 1985, Appleton-Century-Crofts.
21. Fraser, M.W., and others: The community treatment of chronically mentally ill: an exploratory social network analysis, Journal of Psychosocial Rehabilitation 9(2):35, 1985.
22. Gartner, A.J., and Riessman, F.: Self-help and mental health, Hospital and Community Psychiatry 33:631, 1982.
23. Glidewell, J.C.: Priorities for psychologists in community mental health. In Division 27, American Psychological Association, Task Force on Community Mental Health, Issues in community psychology and preventive mental health, New York, 1971, Behavioral Publications.
24. Godin, P., and Wilson I.: Community psychiatry: selling skills, Community Outlook, p. 27, April 1986.
25. Godschalx, S.M.: Effect of a mental health education program upon police officers, Research in Nursing and Health 7:111, 1984.
26. Gold Award: mental health treatment that transcends cultural barriers, Hospital and Community Psychiatry 37(9): 913, 1986.
27. Gold Award: a network of services for the homeless chronic mentally ill, Hospital and Community Psychiatry 37(11): 1148, 1986.
28. Hall, V.: The community mental health nurse: a new professional role, Journal of Advances in Nursing 7:3, 1982.
29. Heath, B.H., Jr., and others: Consumer satisfaction: some new twists to a not so old evaluation, Community Mental Health Journal 20(2):123, 1984.
30. Hoover, R.M.: Medication education: an alliance between inpatient and community mental health center care, Free Association 12(3):5, 1985.
31. Hundert, J.: Community mental health for children: a shift in emphasis, Canadian Mental Health 33(1):2, 1985.
32. Hutton, F.M.: Self-referrals to a community health centre: a three year study, British Journal of Psychiatry 147:540, 1985.
33. Jeger, A.M., and Slotnick, R.S., editors: Community mental health and behavioral-ecology: a handbook of theory, research, and practice, New York, 1982, Plenum Press.
34. Klyczek, J.P., and others: Therapeutic modality comparisons in day treatment, American Journal of Occupational Therapy 40(9):606, 1986.
35. Koldjeski, D.: Community mental health nursing: new directions in theory and practice, New York, 1984, John Wiley & Sons.
36. Lamb, H.R., editor: The homeless mentally ill: a Task Force Report of the American Psychiatric Association, Washington, D.C., 1984, American Psychiatric Association.
37. Lancaster, J.: Community mental health nursing: an ecological perspective, St. Louis, 1980, The C.V. Mosby Company.
38. Lewis, R.: Undesirable neighbors, American Journal of Nursing 86(5):535, 1986.
39. Levy, L., and Rowitz, L.: Ecology of mental disorders, New York, 1972, Behavioral Publications.
40. Manchester, J.: A framework for planning, Nursing Mirror 156(15):34, 1983.
41. Mangen, S.P., and Griffith, J.H.: Patient satisfaction with community psychiatric nursing: a prospective controlled study, Journal of Advances in Nursing 7(5):477, 1982.
42. Mann, L., and Whall, A.: Informed consent and the deinsitutionalized patient, Journal of Psychosocial Nursing and Mental Health Services 22(1):22, 1984.
43. McGuire, J., and others: Attitudes toward mental health professionals in a hospital-based community mental health center, Community Mental Health Journal 22(1):39, 1986.
44. Medders, N.M., and Colman, A.D.: The assisted individual living project: a new model for community care, Psychiatric Annals 15(11):667, 1985.
45. Melen, V.: A response to the American Psychiatric Association report on the homeless mentally ill, Journal of Psychosocial Rehabilitation 8(4):3, 1985.
46. Menolascino, F.J., and others: Issues in the treatment of mentally retarded patients in the community mental health system, Community Mental Health Journal 22(4):314, 1986.
47. Miller, J.C.: Theoretical basis for the practice of community mental health nursing, Issues in Mental Health Nursing 3:319, 1981.
48. Monahan, J., and Vaux, A.: Task force report: the macroenvi-

ronment and community mental health, Community Mental Health Journal 16:14, 1980.

49. Morse, G., and others: St. Louis homeless: mental health needs, services, and policy implications, Journal of Psychosocial Rehabilitation 9(4):39, 1986.

50. Neal, M.T.: Partial hospitalization: an alternative to inpatient psychiatric hospitalization, Nursing Clinics of North America, 21(3):461, 1986.

51. Paolillo, J.G.P., and others: Appointment compliance behavior of community mental health patients: a discriminant analysis, Community Mental Health Journal 20(2):103, 1984.

52. Price, R.H., and others, editors: Prevention in mental health: research, policy, and practice, vol. I, Beverly Hills, Calif., 1980, Sage Publications.

53. Randonsky, V.E., and others: Step ahead—occupational therapy in the community, Occupational Therapy and Mental Health 6(2):79, 1986.

54. Soleman, P.L., Dordon, B.H., and Don, J.M.: Community service to discharged patients, Springfield, Illinois, 1984, Charles C Thomas Publishing.

55. Solomon, P., and others: Meeting community service needs to discharged psychiatric patients, Psychiatric Quarterly 57(1):11, 1985.

56. Solomon, P., and others: An assessment of aftercare services within a community mental health system, Journal of Psychosocial Rehabilitation 7(2):33, 1983.

57. Spence, G.G., and others: Factors affecting the performance of a prescribed community psychiatry role for nurses, Canadian Mental Health 29:36, 1981.

58. Swift, C.: Task force report: National Council of Community Mental Centers task force on environmental assessment, Community Mental Health Journal 18:7, Spring, 1980.

59. Toews, J., and others: The chronic mental patient and community psychiatry: a system in trouble, Canadian Mental Health 34(2):2, 1986.

60. Vonsden, M.: Shared information, Nursing Times 82(49):42, 1986.

61. Wolgrove, N.J.: Mental health aftercare: where is nursing? Nursing Clinics of North America 21(3):473, 1986.

62. Wooff, K., and others: Patient in receipt of community psychiatric nursing in Salford, Psychological Bulletin 16(2):407, 1986.

63. Zelman, W.N., and others: Survival strategies for community mental health organizations: a conceptual framework, Community Mental Health Journal 21(4):228, 1985.

ANNOTATED BIBLIOGRAPHY

Adler, D.A., Drake, R.E., and Stern, R.: Viewing chronic mental illness: a conceptual framework, Comprehensive Psychiatry 25:192, 1984.

A nonmedical conceptual framework for viewing chronic mental illness is adaptation oriented rather than illness oriented. The model emphasizes positive coping capabilities and attitudes of patients, their families, and their communities. Chronic mental illness involves nine interdependent domains: living situation, performance, behaviors, sociocultural environment, fiscal costs, adaptive style, individual attitudes, physical health, and symptoms. Each domain is examined and compared with

assumptions and problems of existing approaches for managing the chronically mentally ill in community settings.

Gonfein, W.: Incentives and intentions in mental health policy: a comparison of the Medicaid and community mental health programs, Journal of Health and Human Behavior 26:183, 1985.

Community mental health programs have been the official policy for care of the mentally ill in this country for more than two decades. One of the rationales stated for instituting this alternative system was to reduce the populations in public mental hospitals and to provide more effective and humane psychiatric care. Inpatient populations in mental hospitals have decreased by 75% during the period noted. However, a major factor in this reduction is the use of Medicaid benefits to effect transinstitutionalization from mental hospitals to nursing homes, and this process has had a greater effect on population reduction than deinstitutionalization through use of community mental health services and programs.

Pardes, H., and Stockdill, J.W.: Survival strategies for community mental health services in the 80s, Hospital and Community Psychiatry 35:127, 1984.

Widespread reduction of financial support for community mental health services from federal and other levels of government has created a concern about whether the community mental health center system can survive. Centers will have to use such strategies as incorporation, alternative services, and innovative funding and will have to become much more active in the political process to survive. In order to retain the values of community mental health, services have to become more efficient and employ business techniques of marketing and finance.

Perlmutter, D.R.: Recent trends and issues in psychiatric-mental health nursing, Hospital and Community Psychiatry 36:56, 1985.

A review of some of the major achievements over the past three decades points out the advances of this special area of practice in role expansion, educational preparation, and research. A trend that is predicted to continue is the expansion of role in clinical nursing practice. An issue that needs attention is the incorporation of more nursing models and concepts in the conceptual bases for psychiatric–mental health nursing practice. More is needed in tests of interventions to determine their effectiveness, and there is a need for research in some of the basic neuroscience areas that have direct relevance to clinical practice in community mental health.

Slavinsky, A.: Psychiatric nursing in the year 2000: from a non-system of care to a caring system. In Bilitski, J.S., and Taylor, M.C., editors: Nursing in the year 2000, Morgantown, W.V., 1983, West Virginia University Press.

The prediction is made that by the year 2000, psychiatric nurses will be in charge of the mental health care system in this country. This decentralized, community-based health care system will be more responsible to client needs, and humane care will be a basic concern. Third-party reimbursement will have ceased to be an issue, and this arrangement will be a general means of payment of mental health services. An issue that will continue to be of concern is that of recruitment to this special area of practice of a sufficient number of nurses to manage the mental health system. A new primary care role for psychiatric nurses will cover three basic functions: assessment, direct patient care, and case management.

CHAPTER 26

CRISIS INTERVENTION

Sophronia R. Williams   Donna C. Aguilera

After studying this chapter the learner will be able to:

Define crisis.

Define crisis intervention.

Describe the historical development of crisis intervention.

Describe selected theoretical models of crisis intervention.

Discuss the characteristics of the crisis therapist.

Discuss the characteristics of crisis intervention.

Apply the nursing process in crisis situations.

Crisis is an inevitable aspect of human existence. Individuals are constantly confronted with potentially crisis-producing events that threaten their level of functioning. The ongoing changes and pressures in today's society test the person's ability to effectively use problem-solving behaviors, and this may result in the individual experiencing a crisis situation that cannot be resolved without professional assistance.

A *crisis* occurs "when a person faces an obstacle to important life goals that is, for a time, insurmountable through the utilization of customary methods of problem solving."[8] Situational supports may help avert the crisis or decrease the intensity of the reaction to the crisis, but in today's mobile society family and close friends may not be accessible to provide support. Individuals then turn to mental health professionals for crisis intervention. *Crisis intervention* is an active entering into the life situation of a person, family, or group who is experiencing a crisis to decrease the impact of the crisis event and to assist the individual to mobilize his resources and regain equilibrium.[39]

Nurses are constantly confronted with clients who are in a potential state of crisis. Regardless of the area in which they are working, nurses are available to implement the concepts and techniques of crisis intervention: with a mother who has given birth to a physically or mentally handicapped child; in the emergency room, for example, with an automobile accident victim; and with families of clients who have had surgery or a heart attack and are told "nothing more can be done."

THEORETICAL APPROACHES
Psychoanalytic

Eric Lindemann's initial contributions[28] to the theory of crisis intervention are based on his scientific investigation of the behavior of people who were experiencing an acute grief reaction. The sample of 101 people studied consisted of disaster victims of the 1942 Coconut Grove fire in Boston and their close relatives, patients with psychoneuroses who had lost a relative during the patient's treatment, relatives of members of the armed forces, and relatives of patients. Lindemann concluded that grief and bereavement in response to a loss by death lead to a crisis in almost all individuals, and most will experience a *normal grief reaction.*

A bereaved person who experiences a normal grief reaction manifests a characteristic syndrome that consists of (1) somatic distress, (2) preoccupation with the image of the deceased, (3) expression of guilt and hostility, (4) disorganization in daily patterns of activity, generally with a decrease in level of activity, and (5) identification with

Historical Overview

DATE	EVENT
1906	First recorded instance of "crisis intervention" concerned Freud's treatment of partial paralysis in a client's arm in six visits.
1940s	Principles and techniques of crisis intervention were derived from the use of supportive techniques to treat soldiers suffering from crises related to combat during World War II. Psychiatrists, on their return home after the war, used the techniques that were effective with soldiers to deal with survivors of civil and military disasters.
1944	Lindemann's classic study of bereaved disaster victims of the Coconut Grove nightclub fire established a format for the study and development of crisis theory and practice.
1948	Lindemann refined his crisis concepts and organized an innovative community mental health program in Boston. Caplan elaborated on Lindemann's model and became known as the father of modern crisis intervention.[33]
1950s	The development of crisis intervention paralleled brief or short-term psychotherapy.
1950s-1960s	Caplan developed his interest in crisis situations out of his early work with immigrant mothers and children in Israel after World War II. Caplan's approach to crisis intervention was set in the format of primary, secondary, and tertiary levels of intervention at the Harvard School of Public Health. Parad, Rapoport, Jacobson, and Aguilera, building on the work of Lindemann and Caplan, refined crisis theory and developed treatment models for crisis in marital and family conflicts and in suicide prevention.
1963	The Community Mental Health Act of 1963 influenced the development of crisis intervention: one requirement of the Act was that community facilities provide emergency services.
Mid-1960s	Crisis intervention became a treatment modality in its own right.
1970s	Caplan focused his attention on natural and mutual support systems in the community that could be used to prevent or ameliorate the destructive aspects of crisis situations.
1980s	Nurses have increased their involvement with crises in a variety of inpatient and outpatient settings.
Future	Rapid, increasingly complex social changes will threaten people's stability and coping behavior, increasing the need for nurses to give priority to crisis intervention as a means of preventing psychiatric problems.

the deceased by some bereaved persons. The duration and intensity of the grief reaction vary among individuals, depending on the extent to which the person successfully completes the grief work.

Normal grief work begins when the individual frees himself from ties to the deceased, readjusts to his social environment, and establishes new and satisfying relationships. Although this process may be accomplished without professional assistance, some individuals with a normal grief reaction need professional help. Lindemann found that with the guidance of a mental health professional in 8 to 10 interviews and within a period of 4 to 6 weeks, these individuals successfully completed grief work.

Lindemann found that survivors of the Coconut Grove disaster who developed serious psychopathological conditions had failed to go through the normal process of grieving. This led him to describe *morbid grief reactions*.

Individuals who experience a morbid grief reaction have either a *delayed* or a *distorted* reaction. People may delay or postpone their reaction to the loss for a few weeks or longer. A distorted reaction may be an immediate response to bereavement and includes overactivity without a sense of loss, taking on symptoms belonging to the last illness of the deceased, the development of a medical problem, and agitated depression.

Lindemann believed that his work with the bereaved was basic to the development of a conceptual framework related to emotional crises. He viewed the birth of a child and marriage as examples of events that could generate sufficient emotional strain to lead to crises. The preventive intervention that is effective with bereavement can also be applied to these events. He believed that when crises are properly managed, prolonged and serious alteration in social functioning can be avoided.

One aspect of crisis theory that Lindemann introduced and that Caplan described in depth is the different types of crises. He acknowledged the influence of Erikson's model[14] of developmental (maturational) and situational (accidental) crises on his theories about life crises.

Caplan defined *developmental crises* as transitional periods in personality development characterized by disturbances in cognitive and affective functioning. These crises are experienced by everyone as they learn to adjust to the new expectations related to the various maturational periods in life. The discussion of Erikson's developmental stages in Chapter 3 includes examples of this type of crises.

A sudden, unexpected threat to or loss of basic resources or life goals is a *situational crisis*. These crises are not as common as the developmental ones and are characterized by periods of psychological and behavioral disorganization that occurs when the individual is unable to cope by his usual behavior. Such crises may by precipitated by fires, floods, earthquakes, and other natural disasters that affect large numbers of people. The Coconut Grove fire is an example of a disaster that led to a crisis. Loss through divorce, the death of a loved one, and a job promotion or demotion are also examples of events that may trigger a situational crisis.

Caplan observed the reactions of clients with psychiatric disorders to changes in life events, such as the death of a significant other, the loss of a job, and becoming a parent, which are types of situational crises. These problems were new to the clients, and their usual coping behavior did not work. Clients who dealt with the problem in adaptive ways seemed healthier after than before the crisis. Based on his observations Caplan concluded that there are universal responses to crises. An individual with a relatively stable personality may change in ways that are unexpected during a crisis; the outcome of the crises may be a positive change in personality, in which case the crisis was a period of opportunity, or the crisis may result in decreased efficiency in the individual's ability to cope. These notions lead to the view of crisis as a transitional period that affords the individual both an opportunity for personality growth and the danger of greater vulnerability. Either response to the crisis is determined by the individual's handling of the situation.

Caplan believed that mental disorders may decrease if individuals are assisted in improving their problem-solving skills, which in turn increases their ability to deal effectively with stress. He considered a crisis a turning point toward or away from mental disorders. He believed that intervention at the point of crisis can prevent later serious mental illness. Caplan viewed crisis intervention as a major technique of *preventive psychiatry*. Preventive psychiatry focuses on using theoretical knowledge and skills to plan and implement programs designed to achieve three categories of prevention: *primary, secondary,* and *tertiary*.

Primary prevention involves decreasing the incidence of psychiatric illness in the community. It is designed to intervene in hazardous situations with the goal of preventing the development of psychiatric disorders. Thus an aspect of primary prevention is the promotion of general mental health. The goals of primary prevention are achieved by such activities as providing educational programs to groups in the community and consultation to school teachers, identifying groups at risk, and designing and implementing programs to prevent psychiatric disorders. For example, sex education for teenagers who are at risk for pregnancy is a type of primary prevention.

The focus of secondary prevention is early diagnosis and prompt and effective treatment to reduce the duration of a significant number of psychiatric disorders. When people in crisis receive early effective intervention and regain equilibrium, their chances for developing a long-term disability decrease. When the first psychiatric illness of a young adult is treated early and effectively, he may not develop a chronic psychiatric problem. Individuals who need treatment for psychiatric problems may be identified through screening large populations referred for treatment. One setting in which screening procedures are conducted is the school. Educating the public to recognize early signs of psychiatric disorders may be effective for secondary prevention. Individuals who require secondary prevention may be hospitalized or may engage in some form of psychotherapy.

Tertiary prevention refers to the reduction of long-term disability that may result from psychiatric disorders. Individuals with chronic psychiatric illnesses benefit from tertiary prevention. Rehabilitation programs are designed for tertiary prevention.

Jacobson and associates classified two types of treatment approaches to crisis: the generic approach and the individual approach.[23] The *generic approach* is based on the premise that certain identifiable patterns of behavior are characteristic of each type of crisis and that psychological tasks specific to the type of crisis are required if the crisis is to be successfully resolved. Treatment of the crisis is focused on the characteristic course rather than the psychodynamics of the particular crisis type. Also treatment is designed for the target group rather than a specific individual. For example, in the crisis of a child with terminal cancer the mother must accomplish the psychological task of accepting that the child will likely die and must prepare for the impending loss.

The client and the therapist participate together in the problem-solving process. The generic approach to problem solving encourages the use of adaptive behavior, includes general support, and allows for manipulation of the environment and anticipatory guidance. Jacobson and associates[23] believed that because of the specificity of the approach, it can be used by nonprofessionals and others not trained in crisis intervention.

The *individual approach* emphasizes assessment of the intrapsychic and interpersonal process of the person in crisis by a mental health professional. The crisis therapist focuses on identification of the precipitating factors and examines reasons the individual's usual coping mechanisms are no longer effective. Once the therapist achieves these goals she determines the intervention that is necesssary to improve the client's coping abilities. The therapist needs to have knowledge of the psychodynamics related to the crisis. Various situational crises that a person experiences may be effectively treated with the individual approach, since this approach is directed toward the individual's unique situation.

Cognitive

An individual in the precrisis state is described as being able to use cognition to process information.[51] The person can think, perceive, evaluate, make decisions, and learn. He is able to select coping strategies to deal with stressful situations. A breakdown in cognitive processes results from a psychological or physical overload, a crisis. At the peak of the crisis there is a cognitive "digestive capacity" in that too much dissonant information has entered the individual's cognitive structure to allow him to use his characteristic problem-solving processes. This crisis situation demands that the individual learn new ways of coping. Initially the individual acquires new information by building new cognitive maps. This process enables him to develop the capacity to learn and select from among coping strategies. The individual may be able to resolve the crisis unassisted by continuing to use existing coping strategies or by developing new ones. Even after the crisis is resolved the person can use the new coping strategies in future crisis situations.

Systems

An aspect of Caplan's work is based on systems theory. He was the first to relate homeostasis to crisis reactions. He recognized that a goal of human functioning is to maintain a homeostatic balance with the environment. The individual is constantly faced with situations that threaten this balance. Usually the individual readily activates habitual problem-solving activities that effectively restore a steady state. However, when faced with a crisis the usual habitual mechanisms are ineffectual in assisting the individual in reestablishing equilibrium within the person's usual time span. When unsuccessful in solving the problem the individual enters the phases of a crisis.

Caplan elaborated on crisis theory by describing four characteristic phases of a crisis. The stages and responses are depicted in Figure 26-1.

Parad[37] introduced the idea that the event that precipitated the crisis must be perceived by the person as stressful before it becomes a crisis. This premise is discussed later in the chapter. Parad and Resnik,[39] using a different approach than Caplan's characteristics of a crisis, described the crisis sequence in terms of time periods: the precrisis, the crisis or upset, and the postcrisis (Figure 26-2). During the *precrisis period* the individual maintains his equilibrium through the use of his usual coping methods. He may have minor stresses, but they are not perceived as threatening to his life goals. A threat to life goals is a hazard to the individual's basic security needs such as body integrity, love, or a sense of security. If the person perceives an event as a threat to life goals and one with which he is unable to cope, he enters the *crisis period*. The crisis period begins at the time of the impact of the crisis.

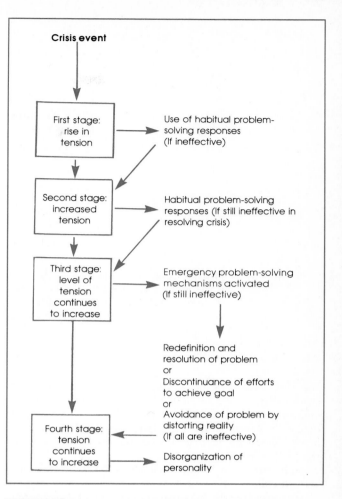

FIGURE 26-1 Caplan's developmental stages of a crisis.

During a crisis the individual experiences disorganization, tension, and anxiety, and uses various trial-and-error responses in an effort to resolve the crisis. *Crisis resolution* is the development of effective adaptive and coping devices based on the client's use of his own resources through the intervention of health care professionals and with assistance from family and significant others.[39]

With resolution of the problem the individual experiences a *postcrisis period*. This period is characterized by a return to the steady state, and the individual may resume his precrisis level of functioning or perhaps a higher or lower state of functioning, depending on the effectiveness of the crisis resolution.

The theoretical approaches are summarized in Table 26-1, p. 495.

CHARACTERISTICS OF CRISIS INTERVENTION
Client Selection

The initial consideration in client selection is the determination that the client is experiencing a crisis. A traditional and still widely accepted criterion for selection is

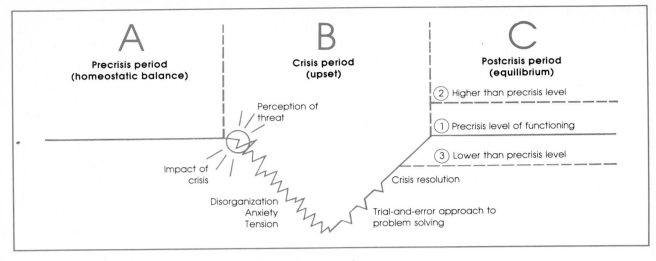

FIGURE 26-2 Crisis sequence diagram. (Adapted from Parad, H.J., and others: In Resnik, H.L.P., Ruben, H.L., and Ruben, D.D., editors: Emergency psychiatric care; the management of mental health crises, Bowie, Md., 1975. Reprinted with permission of Charles Press, Division of Robert J. Brady Co., from the copyrighted work Emergency Psychiatric Care.)

that the client must be dealing with a recent, sudden life situation that requires immediate attention and that the client cannot solve himself. The client must have a clearly defined environmental stress such as the loss of a job, acute bereavement, marital discord, or suicidal gestures that can be resolved rapidly.

Some therapists believe that only clients who are fairly well integrated and who have never had a psychiatric illness can receive the maximal benefits from crisis intervention. Other therapists select clients with previous psychiatric problems who are now experiencing a crisis for treatment. Still others include in the group of clients who are suitable candidates for crisis intervention those experiencing their first psychotic breakdown and those with chronic psychiatric symptoms that are in remission.[27] Janosik believed that chronically depressed clients, alcoholics, individuals with psychoses, and withdrawn persons without reliable social networks are not appropriate candidates for crisis intervention.[21]

It is generally accepted that crisis intervention techniques are effective with individuals in crisis regardless of their socioeconomic background. The client must have the ability and motivation to participate in the problem-solving process. The client's level of motivation is determined in part by the extent to which he shares information and what information he shares. Some therapists expect the client to acknowledge a target problem in two or three sessions or the therapy is terminated.[12]

In addition to individuals, families are suitable candidates for crisis intervention. To be selected for crisis intervention the family must accept the crisis situation as a family problem, regardless of the precipitating event and the family member who is perceived as responsible for the crisis.[12]

The therapist may use her knowledge of *crisis-prone persons* as an aid in the selection of clients. The crisis-prone person has been described as an individual who has no available support system or, if social support, including the family, is available, is unable to use them in his efforts to cope with everyday stress.[39] The person lives a marginal existence and may manifest the following interrelated problems:

1. Difficulty in learning from experience
2. History of frequent crises and unsuccessful resolution of the crisis because of the person's poor coping skills
3. History of previous psychiatric disorders or serious emotional instability
4. Low self-esteem, which the individual may attempt to disguise by provocative behavior
5. Impulsiveness, manifested by taking action before the person thinks through the consequences
6. Poor work history in an unfulfilling job that results in a marginal income
7. Faulty marital and family relationships
8. Alcohol and drug abuse
9. Tendency to have numerous accidents
10. Frequent contacts with law enforcement agencies
11. A tendency to change residence frequently

Therapeutic Settings

Crisis intervention may be provided in a variety of settings. The nurse has many opportunities to perform crisis intervention in formal settings such as emergency rooms of general hospitals. In these settings, the nurse may encounter relatives of accident victims and of clients who may be faced with a serious life-threatening illness, such

TABLE 26-1 Summary of theoretical approaches

Theory	Theorist	Dynamics
Psychoanalytic	Lindemann	Grief and bereavement in response to death leads to a crisis
		The response to death as a crisis may be a normal grief reaction or a morbid grief reaction: a delayed or distorted response
	Caplan	There are developmental and situational crises
		A crises may lead to decreased efficiency in one's ability to function, or may be experienced as an opportunity for growth
		Crises intervention is a major type of preventive psychiatry: primary, secondary, and tertiary prevention
	Jacobson and associates	Generic approach: each type of crisis has identifiable patterns of behavior and characteristics and specific psychological tasks for successful intervention
		Individual approach: emphasizes an assessment of the intrapsychic and interpersonal process of the person in crisis
Cognitive	Taplin	A crisis is a psychological or physical overload
		A crisis results in a breakdown of cognitive functioning that affects problem solving
Systems	Caplan	A crisis is a threat to homeostasis
		The individual's usual problem-solving activities cannot restore equilibrium
	Parad and Resnik	The event that precipitates a crisis must be perceived as stressful by the individual
		There are three time periods in a crisis sequence: precrisis, crisis, and postcrisis

as a heart attack, who are in need of crisis intervention. Rape victims, clients who have made suicide attempts or threats, and individuals with homicidal behavior are possible clients for crisis intervention in the emergency room setting. In some instances, the nurse refers the client to a crisis team in the emergency room after she does a cursory assessment and establishes that the client is possibly in crisis.

Crisis intervention centers and crisis units in community mental health centers are other formal settings in which the nurse conducts crisis intervention. In these settings, ambulatory clients who are making suicidal threats or are experiencing a situation crisis such as a grief reaction in response to a loss, an unwanted pregnancy, or reactions to environmental disasters such as tornadoes and floods are candidates for crisis intervention. Candidates in these settings also include individuals who need assistance with their adjustment to a developmental crisis, for example, adolescent turmoil. The nurse may function in formal agencies for special populations such as adolescents, children, and families when these agencies use crisis intervention as a treatment modality.

Another formal setting in which the nurse frequently intervenes in crises is on units in the general medical hospital. Clients may react to impending surgery with a crisis reaction, especially when the surgery will result in the loss of a body part and other changes in the body image. The stresses associated with any physical illness may precipitate a crisis that will require the nurse to use her knowledge and skills in crisis intervention. Families may need crisis intervention directly after the death of a family member.

Telephone hot lines are semiformal approaches to providing crisis intervention. These hot lines may provide crisis intervention services on a 24-hour, 7-day-a-week basis. Generally, trained nonprofessional volunteers, with consultation from members of a professional mental health staff, operate the telephone services. Among the consultation services provided by way of telephone hot lines are suicide prevention and crisis intervention for rape victims.

Special Characteristics and Process

Most major crisis theorists accept Caplan's premise[9] that a crisis situation is self-limiting, lasting from 1 to 6 weeks. The average crisis lasts 4 weeks. However, the 1- to 6-week time frame for the therapeutic process needs to be flexible, varying according to the needs of the client.

The focus of treatment is the individual's current life experiences that relate to the crisis. The client's previous experiences related to unresolved conflicts are a part of the therapeutic work only to the extent that they influence the current crisis situation.

Balancing factors. Three interrelated *balancing factors* contribute to the production of a crisis and influence the outcome of the crisis.[1] These balancing factors occur between the perceived effects of a stressful situation and the resolution of the problem. The factors are (1) perception of the event, (2) available situational supports, and (3) coping mechanisms. The upper portion of the paradigm in

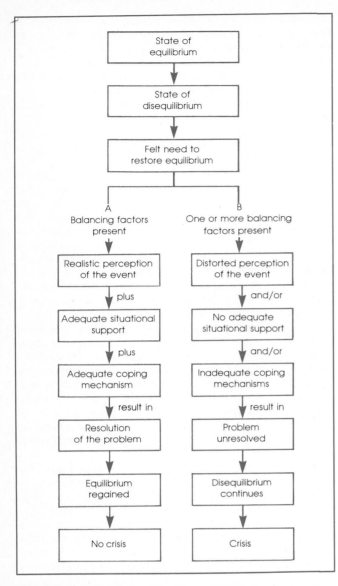

FIGURE 26-3 Paradigm: the effect of balancing factors in a stressful event. (Adapted from Aguilera, D.C., and Messick, J.M.: Crisis intervention: theory and methodology, ed. 5, St. Louis, 1986, The C.V. Mosby Co.)

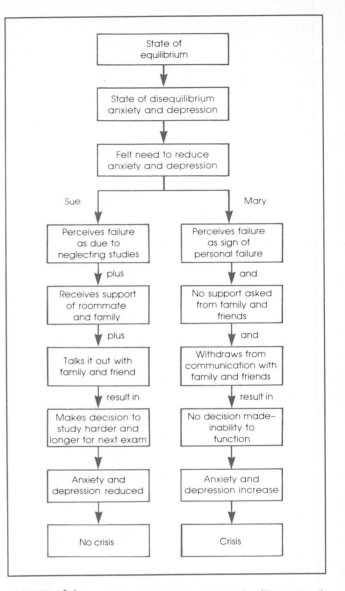

FIGURE 26-4 Paradigm applied to case study. (From Aguilera, D.C., and Messick, J.M.: Crisis intervention: theory and methodology, ed. 5, St. Louis, 1986, The C.V. Mosby Co.)

Figure 26-3 illustrates the "normal" initial reaction of an individual to a stressful event. The presence or absence of these factors can affect the return of equilibrium. In column *A* of Figure 26-3 the balancing factors are operating, and crisis is avoided. In column *B* one or more of these balancing factors are absent. Resolution of the problem may be blocked, thus increasing disequilibrium and precipitating a crisis.

In Figure 26-4 the paradigm is applied to the experiences of two students, Sue and Mary, who were affected differently by the same stressful event. Both students failed a final exmination. Sue is upset about the failure but does not experience a crisis. Mary reacts to failing the ex-

amination with a crisis. What accounts for the differences in their responses to the same stressful event?

Perception of the event. An individual's perception of a stressful event plays a major role in determining the nature and degree of his response to the event. The perception of the crisis event is determined in part by the extent to which the event is a threat to the individual's values and life goals. The crisis event may be perceived as a threat to basic needs that are symbolically related to needs that led to a conflict earlier in life. In this instance the predominant emotional response to the threat is anxiety. The crisis situation may be perceived as a loss. The loss may be real, or it may be experienced as a deprivation. The response to the perceived loss or deprivation is a feeling of depression. Another way the crisis event may be experienced is as a challenge.[43] When the crisis event is experienced as a challenge, the individual mobilizes his energy and engages in purposive problem-solving activities. Examples of challenges may be getting married, job promotions, and parenthood.

The individual's perception of the event may be realistic or distorted. If the person perceives the crisis event realistically, he will recognize the relationship between the event and his feelings of stress. He can then participate in problem-solving activities directed toward successful resolution of the crisis. A distorted perception of the crisis situation leads to continued feelings of tension, and his attempts to resolve the problem are futile. These individuals do not recognize the relationship between the crisis event and their stress.

Differences in Sue's and Mary's perception in terms of the threat of the event to an important life goal account for the diffferences in their response behavior. Sue views failing the examination as the result of not studying enough or of concentrating on the wrong material and decides it will not happen again. Mary, on the other hand, thinks that failing the examination makes her a failure; she feels threatened and believes she will never graduate from college. Sue's appraisal of the situation led her to anticipate success in the future and to use a direct-action mode of coping, such as attack. Mary appraised the situation as overwhelming and resorted to the use of intrapsychic defense mechanisms to distort the reality of the situation.

Situational supports. Situational supports, a second balancing factor, refer to available persons in the environment who can be depended on to help the individual solve problems. The situational supports become the individual's significant others, and from them the individual learns to seek advice and support in solving daily problems in living. Individuals may readily develop dependent relationships with support persons who protect them from feelings of insecurity and thus reinforce their feeling of ego integrity.

Any perceived failure to obtain adequate support to meet one's needs may provoke or compound a stressful situation. Negative support can be equally detrimental to the person's self-esteem. When the self-esteem is lowered by a threatening situation, the individual seeks out situational supports. When there is a loss or a threatened loss of a supportive relationship, the individual feels vulnerable. If faced with a stressful situation when there is lack of situational support, the person may experience a state of disequilibrium and possible crisis.

Sue found someone for support during this stressful event. She talked to her roommate about her feelings over failing the examination; she even cried on her shoulder. She also called home for reassurance from her family. In effect, someone had been found for support during this stressful event. Mary did not feel close enough to her roommate to talk about the problem. She had no close friends she trusted. Fearing their reaction, she did not call home to tell her family about failing. Mary did not have anyone to turn to for help; she felt overwhelmed and alone.

Coping mechanisms. Coping mechanisms comprise the third balancing factor that affects an individual's ability to restore equilibrium after a stressful event. The individual's use of intrapsychic ego defense mechanisms to deal with stress and anxiety is discussed in Chapter 11. Coping mechanisms differ from intrapsychic ego defense mechanisms in that coping mechanisms may be consciously or unconsciously motivated, and they are used to deal with the minor stresses of everyday life. They also are attempts to solve the problem rather than to avoid it by using ego defense mechanisms.

Through the process of daily living individuals are confronted with what Menninger and others[32] referred to as *minor emergencies,* or problems that create disequilibrium. Those individuals, through experience and by learning about their potentialities, develop techniques for dealing with minor external and internal stresses. One way to deal with these stresses is by using the coping mechanisms of everyday living as stabilizers.

Various adaptive and maladaptive coping mechanisms are available when people have minor emergencies or problems. They may try to think out their problems or talk about them with a friend. Some cry or try to get rid of their feelings of anger and hostility by swearing, kicking a chair, or slamming doors. Others may get into verbal battles with friends. Some may react by temporarily withdrawing from the situation to reassess the problem. Each of these mechanisms has been used at some time in the developmental past of the individual, was found to be effective in maintaining emotional stability, and became part of his life-style in meeting and dealing with the stresses of daily living.

Maladaptive coping mechanisms may sometimes resemble ego defense mechanisms. Examples of such mechanisms are excessive fantasy, magical thinking, and withdrawal from reality.

Sue coped by using her roommate to talk it out; this reduced her tension and anxiety. She was able to solve the problem and decided that for the next examination she would study more over a longer period of time. Her tension and anxiety were reduced, equilibrium was restored, and she did not have a crisis.

Mary withdrew. She had no coping skills, and her tension and anxiety increased. Unable to solve the problem and unable to function, she went into crisis.

A person who is in crisis usually seeks crisis intervention within 1 to 2 weeks after the precipitating event occurs. Often the event that led to the crisis has happened within the 24 hours before the individual's arrival for therapy. By the time the client seeks crisis intervention, he is more vulnerable and capable of being influenced by others than when his equilibrium is in balance. Intervention at this point in the crisis can prevent later serious mental illness or the development of maladaptive patterns of behavior. Minimal interaction by the nurse will have maximal effect on the client's coping mechanisms and problem-solving activities. This influence may promote or impede further development of the client's mental health. The client needs immediate attention to his problem. The longer the delay between the time the client requests help and when he receives assistance, the greater the opportunity for the person to distort the crisis event.

The initial phase of crisis intervention is crucial to resolution of the crisis. Sometimes this phase is only one session because with the nurse's assistance the client identifies and resolves the problem. Problem identification and resolution are the crux of crisis intervention. The focus of the therapeutic process is the client's perception of the problem. Anxiety affects the individual's perception of situations and his ability to solve problems. Clients in crisis are often experiencing a severe to panic level of anxiety. Thus their perceptual field is limited and problem-solving abilities become increasingly ineffective.

During the initial phase of therapy and preferably during the first session, the nurse actively guides the client to identify the precipitating event that led to the crisis and the basis for his perception of the event as a crisis. The nurse needs to be persistent in learning the reason the client is seeking crisis intervention at this time. The nurse may ask directly, "What is your reason for seeking help *now* or *today?*" Another question that may be asked is, "What has happened in the last hour, day, or week to upset you?"

During the initial contact with the client the nurse conveys to the client hope that the crisis can be successfully resolved by participating with the client in exploring his problem and clearly defining the goals for treatment and the activities necessary to achieve the goals.[45] The nurse communicates verbally and nonverbally that she will work *with* the client in resolving the crisis and regaining hope. With this support the client can leave the first session with the feeling that he can participate in solving the crisis. In subsequent sessions the nurse plans and implements specific treatment for the client that takes into consideration the client's motivation, strengths, and capabilities. The specific treatment is determined by the precipitating problem. For example, if the crisis is in response to a loss, the nurse guides the client in grief work.

Crisis intervention therapy is terminated when the client has resolved the crisis. Some nurses use the maximum of six sessions as a criterion for termination. If in these instances additional therapy is needed, the client is referred for another type of therapy, such as short-term psychotherapy.[38] Preplanned follow-up interviews are recommended as an aspect of the termination phase. These interviews provide information about the extent to which the crisis is successfully resolved and serve as a safeguard if the client needs additional therapy. The client needs to terminate therapy with the feeling that the therapist is available if needed again.

CHARACTERISTICS OF THE CRISIS INTERVENTION THERAPIST
Qualifications

Many nurses have attended workshops or lectures on crisis intervention and therefore possess the basics of crisis intervention techniques. Nurses who work in community mental health centers and conduct therapy with clients who seek crisis intervention are required to have extensive education and training. In general, to qualify academically to perform therapy with clients in crisis, nurses need to have (1) 2 years of experience in an inpatient psychiatric hospital, (2) a master's degree in psychiatric nursing, and (3) a year of intensive training in crisis intervention at a community mental health center.

An increasing number of paraprofessionals with various levels of basic training and educational preparation are working in crisis centers. They are provided additional education and training that qualify them to perform crisis intervention in the role of mental health worker.

Irrespective of the academic preparation all individuals who perform crisis intervention need to have knowledge and understanding of human behavior. More important, the precarious nature of crisis situations necessitates that all persons working with clients in crisis possess certain personal characteristics. The nurse needs to be a warm and caring person who is able to use herself as a therapeutic tool. Since crisis situations are intense and can be anxiety provoking for the therapist, an ability to tolerate intense painful emotions and keep the focus on the client are important attributes. She needs personal resources for coping with anxiety and other emotions so that she can assist the client.

The nurse needs to be confident in her ability to help the client in crisis. The feeling of confidence helps the client feel secure. A willingness to assume responsibility for the client who may be unable to assume full responsibility for himself is an essential characteristic of the crisis nurse. She needs to be flexible and ready to respond at any time to a crisis situation. This means the nurse must be able to think quickly and achieve goals with little preparation time. Flexibility in the use of various communication techniques is also important. The nurse needs to be sensitive to the client's needs and relate to him positively.

Goals

A maximal goal is to increase the client's functioning above the precrisis level. However, the nurse hopes to achieve a minimum of three basic goals. An immediate goal is to reduce the impact of the crisis. The nurse needs to give immediate attention to the anxiety, the tension, and the feeling of being out of control that the client is experiencing *now*.[39] She intervenes to reduce anxiety and guilt, to prevent further disorganization, and to protect the client from injuring himself and others. The second and third therapeutic goals are to provide an opportunity for the client to deal with the *nuclear problem*, using his previous problem-solving skills, and to assist the client in returning to his precrisis level of functioning. The nuclear problem is the underlying cause of the client's reaction to the precipitating event.

Role

The role of the crisis nurse differs from that of the nurse in traditional therapy roles because of the need to achieve the goals of therapy in a short time. An important role of the nurse is to rapidly establish a therapeutic relationship in which she and the client work to resolve the problem. The active involvement of the client conveys that the client's thoughts and ideas are important and that he has the potential for solving his problems.

The nurses's role includes quickly and accurately assessing the situation and quickly establishing a tentative formulation of the client's problem. She uses the information the client shares amd her understanding of human behavior to fulfill her role in problem identification. At times the nurse needs to make life-and-death decisions within a brief time. Thus quickness and accuracy are crucial for effective and safe functioning.

In crisis therapy, the nurse assumes an active, direct, and involved role. She actively guides the client in an exploration of the problem. Instead of the passive use of reflection that characterizes some traditional forms of therapy, the nurse uses active and direct techniques such as confrontation and interpretation. She shows constructive involvement through empathic understanding of what the client is experiencing. The judicious use of touch is an example of the involvement of the crisis nurse with the client.

Even though the client participates in the process of crisis intervention, the role of the nurse is to demonstrate that she has the situation under control and is able to offer the client direction out of the problem. The nurse uses her role as resource person and teacher to assist in guiding the client toward resolution of the problem. The role of the nurse also includes providing whatever nurturing the client needs to reestablish equilibrium. While enacting this role the nurse avoids fostering unwarranted dependence.

NURSING PROCESS
Assessment

Physical dimension. The physical problems manifested by clients in crisis are generally responses characteristic of depression or anxiety, unless the crisis is precipitated by a physical illness. When assessing the physical dimension the nurse collects data about any alteration of the client's sleep pattern, appetite, and weight. The individual in crisis may have been unable to sleep for a few nights or for a few weeks, depending on the length of time he has been experiencing the crisis. Difficulty falling asleep, restless sleep with frequent awakening during the night, or early morning awakening is a sleep pattern that may be typical for the individual. The client in crisis may have a poor appetite or a complete loss of desire for food. The lack of sufficient food intake may lead to weight loss. A direct result of the sleep disturbances, poor appetite, and weight loss may be changes in the body image. The individual may have dark circles and bags under the eyes. He may also appear debilitated. The effects of sleep disturbances as well as a poor appetite may be a low level of energy and general physical deterioration. The physical symptoms related to anxiety may result in hyperventilation. Other physical manifestations of anxiety are discussed in Chapter 11.

Emotional dimension. The individual's emotional reactions to the crisis experience are varied and need to be carefully assessed. Because individuals often perceive the event that precipitated the crisis as a threat to their survival, anxiety is one of the cardinal signs of a person in crisis. The nurse assesses the level of anxiety to determine the individual's ability to participate in the problem-solving process. Anxiety may range from a moderate to a panic level, and a fear of "going crazy" may be expressed. The client may be in a state of severe emotional upheaval. The manifestations of anxiety described in Chapter 11 are characteristic of the client in crisis.

Depression is another emotional state typically experienced by the individual in crisis because of the frequency with which the crisis is precipitated by a loss. During the first few minutes of the assessment the nurse determines whether the client has engaged in any self-destructive acts such as threatened or attempted suicide. Suicide attempts and threats in conjunction with crisis are common. Even when the likelihood of suicide seems remote, the nurse assesses the person's current thoughts about self-destruction as well as past behavior when he was seriously depressed. The means of suicide are usually more available to this person than to a hospitalized client. If the client has made a suicide attempt, for example, has taken pills, the nurse's first concern is his physical state rather than his emotional state. Rapid assessment of the suicide plan according to the guidelines discussed in Chapter 14 is crucial. The potential for committing suicide is greater when the client has a plan. Thus the nurse asks the client what plan he has for commiting suicide. How he plans to carry out the act helps determine the seriousness of the intent. For example, a plan to use a gun or jump from a building is more serious than taking an overdose of psychotropic medications. The nurse also needs to learn when the client plans to commit suicide. Plans for doing so in the middle of the day while members of the family are up and about may not be as serious as plans to do so after they retire.

In crisis intervention the nurse may need to assess the behavior of a suicidal client on the telephone. The box on p. 500 gives an approach for responding to telephone calls from a suicidal client.

Once the suicidal behavior or potential for it has been assessed, the nurse assesses the depressive behavior. The nurse attends to the severity of the depression to determine whether the client needs to be hospitalized. It is not uncommon for the individual to have profound feelings of despair and dejection. The person in crisis often feels hopeless because of his inability to resolve the crisis and his belief that no one can help him. The client may cry uncontrollably and for prolonged periods, making it difficult for him to provide information. Along with depression the individual may experience guilt and shame. Sometimes the guilt and shame are the client's response to his need to seek professional assistance.

Sometimes the client's crisis is expressed by inappropriate anger directed toward other people, especially those who are trying to help. The anger may be brief but destructive enough to be considered a homicidal intent.

RESPONSE TO CALLS FROM SUICIDAL CLIENT

1. *Establish a relationship during which you maintain contact with the client and obtain information.* Assure the caller of your availability by listening nonjudgmentally. Convey interest and concern.
2. *Identify and clarify the problem.* The caller may be disorganized and confused and may need structure to help him determine what is important.
3. *Evaluate the suicidal potential to determine how close the caller is to harming himself.* Evaluate the information obtained in terms of factors such as age, sex, and suicide plan.
4. *Assess the caller's strengths and resources.* Use the information obtained to develop a therapeutic plan.
5. *Formulate a constructive plan and mobilize the caller's resources and those of others.* The resources available to the client may include family and close friends. Referral to a crisis clinic or recommendation of immediate hospitalization may be indicated. Arrange for these services.

Most homicides occur in the home and may be the culmination of long-standing spouse abuse or parent-adolescent conflicts. The situation that initiated the homicidal ideation may become stressful enough to motivate the individual to seek crisis intervention. A person who has an aggressive, impulsive personality is a likely candidate for carrying out the homicide. When assessing the client's behavior it is important to remember that an act of homicide may not be premeditated. Following are clues to homicidal intent or attempt[42]:

1. Threats made by the aggressor, such as "I will kill you next time."
2. A report that fights are generally limited to the kitchen or bedroom.
3. The presence of weapons in the home, especially guns.
4. An aggressor with impulsive behavior and a bad temper. After striking out, the person may insist that he did not intend to harm the victim.
5. A victim who tends to encourage the fights with belittling remarks.
6. A history of previous fights between the victim and the agressor.
7. Injuries so serious that they might have resulted in death.

Chapter 12 discusses anger more fully.

✳ *Intellectual dimension.* The initial focus when assessing the intellectual dimension is eliciting the individual's perception of the crisis event, which may be realistic. However, because of the intensity of the stress related to the crisis, individuals frequently distort the precipitating event. The opportunity for distortion increases as the client waits for his request for assistance to be met. The less distorted the client's description of the crisis event, the more likely the problem can be solved.

Anxiety causes a narrowing of the individual's perception. When the situation is perceived unrealistically, the individual may resort to the use of intrapsychic defense mechanisms, such as repression and denial, in his efforts to cope. Attack, flight, or compromise are direct modes that may be used to cope when the situation is perceived realistically.

The nurse examines the mental status of the client. The client's ability to recall and to give an account of events leading to the crisis provides information about his intellectual activity. His level of anxiety may be severe and may greatly interfere with his recall of the events. In other instances the client may readily given an account of the situation. When the intellectual functions are intact and the client is alert, he is better able to participate in the problem-solving process.

The clarity with which information is communicated is assessed. In addition to crying, which was mentioned earlier as a possible barrier to verbal communication, the client may be unable to express his thoughts because of muteness. The muteness may result from feeling overwhelmed by the crisis situation. Anger may also interfere with the client's ability to give a logical account of the events that led to the crisis. The client may explode with a barrage of angry questions related to the misinterpretation of the crisis situation. The anger may sometimes motivate the client to work on resolving the crisis situation.

The individual's level of motivation to participate in crisis intervention therapy is assessed in terms of his willingness to help himself. The individual can be asked directly whether he feels able to help work on his problems by performing certain tasks. For example, to assess the level of motivation the nurse can ask the client directly to think about what led to the crisis. She can also elicit the client's willingness to participate in sharing the thoughts and feelings he is experiencing now. When assessing the level of motivation the nurse takes into consideration the emotional state and the intellectual functions that may be affected by the crisis and allows time for the client to respond.

✳ *Social dimension.* An individual in crisis usually experiences noticeable impairments in the social aspects of his life. Relationships with family, friends, and co-workers may change sufficiently that the individual no longer has social supports. Since the availability of social supports is important when making plans to prevent or minimize the recurrence of problems, an assessment of who comprises the client's social network and the accessibility and reliability of social supports is essential. Who comprises the social supports is not as crucial as the accessibility of support.

The dependence needs of a client may be intensified when the client has to turn to another person for assistance. As the client seeks a crisis nurse to help him solve his problems, he may talk about feelings of helplessness and convey a need to be taken care of. In a crisis situation the client is more helpless and more amenable to being helped than at any other time in his life.

Social events that may precipitate a crisis are the discovery of an extramarital relationship and the threat of or

QUESTIONS RELATED TO AN ASSESSMENT OF THE FIVE DIMENSIONS OF A CLIENT IN CRISIS

PHYSICAL DIMENSION

How is your appetite?
When did you first notice a change in your appetite?
What is your sleeping pattern?
How long have you had restless nights?
How much weight have you lost?

EMOTIONAL DIMENSION

What changes have recently taken place in your life?
    Loss of a significant other?
    Loss of a job?
    Job promotion?
    Illness?
    Accident?
How do you feel about having to seek help?
How do you feel about your life situation?
    Scared?
    Anxious?
    Depressed?
    Overwhelmed?
    Fearful you might hurt yourself or someone else

INTELLECTUAL DIMENSION

What does the crisis event mean to you?
In what way is the crisis event going to affect your future?
What do you usually do when you are upset?
    Anxious?
    Depressed?
How did you try to cope with this crisis situation?
If you used your usual method, what are your thoughts about why it didn't work?
What do you think would help you to feel better now?

SOCIAL DIMENSION

With whom do you live?
Where does your closest friend live?
How often do you see your best friend?
Whom do you trust?
Who is your closest friend in your family?
How long have you lived in your present neighborhood?
How do you feel about yourself?

SPIRITUAL DIMENSION

What is your religious preference?
What kind of religious activities do you participate in when you are upset?
How often do you talk with your clergyman?
How has life treated you?

actual occurrence of a divorce. These events may be perceived as a loss or threatened loss and may lead to depression. A crisis may result from the loss of a job, a promotion, or retirement. A job change accompanied by a lower salary may also lead to a crisis.

A change in living arrangements may lead to a crisis. The person may have moved to another city or state or to another place of residence within the same city. In each instance the relocating may necessitate changes such as meeting new neighbors and making new friends. This change may be handled effectively, or the person may experience a crisis when the change is viewed as a loss.

A threat or attack on the self-concept can precipitate a crisis. Since the individual who is in crisis may have a low self-concept, the stress of the crisis will further decrease his self-concept. All of the previously discussed changes in the individual's social life will lower his opinion of himself. The fact that the client has to seek professional help may contribute to his low self-concept.

Spiritual dimension. It is important to learn what religious practices the client upholds. An assessment of how he meets his spiritual needs may provide valuable information to use when planning his care. The role of religion in the client's life needs to be assessed. If the client has thoughts of suicide these feelings may be in conflict with his spiritual orientation and lead to feelings of guilt and shame. At the same time the client in crisis may think that his life is meaningless because he is unable

to resolve the crisis. When the precipitating event is related to a loss, the client may feel isolated and alone. Because of his feelings of helplessness and hopelessness, he may think his God or spiritual leader has forsaken him. The disorganization and loss of control in response to the impact of the crisis may further increase his doubt about his self-worth.

The questions in the box above provide a useful guideline for assessing the five dimensions of a client in crisis.

Analysis

Nursing diagnosis. The following list provides examples of NANDA-accepted nursing diagnoses with causative statements related to crises.

1. Potential for violence to self related to feelings of hopelessness
2. Impaired social interaction related to lack of social support secondary to relocation to another city
3. Sleep pattern disturbance related to anxiety
4. Severe anxiety related to failure in examination secondary to insufficient time for study
5. Alteration in thought processes related to feelings of despair

DSM-III-R diagnoses. There are no DSM-III-R diagnoses for crises. A typical crisis is not pathological; a client may behave in an inappropriate or exaggerated way in re-

TABLE 26-2 Classification of emotional crises

Class	Type	Characteristics	Source	Example
1	Dispositional crises	Caused by distress that arises from a problematic situation in which intervention is not directed at the emotional level	External	Providing information to a mother about parenting classes
2	Anticipated life transition crises	Relates to normal life transitions over which the person may or may not have control	External	Getting married; midlife career changes; retirement
3	Crises resulting from traumatic stress	Precipitated by externally imposed stressors that are unexpected and uncontrolled	External	Rape; sudden death of a family member; sudden loss of job
4	Maturational developmental crises	Relates to an attempt to acheive emotional maturity by completing developmental task; involves a struggle with a deep-seated, unresolved issue	Internal	Emancipation from an overprotective parent
5	Psychopathological crises	Preexisting psychopathological condition precipitates the crisis or complicates resolution of crisis	Internal	Client with severe anxiety disorder, or pathological dependence
6	Psychiatric emergency crises	Severe psychiatric disorder with severe impairment; incompetent; danger to self or others	Internal	Psychosis; drug overdose; acutely suicidal

sponse to a reactivation of earlier unresolved or partially resolved conflicts. Baldwin[3] developed a classification system that describes six general types of crises in relation to the degree of psychopathology, the cause of the crisis, and implications for effective interventions. As each type moves from a lesser to a greater degree of psychopathology, the cause becomes more internal than external. The model is based on the assumption that crisis intervention requires assessing the emotional crisis rather than making a diagnosis in a traditional psychiatric sense. The classification of the crisis, the characteristics, and an example of each type are presented in Table 26-2.

Planning

Table 26-3 provides sample long-term goals, short-term goals, and outcome criteria related to crisis intervention. These serve as examples of the planning stage of the nursing process.

Implementation

Physical dimension. The nurse informs the client that his sleep disturbances will most likely improve after resolution of the crisis. However, until such time he should use such measures as taking a warm bath and drinking warm milk before going to bed. Relaxation exercises may also induce sleep. If sedatives are prescribed to help the client sleep, the amount of medication prescribed needs to be small in the event the client is suicidal. When there is loss of appetite, the nurse suggests that the client prepare his favorite foods and eat as much as he can tolerate at each meal. He may also eat high-caloric snacks between meals to increase his food intake. Once the client is able to sleep restfully and eat sufficient amounts of food, he will regain his weight and the problems with his body image may be resolved.

When the physical symptoms are related to anxiety, the nurse assures the client that the problems will subside after his anxiety is relieved. When the client experiences hyperventilation, the nurse increases the effectiveness of his breathing by providing the client with a paper bag, instructing him to place the bag over his nose and mouth and to breath with the bag in place. The nurse remains with the client until his regular breathing returns.

Emotional dimension. The nurse needs to proceed with caution in establishing rapport with the client who is depressed and is expressing feelings of hopelessness. She allows the client to talk at his own pace and listens for themes related to the precipitating event.

The nurse communicates with the client in a hopeful, empathetic manner. The client often feels some relief when the nurse communicates that she understands his problem. She encourages the client to talk about the loss that may contribute to the depression. She reinforces appropriate behavior the client is using to cope with the loss, such as crying. The client needs privacy when crying and the nurse offers or has available facial tissue for the crying client. Skillful use of verbal and nonverbal communication is supportive for the client coping with a loss. Listening, touch, and the nurse's physical presence are important nonverbal interventions. Empathetic verbal responses are reassuring and comforting for the client in crisis who is dealing with a loss.

TABLE 26-3 Long-term and short-term goals and outcome criteria related to crisis intervention

Goals	Outcome Criteria
NURSING DIAGNOSIS: ANXIETY RELATED TO FAILURE IN COLLEGE COURSE EXAMINATION SECONDARY TO INSUFFICIENT TIME TO STUDY	
Long-term goal	
To arrange work schedule to ensure sufficient time for study within 2 weeks	Verbalizes the amount of time needed for comprehensive study of course materials
	Discusses with supervisor options for work hours
	Selects an option that meets the need for financial income and study of course materials
Short-term goal	
To review lecture materials after each related class	Selects a quiet setting away from dormitory
	Reviews lecture notes after each class for 1 to 2 hours in the early evening
NURSING DIAGNOSIS: IMPAIRED SOCIAL INTERACTION RELATED TO LACK OF SOCIAL SUPPORT RESULTING FROM RELOCATION TO ANOTHER CITY	
Long-term goal	
To become friends with at least 2 people in 6 weeks	Invites neighbors to home for a social event such as coffee
	Joins social organizations of interest
	Participates in social activities involving people at work and at church
Short-term goal	
To use existing situational supports while developing new ones	Telephones relatives or close friends at least once every 2 weeks for 6 weeks
	Shares reactions to new experiences in letters to family and friends

The client may need help to initiate or complete the grieving process after the loss of a significant other. Discussing the steps in the grieving process and related thoughts and feelings enables the client to begin to work through the stages during crisis therapy with the understanding that he can complete grief work. The nurse conveys to the client that depression in response to a loss is seldom resolved in one session. She schedules the client to return for additional sessions. The Research Highlight on p. 504 provides an example of the intervention in grief work.

Because suicide or suicide attempts are more frequent in clients in crisis who are depressed, the nurse is constantly alert for signs of suicide. When the suicidal risk is low, the client can talk about reasons for his feelings and explore alternate coping behavior. The nurse inquires about the family's ability to support the client if he returns home. If people are available and supportive, she gives the client the telephone number for the crisis hotline before he leaves and has him return to the crisis center for additional sessions.

Hospitalization may be indicated if the suicidal client is (1) a high risk for suicide, (2) lacks reliable social supports, or (3) has symptoms so severe that he requires constant observation.

If a client who is suicidal seeks crisis intervention without his family, the nurse accepts responsibility for alerting relatives or close friends. These support persons can assume some of the the responsibility for preventing suicide. A suicidal client needs always to be accompanied by relatives or friends when he leaves the hospital. If hospitalization is indicated the client and family need to be al-

lowed to express their thoughts and feelings about this decision.

The nurse assists the client in expressing his feelings of anxiety, anger, and guilt. Once she assesses the level of anxiety, she implements plans accordingly. The nurse intervenes with the client with a severe to panic level of anxiety by providing a calm environment with limited stimuli. The room should be well lighted to decrease shadows. The nurse explains the approach to treatment used in the crisis setting and orients him to his surroundings to decrease the strangeness of the situation. It is important for the nurse to remain calm and to approach the client in a warm, unhurried manner. The nurse speaks clearly and uses simple language. She communicates to the client that the feelings he is experiencing are normal. The client's painful emotions need to be thoroughly vented before the nurse attempts to obtain the facts of the precipitating event. Expressing these feelings lets the client in crisis gain mastery over his emotions. The nurse skillfully encourages and guides the client toward venting his feelings by using questions and techniques that elicit emotions. For example, when the client says he feels as if he is losing his mind, the nurse may respond, "Describe for me what this feels like." The exploration of statements related to the client's painful feelings help the nurse determine if the client's statement relates to what he is actually experiencing or if the statement is only a figure of speech.

The client who is experiencing guilt should be allowed to express these feelings in an accepting atmosphere. The nurse avoids reassuring the client too rapidly, since such a response may stop the client from expressing his feel-

Research Highlight

Bereavement Crisis Intervention for Widows in Grief and Mourning

R.E Constantino

PURPOSE

The purpose of this study was to compare the levels of depression and social adaptation of widows who received bereavement crisis intervention (BCI) conducted by a mental health–psychiatric nurse with those of widows who did not.

SAMPLE

The sample consisted of seven widows in the BCI experimental group, 10 widows in the control group, and 10 in the socialization group. The widows were assigned to groups based on their willingness to participate in the study and their availability for different aspects of the study. Other criteria for selection were that the spouse died within a 6-month period before the start of the study, the husband's death did not result from malignancy or heart disease, and the widows had no history of psychiatric illness and were not receiving psychotropic medications.

METHODOLOGY

The three groups of widows were administered pretest and posttest questionnaires, which included a consent form, a demographic data sheet, the Depression Adjective Check List (DACL) Form E, and the Social Adjustment Scale Self-Report (SAS-SR). The DACL measured transient depressive mood, feeling, or emotion. SAS-SR was used to measure social adjustment, specifically performance in work, social and leisure activities, relationships with extended family, role as parent, and economic independence. Subjects in the BCI and socialization groups attended group sessions led by two mental health–psychiatric nurses with master's degrees and expertise in crisis intervention and group therapy.

FINDINGS

A planned, time-limited, phase-specific group intervention such as BCI and socialization group led by a mental health–psychiatric nurse and held in a controlled setting is an effective modality in decreasing depression in widows. Change occured in all three groups, but the BCI group had the greatest decrease in both the DACL Form E and the SAS-SR. Although the widows reported increased social activities and decreased feelings of depression, they still were lonely.

IMPLICATIONS

The sample was not randomly selected and assigned to the group. Thus the findings of the study cannot be generalized. However, the results of the study suggest that support for grief and encouragement of mourning in a situation with others who have had the same crisis experience has the potential for increasing a successful outcome of grief work.

Based on data from Nursing Research 30:351, 1981.

ings. Listening attentively and making empathetic responses can assist in alleviating the guilt. The nurse lets the client know that coming for help with his crisis is a sign of strength, not weakness. Thus she readily and actively implements the techniques for anxiety reduction. If none of the techniques reduces the anxiety, the nurse requests an order for antianxiety medication.

The basic principles to apply when intervening in the behavior of the angry client are the same as those discussed in Chapter 12. The nurse needs to give the client permission to express anger suppressed possibly because of feelings of guilt. The client may have a greater fear of losing control in a crisis setting that provides fewer external controls than does an inpatient setting. Thus the nurse conveys confidence in her ability to help the client express his anger within reasonable limits. For example, the nurse verbally communicates to the client that he may express anger appropriately and that she will set limits on the behavior before he hurts himself or another person. Venting, discussed in the intellectual dimension, is effective in helping the client achieve the emotional catharsis that reduces tension.

Intervention in the behavior of a homicidal client needs to be direct. Once the nurse has made an assessment she decides whether the client needs to be hospitalized. As with the suicidal client, if the client requires hospitalization the client and the relatives need to be told. Relatives sometimes assume responsibility for getting the client to the hospital. If the client's homicidal behavior can be treated through crisis intervention, the nurse provides an opportunity for the client to talk about his anger in a controlled, safe environment. She provides general support by active listening and functioning essentially as a sounding board.

Intellectual dimension. With a decrease in the client's emotionality, the nurse focuses on restoring the client's cognitive functioning, which enhances his ability to discuss his perception of the precipitating event.

The nurse directs intervention toward helping the client gain an intellectual understanding of his crisis; the client is guided to examine and understand the here-and-now factors that contribute to the crisis.

Cognitive restoration,[12] a major goal of crisis intervention, is designed to restore cognitive functioning. It is a process by which the nurse communicates to the client in crisis an explanation of the cause of the crisis. The nurse also shares with the client reasons his usual coping behavior were ineffective.

There are two therapeutic techniques for achieving cognitive restoration: causal connecting statements and interpretation.[12] A *causal connecting statement* is the process by which the nurse helps the client relate the cause and effect between two events that are an outcome of the client's specific feelings, behavior, or responses. In essence, the causal connecting statement ties together the cause and effect of the client's related events and responses. Following is an example of a causal connecting statement:

Nurse: What's important for you to talk about today?
Client: Why I feel so hopeless. I can't see how I can get out of it. I just sit and think and think but can't come up with any answer on how to get myself straightened out. But I have to do something. It's very bad.
Nurse: What's bad?
Client: That before I tried to get out of it by cutting my wrist.
Nurse: (Causal connecting statement.) It sounds like you feel helpless to do anything about your feeling of hopelessness and when the pain becomes unbearable you attempt to take your own life.

Causal connecting statements differ from interpretation in that explanations are based on the client's overt communication rather than on unconscious inferences.

The second basic technique of cognitive restoration is *interpretation*. "Interpretation is the crisis therapist's explanation of the unconscious cause and meaning of the client's feelings and behavior for the purpose of the client's self-understanding and reestablishment of cognitive control."[12] The explanations are based on the information the client provides in response to the nurse's questions regarding when and why the crisis occurred. Interpretation restores order and structure to the client's emotional behavior and thus improves his cognitive functioning.

Interpretation enables the client to become conscious of feelings and behavior that are unconscious. He is offered reasons and causes for his behavior. Deep unconscious interpretation is not necessary in crisis therapy. Instead, when cognitive restoration is used in crisis therapy, there are two forms of interpretation: (1) informing the client of behavior of which he is unaware that involves his current life situation, such as interpersonal relationships with significant others or conflicts in goals, and (2) examining with the client the relationship between his past and present behavior. An example of interpretation is as follows:

Client: I need to talk about how to defend myself and not do everything I'm asked to do. At work, I can't say no. I'm always the good guy.
Nurse: I wonder where these feelings about being good come from.
Client: For me, I guess it's in my nature. I grew out of it once, but it came back.

Nurse: Is it possible that when you were a kid, you were expected to be good?
Client: No, I don't think so...but yes, I guess so. I was always being good—at home and at school—and people liked me.

Confrontation is a technique that may be used for intervention in rigidity. This method is used when the client resists facing the reality of the situation, which may include feelings and behavior. The goal of confrontation is to guide the client in accepting some aspects of reality that he prefers not to face. In crisis intervention, supportive measures rather than attack are used with confrontation. The intervention begins slowly with the use of mild confrontation. If the client does not respond to this type of confrontation, a more direct approach is used. For the mild confrontation, the nurse might begin by saying to the client, "For some reason you seem not to want to act on your verbalized desire to change your behavior." If this response is ineffective, the nurse will be more direct and might say, "Knowing that your behavior is interfering with your functioning and you are asking for professional assistance, perhaps you need to look at what is preventing you from working on the problem." If the rigidity continues, the nurse sets limits or takes direct action. An example of a response is, "You will begin working on the problem, or the crisis therapy will be terminated."

Venting is one of the most useful techniques for crisis intervention. Venting allows the client to speak freely about his thoughts and feelings related to the crisis situation. This technique is one of the most effective ways of reducing tension and anxiety. By reliving the crisis experience through active verbalization, the client often perceives the problem in a different perspective and returns to his precrisis level of functioning. Venting involves exploration of the content of the client's communication without controlling the conversation. To explore the communication the nurse may say, "I can see that your marriage was important to you. Describe for me exactly how you feel now that the divorce is final." When the client is extremely depressed or is minimally responsive because of a drug overdose or other reasons, the nurse assumes an active role in which she guides the client to verbally express his thoughts and feelings.

Focused activity serves the purpose of actively focusing the client toward his adaptive coping abilities and away from maladaptive ones. This method may be used with venting. The client is allowed to share his thoughts and feelings with emphasis on his strengths. This technique is useful in crisis intervention, since the nurse needs to learn about the client's adaptive coping abilities within a short time to guide him to capitalize on his strengths as he participates in the problem-solving process.

Another intervention that can be used is *clarification*. Clarification is designed to guide the client to focus on his problem or to recognize that there are inconsistencies or gaps in what he is saying, which the nurse points out. Clarification helps the client expand his perception of the crisis event. Discussing new problems as well as exploring feelings the client did not want to recognize may be outcomes of the use of clarification.

All of the techniques of intervention allow the nurse and client to work on the resolution of the crisis. However, the nurse guides the client in active, deliberate problem-solving activities. The nurse provides the client with knowledge about the steps in the problem-solving process and assists him in examining the effectiveness of his problem-solving behavior.

✳ *Social dimension.* The nurse implements plans designed to restore the client's social functioning to at least the precrisis level. If the crisis was precipitated by the loss of a significant person, the client may need to reopen his social world and meet new people to fill the void. When the client derives support and gratification from the new relationships similar to that which he obtained from the lost one, the new relationships can be especially effective. To avoid possible unrealistic expectations of the new relationship by the client, the nurse clearly conveys that the new relationship will not be the same as the lost one.

The client may need assistance in learning how to strengthen his existing relationships and thus his situational supports. Sometimes the client only needs to develop an awareness of how he can better use the existing support systems. The nurse may use the social worker as a resource when implementing plans for social supports.

The nurse helps the client become aware of and plan to use social activities of interest as a possible resource for meeting people as well as an outlet for reducing tension. If the client once belonged to social organizations in the community, he can resume his involvement in these organizations.

The nurse assists the client in crisis to improve his self-concept by conveying respect for him as a person. Addressing the client by his surname unless he gives you permission to do otherwise is one way to convey respect. Acceptance of the client as a person who deserves the nurse's time will contribute to improving the client's self-concept. The nurse communicates her acceptance to the client, for example, when she reinforces his strengths and conveys her confidence in his ability to participate in the problem-solving process. Also, allowing the client to do what he can for himself contributes to improving his self-concept and decreasing the client's dependence on the nurse. Whatever the outcome of the work on the crisis, the nurse recognizes the client's constructive contributions to these outcomes. Acceptance of the client as a person of worth entails acceptance of his painful feelings regardless of the content.

Environmental modification focuses on making changes in the client's environment that decrease stress and the potential for another crisis. Because changing the client's environment involves other people in his life, the nurse may need to work with the client's spouse, employer, or parents. The client's environment may be modified when he lives alone and is no longer able to carry out his activities of daily living without supervision. Living arrangements may be sought for an adult child who still lives with his parents if the parent-child conflict is perceived as the precipitant of the client's crisis. Sometimes environmental modification means recommending that the client be placed in a hospital for a while because the client's problem was not solved sufficiently for him to function effectively at home. Modification of the environment may involve arranging for the client to have accessible situational supports. Knowledge of community resources, social agencies, businesses, and organizations will contribute to the nurse's effective use of this technique.

Anticipatory guidance is a technique that is useful in helping the client prepare for and adjust satisfactorily to changes in his life. This technique involves assisting the client to anticipate certain events and prepare to cope with them in a constructive and adaptive way. This technique is especially useful for intervention in normal maturational crises. Examples of anticipatory guidance are premarital counseling for the engaged couples and parenting classes for first-time parents.

✳ *Spiritual dimension.* A major intervention related to the spiritual dimension is to work with the client in generating a feeling of hope. Nursing measures for achieving this goal are discussed in Chapter 14. The nurse functions as a stabilizing force and provides external control that may strengthen the client's sense of personal worth as he works toward reestablishing equilibrium and control over his cognitive functioning. Religious organizations and the individual's religious leader may serve as resources in helping him deal with a crisis of bereavement and other losses. The client may arrive for crisis intervention with members of his church or synagogue. He may need a quiet, private place to participate in prayer with these individuals. The therapist takes her cues from the client in terms of how much time and privacy is essential to fulfill his spiritual needs.

Evaluation

The nurse and the client evaluate the resolution of the crisis. They discuss whether the client achieved the goal of returning to his precrisis level of functioning or learned new coping skills that are more effective than those he possessed before the crisis. The nurse needs to discuss with the client realistic plans for the future in terms of his perception of his progress, his support system, and the coping mechanisms he is now using. The nurse reinforces the strengths the client exhibited during his work toward resolution of the crisis. At the same time she and the client explore ways in which he can continue to grow.

If the client did not resolve the crisis within the time frame for crisis intervention, the nurse determines the assistance the client still needs and makes a referral for another type of professional help. Depending on the client's needs the nurse may make a referral for a service such as short-term psychotherapy, long-term psychotherapy, or hospitalization.

BRIEF REVIEW

Lindemann and Caplan were pioneers in the development of crisis intervention as a form of intensive brief therapy, usually consisting of one to six sessions. The therapy was designed for individuals facing a sudden loss of the ability to cope with a life situation. Any change or loss can precipitate a crisis. A crisis may be developmental or situational. Examples of developmental crisis are a child's first day at school, movement into adolescence, and retirement. Situational crisis may be precipitated by such changes as a divorce, a change of job, a promotion, and the loss of a significant other through separation or death.

The focus of crisis intervention is the crisis situation. The goals of therapy are resolution of the immediate crisis and restoration of the individual to his precrisis level of functioning and, it is hoped, to a higher level of functioning. The activity of the nurse is that of an active and direct participant. The client and the nurse work together on solving the immediate problem. They focus on the here and now rather than reflecting on the individual's past.

Nurses are ideally suited to use crisis intervention techniques. They are with clients in hospitals and in the community. They are also adept at problem solving, which is the basis of crisis theory and methodology.

REFERENCES AND SUGGESTED READINGS

1. Aguilera, D.C., and Messick, J.M.: Crisis intervention: theory and methodology, ed. 5, St. Louis, 1986, The C.V. Mosby Co.
2. Allen, N.H.: Homicide prevention and intervention, Suicide Life Threat Behavior 11(3):167, 1981.
3. Baldwin, B.A.: A paradigm for the classification of emotional crises: implication for crisis intervention, American Journal of Orthopsychiatry, 48(3):538, 1978.
4. Ballou, M.: Crisis: recognition and intervention are crucial nursing roles Journal of Practical Nursing, 31(3):25, 1981.
5. Barash, D.A.: Defusing the violent patient—before he explodes RN 47(3):34, 1984.
6. Britton, J.G., and Mattson-Melcher, D.M.: The crisis home: sheltering patients in emotional crisis, Journal of Psychosocial Nursing and Mental Health Services 23(12):18, 1985
7. Brownell, M.J.: The concept of crisis: its utility for nursing, Advances in Nursing Science 6(4):10, 1984.
8. Caplan, G.: An approach to community mental health, New York, 1961, Grune & Stratton, Inc.
9. Caplan, G.: Principles of preventive psychiatry, New York, 1964, Basic Books, Inc. Publishers.
10. Cohen, L.H., Claiborn, W.L., and Specter, G.A., editors: Crisis intervention, ed. 2, New York, 1983, Human Sciences Press, Inc.
11. Danzy, E.S.: Crisis intervention: a response to the mental health needs of children and youth, Emotional First Aid: A Journal of Crisis Intervention 2(4):5, 1985.
12. Dixon, S.L.: Working with people in crisis: theory and practice, St. Louis, 1979, The C.V. Mosby Co.
13. Dubin, W.R., and Sarnoff, J.R.: Sudden unexpected death: intervention with the survivors, Annal of Emergency Medicine, 15(1):54, 1986.
14. Erikson, E.H.: Childhood and society, New York, 1950, W.W. Norton & Co., Inc.
15. Essa, M.: Grief as a crisis: psychotherapeutic interventions with elderly bereaved, American Journal of Psychotherapy, 40(2):243, 1986.
16. Everstine, D.S., and Everstine, L.: People in crisis: strategic therapeutic interventions, New York, 1983, Brunner/Mazel, Inc.
17. Geissler, E.M.: Crisis: what it is and is not, Advances in Nursing Science, 6(4):1, 1984.
18. Glick, R.A., and Meyerson, A.T.: The use of psychoanalytic concepts in crisis intervention, International Journal of Psychoanalytic Psychotherapy, 8:171, 1980.
19. Gross, S.J., and McConville, M.T., editors: Crisis in the family, New York, 1980, Gardner Press, Inc.
20. Hoff, L.A.: People in crisis: understanding and helping, ed. 2, Menlo Park, Calif., 1984, Addison-Wesley Publishing Co., Inc.
21. Jacobs, D., and Mack, J.E.: Case report or psychiatric intervention by mail: a way of responding to a suicidal crisis, American Journal of Psychiatry 143(1):92, 1986.
22. Jacobson, G., Strickler, M., and Morley, W.E.: Generic and individual approaches to crisis intervention, American Journal of Public Health 58:339, 1968.
23. Janosik, E.H., editor: Crisis counseling; a contemporary approach, Belmont, Calif., 1984, Wadsworth, Inc.
24. Johnson, J.: Psychiatric nursing in a crisis center: standards and practice, Nursing Management 17(8):81, 1986.
25. Kaforey, E.C.: Crisis intervention and the new unemployed, Occupational Health Nursing 32(3):154.
26. Kresky-Wolff, M., and others: Crossing place: a residential model for crisis intervention . . . severe psychiatric crises, Hospital and Community Psychiatry 35(1):72, 1984.
27. Lieb, J., Lipsitch, I.I., and Slaby, A.E.: The crisis team: a handbook for the mental health professional, New York, 1973, Harper & Row, Publishers.
28. Lindemann, E.: Symptomatology and management of acute grief, American Journal of Psychiatry 101:101, 1944.
29. Lindemann, E.: The meaning of crisis in individual and family living, Teachers College Record 57:310, 1956.
30. Lopez, D.J., and Getzel, G.S.: Helping gay AIDS patients in crisis, Social Casework 65(7):387, 1984.
31. McGee, R.F.: Hope: a factor influencing crisis resolution, Advances in Nursing Science 6(4):34, 1984.
32. Menninger, K., Mayman, M., and Pruysen, P.: The vital balance: the life process in mental health and illness, New York, 1967, The Viking Press.
33. Morley, W.E.: Theory of crisis intervention, Pastoral Psychology 21(203):14, 1970.
34. Morley, W.E., Messick, J.M., and Aguilera, D.C.: Crisis: paradigms of intervention, Journal of Psychiatric Nursing and Mental Health Services 5:538, 1967.
35. Neville, D., and Barnes, S.: The suicidal phone call, Journal of Psychosocial Nursing and Mental Health Services 23(8):14, 1985.
36. Olivos, G.: Crisis intervention and emergency psychiatric treatment, Emotional First Aid: A Journal of Crisis Intervention 2(4):20, 1985.
37. Parad, H.J.: The use of time-limited crisis intervention in community mental health programming, Social Service Review 40:275, 1966.
38. Parad, H.J.: Crisis intervention. In Encyclopedia of social work, vol. 1, ed. 16, New York, 1971, National Association of Social Workers.
39. Parad, H.J., and Resnik, H.L.P.: The practice of crisis intervention in emergency care. In Resnik, H.L.P., Ruben, H.L., and Ruben, D.D., editors: Emergency psychiatric care: the management of mental health crisis, Bowie, Md., 1975, The Charles Press Publishers, Inc.
40. Parad, H.J., and others: Crisis intervention and emergency mental health care: concepts and principles. In Resnik, H.L.P., Ruben, H.L., and Ruben, D.D., editors: Emergency psychiatric care: the management of mental health crises, Bowie, Md., 1975, The Charles Press Publishers, Inc.
41. Peterson, L.C.: Attribution theory and its application in crisis intervention, Perspectives in Psychiatric Care 22(3):331, 1985.
42. Polak, P.R., Reres, M., and Fish, L.: The management of family

crises. In Resnik, H.L.P., Ruben, H.L., and Ruben, D.D., editors: Emergency psychiatric care: the management of mental health crises, Bowie, Md., 1975, The Charles Press Publishers, Inc.

43. Rapoport, L.: The state of crises: some theoretical considerations, Social Service Review **36:**211, 1962.

44. Rapoport, L.: Crisis-oriented short-term casework, Social Service Review **41:**31, 1967.

45. Rapoport, L.: Crisis intervention as a mode of brief treatment. In Roberts, R.W., and Wee, R.H., editors: Theories of social casework, Chicago, 1970, The University of Chicago Press.

46. Rapoport, R.: Normal crises, family structures, and mental health, Family Process **2:**68, 1963.

47. Ratna, L.: Crisis intervention in psychogeriatrics, British Journal of Psychiatry **141:**296, 1982.

48. Sarner, M.: The family support group as a primary means of crisis intervention for families of psychotic patients, Emotional First Aid: A Journal of Crisis Intervention **2**(3):36, 1985.

49. Sase, S.S.: Grief associated with a prison experience: counseling the client, Journal of Psychosocial Nursing and Mental Health Service **20**(7):25, 1982.

50. Slaby, A.E.: Crisis-oriented therapy, New Directions in Mental Health Services **28:**21, 1985.

51. Stein, D.M., and Lambert, M.J.: Telephone counseling and crisis intervention: a review, American Journal of Community Psychology, **12**(1):101, 1984.

52. Sullivan-Taylor, L.: Policemen and nursing students: crisis intervention team, Journal of Psychosocial Nursing and Mental Health Services **23**(9):26, 1985.

53. Taplin, J.R.: Crisis theory: critique and reformulation, Community Mental Health Journal **7**(1):13, 1971.

54. Valente, S.: The suicidal teenager **15**(12):47, 1985.

55. Waldron, G.: Crisis intervention: is it effective? British Journal of Hospital Medicine **31**(4):283, 1984.

56. Walfish, S.: Crisis telephone counselors' views of clinical interaction situations, Community Mental Health Journal **19**(3):219, 1983.

57. Weisman, G.K.: Crisis-oriented residential treatment as an alternative to hospitalization, Hospital Community Psychiatry, **36**(12):1302, 1985.

58. Wolterman, M.C., and Miller, M.: Caring for parents in crisis, Nursing Forum, **22**(1):34, 1985.

59. Zener, K.A.: Some basic assumptions of crisis intervention, E.F.A. Journal of Crisis Intervention **2**(3):16, 1985.

60. Zizzo, F.: A field experience model for crisis intervention, E.F.A. Journal of Crisis Intervention **2**(4):35, 1985.

ANNOTATED BIBLIOGRAPHY

Aguilera, D.C., and Messick, J.M.: Crisis intervention: theory and methodology, ed. 5, St. Louis, 1986, The C.V. Mosby Co.

The revised edition of this classic book retains the detailed discussion of crisis intervention theory and expands the content on techniques, principles, and processes. Crisis interventions in settings such as the hospital and emergency room are included. Crisis intervention in current health problems such as AIDS and Alzheimer's disease is addressed. This practical book is a valuable reference for the undergraduate student in a variety of health care settings.

Lindemann, E.: Beyond grief: studies in crisis intervention, New York, 1979, Jason Aronson, Inc.

This book contains a collection of Lindemann's papers, including his classical work on the symptoms and management of acute grief. The articles will be of interest to nurses working in various clinical settings, since crisis events such as surgery, ulcerative colitis, and moving are discussed. He also addresses preventive intervention and social changes.

Narayan, S.M., and Joslin, D.J.: Crisis theory and intervention: a critique of the medical model and proposal of a holistic nursing model, Advances in Nursing Science **2:**27, July 1980.

The authors critique Lindemann's and Caplan's theoretical models of crises, emphasizing the problems of the models related to disease and symptom treatment. The holistic nursing model of crisis proposed by the authors is based on depletion of health potential, which is viewed as an aspect of the health continuum. They provide a useful comparison of the medical and holistic nursing models of crisis.

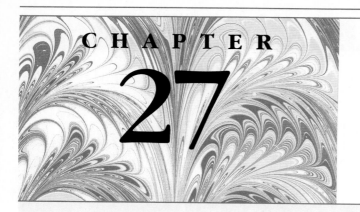

CHAPTER 27

SHORT-TERM PSYCHOTHERAPY

Sophronia R. Williams   *E. Hope Bevis*

After studying this chapter the learner will be able to:

Discuss the historical development of short-term psychotherapy.

Identify theoretical approaches to short-term psychotherapy.

Describe characteristics of short-term psychotherapy.

List criteria for selecting clients for short-term psychotherapy.

Describe qualities necessary for short-term psychotherapists.

Use the nursing process in providing short-term psychotherapy.

Short-term psychotherapy is well established as a brief form of therapy that uses specific criteria for the selection of clients, focuses on a central issue to be resolved, and has therapeutic flexibility. Clients treated with short-term psychotherapy may experience lasting changes in the problems for which they seek help.

Interest has grown in short-term psychotherapy as an efficient, economical means to treat a large number of clients in inpatient and outpatient facilities. This interest is in response to limited financial and staff resources and to the potential effect of diagnosis-related groups, which has led to shorter psychiatric hospital stays. Because fewer nurses are specializing in psychiatric nursing at the master's level, fewer qualified staff are available to meet the growing demand for mental health–psychiatric care. The segment of the population with limited finances and a lack of commitment to long-term psychotherapy may benefit from short-term psychotherapy.

THEORETICAL APPROACHES
Psychoanalytic

A number of specific approaches to short-term psychotherapy have been based on psychoanalytical theory. Although these forms of therapy differ in many aspects, three principal approaches can be identified: (1) the interpretive approach, (2) the empathic approach, and (3) the corrective approach.

Interpretive approach. Of the three approaches, the interpretive approach follows most closely the classic techniques of psychoanalytic therapy. This form of treatment is based on vigorous interpretation of unconscious conflicts. The overall goal of therapy is to have the client understand the relationship between his current problem and his underlying fantasies and conflicts. The works of Malan[38] and Sifneos[57] are most representative of this approach. Sifneos labels his approach *short-term anxiety-provoking psychotherapy,* and Malan refers to his work as *brief psychotherapy.* Because the two approaches are more similar than different, they will be discussed together.

Both Malan and Sifneos choose clients whose current problems reflect unresolved Oedipal conflicts. The immediate goal of therapy is to make clients aware of their conflicts. This is achieved through interpretation of links between the past and the present, clarification of issues, and confrontation of transference phenomena. However, the way in which the two men implement these techniques differs.

Sifneos views himself as an unemotional but involved teacher. He shows little respect for the client's defenses; thus his confrontations and interpretations leave the client little room to maneuver. Through relentless confrontation of the unconscious conflict, Sifneos increases the client's anxiety. This increase in anxiety is at the heart of Sifneos's approach. It leaves the client with three choices: fight, ac-

✿ *Historical Overview* ✿

DATE	EVENT
Late 1800s	Freud performed earliest type of short-term psychotherapy.
Early 1900s	Emphasis switched from short-term to long-term therapy.
Mid-1900s	Alexander and French,[1] in their classical work on brief therapy, planted the seed for the beginning of short-term psychotherapy when they challenged the idea that the depth of therapy is proportionate to its length. The need to treat World War II veterans suffering from emotional trauma led to a treatment approach that used principles of short-term psychotherapy.
1960s	Psychoanalysts in the United States and Europe began studying the theory and techniques of short-term psychotherapy. Malan[38] was one of the first therapists to conduct a study on short-term psychotherapy at Tavistock Clinic in London, while Wolberg[67] was among the first to conduct studies in the United States.
1963	Therapists began publishing a series of major volumes that described and evaluated particular forms of planned short-term psychotherapy.
1970s	Sifneos,[57] Mann,[40] and Davanloo[13] made significant contributions toward refining the theory and techniques of short-term psychotherapy.
1980s	Many nurses who function as independent practitioners are choosing short-term psychotherapy as a treatment approach. With the potential for shorter lengths of stay in inpatient psychiatric settings, nurses began developing conceptual models for short-term nursing therapy.
Future	Nurses will expand their use of short-term treatment approaches that are effective in decreasing the length of hospitalization.

knowledge the truth as Sifneos sees it, or quit therapy. The intensity of treatment propels the therapeutic process and helps shorten treatment time.

Malan's manner is much less intense. He remains more aloof and appears less involved because of the lesser intensity of his confrontations. Like Sifneos, he uses interpretation to help clients achieve insight into their behavior, but he is more controlled and didactic in his approach.

After the client has insight into the unconscious Oedipal conflict, therapy is terminated. The amount of time needed to achieve the goals of *interpretive therapy* is extremely flexible, usually anywhere from 2 to 12 months.

Empathic approach. Mann designed the *empathic approach* to short-term psychotherapy. Similar to the interpretive method in that it deals with unconscious conflict, the empathic approach deals with conflict centering around the experience of loss. Mann believes that the universal central life crisis is the issue of separation and individuation. He further believes that the client's problems in the here and now can be traced to conflicts in the past about dependence, independence, and separation from the mother figure. He postulates that the client clings to the unconscious fantasy of union with his mother and ignores the passing of adult time. A series of 12 treatment

sessions is agreed upon by client and therapist at the first meeting, and the termination date is marked on the calendar. Mann and his followers do not make exceptions to this 12-session format; thus a fixed time for completion of therapy is a distinctive feature of Mann's therapy. Mann believes that mastery of separation anxiety serves as a model for overcoming other neurotic anxieties; thus the goal of therapy is to help the client separate from significant others in the environment and achieve individuation.

Mann believes this goal can be reached through a series of empathic encounters between the client and therapist. He avoids confrontations and interpretations that evoke anxiety. Instead, the therapist consistently identifies with the client's chronic pain through a series of empathic statements while dealing with the reality of separation through the issue of a fixed termination date. As the therapist shares the client's sadness and grief over the impending termination, Mann theorizes that the ability to separate from relationships becomes more successful than in the past, thereby making separation a successful maturational event. This success then translates to other areas of the client's life.

Corrective approach. Alexander and French[1] and Beck[3] are leading contributors to the corrective approach to short-term psychotherapy. Instead of revealing an unconscious conflict as the major source of stress in the client's life, the emphasis in therapy is on resolution of current life problems. Proponents of this approach agree that to develop a treatment plan the therapist must understand the unconscious conflicts the client is experiencing, but need not share this understanding with the client.

The goal of *corrective therapy* is to help the client achieve a feeling of success in the activities of daily living. The techniques used to achieve this goal are more varied than those of the interpretive or empathic approach. Analysis of transference is used as a major tool in helping the client experience success.[1] However, giving suggestions and direct advice are also techniques used to achieve therapeutic goals. Use of these techniques represents a drastic departure from the concepts of traditional analytic psychotherapy. In general the corrective method presents an approach to short-term psychotherapy that least represents the components of classical analysis.

Alexander does not set a specific termination date. He believes that the client's experience itself will determine treatment time. The therapist imposes brief interruptions to wean the client from therapy. Thus there is great flexibility in the number of treatment sessions.

Behavioral

Many short-term psychotherapists incorporate the techniques of behavioral therapy into clinical practice. For example, Beck[3] has extended his psychoanalytic framework by incorporating cognitive and behavioral theory and techniques. Beck stresses the relationship between a person's thoughts and feelings. He tries to provide a "corrective cognitive experience" through a series of detailed instructions and exercises. This facilitates the client's awareness of how distorted thoughts cause a negative evaluation of life experiences. Beck's work provides a clear link between a psychodynamic understanding of the client's conflicts and the incorporation of behavioral techniques to resolve these conflicts. Table 27-1 summarizes psychoanalytic and behavioral approaches to short-term psychotherapy.

CHARACTERISTICS OF SHORT-TERM PSYCHOTHERAPY

The following are distinct characteristics common to all forms of short-term therapy:
1. Use of time
2. Criteria for selection of clients
3. Identification of the central issue—focus of therpay
4. Limited goals
5. Activity of the therapist
6. Flexibility of therapeutic techniques

Use of Time

Most short-term psychotherapists use time in an extremely flexible manner, believing the severity of the client's problems and the client's ego-adaptive capacities necessitate this approach. Therapists who choose a psychoanalytic or behavioral approach to short-term psychotherapy have wide variations in the use of time. Most therapists agree that 25 sessions is the upper limit of brief psychotherapy. Many clinicians recommend a course of treatment lasting from one to six sessions, and some prefer 10 to 25 sessions.

Although therapists differ as to the length of time needed to treat clients, they agree that time itself becomes a primary change agent. The passing of time has long been viewed as having curative power. Short-term psychotherapists maximize the therapeutic effects of time by forcing clients to come to grips with the reality of time in their lives.

A comparison of the use of time in each of the theoretical approaches is presented in Table 27-2.

Client Selection

The selection of clients who would benefit from short-term psychotherapy is one of the most important characteristics of all forms of short-term therapy. Not all clients are suitable candidates for short-term psychotherapy. The therapist looks for the qualities that indicate the client's

TABLE 27-1 Summary of theoretical approaches

Theory	Theorist	Focus of Therapy	Techniques	Goals
Psychoanalytic Interpretive	Malan Sifneos	Oedipal conflicts	Confrontation, interpretation, and clarification of issues	To understand relationship between intrapsychic conflict and present problem
Empathic	Mann	Separation-individuation conflicts	Series of empathic encounters, rigid structure, and use of transference phenomena	To achieve individuation and independence
Corrective	Alexander Beck French	Current life problems	Giving direction, advice, and injunctions	To resolve present problem
Behavioral	Beck	Relationship between thoughts and feelings	Series of detailed instruction and exercises	To provide a corrective experience

TABLE 27-2 Comparison of the use of time in various approaches to short-term therapy

	Sessions		
Theoretical Approach	**Number**	**Length**	**Frequency**
Psychoanalytic theory	5 to 50	15 to 50 minutes for individuals	Daily to weekly
Behavioral theory	1 to 25	1 to 2 hours	Daily to weekly

ability to succeed in therapy. When assessing client suitability, short-term therapists who use a psychoanalytic framework employ the following criteria:

1. Motivation for change
2. Ability to state the major complaint
3. Evidence of ego strength
4. Ability to form meaningful relationships

A high degree of motivation for change is critical for success in therapy. The client needs to be willing to look inward and see that his symptoms are psychological in origin. The motivation for change needs to be more than a simple wish for relief of symptoms. Instead the client needs to desire to alter once and for all the neurotic patterns that bind him to a destructive life-style. This criterion has important prognostic value. Unless lasting change is the motivating factor, little can be accomplished in the time allotted for therapy. However, even change that lasts for 4 years is a realistic expectation for therapy. (See the Research Highlight on p. 513.)

The second criterion for success in therapy involves the client's ability to identify the symptom or complaint that caused him to seek help. Because the time the client will spend in therapy is limited, the issues to be worked through are also limited. If short-term psychotherapy is to be successful, the issues to be resolved in therapy must be limited to one or two. If the client has many symptoms or issues, his ability to establish priorities is of prime importance, especially if the central issue is to be dealt with successfully.

To be suitable for short-term psychotherapy, clients also need to demonstrate sufficient ego strength to withstand the process of therapy. Short-term psychotherapy is primarily a cognitive, insight-oriented form of therapy, so clients need to demonstrate average or above-average intelligence, educational achievement appropriate to their stated age, ability to assume some responsibility for their own actions, and a degree of psychological sophistication. The clients also need to be able to think in psychological terms to understand the interpetations suggested for their thoughts and actions. However, short-term psychotherapists are more flexible with this criterion of client selection than with the two criteria previously stated.

A fourth criterion for consideration in client selection is the ability of the client to form meaningful relationships. The client's past history needs to reflect the presence of at least one meaningful relationship. A history that does not reflect the ability to form relationships suggests an inability on the part of the client to trust others. Be-

cause trust is necessary in any relationship, the client who has problems with trust is not likely to form a therapeutic alliance. The relationship needs to develop quickly, ideally in the first interview, because of the limited time the client spends in therapy. Unless the client is already able to trust, there is very little hope of developing a therapeutic relationship in time to accomplish the goals of therapy.

When the short-term therapist is using a behavioral approach to therapy, the criteria for selection of clients appropriate for therapy are less stringent because insight into behavior is not necessarily a goal of therapy. However, the client needs to be motivated to change his behavior and to participate in identifying the objectives for therapy.

Individuals with the following are unsuitable for most forms of brief therapy:

1. Alcohol addiction
2. Drug addiction
3. Chronic obsessions
4. Phobias
5. More than one course of electroconvulsive therapy
6. Organic or functional psychoses
7. Grossly self-destructive behavior
8. Severe antisocial behavior
9. Inability to function without constant support

The criteria for selection of clients suitable for short-term psychotherapy are extremely helpful because they can be applied to clients throughout the life cycle. These criteria are as valuable in evaluating an adolescent having difficulty in school as in evaluating a 60-year-old with depression. The criteria also allow the therapist to look at clients holistically, because the criteria are not disease oriented.

Identification of the Central Issue

A third element necessary to successful short-term therapy is identification of the central issue at the onset of therapy. Sometimes this is referred to as the *core conflict* or development of the focus of therapy. The therapist needs to keep this central issue or conflict in focus persistently throughout the client's therapy. Short-term psychotherapists believe that identifying the focus of the client's conflict helps him work through the problem and achieve the goals of therapy. This gives the client a sense of mastery, control, and success in life. In addition, identification of the central issue helps keep the therapy brief.

Research Highlight

Evaluation of a Time-Limited Program of Dynamic Group Psychotherapy

B.M. Dick & K. Wooff

PURPOSE

The purpose of the study was to examine the effectiveness of time-limited psychotherapy by comparing a client's use of psychiatric service before and after therapy and to establish the degree of change in attitude the clients experienced.

SAMPLE

Fifty people, 23 men and 26 women, between the ages of 16 and 50, and one client who attended for two periods of therapy during the study constituted the sample. All clients who started therapy at the hospital within a given year and who remained in the area for at least 1 year after discharge were included in the study.

METHODOLOGY

Data to determine the clients use of pre- and post-therapy service were obtained from the Salford Psychiatric Register. The Register included cumulative patient-based demographic, social, diagnostic information, and clients' use of hospital services. The services covered included admission and discharge data from inpatient and day patient care, and outpatient attendances and referrals to and discharges from social work care. Pretherapy service was measured for the 365 days preceding the start of therapy and posttherapy service use was measured for the 365 days after discharge from the unit.

A two-part questionnaire interview was used before and after therapy to measure the clients' satisfaction with themselves and their life situation and attitudes toward their illness. A highly structured questionnaire measured clients' satisfaction in relationships (work and home), work performance (work and home), leisure time, sex life, physical health, self-understanding, self-image, and symptoms. The sec-ond part of the questionnaire was designed to record information on changes in clients' attitude toward the illness before and after therapy. The interviews were conducted the first week of therapy, the final week of therapy, and 3 years after the clients were admitted to the unit.

Clients were required to attend the therapy 5 days a week for 12 weeks (60 sessions). The therapeutic experience consisted of daily small analytical groups with six to eight clients in each group, community meetings, and structured group sessions that included psychodrama, art expression, encounter exercises, video feedback, volleyball, and relaxation groups. The therapeutic experiences were provided concurrently; the analytical group was conducted by the same nurse throughout the therapy period.

FINDINGS

Analysis of data provided evidence that use of all services (days for inpatient and day clients and appointment for outpatient) decreased and the decrease in two of the three types of care was statistically significant ($p < 0.02$) for inpatient days and ($p < 0.001$) for out-patient attendance. Thirty three (82%) of the patients reduced their use of psychiatric services. Seventy percent of the clients had positive changes in attitudes toward their illness. The reduction in use of service was maintained at follow-up 4<5 years later.

IMPLICATIONS

The results indicate that a time-limited structured group psychotherapy program may be a useful modality for preparing hospitalized clients to return to the community and function effectively for at least 4 years.

Based on data from British Journal of Psychiatry **148**:159. 1986.

Limited Goals

All approaches to short-term psychotherapy recognize the importance of setting therapeutic goals. Increasingly, selection of treatment goals is being tied to successful outcomes in therapy.[23,54] The challenge to short-term psychotherapists is to limit the goals of therapy to those which can be realistically achieved during the treatment time. Short-term goals need to reflect the long-term goals and be established through mutual participation between client and therapist. Goals need to be limited to one or two and address the specific problems that prompted the client to seek therapy.

Activity of the Therapist

The nature of short-term psychotherapy requires the therapist to be more verbally active than in traditional psychoanalysis. Because time is limited and the central issue is continuously kept in focus, the therapist cannot take a passive stance. Instead, she needs to consistently direct the session toward resolution of the central conflict through persistent confrontation and interpretation of material presented. When the client attempts to sidetrack the core conflict, the therapist is quick to point out the resistive maneuver and bring the core conflict back into focus. The therapist maintains this active role throughout the course of therapy to protect the therapeutic alliance.

Short-term psychotherapists believe that two major goals may be achieved through an active stance. First, they believe that it reflects the therapist's concern and interest for the client. This helps establish and maintain the therapeutic alliance. Second, actively keeping the central issue in focus maintains a high level of tension and interaction, which in turn propels the course of therapy.

In summary, the active role of the therapist implies consistent application of treatment techniques. This discourages regression and dependence and encourages the ego strength to produce lasting change. Short-term psychotherapy places considerable demands on the therapist, who guides, exhorts, and confronts the client while maintaining the therapeutic alliance.

Flexibility of Therapeutic Techniques

Flexibility refers to the therapist's use of a wide range of therapeutic techniques in short-term psychotherapy and is determined by the theoretical approach the therapist selects. Many short-term psychotherapists find that the therapeutic techniques of analytic and behavioral theories are all applicable within their practice. The following treatment approaches may be useful in achieving an individual client's goals, provided that they are within the scope and training of the therapist:

Confrontation	Medication
Interpretation	Biofeedback
Meditation	Hypnosis
Behavior modification	Cognitive learning
Persuasian	Guided imagery
Psychodrama	Milieu therapy
Recreational activities	Direct counsel

General Characteristics

Some additional, general characteristics are evident in many forms of short-term psychotherapy. First, short-term psychotherapy may be done on either an inpatient or an outpatient basis. Many general hospitals provide a psychiatric unit, and most of these are for short-term care only. Many of these have found short-term psychotherapy to be extremely useful in planning client care.

A course of short-term psychotherapy is also appropriate when clients are treated on an outpatient basis. Most short-term psychotherapy is conducted on an outpatient basis in both the public and private sectors. Although the reasons for this are numerous, economic factors head the list. As with other treatment forms, a setting that provides privacy is required regardless of where the treatment occurs.

Most major proponents of psychotherapy believe that venting emotional tension is an important element of therapy. Short-term psychotherapists believe this needs to be done in an atmosphere that provides a sense of hope and expectation of help.

Short-term psychotherapy differs from other treatment forms, particularly crisis intervention and long-term therapy, but similarities exist among the three approaches. Table 27-3 compares the differential aspects of crisis intervention and short- and long-term psychotherapy.

CHARACTERISTICS OF THE SHORT-TERM PSYCHOTHERAPIST
Qualifications

The first qualification for all short-term psychotherapists is academic preparation at the master's level or above in nursing, psychiatry, psychology, or social work. Each discipline provides opportunities to learn about the theory and practice of short-term psychotherapy. These opportunities may be very brief, such as a lecture on the characteristics of the therapy, or may extend to a formal

TABLE 27-3 Differential aspects of crisis intervention, short-term psychotherapy, and long-term psychotherapy

Therapeutic Aspect	Treatment Modality		
	Crisis Intervention	Short-Term Psychotherapy	Long-Term Psychotherapy
Time	Short, usually 6 sessions or fewer	Intermediate, from 6 to 40 sessions	Long, from 1 to 5 years or longer
Client selection	People in crisis states who may be in danger of decompensating from stress	People with specific problems causing conflict	People who wish to change their personality patterns
Goals	To reduce or remove stress and help the person deal with the crisis	To achieve personal growth and better coping abilities	To reconstruct personality patterns
Identification of the central issue	Crisis situation establishes focus	Clearly defined at onset of therapy because only a limited number of issues can be dealt with effectively	Less clearly defined at onset because many issues may be dealt with
Activity of the therapist	Active-direct	Active-direct, involved	Nondirective, more passive
Therapeutic flexibility	Problem-solving techniques, support approaches	Wide range of techniques, from interpretive to task assignment	Psychoanalytic techniques to explore the unconscious mind

training experience. If a therapist decides to use short-term psychotherapy to treat clients and does not have the expertise to do so, several avenues are available to obtain such expertise. First, the therapist may consult an expert in the field of short-term psychotherapy and receive training through individual supervision. The therapist may also enroll in a course that offers training in short-term psychotherapy. This may be done through academic institutions or through agencies that offer continuing education. Regardless of the avenue taken to receive training, the short-term psychotherapist needs to be thoroughly grounded in a general theory of psychology, psychopathology, and psychotherapy.

A second qualification, identified by some authorities in the field as essential for short-term psychotherapists, is experiential preparation. Mann[41] is representative of short-term psychotherapists who believe that previous experience as a long-term psychotherapist is a prerequisite to practice. Mann and his followers also believe that the short-term psychotherapist needs to have a personal experience in therapy, preferably with a psychoanalytic orientation.

Sifneos[57] is representative of those who believe that any beginning therapist with an open mind who is versed in psychodynamic theory can learn to practice short-term psychotherapy. He believes that a protracted period of training is unnecessary, providing the therapist is treating a suitable client under intense individual supervision.

Other qualifications for short-term psychotherapists include the availability of advanced practitioners for consultation and supervision when necessary and the opportunity to obtain continuing education. In a world with an expanding knowledge base and a rapid development of techniques, the short-term psychotherapist needs to keep abreast of new developments to provide the best service possible to the client. The ability to communicate clearly and succinctly is another important qualification for the short-term psychotherapist. Personal qualities needed include open-mindedness, enthusiasm, empathy, and flexibility. When the therapist reveals these qualities the client views her as a genuine person, not an automated clone. Demonstrating these qualities does not mean that the ethics of a professional relationship are abandoned; what is abandoned is the passivity and formality of traditional analysis.

Roles

The role assumed by the therapist in short-term psychotherapy depends on the treatment approach being used. Given that all short-term psychotherapists assume an active stance in therapy, the therapist may assume one of three roles: teacher, helper, or manager.

The role of teacher is assumed by short-term psychotherapists who use an interpretive approach to therapy. In this method the therapist shows the client how unsatisfactory his solutions have been to his problems. As a teacher, the therapist then tries to present to the client new techniques to solve old conflicts.

In the empathic approach the therapist is seen as a

helper who creates an atmosphere of compassionate empathy. This is extremely important because the client experiences an intense level of emotion in an extremely short period. Therefore the therapist needs to recognize the client's pain and suffering and offer active support to maintain the therapeutic alliance.

The last of the roles that may be assumed by short-term psychotherapists is that of manager. The managerial role is assumed by therapists who use the corrective approach to short-term psychotherapy. As manager, the therapist plans new strategies to solve the client's current problems and frequently gives detailed instructions to the client.

Table 27-1 includes a summary of the goals of the three approaches to short-term psychotherapy.

Goals

The first goal of the short-term psychotherapist, a universal one, is to establish rapport with the client so that a therapeutic alliance can develop. The challenge for the short-term psychotherapist is to establish rapport quickly because the time spent in therapy is limited. Other goals for the therapist include formulating the dynamics behind the central issue and deciding on treatment goals.

A specific goal for the short-term psychotherapist is to make the client aware from the beginning of the limited time available for therapy. In the first session the therapist begins to prepare the client for termination. If a fixed time frame is used, the client is given the exact date that therapy will be terminated. If the therapist is not operating from a fixed time frame, the client is told the approximate time frame with the explicit message that the therapist believes the goals of therapy can be achieved in this amount of time but that the time frame can be renegotiated if the client and therapist deem it necessary.

The initial session is the appropriate time for the short-term therapist to negotiate the treatment contract. The contract includes what services will be provided by the therapist, how much the client will pay for these services, the method of payment, and the time, place, and length of treatment. Some short-term psychotherapists have a formal contract that both parties sign; others prefer a verbal agreement. Whatever the contract format, the negotiated contract further emphasizes to the client that only a limited amount of time is available to achieve the goals of therapy.

TYPES OF SHORT-TERM PSYCHOTHERAPY

As the theory and techniques of short-term psychotherapy have become more familiar to professionals in the field of mental health, many models of brief therapy have been developed. All of the models, regardless of their theoretical orientations, share the identified characteristics of short-term psychotherapy. At present, short-term psychotherapy is being used as a treatment model for individuals, groups, and families.

Short-term psychotherapy also provides a basis for developing types of therapy that can be effective in all phases of the life cycle. In recent years some short-term psychotherapists attempted to choose a type or method of short-term therapy that matches the adult developmental crisis the client is experiencing. This type of therapy uses as a framework the developmental phases of adult life proposed by Erikson. Using the interpretive, empathic, and corrective approaches as the framework for therapy, the therapist assesses the developmental issue the client is struggling with and relates it to one of the three therapy forms:

THERAPEUTIC APPROACH	DEVELOPMENTAL PHASE
Empathic	Identity versus role confusion
Interpretive	Intimacy versus isolation
Corrective	Generativity versus stagnation

NURSING PROCESS
Assessment

Physical dimension. Assessment of the physical dimension is important in short-term psychotherapy, because the client may have a physical illness or the physical symptoms may mask the psychological conflict. A frequent complaint is inability to fall asleep at night, accompanied by feelings of nervousness. Questioning the client about his diet and drinking habits may reveal that an excessive intake of caffeine is causing the problem. After careful assessment of the physical dimension, no apparent organic reason may be found for the physical symptoms. Then further assessment is needed to determine whether the complaints are psychological in origin. Somatization may be a common response to the psychological conflict. However, the nurse needs to do a thorough assessment and should not assume the problem is psychological.

Emotional dimension. Because the client's level of anxiety will increase during the therapeutic experience, the nurse assesses whether the client can tolerate therapy without being flooded with more anxiety than he can tolerate. Clear indications of anxiety may be evident as the nurse assesses the client's central conflicts.

Assessment of the emotional dimension frequently reveals the central conflicts the client is experiencing, as in the following Case Example.

Case Example

A freshman college student came to the nurse's office with vague somatic complaints and low achievement in the academic area. His low academic achievement was of particular concern to him, because he graduated in the upper fourth of his high school class. This was his first experience at living alone, coming from a close-knit family. The nurse noticed that every time the subject of independence directly or indirectly came up in the interview, the client crossed his legs, shook his foot, moved around in his chair, and his voice faltered.

The indications of the anxiety experienced by the client when the subject of independence and role identity came up together with the client's life history gave the nurse clues that the central conflict in this case was separation versus individuation. Having assessed the probable under-lying cause of the young man's anxiety, the nurse may choose to approach the conflict as a developmental crisis and use the empathic approach of Mann as a treatment modality. Once the developmental crisis is assessed, an attempt is made to match the crisis to a particular approach of short-term psychotherapy that most succinctly addresses the developmental issue. In this case the developmental crisis was identity versus role diffusion. Mann's approach, which focuses on separation and individuation, most clearly addresses the client's developmental issues.

The client's anger may become manifest as the nurse challenges the client's resistance or explores painful experiences; thus it is essential that the nurse assess how the client deals with his anger when he feels threatened. A related feeling that the client may experience is sadness, which may be the feeling beneath the anger.

Intellectual dimension. The client's use of grammar, his educational preparation and work experience, and his conception of the problem bringing him to therapy give the nurse an opportunity to assess the client's intellectual functioning. Because all short-term psychotherapy is active and requires the client to do something, the nurse ascertains the client's ability to understand and follow directions. How the client's needs for intellectual stimulation are being met also is assessed, because boredom can lead to symptoms in other areas.

Assessment in the intellectual dimension also provides the opportunity to evaluate the client's ability to understand the problem for which he sought help. Many clients can state the problem clearly and even know why they are having the problem but do not know how to implement change. Other clients can state the problem but do not see any options for solving the problem.

The nurse determines the degree to which the client is motivated to make lasting changes in his behavior. Because motivation is linked to successful outcome of therapy, the nurse stays alert to behavior that suggests motivation. Determining motivation for short-term psychotherapy is difficult. Statements such as, "I can't stand this pain any longer," or "I'm tired of feeling bad, I want to feel good again" are indications that the client is motivated to change. Sifneos[57] suggests that assessment of the client's level of motivation be made using evidence that the client is able to do the following:

1. Recognize that his symptoms are psychological in origin
2. Appear to be introspective and give an honest account of his emotional difficulties
3. Seem willing to participate actively in the therapeutic situation
4. Be actively curious and willing to understand himself
5. Be willing to explore, experiment, and change
6. Have realistic expectations regarding the psychotherapeutic outcomes
7. Be willing to make sacrifices in the service of psychotherapy

Many clients are highly resistant to deal with their painful feeling and use various kinds of defensive maneuvers to avoid doing so. Because resistance is counterproductive to the goals of short-term psychotherapy, the nurse determines the degree of resistance during the initial evaluation. In addition to various defense mechanisms, resistance is manifested by vagueness, regressive behavior, and obsessional behavior.

✿ *Social dimension.* Information about the client's ability to develop and maintain a meaningful relationship can be collected as the nurse assesses the social dimension. This, as well as its connection with the emotional dimension, is seen by most clients as the area of their lives that is most out of balance. The ability to form a relationship is essential to a positive experience in short-term psychotherapy.

The nurse is alert for positive and negative transference as the therapeutic relationship develops. Transference may become manifest during the first session. The transferential feelings may be regressive in nature, with the client expressing a wish to be cared for as a child.

It is essential that the nurse assess the client's degree of dependency, because clients with maladaptive dependency will have difficulty achieving the goals of short-term psychotherapy. The nurse also assesses the extent to which the client's self-esteem has been adversely affected by his inability to solve his problems. The client needs to have confidence in his ability to increase his self-esteem.

Collecting data about the client's family can be significant, because dysfunctional family relationships may be directly related to the client's core conflict. The nurse makes this assessment without delving into the client's childhood experiences in his nuclear family. Learning about the family relationship may provide data about the family as a support system for the client.

It is essential that information related to intimacy and isolation be obtained without probing into the client's past, because reconstruction of the client's personality is not a goal of short-term psychotherapy. Generally the client is able to give a complete history without prompting and direction from the nurse. If necessary, a structured approach with a specific outline or format to follow or a semistructured format may be used in obtaining historical data related to the client's central conflict.

✿ *Spiritual dimension.* The short-term psychotherapist can frequently gain valuable information about the central conflict through assessment of the spiritual dimension. Frequently clients express guilt feelings about their present actions. This guilt may stem from a conviction that what they are doing now or have done in the past is not in harmony with accepted religious principles. Others express a feeling of alienation from God or a supreme being that in turn keeps them alienated from others.

Analysis

Nursing diagnosis. The following list provides examples of NANDA-accepted nursing diagnoses with causative statements related to short-term psychotherapy:

1. Powerlessness related to low self-esteem
2. Ineffective individual coping related to inability to express feelings of anger
3. Impaired social interaction related to pathological dependence
4. Disturbance in self-concept related to fear of being criticized

TABLE 27-4 Long-term and short-term goals and outcome criteria related to short-term psychotherapy

Goals	Outcome Criteria
NURSING DIAGNOSIS: INEFFECTIVE INDIVIDUAL COPING: INABILITY TO CONFRONT EFFECTIVELY RELATED TO LOW SELF-ESTEEM	
Long-term goals	
To develop a more positive sense of self-worth	Rationally verbalizes positive qualities
	Increases number of meaningful relationships
To develop effective confrontation skills in interpersonal situations	Demonstrates effective confrontation skills in and out of therapy sessions
	Decreases overt symptoms after confrontation
Short-term goals	
To attend one social function with a friend	Attends event
	Names friend who also attended
To confront in an appropriate situation	States confrontation skills used
	Has no headache after confrontation
NURSING DIAGNOSIS: INEFFECTIVE COPING RELATED TO FEAR OR ANGER	
Long-term goals	
To develop constructive assertiveness in interpersonal relationships	Discusses situations that evoke anger
	Increases interaction with others
To develop feelings of safety in the environment	Determines causes for feelings
	Increases involvement in activities in the environment
Short-term goals	
To maintain stable and accepting environment to help allay anxiety	Appears to be more at ease
	Has less need for rituals
To increase awareness of anger and triggering events	Is able to describe feelings and link them to certain causes

5. Social isolation related to excessive somatic complaints

6. Anxiety related to irrational guilt

Planning

Table 27-4 provides long-term and short-term goals and outcome criteria related to short-term psychotherapy. These serve as examples of the planning stage in the nursing process.

Implementation

Physical dimension. The nurse refers the client to his family physician for treatment of a physical problem. When the client's physical complaints have a psychological basis, the nurse assists the client in identifying the stressors and exploring measures for alleviating the problems. Appropriate measures the client has used to alleviate pain can be reinforced. The client may benefit from examining what he is thinking and feeling emotionally when he experiences physical symptoms. This activity may help the client gain insight into the relationship between the physical symptoms and the psychological conflict. The nurse can teach the client self-relaxation exercises. A nurse with experience in hypnosis may use this technique to reduce physically exhausting problems such as hyperventilation, vomiting, and hiccups.

Emotional dimension. Allowing the client to experience a *catharsis,* an unburdening of the self, affords him an opportunity to reduce his anxiety through verbal expression. Frequently, verbalizing the life conflict that relates to his anxiety helps the client to put things in a more realistic perspective. Catharsis allows for the creation of an environment conducive to a therapeutic alliance. As the client expresses thoughts and feelings in a nonjudgmental atmosphere, a sense of trust develops between the two parties. Frequently a catharsis is encouraged in the first session to accelerate the therapeutic process. However, the client may be reluctant or unable to experience a catharsis in short-term psychotherapy. (See the Research Highlight below.)

Throughout therapy the client needs to sense that the nurse will consistently provide emotional support, or other more confrontive techniques of therapy will fail. The nurse may collaborate with the psychiatrist regarding drug therapy for the client, if this is necessary, to reduce the client's anxiety to an optimal level for therapeutic work.

Intellectual dimension. The nurse actively keeps the client focused on the central problem and initiates the problem-solving process during the first session by asking questions related to the central conflict. The

---

Research Highlight

A Study of Curative Factors in Short-Term Group Psychotherapy

V. Brabender, E. Albrecht, J. Sillitti, J. Cooper & E. Kramer

PURPOSE

The purpose of this study was to examine the effect of context, such as setting and type of group, on clients' perceptions of curative factors in short-term psychotherapy and the variability in factors identified as useful by the group over time.

SAMPLE

The sample consisted of 84 clients hospitalized at a 192-bed private psychiatric facility. Seventy percent of the clients were female; they ranged in age from 16 to over 60, with 61% between the ages of 21 and 40. The clients had been referred for group therapy by their physician within 4 days of admission, and they voluntarily agreed to participate in the study. The clients had no previous group therapy experience.

METHODOLOGY

The clients in the sample were members of 14 successive groups of 7 to 10 clients. The groups met for eight 90-minute sessions, four times a week for a 2-week period. At the end of each group session the clients completed a critical-events questionnaire that asked the clients to describe in narrative form the most significant event in the session, the group members involved, and the reasons for the significance of the event. The unit of analysis was the frequency with which the various curative factors were identified. The curative factors were catharsis, self-disclosure, learning from interpersonal actions, universality, acceptance, altruism, self-understanding, vicarious learning, guidance, and hope.

FINDINGS

In 23% of the responses vicarious learning was the curative factor that was identified significantly more often than the others ($P < .01$). The other three most frequently mentioned factors were acceptance (9%), learning from interpersonal actions, and universality (8% each). There was no variation in the factors identified as useful over time.

IMPLICATIONS

Learning can be experienced vicariously through mere observation. This may suggest that clients develop limited trust and are thus unwilling to share highly private thoughts and feelings in a short-term group experience.

Based on data from Hospital and Community Psychiatry 34(7):643, 1983.

nurse can give the client homework that requires the use of the problem-solving process between sessions. Role-playing allows the client to actively participate in examining and solving his problems. The nurse may also use homework to help the client realize that his conflict is based on idiosyncratic automative thought—cognitive distortions, not reality. The type of homework depends on the issue being dealt with in therapy. If the issue is low self-esteem resulting from critical thoughts, the client is asked to write down these thoughts in the context in which they happen. At the next therapy session these thoughts are examined for evidence of distortion, and more reality-oriented interpretations are proposed by the nurse. Through this process the client learns to identify and alter distorted life experiences. Assigning homework as a therapeutic technique has proved valuable in the treatment of clients whose conflicts are expressed through the emotional or social dimension but originate in the intellectual dimension. An example is a single woman who comes to therapy ambivalent about a decision to have a child to fullfill her need for mothering. The nurse gives a homework assignment to help deal with her ambivalence and bring the conflict into focus. She is to make two lists, one with advantages and the other with disadvantages, and bring the list of ideas for discussion at the next meeting. The written assignment seems to solidify in the client's mind data for making a decision.

Lowering the client's resistance increases his motivation. Thus the nurse begins dealing with the client's resistive defenses immediately. Confrontation is an excellent technique to use in reducing these defenses. This technique forces the client to confront the underlying issues responsible for his current life conflicts. Frequently the nurse wisely withholds confrontation techniques until after the therapeutic alliance has been established. To use these techniques before an alliance has been established may jeopardize the therapeutic process. Although aggressive confrontation is profitable for a client with a well-integrated ego, a softer form of confrontation may be necessary for others. An example of these two styles of confrontation may be seen in the situation of a client rambling on at great length about how terrible her mother was to her as a child and ending with the following:

Client: *I don't mean to make my mother sound so bad.*
Nurse: *Yes, you do.*

This aggressive confrontation of the issue was used with a client who had a strong ego, and the confrontation forced her to deal with her true feelings about her mother. If the client had had a weaker ego, the following, less confrontational approach could have been used:

Client: *I don't mean to make my mother sound so bad.*
Nurse: *Oh, what do you mean?*

Confrontation techniques can be an effective, productive tool in the hands of a skilled nurse, but if used by a new or unskilled nurse, confrontation can cause premature termination of therapy. Thus the inexperienced nurse

or student needs to work under the supervision of a highly skilled professional.

Hypnosis frequently provides the push a client needs when he "gets stuck" during the therapeutic process. Hypnosis is particularly well suited for clients who are unconsciously resisting the other techniques of therapy. It frequently solves the problem in the least possible time, and the goals of therapy can be achieved in the time allotted.

✿ ***Social dimension.*** Transferential issues are dealt with early in the course of therapy, because of the time limitation. The individual style of the nurse and the theoretical approach determine the manner in which transferential issues are handled. However, in general, transferential material is dealt with explicitly through the use of confrontation and interpretation.

A useful interpretive technique for obtaining clues about transferential material is dream analysis. The client is asked to write down his dreams from the night of the therapy session and the night before the next therapy session. Frequently the client reports dreamlessness. Asking if any particular feeling or picture comes to mind from the previous night frequently helps the client report an entire dream. For example, after some prompting, a client reported the following dream that had taken place the night before:

Client: *It was weird. I was in an operating room, and I was being cut open, but I was awake.*
Nurse: *And you feel exposed and open here in this relationship.*
Client: *Oh, no . . . well, maybe at times.*

As with any therapeutic technique, the use of interpretation is balanced against the client's willingness to receive and benefit from the interpretations. However, in most cases, if the client has met the criteria as an appropriate short-term psychotherapy candidate, interpretations can be made that will help the client acquire an understanding of problems and defenses.

Confronting and interpreting the transference relationship provide a major opportunity for the client to achieve personal growth and insight. Again, the transference relationship is used in an overall atmosphere of compassionate empathy to prevent stalls in the therapeutic process.

The following example demonstrates how transference can be used in short-term psychotherapy. A young man, who viewed his mother as a stern, unloving figure whom he could never please, was telling his nurse, a woman, about a situation that had developed at his place of work.

Client: *You think I should have handled it in a different way?*
Nurse: *Is that what your mother would have thought?*

By interpreting the transference from the past, the client was able to see his distortion of the present, develop a better understanding of his abilities, and begin the process of improving his self-esteem.

✿ ***Spiritual dimension.*** The nurse guides the client to examine any spiritual distress he experiences in terms of its rationality. A skillful nurse may use confrontation and interpretation to intervene in problems related to the client's spirituality, especially religious conflict. However, if empathy is not used along with these techniques, the intervention intensifies the feelings related to religious conflicts. Other measures for intervention in the client's conflicts are discussed in Chapter 13.

Evaluation

The most common reasons for failure to achieve treatment goals include (1) unrealistic treatment expectations on the part of the client, even though appropriate treatment goals were identified, (2) failure of the client to become actively involved in a therapeutic relationship with the nurse, and (3) inappropriately matching client and treatment approach. The last factor identified as affecting the outcome of therapy is the countertransference reaction of the therapist. Negative countertransference seriously interferes with the successful confrontation and resolution of the client's problem.

After assessing the factors responsible for not reaching long-term goals, the nurse and client decide on a course of action. If treatment was established with the understanding that termination would happen on a fixed date, renegotiation of the time frame is impossible. In this case the goals may need to be reevaluated as to their appropriateness within the time frame.

If the nurse is working from an approach that allows for more flexibility in relation to time, renegotiation of the termination date may be the appropriate course of action.

BRIEF REVIEW

Historically short-term psychotherapy is an outgrowth of long-term psychotherapy. Alexander, Malan, Mann, and Sifneos are major contributors to this treatment form.

Three major approaches to short-term psychotherapy are the interpretive, the empathic, and the corrective. All of these approaches are based to some degree on psychoanalytic theory. Behavioral theory has also contributed concepts to short-term psychotherapy but not to the same degree as psychoanalysis.

Although short-term psychotherapy can be approached in several ways, features common to all forms of brief therapy are: (1) use of time, (2) specific criteria for the selection of clients, (3) limitation of the number of therapeutic goals that can be achieved, (4) identification of the central issue, (5) active involvement on the part of the therapist, and (6) flexibility of treatment techniques. Differences among crisis intervention, short-term psychotherapy, and long-term psychotherapy are identifiable.

Academic preparation, experiential preparation, skill in the use of communication techniques, openmindedness, and empathy are qualifications of a short-term psychotherapist. The role of the psychotherapist may be that of teacher, helper, or manager, depending on the approach adopted by the therapist. In all roles, activity is stressed as a vital component. Goals of the short-term psychotherapist are similar to those of other therapists, that is, to es-

tablish rapport, negotiate a contract, and assist the client to resolve the conflict.

Short-term psychotherapy is used in individual, group, and family therapy. Numerous approaches to brief therapy can be used with these three forms of therapy.

By careful assessment in each of the five dimensions, the nurse is able to view the client as a total person and identify the dimension in which the client's conflicts are expressed. Once these conflicts have been identified, the nursing process can be enacted.

REFERENCES AND SUGGESTED READINGS

1. Alexander, F., and French, T.M.: Psychoanalytic therapy: principles and applications, New York, 1946, The Ronald Press Co.
2. Althoff, J.G.: Time limits in and leave from a day treatment program, Hospital and Community Psychiatry **31**:841, 1980.
3. Beck, A.T.: Cognitive therapy and the emotional disorders, New York, 1976, International Universities Press, Inc.
4. Bellak, L., and Small, L.: Emergency therapy and brief psychotherapy, New York, 1965, Grune & Stratton, Inc.
5. Bellak, L.: The therapeutic relationship in brief psychotherapy, American Journal of Psychotherapy **33**:564, 1979.
6. Bellak, L.: Brief psychoanalytic psychotherapy of nonpsychotic depression, American Journal of Psychotherapy **35**:160, 1981.
7. Bowman, C., and Spandoni, A.J.: Assertion therapy: the nurse and the psychiatric patient in acute, short-term hospital setting, Journal of Psychiatric Nursing **19**(6):7, 1981.
8. Brabender, V. and others: A study of curative factors in short-term group psychotherapy, Hospital and Community Psychiatry **34**(7):643, 1983.
9. Bridman, S.H., and others: Advances in brief psychotherapy: a review of recent literature, Hospital and Community Psychiatry **34**(10):934, 1983.
10. Brown, B.M., Binder, M., and Johannessen, K.: Brief psychiatric treatment and symptom improvement in university students, College Health **28**:330, 1980.
11. Budman, S.H., Bennett, M.J., and Wiseneski, M.J.: Short-term group psychotherapy, International Journal of Group Psychotherapy **30**:630, 1980.
12. Danesh, H.B.: The angry group for couples: a model for short-term group therapy, Psychiatric Journal of the University of Ottawa **5**:118, 1980.
13. Davanloo, H.: Basic principles and techniques in short-term dynamic psychotherapy, Jamaica, N.Y., 1978, Spectrum Publications, Inc.
14. Deitz, A.: Time-limited psychotherapy for post traumatic stress disorder: the traumatized ego and its self-reparative function, American Journal of Psychotherapy **40**(2):290, 1986.
15. Drob, S., and others: Time-limited group treatment of genital herpes patients, International Journal of Group Psychotherapy **36**(1):133, 1986.
16. Erickson, R.C.: Small-group psychotherapy with patients on a short-stay ward: an opportunity for innovation, Hospital and Community Psychiatry **32**:269, 1981.
17. Freud, S.: Analysis: terminable and interminable. In Freud, S.: The standard edition of [his] complete psychological works, vol. 23, London, 1962, The Hogarth Press, Ltd. (Translated by James Strachey.)
18. Garfield, S.L.: Research on client variables in psychotherapy. In Garfield, S.L., and Bergin, A.E., editors: Handbook of psychotherapy and behavior change, ed. 2, New York, 1978, John Wiley & Sons, Inc.

19. Gelder, M.G., and others: Specific and non-specific factors in behavior therapy, British Journal of Psychiatry 123:445, 1973.
20. Gillett, R.: Short-term intensive psychotherapy—a case history, British Journal of Psychiatry **148**:98, 1986.
21. Goldberg, R.L., and Green, S.A.: A learning-theory perspective of brief psychodynamic psychotherapy, American Journal of Psychotherapy, **XL**(1):70, 1986.
22. Greer, F.L.: Prognostic expectations and outcome of brief therapy, Psychological Reports **46**:973, 1980.
23. Greer, F.L.: Content of treatment goals and outcome of brief therapy, Psychological Reports **47**:580, 1980.
24. Gustafson, J.P.: An investigation of brief dynamic psychotherapy, American Journal of Psychiatry **141**:935, 1984.
25. Heber, S., and others: The nurse as short-term psychotherapist, Canadian Nurse **80**(6):32, 1984.
26. Hicks, P.S.: Brief family therapy with military families, Military Medicine **146**:573, 1981.
27. Horowitz, M.J., and others: Comprehensive analysis of change after brief dynamic psychotherapy, American Journal of Psychiatry **143**(5):582, 1986.
28. Jensen, S.M., Baker, M.A., and Koepp, A.H.: TA in brief psychotherapy with college students, Adolescence **15**:683, 1980.
29. Jones, E.: The life and work of Sigmund Freud, vol. 2, New York, 1957, Basic Books, Inc., Publishers.
30. Kern, C.D., and others: The effectiveness of brief psychotherapy in an institution PSICO **10-11**(1-2):85, 1985.
31. Kibel, H.D.: A conceptual model for short-term inpatient group psychotherapy, American Journal of Psychiatry **138**:74, 1981.
32. Kinston, W., and Bentovim, A.: Creating a focus for brief marital or family therapy. In Budman, S.H., editor: Forms of brief therapy, New York, 1981, The Guilford Press.
33. Lego, S.: The one-to-one nurse-patient relationship, Perspectives in Psychiatric Care **18**:67, 1980.
34. Leibenluft, E., and others: Guidelines for short-term inpatient psychotherapy, Hospital and Community Psychiatry **38**(1):38, 1987.
35. MacPhail, D.: Brief therapy, Nursing Mirror **14**(11):157, 1983.
36. Magder, D.: The wizard of Oz, Canadian Journal of Psychiatry **25**:564, 1980.
37. Malan, D.H.: A study of brief psychotherapy, New York, 1975, Plenum Press.
38. Malan, D.H.: The frontier of brief psychotherapy: an example of the convergence of research and clinical practice, New York, 1976, Plenum Press.
39. Malan, D.H.: Individual psychotherapy and the science of psychodynamics, Kent, England, 1979, Butterworths.
40. Mann, J.: Time-limited psychotherapy, Cambridge, Mass., 1973, Harvard University Press.
41. Mann, J.A.: A casebook of time-limited psychotherapy, New York, 1981, McGraw-Hill Book Co.
42. Mann, J., and Gold, R.: A casebook in time-limited psychotherapy, Washington, D.C., 1987, American Psychiatric Press, Inc.
43. Marks, I.: Behavioral psychotherapy of adult neurosis. In Garfield, S.L., and Bergin, A.E., editors: Handbook of psychotherapy and behavioral change, ed. 2, New York, 1978, John-Wiley & Sons, Inc.
44. Marmon, J.: Short-term dynamic psychotherapy, American Journal of Psychiatry **136**:149, 1979.
45. Morrison, J.K., and others: Follow-up study of psychotherapeutically induced change in clients' constructs of self, Psychological Reports, **59**(2):537, 1986.
46. Nix, J., and Dillon, K.: Short-term nursing therapy: a conceptual model for inpatient psychiatric care, Hospital and Community Psychiatry, **37**(5):493, 1986.
47. Peplau, H.E.: Interpersonal relations in nursing: a conceptual frame of reference for psychodynamic nursing, New York, 1952, G.P. Putnam's Sons.
48. Piper, W.E., and others: Relationship between the object focus of therapist interpretation and outcome in short-term individual psychotherapy, British Journal of Medical Psychology **59**:1, 1986.
49. Prazoff, M., Joyce, A., and Azim, H.: Brief crisis group psychotherapy: one therapist's model, Group **10**(1):34, 1986.
50. Rasmussen, A., and others: A comparison and critique of Mann's time-limited psychotherapy and Davanloo's short-term dynamic psychotherapy, Bulletin of the Menninger Clinic **50**(2):163, 1986.
51. Reich, J., and Neenan, P.: Principles common to different short-term psychotherapies, **XL**(1):62, 1986.
52. Ross, M.P., and others: Brief psychotherapeutic methods in clinical research, Journal of Consulting Clinical Psychology **54**(1):60, 1986.
53. Rounsaville, B.J., and others: A 25 year follow-up of short-term interpersonal psychotherapy in methodone-maintained opiate addicts, Comprehensive Psychiatry **27**(3):201, 1986.
54. Ryle, A.: Defining goals and assessing change in brief psychotherapy: a pilot study using target ratings and the dyad grid, British Jounal of Medical Psychology **52**:223, 1979.
55. Ryle, A.: The focus in brief interpretive psychotherapy: dilemmas, traps and snags as target problems, British Journal of Psychiatry **134**:46, 1979.
56. Sandell, R.: Influence of supervision, therapist's competence and patient's ego level on the effects of time-limited psychotherapy, Psychotherapy and Psychosomatics **44**(2):103, 1985.
57. Sifneos, P.: Short-term psychotherapy and emotional crisis, Cambridge, Mass., 1973, Harvard University Press.
58. Sifneos, P.E.: Short-term dynamic psychotherapy: evaluation and technique, New York, 1979, Plenum Press.
59. Small, L.: The brief psychotherapies, New York, 1979, Brunner/Mazel, Inc.
60. Strupp, H.H.: Success and failure in time-limited psychiatry, American Journal of Psychiatry **37**:947, 1980.
61. Strupp, H.H.: Toward the refinement of time-limited dynamic psychotherapy. In Budman, S.H., editor: Forms of brief therapy, New York, 1981, The Guilford Press.
62. Thompson, L.: Peplau's theory: an application to short-term individual therapy, Journal of Psychosocial Nursing and Mental Health Services **24**(8):26, 1986.
63. Ursano, R.J., and others: A review of brief individual psychotherapies, American Journal of Psychiatry **1436**(12):1507, 1986.
64. Weissberg, J.H.: The therapeutic relationship in brief focal psychotherapy, Journal of American Academy of Psychoanalysis **14**(2):203, 1986.
65. Wilson, G.T., and O'Leary, K.D.: Principles of behavior therapy, Englewood Cliffs, N.J., 1980, Prentice-Hall, Inc.
66. Winston, A., editor: Clinical and research issues in short-term dynamic psychotherapy, Washington, D.C., 1985, American Psychiatric Press, Inc.
67. Wolberg, L.R.: Short-term psychotherapy, New York, 1976, Grune & Stratton, Inc.

ANNOTATED BIBLIOGRAPHY

Budman, S.H.: Forms of brief therapy, New York, 1981, The Guilford Press.

This book shows how psychodynamic, behavioral, and systems

theory can use the short-term therapy model in the treatment of individuals, families, and groups. It also suggests that short-term therapy in the future will be the norm.

Rush, J.A.: Short-term psychotherapies for depression, New York, 1982, The Guilford Press.

This volume examines behavioral, interpersonal, cognitive and psychodynamic approaches of short-term therapy in treating depression. It offers the practitioner diagnostic tools, an assessment guide for optimal treatment, and specific techniques from these models to use in therapy. Since depression is such a prevalent problem today, this book is essential for short-term therapists.

Winokur, M., Messer, S.B., and Schacht, T.: Contributions to the theory and practice of short-term dynamic psychotherapy, Bulletin of the Menninger Clinic 42:125, 1981.

This article gives a brief review of the important contributions to the field of short-term therapy. It also discusses some of the important principles of brief therapy, such as client selection, effect of time limits, the focal activity, and basic techniques. It is a good overall view of short-term therapy.

Wolberg, L.R.: Handbook of short-term psychotherapy, ed. 2, New York, 1980, Thieme-Stratton, Inc.

This is a detailed discussion of the process and elements of short-term psychodynamic therapy. Particular emphasis is placed on the techniques of treatment.

CHAPTER 28

GROUP THERAPY

Ethel Rosenfeld

After studying this chapter the learner will be able to:

Define group therapy.

Describe the involvement of nursing in group therapy from a historial perspective.

Describe theoretical frameworks for group therapy.

Use the nursing process in group therapy.

Identify types of group therapy available through the life cycle.

Any group—family, school, work, or community—is a collection of individuals who are to some degree interdependent. Groups, then, are naturally appropriate for preventing and treating mental health problems involving interactions with others. Three kinds of groups are discussed in this chapter: group therapy, therapeutic groups, and adjunctive groups. Group therapy focuses on self-awareness, improving interpersonal relationships, and making behavioral changes. Therapeutic groups deal with emotional stress associated with physical illness or developmental crises. An adjunctive group uses special activities to increase socialization, sensory and intellectual stimulation, and orientation to reality. The nurse who is knowledgeable about the different types of groups and group processes increases her effectiveness in working with groups of clients.

GROUP THERAPY

Group therapy is a treatment method in which clients meet at planned times with a qualified therapist to focus on becoming self-aware and self-understanding, improving interpersonal relationships, making behavioral changes, or all three. The group is based on philosophical concepts and theories, with specific content and outcome goals. Positive, creative change is the major purpose. Clients need to want to change some aspect of themselves and be willing to take the necessary steps to change. This may involve recognizing and accepting aspects of themselves

that may benefit from change or learning to make decisions to enhance the quality of their relationships.

Group therapy is generally categorized according to the group objectives. The kind of group reflects the therapist's theoretical framework. This framework also reflects the role the therapist assumes, the terminology used, and the focus of the group.

Groups usually have one or two leaders. The following lists the advantages of both:

ONE LEADER	CO-LEADERS
No clash in leadership style or theory base	Feedback and validation are mutually shared.
	Group strategies are planned together.
Greater autonomy	One leader can assess group as a whole while the other works with one person.
Greater financial gain	Co-leaders relating to each other openly and honestly can be role models.
	When co-leaders are a man and a woman, clients' old feelings about parents may be more readily worked through.
	Dependence on co-leaders is shared.
	If one leader is absent, the other can maintain the group.

Typically, therapy groups are composed of five to ten members. A group of seven or eight members is considered ideal. Therapy groups with fewer than five yields less effective interaction; more than ten means less focus on individuals, diluting group potency and effectiveness. (See Figure 28-1.)

❦ *Historical Overview* ❦

DATE	EVENT
1900s	Joseph Pratt introduced a type of group therapy by his attempts to educate tuberculosis patients, alleviate their feelings of discouragement, and raise their morale. His repressive-inspirational approach used informal discussion, biblical and philosophical readings, and poetry.
	Jacob Morino coined the term *group psychotherapy* and introduced psychodrama as a therapeutic modality.
1940s	The American Group Psychotherapy Association (AGPA) was founded by S.R. Slavson.
	Group therapy flourished during World War II because of the shortage of psychiatrists and psychologists. Treating battle victims in groups was an expedient way of reaching large numbers of clients.
1950s	The effectiveness and economy of treating groups gradually led to the integration of group psychotherapy into the education and practice of nurses, social workers, psychiatrists, and psychologists.
1967	The American Nurses' Association statement on psychiatric nursing practice stated that clinical nursing specialists can function as group therapists when graduate study included theory, supervision, and clinical practice related to group therapy.
1980s	Group therapy is now practiced by many kinds of practitioners, and there are groups for almost everything— to lose weight, to quit smoking, to be a more effective single parent, to cope with divorce or death, to change behavior, to improve management skills, to share common feelings, and so on. Nurses have unlimited opportunities to practice group therapy.
Future	High levels of stress, faulty interpersonal relationships, and rising health care costs will continue to influence the need for nurses to work with groups of clients, scientifically documenting the group's effectiveness and evaluating the outcome of treatment.

The frequency and length of sessions depend on goals and membership. Groups of clients with a short attention span or who withdraw as a way of coping meet two or three times a week for an hour or less; most groups are held weekly. An hour and a half is needed to get beyond the slow starting phase into the working part of the session and to give clients time to deal with specific needs. Some group leaders believe that members use whatever time is alloted—if the time is shorter, participants start to work more quickly. All therapists agree on the importance of beginning and ending on time. If a portion of group work is left uncompleted, it is continued at the next session, or if appropriate, the leader works individually with a member before the next meeting (since the leader is responsible for the emotional safety of the client).

The duration of a group depends on its goals and membership. Groups with a specific task or function may have a set number of meetings, such as once a week for 6 weeks or 6 months. Groups that are intensive and insight oriented may meet for 1 to 3 years. *Marathon groups* meet for several days in a row or an entire weekend.

THEORETICAL APPROACHES
Psychoanalytic

Psychoanalytic groups focus on the analysis and interpretation of transferences, defenses, and resistances. Dreams, slips of the tongue, free associations, and defense mechanisms are seen as clues to unconscious motivation. The overall goal is to reconstruct personality through the development of insight. Through time the therapist focuses on the problems of individual members. Others benefit by recognizing some of these problems as theirs and realizing the need to change patterns of feeling, thinking, and behaving. The group gives support as members grapple with new ideas and choose new life directions.

Transactional Analysis

Transactional analysis (TA) is a unique form of group therapy rooted in psychoanalytic thought. It is a decision model that focuses on learning and doing. It is health oriented rather than illness oriented. Communication among group members is examined, and each member's "script" becomes apparent in all behaviors used during sessions. Each person develops contracts with the therapist to change specific problematic aspects of life. Questions asked by the therapist and other members may include: "How will you make this change? When will you start? How will we know that you have made the change?" When one contract is fulfilled, a new one is made.

Interpersonal

Interpersonal groups emphasize members relating to each other, their perception of the relating, and the im-

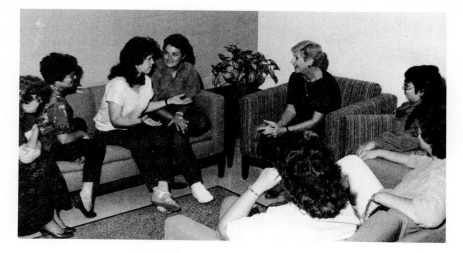

FIGURE 28-1 A group therapy session.

pact of the relating. Anxiety generated by the group experience is a major focus. Sources of anxiety from the client's past and from dynamics in the group are identified. As the anxiety is openly addressed, it becomes less significant. The acceptance of each member as worthy and valuable allows all to develop increased security and self-esteem and strengthens them for the future.

Client- or Group-Centered

The assumption of client- or group-centered groups is that clients have the ability and responsibility to make needed and wanted changes. Each person seeks his true self, and with group support removes his social facade to expose his inner core. Members and therapist are viewed as equals, the therapist being the most experienced member. The therapist relates to the group with genuineness, empathy, and warmth, encouraging all to do the same. Emphasis is on the healthy aspects of the self and on using all of oneself to experience the present reality.

Existential

Clients who lack direction and meaning often find existential groups valuable. They focus on members knowing their inner world, their interpersonal world, and their natural world to bring them together in a meaningful way. Members build emotional strength as they increase awareness by sharing major life events. They are encouraged to be authentic and to involve themselves in living joyously and passionately. Again, the therapist is considered an equal and shares herself openly. The therapist is a role model of authentic relating and deep investment in living.

Gestalt

Gestalt group therapy focuses on becoming a whole person through autonomy, which stems from self-aware-ness. Clients learn techniques and exercises to heighten awareness and assist in recognizing feelings that may be carefully hidden from the self. They are encouraged to fully experience their feelings in the group, thereby resolving incomplete emotional experiences. Gestalt groups seem particularly effective for clients who are depressed or anxious or who have constrained, restricting patterns of living.

General Systems

According to general systems theory (GST), each group member is a system that interacts with other systems to become part of the larger group system. The group develops over time to become relatively stable. Goals for systems groups help members restore or enhance their own autonomy by more effectively opening and closing their boundaries. The therapist monitors and regulates the group and assists with the opening and closing of individual and group boundaries.[29]

Eclectic

Many group therapists combine aspects of more than one theory for an *eclectic approach*. The therapist using this approach is familiar with various theories and blends them purposefully to express her philosophical beliefs and the group purpose. Table 28-1 summarizes groups according to theoretical framework.

Askelepian

Another type of group therapy with a specific theoretical focus is the Askelepian group. The *Askelepian approach* is useful for extremely self-centered, impulsive, and manipulative clients, who do not usually benefit from group therapy as traditionally conducted. In fact, these clients are likely to be destructive elements in the group process. Askelepian (from the Greek *askelapeius,* "place

TABLE 28-1 Organization of groups by theoretical frameworks and theorists

Theory/Theorist	Dynamics	Role of Leader	Focus of Group
PSYCHOANALYTIC			
Sigmund Freud	Personality is determined by biological and environmental forces. Behavior is based on unconscious motivation. Neuroses develop from unmet needs in one's past.	Authority figure; neutral sounding board; active listener; calls attention to group process; challenges defenses; focuses on individuals within the group and also needs of the total group	*General:* Primarily cognitive; insight oriented; expecting reconstruction of personality structure *Specific:* Freeing the libido (positive life energies related to love, energy, and sex) Maintaining a balance among the id, ego, and superego Breaking down defenses against anxiety Dealing with early life and past traumatic experiences and their relationship to current thinking and behavior Transferences and resistances Dream content
TRANSACTIONAL ANALYSIS (TA)			
Eric Berne	Personality is determined by all past experiences. One can be fully in charge of the directions taken in life.	Facilitator; teacher; active or inactive depending on group process; focuses on individuals within the group and also needs of the total group; recognizes and points out ego states in use by group members; assists members to choose more effective modes of behavior; gives permissions and protection to clients in the process of change; relates to group openly and without use of games	*General:* Cognitive, affective, conative, insight oriented; expecting reconstruction of personality structure *Specific:* Ego states used (Parent, Adult, and Child) Transactions used (complementary, crossed, or ulterior) Life script Strokes given and received Games played Congruence in feeling, thinking, and behaving Autonomy Awareness, spontaneity, and intimacy Individual contracts for change Assuming responsibility for self
INTERPERSONAL			
H.S. Sullivan Hildegard Peplau	Behavior is the result of interaction of many forces. Interpersonal security is a basic need. Processes that take place in the interpersonal field are central to understanding human behavior Self-concept is obtained from reflected appraisals from significant people in one's life.	Participant-observer; focuses on group process; catalyst; encourages; strengthens self-esteem of members	*General:* Cognitive, affective; insight oriented; expecting reconstruction of personality structure *Specific:* Interactional patterns of member with family and with group Relationship of past distorted experiences to current problems (transferences) Consensual validation of behavior to correct distortions in growth derived from early anxieties, (parataxic distortion)

TABLE 28-1 Organization of groups by theoretical frameworks and theorists—cont'd

Theory/Theorist	Dynamics	Role of Leader	Focus of Group
CLIENT-CENTERED			
Carl Rogers	Behavior results from self-concept. People are basically good. Wholeness results from becoming fully oneself. Clients have the ability and responsibility to change. Clients and leader are equals.	Nondirective; open; congruent; reflective; "being with" clients with genuineness, empathy, and warmth; focuses on group process and individuals in the group	*General:* Affective *Specific:* Awareness; perceptions of oneself and one's world Here and now Unconditional positive acceptance of oneself and others Self-actualization Responsibility for oneself Empathy, genuineness, and warmth in relating
EXISTENTIAL			
Rollo May Hugh Mullen Josephine Paterson Loretta Zderad	Life is open to choice. Each person is unique and of value. Each person shares commonalities with others. There is mutual growth of self and others through being together and experiencing each other.	Nondirective; guiding; sharing of self; intimate contract with the group as a whole	*General:* Affective; experiencing and relating to others *Specific:* "Being with"; "being here" Themes of death, despair, nothingness, fate, anxiety, guilt, joy, and commitment (the meaning of life) Becoming all that one is capable of being
GESTALT			
Frederick Perls	One needs to live fully in the present. Self-awareness is the avenue to personal autonomy. One can recognize and experience wholeness of self and in one's world.	Active; directs structured exercises; works with one member at a time on the "hot seat"; confronts; supports	*General:* Affective, conative *Specific:* Awareness of feelings and behavior of self and others' responses Completion of unfinished business through fantasies, dreams, experiencing past experiences now, and working through impasses Here and now Authenticity; spontaneity Responsibility for self
GENERAL SYSTEMS			
Ludwig von Bertalanffy	The world is composed of systems, subsystems, and supersystems. Systems function to maintain wholeness, achieve self-regulation, and achieve self-transformation to higher levels of adaptation. Systems achieve the above by opening and closing their boundaries and then exchanging energy and information with their environments. Group members are open systems and the subsystems of the group; in turn, the group is an open, living system. The group is autonomous and capable of changing itself.	Group member; acts in terms of own living structure; a catalyst	*General:* Cognitive and affective *Specific:* Systems of individual personalities composing group Larger system in which group operates; autonomy and determining boundaries Searching for deeper structure Acceptance of uncertainty

of the last resort") groups are held several times weekly. Goals are for members to (1) acknowledge their own behavior, (2) make contracts to change unhealthy behaviors, and (3) put social responsibility above personal wishes and needs. The leader starts by confronting ("indicting") a member about a negative behavior displayed since the last meeting. The other members reinforce the indictment ("rat packing"). The confrontation continues until the member acknowledges the truth of it. The leader then helps the client understand the behavior and to make plans with the client for positive change. If the client is ready, a contract may be drawn up, in which the client agrees to make certain changes, specifying exactly how and when, knowing that the contract will be discussed at the next meeting. This member then proceeds to indict another group member, and the sequence is reenacted. The group continues until all indictments are made and worked through. Leaders are not excluded from indictment. At the end of each session warm, caring verbal and physical responses are shared by group members and leader.

The Askelepian approach seems to work with the hard-to-reach manipulator. The atmosphere is charged with emotion. The leader is a role model of open, honest, confronting, responsible behavior and demonstrates that she is not easily manipulated.

Because these groups are part of a larger therapeutic community (hospitals, halfway houses, and group homes), behavioral change can be assessed daily over a long period by other group members and the leader.

THERAPEUTIC GROUPS

Therapeutic groups deal with emotional stress from physical illness, normal growth and development crises, or social maladjustment.[48] Examples of therapeutic groups are groups for expectant mothers, people who have lost their spouse through divorce or death, the terminally ill, and people with similar health problems. The main purposes are prevention of health problems, as in the groups for expectant and new mothers; education and development of potentials, as in groups for clients with chronic illnesses or disabilities; and enhancement of quality of life, as in groups for the terminally ill. Participants can be inpatients, outpatients, or people in the community. Nurses are commonly leaders of these groups.

Many therapeutic groups are *self-help groups*—groups without leadership by a health professional (although some are led jointly by health professionals and lay people). Almost all self-help groups use the repressive-inspirational approach. They attempt to replace unwanted feelings and behaviors with healthier ones, using group teaching, counseling, and peer support. Some of the major self-help groups are presented in Table 23-2.

ADJUNCTIVE GROUPS

Adjunctive groups deal with selected needs of individuals, such as cognitive stimulation, sensory stimulation, orientation to reality, and socialization. These groups are often adjuncts to group therapy or therapeutic groups (Table 28-3).

Cognitive Stimulation

Bibliotherapy generally is used with chronically ill clients. Articles, books, poems, and newspapers are read to stimulate thinking about events in the real world and to foster relating to one other.

TABLE 28-2 Examples of self-help groups

Type	Purpose or Goal
Alcoholics Anonymous (AA)	To help alcoholics maintain sobriety and to help others abstain from drinking
Al-anon and Alateen	To assist the spouse and children of alcoholics to understand the drinker and to develop healthy lifestyles for themselves despite the problems of the alcoholic
Synanon	To encourage drug-free living by using heavy confrontation in residential centers for drug abusers
Gamblers Anonymous (GA)	To help gamblers stop gambling, using the principles of AA
Neurotics Anonymous (NA)	To assist self-acknowledged neurotics with emotional problems, using the principles of AA
Recovery	To encourage reintegration into community after psychiatric hospitalization, using Low's concepts from "Mental Health through Will-Training"[58]
National Alliance for the Mentally Ill (NAMI)	To help families and friends of the severely or chronically mentally ill understand their illnesses and to give support to each other as care givers and advocates
Parents Anonymous (PA)	To help abusive parents learn healthy parenting and to give support to each other
Parents Without Partners (PWP)	To help single parents improve parenting and to support each other through teaching and social activities
Weight Watchers International	To promote weight loss through peer support while learning and practicing new patterns of eating and more active life-styles

TABLE 28-3 Goals, types, and activities of adjunctive groups

Goal	Type	Activities
To foster cognitive stimulation	Bibliotherapy	Uses articles, books, poems, and newspapers to stimulate thinking and foster relating to others
To foster sensory stimulation	Music, art, and dance groups	Provides outlets for expression of feelings
	Relaxation groups	Focuses on learning relaxation techniques using modalities such as deep breathing, muscle relaxation, and guided imagery
To foster reality orientation and socialization	Remotivation groups	Uses a five-step format to orient withdrawn and regressed clients to reality
	Reality groups	Focuses on *the three, R's*—responsibility, reality, and right and wrong—to help clients meet needs
	Reminiscent groups	Focuses on remembering past experiences, to assign positive meanings to them

Sensory Stimulation

Music therapy involves listening to music, playing in rhythm bands, singing, moving to music for relaxation and enjoyment, and getting in touch with feelings evoked when different kinds of music are heard. *Art therapy* focuses on self-expression and the portrayal of feelings through various forms of art. *Dance therapy* involves the expression of feeling through the rhythmic body movements of dance. All kinds of dance forms are used. Very repressed, rigid clients often "unbend" with this therapy. In *relaxation therapy* clients learn and practice relaxation techniques, such as deep breathing, muscle relaxation, fantasizing about being in a favorite place, fantasizing to music, and guided imagery.

Reality Orientation and Socialization

Reality orientation groups are designed to help regressed or disoriented clients become more aware of present reality (see Chapter 44). *Remotivation groups* are also used for regressed or withdrawn clients to stimulate thinking. Both groups promote social interaction.

CHARACTERISTICS OF THE GROUP THERAPIST
Qualifications

Three areas prepare a person to lead group therapy effectively:

1. Theoretical preparation through lectures, reading, formal courses, and workshops
2. Supervised practice in the role of co-leader and leader
3. Experience as a group therapy member

The American Nurses' Association (ANA) statement on psychiatric nursing practice states that clinical specialists can function as group therapists.[3] Certification by the ANA as a clinical specialist in psychiatric–mental health nursing assures that the nurse is qualified and competent as a group therapist.

The American Group Psychotherapy Association (AGPA) is the principal accrediting organization for group therapists. Membership is open to clinical professionals who have a master's degree level of preparation in the field.

Many nurses lead therapeutic and adjunctive groups. Requirements for these types of groups are specific knowledge of the problems and concerns of the clients, an understanding of the methods used in the specific group, and skill in functioning as leader.

Roles

Task role functions. First the leader identifies the need for a specific group. In an inpatient setting the leader meets with the unit staff members to explain the purposes and plans for the group. The goodwill of unit personnel is important; they can encourage and support the ongoing group or impede its progress if they feel ignored.

The leader also makes room arrangements. The room needs to be quiet, free from distractions, and large enough to hold a comfortably spread circle of chairs, without a table. (A table restricts the ability to see what a member is communicating nonverbally.)

The leader selects group members according to group purpose. She interviews the client to assess needs and behaviors. Clients want to know what they can gain from group involvement and what to expect in the sessions. They need ample time to voice their hopes and fears and to become familiar with the goals of the group.

The leader also decides whether the group will be open or closed. Open groups allow clients to quit when they are ready, while the group itself continues. Open groups are the most common. In closed groups the duration is decided in advance or by consensus of leader and members.

Maintenance role functions. The therapist's maintenance role functions are to continually observe group process, assess levels of anxiety, and establish direction. The therapist is the one person known by all members and therefore can be the mutual supporter of all participants as they begin a new venture together.

In the early stages of group development, many therapists take an active role. They give positive recognition to clients who initiate interactions; they make verbal obser-

TABLE 28-4 Pitfalls and helpful responses for the novice group therapy leader

Pitfalls	Examples	Helpful Responses
A need to structure the group	**Leader:** *(At beginning of each group)* We'll do our usual start of going around the group, telling others who you are and what you feel right now.	Leader quietly waits for group members to begin the session.
Ignoring nonverbal behavior	**Member:** *(Smiles, with eyes tearing)* This week has been so much better for me! **Leader:** That's great! What did you do differently?	**Leader:** Oh? Then what are your tears all about?
A need to give advice from nursing knowledge or personal experiences	**Member:** My foot is hurting today because I have an ingrown toenail. **Leader:** There are several ways you can deal with that. You can lift a corner of the nail and. . .	Leader listens and waits to see how group members move in to respond.
Role reversal: focus of group on leader's needs	**Member:** *(To leader)* You look sad today **Leader:** Well, yes. I heard yesterday that my child is going to need surgery soon.	Leader looks at group members, neither denying nor reinforcing.
Revealing self	**Member:** *(To leader)* Are your married? **Leader:** Yes, for 25 years. I also have three children and four grandchildren who are my pride and joy!	**Leader:** Yes, I am. I wonder what made you think of that right now?
Intellectualizing	**Leader:** Maslow says that. . .	Leader quietly encourages expression of feelings; identifies, where needed, what is occurring; and monitors group process.
A need to be liked by the group members	Leader is primarily reassuring, warm, and protective; encourages, "happy talk."	Leader encourages expression of all kinds of feelings toward leader and other group members.

vations, question, and summarize what has taken place. At times the therapist may purposely remain silent so that members will deal with each other more directly or experience the silences of group interaction. The therapist guides the group but does not control it. Thus the members take responsibility for group actions and reactions and for personal decisions.

New therapists are likely to make some mistakes. Table 28-4 gives examples of common mistakes and helpful leader responses.

CHARACTERISTICS OF GROUP THERAPY
Client Selection

People who profit most from group therapy value and desire personal change, want to know more about their own feelings and to understand others better, and have high expectations for the outcome.[56] Following is a Case Example of someone who benefited from group therapy.

Case Example

Theresa is the only child of a conservative, middle class couple. Her mother taught her from an early age to be personable and outgoing and emphasized the importance of physical attractiveness. Theresa learned her lessons well. She "rarely met a stranger," and she led an active social life in college. Soon after graduation she married a successful businessman. He was very

involved in his work and became more and more disinclined to participate in social and recreational activities with Theresa. She found herself often alone, feeling restless and bored. In time Theresa filed for divorce. Because of her unhappiness with her life, she sought the services of a psychotherapist. After careful assessment of needs, the therapist placed Theresa in group therapy with seven other men and women. In group Theresa appeared outgoing, but her relating was superficial. She was verbal, liked to be the center of attention, and seemed overly concerned with appearances. After a few sessions she was confronted about her behavior. Theresa's response was to cry, sobbing loudly that no one was trying to understand her. The others listened but maintained that her facade was such that she did not allow them to know her as a real person. They pointed out her superficiality and her entertaining or coy remarks that actually served to cover her feelings.

Slowly Theresa began sharing her feelings of loneliness. She asked for help in becoming more a real part of the group. She was encouraged to honestly identify her own feelings in relation to events occurring in the group and to voice them, even when they had a negative connotation. In addition, she agreed to really listen to others responding to her and to accept their concern and caring.

In time, as Theresa continued to participate, she became a role model of open, forthright behavior. She remained in this group for 16 months. She continued to make subtle but increasingly apparent changes in self-esteem and her behavior was more appropriate and deeper when relating to the others.

Theresa's regular mode of relating to others was openly confronted. The group let her know she was a worthwhile individual who did not need to hide behind a facade and encouraged her to try new ways of relating that proved to be more effective. In the process she became a vital group member.

Not everyone is a candidate for group therapy. For example, those who are not "psychologically minded"—who are strongly disinclined or resistant to therapy—do not benefit. Also excluded are psychotic individuals whose autistic thinking, bizarre communication, and short attention span disrupt the group process. Following are reasons used by some people who do not wish to become group members:

1. They are too uncomfortable in groups and may not tolerate the atmosphere.
2. They become irritated with members who have special problems.
3. They are unwilling to share the leader with other group members.
4. They want more time for personal work and do not think they benefit from listening to others.

These people may profit from individual sessions with a therapist or from such sessions concurrent with group therapy. The following Case Example is an example of a person who was not ready for group therapy.

Case Example

Randy was a shy, aloof 20-year-old whose mother brought him to a therapist for help in becoming more comfortable with others. Usually Randy avoided other people whenever possible. In college he was a loner, typically returning to his room immediately after each class. The therapist decided to place Randy in group therapy with six other people who were accepting and welcomed him as a group member. Randy was extremely uncomfortable. He would tremble and shake and would move his chair outside the group circle. When gently confronted about this, he would become agitated. He would then leave the room to pace in the hall until called back in. Because of Randy's increasing anxiety, the therapist decided to remove him from group and see him in individual sessions weekly. The therapist was quiet, warm, and supportive. Gradually Randy responded and talked about his anxieties and feelings of low self-esteem. After 3 months he asked to become a part of the group therapy sessions again.

Randy was not able to respond to the give and take of group process, although the other members were warm and responsive. His anxiety increased until he physically removed himself from the others. However, he was willing to relate to the therapist alone, and in time he acknowledged his anxious feelings and low self-esteem. Moreover, he took the initiative to return to the group, which indicated development of inner strength and readiness for increased risk taking.

The factors of group therapy most commonly identified as beneficial by clients in research studies are (1) encouragement to ventilate feelings (catharsis), (2) close identity with the group, (3) the giving of feedback to other group members, (4) receiving of feedback from other group members, and (5) self-understanding. (See the Research Highlight on p. 532.)

Group membership can be *heterogeneous* (a variety of ages, backgrounds, behaviors, and needs) or *homogeneous* (similar backgrounds, needs, and so on). An advantage of a heterogeneous group is the stimulation created by variety. Values, beliefs, and ways of doing things differ, causing the client to look at options. The anxiety generated can be a catalyst for constructive action, with resultant emotional and behavioral change. However, extreme differences in basic values and behaviors of group members can cause schisms in a group. Also, a balance of behaviors is needed. For example, one or two very depressed individuals may do well in a typical group; they can benefit from the caring and gentle prodding of the others to get reinvolved in living. But several depressed individuals in one group can slow down the process. Such feelings can be contagious. Other members may refuse to identify with the group. A number of hyperactive clients can totally disrupt a group, stimulating each other to a point at which the group goals cannot be met. One hyperactive person in a group may do well.

Homogeneous groups can become cohesive more quickly because of shared feelings and needs. However, most clinicians believe these groups tend to remain more superficial and are ineffective in altering character structure when this is the intent of the group.[70]

Stages of Group Development

Regardless of theoretical framework, all types of group therapy have an orientation phase, a working phase, and a termination phase (Table 28-5). Each of these will be discussed, with emphasis on group behaviors and the tasks of each phase.

In the *orientation phase,* contracts are established. Contracts are the rules, rights, and responsibilities of members and group leaders. They may be written or verbal and need to be understood and accepted by all. Following are examples of contractual components:

1. Awareness of duration, frequency, and length of sessions
2. Commitment to the group, demonstrated by regular attendance, punctuality, and active participation
3. Regular payment of fees or arrangements made for payment
4. Group rules
   a. Confidentiality (Anything occurring in the group is to be kept there; members do not gossip about each other or even divulge each other's names.)
   b. Encouragement of verbal expression of all kinds of feelings
   c. Prohibition of physical violence or use of drugs during sessions
   d. Only one person speaking at a time
   e. Dealing with anxieties engendered by the group process instead of backing away
   f. Taking responsibility for change in themselves.

Contracts may also specificly state expectations of both therapist and members. Clients state what they want to change about themselves, and the therapist states how she can help the client reach these goals. Goals inevitably

Research Highlight

Patients' Perceptions of Curative Factors in Short-Term Group Psychotherapy

R.J. Marcovitz & J.E. Smith

PURPOSE

This study was designed to evaluate the mechanisms of change as perceived by clients in inpatient group psychotherapy. Hypotheses were (1) inpatients' perceptions of curative factors differ from those of outpatients in previous studies who ranked interpersonal input, catharsis, group cohesiveness, and self-understanding of highest value on Yalom's Curative Factor Q-Sort and (2) clients who perceived group therapy as helpful differ in their curative factor rankings from those who did not perceive it as helpful.

SAMPLE

The sample was nine male and 21 female, high-functioning patients in the short-term psychiatric unit of a large teaching hospital. Ages ranged from 24 to 61 years. Almost one third of the sample had previous group experience. Diagnoses were mixed, slightly more than half having a primary affective disorder.

METHODOLOGY

Therapy was based on a psychodynamic model. Participants met four times weekly for 1 hour. Each client was given the Beck Depressive Inventory, the Zung Self-Rating Anxiety Scale within 48 hours of admission and 3 days of discharge, and Yalom's Curative Factor Q-Sort before discharge. Participants were also asked if they had found group therapy helpful.

FINDINGS

The first hypothesis was unsubstantiated. Yalom's Curative Factor Q-Sort revealed high rankings similar to those of Yalom's earlier outpatient rankings—catharsis, group cohesiveness, interpersonal output, self-understanding, and interpersonal input. Altruism was ranked third only in this sample. Eighty-six percent found the group therapy helpful; 10% were undecided; and 4% found it unhelpful. The second hypothesis was discarded because of the small number finding this therapy unhelpful. The Beck and Zung scales measuring depression and anxiety on admission and discharge indicated significant improvement.

IMPLICATIONS

Limitations in this study were the clinical setting's inability to provide random selection of the population; the small size of the sample; and the fact that group members were also receiving other therapies. However, objective measures of symptom improvement lend credence to the client reports of therapeutic benefit from group involvement. Study results also indicate that clients in short-term groups need to help each other by questioning, showing concern, and giving feedback and suggestions. Client perceptions revealed that taking responsibility for their own behaviors and situations was helpful. The study stresses the importance of an early accepting attitude and respect of individual differences by group members. Guidance and instillation of hope have not been validated as critical aspects of short-term groups and require further study.

Based on data from International Journal of Group Psychotherapy **33**:21, 1983.

change as the group progresses, needs are met, and new needs emerge.

Information is given and received, and *group norms* (acceptable group behaviors) are established during the orientation phase. Some members may test other members to determine how much trusting can take place. For example, a member may share some negative personal information, such as having had a child out of wedlock or having abused drugs in the past. Some may test group rules by coming irregularly or late and seeing if they are reprimanded or rejected. Also in this phase conversation may lapse into awkward silences, with frequent stops and starts. The message to the group leader is unspoken but strong: "take over and keep the ball rolling."

The task for group members in this stage is to achieve a sense of identification or belonging to the group. The leader is the catalyst or unifier by spelling out the rules, refusing to control the group, pointing out the process taking place, and encouraging verbalization of all kinds of feelings. The leader's clear message to the group is that this is their group and her strengths, needs, or leadership style do not hold it together. Rather, each member is responsible for all that occurs.

Anxiety is the prominent feeling in this first stage. The newness of the situation is threatening, but the group is a safe place to examine anxiety and what fosters it and to learn to deal with anxiety constructively. The leader is wise to let the group take care of its own anxieties, unless they are excessive. When the group falls silent or otherwise feels tension, each member chooses what response to use to deal with the anxiety. The leader assesses what is occurring and may comment on the group process. She encourages members to be aware of their defenses and to face the threatening situation directly, without their defenses. At these times members are most open to making positive changes in themselves.

Trust cannot develop until group members begin to know each other. Testing takes place until individuals feel

TABLE 28-5 Group phases, leader and member tasks, and group behaviors

Phase	Leader Tasks	Member Tasks	Group Behaviors

Orientation	Serve as catalyst:
	  Encourage verbalization of feelings
	  Summarize process of group
	  Refuse to control group
	  Clarify work and goals of group
		Identify with group
		Develop trust with group
		  Deal with anxiety
		  Verbalize thoughts and feelings
			Relate superficially
			Test group rules
			Test each other
			Stay silent
			Intellectualize
			Depend on leader
			Compete for leader's attention

Working	Serve as role model:
	  Listen intently
	  Respond honestly
	  Support members' exposure of feelings
	  Confront negative behaviors
	  Clarify work and goals of group
		Maintain trust:
		  Expose innermost feelings
		Develop interdependence with group members
		Develop responsibility for own behaviors
			Relate intensely
			Attempt to avoid problem areas
			Manipulative behaviors
			Listen actively
			Confront each other
			Express all kinds of feelings
			Try out new behaviors
			Support positive changes in each other

Termination	Serve as resource person Process group efforts Share perceptions about what is occurring	Offer mutual support Say good-bye	Indicate goals have been met Say good-bye

safe expressing their feelings and needs. If this sense of safety does not develop, the group will not progress to the next stage.

During the *working phase* the group develops some cohesiveness. All kinds of feelings and concerns, positive and negative, are openly addressed. The leader focuses on what is occurring in the group as members confront each other. For example, behaviors that invite others to take care of a member's needs instead of doing this for himself are confronted. (The member becomes tearful when told of any behavior that needs changing, thus suggesting that he is too fragile to be challenged.) Risk taking occurs as group members attempt new behaviors. For example, one client really hears what is said about him. Another, a loner, may reach out to others. Another, who has never dared voice negative feelings, tells someone he is angry about something said or done. Conflict and development of subgroups also need to be confronted and resolved.

Tasks for members at this stage are to maintain trust, develop a sense of reliance on group members and then on oneself, and become responsible for group directions.

The therapist's tasks are to model behaviors, (such as listening intently), respond honestly, and support members as they expose their inner selves. The therapist keeps in mind that controlling activity is not therapeutic. Instead, she comments on the group process. She confronts unhealthy behaviors, such as monopolizing, putting oneself down, misinterpreting, assuming, and ignoring. The therapist does not give advice and insights from personal experience, even though sometimes it seems so obviously excellent. She also continually clarifies the work and goals of the group.

Termination can occur in three ways. In the closed group termination is planned by the group in advance and carried out on schedule. The second kind of termination is by the member who is unsuccessful in meeting his needs (in either a closed or open group). This person usually leaves abruptly without warning or eases out after a brief sojourn. Following are some reasons for premature termination:

EXTERNAL FACTORS	INTERNAL FACTORS
Moving away from the region	Does not feel accepted as a group member
Financial stressors	Has not revealed needs to group
Acute physical disability or illness	Lacks trust or respect for leader or other group members
Obligations that conflict with sessions	Feels overly pressured to participate actively
	Feels too much self-disclosure has occurred

The third kind of termination occurs in the open group when a member has achieved his goals. At first the individual tentatively signals that his goals have been accomplished. He may make statements about feeling good and having made changes. The leader may note that he is less active and more reflective. Others give feedback, stating how they view this member's progress. Sometimes concerns are voiced (such as he still seems depressed), and the member may remain longer to do more individual work.

In many groups members are asked to remain for two or three sessions after making the decision to terminate to deal with the departure adequately. Ambivalent feelings, both sadness and happiness, in anticipation of the future are discussed. Other members also have mixed feel-

TABLE 28-6 Role behaviors

Type of Role	Effect on Group	Examples
Group task roles	Related to completing tasks or goals for which the group convened (group content)	Initiater, coordinator, evaluator, elaborator
Group building or maintenance roles	Related to building group cohesion and maintaining the group itself	Encourager, harmonizer, compromiser
Personal or individual roles	Related to needs of individual group members that do not assist the group task, building and maintenence roles	Aggressor, recognition seeker, dominator, blocker

ings about the termination. They may feel sad, envious, or angry. Usually, everyone has a sense of loss.

In this final stage of the group the therapist is more of a resource person than an active leader. Group members are able to take care of their own needs and to give support to each other. Individual decision making is encouraged; however, the therapist continues to share her perceptions about what is occurring.

Regardless of the reasons for membership, the desired outcome is that the individual has a realistic self-perception, feels good about himself and others; and is ready to be responsible for himself in all areas of living.

Group Dynamics

Group dynamics involves all that takes place in a group from inception to termination, including group content and group process. *Group content* is the specific problems and tasks addressed, or the work of the group. *Group process* is the continuous interaction among members. Both process and content are equally important and occur simultaneously. The novice leader may recognize and work with content and ignore the process, even when it is disruptive. For example, the leader may be so intent on what one member is saying, she will not notice two other members whispering to each other. The constant nonverbal behaviors of group members are valuable clues to what is occurring inside each individual. As members become part of a group, they begin to reveal their usual patterns of behaving and relating. The leader and the other members scrutinize behaviors to identify possible areas for change.

Process refers to the many factors that help or hinder growth of group members. Among the important factors are *role behaviors,* behaviors used repeatedly by members. Role behaviors are divided into three major categories, outlined in Table 28-6.

Bales[5] used these groupings to categorize behaviors that affect process (Figure 28-2). Section *A* lists behaviors mostly conducive to implementing group process. Sections *B* and *C* are behaviors related to group task roles. Section *D* is behaviors that meet individual needs that may also hinder group process.

The Bales categorization is useful in identifying processes in groups. While one co-leader leads the group, the other can act as recorder, using this scale to identify roles taken by the different members. The recorder checks the number of times each of the listed behaviors is used by each of the members. Obviously this scale does not reveal the content of the communication nor does it show the intensity of each behavior.

A method of identifying who talks to whom in a group is drawing diagrams, or *sociograms,* of the group in time sequence immediately after the session ends. For each group there is a series of diagrams, which are accompanied by written capsules of the content of the interactions.

Figure 28-3 illustrates the process during the first 15 minutes of a therapy session. During this time the leader confronts John about his coming 20 minutes late to group 2 weeks in a row. John is apologetic, explaining that he had to drop off mail at the post office on the way and traffic was heavy. Alice sympathizes with John, saying that parking problems also can make it hard to be on time. The leader tells Alice that she is not helping John look at his behavior. Alice breaks into tears, stating that she likes John and was feeling sorry for him. Jean tells John that she feels annoyed with his lateness and excuse making.

Another useful tool for learning how group members interact is the Johari window (see Chapter 6). With it the nurse can become aware of how much of the self is made available to others. She can also identify levels of risk taking as members ask for and give feedback.

Audiotapes of group sessions also help the leader assess group interaction. Voice volume, tone qualities, rapidity and pitch of speech, pauses, and word emphasis give clues to underlying emotions. Of even greater value is videotaping, which gives the extra dimension of direct observation of participants and their nonverbal communication.

Any form of taping needs to be explained to members first, and their written permission is obtained. The leader reassures members that only she and possibly other professionals learning about group therapy will review the tapes and that confidentiality will not be broken. Sometimes tapes are used in the sessions to review or clarify important incidents. Also, individual members may review tapes to gain insight into their group involvements.

Decision making is both a group task and part of group process. Various means are used to make decisions, depending on type of leadership, degree of risk taking, sen-

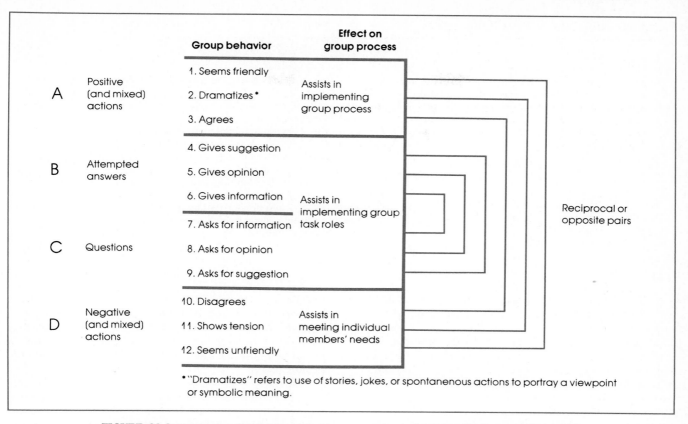

FIGURE 28-2 Categories for interaction process analysis. (Adapted from Personality and interpersonal behavior by Robert Freed Bales. Copyright © 1970 by Holt, Rinehart and Winston, Inc. Reprinted by permission of Holt, Rinehart and Winston.)

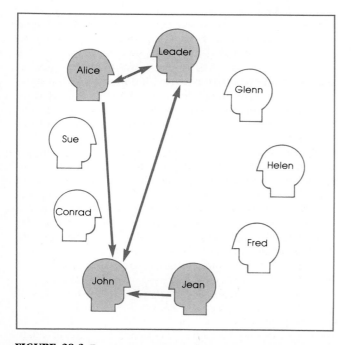

FIGURE 28-3 Process occurring during first 15 minutes of group therapy.

sitivity of the group to needs and wants of individuals and amount of trust. Table 28-7 identifies some helpful and unhelpful methods of decision making.

NURSING PROCESS
Assessment

Physical dimension. When group members have physical problems, such as disfigurement, obesity, or loss of a limb, the relationship to total body image is important to recognize and is appropriate for group focus. For example, the leader may notice that a young woman who is scarred or obese silently compares herself with someone who is good-looking or slender. This client may lash out at the other member or avoid focus on herself. She may attempt to compensate by being overly helpful to other group members (being ingratiating in manner, smiling habitually, and saying and doing what she feels the others want) to avoid negative confrontation.

The nurse needs to assess degrees of openness in acknowledging physical deficits or disabilities by individual members. Also, the nurse assesses how members interact with individuals who put themselves down or use ingratiating behavior because of unresolved feelings about real or perceived physical problems.

TABLE 28-7 Group decision-making procedures

Positive Process	Negative Process
Majority decision: More than half of the group come to agreement, but some disagree or compromise.	*A "plop":* A suggestion is given and it falls flat, usually causing the giver to withdraw.
Consensus (ideal): All group members come to agreement, with concern for both task achievement and persons involved; input is encouraged from all participants.	*Self-authorization:* One member makes a decision and expects it to be carried out regardless of group feelings.
	Hand clasping: Two group members support each other in decision making.
	Minority decision: A decision is made by less than half of the group by vocal and aggressive behaviors.
	Rotten democracy: A decision has already been made by the leader, but the decision-making procedure is carried out anyway.
	"Group think"[36]: Group pressure is imposed on members to be totally united in decision making regardless of individual concerns. Diversity of thought is discouraged.

Emotional dimension. All the emotions felt by group members become part of the group process. Individuals in a group bring their fears, hopes, sadness, anger, and joy with them. These and their multiple attendant feelings create a unique mix in any group. The nurse assesses emotions experienced and expressed by members and the response of the others. The nurse also assesses feeling tones of the whole group. Sometimes a sense of sadness, lethargy, anger, or tension prevails. All are valuable messages about the process.

During group therapy anxiety is exhibited in a variety of behaviors. A member may be late, absent, or simply quiet. Anxiety may be triggered by many things, especially confrontation from other group members.

Anger is a component of group process. Some members are afraid of it, having been taught as children that anger is wrong. The therapist notes which members repress anger to the point where they cannot recognize it. She also notes which members attempt to be peacemakers or avoid angry participants. When anger is escalating, the nurse determines the degree that can be safely handled in the group, then decides how to deal with it constructively.

The nurse assesses feelings of guilt in the group. She observes which members have themes of wrongdoing, making mistakes, neglecting to do things expected of them, or doing something displeasing to others.

Sometimes group members are despondent. They may withdraw, have poor personal grooming and hygiene, feel helpless and hopeless, or say that life is meaningless. Such behaviors frequently dampen the spirits of the entire group. The nurse notes the group's energy level. If she becomes aware of despondence in herself during group process, and it is not from personal concerns, she assesses where it is coming from in the group.

Intellectual dimension. To benefit from group therapy and contribute to the work of the group, individuals need the ability to verbalize well enough to be understood by the others. They also need the ability to think abstractly to deal with ideas and feelings addressed.

Usually the acutely ill are not functional group members. A disoriented person is unable to receive accurate messages from others. An extremely egocentric person may attempt to monopolize the discussion. Membership is postponed until the client is able to both benefit and contribute.

The nurse is aware of how group members communicate with each other. Do they listen, interrupt, belittle, monopolize, use humor? What is the content of messages given? Are some unclear and confusing? Are there repetitive themes? Are there distortions in thinking, such as viewing the therapist as an all-knowing, completely wise and good mother? Perhaps a member views the therapist or another group member as a person from his past, a parent, sibling, or spouse. If so, feelings of resentment, affection, or competition may emerge. These phenomena are important because they indicate unresolved conflicts.

Change in thinking may be gradual and subtle in expression. The group therapist looks for clues such as the client's more active participation in the group; asking for feedback from others; less rigid thinking, indicated by more receptiveness to reasons for behaviors of self and others; giving direct and honest responses instead of devious ones; and improvement in problem solving.

Social dimension. The leader needs to be aware of individual behaviors and their effect on the group as a whole. For example, who are chronic helpers, busying themselves with arranging the furniture or preparing coffee? Who are touchers, and who avoid touch? In each session the leader notes where people sit. Do they sit in the same location each time (territorality)? Are they usually next to specific people? Are they near to or distant from the therapist? Do some attempt to sit apart from the group?

People in newly formed groups are reluctant to reveal sensitive aspects of themselves, because trust has not yet been established. The therapist oberves carefully who interacts with whom and how. As members learn to relate effectively to each other, they can learn to relate to an extended number of people outside of group.

The nurse notes when individuals in the group are taking risks by exposing hidden parts of themselves and assesses if others respond by being accepting and supportive.

The nurse considers all interactions among members. A monopolizer unchecked keeps others from having time to express their needs. A withdrawn member may feel cheated if not recognized and encouraged to participate. Some may attempt to draw attention away from troubling issues because of their own anxieties. Others may act seductively, condenscendingly, or dependently. All of these indicate the members responses outside the group.

Some members actively address needs and concerns of others but are unwilling to share personal thoughts and feelings. In some cultures, however, people do not readily reveal personal feelings or publicly display affection or other feelings. For example, black members in the presence of a white therapist may hide their feelings because of lack of trust. They may be ingratiating and attempt to second-guess the therapist.[32] Latinos and Greeks often favor somatic complaints over emotional symptoms and are often reluctant to participate in "talking therapy."[60] Native American clients may be close to family members in private and diffident to people in public.[49] Mexican and Greek women may be very passive in a group, especially with men, and may perceive the therapist as having magical abilities.[22,67] Minority members in group therapy may also be much less expressive of feelings and thoughts when their native language is not used, even when they are fluent in the second language[60,65] (see Chapter 10). These are generalizations and do not apply in all cases.

Spiritual dimension. The group therapist needs to continually assess possible conflicts in values and beliefs that may interfere with group functioning. How, for example, does the group respond to differences in political, sexual, or religious stances? Does the group accept members who are economically, educationally, or socially different? Do such members feel rejected?

At times in the life of a group, important questions such as "Who and what am I?" "Where am I going?" and "How will I get there?" are addressed. Many persons have adopted values and beliefs from parents and others without much thought. The therapist notes if the group encourages the examination of these values, especially when the seeker's conclusions differ greatly from others' in the group. Is there trust, inclusion, and group cohesiveness despite member differences? What is the clients sense of self-worth?

Analysis

Nursing diagnosis. The behavior of individual members and the total membership is analyzed, and group nursing diagnoses are formulated.

Some examples of nursing diagnoses of group functioning follow:

1. Lack of cohesiveness related to inability of members to compromise
2. Increased anxiety related to perceived unsafe environment
3. Impaired group functioning related to need of member to monopolize
4. Inability to achieve group goals related to hostile members
5. Inability to trust related to lack of confidence in leader
6. Increased group anxiety related to confronting behaviors

Planning

As in other therapeutic methods, plans are made in group therapy to help promote the individual client's well-being. Table 28-8 provides some long-term and short-term goals and outcome critieria related to group therapy. These serve as examples of the planning stage in the nursing process.

Each member is encouraged to set goals for himself and discuss how the group can help him achieve those goals. Group goals depend on the type of group and needs of individual members.

Implementation

Physical dimension. The nurse arranges to use a quiet room, away from traffic flow so that she and group members can hear each other. Neutral or subdued room colors for most adolescent and adult groups is best. Bright colors are preferred for groups of regressed or older clients, who respond best to bright posters or other wall decorations and warm-colored furnishings. A floor-length mirror is useful in many groups for checking grooming and physical appearance. Simple and comfortable furnishings are provided, with chairs placed in a circle. When there are co-leaders, they may sit opposite each other for better observation of all clients. Restrooms are always available.

Clients who are disfigured or disabled are encouraged to talk about themselves when comfortable enough. They may need a chance to share their feelings, if present, and are given time to grieve for what is missing or lost. They also may want to find out if they are perceived as lovable despite deficits.

A major task for all group members is to learn how to take better care of themselves physically and emotionally. This includes a healthy life-style, with a balance of work, rest, and play. Each group member plans how to attain this healthy balance and is expected to enact it. The group gives support as changes are made. The nurse recognizes the improved appearance, increase in energy, and zest for living that accompanies feeling good.

Emotional dimension. In group therapy the universality of negative feelings, such as anxiety, anger, guilt, and despair, is recognized. Expressing negative feelings can be healing. The chance to express these feelings with emotional support from others can allow emotional growth.

People need to face distressing emotional aspects of themselves instead of repressing or circumventing them. For example, group members are encouraged to experience their anxiety—to recall it in detail, relive it, and then, with help from the others, deal with it. Ways of coping with anxiety include risk taking in the group, revealing

TABLE 28-8 Long-term and short-term goals and outcome criteria related to group therapy

Goals	Outcome Criteria
NURSING DIAGNOSIS: SELF-CONCEPT DISTURBANCE: LOW SELF-ESTEEM RELATED TO UNWILLINGNESS TO COMPETE IN SCHOOL WITH SISTER WHO IS "BRILLIANT"	
Long-term goals	
To make vocational plans that mesh with own needs, abilities, and desires.	Joins in group discussions that focus on future vocations and careers.
To feel good about self and sister.	Smiles when complimented.
	Shows self-confidence in speech and body language.
	Tells group that sister and self are two different people, "not better or worse, just different."
Short-term goals	
To participate in group to increase comfort and effectiveness in relating with others.	Is attentive to activities taking place in the group.
	Takes time to reflect before responding to the others.
	Asks for clarification when uncertain about something that is said or done.
	Shares own feelings about what is occurring.
	Listens to responses from others.
	Paraphrases what has been said.
To exchange positive messages with others in group.	Looks directly at the person giving the positive message.
	Thanks the other person and does not attempt to modify what has been said.
	Tells two other persons what is liked about them.
	Describes three things liked about self.

feelings about group interactions, and asking for what is needed and wanted.

The angry group member is encouraged to verbally express the anger when it occurs and to direct it (verbally) to the person with whom he is angry. Members are also encouraged to hear angry messages from others when receiving feedback about behaviors or activities. These responses are useful in developing insight and constructively changing hurtful aspects of the self.

The client who suffers from guilt is encouraged to carefully assess the situations that trigger the feeling. If realistic amends need to be made, he is encouraged to make them. If relationships have been left hanging or activities are uncompleted, the nurse encourages the client with group support to find ways to bring about healthy resolutions. When no known situation causes the guilt, the person is encouraged to look at his past. Past messages may foster the need to feel guilty.

Depressed group members need caring from the others. These members are invited to contact both the therapist and others in the group between sessions if they need support (particularly if self-destruction is a possibility). They are strongly encouraged to attend group meetings even when disinclined and to take an active part. Assignments may be given for life outside of the group—tasks involving physical activity or doing a favor for someone else. Members report the results at the following session.

Depressed people typically focus on what they perceive as negative aspects of themselves and seek criticism from others. The nurse encourages them to accept nurturing from others (compliments and positive messages) as valid. Sometimes when the individual has been deprived of touch or when he feels withdrawn or out of contact with others, hugging or holding is especially healing.

Two messages are central to nearly all forms of group therapy. The first is that all people have a mix of all kinds of feelings, both positive and negative. All feelings are valuable parts of each person; no attempt to eliminate them is made. Group members learn to be in charge of these feelings, instead of being ruled by them. Each is encouraged to use feelings appropriate to the situation to become a more authentic and congruent individual.

The second message is to learn how to recognize and value the goodness in oneself. The nurse may use exercises such as telling the others what one likes about oneself and hearing positive messages from others. Fun and play are important in the development of positive feelings, and members are encouraged to find many things to enjoy. As people learn to feel good about themselves, they will feel good about others.

Group therapy emphasizes that each person accept responsibility for emotions that are experienced. In the following example the therapist attempts to help group members become aware of this:

Therapist: No one can make you feel sad or glad or anxious or angry. You do this for yourself. These are your ways of experiencing and responding to what is happening in your life, inside and outside of yourself.

In all groups an important goal is to learn to feel good about oneself and to express negative feelings constructively.

✳ *Intellectual dimension.* When negative or rigid thinking is encountered during sessions, the therapist encourages clients to acknowledge their mind-set, to look at all sides of issues, and to select new patterns of behavior that will enhance interaction with others and give greater enjoyment (see Chapter 15).

Clients with difficulty distinguishing fantasy from reality may benefit from group awareness exercises. These exercises focus on present reality and assessing the outer environment and one's own physical and emotional responses. Following is an example of an awareness exercise in which an individual alternates between focusing on outer environment and inner feelings:

Group member: I see (in the room) John smiling at me and leaning forward in his chair. . . I feel scared, being the center of this attention. I hear people laughing a little. . . My heart is pounding, and my face feels flushed. . . I see the yellow flowers on the table. . .

This exercise continues until the client is better oriented to self, others, and environment and is relaxed.

Many group members may perceive the therapist as able to read their thoughts and solve their problems if only she were willing. Some even think she has magical abilities to perform miracles in their lives. These beliefs need to be confronted. The nurse verbalizes these perceptions of her omniscience and invites the group to share them with her. Simple denial of owning special powers may also be helpful and may need to be stated many times.

✳ *Social dimension.* One important goal of group therapy is to create a climate in which a client is truly free to address any concern. This cannot occur unless trust has been established; the therapist needs to provide an environment of trust and respect. The group rule on confidentially keeps intimate knowledge about members in the group, thus creating a safe place in which to share such knowledge and work on behavioral changes.

When a member relates to the therapist or another member as someone else from his life experience, transference is taking place. The nurse identifies this phenomenon and deals with the unresolved basic feelings. Sometimes the therapist relates to a group member as someone from personal life experience (countertransference); she needs to recognize this so that her responses in the group are valid for that member.

The therapist confronts avoidance behaviors, and support is given by all for self-disclosure. The therapist can discourage avoidance and encourage disclosure by refusing to be authoritative in leading the group, modeling self-confidence and assertiveness, and supporting group members who reveal inner parts of themselves.

Closeness is fostered in the group when members are allowed to know one another. This means being open and honest with each other. Members are vulnerable when they relate without their protective facade; the therapist

gives support and positive recognition. This encourages other members to risk sharing more of themselves.

Willingness to expose oneself fosters not only a healthier integration of self but also the ability to be intimate with chosen individuals. True intimacy is a common need of group members; in the group, then, people practice intimacy by choosing moments when they disclose the most sensitive parts of their lives. They learn that intimacy leaves one vulnerable to being loved or rejected, is therefore risky, and yet gives intensity and meaning to life.

✳ *Spiritual dimension.* Group members support the sorting of values and beliefs by the following: (1) Recognizing individual uniqueness as well as shared commonalities, (2) Learning more about themselves through experiencing and interacting with other members, and (3) Maintaining and enlarging personal identities while appreciating and accepting differences in others.

As group members share their experiences, the tragedies and pathos inevitable in life may bring tears, while the recognition of shared foolishness and awareness of the world may evoke laughter. Sometimes members experience deep joy as feelings of love are shared, along with the message that no one is alone if he is willing to reach out to others. Individuals also learn that they are vulnerable to life's stressors, yet can be fully in charge of their responses as they are guided by their chosen values.

Evaluation

Subjectively, if group members feel good about themselves and others and have met their personal goals for group involvement, group therapy can be viewed as effective. Objectively, the nurse can evaluate clients who have recently completed their group therapy, noting the degree and nature of the change, the group experiences effecting that change, and the contributions of other factors in the client's life. Indicators of a positive group experience are shown in Table 28-9.

TABLE 28-9 Indicators of a positive group experience

Dimension	Indicator
Physical	Feeling good about one's body image; demonstrating respect for one's physical well-being by improving life-style (eating habits, exercise, rest, work, and recreation)
Emotional	Accepting caring messages from others; being in charge of one's feelings and accepting all kinds of feelings as part of self; feeling good about self and others
Intellectual	Asking for feedback about behaviors; being reality oriented; having expanded awareness of self, others, and environment
Social	Being willing to risk trusting others; sharing self and reaching out to others
Spiritual	Having a sense of being a valued part of the human race

TABLE 28-10 Group therapy through the life cycle

Type	Purpose
CHILDREN	
Activity group therapy	For troubled children ages 7 to 12 to participate in creative and manual activities to increase self-esteem and gain acceptance from others
Activity-interview group psychotherapy	For discussing feelings generated by group interaction
Play group therapy	For disturbed children to increase play experiences and master drives and conflicts through verbal and nonverbal expression of feelings
ADOLESCENTS	
Peer groups	For increasing self-esteem and independence, affirming self-identity, and learning to relate to others
ADULTS	
Growth groups	For establishing interpersonal relationships and intimacy
Groups with a specific focus	For growing emotionally, understanding self, and making behavioral changes
ELDERLY ADULTS	
Remotivation groups	For withdrawn, regressed persons for sensory and intellectual stimulation
Reminiscence groups	For remembering past experiences
Expressive groups	For promoting expression of feelings

GROUP THERAPY THROUGH THE LIFE CYCLE

Table 28-10 outlines specific group therapies available for different age groups (see also Part 5).

BRIEF REVIEW

Theoretical frameworks help determine the approach used in group therapy. Therapists choose theoretical frameworks in accordance with their personal belief systems and the goals of the group.

Groups are classified as (1) group therapy, (2) therapeutic groups, and (3) adjunctive groups. All groups progress in three phases. In the orientation phase anxiety is the dominant feeling and needs to be channeled so that trust can develop and members can identify with the group. The working phase is a time when the major work of the group occurs. Termination takes place when (1) the group reaches its scheduled end, (2) member leaves the group without warning or planning, or (3) member's goals have been reached.

Group dynamics involve all that takes place in a group from inception to termination. Group process and group content are the two equally important components of group dynamics.

Therapy is viewed as effective if group members feel good about themselves and others, have obtained their personal goals, and the achievement is validated by the group.

REFERENCES AND SUGGESTED READINGS

1. Adrian, S.: A systematic approach to selecting group participants, Journal of Psychiatric Nursing and Mental Health Services **18**(2):37, 1980.
2. American Nurses' Association, Division on Psychiatric—Mental Health Nursing: Statement on psychiatric nursing practice, Kansas City, 1967, American Nurses' Association.
3. American Nurses' Association, Division on Psychiatric—Mental Health Nursing: Statement on psychiatric and mental health nursing practice, Kansas City, 1976, American Nurses' Association.
4. August, L., and others: Women's groups: a non-traditional method of mental health treatment, Canadian Nurse **81**:26, 1985.
5. Bales, R.: Personality and interpersonal behavior, New York, 1970, Holt, Rinehart & Winston.
6. Battegay, R.: The value of analytic self-experience groups in the training of psychotherapists, International Journal of Group Psychotherapy **33**:199, 1983.
7. Bellak, L.: On some limitations of dyadic psychotherapy and the role of group modalities, International Journal of Group Psychotherapy **30**:7, 1980.
8. Betcher, W.: The treatment of depression in brief inpatient group psychotherapy, International Journal of Group Psychotherapy **33**:365, 1983.
9. Birckhead, L.: The nurse as leader: group psychotherapy with psychotic patients, Journal of Psychosocial Nursing **22**:24, 1984.
10. Brabender, V., and others: A study of curative factors in short-term group psychotherapy, Hospital and Community Psychiatry **34**:643, 1983.
11. Brende, J.: Combined individual and group therapy for Vietnam veterans, International Journal of Group Psychotherapy **31**:367, 1981.
12. Bumagin, S., and Smith, J.: Beyond support: group psychotherapy with low-income mothers, International Journal of Group Psychotherapy **35**:279, 1985.
13. Butler, R.N., and Lewis, M.I.: Aging and mental health: positive psychosocial and biomedical approaches, ed. 3, St. Louis, 1982, The C.V. Mosby Co.
14. Chutis, L.: Self-help mutual aid groups and community mental health centers: effective partners, New York, 1980, National Self-Help Clearinghouse Center for Advanced Study in Education, The Graduate School and University Center of New York University.
15. Cohen, E., and Rietema, K.: Utilizing marathon therapy in a drug and alcohol rehabilitation program, International Journal of Group Psychotherapy **31**:117, 1981.
16. Collison, C.: Grappling with group resistance, Journal of Psychosocial Nursing **31**:117, 1981.
17. Corder, B., and others: A study of curative factors in group psychotherapy with adolescents, International Journal of Group Psychotherapy **31**:345, 1981.

18. Delgado, M.: Hispanics and psychotherapeutic groups, International Journal of Group Psychotherapy **33**:507, 1983.

19. Dies, R.: Current practice in the training of group psychotherapists, International Journal of Group Psychotherapy **30**:169, 1980.

20. Dube, B., Mitchell, D., and Bergman, L.: Uses of the self-run group in a child guidance setting, International Journal of Group Psychotherapy **30**:461, 1980.

21. Dugo, J., and Beck, A.: A therapist's guide to issues of intimacy and hostility viewed as group level phenomena, International Journal of Group Psychotherapy **34**:25, 1984.

22. Dunkas, N., and Nikelly, A.: Group psychotherapy with Greek immigrants, International Journal of Group Psychotherapy **25**:402, 1975.

23. Durald, M., and Hanks, D.: The evaluation of co-leading a gestalt group, Journal of Psychiatric Nursing and Mental Health Services **18**(12):19, 1980.

24. Durkin, J., editor: Living groups: group psychotherapy and general systems theory, New York, 1981, Brunner/Mazel, Inc.

25. Echternacht, M.: Day treatment transition groups: helping out-patients stay out, Journal of Psychosocial Nursing **22**:11, 1984.

26. Ernst, C., Vanderzyl, S., and Salinger, R.: Preparation of psychiatric inpatients for group therapy, Journal of Psychiatric Nursing and Mental Health Services **19**(7):28, 1981.

27. Fulkerson, C., Hawkings, D., and Alden, A.: Psychotherapy groups of insufficient size, International Journal of Group Psychotherapy **31**:73, 1981.

28. Gartner, A., and Riessman, F.: HELP: a working guide to self-help groups, New York, 1980, Franklin Watts, Inc.

28a. Goldberg, D., and others: Focal group psychotherapy: a dynamic approach, International Journal of Group Psychotherapy **33**:413, 1983.

29. Grojahn, M., Handbook of group therapy, New York, 1983, Van Nostrand Reinhold Co.

30. Hannah, S.: Countertransference in inpatient group psychotherapy for women with a history of incest, International Journal of Group Psychotherapy **34**:257, 1984.

31. Hardy-Fanta, C., and Montana, P.: The Hispanic female adolescent: a group therapy model, International Journal of Group Psychotherapy **32**:351, 1982.

32. Heckel, R.: Relationship problems: the white therapist treating blacks in the south, International Journal of Group Psychotherapy **25**:421, 1975.

33. Herman, J., and Schatzow, E.: Time-limited group therapy for women with a history of incest, International Journal of Group Psychotherapy **34**:605, 1984.

34. Hopper, E.: Group analysis: the problem of content, International Journal of Group Psychotherapy **34**:173, 1984.

35. Hyland, J., and others: The impact of the death of a group member in a group of breast cancer patients, International Journal of Group Psychotherapy **34**:617, 1984.

36. Janis, I.: Group think, Psychology Today **5**:71, 1971.

37. Janosik, E., and Phipps, L.: Life-cycle group work in nursing, Monterey, Calif., 1982, Wadsworth, Inc.

37a. Kahn, E.M.: The choice of therapist self-disclosure in psychotherapy groups: contextual considerations, Archives of Psychiatric Nursing **1**(1):62, 1987.

38. Kaplan, H., and Sadock, B., editors: Comprehensive group psychotherapy, Baltimore, 1982, Williams & Wilkins.

39. Kaplan, R.: The dynamics of injury in encounter groups: power, splitting, and the mismanagement of resistance, International Journal of Group Psychotherapy **32**:163, 1982.

39a. Kapul, R., Ramage, V., and Walker, K.: Group psychotherapy in an acute inpatient setting, Psychiatry: Interpersonal and Biological Approaches **49**(4):337, 1986.

40. King, K.: Reminiscing psychotherapy with aging people, Journal of Psychosocial Nursing and Mental Health Services **20**(2):21, 1982.

41. Klein, R., and Kugel, B.: Inpatient group psychotherapy from a systems perspective: reflections through a glass darkly, International Journal of Group Psychotherapy **31**:311, 1981.

42. Lesser, I., and Friedman, C.: Beyond medication: group therapy for the chronic psychiatric patient, International Journal of Group Psychotherapy **30**:187, 1980.

43. Lesser, I., and Godofsky, I.: Group treatment for chronic patients: educational and supervisory aspects, International Journal of Group Psychotherapy **33**:535, 1983.

44. Leszcz, M., and others: A men's group: psychotherapy of elderly men, International Journal of Group Psychotherapy **35**:177, 1985.

45. Levine, B., and Poston, M.: A modified group treatment for elderly narcissistic patients, International Journal of Group Psychotherapy **30**:153, 1980.

46. Levine, H.: Milieu biopsy: the place of the therapy group on the inpatient ward, International Journal of Group Psychotherapy **30**:77, 1980.

46a. Levitt, D., and others: Group support in the treatment of PMS, Journal of Psychosocial Nursing and Mental Health Services **24**(12):13, 1986.

47. Lieberman, M., and Bliwise, N.: Comparisons among peer and professionally directed groups for the elderly: implications for the development of self-help groups, International Journal of Group Psychotherapy **35**:155, 1985.

48. Marram, G.: The Group approach in nursing practice, ed. 2, St. Louis, 1978, The C.V. Mosby Co.

49. McDonald, T.: Group psychotherapy with native American women, International Journal of Group Psychotherapy **25**:410, 1975.

50. Middleman, R., editor: Activities and action in groupwork, New York, 1983, Haworth Press.

51. Milne, D., and others: The value of feedback: evaluative research in routine community psychiatric nursing, Nursing Times **81**:34, 1985.

52. Moss, N.: Child therapy groups in the real world, Journal of Psychosocial Nursing **22**:43, 1984.

53. Newton, G.: Self-help groups, Journal of Psychosocial Nursing, **22**:27, 1984.

54. Ormont, L.: The leader's role in dealing with aggression in groups, International Journal of Group Psychotherapy **34**:553, 1984.

55. Palmer, J.: A primer of eclectic psychotherapy, Monterey, Calif., 1980, Brooks/Cole Publishing Co.

56. Perls, F.: The gestalt approach and eye witness to therapy, Palo Alto, Calif., 1974, Science & Behavior Books, Inc.

57. Pines, M.: The frame of reference of group psychotherapy, International Journal of Group Psychotherapy **31**:275, 1981.

58. Ringler, K., and others: Technical advances in leading a cancer patient group, International Journal of Group Psychotherapy **31**:329, 1981.

59. Rogers, C.: Carl Rogers on encounter groups, New York, 1970, Harper & Row, Publishers.

60. Ruiz, P.: Group therapy with minority group patients, International Journal of Group Psychotherapy **25**:389, 1975.

61. Schiffer, M.: S.R. Slavson (1890-1981), International Journal of Group Psychotherapy **33**:131, 1983.

62. Stone, W., and Scott-Rutan, J.: Duration of treatment in group psychotherapy, International Journal of Group Psychotherapy **34**:93, 1984.

63. Sullivan, H.S.: The interpersonal theory of psychiatry, New York, 1953, W.W. Norton & Co., Inc.

63a. Tischler, N., and others: Work and defensive processes in small groups: effects of leader gender and authority position, Psychiatry: Interpersonal and Biological Approaches **49**(3):241, 1986.

64. Tozman, S., Hanks, T., and Minkowitz, H.B.: The rap group: a milieu treatment model for the chronically mentally ill in an outpatient setting, International Journal of Group Psychotherapy **31**:233, 1981.

65. Tylim, I.: Group psychotherapy with Hispanic patients: the psychodynamics of idealization, International Journal of Group Psychotherapy **32**:339, 1982.

66. Weiner, M.: Techniques of group psychotherapy, Washington, D.C., 1984, American Psychiatric Press.

67. Werben, J., and Hynes, K.: Transference and culture in a Latino therapy group, International Journal of Group Psychotherapy **25**:396, 1975.

68. White, E., and Kahn, E.: Use and modifications in group psychotherapy with chronic schizophrenic outpatients, Journal of Psychosocial Nursing and Mental Health Services **20**(2):14, 1982.

69. Wolberg, L., and Aronson, H.: Group and family therapy, New York, 1981, Brunner/Mazel, Inc.

70. Yalom, I.: The theory and practice of group psychotherapy, ed. 2, New York, 1975, Basic Books, Inc., Publishers.

ANNOTATED BIBLIOGRAPHY

Loomis, M.: Group process for nurses, St. Louis, 1979, The C.V. Mosby Co.

This is an overview of the group process field using the nursing process as framework. It is nicely organized and readily understandable. Of special interest is the final chapter, which focuses on research questions on group process.

Van Servellen, G. (Marram): Group and family therapy: a model for psychotherapeutic nursing practice, St. Louis, 1984, The C.V. Mosby Co.

Perhaps the best text yet written on group therapy practiced by nurses, intended for the advanced nursing student. Variables of communication, process, and structure are viewed as core components in analysis and intervention with families and groups. A transactional theory is the context for the principles and concepts presented. It is well organized, with a broad yet in-depth focus and excellent references.

Wilson, M.: Group therapy/process for nursing practice, Bowie, Md., 1985, Brady Communications Co.

A perspective on groups is presented by a nurse who is both a clinician and an instructor. Several theoretical frameworks are outlined, and specific issues and themes in groups are identified. Supplemental learning activities are included.

Yalom, I.: Inpatient group psychotherapy, New York, 1983, Basic Books, Inc.

A much needed focus on modifications from traditional group therapy for work with this population is presented. In the inpatient setting autonomy is often lacking when the administrative staff takes on many of the task functions of the therapist. Also, group therapy is but one of several modalities used for client treatment. By necessity it will be of short duration. Yalom suggests in this setting that therapists be active, always supportive, and use a variety of techniques that facilitate the construction of a safe, trusting environment. One should have a here-and-now focus; and high and low functioning clients should be in separate groups. This is a readable and valuable book for all nurses in institutional settings who are providing group experiences for their clients.

CHAPTER 29

FAMILY THERAPY

Ann H. Shealy

After studying this chapter the learner will be able to:

Identify historical events related to family therapy.

Discuss selected theoretical frameworks of family therapy.

Describe characteristic of a family therapist.

Discuss characteristics of family therapy.

Apply the nursing process to clients who are seen for family therapy.

The family can be defined as the traditional two parents with children, a single parent family, or a blended family that results from the marriage of two people who are divorced from previous unions. The family constitutes people who are linked together by blood, affection, loyalty, and time and see their lives as interconnected.

The family is the main force that socializes human beings. Through a prolonged dependency period, children are taught the values, ideals, and political beliefs of their parents. It is often only when children begin school that they become aware of how other families differ from theirs.

Family therapy is that branch of psychiatry that sees an individual's psychiatric symptoms as inseparably related to the family in which he lives. Different theories of family therapy that are based on the theory's origin are used as a framework for defining and intervening in the family problem. Most theorists today perceive the identified client's problems as a symptom of trouble within the family group.

THEORETICAL APPROACHES
Psychoanalytic

Psychoanalyst and child psychiatrist Nathan Ackerman pioneered psychoanalytic family therapy. In 1958, although Ackerman stated that the therapeutic approach to the family was primary and that psychotherapy of individual family members was secondary, he still conceptualized

the client's problems very much from an individual, intrapsychic viewpoint. After an initial psychosocial evaluation of the whole family was undertaken and social support and guidance employed, Ackerman thought the therapy should then be oriented "to the specific dynamic relations of personality and family role and to the balance between intrapsychic conflict and (interpersonal) family conflict."[1] When other family members were brought into therapy, the perceptual distortions caused by the problems of transference and irrational projections between family members were the focus of treatment. Change was thought to occur through a corrective relationship with the therapist, not through a change among the family members.

Basic to the psychoanalytic framework for dealing with dysfunctional families is the belief that illness results from a conflict between the client's need to be connected to the family and the client's desire to separate from them to establish an individual self-identity. *Pseudomutuality,*[38] the total enmeshment of the members of the family through agreement, prevents individual growth or self-identity. *Pseudohostility,* through the defense of quarreling and hostility, denies the need for family connections and closeness. Both defenses deny and distort the need to be close to the family and the need to separate from it.

Psychoanalytic theory as it applies to families was a step away from the therapist's focusing only on the individual client. The pioneers in family therapy conceptualized the problems in individual psychoanalytic terms, but

Historical Overview

DATE	EVENT
World War II	War led to increased concern over treatment of the family as a whole.
1954	Bowen, one of the pioneers in family therapy, began hospitalizing and observing the schizophrenic child and the entire family.
1957	Midelfort's work, *The Family in Psychotherapy,* emphasized the importance of the family's involvement in the therapy of a psychotic member.
1958	Ackerman contributed an important milestone in the development of family therapy with publication of *The Psychodynamics of Family Life.*
1959	Family therapy was becoming nationally known. Jackson formed the Mental Health Research Institute, which served as an arena for research on family problems.
Early 1960s	Minuchin began a research project to study the families of delinquent boys.
1961	Many books and journals on family therapy were published; among these was *Family Process,* founded by Ackerman and Jackson.
1965	Ackerman founded the Family Institute (later renamed the Ackerman Family Institute).
1966	Ackerman's publication, *Treating the Troubled Family,* made the greatest contribution to family therapy as treatment of the whole family to date.
	Committee on the Family of the Group for the Advancement of Psychiatry (known as of 1970 as the Group for the Advancement of Psychiatry) distributed a questionnaire and learned that many theorists were interested in family therapy.
Late 1960s to Early 1970s	Family therapy included as an aspect of the curriculum for master's specialization in mental health–psychiatric nursing.
1979	Beginning of a bridge between child therapy and family therapy.
1970s-1980s	Mental health–psychiatric nurses publishing articles and books on family therapy The family is one of the clients for whom the mental health–psychiatric nurse provides treatment.
Future	Nurses will direct increased attention to intervention in the family system to prevent emotional disorders and mental illness.

they were willing to begin to consider that individual family members did affect each other.

Systems

Two additional theoretical frameworks conceptualize the family as interrelated parts of a system. A change in one member of the family system has an effect on the whole family. For example, if each family member is seen as a member of a delicately balanced mobile, the slightest movement in one member can set off movement in a close member as well as distant but connected family member a generation away. The repercussions of an ill family member and the family's reciprocal response to the illness are demonstrated in the Research Highlight on p. 545.

Structural family therapy. Minuchin[35] was the first theorist to write about structural family therapy. Theorists using a structural family theory model believe that the family with a problem is a system that is in dysfunction and that the problem is sustained by the underlying structure of the family. Family interactions that occur in the presence of the therapist demonstrate to the therapist the dysfunctional structures that have caused the problem. The three most important concepts that Minuchin[35] was concerned with are boundaries, alignments, and power.

The *boundaries* of a subsystem are the rules that say who is in and who is out of the system. Frequently the siblings are defined as one subsystem and the parents as another. Subsystems may also be composed of the older children and the younger, or the girls and the boys. Boundaries are further described by whether they are rigid or diffuse. Rigid boundaries lead to a distance and *disengagement* that promote emotional isolation and hamper communication. Boundaries described as diffuse offer warmth and support from the family, but the ensuing

Research Highlight

Parental Attitude and Adjustment to Childhood Epilepsy

J. Austin, A. McBride & H. Davis

PURPOSE

This study was designed to investigate the relationship between parents' attitudes about epilepsy and how it affected their children's adjustment. Childhood epilepsy is characterized by more emotional disturbances than most chronic childhood illnesses. Negative parental attitudes about a child's epilepsy elicit parenting behaviors that hinder the emotional adjustment of the child.

SAMPLE

The sample consisted of 50 parents whose children were treated for epilepsy on an outpatient basis at a large children's hospital by two private neurologists. The children had a diagnosis of epilepsy, had no other medical problems, were not retarded, and ranged in age from 6 to 14 years.

METHODOLOGY

Parental attitudes were measured using the Fishbein Expectancy-Value Model of Attitudes. An instrument to measure parental adjustment to epilepsy in a child was constructed by the authors. The relationships among attitude, adjustment, length of time since onset of epilepsy, level of seizure control, and the perception of seizure control were studied with a variety of statistical analyses.

FINDINGS

The majority of the parents had both positive and negative attitudes about their child's epilepsy. Interestingly, parents of female children with epilepsy had more negative attitudes. For the mothers in the sample there was a strong positive relationship between parental attitude and the child's adjustment to epilepsy, indicating that the poorer the parental attitude about epilepsy, the poorer the children's adjustment.

IMPLICATIONS

The major impact of epilepsy is on the child's self-concept. Since parental behavior toward the child is the predominant factor in the formation of the child's self-concept, the parents' attitudes toward epilepsy in their child strongly influence both their parenting behaviors and the emotional adjustment of the child.

Based on data from Nursing Research **33**:2, 1984.

---

enmeshment does not allow for individuation and autonomy.

Alignment is a concept that has to do with who takes sides with whom; boundary lines on a family map (Figure 29-1) can make this idea clearer. For instance, in the family map depicted, a very diffuse boundary exists between Susan, Mother, and Grandmother, which indicates that Grandmother and Mother are both attempting to parent Susan, instead of each generation adhering to its age-appropriate roles. Cindy is clearly in conflict with Mother, and Grandmother is not interfering with her. Sam is shown on the family map as having a clear boundary between the female family members and himself. The family map affords the structural family therapist a shorthand method of organizing the membership, boundaries, and alignments of a family.

The goals of structural family therapy are to solve problems by changing the underlying structure that supports them. The therapist accomplishes this by interventions aimed at creating or observing the family's pattern of dysfunctional interactions, joining the family's ecosystem, and then purposefully directing the family members to change their dysfunctional interaction. Structural family therapists are not concerned with the family's having an understanding of the problem. The focus is on the problem as it exists in the present and in finding and changing the underlying family structure that supports the problem's existence.

The structural family therapist intervenes actively to modify the family structure. "Joining" the family is a vital part of all interventions that the structural family therapist employs. Whether the therapist joins by taking sides with a weak parent to provide support in the discipline of a youngster, or directs the child from the sidelines to interact directly with the father without going through the mother, the therapist is in the middle of the family.

After she observes the problematic interactions and "joins" the family, the therapist's next task is to restructure the problematic interventions in such a way that the dysfunctional structure is replaced by a more functional one. There are three broad categories of techniques the structural family therapist uses to modify the problematic interactions: *system recomposition, symptom focusing,* and *structural modification.*[3] A newlywed couple with an overly involved mother-in-law cannot begin the task of making an emotional connection to each other with the mother-in-law between them. System recomposition, by intentionally extracting the mother-in-law from between the couple, would give all of them more opportunities to interact within their designated roles.

Symptom focusing is probably one of the better known techniques of the structural family therapist. Emphasizing the symptom by prescribing that the client increase it is one way the therapist can take control of the symptom. For example, the client who acts depressed and withdrawn is told to become more depressed and withdrawn

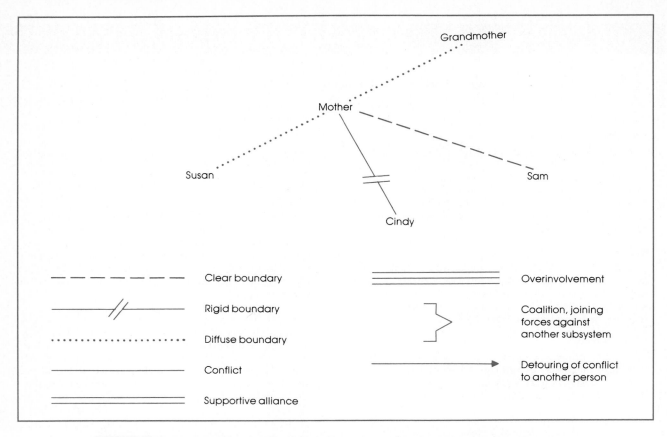

Clear boundary — — — — — — —

Rigid boundary ——//——

Diffuse boundary ·············

Conflict ——————

Supportive alliance ══════

Overinvolvement ═══

Coalition, joining forces against another subsystem

Detouring of conflict to another person

FIGURE 29-1 Mapping. (From Minuchin, S.: Families and family therapy, Cambridge, Mass., 1974, Harvard University Press.)

and to increase the amount of time being miserable by setting aside numerous, specific times each day to dwell on and magnify his condition. The client is willing to follow the therapist's prescription to get better and the family is less upset than before when the client was acting miserable, because now the therapist has prescribed it. The client finds that having to be depressed and withdrawn more of the time is tiresome, which encourages him to seek out alternative ways to get attention from the family.

Structural modification is the third way in which the therapist actively intervenes in the family's interactions. The therapist may observe an overly close alliance between mother and son, conflict between father and son, and a problematic marriage. The therapist may use structural modification in the session by separating the son from his mother's side and sending him to sit with his siblings, and then telling the father to move and sit beside his wife. This is a way of modifying the structure during a therapy session so that appropriate generational boundaries are overtly expressed in the seating arrangements.

When the structural family therapist intentionally "joins" the family she simultaneously maintains enough objectivity to effect change. The therapist gives directions to the family and continuously rediagnoses the interventions, based on the family's response. Although most often

the therapist works with the nuclear family, some structural family therapists may include members of the community if they believe those persons are relevant to the problem.

Bowen theory. The therapist operating from a Bowen theoretical framework conceptualizes the family members as part of a system whose whole is greater than the sum of its parts, as connected to each other, so that a change in one family member affects them all. There are eight concepts in Bowen's conceptualization of how a family operates.[7] This theory postulates that these concepts apply to all families, functional or dysfunctional, and that it is only the intensity of the process that separates the levels of functioning.

The first concept, *differentiation of self,* is the cornerstone of Bowen theory. This concept roughly corresponds with emotional maturity. Differentiation involves the degree to which someone's thinking and feeling are separated from each other, and Bowen saw differentiation as connected to the degree of unresolved emotional attachment to one's family of origin. He developed a scale of differentiation from 0 at the lower end to 100 on the upper end (see Figure 29-2). In reality, no one is totally emotionally mature (differentiated) or immature (undifferentiated), but the scale affords an estimate of the family's functioning over time. Persons on the lower end of

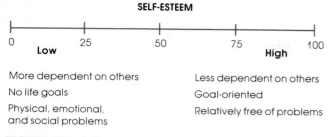

SELF-ESTEEM

More dependent on others   Less dependent on others
No life goals   Goal-oriented
Physical, emotional,   Relatively free of problems
and social problems

FIGURE 29-2 Differentiation-of-self scale.

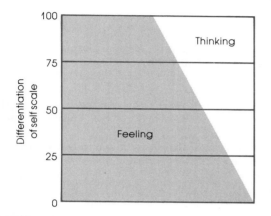

FIGURE 29-3 Conception of balance between thinking and emotional systems as it relates to differentiation-of-self scale. (Concept created by Anne H. Shealy.)

the scale are so ruled by their emotions that decisions are made on the spur of the moment instead of on the basis of thought-out plans and goals. These persons are theoretically the ones with the greatest frequency of psychiatric, social, and physical problems.

The individuals on the upper end of this differentiation-of-self scale base their decisions more on thoughts than on feelings. They are more independent in functioning and have fewer emotional, physical or social problems. People in the midrange have enough basic differentiation for the thinking and feeling systems to function side by side, but when the anxiety gets high, the emotionally based automatic circuits will most likely dominate decision making. Figure 29-3 shows a conception of how the balance between thinking and feeling fits with the differentiation-of-self scale.

Another part of the differentiation of self-concept relates to the levels of *pseudo-self* and *solid-self*. The pseudo-self is that part of a person that can be persuaded to change its beliefs, shifts with the emotional tide of the moment, and is available to fuse with another pseudo-self. Solid-self, by comparison, includes those parts of self that are not negotiable and that are thought-out beliefs and convictions that are not shifted, even under pressure from others. Solid-self, pseudo-self, and levels of differentiation are difficult to estimate except over time, because acute,

intense anxiety can make someone who is relatively high on the differentiation-of-self scale appear dysfunctional, and periods of calm can cause a relatively dysfunctional person to appear to be at a higher level of functioning than is actually true overall.

The *triangle* is a second concept of Bowen theory. It is "the smallest stable relationship system" and is the basic building block of any emotional system.[6] A triangle represents two people avoiding an issue by pulling in an outside person or issue. When two people spend time together and are close, one of them may begin to be uncomfortable with the closeness and may "triangle in" another subject or another person. The triangle discourages a personal relationship between the two because the conflict or fears of overcloseness are not dealt with directly: a third person or issue becomes the focus.

In a period of calm between two persons when they are feeling close, the uncomfortable third person is the one left out. When conflict develops between the two, the comfortable person is the one on the outside of the conflict.

The term *nuclear family emotional system* describes how a single generation of a family deals with their level of differentiation. Two persons enter a marriage with two individual levels of differentiation from their families of origin. If the individual levels of differentiation of the two spouses are low, the level of differentiation in the new union will also be low. There are four mechanisms used by the couple and by all families to deal with the anxiety caused by the fear of fusing into the other person and losing one's self completely. A universal way of dealing with the anxiety of fusion is by emotional distancing. Taking this anxiety from between the spouses and projecting it onto a child is a second way. Two other ways of dealing with the anxiety of fusion include the spouses handling this anxiety through intense conflict or one spouse's compromising his or her functioning to preserve the peace. The more fusion that is present, the more likely that the spouses are willing to do what the other one wants and allow the other to make all the decisions. As this pattern repeats itself and becomes fixed, one spouse assumes the dominant role, and the other the adaptive role. These fixed positions in the marriage taken by the undifferentiated spouses are determined by each spouse's position in his or her own family of origin.

Most families use all four ways of dealing with the anxiety aroused by the fear of fusion, but the less differentiated the spouses are to begin with, the more fusion there is. It is when one of the mechanisms is consistently used to the exclusion of others that problems arise. Psychiatric or physical symptoms are seen in those families that consistently use only one of the mechanisms.

When spouses deal with the anxiety caused by their fear of fusing by projecting that anxiety onto a child, it is called the *family projection process,* which results in serious emotional impairment in the child. There is no way to predict which child will receive the focus of this parental intensity, but it is related to the level of differentiation each spouse brought to the marriage and to the circumstances surrounding this child's conception and birth. For instance, a youngster born on a beloved grandfather's birthday may become the child who is the focus of parental intensity, or a child with physical handicaps may be the main object of parental interest and grow up less differentiated than the siblings.

When the family projection process goes through successive generations, it is called the *multigenerational transmission process*. In any nuclear family there may be one special child who is the focus of parental anxiety and grows up more emotionally immature (less differentiated) than the rest. With parental anxiety invested in the child to avoid dealing with the issues between the parents, this child gets overprotected and has limited opportunities to function independently. That child grows up and marries a person with a similar level of differentiation, and the multigenerational transmission process continues into the next generation.

Sibling position is a concept in Bowen theory that is related to the behavioral characteristics of ten sibling positions. After years of research with functional families, Toman[44] was able to describe sibling profiles and the characteristics common to each one. Bowen found Toman's work useful in his theory as a way of hypothesizing the presence of the multigenerational transmission process by observing whether an individual differed significantly from his expected sibling profile. For instance, if the oldest male in the family behaved in a manner more typical of a youngest sibling, and the parents had little marital conflict and neither parent was physically or emotionally ill, then this oldest male's deviation from his expected sibling profile would be hypothesized to be the result of the family projection process that focused the majority of the parental anxiety on this atypical oldest.

Emotional cut-off is a concept in the Bowen theory that deals with how adult children separate themselves from their parents to start an independent life. In an emotional cut-off, the pain of separation is handled by either physically establishing distance or emotionally cutting the parents off and denying any meaningful connection. This emotional cut-off mechanism learned in one's family is then used in other times of painful separations, as in divorce.

The last of Bowen's concepts is called *societal regression*. Bowen theory hypothesizes that intense anxiety prompts reactive, emotionally based decisions. As anxiety in society escalates in response to such stressors as the limited food supply and threat of a nuclear holocaust, more and more of society's decisions will be emotionally based and will lead to societal regression. Bowen believed that the family experiences societal regression when it is subjected to chronic anxiety. In response to the anxiety and in an effort to allay the anxiety, the family's decisions become more and more emotionally instead of intellectually determined. The emotional approach to decision making results in symptoms of societal regression in the family and eventually regression to a lower level of family functioning and emotional illness.

The primary goal of family therapy, from a Bowen theory framework, is differentiation from one's family of origin, which is accomplished through reopening family ties and efforts aimed at detriangulation. The family system, not an individual person, is the focus of treatment. Because the triangles in any family are interlocking, it is believed that modification in this primary triangle of the marital couple and the therapist will prompt changes throughout the system. This modification is accomplished by the therapist's becoming the neutral third leg in that triangle so that the spouses can begin detriangulation and differentiation. The therapist avoids being emotionally triangulated with the couple and thereby forces the couple to deal with each other and clarify the issues between them. The therapist asks questions that promote thinking instead of feeling. The therapist continually endeavors to remain neutral and objective and to avoid getting embroiled in the fighting and blaming that increases emotionality.

To enable each spouse to begin to define a more differentiated self, the therapist takes "I" stands—that is, statements about what the therapist is and is not willing to do. The more the therapist is able to state beliefs and convictions, the easier it is for the couple to begin doing so in regard to each other. This process takes place in small steps and has setbacks as each spouse responds to his partner's efforts at differentiation by attempting to reinstate the old behaviors. If these efforts are met with calm resolve, both partners can move toward a higher level of differentiation.

Throughout the therapy, when anxiety is lower, the therapist is teaching the couple how emotional systems operate. Beginning to understand the principles of triangles and differentiation and having a coach who offers information about how to explore a personal relationship with members of one's family of origin give the couple tools for use outside the therapist's office. When tension begins again, these concepts enable them to continue work on their families between each session and after family therapy has been discontinued.

The therapist who uses Bowen's framework maintains an objective distance from the family while simultaneously maintaining emotional contact. This therapist intentionally does not side with one family member against another but maintains neutrality. Instead of becoming involved emotionally in the family, the therapist is on the sidelines as a coach and as a teacher of how emotional systems operate. She intentionally avoids becoming as important to the family members as they are to each other.

It is difficult for the therapist to maintain this stance of neutral objectivity or to coach the members toward differentiation steps within their own families of origin without ongoing work by the therapist in the therapist's family of origin. Unless she gains direct knowledge of the struggles and pleasures involved in efforts at differentiation in her own family, the therapist cannot be useful to the client family. Besides work in the therapist's own family, a second requirement for the role of a therapist using Bowen's theory is ongoing supervision. Without an occasional outside opinion when problems arise in working with client families, the therapist is at risk of getting triangled into the family as a result of unresolved issues from the therapist's own family.

Humanistic

Communication. Virginia Satir conceptualized treating dysfunctional families from a group therapy framework. She intentionally focused on communication among family members as the area in the family that needs the therapist's attention. The goal of therapy is to improve communication, making it clear, accurate, and meaningful to the family.[20]

The therapist who supports a communication framework accepts several principles.[38] First is the assumption that there is no way not to communicate, because communication occurs on a behavioral and emotional level even when someone is silent. Second is the assumption that communication is an exchange of information in a family that becomes repetitive and predictable and is governed by unspoken family rules about what is to be discussed and by whom. Because the family is seldom aware of their unspoken rules of communication, the therapist observes the behavior that supports the rule and verbalizes it for the family to consider. For example, if Susan asks Mother for money for a new dress, Mother may tell her that Father says the money is not available. The rules may be that Mother protects the children from Father. The therapist may comment on this rule, allowing family members the option of dealing with each other more directly.

Another aspect of Satir's communication theory of dealing with troubled families examines how a person's style of nonverbal communication fits with his self-esteem. She stated that the postures of the placater, the blamer, and the computer show how he feels about himself. For example, the placater is always trying to please someone else, and his posture looks as if he were begging for the merest crumb of acknowledgment or recognition.[40] The placater's words are full of agreement and his goal seems to be to constantly please his audience, because he sees his own opinion as worthless.

On the other end of the scale is the blamer. The blamer's stance complements that of the placater. The blamer is always criticizing everyone and has a tight facial expression and pointing finger to go with this blaming stance. The blamer acts superior but inside is actually feeling scared, lonely, and probably unsuccessful.

The computer appears ultrareasonable and as if everything is under control. His posture is reserved, cool, and collected, and he reveals no emotion through facial expression. He uses big words in a drawn-out monotone, attempting to impress others with his vocabulary and intelligence. The person who maintains a computer stance is like someone with a steel rod down his back, who cannot move his head, and who must talk slowly to keep from making a mistake.

From a Satir communication theory point of view, the therapist has several goals: (1) Helping the family make implicit rules explicit, (2) helping each family member become aware of his posture and how it communicates messages to others on a nonverbal level, and (3) helping family members begin to see that other members are not malicious or full of ill intentions but that their communications are not clear.[20] To accomplish these goals, the therapist "does not enter the family system, but acts as a corrective feedback mechanism to disturb the present dysfunctional communication"[19] and as a role model of clearer, more congruent communication.

Table 29-1 presents a summary of the theoritical approaches.

TABLE 29-1 Summary of theoretical approaches

Theory	Theorist	Goal	Role	Focus of Treatment
Psychoanalytic	Ackerman	Corrective relationship with the therapist	Neutral; nondirective; makes interpretations of individual and family behavior	Specific dynamics of the individual's personality and role in the family; the perceptual distortion between family members
Humanistic Communication	Satir	Assists family to make explicit rules, to become aware of their nonverbal communication, and to recognize that ill feelings in the family are due to unclear communication	Intervenes in dysfunctional communication by acting as a corrective feedback mechanism (to role model clear and congruent communication)	Communication among family members
Systems Structural	Minuchin	To change the underlying structure of the family organization that maintains dysfunctional family interaction	Actively joins family; directs and realigns family interaction	Family boundaries, alignment, power, and coalitions
Bowenian	Bowen	Self-differentiation of each member from family of origin	Neutral; coaches and teaches the family how to become differentiated and detriangulated	The entire family system over several generations; may work with one partner for a period of time

CHARACTERISTICS OF THE FAMILY THERAPIST
Qualifications

Currently no universally accepted training is required to become a family therapist, but all therapists have preparation at least at the graduate level in the mental health field, with family theory classes and clinical supervision of practice. Although there are psychiatrists who do family therapy, most often they have been primarily exposed to a medical model of psychiatric illness that supports dealing with the family in a limited way. Psychologists, psychiatric social workers, and mental health–psychiatric nurses have had graduate psychiatric programs in formal family therapy training and supervision, although psychiatric social workers and psychiatric nurses often have had a broader base in this area because of their frequent family contacts.

The primary skill for a family therapist, as in all areas of psychiatric intervention and treatment, is self-awareness. The ability to observe one's own thinking, feeling, and behaving is a prerequisite to being able to help a family deal with a problem. A second requirement is ongoing supervision. Maintaining a stance that is objective enough to get a different perspective on the family's problem while staying in emotional contact with the family is difficult without ongoing peer support, feedback, and supervision.

Roles

The specific roles of the family therapist depend on that therapist's way of conceptualizing the family's problems, as presented in the preceding discussion of theoretical approaches. Some therapists intentionally "join" the family, while others maintain a more objective distance. In general, any family therapist may function as a role model, an educator, or as a feedback mechanism, depending on the therapist's theoretical orientation. Some schools of family therapy regard the family's gaining insight into the problem as essential, whereas others change the family structure to remove the presenting symptom and have no interst in the family's achieving insight.

CHARACTERISTICS OF FAMILY THERAPY
Client Selection

The family may refer itself for therapy. It is not uncommon for self-referral to occur in response to a problem with a child in the family. Families may be referred for treatment by agencies such as the school system, welfare board, parole officers, and judges. The family may not agree that a problem exists and may feel coerced into therapy. For example, when abuse has taken place, the judge may order parents to enter family therapy as a condition for leaving the child in the home. Some families are referred for therapy from emergency room psychiatric services after a visit caused by a crisis in the family such as a drug overdose. Upon discharge from a psychiatric hospital a client and his family may be referred for family therapy. Ministers, private physicians, and families who have experienced family therapy may make referrals.

Family therapy is the treatment of choice when there is marital problem or sibling conflict. Situational crises such as the sudden death of a family member and maturational crises such as the birth of the first child may cause sufficient stress that family therapy is indicated. When there is fusion or overcloseness of family members, family therapy may be beneficial. Family therapy may be indicated when problems are caused by using one child as the scapegoat.

Types of Family Therapy

The therapist may help the family in several ways. The type of therapy is usually determined by the therapist's training, or the therapist may be comfortable with several approaches and decide after the first interview with the family the method that is best suited for that particular family.

Individual family therapy. With individual family therapy each family member has a single therapist. The family as a whole may meet occasionally with one or two of the therapists to see how the members are relating to one another and work out specific issues that have been defined by individual members. This model works well with individual growth and the development of the individuality of each family member who is in therapy. Direct effect on the family system to facilitate the interactional and connective process with the unit as a whole is minimal. The family becomes the reference point for what is happening and is not the primary focus of the process.

Conjoint family therapy. The most common type of family therapy is the single-family group, or conjoint family, therapy. The nuclear family is seen, and the issues and problems raised by the family are the ones addressed by the therapist. The way in which the family interacts is observed and becomes a focus of therapy. The therapist helps the family deal more effectively with problems as they arise and are defined. Both the family and the therapist define the goals. These goals change as the problems are redefined. The integrity of the family system and its individual members is supported. Communication patterns are continually addressed to facilitate more effective relationships between family members.

Couples therapy. Couples often seek assistance and are seen by the therapist together. The couple may be planning to marry and may want to examine and strengthen their relationship. In some cases, the couple is married or unmarried and living together and having difficulties. In couples therapy, the spouses may begin to work together to seek resolution or to facilitate their separation. Family patterns, interactional and communicational styles, and each spouse's goals, hopes, and expectations of each other are examined. This examination enables the couple to find a common ground in resolving conflicts by recognizing and respecting each other's similarities and differences. Couples therapy is discussed in detail in Chapter 23.

Multiple family group therapy. In multiple family group therapy four or five families meet weekly to confront and deal with problems or issues they have in common. Ability or inability to function well in the home and community, fear of talking to or relating to others, abuse, anger, neglect, the development of social skills, and responsibility for oneself are some of the issues with which these groups deal. All of the families in these groups have problems coping with change. Most of the families in these groups are isolated and have difficulty forming relationships outside their nuclear family.

Because four or five families make up the group, a larger and different social network is formed. This network enables these families to begin or further develop the skills needed for more effective communication. Over time the levels of fear the people in these families have is reduced. Often family members in these groups have lived in constant crisis because of the feeling that they were alone and no one was there for support. These feelings change in the groups. The multiple family group becomes the support for all the families, and the number of times crises continue to occur and overwhelm these families is significantly reduced. This happens because these families form a sustaining network that in many cases is able to move into their homes. The network also encourages each person to reach out and form new relationships outside this group. These families become more effective in dealing with change as their need for adaptation increases.

Multiple impact therapy. Therapists can also bring families together for intensive work, usually over a three-day weekend or week-long encounter. In multiple impact therapy several therapists come together with the families in a community setting. They live together and deal with pertinent issues for each family member within the context of the group. Multiple impact therapy is similar to multiple family group therapy. However, it is more intense and time limited. Like multiple family group therapy, it focuses on developing skills of working together as a family and with other families.

Multiple impact therapy groups are goal oriented and always deal with immediate issues of problem solving. Reactions, feelings, and confrontation are important aspects of this type of therapeutic encounter. Because of the intensity of the encounter, this approach should not be used in families with a psychotic member.

Network therapy. Network therapy is conducted in people's homes. All persons interested or invested in a problem or crisis that a particular person or persons in a family are experiencing take part. This gathering includes family, friends, neighbors, professional groups or persons, and anyone in the community who has an investment in the outcome of the current crisis. People who form the network generally know each other and interact on a regular basis in each other's lives.

The network group is called together by its members under the guidance of the therapy team. The team enters the home to assist the network in solving the immediate problem. A network may include as many as 40 to 60 people, all of whom are interested in and invested in making things better for the person or family in crisis.

The rewards are great when all persons involved mobilize energy and management. The power is in the network itself. The network team only guides the process.

The answers to each problem come from the network and how people in the network decide to manage each issue as it arises. The therapists serve as guides to clarify issues, manage the process of each major network meeting, reinforce the importance of and need for the network toward its members collectively and individually, and assist in the development and effective management in the evolution of the problem resolution.

The network determines how often it meets. Generally it meets formally with the network team only three to six times before it accomplishes its goal. In the intervals between the formally called meetings, network members often encounter one another informally. Issues and problems are dealt with realistically as they occur. This method is very powerful. It supports people's strengths and abilities to help themselves. They are much less dependent on professionals to continually give them answers about issues that arise. The network members must come up with their own answers.

Because of the familiarity, intimacy, and interest this group has and continues to have in each other's lives, a renewal of the concept of community and home is discovered by all who participate in the network.

NURSING PROCESS
Assessment

Physical dimension. A dysfunctional family may encounter problems meeting the physical needs of its members: sufficient food, shelter, or protection from common physical dangers. The nurse may observe indications of physical neglect, incest, and physical abuse. The adults may fail to meet the family's needs because of limited finances, lack of knowledge, disinterest or for other reasons. Spouse and child abuse are common occurrences in some troubled families. The nurse observes for physical signs, such as bruises, that may indicate abuse. She also notes the family members' response to arguments, because abuse may follow arguments.

When doing an assessment the nurse may learn that various members of the family have physical problems in response to family conflict. As the nurse collects a thorough history of the family's physical functioning, it may be revealed that the use of physical symptoms to cope with stress is genetically determined.

The physical dimension is tracked with a genogram—a pictorial representation of at least three generations of a family (Figure 29-4). The entire family's physical complaints and illnesses are placed on the genogram, usually clearly demonstrating that the person with the identified complaint is not the only person experiencing distress. The genogram also helps the therapist and the family to observe that physical acting-out often follows or coincides with a significant physical diagnosis in the family. For example, an adolescent may be expelled from school for fighting on the same day his grandmother is scheduled for a radical mastectomy for cancer. If the only focus of treatment is this disruptive youngster, the whole family's anxiety and pain about grandmother's cancer can easily be overlooked.

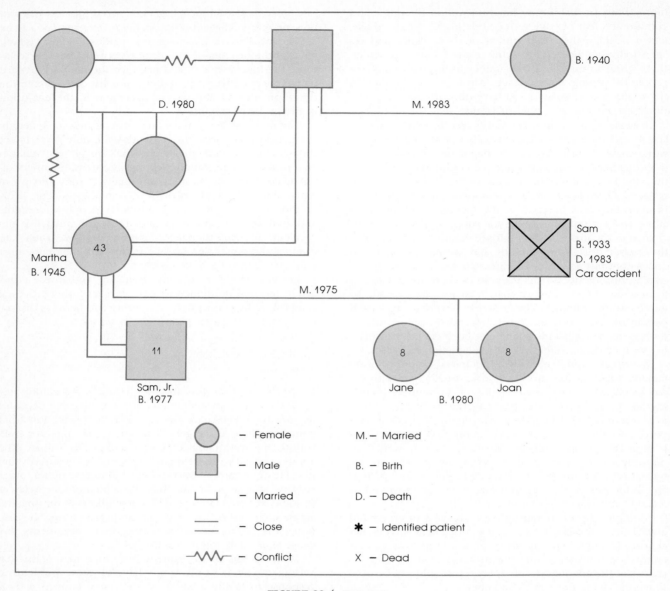

FIGURE 29-4 Genogram.

Emotional dimension. The focus of family problems may be losses or change experienced as a loss: illness, death, job loss, destruction of home by fire or a natural disaster. Such losses may be sufficient to shift the delicate balance in a dysfunctiional family and motivate them to seek therapy. The family's ability to grieve in response to the losses needs to be assessed. The family as a whole may be unable to express grief and they may disallow a specific member from doing so by blocking any discussion of feelings about the loss.

The nurse may note a problem in the expression of any feelings between family members and in the degree and quality of the emotional involvement that family members have in each other's needs, interests, and activities. The emotional expression may be too intense or too little; excessive emotional closeness prevents the family members from having the autonomy they need. When the family is emotionally distant, members may not receive sufficient emotional support.

Family members may experience guilt when a member resents assuming additional responsibility because of the illness of another member or because a member does not carry his share of responsiblility for tasks. A child in the family may experience guilt when told his behavior is the cause of the family's problems. Feelings of inadequacy in a situation—for example, caring for a new baby—may give rise to feelings of guilt. The guilt that one member experiences affects the whole family system. The family may be aware of the guilt and use secrecy in an effort to conceal the feeling from the nurse. The nurse listens for indications of a need for punishment, overly apologetic behavior, and scapegoating. The absence of a reasonable expression of anger may be an indication of guilt (see Chapter 13).

Some families' emotional response to stress is not evident. The nurse discerns these feelings by observing the family's response to stress-related words such as guilty, anger, or upset. She also listens for accounts of experiences associated with feelings—for example, "I was worried when . . . ." Encouraging the family members to engage in storytelling about illness or other stressful experiences may provide valuable information about anxiety, guilt, or other feelings. The nurse may learn about the family's true emotions by attending to their attempts to gain sympathy or emphasize negative experiences.

Triangulation is another part of the family's emotional process that the therapist tracks during the assessment phase. Pivotal family issues that often lead to potential conflict and triangling are discipline, sex, money, religion, and in-law relationships, but each family has its own "toxic" issues that prompt emotionality, conflict, and triangulation. Identifying and observing triangles in the family show the nurse which family members are the closest and which issues cause the most distance and conflict.

Intellectual dimension. The intellectual dimension of the whole family is assessed as the nurse observes the family's ability to separate thinking and feeling. Some families may appear to be intellectually duller than they actually are because of the long-term effects of chronic anxiety. An elderly family member with disorientation or confusion may be viewed as the cause of the problem. The nurse, after many questions, may be able to ascertain that the "confusion" is primarily a problem when certain toxic issues are addressed, or that the "disorientation" is much more apparent with some family members than with others. These kinds of findings during a family assessment may indicate that the intellectual functioning (confusion) of the elderly family member is more related to family problems than to organic brain changes.

The nurse assesses the family's ability to change. The dysfunctional family is likely to be inflexible and unable to shift roles and levels of responsibility. The family may seek therapy because of the members' inability to deal with developmental changes in the family, such as the birth of children, departure of children to school, children entering adolescence, and young adults leaving to make their own home. A change brought about by a promotion for the breadwinner of the family may create problems. Some families cope well with certain stages of the family's development; however, during a period when there is considerable change in the family's rules and roles, the family may become dysfunctional.

Families' rules are often rigid and do not allow for any flexibility for its members. The rules are likely to be implicit, yet family members assume that the rules are known and understood by all members. The family may have myths that conflict with reality. *Family myth* refers to a family's beliefs about their family that are fairly well integrated and shared by all members.[14] These myths concern each family member and his position or role in the family. Well-functioning families have myths that are changeable and explicit. Dysfunctional families have myths that conflict with reality. For example, the family believes "we would be okay if people didn't pick on us." In reality, the son is a bully and the father often picks a fight with the neighbor after a few drinks. Such myths deny the problems the family has and make it difficult for family members to realistically assess their own behavior and be responsible for it. These beliefs are not challenged by family members, even though the myths imply a distortion of reality.

The nurse may learn that the dysfunctional family does not know how to problem solve. Their handling of problems is based on reaction rather than on a constructive approach. The problem-solving may also be a type that reduces complex problems to simple solutions. Ineffective problem-solving abilities may be evident when family members quarrel without identifying the basis for the argument or offering an alternative solution to verbal fighting.

The power between the husband and wife in the family frequently is not balanced in a troubled family, and this may lead to conflict that affects the family system. The nurse assesses the power in the family by noting who makes the decisions in the family. The nurse can ask family members directly who makes decisions and how they are made. This information helps the nurse determine who has the most and least power in the family system and whether decisions are made impulsively, with little thought, or with so much thought that indecision is the result. The nurse may learn that the power for decision-making has changed during the life of the family—for example, the father made decisions early in the marriage and now the wife does. Other means for assessing who makes decisions include the following: observing the interaction between spouses, between parents and children, or between siblings and the family as a whole; self-reporting; and asking such questions as "Who has the last say about important issues?" and "Who wins when there is disagreement?"

Social dimension. Many families who come for therapy have problems in verbal and nonverbal communication. The nurse attends to the family's communication pattern to determine whether their pattern is functional or dysfunctional, because breakdown in communication is a clue to trouble in the family. Communicative behavior such as poor eye contact, interruptions, changing the subject, and speaking for one another are indications that the family has a communication problem.

The family's communication may be insufficient to provide family members with enough information to function well as a family. Because of vague or ambiguous communication, family members may not get a clear message as they communicate. *Double bind communications,*[6] conflicting messages given simultaneously, may be the predominant communication pattern in a dysfunctional family. The nurse determines whether the communication is direct or indirect. Direct communication in which the message is sent to the family member intended, is seen less frequently in the dysfunctional family than is indirect communication. Indirectly, the family members may send messages to the intended member by another family member and sometimes members outside the home. Such a communication pattern leads to misunderstanding, mistrust, and greater distortion of communication in the family.

Communication patterns provide information about relationships in the family. Often the way family members sit in the session provides nonverbal information about their relationships. For example, a member may sit across from the person from whom he seeks validation for his ideas. As family members interact, the nurse notices who talks to whom, who interrupts, who gives help and confirms what another member says. This information provides clues to who is close to whom and the dyads and triads in the family.

The family that seeks therapy is likely to have problems in performing their roles. Roles may not be clearly defined or there may be a lack of agreement as to who fulfills certain roles. Frequently the dysfunctional family has never openly discussed roles and who performs each of them. The roles may be rigid, and the family members may be unable to shift roles to meet the needs of the family members. The nurse inquires about the roles the various members are assuming and whether they meet the needs of the family members.

In an effort to deal with stress, the family members may unconsciously assign the role of *scapegoat* to one of its members.[44] A scapegoat is one who bears the blame for the family problem. This member, usually a child, shows symptoms of the family disturbance and thus keeps the family from focusing on the problem as a family problem. The scapegoat serves the function of keeping the rest of the family united. Often this focus on the scapegoat is the only thing the family can be united about. When doing an assessment the nurse may note that the family presents the scapegoat as the identified client.

The nurse may observe the role of "parental child" in the family.[43] In this role the older child is given parental responsibilities for younger children and sometimes the parent. For example, a father may not fulfill aspects of his role because of alcoholism or another problem, and the mother may place the oldest boy in the role of "man of the house."

The nurse observes the patterns of interaction between family members and family interactions with the outside world. Within each family are specified reciprocal roles that delineate how members behave toward each other. The obvious roles of mother-daughter and brother-sister need little explanation, but more subtle roles are also assessed.

The family system may be very closed and have little interaction with the community and rely entirely on nuclear family members for emotional sustenance. A family that functions as a tightly closed system is in a precarious position because it does not have outside sources of support. When a crisis occurs, the family members in a closed system are more reactive and more easily become dysfunctional physically, emotionally, or socially because of limited emotional resources.

An open family system allows and encourages contact outside the family and is less vulnerable. Crises occur in all families, but the family members in an open family system are able to rely on people outside of their family and therefore have more emotional support during crises.

Spiritual dimension. It is useful to inquire about the family's spiritual beliefs, as well as how differences about spiritual beliefs are handled. If differences exist, there may be tension. In some instances the children are in conflict when the parents have different religious affiliations and each parent wants the child to practice his or her faith. A dysfunctional family may disallow a discussion of ethical and religious issues and values. Some families are very antagonistic toward someone who married "outside the faith" or toward someone who espouses religious beliefs but behaves in an immoral way. Other families are unconcerned about these issues, but it is useful for the therapist to know not only what the spiritual beliefs are, but also how and in what context religion is an issue in the family.

In dysfunctional families value systems may be rigid and chaotic. The family members may adhere to their val-

ALTERATION IN FAMILY PROCESSES

DEFINITION

Disruption in the effective functioning of a normally supportive family in response to stress.

DEFINING CHARACTERISTICS

Physical Dimension
- Family system cannot or does not meet physical needs of all its members
- *Numerous physical illnesses
- *Physical abuse

Emotional Dimension
- Family system cannot or does not meet emotional needs of all its members
- Family system cannot or does not express or accept a wide range of feelings from other family members
- *Guilt

Intellectual Dimension
- *Inability to shift roles
- *Ineffective problem solving
- *Ineffective decision making

Social Dimension
- Family system cannot or does not seek or accept help appropriately
- Family system cannot or does not adapt constructively to crisis
- Ineffective communication between family members
- *Scapegoating

Spiritual Dimension
- Family is unable to meet the spiritual needs of all its members
- *Preoccupation with their supreme being
- *Conflictual religious beliefs

Adapted from North American Nursing Diagnosis Association Classification of Nursing Diagnosis: Proceedings of the seventh conference, St. Louis, 1987, The C.V. Mosby Co.

*Defining characteristics in addition to those defined by NANDA.

ues so rigidly that they become preoccupied with religion and a supreme being. The family may not participate in therapy because of their belief that a supreme being will solve the problems, if it is His will.

Analysis

Nursing diagnosis. Alteration in family processes and ineffective family coping are nursing diagnoses approved by NANDA that apply to family therapy. The defining characteristics of these diagnoses are listed in the box on p. 554 and below.

The following Case Example illustrates characteristics of alteration in family processes; the second Example demonstrates ineffective family coping.

INEFFECTIVE FAMILY COPING

DEFINITION

A state of coping wherein the family typically manifests a pattern of destructive behavior in response to the inability to manage internal or external stressors as a result of inadequate resources (physical, psychological, cognitive, and/or behavioral).

DEFINING CHARACTERISTICS
Physical Dimension
  Physical abuse
  Nelgect of client's basic human needs
  Neglect of client's illness-related treatments
  Hyperactivity
  *Physical illnesses
Emotional Dimension
  Unresolved anger, depression, hostility, and aggression
  *Guilt
  *Dysfunctional grieving
Intellectual Dimension
  Distortion of reality regarding the client's health problem
  Prolonged denial and reality
  *Rigid family rules
  *Family myths that conflict with reality
  *Ineffective decision making
Social Dimension
  Neglect of family member through activity such as abandonment or desertion
  Helpless, inactive dependency of client
  *Faulty family relationships; overly close or overly distant
  *Dysfunctional communication; double bind, indirect, insufficient
  *Unrealistic role expectations of children
Spiritual Dimension
  *Rigid spiritual beliefs
  *Conflicting religious affiliations
  *Overdependence on supreme being

Adapted from North America Nursing Diagnosis Association Classification of Nursing Diagnosis: Proceedings of the seventh conference, St. Louis, 1987, The C.V. Mosby Co.
*Defining characteristics in addition to those defined by NANDA.

Case Example

Mrs. Raney was referred to the nurse for family therapy because she felt that her home life had fallen apart since her husband's death four months earlier. Other members of the family are a 16 year old son and a 13 year old daughter. The daugher was very close to her father and has become increasingly withdrawn since his death. The son was supportive of the mother shortly after his father's death. Now the son is spending most of his time away from home; he no longer does chores unless his mother tells him to do so and then he rebels. Mrs. Raney has developed various physical complaints since her husband's death and reported that she feels overwhelmed with family responsibilities and the financial crises she faces now that the family's savings are gone. She admits to difficulty managing the children and her physical health. With much encouragement she agreed to attend family therapy.

Case Example

The Barnes family came to the mental health center because of Mrs. Barnes' concerns about her 12 year old son's failing performance in school and her inability to discipline him. Other members of the family are Mr. Barnes, a 13 year old son, and two daughters ages 9 and 7. Mr. Barnes is frequently out of work and the family is on welfare. Often the children do not have adequate food and clothing because the money the family receives is used to pay the rent. When Mr. Barnes earns a small amount of money, it is not unusual for him to spend it on gambling or alcohol. During the interview Mr. Barnes was loud and aggressive and the rest of the family seemed fearful of him. It was disclosed that he sometimes physically abuses the children in an effort to discipline them, especially the boys, and that he sometimes hits Mrs. Barnes. The 12 year old son is blamed for the family problems; the other children are considered "good kids."

The following list provides examples of other NANDA-accepted diagnoses with causative statements that are appropriate for family therapy:
1. Impaired verbal communication related to insufficient sharing of information
2. Diversional activity deficit related to lack of interaction with the community
3. Powerlessness related to inability to make decisions.
DSM-III-R diagnoses. The following DSM-III-R classifications apply to family therapy:
1. V61.80 Other specified family circumstances: Classification that can be used when a family response is to an aged in-law or when sibling rivalry is present
2. V62.89 Phase of life problem or other life circumstance problem: Classification that can be used when the focus of treatment is related to a family's developmental life cycle problem

Planning

Table 29-2 provides some long-term and short-term goals and outcome criteria for family therapy. These serve as examples in the planning stage of the nursing process.

Implementation

Physical dimension. The nurse recommends that all family members have complete physical exami-

TABLE 29-2 Long-term and short-term goals and outcome criteria related to family therapy

Goals	Outcome Criteria
NURSING DIAGNOSIS: POWERLESS RELATED TO DIFFICULTY IN MAKING DECISIONS THAT AFFECT FAMILY FUNCTIONING	
Long-term goal	
To recognize the effect of decision making on feeling of power	Discusses knowledge of relationship between decision making and power
	Identifies feelings related to decision making
	Examines the effects of decisions made on family members and self
	Takes credit for sound decisions
	Takes blame for ineffective decisions
Short-term goal	
To become comfortable making decisions	Appear more at ease when making decisions
	Shows williness to make decisions
	Tolerates family's lack of agreement with decisions
	Uses different approaches to decision making
NURSING DIAGNOSIS: IMPAIRED VERBAL COMMUNICATION RELATED TO SHARING OF INSUFFICIENT INFORMATION	
Long-term goal	
To recognize factors that interfere with sharing sufficient information	Initiates and accepts feedback from family about nature of communication
	Notes own and family's nonverbal behavior while communicating
	Verbalizes knowlege of deterrents to sharing adequate information
Short-term goal	
To increase ability to share adequate information	Shares information spontaneously
	Seeks feedback from others
	Determines what is sufficient information for a given situation

nations if physical problems are present. She emphasizes the importance of adhering to their medical and nursing regimens for the physical problems. If the nurse determines that the family has insufficient finances for proper food and shelter, she refers them to social services. The nurse secures a protective environment for any abused member in the family and discusses the abusive behavior in the family sessions (see Chapter 36). To deal with any problem that is genetically determined, the nurse refers the family for genetic counseling. The nurse educates the family about the problem, using the genogram to explain to the family how family problems may be passed down through each generation.

🔆 *Emotional dimension.* The nurse assists the family in resolving grief without distancing the grieving member or members from the rest of the family. There are four stages for family grief work: family announcement, family acknowledgment, family mourning, and family renewal.[16] In family announcement the goal is to facilitate open expression of feelings and an announcement of the death by all family members. The family members relive the emotional aspects of their experiences related to the loss. The nurse makes certain that each member participates, asking each member to share his thoughts about the loss and the family's emotional response. Family acknowledgment is realization by all family members that the loss has occurred and cannot be changed. The nurse intervenes in any family denial by asking each member to share his experience of the death and its meaning to him. With acknowledgment the family can enter the stage of

mourning. Family mourning occurs when each family member directly shares and manifests his feelings. As the members recognize similarities of their expression, they empathize with each other and recognize their mutual pain. During this experience, the family members learn about each other within the context of death and can transfer this knowledge to future family problems. Family renewal involves finding alternative means for meeting the psychological needs that were previously met by the deceased. The effectiveness of the renewal process depends on how well the family achieved the preceding stages. If the family was able to share feelings and experiences, they may now function at a higher level than before the death.

The nurse respects the family's need to experience guilt. She guides the family to elaborate and explore their feelings. It is helpful for the nurse to respond neutrally as a family describes feelings of guilt. With knowledge of what is causing the guilt—for example, feelings of inadequacy in a new role—the nurse explores with the family member realistic expectations without negating the member's feelings.

🔆 *Intellectual dimension.* The nurse assists the family with problem-solving by guiding the family through the steps of the problem-solving process, using one of their pressing problems. The nurse may need to first teach the family to identify problems and help them state the problem in a way that is understood by all family members. The nurse lets the family go through the problem-solving process during a session and then she gives them homework to solve a problem between sessions. At the next session, the family disucsses the problem-solving approach used and the outcome.

Role-playing can be useful when the family handles the problems on an intellectual level. For example, the family might be asked to act out what happens when the mother asks them to do household chores, if this has been a problem. The nurse begins the role-playing with a simple, non-threatening situation. Role-playing brings the reality of the family's life into the family session and provides the nurse with something concrete to work on.[5]

❀ ***Social dimension.*** The nurse uses clarification as a technique for intervention in the family's dysfunctional communication. Clarification allows the family to recognize discrepancies between (1) what they are saying and what others are hearing, what they are hearing and what others are saying, and (3) what both the individual and others mean, but are not saying in a clear and congruent way.[29]

The nurse redirects the family's indirect communication through her behavior. For example, when a family member talks to her about a family member, she directs the message to the intended family member. She tells the family member of the expectation that they will talk to one another and then actively directs them to do so. The nurse gives the family homework based on the expectation that they practice talking directly to each other in the home; they discuss how well they achieved this goal at a subsequent family session.

The nurse intervenes in problems in role by labeling the roles or having the family members label them, with assistance from the nurse; then the nurse develops a plan for changing nonfunctional roles.[5] For example, if the father is uninvolved in the care of the children and in family activities, the nurse may actively bring him into a discussion of these matters during a family therapy session and have the whole family share thoughts about ways he can become involved. The nurse can also give the father homework that requires his active family participation.

Changing the role of scapegoat is difficult and long term. The family is made aware of their behavior regarding this family member. As the family works toward resolving their problem, the role of scapegoat will no longer be needed to maintain the family's stability.

Evaluation

Evaluation of the outcome of therapy is seen primarily from the family's perspective. Often what the therapist sees as minor improvement may be beneficial from the family's point of view. Because it is the family and not the therapist who has to live with the problem and the outcome, the ideal outcome becomes one that is seen as satisfactory by the family.

Brief Review

The field of family therapy is relatively new to psychiatry. Initial interest and research with families began in separate parts of the United States as therapists either became frustrated in attempting traditional psychoanalytic therapy

with schizophrenics or came in contact with dysfunctional families through the problems of an emotionally disturbed child.

Psychoanalytic, Systems, and Humanistic schools of family therapy were discussed, although other branches exist. Many of the family therapy theoretical frameworks conceptualize the family as a system in which a disturbance in one member affects all members. The communication branch of family therapy believes it is incongruent communication processes that cause a family to have pain. The structural family therapy approach also observes how the family members interact with each other and with the goal of treatment to change the underlying structural arrangement of the family to improve the family's functioning. Differentiating from one's family of origin by establishing a one-to-one relationship with each family member is the goal of Bowen theory therapy.

The family therapist gathers data and plans interventions according to the chosen theoretical framework. The goals of treatment and the role of the therapist depend on what the therapist and family believe caused the problem. Identifying and dealing with the issues in the therapist's own family and ongoing supervision are essential for the professional practice of family therapy.

REFERENCES AND SUGGESTED READINGS

1. Ackerman, N.: The psychodynamics of family life, New York, 1958, Basic Books, Inc.
1a. Ackerman, N.W.: Treating the troubled family, New York, 1966, Basic Books, Inc.
2. American Psychiatric Association: Diagnostic and statistical manual of mental disorders, (DSM-III), Washington, D.C., 1980, The Association.
3. Aponte, H.J., and Van Deusen, J.M.: Structural family therapy. In Gurman, A.S., and Kniskern, D.P., editors: Handbook of family therapy, New York, 1981, Brunner/Mazel.
4. Austin, J., McBride, A., and Davis, H.: Parental attitude and adjustment to childhood epilepsy, Nursing Research **33**:92, 1984.
5. Barker, P.: Basic family therapy, Baltimore, Md., 1981, University Park Press.
6. Bateson, G., and others: Toward a theory of schizophrenia. In Howell, J.G., editor: Theory and practice of family psychiatry, New York, 1978, Brunner/Mazel, Inc.
7. Bowen, M.: Family therapy in clinical practice, New York, 1978, Jason Aronson, Inc.
8. Bowen, M.: Theory in the practice of psychotherapy. In Guerin, P.J., Jr., editor: Family therapy, theory and practice, New York, 1976, Gardner Press, Inc.
9. Cain, A.D.: Family therapy: one role of the clinical specialist in psychiatric nursing, Nursing Clinic of North America **21**(3):483, 1986.
10. Carpenito, L.: Nursing diagnosis application to clinical practice, Philadelphia, 1983, J.B. Lippincott Co.
11. Carter, E.A., and McGoldrick, M.: The family life cycle, New York, 1980, Gardner Press, Inc.
12. Collison, C.R., and others: The role of family re-enactment in group psychotherapy, Perspectives in Psychiatric Care **23**(2):74, 1985.
13. Committee on the Family: The field of family therapy, vol. VII, Report No. 78, New York, 1970, Group for the Advancement of Psychiatry.
14. Ferreira, A.: Family myths and homeostasis, Archives of General Psychiatry **9**:457, 1963.

15. Goldstein, M.Z.: Family involvement in the treatment of schizophrenia, Washington, D.C., 1986, American Psychiatric Press, Inc.

16. Greenberg, L.: Therapeutic griefwork with children, Social Casework **56**:396, 1975.

17. Guerin, P.J.: Family therapy: the first twenty-five years. In Guerin, P.J., Jr., editor: Family therapy, theory and practice, New York, 1976, Gardner Press, Inc.

18. Guerin, P.J., Jr., editor: Family therapy, theory and practice, New York, 1976, Gardner Press, Inc.

19. Gurman, A.S., and Kniskern, D.P., editors: Handbook of family therapy, New York, 1981, Brunner/Mazel.

20. Hansen, J.C., editor: Health promotion in family therapy, Rockville, Md., 1985, Aspen Systems Corp.

21. Hardesty, F.: Dinner with the family as an effective assessment method, Nurse Practitioner 9(9):57, 1984.

22. Jones, S.: Techniques of family therapy. In Lego, S., editor: The American handbook of psychiatric/mental health nursing, Philadelphia, 1984, J.B. Lippincott Co.

23. Jones, S.: Family therapy as a psychiatric nursing intervention, Advances in Psychiatric Mental Health Nursing **1**:1, 1982.

24. Jones, S., and Dimond, D.: Family theory and therapy models: comparative review with implications for nursing practice, Journal of Psychiatric Nursing and Mental Health Services **20**:12, 1982.

25. Kerr, M.: Family systems theory and therapy. In Gurman, A.S., and Kniskern, D.P., editors: Handbook of family therapy, New York, 1981, Brunner/Mazel, Inc.

26. King, J., and others: A nursing family assessment program, Canadian Journal of Psychiatric Nursing 27(3):12, 1986.

27. Kolevzon, M.S., and Green, R.G.: Family therapy models, New York, 1985, Springer Publishing Co.

28. Lansky, M.R.: Family approaches to major psychiatric disorders, Washington, D.C., 1986, American Psychiatric Press, Inc.

29. Lantz, J.E.: Family and marital therapy: a transactional approach, New York, 1978, Appleton-Century-Crofts.

30. Lasky, P., and others: Symposium: development of a research group—developing an instrument for the assessment of family dynamics, Western Journal of Nursing Research 7(1):40, 1985.

31. Leavitt, M.B.: Families at risk: primary prevention in nursing practice, Boston, 1982, Little, Brown & Co.

32. Morrissette, P.: Avoiding the coalition trap: recognizing the centricity and vulnerability of the psychiatric nurse in the realm of family treatment, Canadian Journal of Psychiatric Nursing 27(2):14, 1986.

32a. Midelfort, C.F.: The family in psychotherapy, New York, 1957, Blakiston Publishing, Division BK, McGraw-Hill Book Co.

33. Miller, J.R., and Janosik, E.H.: Family-focused care, New York, 1980, McGraw-Hill Book Co.

34. Miller, S., and Winstead-Fry, P.: Family systems theory in nursing practice, Reston, Va., 1981, Reston Publishing Co., Inc.

35. Minuchin, S.: Families and family therapy, Cambridge, Mass, 1974, Harvard University Press.

36. Nichols, M.: Family therapy, New York, 1984, Gardner Press, Inc.

37. Oliveri, M.E., and others: Family concepts and their measurement: things are seldom what they seem, Family Process **23**(1):33, 1984.

38. Phipps, L.B.: Theoretical frameworks applicable to family care. In Miller, J.R., and Janosik, E.H., editors: Family-focused care, New York, 1980, McGraw-Hill Book Co.

39. Rose, L.E.: Responses of families to the treatment setting . . . a psychiatric hospital, Nursing Papers Perspectives in Nursing 17(2):72, 1985.

40. Satir, V.: Conjoint family therapy, Palo Alto, Calif., 1967, Science and Behavior Books.

41. Sebastian, L.: Use of multi-family therapy groups in nursing, Kansas Nurse 61(12):1, 1986.

42. Siegel, E.: Scapegoating: manifestations and intervention, Journal of Psychiatric Nursing **19**:11, 1981.

43. Skynner, A.C.R.: Systems of family and marital psychotherapy, New York, 1976, Brunner/Mazel, Inc.

44. Toman, W.: Family constellation, ed. 2, New York, 1969, Springer Publishing Co., Inc.

45. Vogel, E.F., and Bell, N.W.: The emotional disturbed child as the family scapegoat. In Bell, N.W., and Vogel, E.F., editors: A modern introduction to the family, Glencoe, 1960, Free Press.

46. Whall, A.L.: In search of holistic family assessment: an investigation of a clinical instrument . . . Watzawick's structural family interview (SFI), Issues in Mental Health Nursing 6(1/2):105, 1984.

47. Whall, A.L., editor: Family therapy theory for nursing: four approaches, New York, 1986, Appleton-Century-Crofts.

48. Williams, M.: Use of a concluding process to assist grieving families, Journal of Emergency Nursing 10(5):254, 1984.

49. Williams, P.: Family feeling, Community Outlook **1**:9, 1987.

50. Wright, L.M., and Leakey, M.: Nurses and families, Philadelphia, 1984, F.A. Davis Co.

ANNOTATED BIBLIOGRAPHY

Committee on the Family: The field of family therapy, vol. VII, Report No. 78, New York, 1970, Group for the Advancement of Psychiatry.

Although more than 15 years old, this is an exceedingly useful reference because of its historical value. One chapter, "Premises About Family Therapy," classifies family therapists on an A-to-Z continuum, with A therapists having an individual focus and Z therapists operating exclusively from a family system orientation.

Gurman, A.S., and Kniskern, D.P., editors: Handbook of family therapy, New York, 1981, Brunner/Mazel.

This comprehensive book compares and contrasts the major current clinical theories in family therapy. Critically reviewing the works of the divergent approaches has been aided by the editors' requirements that each author who contributed attempt to follow the same format.

Miller, J.R., and Janosik, E.H.: Family-focused care, New York, 1980, McGraw-Hill Book Co.

This book provides a theoretical foundation for the clinical use of family-focused care, whether with physical illness or mental illness. Clinical cases are given to aid the reader in understanding the theories discussed. The editors and many of the contributors are nurses.

CHAPTER 30

MARITAL THERAPY

Ellen A. Andruzzi

After studying this chapter the learner will be able to:

State three factors that have influenced the historical development of marital therapy.

Describe the concepts of three major theorists in the field of marital therapy.

Discuss characteristics of a marital therapist.

Use the nursing process to provide care to clients in marital therapy.

Marital therapy is a mental health service for married couples or unmarried couples living together who experience difficulties within their relationship and are unable to achieve a satisfactory solution. The goal of therapy is to ameliorate problems of the couples. Various psychodynamic, sexual, ethical, and economic aspects of the couple's lives are considered. Husband and wife are seen individually or together. A broader term is "couples therapy," which encompasses unmarried couples.

At times problems in the marriage lead to psychosocial problems in the child and motivate the parents to seek help. If the therapist's assessment indicates that the problems originate in the spouses, marital therapy will be recommended.

Serious prolonged physical health problems in either spouse significantly affect the other spouse and the marriage. Marital therapy can help such spouses enhance their abilities to cope with the stressors induced by these health problems. Marital problems may be expressed as physical or mental symptoms. Medical, surgical, and individual psychiatric treatment may be tried to little avail, and the symptoms may not disappear until both spouses engage in marital therapy.

THEORETICAL APPROACHES
Psychoanalytic

When psychoanalytic theory is used in marital therapy, the assumption is that unconscious factors influence all aspects of the marital relationship: choice of marital partner, the problems that characterize the relationship, and how the problems are resolved. A transference neurosis that evolves from past and present unconscious infantile and childhood conflicts is the central focus in the therapeutic work with the goal of bringing about personality changes. Some psychoanalysts see each of the spouses alone; others see each spouse alone and then both spouses together. The focus of treatment is likely to be the spouse who exhibits symptoms, the Identified Patient. Usually the treatment is long.

The aspect of psychoanalytic theory that is particularly useful for application to marital functioning and therapy is *object relations,* which focuses on the link between the marital object and the couple's early object relations in the family or origin. Object relations refer to the emotional bonds between two persons. To achieve a healthy adult level of object relations, the individuals achieve separation from early, infantile object relations. This separation, referred to as separation-individuation, or differentiation, begins in infancy and is refined throughout adolescence. When this process has occurred, the marital relationship consists of spouses who have reached a level of maturity and are fully differentiated individuals.[11] When the process of separation-individuation does not occur or is incomplete, the individual carries an impaired sense of self into adult life. The adult either has a pattern of depending on others to tell him what to do and how to do it or of depending on others to express his feelings. The person with an impaired sense of self may alternate between the patterns described above, depending on the sit-

Historical Overview

DATE	EVENT
1890	Social workers were providing counseling to married couples.
1910	Adler[1] and Jung[54] recognized the effect of the marital pair on the children's development in their writings on socially rooted theories in psychodynamics.
1924	Earnest R. Groves taught a noncredit course on marriage at Boston University.[35]
1930	Marriage counseling centers were started in Los Angeles by Paul Popenoe and in New York by Abraham and Hannah Stone.
1938	Psychoanalytically oriented therapists did advanced work in examining the nature of marriage and marital dysfunction.
1938	Marital therapy began as a specialized professional approach.
1939	"Marriage and Family Living" was begun as the official organ of the National Council of Family Relations.
1942	Family life educators, counselors, and a social hygienist first discussed forming a professional organization of marriage counselors.
1945	The American Association of Marriage Counselors was established.
1947	Fifteen nationally recognized centers for marriage counseling were operating in the United States.[35]
1956	Three accredited training centers were recognized in the United States.
1959	Don Jackson coined the term "conjoint therapy" to describe a therapist meeting conjointly with a husband and wife.
1960s and 1970s	Professional disciplines published works on marital therapy in journals of their primary professions.
1963	California became the first state to pass a licensing law for marriage and family counselors.
1970	The name of the American Association of Marriage Counselors was changed to American Association of Marriage and Family Counselors (AAMFC).
1970s	Psychiatrists gradually increased the use of conjoint therapy instead of individual therapy with marital pairs.
1975	The "Journal of Marriage and Family Counseling" was initiated by AAMFC.
1978	The name of AAMFC was changed to American Association for Marriage and Family Therapy (AAMFT).
1979	The name of the journal was changed to "Journal of Marriage and Family Therapy."
1980	The Commission on Accreditation for Marriage and Family Therapy Education of the AAMFT was approved for inclusion on the list of recognized accrediting agencies by the U.S. Department of Health, Education and Welfare.[4]
Future	As more nurses enter independent practice, they will become more active as marital therapists.

uation. This process influences mate selection, the marital relationship, and parenting as the person seeks to act as an adult but relates to the object on an infantile level. Relating to a marital partner on an infantile level involves *collusion,* an active process by which each mate uncon-sciously chooses a partner based on his unmet infantile needs with the expectation that the partner chosen will meet the needs.[23] Each partner unconsciously forms an implicit *contract* to meet the mate's unfulfilled infantile needs.

Object-relations theory assumes that the child develops a "heterosexual sense of reality" or "family image" as a part of normal development.[87] This development encompasses three simultaneous processes that affect the marital relationship:

1. The recognition of an internal triangle, including the "parental dyad" as an "object organism."
2. The identification, over time, of the roles assumed by each parent as marriage partners and as parents, roles the child may assume or experience as an adult.
3. An increasing awarenes of the child's role, his separateness, and his lack of genital fulfillment in relation to the parental dyad.

A marital partner who has not mastered the developmental processes may idealize the partner early in the marriage and devalue and blame later in the union. The blaming often results in conflict, and the couple may decide to seek therapy or separate.

Self-distortion may occur in persons in marital therapy; for example, a wife who mistrusts her husband without foundation has projected on him her distrust of her father. Such a projection is unconscious and can be resolved when the wife becomes aware that she is relating to her husband as if he were her father.

In psychoanalytic theories the therapist's role is nondirective. The therapist listens neutrally to each of the partners.[87]

Sager[81] uses the term *contract* to refer to the separate, unspoken, unconscious understanding of expectations within the relationship that exist between mates who join in a committed relationship. Problems arise as each mate relates to the other as though the terms of the contract are consciously known and agreeable. Since they are not known and agreeable, each spouse is disappointed when the contract is not fulfilled.

Sager supports conjoint therapy with couples so that both the conscious and unconscious aspects of each spouse's contract can be explored and revealed (see box below). Then the contracts are available so that the couple can negotiate a unitary contract. During negotiations the husband and wife enhance their awareness of the interactional component of the contract. This component includes the conscious and unconscious ways in which they cooperate or sabotage each other as they seek to fulfill the terms of their separate contracts.

Sager's theory recognizes that the complaints couples bring to marital therapy are symptoms. The therapist seeks the underlying difficulties in the expectations of the marriage or in the biological and psychological parameters of the spouses. In Sager's theory the therapist's role is to teach partners how to negotiate because the terms of their contract and the goals of their marriage fluctuated to reflect changes in their life situation.

Behavioral

Jacobson's[50,53] behavioral marital therapy (BMT) is more complex than changing problematic behaviors by means of new learning. Although Jacobson gives credit to behavioral theory evolving from operant conditioning with children, he recognizes that conditions are different between spouses and that these conditions require the spouses to negotiate.[53] He therefore added communication and problem-solving skills to operant programs. Successful couples adapt effectively to the requirements of day-to-day intimacy. In particular they influence their spouses actions by acknowledging desired behaviors in new, rewarding ways.[50] BMT assumes that the enduring success of a marital relationship depends primarily on the characteristics of the partners' exchanges and the environmental forces that impinge on them rather than on any preordained personality characteristics. Marital satisfaction is thought to be directly related to spouses' abilities to maximize individual rewards and minimize individual costs, both of which are highly individualized, in their ongoing interactions. A high correlation between rewards given and received over time is consistent with a high level of marital satisfaction.

The role of the therapist in BMT is to assess the marital problems and to select appropriate behavioral interventions. The therapy is directive and involves teaching as a major tool. The therapist uses a variety of assessment methods. In addition, the therapist selects behavior models that can be taught to the couple. Usually the goal is to minimize marital conflict and to direct the couple so that there is a better balance between rewards and punishments than the couple has experienced before therapy.

Systems

Bowen[17-19] is one of the first theorists to relate systems concepts to marital therapy. The marital couple is perceived not only as a nuclear family but as a couple systematically linked to the families of origin and the extended families for multiple generations.

Central to Bowen's theory[19] is the *emotional system,* the emotional chain reactions that occur among family

---

REMINDER LIST FOR MARRIAGE OR COUPLE CONTRACTS

EACH "CONTRACT" HAS THREE LEVELS OF AWARENESS:

1. Verbalized—these parts of your contract are discussed with each other, although not always heard by the receiver.
2. Conscious but not verbalized—these are parts of your contract that you are aware of but do not verbalize to your spouse because you fear anger, disapproval, or embarrassment.
3. Beyond awareness, or unconscious—these aspects are beyond your usual awareness. You may have an idea what some of these are. They are often felt as a warning light in your head or a fleeting feeling of concern that gets pushed away.

Adapted from Sager, C.J.: In Gurman, A.S., and Kniskern, D.P., editors: Handbook of family therapy, New York, 1981, Brunner/Mazel, Inc., p. 88.

members and tie the emotional functioning of one family member integrally to that of another. Awareness of the emotional system is essential to understanding the development and course of symptoms in the marital pair, whether they are symptoms of physical illness, mental illness, or social acting out behavior.

Another important aspect of the system is that it can exist in a state of equilibrium or disequilibrium. Increasing anxiety drives a balanced marital system toward imbalance or disequilibrium. Short-term symptoms can have a balancing effect, but long-term symptoms can cause severe disequilibrium. Bowen[19] identifies two primary life

forces that counterbalance each other in the emotional system: a force toward individuality or *differentiation* and a force toward togetherness or *fusion* (undifferentiation). A disturbance in the balance of these forces can generate anxiety and lead to symptom development. There is great variation in the characteristics of these forces within persons, families, and other groups. What constitutes imbalance in one circumstance may be balance in another. A person who grows up in a family in which the balance is strongly toward togetherness may be programmed for fusion[29] and thus poorly differentiated.

The process of fusion (undifferentiation) is shown in Figure 30-1, in which the square represents the husband and the circle the wife. In the process of fusion the spouses are not separate, but each blends some identity with the other. The adult who was fused to a parent as a child carries the characteristic of fusion into relationships outside the family, including the marital relationship. The fused person is apt to select a mate who is at the same level of differentation. When the intensity of the fusion becomes too great to tolerate, emotional distance is used to cope with the increased anxiety. In Figure 30-2 the

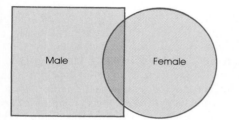

FIGURE 30-1 Fusion.

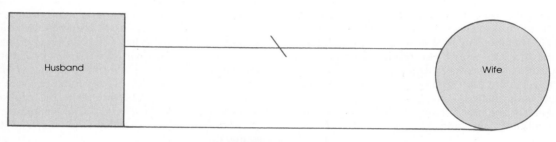

FIGURE 30-2 Distancing.

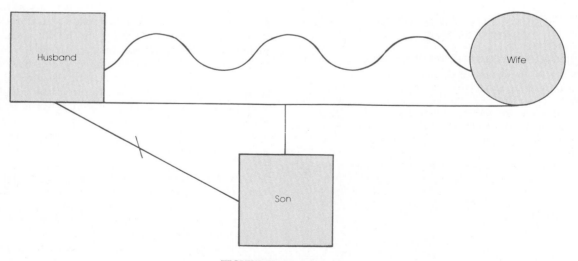

FIGURE 30-3 Triangling.

space and the line with a slash represent the *emotional distance,* or the effort of the spouses to move away from each other. Fusion and *distancing* are two sides of the same coin. Emotional conflict allows intense relating to the spouse and maintaining emotional distance at the same time.[56]

The term *fusion-exclusion* describes a third compensatory mechanism. Bowen originally used the term *triangle* to refer to the emotional process of fusion-exclusion.[29] The fusion-exclusion mechanism is shown in Figure 30-3. The wavy line denotes conflict; the straight line, closeness; and the straight line with a slash, cutoff. The emotional process symbolized is fusion in the husband and wife subsystem. This is compensated for by conflict between the spouses. The wife and son are close to each other and the husband and son are cut off from each other. Through this mechanism two people can stay in close contact with each other and avoid fusion-generated anxiety either by excluding a third person from their relationship or by focusing their energies on a third person, sometimes a child.

In the fourth mechanism, *pseudoposition,* the spouses assume "pretend" polarized postures, for example, dominant-submissive, overresponsible-underresponsible, and overadequate-inadequate. One persons acts and feels strong, and the other acts and feels weak. These mechanisms maintain equilibrium; problems occur when additional stress strains minimal coping reserves.

In an effort to maintain equilibrium, one spouse develops symptoms, which replace the direct expression of emotions. Alcoholism, obesity, physical illness, mental illness, and even criminal behavior at their extremes are symptoms that reflect a significant lack of differentiation.[56] Better-differentiated persons and marital systems can have the same problems, but they are likely to be in a milder form. These illness patterns can be seen in several generations, with the more fused generations having the more severe problems.

The therapist's role in Bowen's theory is to assess the needs of the couple, to estimate the level of differentiation of each spouse, and to work with the couple as members of a multigenerational family system so that each person reaches a higher level of differentiation. Any profile of persons at various levels of differentiation is more hypothetical than real; that is why the profiles of differentiation given in Table 30-1 are for guidance only and are to be used cautiously.

According to Bowen[19] three main clinical approaches have been effective when the client's goal is differentiation of self: (1) psychotherapy with both spouses, (2) psychotherapy with one family member, and (3) psychotherapy with one spouse in preparation for a long-term effort with both spouses. Usually the therapist meets with the client or clients approximately monthly, thus allowing time to work on the problems between sessions. The therapist adjusts the focus from feelings to thinking and consistently implies that the marital partners own the problems and that the problems are theirs to solve.

In the first approach the therapist listens to one spouse while the other spouse listens. The therapist asks many questions about the problems and what each member of

TABLE 30-1 Profiles of differentiation

Level of Differentiation	Characteristics
Moderate to good	Emotional and intellectual systems function cooperatively.
	Use factual knowledge to make decisions that can overrule the emotional system in situations of anxiety and panic.
	Can live freely with emotional system using logical reasoning when need arises.
	Able to follow independent life goals.
	Marriage is a functioning partnership.
	Are responsible for selves.
Pseudoself	Some beginning differentiation of emotional and intellectual systems.
	Life guided by emotional system.
	If anxiety is low, functioning resembles moderately differentiated self.
	Life energy directed to winning friends and approval.
	Self-esteem dependent on others.
	Lack solid self-convictions; refer to authority.
	Personal lives in chaos.
	May be conforming disciples or rebels.
	Have intense versions of overt feeling.
	Develop high percentage of human problems such as physical illness, social dysfunction, and emotional illness.
Low	Dysfunctional.
	Anxious.
	Live in a feeling-dominated world.
	Do not distinguish feeling from fact.
	Totally relationship oriented.
	No energy for life-directed goals.
	Seek approval; often experience failure to have approval, leading to withdrawal or fighting in the relationship system.

Based on data from Bowen, M.: In Olson, D., editor: Treating relationships, Lake Mills, Iowa, 1976, Graphic Publishing Co., Inc.

the couple has been thinking. The therapist *detriangles* situations as they arise, often by confronting the phenomenon and questioning its value to each spouse. The genogram is used during this process (Figure 30-4).

Frequently the spouses are pleasantly surprised at the quality of their mates' thinking. The therapist supports each person's expression of thoughts while differentiating thoughts from feelings. The therapist encourages each spouse to listen to the other's expressed thoughts, to think about the thoughts, and to respond with related ideas. The effect is to calm the anxiety in the relationship.

The teaching aspect of Bowen's marital therapy is operational when intramarital tension has become low. At this point the twosome can hear the teaching. Comments are made from the "I" position, for example, "I have had some experience with other couples that may be useful for you to know about or may not suit you. I do not want you to adopt it as it's described, but, if you want to use it,

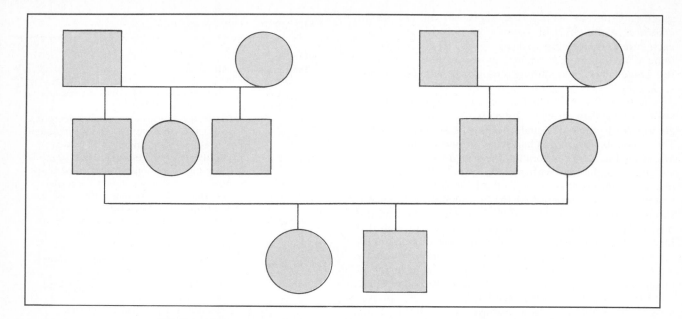

FIGURE 30-4 Family map, or genogram. *Squares,* males; *circles,* females.

you can adapt it to your own situation." The therapist uses *coaching* as a way to share ideas that may be useful. This method engages the spouses in dialogue about alternative actions while leaving the choice to clients.

In the second approach, when only one spouse comes for marital therapy because of the other's aversion to the image of psychotherapy, the therapist proceeds as for one family member. In the third approach, eventually the spouse is impressed with the changes made by the spouse receiving therapy and may ask to join the sessions. At this point therapy proceeds as for spouses together.

Using the *genogram* the therapist points out the relationships across the generations. The spouses are assigned to study the patterns of their extended families and of themselves and to then identify what they want to change or retain. The therapist coaches the clients as they take steps to change their relationships with selected family members.

Existential

Whitaker's approach to marital therapy[98,99] is known as existential marital therapy and is a subsystem of existential family therapy. The therapy espouses three values—experience, reality, and growth—and relies on the immediate experience of the moment in all its fullness. Emphasis is on reality and the facts of life. The aim of the therapy is helping people grow, in contrast to helping people adapt.[99]

Whitaker[98] addresses premarital and marital myths. An example of a premarital myth is the expectation of unconditional positive regard, which does not occur after infancy. An example of a marital myth based on Whitaker's theory is "If you're going to run around with somebody

else, don't tell me." Infidelity, which always involves a triangle, is usually bilateral and preplanned by both partners, and both want it that way, according to Whitaker. The "someone else" may be a lover, money, school, or a house.

Whitaker calls attention to two concurrent processes in a marriage, the legal commitment and the feeling experience, the binding and the bonding. The feeling level is unstable and, as each partner grows, always changing, with peaks of love and hate. Each partner behaves in a way to maintain balance. The more one or both get stuck in a fixed role, the more each loses his humanness.

The couple is most likely to change at crisis points such as the honeymoon, pregnancy and birth, extramarital affairs, absences and reentries. A noteworthy phenomenon is the 10-year impasse syndrome, at which time the couple has an opportunity to establish a wholehearted marriage or to provoke hostility.

The therapist has Whitaker's typology of marriage available as a guide to observing and evaluating the couple's behavior in the therapy session and to understanding their descriptions of their ongoing interactions:

1. Stable and dead, with the relationship frozen into pseudomutual politeness or hostility
2. Unstable and growthful, which can provide optimal conditions for continual individual and marital growth
3. Stalemated chaos in which the system lacks well-defined limits; partners are locked into interactions that are non-growth-producing

Whitaker recognizes the multigenerational system and its influence on the marital dyad. When necessary he directs one spouse to arrange for parents or siblings to attend the session. Whitaker accepts no excuses and does

TABLE 30-2 Summary of theoretical approaches

Theory	Theorist	Goal	Role
Psychoan-alytic		Separation-individuation (to achieve separation from early infantile object relations)	To assist partners to achieve a healthy adult level of object relations
	Sager	To determine the conscious and unconscious aspect of each spouse's contract (expectations in the marriage)	To teach partners how to negotiate a unitary contract
Behavioral	Jacobson	To minimize marital conflict and to direct the couple to achieve a better balance between reward and punishment than experienced before therapy	To assess the marital problems and select appropriate behavioral interventions
Systems	Bowen	To assist the couple to reach a higher level of differentiation	To teach, coach and assess the needs of the couple; to estimate the level of differentiation; to work with the multigenerational system
Humanistic-existential	Whitaker	To observe, evaluate, and understand the couple's behavior in the session	To free the couple from the multigenerational system so that they can proceed with the growth and development of their marital relationship

not hold the session until the other family members are present. Thus many multigenerational problems are solved, freeing the couple to proceed with their own growth and the development of their marital relationship. See Table 30-2 for a summary of the theoretical approaches.

CHARACTERISTICS OF THE MARITAL THERAPIST
Qualifications

Some states require that marital therapists be licensed. In those states the qualifications are defined. For the majority of states the standards of the American Association for Marriage and Family Therapy (AAMFT) are applied. The AAMFT standards set minimal requirements as a master's degree in either marital and family therapy from an accredited institution or a master's degree in an allied mental health profession. In addition, the therapist is required to have 1,500 hours of clinical experience (defined as face-to-face contact) in marriage and family therapy, with 200 of those hours supervised. It is essential that marital therapists be persons of integrity with high ethical standards, since they are working with vulnerable persons who are often in great need of objective assistance and support. The therapists' training ideally has enabled them to differentiate their own biases from those of their clients.

Goals

The goals of the therapist depend on the therapist's theoretical orientation and were discussed under theories of marital therapy. In addition, the goals may be to treat pathological disorders, to enable the spouses to solve specific problems, and to foster healthy, satisfying relationships within the marriage.

Role

The role of the therapist is defined largely by the theoretical framework the therapist uses. Specific roles have been presented in the discussion of the theories. All marital therapy involves a certain amount of teaching. The therapist makes recommendations for action based on the therapist's theoretical knowledge and the couple's goal. In some therapy (for example, behavioral) teaching is a major goal.

The therapist assumes a certain level of activity appropriate for her theoretical orientation. Some therapists are active and use a directive approach in guiding the couple to resolve the marital conflict. Often therapists are nondirective while listening attentively to what each spouse has to share. With the latter approach, which is more typical of psychoanalytic therapy, the therapist believes the couple needs to make decisions based on their own conscious and unconscious motivations. Some marital therapists work alone and others work in teams. Some advocate a male-female cotherapy team to avoid the appearance or occurrence of biased alliances that cause hostility and an impasse. Others advocate a marital pair as therapists, believing that the actual resolution of problems that therapists achieve in their own lives serves as a role model as well as a continuing demonstration of problem solving in a couple.[2a]

Haley[38] believes that cotherapists complicate therapeutic efforts and that the most effective interventions can be made directly by one therapist. For persons training in strategic therapy, (the problem-solving therapy developed by Haley) the supervisor is behind the one-way mirror and is thus readily available to the trainee.

The choice of one therapist or cotherapists is often based on economic considerations. Cotherapy may be economically feasible in facilities with training programs, such as hospitals and clinics. In addition, cotherapy offers the opportunity for in vivo training. Many nurses are employed in settings in which cotherapy may be used in the training program and thus have the experience of serving as mentors to marital therapy trainees. In private practice or in other settings in which funds are limited, cotherapy may prove to be too expensive.

CHARACTERISTICS OF MARITAL THERAPY
Client Selection

Various types of crises may create a need for marital therapy. Many clients seek help because of the conflict or distance that troubles one or both of the partners. Some clients are self-referrals, and others are referred by social service agencies, attorneys, or their clergy or physicians from whom they initially sought guidance. Marital therapy is the treatment of choice when marital conflicts lead to spouse or child abuse. Often these couples are referred for therapy by the local police or a treatment service for victims of abuse. The age range of clients is from the middle teens (15 to 16 years of age) to the seventies, with the majority of couples falling between the late twenties and early forties. Suitable candidates for marital therapy generally are ambulatory and are sufficiently in touch with reality to participate actively in the therapy session and report problems that they seek to solve. Some therapists provide marital therapy for clients with a diagnosed psychotic disorder.

Some therapists think an appropriate time for marital therapy is when spouses need assistance in getting a separation or divorce. Others reject couples for therapy when the marriage is beyond repair and separation or divorce is imminent.

Stages of Marital Therapy

Marital therapy has three stages: beginning, middle, and termination. At the beginning the therapy is aimed at relieving the problems and symptoms of each spouse. As a result of the therapeutic interventions utilized during the beginning stage and the clients' changes in affect about their situation, anxiety is relieved and each of the spouses can think more clearly about options and solutions to the problems. During the middle phase the therapy moves more slowly, and each change is accompanied by a recurrence of an old behavior as each of the spouses struggles to use in daily life the learning that has occurred in the therapy sessions. Personal change and system change are deeper than in the beginning stage. As tension is expressed in the therapy session, this is related to the families of origin and to the early experiences of the spouses. Each partner is coached about alternative ways to relate to family members and to each other. During the termination stage the couple continues to practice the changed thinking, feeling, and behaving that they have developed as the therapy has progressed. They use the termination time to consolidate their gains and to obtain assistance from the therapist in polishing their skills at problem solving and improving relationships.

NURSING PROCESS
Assessment

Physical dimension. The nurse maintains awareness of the physical condition and complaints of both spouses. She collects data about the health history, including current health problems, medications prescribed, and use and abuse of over-the-counter drugs as well as various addictive substances such as alcohol and illicit drugs. Decreased marital satisfaction may result when the couple is investing much time, energy, and money on chronic medical problems. Often the medical problem becomes the focus of their lives, causing the interpersonal problem between the spouses to assume a secondary role. When either or both spouses are receiving medication, the nurse considers the therapeutic effects and side effects in assessing behavior and symptoms. Marital discord often occurs in a marriage in which drug or alcohol dependency is a factor. The nurse also needs to determine if one or both spouses use chemical substances before or in response to the marital distress.

The marriage may have become dysfunctional after the birth of a child with a genetic defect. Each spouse may blame the other for the child's problem and be unable to openly discuss the problem.

Changes in either spouse's body image as a result of surgery, hysterectomy, mastectomy, pregnancy, or weight gain may strain the marriage. Often persons are reluctant to openly discuss their thoughts on these subjects. During the assessment the nurse may become aware of changes in sexual activity that result from physical health problems such as cardiovascular disease or diabetes.

Signs of physical abuse may be evident during the assessment. Regardless of education, occupation, or social status, some couples have constant arguments that end in spouse or child abuse.

Emotional dimension. The nurse pays close attention to the emotions expressed by the couple. She also observes any difficulties they have in expressing emotion. Sometimes one spouse withholds expression of feelings until he is provoked to express accumulated feelings and then he may explode and become violent. The therapy session is a crucial time to look for positive feelings between the spouses. Few couples lack positive feelings for each other; as they express and share their positive feelings, their outlook becomes more optimistic.

The presence of the couple in the therapeutic setting for marital therapy may be evidence that they hope and care enough about each other to try to resolve the marital conflict. However, when doing an assessment the nurse may learn that the caring is masked by strong emotions such as anger, anxiety, hate, fear, and depression. Many couples in marital therapy have a history of unresolved anger and anxiety.

Anger is a fundamental cause of marital failure. Anger may be in response to one's spouse's unconscious or unverbalized infantile expectation for need satisfaction. Anger may result from hurt feelings and the fear of further hurt. Over time the anger becomes so intense that it disrupts the marital relationship.

The anxiety that the nurse observes during the first few sessions may be in response to discomfort in the therapy situation. However, uncertainty about their futures should the marriage not continue can also be a source of anxiety for one or both spouses. In addition, either spouse may experience anxiety about the other's complaining, blaming, and emotional distance.

The nurse's assessment includes determining how the partners feel about seeking therapy. Sometimes one person has threatened the other one with divorce if he does not attend marital therapy. The partner who is threatened may respond with anger and remain disengaged from the therapeutic process. If the problems are not resolved the partner who initiated the therapy may feel guilty. One or both spouses may experience guilt feelings because each feels responsible for the dysfunctional marriage. A spouse who wants to keep a secret, such as infidelity, may think that his secret decreases the effectiveness of the therapy and may feel guilt.

In the assessment the nurse is alert to symptoms of despair, depression, and potential suicide. Because depression is common for one or both spouses when there is marital discord, the nurse needs to ask directly if either spouse or any member of the immediate family has made a suicide attempt or thought about committing suicide. Any major change may trigger depression and the potential for suicide: illness, death of a significant other, geographical relocation, job instability, or potential for a divorce or separation.

Temporary absences and reentries occur in some marriages, such as because of a job or military assignment. At times a crisis occurs when the spouse reenters the couple's system, the imbalance in the system is sufficient to create marital discord, and one or both spouses experience anxiety and depression.

✳ ***Intellectual dimension.*** Assessment of the intellectual dimension is often accomplished in marital therapy by inferences that the therapist draws from the clients' vocabularies, levels of education, socioeconomic status, and feedback each gives about understanding the information that the therapist supplies. Attention is paid to the congruities and incongruities in the partners' functioning as spouses, as in the following Case Example.

Case Example

Tim thinks in concrete terms, has a cognitive style that is deliberate and measured, and expresses his ideas in visual terms such as "I see" or "Let's have a look at the problem." Agnes, on the other hand, conceptualizes well, uses more abstract thinking than Tim does, has a cognitive style that is quick and somewhat distractible, and expresses ideas in kinesthetic terms such as "I feel like that might happen."

In the preceding example it is better to use Tim's style with him and Agnes's style with her to first establish rapport and then to help each to understand the other's cognitive and expressive styles. The Research Highlight on p. 568 describes cognitive styles.

When the educational level is assessed the nurse may determine the appropriate type of intervention. People with less education may need more direct and active intervention. For example, the spouses may request direct answers instead of engaging in problem solving. A difference in the spouses' educational level may be a problem, especially when the woman's level of education is higher than the man's. Even when the spouses discuss the differences in educational level before marriage, the husband may feel threatened by a wife with a higher level of education. The wife is less likely to be concerned if the husband has a higher educational level; however, problems do emerge. The wife may think she does not fit in with his friends.

The expressiveness of each spouse is another important function to assess. Inadequate, incomplete, and misperceived communications are often a source of marital discord. In response to the statement, "I know that you hear what I said, but do you know what I mean?" too many couples would say, "No." The assessment of expressiveness is a continual process during therapy and is discussed later in the chapter.

The therapist assesses each spouse in terms of flexibility and rigidity, as discussed in Chapter 15. For some spouses, rigid adherence to rules and their established values is essential and flexibility is perceived as weakness.

Case Example

Bruce has a rigid requirement that established table manners be scrupulously observed at the family dinner table. Sandra, his wife, believes that the dinner table is a place for relaxed, informal family visiting. When either of their sons, 10 and 12 years old, breaks a rule, Bruce reprimands the boy. Sandra says nothing at the time but is offended and adds this act to her grievance collection about Bruce. In therapy Bruce is emphatic that he will not modify his behavior. His rigidity and Sandra's flexibility are both areas of disagreement in their marriage.

One or both spouses often use projection and displacement to deal with marital distress. The spouses may verbalize their belief that the marital problem is entirely due to the other mate. Some spouses anticipate rejection if they share their problems, feelings, and secrets and may use denial. It is common for denial to be accompanied by resistance. Some of the ways the couple may manifest resistance is by missing sessions, arriving late for sessions, and using long periods of silence during the session. These behaviors are an attempt to deal with some threat and are necessary for coping.

Because of anxiety, fear, lack of experience, or disagreement as to the actual problem or what approach to use, a couple may be unable to use effective problem-solving skills. When doing an assessment the nurse may observe that the spouses attempt to change behavior by coercion instead of problem solving and thus contribute to the marital conflict.

�֎ ***Social dimension.*** The nurse assesses the degree of dependence-independence in the couple's relationship by asking them about their styles of relating and

Research Highlight

Spouses' Cognitive Styles and Marital Interaction Patterns

L.W. Tyndall & J.W. Lichtenberg

PURPOSE

This study explored the relationship between spouses' cognitive styles and interaction patterns that were characteristic of their marriage. Three measures of cognitive style and one measure of relational interaction patterns were used.

SAMPLE

Sixty married couples (N = 120), solicited through announcements and bulletins at local churches and work settings, volunteered to participate. The solicitation for volunteers specified that couples were to have been married for at least 1 year, and spouses had to be at least 18 years of age. The mean age for husbands was 36.1 years (SD = 9.77); for wives it was 33.7 years (SD = 9.18). The average difference in age between husbands and wives was 3.14 years (SD = 2.46).

The range for duration of marriage in the sample ran from 1 to 33 years, with an average length of marriage of 11.3 years (SD = 8.92). Of the 120 subjects 15 (eight husbands and seven wives) had been married previously; none had been married more than twice. Twelve of the marriages were second marriages for at least one partner.

The median combined annual income of the couples was approximately $30,000. No significant influence on scores was found from the level of education or the religious orientation of the subjects.

METHODOLOGY

The researcher met with couples individually to explain the instructions for the five tests and to answer questions. All spouses signed a consent form before completing the tests. They were asked to work independently and not to discuss the tests before returning them to the researcher.

The following instruments were used. Numbers 2, 3, and 4 measured cognitive complexity; number 5 measured interaction patterns.

1. Demographic questionnaire: Included 19 items deemed potentially relevant to the cognitive style of the subjects and to issues involving interaction patterns in marriage and was used to develop a demographic profile of the sample as a whole.
2. Intolerance of Ambiguity Scale (IA): Intolerance of ambiguity is the "unwarranted imposition of structure when the situation is unstructured." Such situations are often perceived as threats by individuals with a low tolerance for ambiguity.
3. Category Width Scale (CWS): Taps an underlying process of discrimination; scores on the CWS are a measure of the number and types of stimuli individuals may include in a given category or concept.
4. Bierri's Modified Role Construct Test (BMRT): Measures cognitive complexity.
5. Relationship Style Inventory (RSI): Designed to measure the degree to which a given relationship manifests parallel, complementary, and symmetrical interaction patterns.

Data from the instruments were analyzed using multivariate procedures plus a canonical correlation analysis to clarify the nature of the relationship between cognitive style and interaction style variables and to identify any patterns underlying these constructs that might help explain the relationship.

FINDINGS

The findings suggested that individuals who were more tolerant of ambiguity (that is, cognitively flexible) were likely to report a greater occurrence of more parallel interactions (behavioral flexibility) in their marriage and vice versa. The scores on the IA and the correlations with the RSI suggested that individuals who were less tolerant of ambiguity were more likely to report rigid relational patterns in their marriage (that is, complementary or symmetrical interactions) than were spouses who were more tolerant of ambiguity.

IMPLICATIONS

These results highlight the need for therapists to consider the relationship of cognitive rigidity to marital interaction patterns (especially the rigidity of those patterns). The flexibility-rigidity dimension has been suggested as an important component of family relational structures. So flexibility-rigidity may be used to assess the ease with which the couple can shift their organization to adapt to changing environmental circumstances. These considerations may have implications in structural and strategic therapies. Both techniques are based on the cognitive belief that clients' problems are largely a consequence of their categorical and inflexible views, opinions, and values regarding roles and relationships, which in turn affect their interactive behavior.

Based on data from Journal of Marital and Family Therapy **11**:193, April 1985.

by listening to their speech patterns, such as speaking for the other or looking to the other before replying. Assessment of this behavior is a clue to the level of differentiation. Frustration of dependence needs may be a complaint expressed by both spouses. The nurse may observe that each spouse has the conscious or unconscious expectation that dependence needs will be met by the other spouse. Often the dependence needs of spouses who seek marital therapy are at an infantile level and thus maladaptive. When the needs are not met to the satisfaction of the spouse, the mate may question the spouse's fidelity.

The nurse assesses the level of trust between the partners as well as between each spouse and the nurse. Often this aspect is revealed directly as the spouses interact in the assessment session. Candor or guarded statements, expressions of suspicion, and periods of silence can all be clues to the level of trust-mistrust. Mistrust may be in response to a family secret.

The couple's self-esteem and self-respect may be damaged by the time they come for therapy. The nurse attends to statements spouses make about each other and themselves to get some indication about their self-esteem. In anger the spouses may denigrate each other.

Both spouses are highly vulnerable to decreased self-esteem in response to masculine and feminine sex concepts. One spouse may belittle the other because of sexual biases. For example, some men believe that women are inferior physically and intellectually. The nurse assesses how closely the spouses adhere to the traditional relationship expectations that the man be the breadwinner and the woman assume the role of housewife and mother. If both spouses work outside the home, the nurse is alert for clues to role conflict. For example, does the man expect the woman to also be a full-time mother and housewife or does he share the housework? If the man assists the woman with what are traditionally considered her responsibilities does she disparage his efforts?

The couple may request assistance in resolving conflict related to sexual adjustment. During the initial interview the nurse inquires about when the problem began and the nature of the sexual dysfunction. Sometimes the sexual maladjustment caused the conflict, and at other times the problem is a result of the marital distress; the two are often interrelated since it is common for spouses to unconsciously displace other tensions into the sexual area. As the couple relates their marital distress the nurse may learn that they really have a relationship problem. Some couples will not directly talk about sexual concerns but the nurse gets clues to problems when a couple talks about such topics as sleeping in separate beds and sometimes different bedrooms or allowing children to sleep with them (see Chapter 31).

Typically a couple who marries expects that their social relationships will endure. This expectation increases the pressure to have mutually acceptable interactions. When the nurse assesses the couple's social interaction she may observe that they have limited or no other social relationships in the community and thus relate to each other intensively. This type of situation may be a factor in one spouse distancing and the other becoming dysfunctional; it may also lead to marital conflict followed by physical abuse. Distancing may be in response to personal space needs, as described in the Research Highlight on p. 570.

On the other hand, the nurse may learn that the marital conflict is triggered by one or both spouses spending increasing time outside the marriage. Examples of "rival" interests are a job, a favorite sport, community activities, alcohol or drugs, or care of an aged parent. The woman is more likely than the man to be involved in community activities. This may be her attempt to convey to her spouse that she does not need him, especially if he spends much time with his job. If the nurse examines the various community activities in which the woman is involved she

may find that even though the woman is active, she is isolated and lonely.[51]

The nurse may pick up clues that an extramarital relationship decreases the time the couple spends together. According to surveys infidelity ranks third as the cause of marital conflict; one half of clients who seek marital therapy have a problem in this area.[41] More men than women seek intimate companionship outside the family. A woman may accuse her husband of infidelity after a vasectomy, and the man may make the same accusation about the woman after she has a hysterectomy, because each procedure eliminates the risk of pregnancy in extramarital sex. Infidelity does not necessarily mean the spouse no longer loves the mate. Boredom, revenge, and testing sex appeal are some of the reasons for extramarital affairs. If an extramarital relationship is the present problem, the spouses may be more candid if the nurse interviews them separately and promises confidentiality.

One of the first problems mentioned by the majority of couples who seek marital therapy is lack of effective communication. As the nurse listens to the couple she may hear the following complaints about communicating:[34]

1. A narcissistic partner who is self-centered instead of attending to the marital relationship
2. Indifference in which the partner shows lack of concern through a negative approach toward the mate's feelings, needs, and wishes
3. Inability to reinforce and support the partner
4. Inflexibility as evidenced by rigid attitudes and values
5. Inexperience in positive and meaningful relationships
6. Crossed transactions that reflect a limited relationship between verbal and nonverbal communication
7. Avoidance maneuvers in which the mate communicates rejection by withdrawing
8. Distortion in which messages are sent to the partner but not received

The nurse determines the reasons for blocked communication. The most common reason is the presence of a secret that causes the partner to anticipate rejection by the nurse.[61] The four most frequent secrets that impede communication are: extramarital affairs, homosexuality, incestuous experience, or racial or religious prejudices.

Spiritual dimension. The following are considered when assessing the spiritual dimension. What are each partner's beliefs? Are their beliefs congruent with or complementary to each other's, or are they a source of conflict? Does each spouse's philosophy of life include a sense of commitment to the marital relationship and to the other? When it does, it may be a powerful motivator to solve marital problems.

The spiritually healthy spouse has the inner resources to experience the stresses that occur in a marriage and to transform them into growth experiences. Those whose spiritual health is limited are faced with threatening questions about the meaning of their lives. A wife may say, "If my mariage is over, it's the end of me!" Spouses who become aware of their expanded states of consciousness may find that awareness to be a source of strength.

Research Highlight

Personal Space: An Objective Measure of Marital Quality

D.R. Crane & W. Griffin

PURPOSE

The purpose of this study was to test the relevance of the personal space concept when applied to the marital relationship. Positive results would yield preliminary data on an objective measure of marital quality.

SAMPLE

Subjects were 24 married couples recruited primarily from clients (22) of marital therapy practicum students.

METHODOLOGY

The subjects were tested on three tests of marital adjustment:

1. The Marital Status Inventory (MSI) is a Guttman type of scale designed to evaluate a couple's divorce potential. Scores on this true-false inventory range from 0 to 14, with higher scores meaning greater instability.
2. The Locke-Wallace Marital Adjustment Test (MAT), a widely used measure of a couple's marital adjustment, has been used to distinguish distressed from nondistressed couples.
3. The Areas of Change (AOC) questionnaire yields an amount-of-conflict score (range 0 to 68) with 15 believed to discriminate distressed from nondistressed couples.

The couples were also asked to participate in two validated and widely used measures of space. The first was the Couples' Stop-Distance Space Measure, which is taken by asking each couple to stand some distance apart and then approach each other and stop at "a comfortable conversation distance." The distance between the couple's closest toes was then measured. The second space measure was the Couples' Chair Placement Space Measure, which is done by having the couple remove two chairs from a larger stack and place them on the floor. Then the distance between the chairs was measured after the couple left the room.

As each couple arrived for testing, they were given the packet of instruments, shown to the assessment room, and asked to take a seat and to complete the instruments independently. The couples' Stop-Distance Space Measure was taken nonrandomly before (13 couples) and after (11 couples) testing, primarily to ease the overflow of couples in the waiting area.

The couples' space measures were also tested to see if they could reliably differentiate between distressed and nondistressed couples. Two tests were conducted using previously established criterion measures. In the first test, couples were grouped using a 100 (couple mean) MAT score as the criterion. In the second test, couples were grouped using the AOC score of 15 as the criterion.

FINDINGS

The two measures of couples' space were found to correlate with the (MAT) in the expected direction. That is, the larger the space between the spouses, the lower the marital adjustment. In terms of the other dimensions of marriage, the results were mixed. The stop-distance measure correlated with the AOC but not the MSI. The chair placement measure correlated with the MSI but not the AOC.

In both tests the stop-distance measure was able to differentiate between distressed and nondistressed couples. The MAT-based test yielded a mean distance of 9.79 inches for nondistressed couples and 16.95 inches for distressed. The AOC-based test yielded similar results, 9.40 and 18.30, respectively. However, no difference in distance was found on the chair placement measure.

IMPLICATIONS

The personal space concepts seem to logically apply to marital therapy concepts. The results of the study support the value of applying the concept of personal space to marital research. The correlations between space and marital measures are consistent but not strong. Additional work in refining the personal space measures, studying the influence of other variables (for example, culture and intimacy level), and using larger samples is necessary before valid generalizations can be made.

Based on data from Journal of Marital and Family Therapy 9(3):325, 1983.

Many modern couples have a firm faith in God or a supreme being and find that their shared faith assists them in tolerating the irritations of their life together. Others, who may have had religious education and participated in the religious rituals appropriate to their age and maturity, may drop out of organized religion. They may retain some faith in a Supreme Being or a higher power, but the belief may have limited influence on their life-styles. Such couples may be wed in a civil ceremony. Later, when conflict occurs, instead of having a strong desire to solve the problems, they may choose to dissolve the marriage.

The couple's religious beliefs also influence other decisions. In some faiths children are perceived as the purpose of a marital union and no efforts to limit family size are permitted. In other faiths various birth control measures and abortion are permissible. As long as the couple's practices are congruent with their religious beliefs and each spouse's beliefs are in harmony with the other's, marital conflict may not occur. When there is dissonance, serious marital problems may result.

Strongly held, incompatible beliefs may support increased distance and blaming, as in the following Case Example.

Case Example

Mamie was reared in a particular religious faith, was a devout follower, and wanted her two children to attend worship services with her. Roland, her husband, had a very strong faith in a different religious belief that taught him that only those faithful to that belief could achieve salvation. Roland insisted that their children attend worship services with him and was extremely disapproving of Mamie because she would not convert. Mamie complained of feeling deeply depressed most of the time.

At times one or the other spouse may be very creative and feel an intense need to be free to make choices. When the other spouse supports the creativity and freedom, the marriage relationship is helped to flourish. Likewise, when there are restrictions placed on the creative spouse's freedom, the person may become dysfunctional, may distance himself from the other, or may rebel and generate conflict.

Analysis

Nursing diagnosis. The following list provides examples of NANDA-accepted nursing diagnoses with causative statements that apply to marital therapy:

1. Impaired verbal communication related to failure to listen
2. Ineffective individual coping related to marital discord
3. Sexual dysfunction related to extramarital affair
4. Impaired social interaction related to overinvolvement in community activities

DSM-III-R diagnoses. The DSM-III-R diagnosis related to marital therapy is V61.10, marital problem. There are no defining features or manifestations for this disorder. This category may be used when the marital problem is not caused by a mental disorder—for example, marital conflict related to infidelity or divorce.

Planning

Table 30-3 provides long-term goals and short-term goals and outcome criteria related to marital therapy. These serve as examples of the planning stage of the nursing process.

Implementation

Physical dimension. When the couple is experiencing marital discord related to chronic medical problems, the nurse refers them to social services if the problem is financial. A community health nurse may be another useful source for services. The couple is informed that since physical problems sometimes mask interpersonal difficulties, they need to make an effort to resolve medical problems to have energy to work on the other factors causing marital stress. If one or both spouses have a chemical dependence problem, the nurse refers them to Alcoholics Anonymous, Alanon, or a drug treatment program. Also ground rules are established at the first sesison that neither spouse can attend the marital therapy session if inebriated or on illicit drugs.

TABLE 30-3 Long-term and short-term goals and outcome criteria related to marital therapy

Goals	Outcome Criteria
NURSING DIAGNOSIS: MARITAL DISCORD RELATED TO HUSBAND'S EXCESSIVE DRINKING	
Long-term goals	
To decide whether to continue the marriage	Sees a marriage therapist.
	Discusses reasons for and against continuing the mariage.
	Both partners make a commitment to the decision made.
	Talks about problems that drinking brings about.
For wife to experience satisfactions with other relationships	Spends time with family and friends.
	Participates in activities that are pleasurable for her.
	Makes statements that reflect pleasure.
For husband to decrease drinking sprees	Spends time with wife without drinking.
	Drinks without getting drunk.
	Seeks help to control drinking (counseling, AA).
Short-term goals	
To deal with negative feelings constructively	States negative feelings to therapist and spouse using "I" statements.
	Makes eye contact when speaking.
	Identifies causes of negative feelings.
	Accepts negative feelings as each partner's own.
	Engages in physical activity to use the energy.
To know that each partner can choose other ways to respond	States other ways to respond to partner's behavior.
	Practices other ways of responding.
	Talks about what it feels like to receive different responses.
To express positive feelings to partner	States things liked about each other.
	Plans ways to increase enjoyable times together.
To agree to refrain from blaming and name-calling	States mutual agreement.
	Refrains from blaming and name calling.

Genetic counseling may be indicated if the couple has a child with a genetic defect. The couple needs to discuss thoughts and feelings related to the child in the marital therapy sessions.

The nurse provides an opportunity for the couple to discuss changes in body image and physical illnesses that have affected their marital relationship, including sexual functioning. The nurse may need to do some teaching about limitations in sexual activity. (See Chapter 31 for additional interventions in sexual dysfunction.)

❋ *Emotional dimension.* Early in the therapy the nurse shares her observations of and reinforces any positive feelings the partners have for each other. This intervention may increase their awareness of feelings they thought no longer existed. If the negative feelings are not overwhelming, the nurse may gently encourage but not force each spouse to share a positive feeling he or she has for the other mate.

The couple needs to know early that beneath the anger may be unresolved hurt and that once the anger is resolved, they may experience increased intimacy. L'Abate and L'Abate[60] describe five steps as guidelines for couples to deal with anger:

1. When there is anger, recognize that there is also hurt.
2. Address these hurt feelings and express them to the spouse in terms of "I feel . . . ." Or "It hurts me when you . . . ."
3. Avoid projecting feelings onto the other spouse and assume responsibility for your own hurt.
4. Forgive yourself for trying to be perfect and invulnerable by trying to deny awareness of hurt feelings.
5. Redefine the self, in terms of errors and weaknesses, as human, not "crazy." Do not demand invulnerability (superman and superwoman) of yourself.

With guidance from the nurse, the couple uses these guidelines to examine and resolve anger and hurt.

The nurse can instruct the couple to keep a separate written record of any situation or behavior that causes anger or anxiety and bring it to the session for discussion. The nurse asks them to keep the information confidential until they get to the session so that they can compare similarities and differences in their experiences.[34]

It is important that the nurse allow the couple to ventilate feelings and experience some relief at the first session. The nurse clearly states to the couple that physical violence is not allowed. This rule may help lessen the couple's fear that they will lose control of their emotions, especially anger.

By having both spouses identify and label feelings, the nurse assists them to become responsible for learning means to cope with the feeling. Once feelings are expressed constructively guilt may decrease.

If one of the spouses is depressed, as the couple begins resolving the marital conflict the depression may lift. When the depression is severe, measures discussed in Chapter 14 may be used.

✺ *Intellectual dimension.* The nurse guides the couple to recognize and examine their defense mechanisms. Confrontation is used as she assists them to face reality. The nurse may use a moderately directive approach and provide information about the problem that she discerned during the assessment.

The couple is guided to explain what is interfering with their ability to solve problems. If necessary they are taught the problem-solving process. The nurse discusses the steps in the process, and sometimes homework can be useful in this effort. The couple is directed to arrive at some consensus about a problem and to discuss the problem solving approach they used at the next session.

✻ *Social dimension.* Once a secret is revealed, the nurse lets the spouse decide whether to share the secret with the other spouse. Revealing a secret can clear the air, and therapeutic work can continue.[34]

Initially the nurse intervenes in the dysfunctional communication by concentrating on the process of communication between the partners. After a positive two-way process is established, she focuses on the content of the couple's messages. Each partner is assisted to think about what he wants to say, say it accurately, and check to see if the partner got the messages. The nurse guides the spouses to rephrase, restate, and clarify unclear issues. She teaches and models appropriate and open communication. She can have the couple use role-playing to share their perception of the dysfunctional communication and learn new ways to communicate their needs. They are guided to listen, make eye contact, and speak one at a time. The nurse discusses the role-playing and helps each spouse see how he contributes to the problem. The partners learn to take responsibility for accuracy in their communication by using "I" statements instead of "It." The couple also learns to make statements instead of asking questions. Gradually each spouse assumes responsibility for the communication problem and learns to communicate more clearly and accurately.

When the partners have limited social contacts and spend too little time together, they can be guided to talk with each other about their favorite activities and make arrangements to alternate activities so that each one has a chance to have fun with the other. They can also be encouraged to seek social opportunities and to make new friends.

✳ *Spiritual dimension.* When both spouses view their spirituality as a source of strength, the nurse reinforces their belief and helps them explore ways this strength may be used to resolve the marital conflict. She guides the couple in a discussion of similarities and differences in their religious beliefs, and when incongruent, she guides them to explore compromises. If the couple did not seek counseling from their religious leader before coming for marital therapy, the nurse can refer them to that person. This intervention may be especially helpful when the couple is considering separation or divorce against their religious teaching. Referral to a religious leader may also be appropriate when the spouses values about birth control are in conflict.

Evaluation

When the therapeutic experience is effective, the spouses have improved their coping skills, communicate with each other effectively, and feel confident about their problem solving. Often their feelings for each other are warmer and they are more effective in expressing tenderness and affection. They have found ways to appreciate each other's values, to exchange ideas objectively, and to share joy as well as sadness and disappointment. The couple is able to recognize the need for and seek assistance in the future before problems becoming overwhelming.

BRIEF REVIEW

Marital therapy is a treatment modality directed toward ameliorating the problems of couples, irrespective of their marital status. Theoretical approaches to marital therapy include psychoanalytic, behavioral, systems, and humanistic-existential. Object relations is the aspect of psychoanalytic theory that can be most effectively applied to marital therapy.

The specific role and goals of the marital therapist are dictated by the therapist's theoretical orientation. All marital therapists assume the role of teacher and educator. There are pros and cons regarding the use of cotherapists. Clients for marital therapy are primarily self-referred; however, they may be referred by the court or persons such as ministers, lawyers, and teachers. In the treatment of couples the nurse selects interventions that are appropriate to the clients and their life circumstances.

REFERENCES AND SUGGESTED READINGS

1. Adler, A.: The neurotic constitution, New York, 1917. Moffat, Yard & Co. (Translated by B. Blueck and J.E. Lind.)
2. Alexander, J., and Cohen, J.: Customs, coupling, and the family in a changing culture, American Journal of Orthopsychiatry **51**(2):307, 1981.
2a. Alger, T.: Multiple couple therapy. In Guerin, P.J., Jr., editor: Family therapy, New York, 1976, Gardner Press.
3. American Association for Marriage and Family Therapy: Membership standards, Uplands, Calif., 1978, The Association. (Pamphlet.)
4. American Association for Marriage and Family Therapy Commission on Accreditation receives Dept. of Education approval, AAMFT Newsletter 12:1, January 1981.
5. American Institute of Family Relations: Final program: The 100th Conference of the American Institute of Family Relations on the Successful Family, October 4-5, 1940, at Occidental College, Los Angeles, The Institute.
6. American Psychiatric Association: Diagnostic and statistical manual of mental disorders, Washington, D.C., 1987, The Association.
7. American Psychiatric Association: A psychiatric glossary, ed. 5, Boston, 1980, Little, Brown & Co.
8. Bader, E., and others: Do marriage preparation programs really work? Journal of Marriage and Family Therapy **6**(2):171, 1980.
9. Bagarozzi, D.A., Jurich, A.P., and Jackson, R.N., editors: In marital and family therapy: new perspective in theory, research and practice, New York, 1983, Human Sciences Press, Inc.
10. Ball, J.D., and Henning, L.H.: Rational suggestions for premarital counseling, Journal of Marriage and Family Therapy **7**(1):69, 1981.
11. Baruth, L.G., and Huber, C.H.: An introduction to marital therapy and theory, Monterey, Calif., 1984, Brook/Cole Publishing Co.
12. Berman, E., Lief, H., and Williams, A.M.: A model of marital interaction. In Sholevar, G.P.: A handbook of marriage and marital therapy, Jamaica, N.Y., 1981, Spectrum Publications, Inc.
13. Bjorksten, O.J.W.: New clinical concepts in marital therapy, Washington, D.C., 1985, American Psychiatric Press.
14. Black, C.: It will never happen to me, Denver, 1981, M.A.C., Printing and Publications Division.
15. Bloom, B.L., and others: A preventive intervention program for the newly separated: final evaluations, American Journal of Orthopsychiatry **55**(1), 1985.
16. Bodin, A.M.: The interactional view: family therapy approaches of the Mental Research Institute. In Gurman, A.S., and Kniskern, D.P., editors: Handbook of family therapy, New York, 1981, Brunner/Mazel, Inc.
17. Bowen, M.: Family therapy and family group therapy. In Olson, D., editor: Treating relationships, Lake Mills, Iowa, 1976, Graphic Publishing Co., Inc.
18. Bowen, M.: Theory in the practice of psychotherapy. In Guerin, P.J., Jr., editor: Family therapy, New York, 1976, Gardner Press.
19. Bowen, M.: Family therapy in clinical practice, New York, 1978, Jason Aronson, Inc.
20. Bowman, H.: Marriage education in college, New York, 1942, McGraw-Hill Book Co.
21. Broderick, B., and Schrader, S.S.: History of professional marriage and family therapy. In Gurman, A.S., and Kniskern, D.P., editors: Handbook of family therapy, New York, 1981, Brunner/Mazel, Inc.
22. Clark, T.E.: Marital therapy and mental health, AAMFT Newsletter **8**(4):10, 1977.
23. Dicks, H.: Marital tensions, New York, 1967, Basic Books, Inc., Publishers.
24. Epstein, N., and Williams, A.M.: Behavioral approaches to the treatment of marital discord. In Sholevar, G.P., editor: The handbook of marriage and marital therapy, Jamaica, N.Y., 1981, Spectrum Publications, Inc.
25. Fairbairn, W.R.D.: An object-relations theory of personality, New York, 1952, Basic Books, Inc., Publishers.
26. Fine, M., and Hovestad, A.J.: Perceptions of marriage and rationality by levels of perceived health in the family of origin, Journal of Marital and Family Therapy **10**(2):193, 1984.
27. Fish, R.C., and Fish, L.S.: Quid pro quo revisited: the basis of marital therapy, American Journal of Orthopsychiatry **56**(3):371, 1986.
28. Fogarty, T.F.: Marital crisis. In Guerin, P.J., Jr., editor: Family therapy, New York, 1976, Gardner Press.
29. Fogarty, T.F.: Fusion, The Family **4**(2):49, 1977.
30. Fogarty, T.F.: The distancer and pursuer, The Family **7**(1):11, 1979.
31. Freud, S.: Analysis: terminable and interminable. In Strachey, J., editor: Collected papers, vol. 5, New York, 1959, Basic Books, Inc., Publishers.
32. Gilbert, R.: The public health nurse and her patient, Cambridge, Mass. 1951, The Commonwealth Fund.
33. Gravitz, H., and Bowden, J.: Guide to recovery: a book for adult children of alcoholics, Holmes Beach, Fla., 1985, Learning Publications, Inc.
34. Greene, B.L.: A clinical approach to marital problems: diagnosis, prevention, and treatment, ed. 2, Springfield, IL, 1981, Charles C Thomas, Publisher.
35. Groves, E.R., and Groves, G.H.: The contemporary American family, Chicago, 1947, J.B. Lippincott Co.
36. Gurman, A.S.: Dimensions of marital therapy: a comparative analysis, Journal of Marriage and Family Therapy **5**(1):5, 1979.

37. Gurman, A.S., and Kniskern, D.P.: Research on marital and family therapy. In Garfield, S.L., and Bergin, A.E., editors: Handbook of psychotherapy and behavior change: an empirical analysis, ed. 2, New York, 1978, John Wiley & Sons, Inc.

38. Haley, J.: Problem-solving therapy, San Francisco, 1976, Jossey-Bass, Inc., Publishers.

39. Hamburg, S.R.: Leaving the consulting room to provoke enactment in marital therapy, Journal of Marital and Family Therapy 11(2):187, 1985.

40. Humphrey, H.G.: Presidential address for American Association of Marriage and Family Therapists, Houston, October 1978.

41. Humphrey, F.G.: Marital therapy, Englewood Cliffs, N.J., 1983, Prentice-Hall, Inc.

42. Im, W., Wilner, R.S., and Breit, M.: Jealousy: interventions in couples therapy, Family Process 22(2):211, 1983.

43. Jackson, D.D.: The question of family homeostasis, Psychiatric Quarterly Supplement 31:79, 1957.

44. Jackson, D.D.: Family interactions, family homeostasis, and some implications for conjoint family therapy. In Masserman, J., editor: Individual and family dynamics, New York, 1959, Grune & Stratton, Inc.

45. Jacobson, N.S.: Specific and non-specific factors in the effectiveness of behavioral approach to the treatment of marital discord, Journal of Consulting and Clinical Psychology 42:203, 1974.

46. Jacobson, N.S.: Training couples to solve their marital problems: behavioral approach to relationship discord. I. Problem-solving skills, International Journal of Family Counseling 5(1):22, 1977.

47. Jacobson, N.S.: Training couples to solve their marital problems: behavioral approach to relationship discord. II. Intervention strategies, International Journal of Family Counseling 5(2):20, 1977.

48. Jacobson, N.S.: A stimulus control model of change in behavioral couples' therapy: implications for contingency contracting, Journal of Marriage and Family Counseling 4(2):51, 1978.

49. Jacobson, N.S.: Increasing positive behavior in severely distressed marital relationships: the effects of problem-solving training, Behavior Therapy 10:311, 1979.

50. Jacobson, N.S.: Behavior marital therapy. In Gurman, A.S., and Kniskern, D.P., editors: Handbook of family therapy, New York, 1981, Brunner/Mazel, Inc.

51. Jacobson, N.S., and Gurman, A.S., editors: In Clinical handbook of marital therapy, New York, 1986, The Guilford Press.

52. Jacobson, N.S., and Margolin, G.: Marital therapy: strategies based on social learning and behavior exchange principles, New York, 1979, Brunner/Mazel, Inc.

53. Jacobson, N.S., and Weiss, R.L.: Behavioral marriage therapy. III. The contents of Gurman et al. may be hazardous to your health, Family Process 17:149, 1978.

54. Jung, C.: The association method, American Journal of Psychology 21:219, 1910.

55. Justice, B., and Justice, R.: The abusing family, New York, 1976, Human Sciences Press.

56. Kerr, M.: Bowen theory and therapy. In Sholevar, G.P., editor: The handbook of marriage and marital therapy, Jamaica, N.Y., 1981, Spectrum Publications, Inc.

57. Kim, M., McFarland, G., and McLane, A.M.: Classification of nursing diagnoses, St. Louis, 1984, The C.V. Mosby Co.

58. Kubie, L.S.: Psychoanalysis and marriage: practical and theoretical issues. In Eisenstein, V.W., editor: Neurotic interaction in marriage, New York, 1956, Basic Books, Inc., Publishers.

59. L'Abate, L.: Skill training for couples and families. In Gurman, A.S., and Kniskern, D.P., editors: Handbook of family therapy, New York, 1981, Brunner/Mazel, Inc.

60. L'Abate, L., and L'Abate, B.L.: The paradoxes of intimacy, Family Therapy 6:175, 1979.

61. L'Abate L., and McHenry, S., editors: Handbook of marital interventions, New York, 1983, Grune & Stratton, Inc.

62. Leahey, M.: Findings from research on divorce: implications for professional skill development, American Journal of Orthopsychiatry 54(2):298, 1982.

63. Lester, G.W., Beckham, E., and Buncom, D.: Implementation of behavioral marital therapy, Journal of Marriage and Family Therapy 6(2):189, 1980.

64. Lieberman, E.J.: Couples group psychotherapy. In Simpkinson, C.H., and others, editors: Synopsis of the first annual Maryland/District of Columbia/Virginia Network Symposium, Olney, Md., 1978, Family Therapy Practice Network.

65. Lieberman, E.J.: Essay review: the first thirty years of family therapy, Journal of Marriage and Family Therapy 7:395, 1981.

66. Mace, D.R.: Marriage guidance in England, Marriage and Family Living 7:1, 1945.

67. Markowitz, M., and Kadis, A.L.: Short-term analytic treatment in a group by a therapist couple. In Sager, C.J., and Kaplan, H.S., editors: Progress in group and family therapy, New York, 1972, Brunner/Mazel, Inc.

68. McGoldrick, M., and Preto, N.G.: Ethnic intermarriage: implications for therapy, Family Process 23(3):347, 1984.

69. Mikesell, R.: Therapy with couples living together. In Simpkinson, C.H., and others, editors: Synopsis of the first annual Maryland/District of Columbia/Virginia Network Symposium, Olney, Md., 1978, Family Therapy Practice Network.

70. Morofka, V.: Marital therapy from a systems approach, Perspectives in Psychiatric Care 22(4):145, 1984.

71. Mudd, E.H., and Fowler, D.R.: The AAMC and AAMFC: nearly forty years of form and function. In Ard. B.N., Jr., editor: Handbook of marriage counseling, ed. 2, Palo Alto, Calif., 1976, Science & Behavior Books, Inc.

72. Mudd, E.H., and others, editors: Marriage counseling, a casebook, New York, 1958, Association Press.

73. Nadelson, C.C., and Polonsky, D.C., editors: Marriage and divorce, New York, 1984, The Guilford Press.

74. Nelson, J.C.: Family treatment: an integrated approach, Englewood Cliffs, N.J., 1983, Prentice-Hall, Inc.

75. O'Leary, K.D., and Turkewitz, H.: Marital therapy from a behavioral perspective. In Paolino, T.J., and McCrady, B.S., editors: Marriage and marital therapy: psychoanalytic, behavioral and systems theory perspectives, New York, 1978, Brunner/Mazel, Inc.

76. O'Leary, K.D., and Turkewitz, H.A.: A comparative outcome study of behavioral marital therapy, Journal of Marriage and Family Therapy 7(2):159, 1981.

77. Papp, P.: Staging reciprocal metaphors in a couples group, Family Process 21(4):453, 1982.

78. Pittman, F.S., III, and Flomenhaft, K.: Treating the doll's house marriage. In Sager, C.J., and Kaplan, H.S., editors: Progress in group and family therapy, New York, 1972, Brunner/Mazel, Inc.

79. Price-Bonham, S., and Murphy, D.C.: Dual career marriages: implications for the clinician, Journal of Marriage and Family Therapy 6(2):181, 1980.

80. Rappaport, A.F., and Harrell, J.A.: A behavioral-exchange model for marital counseling, Family Coordinator 21:203, 1972.

81. Sager, C.J.: Marriage contracts and couple therapy; hidden forces in intimate relationships, New York, 1976, Brunner/Mazel, Inc.

82. Sager, C.J.: Couples therapy and marriage contracts. In Gurman, A.S., and Kniskern, D.P., editors: Handbook of family therapy, New York, 1981, Brunner/Mazel, Inc.

83. Sager, C.J., and others: The marriage contract. In Sager, C.J., and Kaplan, H.S., editors: Progress in group and family therapy, New York, 1972, Brunner/Mazel, Inc.

84. Schaefer, M.T., and Olson, D.H.: Assessing intimacy: the PAIR inventory, Journal of Marriage and Family Therapy 7(1):47, 1981.

85. Skynner, A.C.R.: An open-systems, group-analytic approach to family therapy. In Gurman, A.S., and Kniskern, D.P., editors: Handbook of family therapy, New York, 1981, Brunner/Mazel, Inc.

86. Sluzki, C.: Marital therapy from a systems theory perspective. In Paolino, T., and McCrady, B., editors: Marriage and marital therapy: psychoanalytic, behavioral, and systems theory perspectives, New York, 1978, Brunner/Mazel, Inc.

87. Sonne, J.C., and Swirsky, D.: Self-object considerations in marriage and marital therapy. In Sholevar, G.P., editor: The handbook of marriage and marital therapy, Jamaica, N.Y., 1981, Spectrum Publications, Inc.

88. Spark, G.M.: Marriage is a family affair: an intergenerational approach to marital therapy. In Sholevar, G.P., editor: The handbook of marriage and marital therapy, Jamaica, N.Y., 1981, Spectrum Publications, Inc.

89. Stanton, M.D.: Marital therapy from a structural/strategic viewpoint. In Sholevar, G.P., editor: The handbook of marriage and marital therapy, Jamaica, N.Y., 1981, Spectrum Publications, Inc.

90. Steinglass, P., Tislenko, L., and Reiss, D.: Stability/instability in the alcoholic marriage: the interrelationships between course of alcoholism, family process, and marital outcome, Family Process 24(3):365, 1985

91. Stone, A.: Marriage education and marriage counseling in the United States, Marriage and Family Living 11:38, 1949.

92. Strayhorn, J.M.: Behavioral concepts and methods for dyads, workshop presented at Associated Catholic Charities Marital Therapy Seminar, Baltimore, November 6, 1981. (Slides.)

93. Stuart, R.B.: Operant interpersonal treatment for marital discord. In Sager, C.J., and Kaplan, H.S., editors: Progress in group and family therapy, New York, 1972, Brunner/Mazel.

94. Watzlawick, P., Brown, J., and Jackson, D.: Pragmatics of human communication, New York, 1967, W.W. Norton & Co.

95. Wegscheider, S.: Another chance: hope and health for the alcoholic family, Palo Alto, Calif., 1981, Science and Behavior Books, Inc.

96. Weinstein, R.K.: Bowen's family systems theory as exemplified in Bergman's "Scenes from a Marriage," Perspectives in Psychiatric Care 19(5 and 6):157, 1981.

97. Wells, R.A., and Giannetti, V.J.: Individual marital therapy: a critical reappraisal, Family Process 25(1):43, 1986.

98. Whitaker, C.A.: Making marriage work, Chicago. 1970. Instructional Dynamics. (Ten cassette audiotapes.)

99. Whitaker, C.A., Greenberg, A., and Greenberg, M.I.: Existential marital therapy: a synthesis, a subsystem of existential family therapy. In Sholevar, G.P., editor: A handbook of marriage and marital therapy, Jamaica, N.Y., 1981, Spectrum Publications, Inc.

100. Willi, J.: The concept of collusion: a combined systemic-psychodynamic approach to marital therapy, Family Process 23(2):177, 1984.

101. Williams, A.M., and Miller, W.R.: Evaluation and research on marital therapy. In Sholevar, G.P., editor: The handbook of marriage and marital therapy, Jamaica, N.Y., 1981, Spectrum Publications, Inc.

ANNOTATED BIBLIOGRAPHY

Jacobson, N.S.: Behavioral marital therapy. In In Gurman, A.S., and Kniskern, D.P., editors: Handbook of family therapy, New York, 1981, Brunner/Mazel, Inc.

Behavioral theory evolved from operant conditioning with children. Jacobson recognized that conditions for adults were different and required the spouses to negotiate with one another. Patterson and Hops[98] and Jacobson and Weiss [70] added communication and problem-solving skills to operant programs. They have named the method *behavioral marital therapy* (BMT). The model is the social learning model. BMT assumes that maintenance and enduring success of a marital relationship depend primarily on the characteristics of the partners' exchanges and the environmental forces that impinge on them rather than on any preordained, historically shaped personality characteristics.

Magran, B.: Transactional analysis in marital therapy. In Sholevar, G.P., editor: The handbook of marriage and marital therapy, Jamaica, N.Y., 1981, Spectrum Publications, Inc.

Transactional analysis theory for marital therapy combines rational, emotional, and behavioral approaches. Theories were developed by Eric Berne, a psychiatrist. The therapy is contractual, involving a clear, succinct statement of each partner's treatment goals. It is based on ego states, transactions, strokes, games, and scripts. The goal is to enable the couple to have an honest, open, and intimate relationship.

Pollack, O.: Discussion of psychodynamic theories of marital therapy. In Sholevar, G.P., editor: The handbook of marriage and marital therapy, Jamaica, N.Y., 1981, Spectrum Publications Inc.

This chapter is an overview and critique. Pollack calls attention to our debt to psychoanalysis and observes that the therapeutic goal setting is different. In psychoanalysis Freud was not exactly optimistic, and his goal was to help neurotics to achieve what normal people accomplish for themselves without help.[44] In marital therapy the clients and therapists are optimistic and their goal is a better life.

Sager, C.J.: Couples therapy and marriage contracts. In Gurman, A.S., and Kniskern, D.P., editors: Handbook of family therapy, New York, 1981, Brunner/Mazel, Inc.

Sager describes a schema in which he asserts that individual intrapsychic factors determine the system and in turn are affected by the interaction in the system of the couple. In addition, Sager alerts the therapist to consider determinants of interactions. He includes a typology of marriages and uses an eclectic therapeutic approach.

Individual contracts, as described by Sager, are verbalized and conscious. The parameters may be based on the expectations of marriage, on intrapsychic and biological needs, or on external foci. Sager's typology of marriage is presented in seven profiles of couples and in two-partner combinations.

Sholevar, G.P., editor: The handbook on marriage and marital therapy, Jamaica, N.Y., 1981, Spectrum Publications, Inc.

This book is a collection of excellent chapters on theory and techniques of marital therapy. The contributors include many highly respected therapists, educators, and authors. Among them are Ivan Boszormenyi-Nagy, Norman Epstein, Florence Kaslow, Michael Kerr, Stephen B. Levine, E. James Lieberman, Harold Lief, William R. Miller, Clifford Sager, Jong C. Sonne, Geraldine Spark, M. Duncan Stanton, and Carl A. Whitaker. The chapters cover 11 theoretical approaches and 12 descriptions of techniques. It is an extremely valuable reference for students and marital therapy practitioners.

C H A P T E R
31

SEX THERAPY

Rose Therese Bahr

After studying this chapter the learner will be able to:

Discuss the historical development of sex therapy.

Define sex therapy.

Discuss theoretical approaches to sexual dysfunctions.

Describe the qualifications, goals, and role of the sex therapist.

Apply the nursing process to management of sexual dysfunctions.

Identify current research findings on sexual dysfunctions.

Human *sexuality* is sexual orientation plus the sensations, attitudes, thoughts, beliefs, feelings, and actions related to that orientation and their effects on personality and relationships. The sexual self is composed of *gender identity* and *gender role*. Gender identity is an internal sense of sexual self—that one is male or female. Gender role is an expression of maleness or femaleness and is learned.

The sexually healthy person has the ability to enjoy and control sexual behavior according to personal and social ethics. He is also free from physical disease impairing sexual function; from fear, shame, and guilt; and from misconceptions hindering sexual relationships and responses.

Problems with any aspect of sexuality are *sexual dysfunctions;* treatment is *sex therapy.* A knowledgeable and competent sex therapist facilitates identification of the problem and its resolution.

An estimated 50% of couples in the United States experience some type of sexual dysfunction during their life.[12] Some may need only information or education on communicating better. Others may need brief psychotherapy to promote behavioral change. Others may benefit from more in-depth therapy, long-term psychoanalysis, or sex therapy.

THEORETICAL APPROACHES
Psychoanalytic

Freud[13] was the first to call attention to the importance of sexual conflict in human behavior. He believed that sexual conflicts are the root of all psychopathological conditions. He described sexual disturbances as an unconscious conflict between enjoying sexual satisfaction and fear of punishment and guilt. This fear is learned as a child and reevoked by adult sexual experiences.

Freud stated that the unconscious component of the psyche contains repressed sexual thoughts, which are intolerable to the ego and therefore pushed into the unconscious. Although the thought or wish is unconscious, it seeks expression. Forbidden sexual wishes strive for satisfaction in ways the individual is unaware of and may lead to sexual dysfunctions. Therapy attempts to make the unconscious conscious, overcome resistances, reveal ways that sexual conflicts are kept from awareness, and help redirect energy to more appropriate and less self-defeating ways of satisfying needs. (See Chapter 3 for a further discussion of Freud's theory of psychosexual development.)

Erikson[11] addressed sexuality specifically in the adolescent developmental stage of identity versus role confusion. Adolescent love is an attempt to define self by projecting bits of identity onto a partner. Through the partner's responses the adolescent gradually clarifies the

🍇 *Historical Overview* 🍇

DATE	EVENT
Early 1900's	Until the 1940s sexual dysfunctions were considered symptoms of deep-seated disturbances from early childhood trauma. Treatment was lengthy psychoanalysis.
1948	The Kinsey Reports on sexual behavior in men and women startled readers with their explicit reports.
1950s	Behavioral therapy used directive approaches to sexual problems successfully. It focused on current behavior rather than past causes.
1960s	Sex researchers Masters and Johnson combined psychoanalysis and behavioral and educative approaches to manage sexual problems with the couple as the client. Their studies on human sexual response opened the door for sex therapy.
1970s	Sex therapy became a full-fledged discipline, and literature on human sexuality proliferated. The Sex Information and Educational Council of the United States (SIECUS), formed in 1972, became a highly influential agency for sex education.
1976	The Hite Report proposed a new theory of women's sexuality.
1980s	Literature abounds on the sexual issues of women; the aged; persons with illnesses, injuries, and handicaps; and persons with alternative life-styles. The openness and permissiveness toward sexual activity today contributes to the recognition of sexual dysfunctions and the acceptance of sex therapy as a treatment for reestablishing, maintaining, and enhancing sexual functioning.
Future	The current escalation of sexually transmitted diseases such as herpes and AIDS may contribute to people altering their sexual lifestyles, and nurses will be called on increasingly for sex education, counseling, and therapy.

relationship, and a more complete identity evolves. When identity is not clarified, identity confusion results. The individual expresses doubt about his sexual self and his role in society.

Intimacy and sharing emerge in the young adult developmental stage, according to Erikson. Relationships with the opposite sex provide opportunities to develop a long-term relationship with another. Frequently sexual expression emerges prematurely. An adolescent not ready for sexual activity may experience marked confusion. For example, many feel pushed into sexual activity in the belief that they can "find themselves" in another. However, the experience does not lead to resolution of identity needs, and more serious problems may result, such as pregnancy, premature marriage, or sexual dysfunctions in later life.

When a young adult fails to learn intimacy, isolation may occur. He feels incompetent, unattractive, stupid, and awkward. If the feelings persist, he may withdraw or fantasize excessively.

Developmental

Havighurst[16] related various developmental tasks to sexual behavior through the life cycle. As one successfully completes tasks at each stage, he is able to feel pleased with himself and his life.

One task of infancy and early childhood is to learn sex differences. The child has no clear concept of "boy" or "girl" until he sees genital differences. Observations usually occur at 2 or 3 years of age, depending on contacts with parents, siblings, and other children. The child's increasing interest in sex is part of his natural curiosity. He is actively interested in toilet activities and explores his body and others'.

Learning an appropriate masculine or feminine role is the task of middle childhood. Gender identity and role are solidified through peer associations during school years. Boys and girls adopt exclusive rules and games that reinforce masculine and feminine roles.

The tasks of adolescence are to achieve new, more mature relationships with both sexes and a masculine or feminine social role. The peer group is a forum for exploring thoughts and feelings about sexuality and roles. It eases the transition into adulthood by providing security while the adolescent withdraws from emotional dependence on his family. Armed with the new security, the adolescent moves into new relationships with both sexes.

When these tasks are mastered, early adulthood becomes a time for selecting a sex partner, learning to live with the partner, and often rearing children. When these tasks are not mastered, problems with sexual identity, relationships, and sexual functioning may occur.

Learning

Kaplan[22] viewed sexual dysfunctions as the result of an earlier negative sexual experience. Dysfunctional symptoms are learned inhibitions, acquired from conditioning and reinforcement. This process occurs entirely outside the person's awareness, and once the conditioning response is established, it is often beyond conscious control. For example, an *erection* in response to penile stimulation is a natural reflex. However, if it is followed by fear or guilt, the individual learns to inhibit this response.

Kaplan believed that sexual dysfunction arises from an antierotic environment created by the couple that is destructive to the sexuality of one or both partners. Openness and trust allow partners to abandon themselves fully to sexual experience. But anxiety, fear of failure or rejection, unstimulating sexual behavior, or lack of communication create an environment not conducive to adequate sexual functioning. He emphasized that sexual differences are not expressions of one person's conflict but products of the relationship. Therapy involves both partners. Relationship problems include partner rejection, lack of trust, tension between partners' roles or expectations, transferences, power struggles, contractual disappointments, sexual sabotage (such as making oneself repulsive), and inadequate communication.

Kaplan also saw deeper kinds of sexual conflicts rooted in culture that predispose an individual to sexual dysfunction. Negative attitudes and restrictive child-rearing practices contaminate the pleasure-seeking sexual instinct and impair sexual functioning.

Kaplan believed that modifying the immediate causes of dysfunction is essential for relieving the target symptoms. Although deeper psychological and interpersonal influences may underlie the symptoms, the focus is on relieving the client's dysfunction and ensuring that the disability does not recur. Psychoanalytical and transactional material is interpreted and neurotic behavior modified if they directly influence the dysfunction or create obstacles to treatment.

Kaplan's approach is a combination of prescribed sexual exercises and psychotherapy. Kaplan[36] noted that 80% of clients with sexual dysfunction are freed of symptoms when psychotherapy is coupled with sexual exercises. Through psychotherapy immediate and deeper causes of dysfunction can be overcome. The crucial ingredient of the therapy is the partner's participation in sexual exercises to arouse each other. The tasks include unlearning destructive behavior, becoming conscious of one's own sensuous feelings, resolving fear, enhancing sexual pleasures, and learning new positive behaviors. When the partners resolve their defenses against sexuality or resistance to the treatment process, dysfunction is overcome.

Effective sexual experiences from Kaplan's approach have the following rationale: (1) the prescribed sexual experiences change the destructive sexual system and create a sexual environment in which the couple makes love in a freer, more enjoyable way; (2) when previously avoided sexual acts are carried out, resolution of the underlying conflict is facilitated; and (3) the sexual tasks bring out unconscious interpersonal and psychological conflicts for discussion and resolution in psychotherapy.

Masters and Johnson[28,29] believe the sexual response is a natural response. Therapy consists of (1) ruling out any pathophysiological conditions in a thorough physical examination and (2) identifying basic psychosocial aspects that might affect sexual functioning such as anxiety, depression, or physical stress. A basic assumption is that sexual behavior is learned, but the potential to respond to sexual stimuli is instinctual. When there are barriers to this biological potential, disruptions of the natural physiological functions occur, creating obstacles to sexual functioning. Negative attitudes need to be replaced with positive ones and an environment made conducive to healthy response. When these obstacles are withdrawn or modified, natural functioning can take place.[28,29]

Several basic treatment elements form the basis for Masters and Johnson's sex therapy: (1) clients can learn to overcome negative attitudes toward sexual response,

TABLE 31-1 Summary of theories of sexual dysfunction

Theory	Theorist	Dynamics
Psychoanalytic	Freud	Unconscious sexual conflicts are the root of sexual dysfunction.
	Erikson	Failure to master the developmental stage of identity versus role confusion contributes to doubt about sexual self and role. Failure to master the developmental task intimacy versus isolation results in withdrawal from intimate relationships and may impair sexual functioning.
Developmental	Havighurst	Successful completion of developmental tasks contributes to sexual adequacy. At 2 to 3 years the child distinguishes girls from boys by observing genital differences. During middle childhood masculine and feminine roles are learned. Gender identity and role are solidified through peer associations during school years. Sexuality and sex roles are mastered during adolescence.
Learning	Kaplan	Sexual dysfunction is a result of early negative sexual experiences. Symptoms are learned inhibitions. Immediate causes of sexual dysfunction arise from antierotic, sexually destructive environment created by the couple. Culture may predispose to deeper psychological conflicts and result in sexual dysfunction. Sexual differences may be rooted in the relationship.
	Masters and Johnson	Sexual functioning is a natural response and barriers (such as negative attitudes and lack of sexual knowledge) create sexual dysfunction.

(2) the couple is the client in therapy, (3) a mixed gender therapy team treats the couple, (4) factual information on sex relieves a significant amount of dysfunction, and (5) dysfunction is related to interpersonal relationships.

With these tenets in mind, Masters and Johnson state that satisfactory sexual activity is possible through enhanced communication between partners. Because sex in itself is a form of communication, Masters and Johnson note that a variety of nonverbal techniques during sex communicate warmth and caring and each touch enhances communication. Thus emphasis is on touching to learn more about the partner's sexual needs, what pleases the partner, and how one can perform to the other's satisfaction. When nonverbal techniques are combined with verbal communication, the couple's sexual feelings toward each other and sexual activity are enhanced. Masters and Johnson require their clients to come to their laboratory daily for 2 weeks to accomplish the goal of the therapy: enhancement of the enjoyment of sexual activity.

Table 31-1 summarizes the theories of sexual dysfunction.

CHARACTERISTICS OF THE SEX THERAPIST
Qualifications

The sex therapist is qualified through a variety of educational programs. The initial training in the chosen profession lays the groundwork for becoming a sex therapist. For example, the professional nurse with basic preparation provides sex education to a client. The professional nurse with postgraduate training in sex education and counseling provides sex education and counseling for problems such as sexual fears after a heart attack or childbirth. Health professionals trained as sex therapists through a formal sex therapist training program are qualified to initiate sex therapy on an individual or group basis. They are highly skilled, knowledgeable persons who understand the psychosocial and physical developments of a client, with particular emphasis on sexuality.

The sex therapist is comfortable discussing sexual matters. Because of the highly sensitive, personal nature of sexual conflicts, it is important for the therapist to have the self-assurance and confidence to convey that whatever is shared will be accepted. Licensing by the American Association of Sex Educators, Counselors and Therapists (AASECT) assures competence and contributes credibility to the practice of sex therapy.

Role

The role of the nurse as sex therapist includes the following[21]:

1. Taking a history, cognizant that anxiety may be present
2. Listening, watching nonverbal communication, and refraining from note taking if possible to alleviate further anxiety
3. Providing privacy and assuring confidentiality
4. Allowing sufficient time to discuss and explore all aspects of the client's concerns, including anxieties, needs, values, attitudes, expectations, fears, feelings, problems, and practices
5. Being open, nonjudgmental, unembarrassed, respectful, warm, nonevasive, frank, objective, empathic, and reassuring
6. Clarifying vocabulary with special consideration of the clients' choice of words to describe their sex life
7. Helping clients arrive at their own answers when exploring moral issues
8. Being aware of anxiety as indicated by silence, testing, trying to please, covert complaints, distortions, and jokes
9. Mindful that several interviews may be necessary to complete the history and initiate sex education

Goal

The goal of sex therapy and the therapist is primarily the resolution of the sexual conflicts that hinder normal sexual functioning. It is accomplished through individual counseling sessions, in which the client or couple develops plans for conflict resolution. Resolution can also be achieved in group settings with group goals.

Client Selection

Each client is unique in sexual functioning. A specific treatment modality is required to resolve the highly complex conflicts or dysfunctions in sexual behavior. Dysfunctions that cause clients to seek help include (1) ignorance of sexual techniques or misinformation, which requires sex education and counseling; (2) fear of failure or loss of control, performance anxiety, rejection, or interpersonal conflicts, which require in-depth counseling; and (3) lack of communication skill between sex partners, which requires brief sex therapy to add depth of meaning to and satisfaction in sexual activity.

Some clients may be unaware of or reluctant to discuss sexual conflict. When this occurs, it is important for the nurse to take the cue from the client in addressing the sexual problem. The nurse is in a key position to identify clients who may profit from sex education or therapy.

NURSING PROCESS
Assessment

✦ ***Physical dimension.*** The first step in assessing a client is to obtain a thorough sexual history, including an in-depth identification of the problems. Histories are taken from anyone who has reached the age of puberty. When the client is a couple, both partners state their perception of the problem.

The nurse collects the sexual data; the primary complaint, the time of onset, the major concern, and its degree of difficulty for the client. To help the client feel comfortable, the nurse starts with less personal subjects and proceeds to the emotional and sexual problems. The sexual history helps in identifying needs, concerns, misconceptions, problems, reassurances, and questions.

TABLE 31-2 Reactions during sexual response cycle

Phase	Male	Female
Excitement	Penile erection (in 3-8 seconds); thickening, flattening, and elevation of scrotal sac; partial testicular elevation and size increase; nipple erection (25%)	Vaginal lubrication (in 10-30 seconds); thickening of vaginal walls and labia; expansion of inner two-thirds of vagina and elevation of cervix and corpus; tumescence of clitoris; nipple erection (consistent); sex tension flush
Plateau	Increase in penile circumference and testicular; tumescence (50-100% enlarged) full testicular elevation and rotation (orgasm inevitable); purple hue on corona of penis; mucoid secretion from Cowper's gland; sex-tension flush (25%); generalized skeletal muscle tension; hyperventilation; tachycardia (110-170 beats per minute)	Orgasmic platform in outer one third of vagina; full expansion of two-thirds of vagina, uterine and cervical elevation; "sex skin" or discoloration of minor labia (constant if orgasm is to ensue); mucoid secretion from Bartholin's gland; withdrawal of clitoris; sex-tension flush (75%); hyperventilation; tachycardia (100-160 beats per minute)
Orgasmic	Ejaculation; contractions of accessory organs of reproduction (vas deferens, seminal vesicles, ejaculatory duct, prostate); relaxation of external bladder sphincter; contractions of penile urethra; anal sphincter contractions; specific skeletal muscle contractions; hyperventilation; tachycardia (100-180 beats per minute)	Pelvic response (vasocongestion); contractions of uterus from fundus toward lower uterine segment; minimal relaxation of external cervical opening; contractions of orgasmic platform; external rectal sphincter contractions; specific skeletal muscle contractions; hyperventilation; tachycardia (100-180 beats per minute)
Resolution	Refractory period with rapid loss of pelvic vasocongestion; loss of penile erection in primary (rapid) and secondary (slow) stages; sweating reaction (30-40%); hyperventilation; tachycardia (150-180 beats per minute)	Ready return to orgasm with retarded loss of pelvic vasocongestion; loss of "sex skin" color and orgasmic platform in primary (rapid) stage; loss of remainder of pelvic vascongestion as secondary (slow) stage; loss of clitoral tumescence and return to position sweating reaction (30-40%); hyperventilation; tachycardia (150-180 beats per minute)

From Woods, N.: Human sexuality in health and illness, 1984, St. Louis, The C.V. Mosby Co.

A complete physical examination after a thorough history reveals any physiological deviations. The examination particularly focuses on physical dysfunctions in the reproductive system that may interfere with sexual functioning.

An assessment of the client's sexual arousal pattern also uncovers areas of sexual difficulties. The sexual response cycle, with orgasm at the peak,[51] is described in Table 31-2.

Many physical factors affect sexual functioning: stress and fatigue; health problems, such as diabetes, debilitating illnesses, hepatic disease, neurological disease (for example, multiple sclerosis and spinal cord injury); and surgical procedures (for example, prostatectomy, colostomy, hysterectomy, sterilization, and mastectomy). The impact of mutilating surgery on the client's body image is an important assessment factor. The nurse assesses illnesses and diseases that impair general muscle tone and specifically perineal muscle tone and responsiveness that may weaken the muscle contractions needed for orgasm. Endocrine imbalances that lower the androgen level may also contribute to sexual dysfunctions.

The nurse assesses medications that the client is taking. Medications known to affect sexual functioning are the following:

Antihypertensives
    Guanethidine (Esimil)
    Reserpine (Serpasil)
    Spironolactone (Aldactone)
    Methyldopa (Aldomet)
    Propranolol (Inderal)
Antidepressants
    Imipramine (Tofranil)
    Amitriptyline (Elavil)
    Phenelzine (Nardil)
Antihistamines
    Diphenhydramine (Benadryl)
    Chlorpheniramine (Chlor-Trimeton)
Antispasmodics and anticholinergics
    Glycopyrrolate (Robinul)
Antipsychotics
    Chlorpromazine (Thorazine)
    Thioridazine (Mellaril)
    Haloperidol (Haldol)
Oral contraceptives
Narcotics
    Heroin
    Morphine
    Meperidine (Demerol)
Chemotherapeutic agents
Estrogen
Diuretics
    Furosemide (Lasix)

The nurse also asks about alcohol intake and use or abuse of medications and drugs such as marijuana and narcotics.

Sexual functioning is impaired when intercourse is painful, as in *vaginismus.* The client is checked for endometriosis, pelvic inflammatory disease, vaginal atrophy, relaxed supportive uterine ligaments, pelvic tumors, pathological conditions related to childbirth, and vaginal stenosis.

For some, physical attractiveness enhances sexual functioning. Weight, hairstyle, and clothing enhance appeal. A partner can destroy sex appeal by becoming fat, smoking, failing to bathe, brush his teeth, or use deodorant. Clients are sometimes unaware of the impact of this behavior in a partner's sexual arousal. Addressing this issue can easily arouse defenses unless handled with utmost sensitivity.

Emotional dimension. Anxiety is a major contributor to sexual dysfunctions. Frequently anxiety about performing satisfactorily results in an inability to perform. Men highly vulnerable to stress respond with anxiety, and pressure from his partner may result in acute anxiety and impotence. An assessment of the client's fears—fear of failure, rejection, abandonment, punishment, loss of control, intercourse, pregnancy, or asserting independence (particularly women)—helps the nurse understand the client's anxiety. Fears of a specific aspect of the partner (genitals, secretions, or aroma) may be of phobic intensity. Strong negative emotions, such as anger, guilt, and depression, disrupt sexual arousal and may lead to dysfunctions. When one partner is angry or frustrated with the other, arousal may be impaired. Clients may be frightened by the intensity of sexual feelings. They may feel shame or guilt about intercourse or past sexual experiences, resulting in fear of punishment that may hinder functioning. Depressed clients lack interest in sex and frequently are unable to function sexually.

Other important affective states are absence of sexual feeling (frigidity); inability to abandon oneself to sexual feelings because of fears; and ambivalence, commonly seen in men harboring intense hostile feelings toward their partners. The ambivalent client may enjoy intercourse but *ejaculate* prematurely, thereby depriving his partner of sexual pleasure. Other clients may be exceedingly sensitive to *erotic* sensations and ejaculate prematurely.

Intellectual dimension. Clients may not have a sound knowledge of sexuality. Myths abound about techniques, contraception, sexually transmitted diseases, arousal, and responses. Ignorance and misunderstanding may lead to fear and avoidance of sex. The nurse gathers information about the client's knowledge by asking where and from whom information was obtained. Questionnaires or interviews with the sex partner are also useful.

The nurse assesses the client's ability to communicate sexual concerns. She listens to his expressions of thoughts and feelings and assesses his response to her open, honest mode of communication. The nurse is attentive to the client's language and meaning. For some, "having sex" means intercourse; for others, it may mean oral sex. The nurse assesses the couple's ability to openly and sensitively communicate their needs to each other, to tell each other what feels good and what does not.

The nurse assesses the client's attitudes toward sex. Strong negative attitudes, sometimes culturally induced, about the partner or sex in general may contribute to dys-

function. The nurse explores these attitudes with the client. Other attitudinal problems may be deeply rooted in fears of rejection, competitiveness, and power struggles. Sexual dysfunction may occur when symbolic meanings are attached to sex and evoked by the erotic feelings. On the other hand, some clients sublimate and suppress their sexual needs without psychological damage.

Clients may have unconscious, unresolved deeply embedded sexual conflicts reevoked by sexual experiences. It is beyond the scope of this chapter to assist the nurse in uncovering these.

Social dimension. The quality of the couple's relationship needs to be assessed. Troubled or destructive relationships may promote sexual dysfunctions. Subtle rejections or power struggles can be identified by the astute nurse. For example, if the female becomes more assertive in her relationship with her partner and more in control of her sexual body she may demonstrate sexual aggression. The male, as a result of this aggression may experience sexual dysfunction. Past sexual trauma, such as rape, sexual abuse, child molestation, incest, *exhibitionism,* or exploitation, is explored. Infidelity is also a traumatic event. Any of these problems may have devastating ramifications for the establishment of healthy sexual relationships.

Each couple represents a unique relationship in degree of involvement, closeness, self-disclosure, and intensity of emotion expressed.

For example, a newly married couple may be highly physical and intense because of the newness of the relationship, whereas a couple married many years may be less physically involved but more caring and loving in other ways (See Figure 31-1). Therefore the nurse consid-

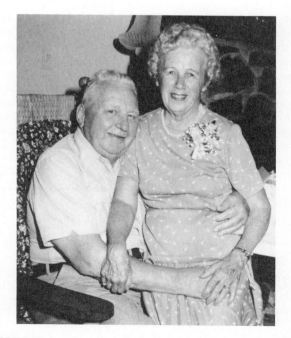

FIGURE 31-1 Affection and a sense of humor are evident in this couple celebrating their sixtieth wedding anniversary.

ers the length of the relationship, the amount of energy generated from the relationship, and the quality of caring and intimacy. A meaningful sexual relationship develops best when there is trust. Signs of mistrust are suspiciousness, jealousy, and rash judgment of the partner's behaviors. Lack of emotional intensity in the relationship may be a sign of ambivalence about it. The nurse explores the client's depth of commitment.

The nurse assesses dependence and independence in the sexual relationship. Long-lasting relationships may generate dependence, and the partners may begin to magnify each other's flaws, creating sexual problems. Increased independence of one partner may create sexual difficulties when the couple fails to communicate needs and desires and takes the relationship for granted.

Environment is an essential element to assess. Does it afford the privacy necessary for sexual activity? Are other people constantly present, making sexual expression and private communication between partners either difficult or impossible?

The socialization process by which each of the partners learned sexual behavior is an important area to be explored. Is one from a large, close, loving family, while the other is a single child raised in an undemonstrative family? These factors have deeply rooted implications for the sexual relationship.

The nurse also assesses the understanding of sex roles of each partner. How does the man perceive the woman's role in terms of work and home? How does the woman view the man's role? These social factors influence the sexual relationship.

Many aspects of the sexual behavior are influenced by cultural norms. Examples are the preferred position for intercourse, whether the female plays an active or passive role, and the length and type of foreplay. Kissing is accepted in the United States, but some societies believe it is unsanitary. Circumstances for intercourse vary. Some groups prohibit sex during menses, lactation, or pregnancy. Conflicts in these areas may cause sexual disturbances. The sexual life-style of the client is vital to assess because of the various problems associated with different life-styles and the alarming increase in sexually transmitted diseases, such as herpes and AIDS. (See the Research Highlight on p. 583.) Different sexual life-styles are listed in the box below.

DEFINITIONS OF VARIOUS SEXUAL LIFE-STYLES

SEXUAL LIFE-STYLE	DEFINITION
Heterosexual	Prefers sexual relations with someone of the opposite sex
Homosexual	Prefers sexual relations with someone of the same sex
Bisexual	Prefers sexual relations with both sexes
Transsexual	Wishes to be or believes one is a member of the opposite sex

---

Spiritual dimension. The nurse assesses the client's personal beliefs about what is "right" and "wrong" in sexuality. Beliefs about techniques, frequency of masturbation, oral sex, permissiveness, open marriage, celibacy, and sexual life-styles are highly charged issues subject to conflicting views. An assessment of these beliefs helps determine the areas of conflict both within the client and within the relationship. For example, does the client find oral sex exciting, while his partner thinks it is wrong and unnatural?

The nurse and client also explore the aspects of the sexual relationship that the client values and that add meaning and enrichment to his sense of personal worth. Following are some questions to consider when assessing the client:

1. What activities increase sensuousness? For some, walking barefoot through warm sand, smelling fresh cut grass, stroking a cat, and admiring a sunset are as appealing and delightful as a sexual experience. For others, physical contact is important—touching, cuddling, massaging, and hugging.
2. Where is the focus of the sexual experience? The client may narrowly concentrate on the genitals for sexual satisfaction or may find expression of sexuality in a much broader capacity—in the pleasure of the whole body and person.
3. What purpose does sex serve? Sex fulfills several different desires: to feel physical release, share sexual pleasures, express deep emotional connection, overcome loneliness or boredom, feel alive, satisfy curiosity, seek adventure, obtain status, bolster self-worth and competence, express power, exploit, or express rebellion against parents or society. Everyone has his own belief of what is acceptable and what is not.
4. How important is sexual functioning for the client to live a productive and satisfying life? Knowing this helps the nurse plan care based on the client's personal beliefs and values.
5. How does the client respond to conflicts in sexual values? He may deny the conflict and withdraw, suppress it, smooth it over, use power or dominance, compromise, or negotiate. The nurse observes the client's manner of response.

Differences in religion are discussed. Some clients with strict religious upbringings maintain rigid, restrictive attitudes and beliefs that generate anxiety and guilt about sex. In some religions masturbation is considered a sin against God, sexual fantasies are impure, sexual experimentation in adolescence is strictly forbidden, and sex is saved for marriage. Those who experiment sexually may feel guilty about their sexual behavior and may later experience dysfunction.

Analysis

Nursing diagnosis. The defining characteristics of the NANDA-accepted nursing diagnosis altered sexuality patterns are listed in the box on p. 583.

The Case Example on p. 584 demonstrates the characteristics of the nursing diagnosis of altered sexuality patterns.

Research Highlight

Premarital Sex: Attitudes and Behavior by Dating Stage

John P. Roache

PURPOSE

The purpose of this study was to assess premarital attitudes and reported sexual behavior to make a judgment as to the direction of the "sexual revolution" in the 1980s. The fear of contracting herpes simplex II is said to be causing young adults to think twice before engaging in premarital sex, thus supporting the suggestion of a new conservatism in sexual behavior.

SAMPLE

The study was based on a sample of 280 college students enrolled in a social science class at a state college in New England during the spring of 1983. The sample included a high percentage of commuter students, Roman Catholics, and persons of urban, ethnic, and working-class backgrounds. In addition, 76 nonstudents (acquaintances of the college students but not close friends) were included in the sample.

METHODOLOGY

Respondents were asked what they considered proper dating behavior for five identified premarital dating stages: stage 1, dating with no particular affection; stage 2, dating with affection but not love; stage 3, dating and being in love; stage 4, dating one person only; stage 5, becoming engaged. Respondents were also asked which dating behavior was appropriate for each dating stage, ranging from the least to the most intimate. Questionnaires were filled out anonymously in the classroom. Acquaintances filled out questionnaires anonymously and mailed them back to the researcher.

FINDINGS

The findings indicated that as a couple becomes more emotionally involved, a more sexually active intimate relationship is regarded as appropriate. Males appear more permissive in their attitudes as to what is proper sexual behavior in the first three stages and in all areas of intimacy. By stage 4 there is no difference in sexual conduct between males and females. Findings also indicated that males expected sexual intimacy sooner and females tend to tie sexual intimacy to love and commitment. Further analysis of the data indicates a high level of premarital sexual activity.

IMPLICATIONS

The study suggests that the "sexual revolution" shows no signs of abating. Sexual permissiveness continues even with the threat of contracting a sexually transmitted disease.

Based on data from Adolescence **21**(81):107, 1986.

ALTERED SEXUALITY PATTERNS

DEFINITION

The state in which an individual expresses concern regarding his sexuality.

DEFINING CHARACTERISTICS
Physical Dimension

Altered body structure or function
Physical disease
Obesity
Lack of privacy
Pain
Alcohol ingestion
Medications
Altered body image
Aging
Pregnancy
*Decreased libido

Emotional Dimension

*Anxiety
Fear of pregnancy or of acquiring a sexually transmitted disease
*Anger
*Guilt
*Depression

Intellectual Dimension

Reported difficulties, limitations, changes in sexual activity or behavior
Knowledge/skill deficit about alternative responses
*Verbalization of problem
*Change of interest in self or others
*Job, financial worries

Social Dimension

Dissatisfaction with sex role
Changed relationship when separated, divorced, or after partner's death
Lack of significant other
*Abusive partner

Spiritual Dimension

Conflict in sexual values, orientation

Adapted from North American Nursing Diagnosis Association Classification of Nursing Diagnosis: Proceedings of the seventh conference, St. Louis, 1987, The C.V. Mosby Co.
*Indicates characteristics in addition to those defined by NANDA.

Case Example

Mary, a mother of two children, is a full-time housewife. Her husband, Joe, is an executive officer in a large corporation, which demands more and more time away from the family. As a result of his absence and because Mary must assume responsibility of the household decisions without input from her husband, social distancing has occured, and sexual functioning is affected. Mary feels trapped in a relationship that cannot be discussed with her very busy husband. The conflict continues to grow. She turns her full attention to the children and her social life without him.

DSM-III-R diagnoses. The sexual disorders, as described in the DSM-III-R categories, are listed in the box below.

The paraphilias are characterized by sexual arousal in response to objects or situations that are not part of nor-mal arousal activity patterns and that may interfere with the capacity for reciprocal, affectionate sexual activity (Table 31-3). Sexual dysfunctions are characterized by inhibitions in sexual desire or the psychophysiological changes that characterize the sexual response cycle (Table 31-4). Other sexual disorders are a residual category for disorders in sexual functioning that are not classifiable in any specific category.

Planning

Table 31-5 lists examples of long-term and short-term goals and outcome criteria related to sexual disorders. These serve as examples of the planning stage of the nursing process.

Implementation

Physical dimension. When physical conditions such as illness, disease, obesity, impairment from surgical procedure, or trauma affect sexual functioning, the nurse and client explore alternative methods for sexual gratification. New positions for intercourse may be helpful, or new areas of erotic sensations may be developed (especially for paraplegic clients). Lubricants are useful when vaginal lubrication is insufficient and vaginal walls lose their elasticity.

DSM-III-R CLASSIFICATION RELATED TO SEXUAL DYSFUNCTIONS

SEXUAL DISORDERS
Paraphilias

302.40	Exhibitionism
302.81	Fetishism
302.89	Frotteurism
302.20	Pedophilia
302.83	Sexual masochism
302.84	Sexual sadism
302.30	Transvestic fetishism
302.82	Voyeurism
302.90	Paraphilia not otherwise specified

SEXUAL DYSFUNCTIONS
Sexual Desire Disorders

302.71	Hypoactive sexual desire disorder
302.79	Sexual aversion disorder

Sexual Arousal Disorder

302.72	Female sexual arousal disorder
302.72	Male erectile disorder

Orgasm Disorders

302.73	Inhibited female orgasm
302.74	Inhibited male orgasm
302.75	Premature ejaculation

Sexual Pain Disorders

302.76	Dyspareunia
306.51	Vaginismus
302.70	Sexual dysfunction not otherwise specified

Other Sexual Disorders

302.90	Sexual disorder not otherwise specified

Adapted from American Psychiatric Association: Diagnostic and statistical manual of mental disorders, (DSM-III-R), Washington, D.C., 1987, The Association.

TABLE 31-3 Types and definitions of paraphilias

Paraphilia	Definition
Exhibitionism	Repeated acts of exposing the genitals to unsuspecting stranger to achieve sexual excitement
Fetishism	Repeated use of inanimate objects to achieve sexual excitement
Frotteurism	Sexual excitement achieved by touching or rubbing against a nonconsenting person
Pedophilia	Act or fantasy of engaging in sexual activity with prepubertal children
Sexual masochism	Sexual excitement produced by being humiliated, bound, beaten, or made to suffer
Sexual sadism	Infliction on another of physical or psychological suffering to achieve sexual satisfaction
Transvestic fetishism	Recurrent cross dressing by a heterosexual male to achieve excitement
Voyeurism	Repeated observation of unsuspecting persons who are naked, in the act of disrobing, or engaging in sexual activity

The nurse assists the client with body image distortions (following surgery or trauma) to foster a more positive view of himself. Focusing on the client's strengths and positive qualities may lessen the sting of having only one breast or being unable to reach orgasm. Clients can learn to accommodate changes in sexual functioning by accepting lovemaking techniques that enhance their body image rather than negate it.

The client's medication regimen is evaluated to balance the medication's desired effects with its adverse reactions, such as impotence. When the illness is life-threatening (such as hypertension), the client needs to accept the adverse symptoms. In some cases a different antihypertensive may not affect sexual functioning.

A variety of techniques can be used for arousing sexual feelings and enhancing pleasure: kissing, touching, fondling, caressing, scratching, and gentle slapping of various sensitive body parts, such as lips, neck, earlobes, breasts, insides of thighs, fingertips, palms, and genitalia. Arousal is also heightened by oral genital stimulation, although some persons may consider this inappropriate.

When it is important for partners to be attractive and well groomed, the nurse tactfully confronts the individual about the physically repulsive behavior.

Helping clients express likes and dislikes about the sexual relationship opens communication between partners. When partners know what pleases during sex, they tend to respond positively.

Two specific techniques known to alleviate certain sexual dysfunctions are *Kegel's exercises* and *Seman's stop-*

TABLE 31-4 Sexual dysfunctions

Dysfunction	Definition
Hypoactive sexual desire disorder	Persistent, pervasive inhibition of sexual desire; age, sex, health, intensity and frequency of sexual desire, and environment considered
Sexual aversion disorder	Persistent and extreme aversion to and avoidance of almost all genital sexual contact with a sexual partner.
Female sexual arousal disorder	Persistent failure to attain the lubrication swelling response of sexual excitement or a lack of pleasure during sexual activity.
Male erectile disorder	Persistent failure to attain or maintain an erection until completion of the sexual activity.
Inhibited female orgasm	Recurrent, persistent inhibition of female orgasm, manifested by delay or absence of orgasm
Inhibited male orgasm	Recurrent, persistent inhibition of male orgasm, manifested by delay or absence of ejaculation
Premature ejaculation	Ejaculation with minimal sexual stimulation sooner than desired
Dyspareunia	Intercourse associated with persistent genital pain
Vaginismus	Recurrent, persistent involuntary spasm of the musculature of the outer third of the vagina, which interferes with intercourse

TABLE 31-5 Long-term and short-term goals and outcome criteria related to altered sexuality

Goals	Outcome Criteria

NURSING DIAGNOSIS: ALTERED SEXUALITY PATTERN RELATED TO INABILITY TO ACHIEVE ERECTION

Long-term goals

Goals	Outcome Criteria
To develop a more meaningful relationship with spouse	Makes consistent statements that are positive toward spouse
	Has daily harmonic communication with spouse to enhance sexual endearment statements
	Demonstrates pleasure regarding continued sexual activity in connection with spouse
To develop a positive self-image	Consistently expresses confidence
	Is able to see self as attractive sex partner
To establish a satisfactory erection for sexual activity	Remains free of anxiety regarding sexual performance
	Enjoys *foreplay* with sexual partner
	Achieves erection to the degree needed for penetration of vaginal area
	Maintains erection for a satisfactory length of time

Short-term goals

Goals	Outcome Criteria
To establish rapport with nurse	Demonstrates an openness and trust in sharing concern
	Speaks freely of impotence
	Provides history of difficulty
To identify any physical barrier to sexual performance	Agrees to physical examination without hesitation
	Allows nurse to perform thorough health examination
	Demonstrates appropriate attitude toward health status when physical examination is performed
	Listens carefully and attentively to report on physical status
	Agrees to referral for medical treatment if physical problem is discovered

Continued.

TABLE 31-5 Long-term and short-term goals and outcome criteria related to altered sexuality—cont'd

Goals	Outcome Criteria
NURSING DIAGNOSIS: ALTERED SEXUALITY PATTERN RELATED TO MARITAL CONFLICTS	
Long-term goals	
To develop more positive regard for spouse	Makes statements that describe positive attributes about spouse
	Views spouse as attractive and pleasant—a friend
To establish satisfactory communication patterns with spouse	Is able to initiate conversation with spouse in unthreatening way
	Engages in established pattern of communication in which feelings are expressed
To demonstrate openness and continued growth in conflict resolution	Initiates a rapport of trust and openness to allow venting of feelings by spouse; does not retaliate with verbalized anger
	Has resolved conflict as demonstrated by adaptive relationship established with spouse
Short-term goals	
To verbalize anxiety over difficulty with spouse	Repeats statements of anxiety less frequently
	Is increasingly adaptive in behavior toward spouse
To clarify distorted perceptions of conflicts with spouse	Validates perceptions with objective person
	Deliberately chooses adaptive behavioral strategies rather than reacting impulsively
To respond to nurse therapist	Establishes a nurse-client relationship
To have positive regard for self	Demonstrates consistent adaptive behavior and makes statements reflecting strengthened sense of identity, trust, self-worth, and positive self-perception

start technique. Poor pubococcygeal muscle tone in women, which contributes to sexual inadequacy, can be improved by Kegel's exercises—the tightening and relaxing of the pubococcygeal muscle, a technique useful in initiating orgasm.[22]

Seman's technique for preventing premature ejaculation prolongs the reflex mechanism by extravaginal stimulation by the partner during erection until the sensation before ejaculation is experienced. Stimulation is then stopped until the sensation disappears, at which time stimulation is resumed. When the client can tolerate the stimulation, premature ejaculation is cured. Methods that repeatedly focus the man's attention on the sensation preceding orgasm are dramatically effective in ejaculatory control. Masters and Johnson expanded this technique with their "squeeze technique," in which the partner squeezes the erect penis just below the rim of the glans when he perceives orgasm to be imminent. Stimulation is resumed, and the procedure is repeated several times before ejaculation.

Emotional dimension. Reducing performance anxiety is a primary treatment focus. Couples are given instructions, such as to touch and caress each other without intercourse, to reduce the pressure to perform. The teasing, enticing, and gentle stimulation along with the prohibition of intercourse removes the pressure and lessens the fear of failure. Partners are provided with evidence that erection can occur spontaneously under certain circumstances, and confidence is restored as a successful and satisfying sexual experience occurs.

To dispel fears that inhibit sexual functioning, a client is instructed to focus on erotic sensations and make a conscious effort to stop distracting thoughts by detaching himself from the situation and withdrawing into a favorite sexual fantasy.

Fears of rejection, abandonment, and guilt often promote overconcern for a partner and impair sexual functioning. Clients are helped to realize that sexual enjoyment depends largely on the ability to abandon oneself to erotic feelings to the temporary exclusion of everything else. The ability to give and receive pleasure allows the client to do this and still be secure in the knowledge that his partner, too, will have a turn at giving and receiving pleasure.

Strong negative emotions, such as anger, hostility, and resentment, need to be dealt with. The nurse helps the couple become aware of how these negative emotions inhibit sexual functioning and how they are used to avoid and sabotage sexual encounters (see Chapter 12). Psychoanalysis may help uncover and resolve the client's unconscious sexual conflicts, although it may take a long time.

The absence of sexual feelings (frigidity) can be treated with *sensate focus* exercises.[22] The couple forgoes intercourse for a time and limits their sexual activity to touching and caressing. The woman is instructed to caress her partner's body first if she is inorgasmic to counteract her guilt for receiving something for herself and to alleviate her fear of being rejected. Once sexual feelings are experienced, the exercise is expanded to include genital stimulation. As genital stimulation increases sexual responsiveness, intercourse follows. During these exercises partners become more perceptive and sensitive to each other's sexual needs and reactions. The woman realizes that her partner enjoys making her happy, that he will not reject her when she actively seeks sexual pleasure, and her defenses against the sexual experience are dissolved.

✳ ***Intellectual dimension.*** Incorrect or lack of information about sexuality is clarified. Knowledge of the human sexual response, sexual dysfunctions, the effects of illness and medications on sexual functioning, sex terms, and the reproductive systems can be given formally in sex education classes or informally as situations arise. Because many clients are reluctant to discuss their sexual concerns, it is the nurse's responsibility to initiate the discussion. Sex education in groups has advantages, as it exposes clients to attitudes and feeling of others and enables them to voice their concerns.

Clients need to learn to communicate their sexual needs to their partners openly and comfortably. The nurse can help by desensitizing clients to the words used in the expression of sexual functioning and by comfortably discussing sexual concerns herself.

Negative attitudes or irrational thoughts that impair sexual satisfaction are voiced. A statement such as, "Many people *masturbate* after the loss of their spouse," helps the client to explore his attitude toward masturbation in the light of new information.

The nurse may suggest engaging in *sexual fantasies* to enhance satisfaction. This is best done after the notion of sexual fantasies is discussed, because sexual fantasies may not be acceptable for some (see the Research Highlight on p. 587).

✤ ***Social dimension.*** Because sexual difficulties are products of couples' interactions, treatment to build and maintain healthy relationships is offered. Marital discord can be treated by a therapist with expertise in the dynamics of marital relationships. The marital therapist identifies transferences, promotes feelings of trust and security, analyzes power struggles, confronts sexual sabotage, and examines marriage contracts. Referral to a marital therapist is considered when relationships are destructive (see Chapter 30).

The nurse needs to help couples find the privacy needed for adequate sexual functioning. Clients at home, in the hospital, and in nursing homes may need "Do Not Disturb" signs on their doors.

Sexual problems arising from a woman's independence or lack of it may affect both partners. In many cases the inner conflict between dependence and independence is resolved when the woman becomes aware of it and takes

---

Research Highlight

Sexual Fantasies and Sexual Satisfaction: An Empirical Analysis of Erotic Thought

J. Davidson & L. Hoffman

PURPOSE

The study was designed to explore the meaning and function of sexual fantasizing for married women.

SAMPLE

The sample was 212 married undergraduate and graduate female students, ages 18 to 40 (mean, 28.1) years, in a midwestern commuter college of 5500 students.

METHODOLOGY

A questionnaire of 35 open- and closed-ended questions was given. A checklist of 49 sexual fantasies was administered to assess the variety and type of sexual fantasies. The variable "satisfaction with current sex life" was recorded on a five-category scale from very satisfied to very dissatisfied.

FINDINGS

Eighty-eight percent admitted to engaging in sexual fantasies. Daydreaming was the most common context. The most commonly expressed fantasies included extramarital affairs, reliving a sexual experience, different position for intercourse, sex with current sex partner, sex in rooms other than bedroom, sex with a new partner, more affectionate sex partner, and sex on carpeted floor. Engaging in sexual fantasies was not related to dissatisfaction with current sex life and did not suggest marital discord. The data do suggest that sexual fantasies for some married women help achieve sexual arousal or orgasm, irrespective of satisfaction or dissatisfaction with their current sex life. The findings do not support previous arguments that sexual fantasies may be undesirable for mental health.

IMPLICATIONS

Sexual fantasies for some married women represent very personal experiences to be enjoyed, not detriments to their overall sexual adjustment. Thus sexual fantasies may be a therapeutic experience for women having difficulty in achieving orgasm or sexual satisfaction. The study raises the question of cultural influences on sexual fantasies as an area for consideration when suggesting fantasies as a therapeutic technique.

Based on data from The Journal of Sex Research **22**(2):184, 1986.

steps to resolve her dependence needs. Her partner's acceptance of her independence is essential for satisfying sexual activities.

✖ *Spiritual dimension.* Since the focus of sex therapy is on immediate symptoms, interventions for conflicts in values center on clarification. Helping a client clarify personal morals, beliefs, and values about sexual functioning assists him to sort through his dilemmas and to make responsible choices acceptable to him (see Chapter 45).

Conflict resolution is a method of working through problems couples may have when conflicting beliefs and values interfere with sexual functioning. The nurse helps identify the source of the problem, and the couple carefully examines it using clear communication. Tense emotions are dealt with before problem-solving can begin. The couple needs to remain rational by avoiding insults, hearing the other partner's argument, and stating views and feelings.

When sexual conflicts result in guilt from strict religious upbringing, specific experiences can help free the client from rigid attitudes. For example, touching a partner's genitals may bring back strongly embedded feelings of sin and guilt and generate anxiety. Specific exercises that gradually promote this touching may be prescribed. Confronting the client with avoided feelings, helping him get in touch with the loving aspects of himself from which he is alienated, and encouraging him to behave differently are helpful.

Treatment of sexual dysfunction encompasses all aspects of the client. When treatment is effective, attitudes are broadened, conflicts are resolved, and values are clarified, often resulting in a more intimate relationship between partners and leading to a more satisfying and enriching life for both.

Evaluation

When the symptoms of sexual dysfunction are alleviated, the treatment is considered effective. Improved sexual functioning may result in profound changes in the client's emotional status. Similar results may be achieved when the client resolves basic conflicts about sexual difficulties. The anxious or guilty client learns to be free and more accepting of himself. He may feel an enhanced sense of self-esteem and be more open in his relationships. Enhanced self-esteem accompanying restoration of sexual capacity also affects general emotional functioning. With increased confidence, relationships with others may be less competitive, and the client may become a more productive and creative person. Improved sexual functioning potentially benefits all aspects of behavior.

BRIEF REVIEW

Sex therapy is the treatment of sexual dysfunction. Treatment focuses on the resolution of sexual conflicts that impair functioning. Causes of sexual dysfunction that require clients to seek sex therapy include ignorance of

sexual techniques, misinformation, performance anxiety, and interpersonal conflicts. Sexual disorders include gender identity disorders, paraphilias, sexual dysfunctions, and other sexual disorders.

Freud believed that sexual conflicts are the root of all psychopathological conditions. Erikson focused on the adolescent developmental task of intimacy in relationships as a basis for satisfactory sexual functioning in adulthood. Havighurst identified stages of development that required successful completion for sexual adequacy. Kaplan and Masters and Johnson believe that sexual response is a natural response and emphasize psychosocial aspects that may affect sexual functioning. They combine psychotherapy with sexual exercises to restore sexual functioning.

The professional nurse may assume the role of sex therapist. Formal sex therapy training, graduate education, and licensure by the American Association of Sex Educators, Counselors and Therapists provide appropriate qualifications. Skill, knowledge, comfort, and rapport are needed by the nurse working as a sex therapist.

Assessment of sexual dysfunction involves a full examination of the client, including physical examination and consideration of general health, past traumas, medications, negative emotional and attitudinal states, knowledge of sexuality, ability to communicate sexual concerns, sex role perception, cultural sex norms, sexual life-style, and sexual values. The defining characteristics of the nursing diagnosis of sexual dysfunction and the essential features of the DSM-III-R classification of sexual dysfunction are listed. Goals for planning and implementing care are also described, with a discussion of methods for evaluating clients with sexual dysfunction.

REFERENCES AND SUGGESTED READINGS

1. American Psychiatric Association: Diagnostic and statistical manual of mental disorders, ed. 3, Washington, D.C., 1980, The Association.
2. Anderson, M.L.: Talking about sex—with less anxiety, Journal of Psychiatric Nursing and Mental Health Services 18(6):10, 1980.
3. Assey, J., and Herbert, J.: Who is the seductive patient? American Journal of Nursing 83(4):531, 1983.
4. Bachman, R.: Homosexuality: the cost of being different, Canadian Nurse 77:20, 1981.
4a. Bioder, R.L.: Why women don't report sexual assault, Journal of Clinical Psychiatry 42:437, 1981.
5. Bogen, I.: Sexual myths and politics, Journal of Sex Education and Therapy 7(1):7, 1981.
6. Brick, P.: Sex and society: teaching the connection, Journal of School Health 51:226, 1981.
7. Bullard, D., and Knight, S.: Sexuality and physical disability: personal perspectives, St. Louis, 1981, The C.V. Mosby Co.
8. Burgess, A.W., McCausland, M.P., and Wolbert, W.A.: Children's drawings as indicators of sexual trauma, Perspectives of Psychiatric Care 19(2):50, 1981.
8a. Crosby, J.F.: Sexual autonomy: toward a humanistic ethic, Springfield, Ill., 1981, Charles C Thomas, Publisher.
9. De Moya, D., De Moya, A., and Lewis, H.: RN's sex q and a, Oradell, N.Y., 1984, Medical Economics Books.

10. Edelwich, J., and Brodsky, A.: Sexual dilemmas for the helping professional, New York, 1982, Brunner/Mazel, Inc.
11. Erikson, E.: Childhood and society, New York, 1963, W.W. Norton & Co., Inc.
12. Fogel, C.I., and Woods, N.F.: Health care of women: a nursing perspective, St. Louis, 1981, The C.V. Mosby Co.
12a. Frank, D., Downard, E., and Lang, A.: Androgyny, sexual satisfaction and women, Journal of Psychosocial Nursing and Mental Health Services 27(7):10, 1986.
13. Freud, S.: Three essays of the theory of sexuality, Ed. 3, London, 1962, Hogarth Press. (Originally published 1905.)
14. Furstenburg, F.F., Lincoln, J.M., and Merken, J.: Teenage sexuality, pregnancy, and childbearing, Philadelphia, 1981, University of Pennsylvania Press.
15. Guarino, S.C.: Planning and implementing a group health program on sexuality for the elderly, Journal of Gerontological Nursing 6:600, 1980.
16. Havighurst, R.: Human development and education, New York, 1953, Longman Inc.
17. Higgins, L., and Hawkins, J.: Human sexuality across the life span, Montery, Calif., 1984, Wadsworth Health Sciences Division.
18. Hogan, R.M.: Human sexuality: a nursing perspective, New York, 1980, Appleton-Century-Crofts.
19. Hyde, J.: Understanding human sexuality, Ed. 3, New York, 1986, McGraw-Hill, Book Co.
20. Jordheim, A.: Non-professional ethnic treatment of sexual dysfunctions, Journal of Sex Education and Therapy 9(1):57, 1983.
21. Kaluger, G., and Kaluger, M.F.: Human development: the span of life, ed. 3, St. Louis, 1984, The C.V. Mosby Co.
22. Kaplan, H.S.: The new sex therapy, New York, 1974, Brunner/Mazel, Inc.
23. Kim, M., and Moritz, D.A.: Classification of nursing diagnoses: proceedings of the fifth national conference, New York, 1985, McGraw-Hill Book Co.
24. Kirkpatrick, M.: Women's sexual development: exploration of inner space, New York, 1980, Plenum Press.
25. Leach, A.: Threat to the nurse's sexual identity. In Haber, J., and others: Comprehensive psychiatric nursing, ed. 2, New York, 1982, McGraw-Hill Book Co.
26. Leiblum, S.R., and Pevuin, L.A.: Principles and practices of sex therapy, New York, 1980, The Guilford Press.
27. Lion, E.: Human sexuality in nursing process, New York, 1982, John Wiley & Sons.
28. Masters, W., and Johnson, V.: Human sexual response, Boston, 1966, Little, Brown & Co.
29. Masters, W., and Johnson, V.: Human sexual inadequacy, Boston, 1970, Little, Brown & Co.
30. Masters, W.H., and Johnson, V.E.: Homosexuality in perspective. Boston, 1979, Little, Brown & Co.
31. Masters, W., Johnson, V., Kolodny, R., and Weems, S.: Ethical issues in sex therapy and research, Boston, 1980, Little, Brown & Co.
32. McDonald, A.: A little bit of lavender goes a long way: a critique of research on sexual orientation, Journal of Sex Research 19:95, 1983.
33. McIntosh, D.: Sexual attitudes in a group of older women, Issues in Mental Health Nursing 3:109, 1981.
34. Miller, V., and Mansfield, E.: Family therapy for the multiple-incest family, Journal of Psychiatric Nursing and Mental Health Services 19(4):29, 1981.
35. Mims, F.H., and Swenson, M.: Sexuality: a nursing perspective, New York, 1980, McGraw-Hill Book Co.
36. Moses, A.E., and Hawkins, R.O., Jr.: Counseling lesbian women and gay men: a life-issue approach, St. Louis, 1982, The C.V. Mosby Co.
37. Nadelson, C., and Marcotte, D.: Treatment interventions in human sexuality, New York, 1983, Plenum Press.
38. Penland, L.R.: Sex education in 1900, 1940, and 1980: an historical sketch, Journal of School Health 51:305, 1981.
39. Prince, J.: Father-daughter incest: an attempt to maintain family to meet human needs, Family and Community Health 4:35, 1981.
40. Pulvino, C.J., and Calangelo, N.: Counseling for the growing years: 65 and over, Minneapolis, 1980, Educational Media Corp.
41. Roesel, R.: The nurses' role in primary prevention in sexual health, Imprint 27:27, 1980.
41a. Salisbury, D.: Aids: psychosocial implications, Journal of Psychosocial Nursing and Mental Health Services 24(12):13, 1986.
42. Sandler, J., Myerson, M., and Kinder, B.: Human sexuality: current perspectives, Florida, 1980, Mariner Publishing Co., Inc.
43. Schaffer, K.F.: Sex-role issues in mental health, Reading, Mass., 1980, Addison-Wesley Publishing Co, Inc.
44. Sha'Ked, A.: Human sexuality and rehabilitation medicine: sexual functioning following spinal cord injury, Baltimore, 1981, The Williams & Wilkins Co.
45. Silbert, D.T.: Human sexuality growth groups, Journal of Psychiatric Nursing and Mental Health Services 19(2):31, 1981.
46. Smith, P.B., and Mumford, M.: Adolescent pregnancy: perspectives for the health professional, Boston, 1980, G.K. Hall & Co.
47. Strecker, I.J.: Proper vision of human sexuality enriches person, society, and family, The Leaven 2:3, 1981.
48. Thomas, J.N.: Symposium on child abuse and neglect: sexual abuse of children—case finding and clinical assessment, Nursing Clinics of North America 16:179, 1981.
49. Weinberg, J.: Sexuality: human needs and nursing practice, Philadelphia, 1982, W.B. Saunders Co.
50. Weller, R., and Halikas, J.: Marijuana use and sexual behavior, The Journal of Sex Research 20(2):186, 1984.
51. Wolman, B., and Money, J.: Handbook of human sexuality, Englewood Cliffs, N.J., 1980, Prentice-Hall, Inc.
52. Woods, N.F.: Human sexuality in health and illness, ed. 3, St. Louis, 1984, The C.V. Mosby Co.
53. Yoselle, H.: Sexuality in the later years, Topics in Clinical Nursing 3:59, 1981.

ANNOTATED BIBLIOGRAPHY

Bancroft, J.: Human sexuality and its problems, New York, 1984 Churchill Livingstone, Inc.

This text for health professionals emphasizes the variety of factors and complexity of their interactions that are taken into account when attempting to understand human sexuality. Issues and concepts related to sexuality and the influence of personal values are also discussed.

Haas, K., and Haas, A.: Understanding sexuality, St. Louis, 1987, The C.V. Mosby Co.

The authors explore the growth and evolution of sexual awareness. Development of sexuality is discussed in children, adolescents, adults, and the elderly. Special attention is given to those who are single, separated, or divorced. Homosexuality is discussed as well as the impact of AIDS and nonmarital sexuality.

Hawton, K.: Sex therapy, New York, 1985, Oxford University Press.

This text discusses the variety of ways in which sexuality can be impaired and the innovative approaches available to help persons with sexual problems. References substantiate research findings.

Woods, N.F.: Human sexuality in health and illness, ed. 3, St. Louis, 1984, The C.V. Mosby Co.

This text focuses on human sexuality from a holistic perspective, emphasizing the role of the nurse in sexual health and health care of clients. Clinical aspects of human sexuality are examined in light of nursing practice.

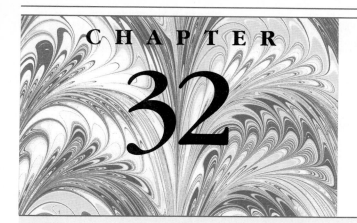

CHAPTER 32

THERAPY WITH CHRONICALLY DISTRESSED CLIENTS

Sharon Elizabeth Byers

After studying this chapter the learner will be able to:

Describe the development of the current political, social, and legal status of the chronically distressed client.

Discuss the development of the career of the chronically distressed client, according to symbolic interactionism.

List characteristics and roles the nurse assumes when working with chronically distressed client.

Use the nursing process to provide care to chronically distressed clients.

All chronically distressed clients have certain characteristics in common, no matter what the nature of their health disruption. Clients who are chronically ill tend to feel isolated from the rest of society and to take on a new identity related to the stigma society has placed on their illness.

Chronicity, therefore, is the continuation of a health disruption until it has a possibly permanent impact on the overall identity and life-style of the client. This process results in distinguishable changes in one's world view, habits of relating, view of self, and ability to carry out self-care functions. However, even very entrenched life patterns can be changed in the presence of the "right" conditions, which may only be defined by the client. It is essential to maintain hope for an improved quality of life for clients without imposing expectations for change according to the nurse's personal goals or timetables.

A chronically mentally distressed client is to some extent dependent on the mental health system or a supportive network of family or friends. This dependency is the result of troublesome behaviors, maladaptive coping patterns, or disturbed patterns of thought that interfere with the client's ability to care for himself and maintain a useful role in society. Chronically mentally distressed clients may or may not appear different from other people. Some of these clients meet the stereotypical images people have of "mental patients," such as the street person or the "bag

lady," the bizarrely dressed, ill-groomed man or woman with rambling speech or uncanny expressions and mannerisms.

Some clients have been acculturated into the life-style of the very regressed client since the days when all psychiatric patients were institutionalized. These clients may have never learned how to function on the "outside." Other chronically distressed clients have spent very little time in any hospital and appear to function at a higher level. They avoid societally imposed relationships, responsibilities, and realities by traveling constantly. They work only enough to stay alive and stay moving and are hospitalized only when they get into conflicts involving the police.

Chronically distressed psychiatric clients who have families to offer them emotional and financial support are rarely hospitalized in the larger public facilities but may enter private hospitals for brief stays several times a year. These clients may have much trouble negotiating with society at large, but they have social skills that remain intact except during acute episodes of psychosis.

Some chronically distressed clients, for various reasons, may be only rarely hospitalized but come to an outpatient mental health center for frequent visits such as for individual therapy, medication checks, and group or family therapy. During acute periods of psychosis, they may come in daily. These people may have minimal social skills, but,

591

Historical Overview

DATE	EVENT
Pre-1950	The chronically distressed client was institutionalized in long-term treatment facilities and received primarily custodial care.
1950s	With the introduction of chlorpromazine the chronically distressed client with a poor diagnosis was differentiated from the acutely disturbed client with a good diagnosis.
1960s	Because of drug therapy, some psychotic clients were able to leave the hospital permanently.
	The image of the mental patient changed as hope and sophisticated therapies began to replace blanket labeling and custodial care.
	An examination of all state mental health facilities by a presidential committee resulted in a directive to reduce the population of state hospitals and to limit admission to these facilities to clients posing an imminent danger to themselve and others.
	The presidential directive called for community-based outpatient mental health facilities for treatment of the chronically mentally ill.
	Chronically distressed clients became a target population for care and were viewed as unable or unwilling to learn necessary skills for survival out of the hospital.
	Nurses were given more independence in their work with the chronically distressed.
1970s	A new group of chronically mentally ill clients, composed of individuals who were born in the 1950s and first hospitalized after the deinstitutionalization movement, was identified.
1978	The President's Commission on Mental Health recommended a national plan for defining the chronically mentally ill and evaluating their needs and problems. This plan was to be implemented through national study and research as well as state level tracking of persons entering and leaving state mental health facilities.
1980s	Professionals of all disciplines are seeing the importance of assigning experienced nurses to work with chronically distressed clients.
Future	With increased focus on the needs of chronically distressed clients, nurses will be more involved in planning nursing care for these clients.

with support and guidance, are able to take care of themselves, work, marry, and have children.

Chronically distressed clients may function on a high level, perhaps for several years. This phase may be followed by several years of chaos during which the clients are in and out of the hospital constantly, unable to care for themselves. Friends and family blame first themselves and then the disorganized client for these erratic changes. Anger may generate long-term hostility and become a barrier to love and understanding. Many times this anguish can be prevented if families learn early about the nature of the mental illness. Friends and family members need ongoing support to process all the crises, trials, and anxieties they experience while offering support to the chronically distressed client.

THEORETICAL APPROACHES
Sociocultural

Chronic mental distress is a set of behaviors representing a role created by society as a result of observations of individuals exhibiting behaviors troublesome to society, and labeled "mentally deviant." Society reinforces the role and the individual internalizes the expectations inherent in this role. New behaviors are either not recognized, or are interpreted as characteristic of the mental illness. The individual's character is seen only in the context of mental illness, as a result, healthier aspects are ignored or extinguished.

Symbolic interactionism offers a perspective that explains the role of society, social learning, cognition, and choice in the development of a chronic mental illness. Symbolic interactionism asserts that individuals interact by assuming a series of roles. They choose these roles according to their perceptions of the environment, their understanding of other people's expectations of them and their understanding of the roles from which they may choose. If people are flexible and adaptive, they pass quickly through many roles according to their perceptions of the environment. If they are inner directed as well, individuals maintain an inner view of self, based on the combined successes and failures of all their roles. People who are not so flexible may strain a role to fit in with an environmental change. They may tenaciously cling to a role as if it were a complete identity, ignoring cues from the environment that tell them to develop a new role. A rigid person may assume a role and make few adaptations despite the expectations of those around them.

The development of chronic mental illness, according to symbolic interactionism, assumes that there is initially a healthy self. Organic or psychodynamic influences result in behaviors that are considered by society to be characteristic of mentally ill persons. For a period of time, referred to as the "acute illness state," the unhealthy behaviors (the role) create the primary identity of the individual as mentally ill. In the therapeutic environment of the hospital, the client is helped to develop more adaptive behaviors and assume roles that will be more acceptable in society.

The client next leaves the therapeutic environment. In society, he may find that many people behave as if he were still mentally ill. People around the "ex–mental patient" may respond to his behavior based on their understanding of the mental patient role. In this case, the individual finds that it is no longer easy to reassume a "healthy identity." The easiest, most acceptable role for him to assume is that of a mentally ill person.

As the individual forms his new role, he takes information from the environment. He bases a self-concept on how others in the environment seem to perceive him. People in the environment may verbalize their support for an independent life-style for him, but the way they behave indicates that they expect him to assume the role of a chronically mentally ill person. These expectations are internalized by the individual, and the role of the chronically mentally ill person is assumed. The individual is now stigmatized.[19] Society sees the individual as a "mental patient" and will observe only those characteristics of the individual which fit with that image. In turn, the individual expects the characteristics of a "mental patient" to be his primary behaviors.

In this manner, the individual has chosen the career of a chronically distressed client. His future goals as well as current realities are viewed from this perspective. The individual expects to be dependent on the health care system. To fight this role is to expose himself to uncertainties and new experiences that in the past have resulted in failures. The perceptions and expectations of those around him have reinforced his initial suspicion that he is chronically mentally ill. To challenge these perceptions and expectations is to challenge an entire power structure, and according to symbolic interactionism, the pessimistic view society holds of mental illness has already been internalized by the individual. The individual now expects only the life of a chronically mentally ill person and, in many ways, engineers his life to fulfill these prophecies.

The role of the chronically mentally ill person is learned from society and then refined through interactions with other people labelled as chronically mentally ill. These people comprise a subculture or perhaps several subcultures within society. These subcultures are probably complete with their own mores, values, and nonverbal

STEPS IN THE DEVELOPMENT OF CHRONIC MENTAL DISTRESS ACCORDING TO SYMBOLIC INTERACTIONISM

1. The self is born healthy, with genetic and/or environmental predispositions for the development of a mental illness.
2. Environmental and/or organic stressors occur.
3. The individual develops behaviors that society has labeled as the role of the mentally ill.
4. The individual is identified as unsafe in society and placed in a therapeutic environment.
5. The individual's maladaptive behaviors are controlled or extinguished, and he is again returned to society.
6. If he can be properly supported to reenter the normal role of a competent individual, the cycle is interrupted.
7. If the individual finds that society treats him as if he were still displaying behaviors associated with mental illness, the cycle continues.
8. People around the individual interpret his behavior as if he were still mentally ill.
9. The individual finds that he can no longer reassume a "healthy identity."
10. The individual finds that the easiest and most acceptable role to assume is that of a mental patient.
11. The individual hears people tell him he is supported and encouraged to adopt the role of a "normal," but he sees people behave in such a way as to indicate they expect him to assume the role of the mentally ill person.
12. These expectations of society are internalized by the individual.
13. The individual is stigmatized.[4]
14. The individual and society see the individual primarily according to the "mental illness" aspect of his personality.
15. Only those behaviors characteristic of a mentally ill person are observed by society and by the individual.
16. All of the individual's behaviors are seen in the context of mental illness.
17. The individual sees his goals and current realities within the perspective of his chronic mental illness.
18. The individual expects to be dependent on the health care system, because he sees this as part of the role of the mentally ill person.
19. The individual is afraid to challenge this perception of himself, because such a challenge represents uncertainty and has in the past been met with negative reactions by others.
20. The individual internalizes society's pessimistic view of mental illness, which is "once mentally ill, always mentally ill."
21. The individual engineers his life to fulfill society's expectations of chronic mental illness and thus fulfills the negative expectations.
22. The individual sees other people in various treatment centers who are also labeled chronically mentally ill.
23. These people represent a subculture with unique values, mores, and systems of nonverbal communication.
24. The individual's interactions within this subculture strengthen his role as chronically mentally ill and widen the gap between the individual and the norm.

TABLE 32-1 Determination of treatments according to level of functioning

Level of Functioning	Description	Setting for Treatment	Individual Treatment Strategies	Group Strategies	Family Strategies	Couple Strategies
Low	1. Shows obvious residual signs of mental illness 2. Dependent in all or most personal care	1. Day hospital 2. Inpatient 3. Day activity program	1. Behavioral approaches 2. Supportive problem solving 3. Skills training	1. Clinican-led group 2. Skills training 3. Reality groups	1. Support 2. Teaching	1. Support 2. Information
Moderate	1. Requires consistent support to maintain motivation to complete personal care 2. Unable to live independently but requires only supportive assistance	1. Brief hospitalizations 2. Outpatient therapy	1. Consultant/peer approach 2. Individual therapy to strengthen healthy defense	1. Social network group 2. Peer-led group	1. Support 2. Communication therapy 3. Supporting boundary	1. Communication therapy 2. Supporting boundary
Independent	1. Able to live independently much of the time 2. Demonstrates basic skills of differentiating thoughts and feelings 3. Recognizes personal responsibilites in some situations 4. Is able to formulate own problem list and treatment plan with assistance (The nurse clinician offers insight-oriented and/or confrontive approaches if the client requests to work on issues regarding early life or changing life patterns. If the client does not request such work, the nurse plays a more passive role as consultant.)	1. Self-help programs 2. Liaison with outpatient programs 3. Outpatient clinics	1. More in-depth, insight-oriented approaches 2. Consultant/peer approach	1. Peer-led group 2. Therapy groups 3. Insight-oriented	1. More in-depth, "uncovering" therapy 2. Insight-oriented	1. Uncovering therapy 2. Insight-oriented

communication signals. These all may be easily seen in the population of a large state hospital.

Development of the career of a chronically distressed client is summarized in the box on p. 593.

Much recent study, categorization, and development of new treatment approaches has concentrated on the "new" young population of chronically distressed persons between 18 and 35 years of age.[4,32a,35] They represent a group of clients who were not exposed to the influences of long-term institutionalization and custodial care. They are from the "baby boom" era of the 1950s and later. Sheets and others[35] hypothetically subdivided this population into three groups to show the distinct categories of their needs. (See Table 32-1.)

One group may be called the "low energy, low demand" group, characterized by passivity and low motivation. They are dependent on the mental health system, and despite their lack of years of experience in the large state hospitals, they are well socialized into the patient role.

Another group is the "high energy, high demand" group. They are also fairly dependent on mental health workers, but are also aggressively demanding, impulsive, and impatient in their dealings with counselors and case managers. They push away those who try to help them and often move around from place to place, float in and out of jobs and public assistance, and go through sexual relationships quickly and dramatically. They are characterized by their high energy and their expectations of self-reliance, which are often frustrated. This group also includes the eccentric street people and the "revolving-door" patients who arrive on the hospital doorstep when times are hard.

A final group is called "high functioning, high aspiration." They tend to function fairly well most of the time and sometimes appear much healthier than they are. They may also be better educated and come from higher income families than those of the other groups. They frequently consider traditional mental health activities to be unappealing and avoid anything that leads anyone to label them mentally ill. They wish to blend smoothly in with society and have well-established goals for success.[35]

These groups are not official classifications, but they do help point out the variety of needs and problems seen in the population considered chronically mentally distressed. The needs of younger psychiatric clients are also inherently different because of societal changes, including greater overall mobility, general loosening of family ties, increased availability of street drugs, and changes in the approach to rehabilitation of mental illness.[4]

A summary of the dynamics of the theory is presented in Table 32-2.

QUALIFICATIONS OF THE THERAPIST

The chronically distressed client is viewed by many nurses as more than an ordinary challenge. The nurse needs to have patience and realistic expectations of the client to work effectively with the chronically distressed client. Nurses avoid imposing their personal goals on the

TABLE 32-2 Summary of the dynamics of the theoretical approach

Theory	Theorist	Dynamics
Sociocultural (Symbolic interactionism)	Goffman	The formerly mentally ill person internalizes and assumes a role that is perceived and reinforced by society as that of a mentally ill person.
	Sheets and others	There are three groups of young adult, chronically distressed clients: low energy, low demand; high energy, high demand; and high functioning, high aspiration.

client or promising the client more nurturance than they can practically provide in a professional role. The nurse has knowledge of general psychodynamics, psychopathology, and personality development, as well as counseling skills. The nurse also has a personal interest in chronically distressed people and considers them worthwhile and deserving of high-quality work with experienced expert nurses.

The nurse is understanding of the nature of the client's chronic problems as well as his abilities and strengths. The nurse understands how extensive limitations can exist in a creative, spontaneous, holistic person. The nurse sees the client as an individual and is not overwhelmed by the long-standing nature of the client's problems.

The nurse understands that the client's symptoms appear in cycles that frequently are little influenced by external factors. The nurse also maintains hope that the client can reach an optimal level of development while not expecting the client to follow a timetable or respect traditional goals and norms of society. The nurse maintains a patient and honest presence while awaiting the client to develop trust, test limits, frequently misunderstand the nurse's role, and finally accept the relationship with the nurse in the client's unique manner.

The nurse working with chronically distressed clients is an expert in congruent and concrete communication. Clear communication, verbal and nonverbal, conveys the nature of the relationship and is necessary in assisting the client to recognize and cope with reality and personal responsibility. The nurse also uses clearly defined social skills and serves as a role model while helping the client to define the relationship.

The nurse is creative in both accepting and assisting the client. A client who is chronically distressed may have well-developed patterns of dysfunction. These patterns may be delusional systems or faulty habits of relating. If the nurse focuses on challenging such entrenched habits, she is, in effect, rejecting the most delicate aspects of the client's being. It is usually best to accept the client with his dysfunction, learn the overall nature and limits of use of such patterns, then gently help the client to incorporate more functional habits of living. Assisting the client creatively may mean being willing to share oneself while still maintaining a professional role and remaining aware of one's own limitations. Over time and with the client's help, the nurse may find new, creative therapy approaches that work well.

Role

Generally the nurse's role is to help the client adapt and thus live more successfully. This means the nurse focuses on the everyday tasks at hand, assisting the client to approach life and daily problems in a more realistic, responsible, and task-oriented manner. The nurse's problem-solving skills assist the client to function better, and it is hoped the client will learn these skills for more independent living.

The nurse maintains a variety of professional roles with the client, depending on the client's needs. In the surrogate mother role, the nurse assists the regressed client to reach out and begin to trust. As the surrogate mother she also accepts the client's dependence while remaining mindful of growth cues. These are signs in the client's behavior that alert the nurse to encourage more responsibility or more individuation without risking decompensation or withdrawal. Growth cues are responded to by support during intimidating trials and mistakes.

If a beginning level of trust and individuation is stabilized, the nurse assumes a role closer to that of teacher by instructing the client in means of adaptive behavior. The client frequently accepts the nurse as a role model and may temporarily mimic or at least adopt superficial habits of the nurse.

As the client progresses in goal attainment, the nurse may recognize temporary stability in the chronically distressed client's behavior. At such times, the most therapeutic role may be that of a peer or partner in problem solving. The client may better accept the nurse's assistance if it is offered as suggestions rather than directives, limits, or advice.

During periods of remission or adaptive functioning, the client is still faced with the stigma of chronic mental illness in an increasingly complex society. Armed with appropriate skills and habits, the chronically distressed client may still need an advocate. This person assists the client to understand social systems, societal boundaries, and how to move smoothly within society.

Goals

The client at times may be able to set appropriate goals, independently or with the help of the nurse. At other times the nurse may need to set goals for the client, preferably with the client's permission. The nurse plans interventions to assist the client to meet these goals, watching for signs that the client may be ready to independently accept and strive for them. Such goals include increased independence in daily living. For some clients a reasonable goal may be decreased time in the hospital.

Chronically distressed clients may sometimes be unable to tolerate adult relationships or any form of closeness with others. But during less vulnerable times, such clients seem to do better if they are a part of a safe, reliable social network. This may consist of family, old friends, or other people struggling with a chronic disturbance. Establishment of such a network is a reasonable goal for many clients.

The clinican also remains mindful of the client's need to understand himself. At many times self-awareness may be an overwhelming and frightening thing for the client. However, during levels of adaptive functioning, it is best for the client to learn about the special needs he may have, both as a unique human being and as a chronically distressed person. It is also essential for the client to learn about his strengths and special attributes. The therapeutic relationship hopefully reflects such knowledge.

One goal for the chronically distressed client is to learn to have greater trust in himself. He needs to believe himself worthy of kindness, warmth, and acceptance of others. The client learns to accept and care about himself in order to really know how to care for himself. The client needs to develop a positive self-esteem to negotiate successfully in society.

The nurse remembers that the client needs to see a goal as better than his current state of functioning. This goal needs to appeal to the client according to the client's value system, and the nurse remembers that the chronically distressed client usually does not maintain the value system of society at large. To reach a goal, the client needs to develop motivation. To have motivation, the client has to feel uncomfortable in the present and maintain hope for the future. At times such sensations are impossible or intolerable for the client. The nurse, therefore, needs to have a sense of timing and sensitivity to the client's changing abilities, to accept current reality, and to believe in the possibility of a different level of functioning. Helping the client find motivation to pursue a goal is probably the greatest challenge the nurse has with the chronically distressed.

CHARACTERISTICS OF THERAPY

The chronically distressed client frequently seems to respond to therapy modalities differently than clients with acute, short-term problems. To some extent this difference results from the nature of the chronic client's disturbance. Also, long-term clients become therapy-wise, skillful in eluding the positive effects of therapy, but able to talk as if real learning and integration are occurring. Long-term clients usually have deeply entrenched dysfunctional patterns that have become integral parts of their personality. To confront such patterns directly, as the nurse may with a client who has a short-term illness, would be asking the client to give up too much of himself. These patterns are an important source of defense, and the nurse offers nothing safe with which to replace the personality pattern. Therefore the nurse frequently varies the manner in which therapeutic modalities are used with the chronically distressed client so as to focus on the positive goals of developing new functional behaviors without directly addressing the dysfunctional ones. The nurse may help create an environment or experience in which the client sees a clear personal advantage in giving up a dysfunctional pattern.

Many chronically distressed clients who are regressed in their social skills respond better to behavioral approaches than they may to approaches requiring emphasis on communication skills. Behavioral approaches offer the client well-bounded and clearly defined expectations. Consistency, as is seen in behavioral approaches, assists the confused or disoriented client in reality orientation. Such approaches may be as complex as a token economy system, in which the client "buys" privileges with tokens earned by meeting expectations of self-care or social responsibility. Behavioral approaches more likely seen with chronically distressed clients include use of "time out" rooms when the client loses control, giving the client extra privileges when self-care behaviors are completed correctly, or commenting regularly on the client's good appearance. All behavioral approaches are carried out with respect for the client and with an attitude that conveys that the client is accepted unconditionally while attempting to modify specific behaviors of the client.

The therapeutic relationship with the chronically distressed client is commonly a long-term and intense relationship. The nurse has perhaps followed the same client through many periods of decompensation, regression and hospitalization. This nurse may have also assisted the client to enjoy brief periods of independence and adaptive functioning. The nurse keeps a healthy perspective on the appropriate professional role with this client with varied and changing needs. The nurse stays flexible to encourage the client to maintain hope while assisting him to recognize realistic limitations.

An additional individual therapy approach frequently helpful with the chronically distressed client is the consultant or peer approach. This approach is best used with the client who is well stabilized, has learned how to meet his basic needs consistently in an adaptive fashion, and simply needs positive reinforcement and problem-solving assistance. Such clients are frequently mistrustful of traditional roles of the nurse and client and wish to maintain as much independence as possible. In these situations, the nurse avoids any type of authoritative or parental role and offers the client complete feedback in a nonjudgmental, nonpersuasive manner. Sometimes chronically distressed clients with bizarre but well-contained (ego syntonic) delusional systems respond well to this approach. Also, the matter-of-fact approach of the consultant, which avoids confrontation or challenge of the client's reality, assists the client to be more trusting and accepting of therapeutic assistance. Acceptance by the nurse also helps the client begin to adopt new behaviors and accept the risk of breaking old patterns.

Insight-oriented approaches are generally least helpful with chronically distressed clients. The focus with these clients is on building and reinforcing healthy defenses, not breaking down unhealthy ones. In addition, the chronically distressed client frequently lacks motivation to withstand the stresses of confrontive approaches. A client who is chronically distressed but well stabilized and who demonstrates a consistent sense of self and of his own strengths and limitations may be an appropriate candidate for more insight-oriented approaches. This may include confrontive psychotherapy if the client is motivated to request such "uncovering" therapy approaches.

Similarly, group therapy approaches are usually found to be effective with chronically distressed clients. Such groups focus on problem solving, skill building, and support rather than a confrontive or insight-oriented approach. Chronically distressed clients are more likely than other clients to have confused personal boundaries, which make it difficult for them to benefit from group therapies. However, a skilled nurse can create a learning environment for clients with confused personal boundaries by offering structure for the clients, encouraging verbal participation without requiring it, and modeling clear social skills. The nurse also enters the group with an attitude that conveys that the group is fun to be in but does not draw attention from the more serious therapeutic goals of the group therapy process.

After such positive therapist-led group experiences, the more motivated clients may prefer to participate in peer-led groups. These may be support groups or involve skills training, in the way that Alcoholics Anonymous groups teach skills to recovering alcoholics. Such groups offer the client a method of finding a family or "we group," a group of people who understand because "they've been there." The "we group" offers the client support and peer guidance while reinforcing a positive identity, a belief in the self as worthy and lovable.[9]

Social network groups for the chronically distressed client again offer an opportunity for development of the "we group." The focus is on providing the client with safe opportunities to socialize with others who are familiar with the problems of chronic mental illness. If organized and structured by a nurse, the group provides opportunities for trying out new social behaviors and roles for the regressed client. The client with a higher level of functioning commonly prefers peer-led groups.

Family therapy is necessary to ensure the family's continued support of the chronically distressed client. With family therapy, as in other therapy approaches with chronically distressed clients, the therapist avoids confrontation or even family restructuring unless the family and client are prepared and strong enough emotionally. Instead, the focus may be on the therapist offering information and support to family members who are attempting to support the client. The therapist also attempts to teach the family members and the client how to give and receive support among themselves. Other topics, as in any family therapy, include boundaries, communication, and family roles.

Couples therapy, when one member of the couple is a chronically distressed client, may focus on giving support and information to the spouse or partner of the client. The client in an intimate relationship will often require much support as well as assistance in clarifying boundaries. Maintaining clear communication is an important goal with the chronically distressed client. The client may also require support in bearing the pain associated with any intimate relationship. In couples therapy the nurse has even more responsibility than usual to offer strong support to both partners, supporting the relationship if it shows signs of becoming a healthy, growth-producing one.

In many cases, chronically distressed clients come from dysfunctional family systems that offer less than adequate training for intimate relationships; such a client needs more skill training than other clients. If the relationship is an unhealthy one, the client needs extra support to get through the process of deciding to separate, and through the separation itself. The chronically distressed client has fewer internal—and usually also fewer external—resources to call on in such a crisis. The loss of a relationship commonly means abandonment for the chronically distressed client, even if he was the one to withdraw from his partner. Abandonment can bring up many unresolved wounds from unmet childhood needs, and the client responds by regressing to an earlier level of development. The nurse maintains patience through this regression and continues to offer understanding and hope, while allowing the client to increase his dependence temporarily.

NURSING PROCESS
Assessment

The assessment process with the chronically distressed is no less important because the client has been diagnosed many times in the past. Even if the nurse has assessed the client during past hospitalizations, she makes assumptions based on the client's current status instead of on past assessment data.

The client may be fairly hardened to the assessment process. The nurse may face responses such as "It's in my old charts" and "You know all this stuff anyway." Historical information may be gathered from old records, and the nurse may wish to spread the assessment over several sessions to avoid overwhelming the client.

✦ *Physical dimension.* If the client is being seen on an outpatient basis, the best place for the assessment is his home. This enables the nurse to assess the client's self-care abilities, among other things. In a residential treatment center, a visit to the client's room may also be enlightening. His housekeeping skills are noted, as is the level of stimulation the environment offers. For example, are there windows with curtains open, or is the room dark? Are the walls bare? Are there any indications that the client has given his room a personal touch? Also, the client's perspective on his neighborhood and neighbors is ascertained. Does he feel accepted and safe?

The client's hygiene habits are also examined to indicate his general physical health. How well or poorly groomed is the client and how appropriate is his dress for the weather and occasion? The nurse can get an idea about how typical the client's habits of self-care and dress are. She can also observe the client's posture and gait; many chronically distressed clients shuffle and slouch. This may be related to a mental illness, a medication reaction, or self-esteem. The nurse also observes how spontaneously the client moves. A severely distressed client may have stiff or mannequin-like physical motions. In extremely regressed clients, control of body functions, bowel and bladder, are also monitored to give an indication of physical health as well as dependency needs.

Caregivers, such as family or regular residential staff members, can provide information about the client's abilities to control bowel and bladder and to complete hygiene tasks. Such caregivers can give important information about any variations from the norm in the client's behavior. The establishment of norms is essential to enable the nurse to appreciate the severity of the client's state of distress and to set more reasonable goals with him.

Chronically distressed clients are sometimes found living in precarious situations; they may have been exposed to the elements and poorly nourished for months. The possibility of disease or ingrained but maladaptive personal care patterns is great in these clients. Some clients who have been living on the street have pain and troublesome diseases for which they have no skill to self-diagnose nor motivation to seek relief.

The client's current and normal states of physical health are assessed. The nurse notes any pain or chronic physical discomfort and gathers information about the client's cycle of activity and rest, past and current. The client's eating habits during periods of regression and higher functioning are assessed, lending clues to his overall level of nutrition.

The client's needs for assistance in obtaining proper health care is assessed. The nurse assesses the client's system of reminders to keep prescriptions filled, appointments kept, and medications taken regularly. The client may need help in recognizing when an extra health care appointment is needed. The nurse may observe the client's ability to make doctor's appointments or seek general health care as needed. The nurse assesses the client's knowledge of proper care for minor illnesses and injuries and observes his supply of first aid materials.

It is helpful to determine if other people in the client's family have been chronically distressed. Such information may lead one to the recognition of a genetic predisposition for the development of chronic mental distress, or may indicate the client's socialization by a family role model.

The client's body image is important to assess. Again, past and current patterns are essential to note. The first assessment is how the client perceives his body and how realistic this perception is. How does the client perceive other people's reactions to his body?

An important aspect of body image is sexual image. The chronically distressed client's sexual behavior may vary between when he is regressed and when he is functioning at a higher level. The nurse assesses the client's sexual preference, image of himself as a sexual being, and level of sexual activity. Direct questions related to areas such as body image and sexuality may increase the anxiety level of the chronically distressed client. Some level of trust needs to be developed before a client can comfortably reveal this sort of information.

A checklist assessing how the client copes in his environment offers a matter-of-fact approach if the nurse main-

---

SAMPLE CHECKLIST OF ACTIVITIES OF DAILY LIVING TASKS

PERSONAL HYGIENE

Brushes teeth daily
Combs hair
Bathes daily
Shampoos hair three times weekly
Uses deodorant daily
Wears clean clothing
Keeps nails clean and trim
Dresses appropriately for activity and weather

HOUSEKEEPING AND FOOD MANAGEMENT

Keeps kitchen clean and properly cares for garbage
Does laundry as needed
Keeps bathroom clean
Keeps living areas clean and straightened
Prepares adequate, nutritious meals
Varies daily menus
Stores and cares for food properly
Keeps refrigerator and cupboards free of spoiled foods
Keeps entire area smelling fresh

MONEY MANAGEMENT

Budgets money for the month
Plans all expenditures; makes lists before shoppng
Uses food stamps and coupons as much as possible
Pays bills on time and with checks or money orders
Keeps receipt of bills paid
Looks for bargains for major expenditures

HEALTH CARE

Has basic first aid supplies and uses them when needed
Keeps prescriptions renewed and filled as needed
Keeps schedule for all daily and weekly medications
Keeps schedule of regular health care appointments
    and makes additional ones as needed
Cares for minor illnesses appropriately
Asks for assistance or advice when needed

---

tains a nonjudgmental attitude in responding to the client. The client may be asked to complete such a questionnaire checklist, or the nurse may ask the client to review the checklist. The nurse then completes the questionnaire following several interactions and periods of observation. The Sample Checklist above is an example of such an approach.

The chronically distressed client's income is generally low, and the nurse assesses the skills the client has to increase his income. The nurse learns about the client's ability to prepare and follow a budget as well as his use of coupons and food stamps. The nurse collects information about the client's ability to plan every expenditure, use shopping lists, and seek bargains. She assesses the client's ability to launder and repair clothes and to store and prepare foods.

✳ ***Emotional dimension.*** When assessing the emotional dimension, the nurse observes first the pri-

mary emotion the client is experiencing. Emotions to assess include anxiety, anger, grief, despair, guilt, fear, joy, and hope. Chronically distressed clients may disassociate their feelings and may not report experiencing emotions. Also, clients may be unsophisticated regarding emotions and may not know what is meant by the term anxiety or even anger. The client may deny the experience of an emotion because he believes such an emotion is too painful, too difficult to control, or too shameful to admit. Limited trust in the early stages of the relationship may prevent the client from revealing information about his emotions during the assessment process.

The nurse assesses how intensely the client experiences various emotions and how the client's current affective state differs from his norm. Also important to assess is the client's ability to control his emotions and the degree of congruence between the client's emotional reaction and the situation to which the client is reacting. Chronically distressed clients may express one emotion while actually experiencing another. The nurse clarifies what emotion the client is experiencing, any stimulus for the reaction, and the intensity of the affect displayed. The client's general degree of emotional or affective lability is also assessed and noted.

✳ ***Intellectual dimension.*** Assessment of the intellectual dimension usually reveals variations in a client's abilities between periods of regression and higher functioning. It is helpful to know the client's basic, healthy intellectual capacity rather than rely on assessments made during acute episodes. Formal testing during such an acute period may be of little assistance, but the nurse assesses the client's current intellectual capacity through the mental status examination and general observation. This information aids the nurse in planning care as well as in assessing the client's degree of disorganization.

During an acute period the client may also exhibit unusual content of thought, such as bizarre thoughts or inability to control his thoughts. The nurse determines whether these problems are also present during periods of higher functioning. The nurse assesses the client's flow of thought, observing for periods of thought blocking and disruptions caused by hallucinations or delusions. The nurse also needs to differentiate disrupted or emotion-laden speech from abnormal thought. The chronically distressed client may or may not accurately represent his thoughts in ordinary speech. He may use grandiose or unusual speech because of his heightened emotions or illogical thinking. The nurse may wish to try to help the client focus his thoughts and clarify his vague or unusual speech to further assess intellectual function.

The nurse needs to assess how the client actually perceives his environment. How is the client responding to ordinary physical sensations, such as fatigue, warmth or cold, and bright or dim light? How do these perceptions differ from the norm for that client? In-depth assessment to differentiate long-standing from acute delusional systems helps the nurse plan more appropriate interventions.

The client's ability to retain and recall information, in both the short- and long-term, is assessed and compared to his norm. This information helps the nurse determine the client's ability to benefit from various types of therapeutic interventions. When possible, observations rather than direct questions are used for such assessments. This approach is used because chronically distressed clients become easily irritated and confused in response to direct mental status questions when they are in an acute or regressed period.

Because the chronically distressed client may have enough compensatory social skills to mask cognitive dysfunction, it is necessary to assess abstract and concrete thinking directly, such as by asking the client to interpret a proverb. Orientation also is not assumed from conversation but rather assessed through direct questioning. Such direct questions may be less offensive if introduced in a nonthreatening manner. For example, the nurse may say, "I'm going to ask you some questions now that will sound pretty silly but are important for me to be able to know how you think."

Many chronically distressed clients are noted to be rigid in their thinking. Such rigidity may be reflected in a simplistic right-wrong or good-bad view of the world. In contrast to the client with extremely rigid thinking is the client who has weak ego structure resulting in overflexibility. This client may follow any lead; he may adopt the mannerisms and values of others quite readily and may be overly distractible. Again, it is essential to assess this behavior against the client's baseline.

Another variation in thinking commonly seen in chronically distressed clients is reflected in abnormally fast or slow speech. The nurse ascertains whether the client's rate of speech is slower or faster than his rate of thinking. The client may also exhibit overwatchfulness or unusually detailed thought and speech. Focusing on details prevents a client from perceiving the whole picture, which is reflected in behavior.

Chronically distressed clients may have little or no insight, lack appropriateness of judgment, and possess limited knowledge about the world and current events. Information related to these areas may be assessed through the general interview. Questioning may focus on the client's understanding of his illness and his need for assistance. The nurse may also ask the client how he handles his own emergency needs. Casual conversation about current events seen widely in the newspaper and on television helps the nurse assess the client's general fund of knowledge. When assessing the client's speech the nurse may observe aberrations of speech, including bizarre speech, word salad, use of rhyme, and unusual voice tones. Nonverbal as well as verbal communication used by the chronically distressed client may be idiosyncratic during periods of higher functioning and frankly bizarre during periods of decompensation. For example, the client may normally use rhyme, a singsong voice, or ritualistic head nodding and shrugging. This would differ from the frankly bizarre behaviors of shouting, extreme grimacing, watchful scanning of the environment, or reaching out in a threatening manner to others.

In all of these areas, the nurse assesses how much and in what ways the client's unusual patterns of thought and behavior actually affect his ability to function in the world. The behavior may be troublesome to others but would otherwise not interfere in the client's quest for independence. An example may be an unusual need for constant reassurance and direction. The client may actually know what to do but be afraid to proceed. Another example is muttering or making clicking noises with the mouth. Such behaviors may need to be addressed to ensure employment, but do not indicate inability to function appropriately.

Vocational skills are also assessed by the nurse. The client needs to be able to concentrate on a task for an extended period of time to benefit from vocational training or placement in a job. Vocational rehabilitation professionals assess for ability to work or be trained for work, but the nurse can assess general areas to know when to make a vocational assessment referral. The nurse assesses the client's ability to concentrate for extended periods and his ability to be punctual, courteous, and reliable in following directions. The nurse assesses the client's vocational motivations and interests as well as his ability to control idiosyncratic mannerisms that may be annoying to others.

Social dimension. It often seems that chronically distressed clients have failed to integrate their social knowledge. In the interview and during observations of the client's interactions with others, the nurse may note the client's awareness of the social expectations of others and his ability to choose appropriate responses to others. Eating habits, communication patterns, body language, and respect for others' personal space all reflect social awareness and skill in some manner. A related factor is the client's ability to live in close quarters with others without violating their privacy or basic rights. The nurse assesses social skill by observing the client's tolerance of emotional closeness or intimacy, because the chronically distressed have trouble tolerating close relationships. The number of friends or socially supportive people the client knows reflects the client's social abilities.

The nurse assesses the way in which the client uses vocabulary, expresses thoughts, and conveys emotions, in addition to any unique patterns of communication with family or friends. The client's family communications may include double messages, statements that invalidate the feelings of the client or other family members, or communication that is otherwise vague or global. The nurse observes the family's interactions with the client for signs of unusual or inappropriate expressions of emotions. The family members may seem underemotional; appearing to deny or hide their emotions, or highly overemotional, reacting to seemingly insignificant occurrences with dramatic emotional displays.

Chronically distressed clients tend to have low self-esteem, so assessment includes how the client values himself, what ideal self he imagines as a goal, and how he identifies himself. Noted is the way the client communicates his self-esteem to others and how what he conveys compares to his actual self-esteem. The nurse observes whether or not the client identifies with the stereotype of the "chronically mentally ill" and how this affects his perceptions and functioning. The nurse may observe that the client who was institutionalized for a long period is likely to view himself as chronically mentally ill and believe he is a failure. The "new" chronically mentally ill person is less likely to perceive himself in the role of patient. Instead, the nurse may observe that these clients assume or wish to assume roles such as caretaker, leader, or spouse and make an effort to fit into the community.

The client with chronic mental illness tends to fluctuate between dependence and independence. The nurse assesses how dependent the client is on others, how dependence influences his overall functioning, and how aware he is of his dependence. Similarly, the nurse observes and notes areas of independence. The nurse assesses how the client responds to authority figures, peers, and subordinates. These patterns refer to the client's interdependence and sharing, and giving and taking of power with others. The client's ability to trust himself and others may also be reflected in his behaviors of dependence and independence. The chronically distressed client may have had few successes in the world to aid development of trust. The nurse collects information about the client's experiences that are a basis for the trust-related behaviors he has acquired and may display during the interview.

Spiritual dimension. The chronically distressed client may have difficulty with questions about his values, how he learned them, and how he makes moral and ethical decisions. This difficulty results from concrete, overly abstract, or dichotomized thinking (seeing the world as only good or bad, rather than using broader judgment and considering specific situations). Other questions that need to be asked concern a belief in a higher power, in an organized religion, and in a purpose for life in general or the client in particular. The chronically distressed client may have been offered few opportunities to consider such topics for himself. The client may be too self-absorbed to have considered spiritual questions. If the client is unable to articulate his beliefs and opinions, the nurse gains useful assessment information in this area through observation of the client.

ALTERATION IN HEALTH MAINTENANCE

DEFINITION

Disruption in health status because of inability to identify, manage, and/or seek out help to maintain health.

DEFINING CHARACTERISTICS

Physical Dimension
- *Lack of necessary equipment to meet health needs
- *Frequent use of over-the-counter medication

Emotional Dimension
- Apathy
- Chronic fatigue
- Frequent feeling of being overwhelmed
- Belligerence
- Emotional fragility

Intellectual Dimension
- Compulsiveness
- *Lack of knowledge about basic health practices
- *Lack of motivation
- *Lack of awareness in difference in ill and non-ill behavior

Social Dimension
- *Dependence
- *Impairment of personal support system
- *Lack of adaptive behaviors to internal or external environmental change
- *Inability to take responsibility for meeting basic needs
- *Lack of health-seeking behavior
- *Lack of financial resources

Spiritual Dimension
- *Belief that ill health is God's will

Adapted from North American Nursing Diagnosis Association Classification of Nursing Diagnosis: Proceedings of the seventh conference, St. Louis, 1987, The C.V. Mosby Co.

*Indicates characteristics in addition to those defined by NANDA.

IMPAIRED HOME MAINTENANCE MANAGEMENT

DEFINITION

Inability to independently maintain a safe home environment.

DEFINING CHARACTERISTICS

Physical Dimension
- Presence of unwashed dishes and clothes
- Offensive odors
- Repeated infections
- Lack of necessary equipment for maintaining home
- Accumulation of food, waste, and dirt
- Poor hygienic practices
- Presence of rodents or vermin

Emotional Dimension
- *Anxiety
- *Generalized discomfort
- *Exhaustion

Intellectual Dimension
- Requests assistance with basic home maintenance
- Expresses difficulty in maintaining a comfortable home environment
- Lack of knowledge about maintaining a safe home environment
- *Inability to identify the need for home repairs

Social Dimension
- *Insufficient finances
- *Dysfunctional family relationships
- *Unavailable support system

Spiritual Dimension
- *Lack of belief in a supreme being
- *Hopeless life situation

Adapted from North American Nursing Diagnosis Association Classification of Nursing Diagnosis: Proceedings of the seventh conference, St. Louis, 1987, The C.V. Mosby Co.

*Indicates characteristics in addition to those defined by NANDA.

Analysis

Nursing diagnosis. Impaired home maintenance management and alteration in health maintenance are examples of nursing diagnoses approved by NANDA that apply to chronically distressed clients. The defining characteristics of these nursing diagnoses are listed in the boxes on p. 601. The following list provides examples of other nursing diagnoses with causative statements appropriate for the chronically distressed client:

1. Impaired decision making related to cognitive dysfunction
2. Impaired social interactions related to withdrawal from external world
3. Alteration in thought processes: delusion related to inability to evaluate reality
4. Social isolation related to withdrawal from others
5. Powerlessness related to low self-esteem

The following Case Example illustrates the defining characteristics of alteration in health maintenance.

Case Example

Mr. Jamison, age 65, suffers from chronic mental illness. A neighbor brought him to the emergency room stating that for the past several weeks, he has been apathetic and complaining of exhaustion. The neighbor reported that when she asked Mr. Jamison about his medication (psychotropic), he said he didn't need the medication and that he felt fine. During the intake interview, Mr. Jamison was belligerent and repeatedly said, "Leave me alone, I'm fine." He has not been eating balanced, nutritional meals and has some difficulty sleeping. Mr. Jamison told the nurse that his daughter, who he depends on, recently moved to another city. He reported that his daughter took care of his meals and other basic needs and he does not know how to do these things for himself. Mr. Jamison has no other children. With Mr. Jamison's approval, the nurse arranged for one of his sisters to live with him. The nurse will also teach Mr. Jamison some basics about his physical needs and his medication.

The following Case Example illustrates the defining characteristics of impaired home maintenance management.

Case Example

Mrs. Brazzel, age 65 and widowed, was hospitalized for 25 years with a diagnosis of schizophrenia. For the past 20 years she has lived in a small apartment. On and off, she has had some difficulty carrying out her activities of daily living and maintaining the apartment. However, with some assistance she was able to regroup and resume the tasks. Lately, when Mrs. Brazzel attends the after-care program at the community mental health center, she complains of feeling anxious and exhausted. She says she has no energy or interest in keeping her apartment clean. When the nurse visited Mrs. Brazzel's apartment, it was dirty and there was an accumulation of boxes and other material that she hoards. The nurse noted that the kitchen faucets leaked and the tiles in the floor were loose. Mrs. Brazzel seemed unconcerned about safety hazards in the apartment. Her situation indicated that she was no longer able to live independently. Because of her limited finances and the lack of contact with her son and daughter for 15 years, the nurse arranged for Mrs. Brazzel to live at a supervised group living home that charges a nominal fee. She received sufficient social security to pay the fee of the home.

DSM-III-R diagnoses. The DSM-III-R diagnostic categories associated with chronic distress are the organic mental disorders, schizophrenic disorders, paranoid disorders, affective disorders, other psychotic disorders, and personality disorders. Anxiety disorders, disorders of impulse control, or dissociative disorders may, in extreme cases, result in long-term dysfunction to the point of chronic distress, but these categories are not generally considered to represent the total life disruption of chronic distress.

Conversely, many individuals labeled as psychotic, paranoid, schizophrenic, manic-depressive, or borderline do not demonstrate the pervasive life disruption of the chronically distressed client. The personality disorders most likely to result in long-term dysfunction are schizoid, schizotypal, and borderline. The borderline personality is the most likely of the three to be chronically distressed.

Planning

Table 32-3 presents long-term and short-term goals and outcome criteria related to therapy with the chronically distressed client. These serve as examples of the planning stage in the nursing process.

Implementation

Physical dimension. Clients who have lost bowel and bladder control are placed on a toileting schedule. Punitive measures or any type of subtle confrontation in this area is counterproductive. The client responds best to regularity, consistency, and a calm approach.

Improved body image is encouraged by helping the client focus more on his body. A mirror may be used on an inpatient ward during supervised time to allow clients to assess themselves physically. Exercise programs often help clients get in touch with their physical functioning in a more realistic manner. Making clear, matter-of-fact comments to the client about positive physical attributes gives the client useful feedback.

When assisting the client to learn hygiene skills, a concrete behavioral approach may be of greatest help. The nurse starts with very basic behaviors such as teaching the client to comb his hair, brush his teeth, or button his shirt. The nurse reviews these skills with the client and has him perform the behaviors. Next, the nurse tells the client when these behaviors are expected. A chart placed in the client's room is usually a helpful reminder. The client may at first require supervision, then only a reminder. After completion of each behavior, the nurse praises the client. Also, comments on improved appearance are rewarding feedback. Eating habits may be shaped through a similar behavioral program. Nondisruptive mealtime behavior may be rewarded with nutritional treats or special privileges.

Chronically distressed clients usually have a higher level of functioning in all dimensions when they take med-

TABLE 32-3 Long-term and short-term goals and outcome criteria related to the chronically distressed client

Goals	Outcome Criteria

NURSING DIAGNOSIS: ALTERATION IN HEALTH MAINTENANCE RELATED TO INABILITY TO USE SOUND JUDGMENT

Long-term goal

To recognize early changes in health state and take appropriate action	Gets more rest and increases fluid intake when he has a cold. Recognizes signs of a fever, takes temperature appropriately, and reports any elevation to visiting nurse. Makes appointment to see his physician if health disruption persists or worsens.

Short-term goal

To take medications only as ordered	Makes lists of medications with scheduled times. Pays attention to directions of taking medication before or after meals, or any other specific directions, and includes these with time schedule. Reminds physician when prescription renewals are needed. Keeps prescriptions filled so no doses are missed.

NURSING DIAGNOSIS: IMPAIRED HOME MAINTENANCE MANAGEMENT RELATED TO LACK OF KNOWLEDGE

Long-term goal

To recognize in advance need for home maintenance work and plan for this pragmatically	Recognizes slowed drainage in sink and notifies landlord. Keeps sidewalks and outdoor stairs free of ice and snow for safe walking. Investigates faucet drips and toilet leaks when possible, and notifies landlord if problem is complicated.

Short-term goal

To keep home free of clutter, clean, and odor free	Does laundry frequently to avoid piles of dirty clothes. Does dishes after every meal. Cleans bathroom fixtures weekly.

ications properly. The nurse's first task may be to help the client recognize differences in his personal function while he is on and off medication. Clients may be impressed by "before-and-after" photographs, audiotapes, or feedback from family, friends, and staff. The client is helped to accept the necessity of his medication regimen as a current reality. If the client experiences more freedom and success while taking medications, he may be motivated by support and reminders to continue.

Chronically distressed clients usually display cues before they lose control or begin acting out. When cues of impending loss of control are observed, the client is removed to a less stimulating environment. Confrontations by the nurse are avoided when the client is losing behavioral control. Nurses need to avoid entering into power struggles with the client who is in danger of losing control by setting only necessary limits for the client's safety, ignoring minor infractions, and using extra care to enforce necessary limits with a matter-of-fact, nonintrusive manner. While the client is demonstrating potential for loss of control, it is safest for him to remain in his room or alone in a quiet room. Staff check on the client frequently to let him know of their presence. In general, the physical presence of alert staff serves as external control and reduces acting-out episodes.

The client's physical environment may be found to be unstimulating, chaotic, or otherwise unconducive to health. The nurse may wish to suggest or assist in improvements. Any cooperation or improvement is praised. The nurse may suggest changes in the client's environment that would better reflect the client's own desires.

Eating and sleeping are made more pleasant to the client and are thus encouraged. The client is assisted to relax before meals or bedtime. Areas for dining or sleeping are used only for these purposes and are made attractive and comfortable. Clients with high levels of anxiety may require reassurance and support to relax enough to eat or sleep.

Chronically distressed clients sometimes exhibit negative patterns of communication. Such clients complain constantly of inability to do anything from opening their eyes to walking. A behavioral approach to this problem is to politely ignore such statements when they are repeated. The nurse diverts the client's attention through a firm, matter-of-fact change of topic or directive. If the client says "I can't walk," the nurse might say, "Take my hand and we'll walk down the hall." The nurse avoids trying to reason with chronically distressed clients; they may continue in their negativity even after their behavior has improved. As the client acquires more pleasant thoughts to occupy his time, such statements decrease.

✳ *Emotional dimension.* Interventions in the emotional dimension begin with helping the client understand that he can bear uncomfortable emotional experiences. The client may be taught, with support and patience from the nurse, how to tolerate higher levels of anxiety and greater sadness, as well as more intense anger.

Such tolerance of emotions develops after the therapeutic relationship is established, when the client trusts the nurse sufficiently to discuss difficult emotions. When the client experiences intense emotions, the nurse reassures him and suggests safe methods of decreasing anxiety or assists the client to defuse the situation by focusing on thoughts instead of feelings. The nurse accepts the client's emotional outbursts, sets limits in time to prevent harmful escalation, and allows the client to return to his activities without guilt or shame when the client's behavior is under control.

The client first learns the relationship between his physiological experiences and his thoughts and behavior. The nurse assists the client in recognizing how this experience relates to the situation or the problem that resulted in such intense emotions. For example, the client learns how his body feels when he is angry. The nurse guides him to examine the thoughts he has with anger, such as "That person was unfair to me," or "That person did not listen to me and acted as if I weren't there," or perhaps "I need to get even with that person." The client then learns that the stimulus was his perception of being ignored or overlooked by another person. The client's perception may have been inaccurate; the person involved may not have seen or heard him. Even if the client is not motivated enough to understand why certain situations result in such strong reactions, he can learn to minimize acting-out behaviors in response to intense emotion. This is done by learning that the intense emotions are not always real cues to action and by learning to think through the situation before acting.

With time, experience, and support, the client frequently learns to become aware of his experience of intense emotions. These emotions may serve as cues for the client, indications that he needs to seek therapeutic assistance, resume taking psychotropic medications, or otherwise reduce stress and seek support. The client may also learn to decrease his emotional reactions to hallucinations, delusions, or bizarre thoughts. Even if such experiences continue, they need not interfere in the client's functioning by resulting in intense emotional reactions.

The nurse uses well-timed feedback, reassurance, and modeling, as well as didactic information, to teach the client new attitudes about emotions. The client is assisted to see that unpleasant emotions can be accepted and that they will not destroy the client or the nurse.

✳ ***Intellectual dimension.*** The area of motivation is always addressed with the chronically distressed client. The question is, how can the client be helped to see a change of behavior as desirable? Staff approval or attention will not usually contribute to long-term change, because clients are inclined to just "act nice" for specific staff members rather than for themselves or their own goals. With some clients, a specific reward, such as a nutritional snack or a favorite activity, is helpful in maintaining progress. As their self-esteem and self-image grow, clients may wish to change simply to please themselves. However, clients frequently regress when the actual attainment of a goal is in sight because of their anxiety about changing and assuming new roles and responsibilities.

Reaching a goal, such as independent placement or a job, may mean that the client's image to others and himself will change. New expectations will be placed on the client by himself and others. The client may need a total rearrangement of plans and goals if he really did not expect to attain his goal. Carrying a self-image of "helpless" or "incompetent" may not be pleasant, but it is at least familiar. Changes in self-image and behavior are closely supported and constantly reinforced by the nurse. The client may be discouraged easily if accepting the change in status means increased frustration. At such times the nurse strongly encourages the client to continue in his effort; too much confrontation makes the goal the nurse's

rather than the client's. This necessarily results in withdrawal, anger, or both. The nurse always works with the client—not for or on the client. The motivation is ultimately the client's.

The client learns to accept the nature of delusions and hallucinations. It is usually not possible for a client to accept such perceptions as false, but it may be possible for him to accept them as meaningless, harmless, and better to be ignored. The client may learn through a trusting relationship with the nurse that the hallucinations and delusions are not reality to other people. The client may also learn how to avoid revealing to others that he experiences perceptions that other people do not. This is conveyed to the client in a way to avoid shaming him. The client needs to recognize that the nurse honestly accepts these perceptions as very real to the client, though not to the nurse.

The client's ability to express himself can be improved through clear, consistent, and repeated feedback. The client is also asked to clarify global, confused, or bizarre communications when the nurse observes that the client is able to tolerate such confrontations. During acute states, requesting clarification may be necessary, but only to facilitate basic communication.

The nurse gives the client clear, consistent feedback regarding his communications by requesting clarification or assisting in focusing the conversation. The nurse also asks the client to verbalize his understanding of what she has said. The nurse does the same in response to the client's communications. These checks for distortions of perception also emphasize for the client the importance of clear communication between people.

Orientation, memory, and basic cognitive skills can be developed within the nurturance of a therapeutic relationship. Time is set aside daily for the nurse to orient the client if he is disoriented on any sphere. Games, storytelling, current events groups, and general conversation stimulate the client intellectually and eventually help him improve cognitive function. As cognition improves, the client may find it easier to focus attention more on reality and goal-setting and less on hallucinations or delusions. The dysfunctional perception will not be "extinguished" in this way, but the client may choose to focus on something else.

Judgment will generally improve with life experiences, especially successful experiences. Chronically distressed clients tend to gain such maturity slowly and at great costs. They may never achieve real insight. A reasonable goal in this area is for the client to accept his own limitations, needs, and abilities. The client, as well as his health care providers, may never know why such limitations exist. Motivation to achieve any insight probably comes from a supportive relationship, a realistic role model, and a consistent, patient approach.

✺ ***Social dimension.*** The chronically distressed client is likely to require external motivation to develop new social behaviors. Motivators are found for the client's specific interests. He will probably not be impressed with a simple plea to display "appropriate" behavior. The client may not desire closeness with others or a supportive relationship and may therefore lack the ordinary motivators to adopt socially "appropriate" behavior. At the same time, social skills ultimately determine the client's chances of independence.

For many reasons, the chronically distressed client is frequently not motivated to carry out socially accepted behaviors that may increase self-esteem. The client may learn to understand and accept himself, however, if the nurse expresses understanding and acceptance of him. If the nurse can genuinely accept the client's unpredictable course of disease, occasionally disruptive behavior, and sometimes bizarre communication and appearance, the client may accept his experiences and behaviors and see how to make realistic changes.

A client experiencing severe regression responds best to consistent, one-to-one interactions with the nurse. Initially, the "honeymoon effect" of increased attention from another person will improve behavior. This effect occurs most often in clients who have not been involved in a therapeutic relationship before. The client sees the relationship in a grandiose manner as a means of solving all problems, as if the acceptance and warmth of the relationship alone can motivate any necessary change. The client may begin to mimic the nurse's behaviors, and the nurse becomes a powerful role model in teaching social skills that, hopefully, may outlive the therapeutic relationship. An approach to teaching social skills is described in the Research Highlight box below.

The client frequently regresses after an initial period of increased responsivity as a result of anxiety about change. However, a skillful nurse can make effective use of the "honeymoon" period by encouraging as many new activi-

ties as the client can tolerate. The hope is that during a period of increased responsivity to the nurse the client is exposed to an activity or interaction that becomes a real, internal source of motivation. During such a responsive period, the nurse may find the client to be unusually open to feedback regarding his hygiene habits or social skills. If other people in the environment praise the client's newly formed skills or improved habits, such behaviors may continue. The goal is for the client to find more pleasure in displaying socially acceptable behavior than withdrawn or regressed behavior.

Within the relationship, the nurse assists the client to examine his self-image and self-esteem. The client has support from the nurse that allows him to look at his self-image and measure how accurately he sees himself. The client also examines how well he likes himself and looks at how unfair and harmful his self-dislike is. The nurse emphasizes some points about self-image and self-esteem, using reflection and active listening, to make apparently social conversation a therapeutic measure. The chronically distressed client, usually very therapy-wise, may respond better to "apparently social" interactions than to analytical, confrontive, or otherwise "professional" interactions with the nurse. The nurse maintains a professional role, but in perhaps a more "human," less objective, and less removed manner.

Appropriate sexual behaviors are perhaps more difficult for nurses to foster because of their own discomfort with the subject. Again, specific behavioral expectations are clarified with the client. It is generally helpful to allow the client to ventilate his feelings about sexual issues and to

---

Research Highlight

Social Dramatics: Social Skills Development for the Chronically Mentally Ill

W.R. Whetstone

PURPOSE

This study investigated the use of dramatics in a social context as a clinical means of teaching social skills to chronically mentally ill inpatients in a state facility.

SAMPLE

The subjects were 15 men and women between 20 and 55 years old who met the DSM-III-R criteria for having schizophrenia. The subjects were free of physical disabilities, physical illness, organic syndromes, and marked hallucinations or delusions; at the initiation of the study the subjects were stabilized on a regimen of psychotropic medications.

METHODOLOGY

The design was quasiexperimental. The Randomized control group was given only a posttest. The experimental group was exposed to the treatment effects of social dramatics. The

Nurses' Observation Scale for Inpatient Evaluation (NOSIE-30) was used to measure changes in social skills. The NOSIE-30 measures social competence, social interest, personal neatness, irritability, manifest psychosis, and psychotic depression.

FINDINGS

Only social competence was seen to change significantly. There were no significant differences on the total NOSIE-30 score.

IMPLICATIONS

The approach used, Orem's construct of social interaction, with social dramatics and videotape feedback, appeared to be relevant for therapeutic effectiveness. A need to use better control procedures and to gather more follow-up data in future research was indicated.

Based on data from Journal of Advanced Nursing 2(1):67, 1986.

offer sincere understanding of the problems he has in controlling his behavior. The nurse needs to help the client understand the consequences he may face from sexual acting out. It is important that nurses do not criticize the client's value system or moral character. Decisions about sexual behavior, especially when the client is viewed as competent, are ultimately left to the client. For example, a client may choose to begin a sexual relationship with another client in an outpatient therapy program. Unless the program has regulations stating that clients cannot develop sexual relationships among themselves, this is the decision of the two clients involved. Another example is the client who has a homosexual relationship. This may seem inappropriate to some staff but may be the client's choice. Most inpatient settings do not permit sexual activity among clients, but it may still occur, especially when the clients are off the premises. The nurse may intervene only to offer information or to aid in decision making that would reduce the likelihood of harm to the client or others. In inpatient settings, calm, matter-of-fact vigilance by staff will generally prevent sexual acting-out behaviors.

Struggles concerning dependence and independence may be the nurse's greatest challenge. The nurse need not be afraid to offer needed support and nurturance, but as the client progresses, the nurse takes a more supportive role than that of a nurturing surrogate mother. Slowly, in response to cues of growth, the nurse becomes more of a peer consultant and helps the client find additional and appropriate means of meeting his dependence needs. Decreasing dependence on the nurse is a frightening process for many chronically distressed clients; they may regress when faced with the possibility of real independence, such as separation from the nurse. The nurse anticipates the regression and offers support and acceptance, but always keeps the goal of independence at the center of the relationship.

Throughout all of these struggles, the client occasionally tests the nurse. Such testing continues throughout relationships with chronically distressed clients, because trust is very difficult for them. The nurse cannot expect rapid trust or complete trust—the client may have a lifetime of evidence indicating that trust is impossible or unwise. The nurse respects the client's need to test and recognizes behavior management problems as such. During periods of testing, it is therapeutic for the nurse to use an intellectual or rational approach to the client, because emotional approaches may be too threatening.

Clients who are progressing toward independence frequently benefit most from interactions with their peers. Group interactions may offer structured opportunities to try new social behaviors. Discussion groups with their peers help chronically distressed clients examine their past, current, and future roles as members of society. Such conversation helps clients reaffirm the reality of their perceptions, thoughts, and feelings. Clients may discuss society's influence in their labeling as mentally ill and even institutionalization. Such a discussion creates an opportunity to express anger in an appropriate context. This group experience also helps create a "we group" from which the client gains support. The client is encouraged to find a healthy we-group with which to relate.

The group assists the client to create a new role for himself. This role prepares the client to accept the rejection by society. The client is taught to "fit in" with society without losing his true identity. The client is encouraged to view his limitations and strengths realistically. Goals of independence and higher adaptive functioning are valued in this sort of group. The internalized role is a flexible, adaptive one based on realistic appraisal of self.

Spiritual dimension. If the client is able to think abstractly and concretely and still maintain a realistic view of life, he may benefit from conversations with the nurse focused on the identification of his belief system, values, morals, and ethics. The chronically distressed client may have been unable to integrate such information during his adolescence because of disturbances in his behavior or cognition. Such a client requires an opportunity to explore concepts of values and personal ethics as part of the process of differentiation and individuation. Concepts of hope and faith assist the chronically distressed client to withstand the society's pessimism regarding his own goals and aspirations. Spiritual inquires aid the chronically distressed client in finding his own place from the perspective of the struggles of all people, and thus reducing his isolation and alienation.

Some chronically distressed clients have such problems with abstract and concrete thinking that they misinterpret the intent of spiritual discussions and are unable to approach spirituality in a realistic or meaningful manner. Some clients have delusions that center on religious rituals or mysticism and are guided by staff to avoid religious topics as a means of controlling psychotic thinking. The nurse ascertains the client's ability to benefit from discussions of spirituality before entering into discussions of a religious or spiritual nature. If the nurse does pursue a discussion regarding spirituality, she needs to be clear on her own beliefs and biases so as to not adversely affect the client's thinking or influence the development of his belief system away from his own natural inclinations.

Evaluation

The chronically distressed client frequently offers the greatest challenge to the creativity of the nurse. Evaluation conferences may reveal that the client has managed to avoid the therapeutic intention of the treatment plan. Evaluation conferences are then the time to use personal ingenuity along with professional experience and knowledge to determine whether progress is being made and, if not, to suggest approaches the client is more likely to benefit from. Although the client is frequently adept at foiling attempts to create real progress, the nurse does not blame him for this behavior; it is normal for a chronically distressed client. However, the nurse also maintains an understanding of the client's responsibilities as well as his rights to make choices about his behavior.

The client may be more comfortable if close friends or family are present for a conference. Family and close friends are also useful sources of evaluation data. These people are an integral part of the client's treatment, because they form the necessary support system. Staff need to listen to family and friends regarding their impressions of the client's progress. The client may hide much from staff members that his family does not miss. Also, the family can give a better impression about whether the changes the nurse sees will last.

SPECIAL ISSUES

The long-term client requires a flexible system of health care delivery that offers continuity of care. Two special issues are the case management system and the ethical and legal dilemma of patients' rights to freedom and treatment.

Case Manager System

The chronically mentally ill have been designated by governmental studies as a "target population" to receive extra funding as it is available and to be observed as they move in and out of society at large.[34] A study of the failures of the past has resulted in the following suggestions for this target population:

1. Case management services.
2. A coordinated delivery system.
3. A spectrum of residential facilities.[32]

The first two suggestions can both be approached through the institution of a well-planned case management system. The third refers to the need for an ample supply of different residential arrangements. These include government-subsidized partially and completely independent living apartments, adult foster care homes, board and care houses, supervised board and lodging houses, and short-term crisis homes.

The case management system required is a centralized, well-coordinated, and well-planned system. Any client designated as "chronically mentally ill" enters a statewide list and is assigned for case management on a county level. Only one case management system is networked state-wide so that duplication of services does not occur. The case manager serves the client by helping to coordinate all levels of mental health treatment and daily care.[34] This coordination would ensure that clients are assisted to function at their maximum level of independence with a minimum of outside interference or restriction.

Much of the case manager's work is to link the client with available services, such as day treatment programs, home-delivered meal services, or homemaker services, as needed and accepted by the client. The case manager also serves as the client's advocate to make sure the client's rights are being respected and his needs recognized properly by service providers. The case manager works with the client as he goes in and out of hospitalizations and in some cases may even provide clinical therapy. The case manager assists in finding housing for the client, making sure he has food and is eating and that he is safely functional in the least restrictive environment possible, and overseeing his rehabilitation. The case manager also assists the client with clothing, income, all areas of health care, and legal, vocational, educational, and family needs and problems.

Case managers need manageable caseloads to be able to so thoroughly assist their clients. The case managers have to be knowledgeable about and have timely access to all kinds of resources as the client's needs are known. The role of case manager carries some authority within the area's legal, fiscal, and health care systems.

The case management system is only successful insofar as the factors listed here are present. This approach does not solve all the problems posed by chronic mental illness, but it offers a well-coordinated attempt to assist the client to function within society.

Patient Rights

Patients' rights, especially those of the severely dysfunctional, chronically distressed client, will require more attention in the future. Chronically distressed clients have the right to accept or reject assistance and to make their own decisions, even if their decisions do not seem to be based on sound judgment. Only if the client is seen to be imminently dangerous to himself or others can interventions be made without the client's consent.

Additionally, though many chronically distressed clients are seen as unlikely to benefit from any treatment approaches, some of these have treatment forced on them. Some chronically distressed clients do respond to legally forced treatment and are released to pursue their usual, hazardous, marginal life-styles, refusing the availability of therapeutic services. Many clients recognize that they have to "get along" with the mental health system to survive and maintain what independence they have; yet they frequently feel bitter after receiving legally forced treatment, feeling as if their rights and bodies were violated. Obviously, this situation is not likely to breed trust and goodwill. All this is part of the reason that chronically distressed clients present such a challenge to nursing staff, who generally believe trust to be necessary for personal change.

The problem is complex. The chronically distressed client may "look normal" but be dangerous to society or himself, or he may fit the stereotype of a psychotic person and be perfectly capable of caring for himself and perhaps even nurturing others. These clients may distance health care professionals so that they are unable to assess what they think they see. Clients have the right to choose this distance if they desire.

BRIEF REVIEW

The theoretical perspective for understanding the development of the life-style of the chronically distressed client is symbolic interactionism. The chronically distressed client demonstrates widely varying degrees of functioning. The client is assessed according to his own norms, and treatment approaches are developed according to his specific level of independence at any time. The nurse allows the client to set the pace for the therapeutic relationship but watches carefully for growth cues and includes the client in all stages of the nursing process.

Two special issues that influence the nursing care of the client are the case management system and the patient's rights.

REFERENCES AND SUGGESTED READINGS

1. Aiken, L.H., Somers, S.A., and Shore, M.F.: Private foundation in health affairs: a case study of the development of a national initiative for the chronically mentally ill, American Psychologist 41(11):1290, 1986.
2. Abramson, N.S.: Continuum of care for the chronically ill elderly, New Directions for Mental Health Services 29:33, 1986.
3. Bachrach, L.: Dimensions of disability in the chronic mentally ill, Hospital and Community Psychiatry 37(10):981, 1986.
4. Backrock, L.: Young adult chronic patients: An analytical review of the literature, Hospital and Community Psychiatry 33:3, 1982.
4a. Baier, M.: Case management with the chronically mentally ill, Journal of Psychosocial Nursing and Mental Health Services 25(6): 17, 1987.
5. Barnes, G.E., and others: Mental health professionals' knowledge in the field of caring for chronic mental disorder, Social Science and Medicine 21(11):1229, 1985.
6. Britton, J.G., and others: The crisis home: sheltering patients in emotional crisis . . . chronically mentally ill clients, Journal of Psychosocial Nursing and Mental Health Services 23(12):18, 1985.
7. Brunger, J.B.: The young chronic client in mental health, Nursing Clinics of North America 21(3):451, 1986.
8. Burd, S., and Marshall, M.: Some clinical approaches to psychiatric nursing, New York, 1963, Macmillan Publishing Co.
9. Carlson, C., and Blackwell, B.: Behavioral concepts and nursing intervention, ed. 2, Philadelphia, 1978, J.B. Lippincott Co.
10. Chacko, R.C.: The chronic mental patient in a community context, Washington, D.C., 1986, American Psychiatric Press, Inc.
11. Conklin, J.J.: Therapy for deinstitutionalized patients, Journal of Psychosocial Rehabilitation 10(1):49, 1986.
12. Cutler, D.L.: Clinical care update: the chronically mentally ill, Journal of Community Mental Health 21(1):3, 1985.
13. Davidhizar, R.: Beliefs and values of the client with chronic mental illness regarding treatment, Issues in Mental Health Nursing 6(3/4):261, 1984.
14. Drake, R.E., and others: Inpatient psychosocial treatment of chronic schizophrenia: negative effects and current guidelines, Hospital and Community Psychiatry 37(9):897, 1986.
15. Ferree, M.M., and Smith, E.R.: A cognitive approach to social and individual stigma, The Journal of Social Psychology 109:87, 1979.
16. Flaskerud, J.H.: Profile of chronically mentally ill psychotic patients in four community mental health centers, Issues in Mental Health Nursing 8(2):155, 1986.
17. Gallop, R., and others: Difficult young adult chronic patients: reevaluating short-term clinical management, Journal of Psychosocial Nursing and Mental Health Services 24(4):8, 1986.
18. Gerber, K.E., and Nehemkis, A.: Compliance: the dilemma of the chronically ill, New York, 1986, Springer Publishing Co.
19. Goffman, E.: Stigma, Englewood Cliffs, N.J., 1963, Prentice-Hall, Inc.
20. Gold Award: a network of services for homeless chronic mentally ill, Hospital and Community Psychiatry 37(11):1148, 1986.
21. Goldman, H., Gattozzi, J., and Taube, C.: Defining and counting the chronically mentally ill, Hospital and Community Psychiatry 32:1, 1981.
22. Gomez, E.A., Adams, G.L., and Chacko, R.C.: A prognosis minority: chronic patients and mental health care, American Journal of Social Psychiatry 3(2):63, 1983.
23. Jones, B.E., editor: Treating the homeless; urban psychiatry's challenge, Washington, D.C., 1986, American Psychiatric Press, Inc.
24. Kim, M.J., McFarland, G.K., and McLane, A.M.: Classification of nursing diagnoses: proceedings of the Fifth National Conference, ed. 2, St. Louis, 1987, The C.V. Mosby Co.
25. Kraus, J.B., and Slavinski, A.T.: The chronically ill psychiatric patient and the community, Boston, 1982, Blackwell Scientific Publications.
26. Liberman, R.P., editor: Psychiatric rehabilitation of the chronic mental patient, Washington, D.C., 1987, American Psychiatric Press, Inc.
27. Ludwig, A.M.: Treating the treatment failures: the challenge of chronic schizophrenia, New York, 1971, Grune & Stratton, Inc.
28. Macmick, C.G., and Macinick, J.: Hope for the chronic mentally ill, Issues in Mental Health Nursing 6(3/4):255, 1984.
29. Miller, J.F.: Inspiring hope, American Journal of Nursing 85(1):22, 1985.
30. McCausland, M.P.: Deinstitutionalization of the mentally ill: oversimplification of complex issues, Advances in Nursing Science 9(3):24, 1987.
31. Morrison, J., and others: An attempt to change the negative stigmatizing image of mental patients through brief reeducation. Psychological Reports 47:334, 1980.
32. Norwind, B.: Developing an enforceable "right to treatment" therapy for the chronically mentally disabled in the community, Schizophrenia Bulletin 8:4, 1982.
32a. Pepper, B., Kirshner, M.C., and Ryglewicz, H.: The young adult chronic patient: overview of a population, Hospital and Community Psychiatry 32:463, 1982.
33. Scheff, T.: Labeling madness, Englewood Cliffs, N.J., 1975, Prentice-Hall, Inc.
34. Schwartz, S., Goldman, H., and Churgin, S.: Case management for the chronic mentally ill: models and dimensions, Hospital and Community Psychiatry 33:3, 1982.
35. Sheets, J.L., Prevost, J.A., and Reihman, J.: Young adult chronic patients: three hypothesized subgroups, Hospital and Community Psychiatry 33:3, 1982.
36. Skepple, I.V.: A profile of the new young chronic patient: implications for psychiatric nursing for the 90's, Canadian Journal of Psychiatric Nursing 26(4):13, 1985.
37. Staats, G.R.: Images of deviants: stereotypes and their importance for labeling deviant behavior, Washington, D.C., 1978, University Press of America, Inc.
38. Test, M.A.: Effective community treatment of the chronically mentally ill: what is necessary, Journal of Social Issues 37:3, 1981.
39. Weisman, G.: Crisis Houses and lodges: residential treatment of acutely disturbed chronic patients, Psychiatric Annals 15(11):642, 1985.
40. Whetstone, W.R.: Social Dramatics: social skills development for the chronically mentally ill, Journal of Advanced Nursing 2(1):67, 1986.

ANNOTATED BIBLIOGRAPHY

Krauss, J.B., and Slavinsky, A.T.: The chronically ill psychiatric patient and the community, Boston, 1982, Blackwell Scientific Publications.

This is a well-written, thorough exploration of nursing's perspective on chronic mental illness. The book is divided into three parts. Part One is a historical and theoretical overview. It includes descriptions, definitions, and discussions of the nature of chronic psychiatric illness, the new era of community treatment focus, and changing patterns of care.

Part Two, the treatment section, discusses community placement, assessment, managing episodes of both crises and stability, supportive therapies, psychiatric rehabilitation, family treat-ment, and the difficult legal, ethical and fiscal aspects of treatment.

Part Three discusses past, present, and future nursing roles in working with the chronically distressed client. It includes the history and development of the role of the nurse in the therapeutic relationship and milieu. Community support networks are also discussed within the context of the nursing role.

The great merit of this book lies in the author's discussion of the episodic nature of chronic mental illness. The nurse is encouraged to be patient, sensitive to growth cues, and adept at rehabilitation. There is also an excellent discussion of the nature of chronicity in mental illness.

CHAPTER 33

THERAPY WITH CLIENTS WITH ORGANIC MENTAL DISORDERS

Judith R. Lentz

After studying this chapter the learner will be able to:

Discuss the historical development of ideas related to organic mental disorders.

Identify major theories related to the etiology of organic mental disorders.

Implement the nursing process with clients with organic mental disorders.

Discuss research related to the care of clients with organic mental disorders.

Organic mental disorders (OMD) are a general category of diseases, syndromes, and conditions characterized by an observable disturbance in previously unimpaired mental functioning. They result from innumerable environmental, physical, or emotional impairments of brain functioning and are among the prevalent reasons for disturbances in an individual's behavior, judgment, and intellect. The presence of OMD often comes to the attention of caregivers when the family can no longer cope with an individual's deteriorating behavior and judgment.[20,57] Among professional caregivers, treatment of isolated symptoms—confusion, hallucinations, hysterical behavior, paranoid delusions, nighttime agitation, refusal to cooperate, and poor judgment—often precedes the consideration of OMD.[19,28,42]

Organic mental disorders constitute a major public health problem and a major mental health problem among the elderly. OMD are by no means inevitable with aging, but the elderly are more vulnerable to them. Chronic illness, diminished hearing and sight, poor nutrition, social isolation, and drug reactions not only complicate but cause cerebral impairments. Physical illnesses, especially multiple conditions typical of older, more gravely ill clients, also seem to predispose to the development of OMD.[37,50]

Client management problems are common. Individuals who overreact, become agitated and confused, wander off,

or become unusually anxious or depressed are commonly seen by their families and caregivers as disruptive and problematic. Such behaviors often disrupt usual social and interpersonal relationships. Caregivers, especially family members, are often overwhelmed trying to meet the individual's enhanced needs as well as compensate for his unmet role and responsibilities. Caring for a seriously impaired individual is not only physically and emotionally demanding but often socially isolating and unrewarding.

THEORETICAL APPROACHES
Biological

The term *organic mental disorder* denotes a disturbance in previously normal or unimpaired cortical structures or mental functions. OMD is manifested as acquired disorders in perceptions cognitions, and emotions. These disorders arise from physical or chemical insult, immobilization, sensory deprivation or monotony, sleep or dream deprivation, sensory or emotional overload, or a combination of these.[48]

Until recently, acute OMD was generally understood to be the dramatic but reversible changes in consciousness and behavior that accompanied acute illnesses such as infections, trauma, surgery, or rapid onset metabolic disturbances. In contrast, chronic mental syndromes were understood as irreversible changes in brain tissue charac-

Historical Overview

DATE	EVENT
1500	René Descartes provided the conceptual basis for perceiving the mind as separate from the body.
1700-1800	The idea that psychological functions have a specific location and biological correlates was elaborated.
Late 1800s	Huling Jackson disputed the locational correlates theory, which viewed cerebral organization and psychological functioning as determined by location, and advocated a holistic, integrated theory of brain organization and function.
1900s	Psychology and neurology became separate medical specialties.
1940s	Goldstein and Luria documented the effects of brain damage on personality and social adjustment.
1950s	Luria documented that a lesion in a circumscribed area of the brain rarely led to complete loss of a function. He proposed that neurological organization is based on a vertical hierarchy of neurological function.
1960s	Extensive psychobiological research provided a scientific basis for overcoming the mind-body dichotomy. Technological advances gave researchers and physicians a new view of the brain.
1970s-1980s	Neurobiological aspects of psychological functions were better defined. Lipowski documented physiological changes associated with delirium. Sociopsychological factors are increasingly implicated in the roles of cerebral organization and organic function previously thought to be physical.
Future	As people live longer with various neurological impairments and diseases, nurses expect to be involved in the identification and treatment of neurological disorders and the management of lives irrevocably changed by neurological injuries or diseases.

terized by progressive global deterioration in intellectual function and social behaviors. This deterioration was often associated with aging and attributed to the presence of specific syndromes, such as Huntington's chorea, Pick's or Alzheimer's disease, and arteriosclerosis.

As information about OMD accumulated, gross differentiations between acute and chronic became insufficient. It was clear that a particular incident, such as head injury, stroke, or encephalitis, often had both acute and chronic characteristics. The nature of onset and probability of recovery were no longer considered the best way to categorize observable symptoms.

The new diagnostic categories in the DSM-III-R categorize OMD by their most prominent psychological change, whether in consciousness, intellect, affect, or sociability. This diagnostic system facilitates the recognition of additional types of OMD. DSM-III-R is particularly useful in cases of OMD with no discernible pattern of onset or progression of symptoms. The notions of "acute" and "chronic," however, remain important medical diagnostic considerations. Acute OMD are now typically referred to as delirium; and chronic mental syndromes are referred to as dementia. Additionally, the expansion of categories and changes in terminology have removed the implicit dichot-

omy between acute and chronic OMD, facilitating better recognition and management of individuals who exhibit symptoms of both delirium and dementia. Delirium and its causes are often overlooked in individuals known to have dementia.[50]

Delirium is a syndrome characterized by clouding of consciousness, failure of attention, memory deficits, emotional turmoil, and disorientation, especially to time and place. The principal feature is clouding of consciousness[23,39] which results in fluctuations in awareness. The individual often has erratic periods of lucidity followed by episodes of somnolence. Intermittently these clients can be fearful, irritable, and prone to visual hallucinations. Disorientation is particularly marked, and present and recent past memories are greatly disturbed. Neurological findings such as headache, *dysarthria*, EEG abnormalities (particularly slow waves), *myoclonus, asterixis*, and tremulousness are often evident.[39] However, personality changes, inappropriate behaviors, and fragmented, disordered thought are the signs that draw attention to the client.

Pathophysiological processes that result in hypoxia, toxicity, or changes in blood glucose level often cause delirium.[15,44] The demands of brain cells for oxygen make the brain particularly susceptible to changes in the body's internal environment. Of particular significance are changes in the availability of oxygen to the brain and the cortical tissue's ability to use available oxygen. Hypoxia-induced delirium is known to arise from four major sources:[44]

1. Inability to transport oxygen to cerebral cells
2. Inability of cells to absorb/metabolize oxygen
3. Inability of the body to take in sufficient oxygen
4. Obstruction of blood flow to or in the brain

Anemic hypoxias are typically found in clients who have insufficient red blood cells or hemoglobin. The most obvious and dramatic cause of these hypoxias is hemorrhage or transfusion with noncompatible blood. If blood loss results from cortical trauma (cerebrovascular accident, surgery, injury), the secondary inflammation worsens the hypoxia, exacerbating confusion, and/or diminishing the level of consciousness. More insidious causes of anemic hypoxia include gradual blood loss from an irritated or ulcerated gastrointestinal tract and nutritional deficiencies, especially iron-poor or protein-deficient diet. Pernicious anemia, a folic acid deficiency associated with excessive alcohol or lack of fresh fruits and vegetables in the diet, can cause confusion, loss of sensation, and motor difficulties.

Dehydration is a common cause of hystotoxic anemia.[44] This problem is likely to occur if other physical or environmental problems interfere with the individual's ability to acquire or retain fluid. At high risk are those who are not mobile enough to obtain fluids, those taking diuretics, those with chronic gastrointestinal disturbances, those who do not perceive thirst, and those exposed to extreme temperatures. The very young and the very old are particularly prone to dehydration, and the elderly are most likely to experience delirium when dehydrated.[23]

Hyperthermia and hypothermia appear to interfere with an individual's ability to acquire and metabolize oxygen. Especially in the elderly, a temperature of 100° F is known to cause hallucinations. Questions are now being raised about the implications of body temperatures below 97° F[54]. Restless, unresponsive, or apathetic older people are often labeled confused; unfortunately, the possibility of hypothermia as a cause for these symptoms is rarely entertained.[54]

Ventilatory failure and hystotoxic hypoxia are increasingly common causes of mental confusion. Over time, industrial pollution, cigarette smoking, chronic respiratory infections, environmental dust, and aging decrease the capacity to take in adequate oxygen. With age the chest wall becomes more rigid, the excursion of the diaphragm decreases and the lungs expand less completely. These anatomical changes make the inactive or immobilized individual increasingly prone to fluid accumulation in the lungs, thereby increasing the risk of pneumonia and insufficient oxygenation of the blood. When breathing and oxygenation are further compromised by significant damage to the lung tissue itself (for example, from emphysema, pulmonary edema, lung cancer, or brown or black lung), confusion and disorientation are not only more likely to occur but also the symptoms are likely to be more severe.

Metabolic changes from infections and organ dysfunction and the toxic effects of drugs can adversely affect the metabolism of neural cells and/or the function of neural systems.[23,54] With infection, emotional and intellectual symptoms may precede a fever, occur during a fever, or after the temperature has returned to normal (postfebrile delirium). In the case of kidney or liver failure the metabolic toxins seem to affect metabolism of cortical cells directly. The mental changes associated with arteriosclerosis and cardiac decompensation, however, may result from disturbances in the cerebral capillaries. Deterioration or changes in the permeability of the cerebral capillaries can disturb the transfer of oxygen and nutrients into and metabolic wastes out of the cortical cells.

Drugs are another common but overlooked source of toxicity. Oral antibiotic agents can cause hypoglycemia, and diuretics often deplete electrolytes (particularly K^+) and cause dehydration. Hypertensive agents can reduce blood pressure so much that hypostatic hypotension occurs or insufficient oxygenated blood reaches the brain. Other commonly prescribed drugs associated with episodes of disorientation and confusion include digitalis, phenothiazenes, psychotropic medications, urinary antiseptics, analgesics, and antibiotics.[19,44] In the case of drugs or metabolic or bacterial toxins, however, it is important to remember that despite the specificity of the toxin, its effects on nervous tissue or behavioral symptoms are highly variable.

Most recent attempts to link observed delirium with physiological and neurological mechanisms have concentrated on the reticular activating system that comprises multiple structures of the brainstem and has numerous diffuse connections in the cerebral cortex (Figure 33-1). This system regulates the tone of the cortex, influencing individual functions of awareness, attention, vigilance, and consciousness.[22] At higher cortical levels, disturbances in the reticular activating system interfere with selective attention. Failure to attend selectively results in disorganized, non-goal-directed behavior, because everything equally commands the client's attention, he moves erratically from one topic, activity, or stimulus to another. He cannot select his actions nor distinguish time—hence his loss of orientation. Inability to filter out irrelevant stimuli and the decreased level of alertness combine to produce mental confusion and confabulation.

Explanations of delirium based on impairment of the reticular activating system go a long way toward explaining how so many diverse injuries and metabolic malfunctions can produce the same symptom complex. In addition, this approach explains why symptoms vary so greatly in degree and actual expression.

Dementia is a chronic, progressive, and usually nonpsychotic deterioration in mental functioning. The onset of symptoms is often insidious, typically including progressive global impairment of intellect caused by changes in brain structure. Dementia is more common after age 65 and affects 20% of people over 80.[58] Deterioration in intellectual functioning is recognized as a clinical syndrome when occupational or social performance becomes prob-

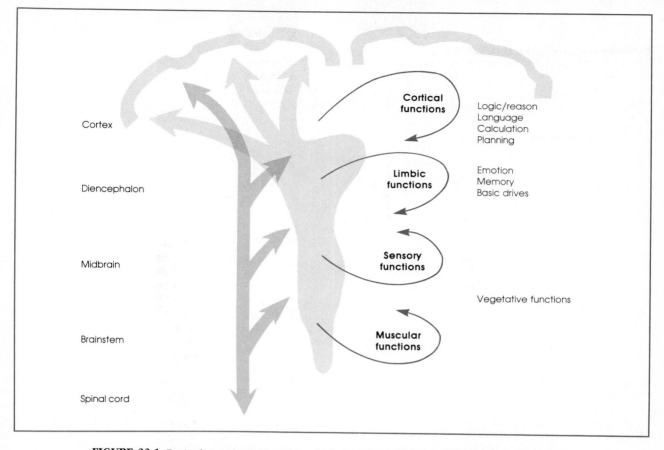

FIGURE 33-1 Reticular activating system. (Adapted from The working brain by A.R. Luria. © Penguin Books, Ltd., 1973, Basic Books, Inc., Publishers. Reprinted by permission of the publisher.)

lematic.[7,41] The actual amount of physical change necessary to cause observable or measurable deterioration in intellectual function is relative. It depends on a variety of factors, including physical and emotional stress, preexisting knowledge and skills, and the complexity of the task at hand. Clients with dementia have increasingly less tolerance for any kind of stress and less ability to recover from its physical and emotional effects. The marginality of their condition makes them susceptible to drug reactions, dramatic complications from minor physical symptoms such as constipation, and minor emotional or social disruptions. In time the progression of the disease affects the individual's ability to perform the most basic tasks.[58] Some become totally dependent, noncommunicative, and bedridden before death.

The most common type of dementia is senile dementia of the Alzheimer type. Alzheimer-type diseases are characterized by the appearance of abnormal structures such as senile plaques, neurofibrillary tangles, and granulovascular structures in the cerebral cortex and limbic system (hippocampus). These cortical dementias are characterized by impaired cognition, amnesia, aphasia without im-

paired speech, social inhibition, apathy, and normal motor function (until late stages). Cortical Alzheimer-type dementias need to be differentiated from subcortical dementias that involve lower brain structures (basal ganglia, thalamus, brainstem) and are often more amenable to treatment with surgery or drugs.[49] Common causes of subcortical dementia include Huntington's disease, hydrocephalus, chronic toxic-metabolic disturbances, and Parkinson's disease. Unlike cortical dementias, these diseases are often characterized by a depressed mood, speech dysarthria, and movement disorders.[41]

Typically cortical dementias are insidiously progressive and are not particularly amenable to medical interventions. The physical changes that cause these dementias usually are not directly observable until after the person has died. The key to identifying, understanding, and managing the client with cortical dementia lies in recognition and interpretation of changing patterns of expression and behavior. The clinical picture of dementia is usually dominated by a generalized intellectual deterioration, beginning with impairment of recent memory and progressing to difficulty with judgment, discrimination, and abstract

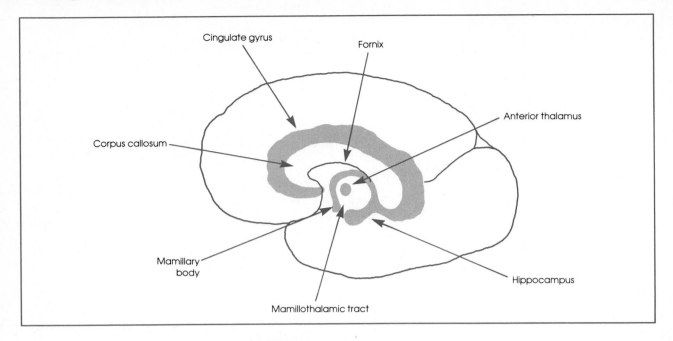

FIGURE 33-2 Limbic system.

reasoning. The final stages are typically characterized by overt disorientation and inability to cooperate with even the closest caregivers.

Korsakoff's syndrome usually appears with the thiamine deficiency of alcoholism, but similar memory defects result from lesions in midbrain and limbic structures (Figure 33-2). Lesions or malfunctions in the mamillary bodies, anterior thalamus, fornix, hippocampus, and medial zones of the hemispheres are particularly associated with gross disturbances of memory. These brain structures appear to play an important role in selective retention and recall of sensory impressions and experiences.

Relatively mild lesions of the deep medial zones tend to be evident only when a client is required to retain and subsequently recall a complex series of isolated bits of information such as random numbers. The client does not have trouble recalling organized information such as sentences or stories. The client with massive lesions is unable to retain information or inhibit the intrusion of interfering stimuli. His deficit is not so much in an initial comprehension as in selective retrieval of memory traces in the face of other stimuli. However, traces of the "forgotten" information can suddenly reappear in another setting. The client may appear to remember when and what he wants to remember. Careful assessment, however, often reveals that specific memories are evoked spontaneously by environmental stimuli and that the client has lost voluntary access to, and control of, his memories.

RELATING TO THE CLIENT

Caring for the client with an OMD may be difficult and frustrating for the nurse. These clients are often unpre-

dictable and hard to control, and frequently need inordinate amounts of attention and supervision. Their propensity to react with rage or uncontrolled sobs often leaves their family and caregivers emotionally exhausted. Incidents of self-exposure, lewd jokes, and even overt propositions produce immense embarrassment. The physical work necessary to care for these clients is also demanding, especially when the only reasonable goals are to maintain an individual in an obviously deteriorated state and to slow inevitable future deterioration.

To complicate the situation, allocations of personnel, facilities, and funds are often insufficient to provide for a growing population of individuals who probably will not be cured. Clients with OMD often are left with their needs unmet, and caregivers are frequently frustrated by the overwhelming demands and angered and depressed by the apparent lack of appreciation for their efforts. This situation causes caregivers and families to conclude that there are no rewards or purpose to caring for the organically impaired client.

This perception is too common. Caring sensitively for clients with OMD demands a great deal of professional knowledge, personal maturity, and wisdom. Most of these individuals are not so impaired that they are unable to perceive another's presence and care. For nurses the first step in establishing a therapeutic relationship is to believe that their role and knowledge are vital to assessment and that the care they provide to the client makes an important difference.

Because the initial symptoms of so many illnesses are characterized by changes in behavioral and emotional expression, alertness to such changes often facilitates the timely and appropriate treatment. In addition, the nurse's alertness to diminished capacity for judgment and discrimination may facilitate the institution of measures that protect the clients from inadvertently harming themselves or others or from making decisions when the consequences of the decisions cannot be anticipated or understood.

The nurse's skills in managing these clients, especially those with permanent, progressive disease, can often improve the most difficult situations. By understanding the client's fragmented communication or anticipating his needs, the nurse may improve both the client's behavior and others' ability to cope effectively with him. In addition, skillfull nurses carefully note not only the client's reactions but also their own. The nurse's concern about emotional lability or hysterical behavior is frequently unconscious, acted on only by avoiding the client's troublesome requests and questions. Nurses' concern about angry or depressed clients is often the result of fear that an individual is likely to lose control of emotional expressions.

NURSING PROCESS
Assessment

✦ Physical dimension. Delirium is an inherent part of many illnesses. Some of the more common causes of delirium are listed in the box at right. Because the individual is often obviously sick, recognizing delirium is relatively easy. A careful assessment generally reveals some obvious disorder or disease process. Fevers, disturbances of heart rhythm and rate, hyperventilation or hypoventilation, and electrolyte disturbances are common. The individual is restless, sometimes agitated, and sleeps fitfully, giving reports of wild, frightening, and vivid dreams. Pain or discomfort often accompanies and complicates delirium.

A careful history and complete physical and laboratory studies are essential to identifying the underlying pathological condition that causes delirium. The history is helpful in identifying the individual's usual patterns and habits but more significantly recent changes or deviations from usual reactions and behaviors. The history also provides an idea about how this illness is like or unlike previous illnesses. Areas of particular interest include the person's past medical history; baseline or usual patterns of use of medications, drugs, and alcohol; usual dietary patterns and intake; opportunity for exposure to infection and toxic substances and a careful overview of the onset of the current episode. Table 33-1 is a suggested format for taking a history of a client with an OMD.

Because there is little relation between the specific pathological condition and the occurrence of delirium, the initial physical examination needs to include a review of all physical systems, including a complete neurological review. If a client has positive neurological findings, head injury, or marked intellectual or personality changes, more extensive and more specific diagnostic tests are routinely performed.

The ongoing assessment of an individual who shows

COMMON CAUSES OF DELIRIUM

INFECTIONS
  Systemic (pneumonia, typhoid fever, malaria, and septicemia)
  Intracranial (meningitis and encephalitis)

POSTOPERATIVE STATES
  Open heart surgery
  Transplant surgery

NEUROLOGICAL CAUSES
  Postseizure effects
  Post–head trauma effects
  Post–cerebrovascular accident effects
  Focal diseases (right parietal lobe and inferomedial surface of the occipital lobe)

INTOXICANTS
  Alcohol
  Sedatives
  Anticholinergics
  Opiates
  Stimulants
  Hallucinogens
  Levodopa
  Digitalis
  Heavy metals

METABOLIC DISORDERS
  Hypoxia, hypercapnia
  Hypoglycemia
  Diseases that produce encephalopathy (hepatic, renal, vitamin B_1 deficiency, and hypertensive endocrine disorders)

---

signs of an altered state of consciousness or mental confusion includes the following:
1. Assessment of the client's fluid and electrolyte balance
   a. Indication of dehydration
   b. Changes in urinary output and consistency
   c. Indications of blood viscosity
   d. Change in vital signs
   e. Evidence of muscle flacidity or tetany
   f. Change in electrolyte or blood laboratory reports
   g. Vomiting, diarrhea, or edema
   h. Evidence of twitching, hyperirritability, seizures, or mental disturbances, especially hallucinations or delusions
2. Assessment of the client's cardiac and respiratory status
   a. Evidence of extremely rapid (greater than 100) or slow (less than 60) or irregular heart rate

    b. Rales or rhonchi in lungs

    c. Bruits (pounding sounds against the arterial wall)

    d. Increased venous pressure

    e. Pupil dilation

    f. Decreased peripheral circulation

3. Assessment of the individual's nutritional status

    a. Appetite

    b. Ability to sustain sufficient food intake

    c. Weight loss, dropping hematocrit and hemoglobin values, and status of serum proteins

4. Assessment of indications of secondary infections

    a. White blood cell count, temperature, pulse, and respiration

    b. Sudden, noticeable deterioration in mental status

    c. Contact with others who appear to have infections

Even when the primary disease process is cured or controlled, residual symptoms of delirium may remain.

Symptoms of marked fatigue, which may resemble depression, are common. Objective indicators such as vital signs, laboratory tests, bacteriological studies, and organ function testing may return to "normal," yet the individual may continue to require considerable nursing care and environmental support. Bathing, changing clothes, and eating breakfast may leave the individual exhausted. Active participation in even the most usual or routine activities returns slowly, and interest in family, home, work, or community activities returns even more slowly.

The nurse needs to carefully assess the client's mental and physical energy, because pushing the individual to resume activities and responsibilities may predispose him to physical complications or establish interpersonal conflicts. Quickness to tire, dozing at inappropriate times, inattention, and apathy suggest the client may still be ill. His interest and energy usually increase over several weeks. When they do not, depression or malingering may be considered; however, the possibility of an unrecognized phys-

---

TABLE 33-1 History format for clients with OMD

Data Collection	Description
Past medical history	History of trauma, severe infections, seizures, chronic illness, violent or uncontrolled behavior, learning disabilities, fighting when intoxicated, hyperactivity, frequent auto accidents or traffic violations, and sexual or physical assaults; list of previous physicians and hospitalizations and their phone numbers and addresses
Medication	Use and patterns of use of any medication or drugs
	Use and patterns of use of alcohol
	Type and amount of drugs used in the past 24 to 72 hours, noting any change from usual patterns of consumption
	Use of herbs or folk remedies
	Use of mind-altering drugs or techniques (for example, yoga, spiritual experiences, or meditation)
Infection	Exposure to individuals known to have had an infection or contact with the blood, brain, or organs of an infected individual
	Travel, especially outside the United States, Canada, or Western Europe
	Recent symptoms of illness, such as rash, fever, vomiting, diarrhea, respiratory congestion, or pain
Toxic substances	Work responsibilities and environment—toxic chemicals or metals
	Home environment—peeling paint, toxic building insulation, environmental pollution or toxic waste products; also, new hobbies
	Air pollution, especially prolonged periods of stagnation or smog
Nutrition	Usual diet and dietary habits
	History of diarrhea, vomiting, skin rashes or eruptions, burns, or bleeding gums
	Food allergies
	Diet and dietary restrictions
	History or indications of fasting or binge eating
	Food cravings or excessive thirst—if so, what and when?
Onset of symptoms	What does the individual think is wrong, how do the client and family members describe the problem(s); to what do they attribute them?
	Has the individual undergone surgery, or extensive medical tests or treatments? What were the effects on the body systems, length of procedure, exposure to anesthesia, complications, and other effects?
	When did the individual first feel sick? When was the illness or change of behavior apparent to others? Describe. What was the progression of symptoms?
	Has the individual ever acted or felt like this previously? If so, describe circumstances and symptoms in detail.
	What other things was the individual doing?
	Describe especially new or unusual activities, associations, or personal or environmental events.
	How have the current symptoms affected the individual's capacity and ability to engage in usual activities, responsibilities, and relationships?

ical problem or unexpected complication is more likely. If the individual remains unable to resume prior intellectual function or social roles, dementia is a possibility.

Dementia is usually characterized by intellectual and emotional deterioration, but these changes are often caused by global or focal brain damage. In general, individuals in the early stages of a global dementia are most likely to seek health care for somatic complaints or nonspecific anxiety and malaise.

Common causes of dementia are listed in the box below. Complaints often center around uncomfortable but not necessarily intolerable feelings of fatigue, uneasiness, or difficulty concentrating. The individual may try to rationalize, attributing his feelings to identifiable physical, social, and environmental situations. When the symptoms persist or worsen, the individual seeks medical relief. Even then he may try a series of home remedies and over-the-counter drugs before seeking professional help.

COMMON CAUSES OF DEMENTIA

DEGENERATIVE DISORDERS

Alzheimer's disease
Pick's disease
Huntington's chorea
Idiopathic cortical
   atrophy

MECHANICAL DISORDERS

Trauma*
Normal pressure
   hydrocephalus
Subdural hematoma

METABOLIC DISORDERS

Hypothyroidism
Hyponatremia
Hypercalcemia
Hypoglycemia
Porphyria
Hypoxia
Wilson's disease
Chronic anoxia
Uremia
Hepatic coma
Carbon dioxide narcosis
Disturbed protein metab-
   olism
Electrolyte disorders

EXOGENOUS POISONS

Heavy metals (lead, arsenic,
   and thallium)
Bromides
Alcohol
Belladonna alkaloids
Organic phosphates
Hallucinogens
Idiosyncratic drug reactions

VASCULAR DISORDERS

Arteriosclerosis
Cerebrovascular accidents
Aneurysm
Collagen disease

NEOPLASTIC DISORDERS

Gliomas
Meningiomas

INFECTIONS

Abscess
Chronic meningitis
Subacute encephalitis
Creutzfeldt-Jakob disease†
AIDS
Syphilis

VITAMIN DEFICIENCY

B_1
B_6
B_{12}
Niacin
Folate

---

*Potentially reversible at least to some degree with medical or surgical treatment.

†Presenile dementia has been linked to a slow virus.

Clients with progressive global dementia have low physical energy or tolerance. They are unable to complete tasks and often doze off during extended social encounters. They may be exhausted by the activities of daily living, so they are often poorly groomed. Nutritional deficits, anemia, and dehydration are common, along with other signs of neglect such as leg ulcers, cellulitis, and chronic diarrhea.

Physical tolerance for any type of extreme temperature is significantly diminshed. Thermostat settings are constantly changed and complaints about being too hot or too cold become more frequent. Susceptibillity to heatstroke or heat exhaustion without exertion can also indicate reduced physical tolerance and an OMS.

Changes from an established baseline are especially important to the assessment. When physical changes occur slowly, as in the case of a slow-growing tumor, the body adjusts or adapts to its altered metabolic state. Only under stress do the symptoms of physical or emotional impairments become evident. Consequently individuals with nonspecific symptoms at their initial visit need to have a physical evaluation.

Emotional dimension. The individual with delirium has trouble controlling the meaningful expression of his emotions. His ability to understand or comprehend the meaning of other people's emotional experiences, especially how he influences others' feelings, is also impaired. Loss of emotional control varies from barely recognizable to obvious and dramatic. Individuals with delirium generally have difficulty initiating an emotional response, but once the response begins, the individual is less able to either modulate or terminate it. Consequently the client may appear to overreact or to be insensitive.

If the individual's mood is frequently fearful and suspicious, he may perceive his caregivers as dangerous and his care as harmful. He may flee or resist treatment, often pulling at tubes and dressings or forcibly removing monitoring devices. The client has little or no comprehension of purpose, only recognition of his irritation.

The delirious client's mood tends to be irritable. Unavoidable inconveniences or minor provocations can evoke tirades of criticism and abuse. Tolerance for discomfort is minimal. Physiological urges and drives require immediate satisfaction, and social conventions exert only the most basic restraint. Consequently the client may often seem impatient, demanding, insensitive, and even crude.

The particular mood disturbances exhibited by the delirious client are often influenced by the following interrelated factors:

1. Premorbid personality
2. Nature and cerebral location of the specific disease process
3. Nature of the environmental stimuli
4. Individual's understanding of environmental stimuli and the social relationships involved

The box on p. 618 presents conditions that tend to exacerbate the mood disturbances and agitate the behavior of a delirious patient.[8]

FACTORS THAT EXACERBATE DELIRIUM

SENSORY VARIABLES

Overload
   Visual: flashing lights, constant lighting
   Auditory: hissing, chatter, vibrations
   Tactile: pain, rough or excessive handling
   Taste: forced feeding, tube feeding
Deprivation
   Visual: obscured vision, medication blur, eye patch
   Auditory: mumbling, silence
   Tactile: overmedication, numbness, no physical contact
   Taste: npo status, intravenous fluids, tube feeding

MOVEMENT

Overload: total restraint
Deprivation: exhaustion, inability to move

MILIEU

Overload
   People: too many visitors, overemotional, noisy
   Physical: confusing stimuli, changing rooms
Deprivation
   People: absent or affectually unrelated people
   Physical: unfamiliar or unstimulating

COMMUNICATION

Overload
   Verbal: professional jargon, incomprehensible explanations, foreign language
   Affect: overreactions, particularly anger, anxiety of others
Deprivation
   Verbal: respirators, tracheostomy
   Affect: suppression of affectual responses, aloofness

ACTIVITY

Overload: endless diagnostic tests, frequent procedures
Deprivation: no meaningful activity, endless television watching, confinement to bed and/or home

CONTROL OF ENVIRONMENT

Overload: expectations beyond capabilities, need to unduly monitor own care to avoid error or neglect, need for emergency or unscheduled procedures
Deprivation: lack of reliable information about one's condition, unable to control personal space or belongings, no expectations or meaningful activities

SOCIAL CULTURAL VARIABLES

Overload: excessive social and family demands, financial worries, continued occupational demands
Deprivation: lack of interests, social isolation, foreign language, withdrawal of family and friends

---

If the onset of symptoms is gradual, as is typical of dementia, the individual's premorbid patterns of emotional reaction and expression are especially important in assessing changes in emotional expression.

Initial changes in emotional expression are usually exaggerations of characteristic responses. Individuals who were typically energetic and excitable may appear cynical, hysterical, and even manic; persons who were shy and withdrawn are more likely to appear depressed or suspicious. The individual who becomes anxious easily may become even panicky when confronted with a new or distressing situation. A complete personality reversal, although known to occur, is atypical. Most reports of this phenomenon involve highly controlled, rigid individuals. For this group, the brain's functional processes are depressed enough that they appear to respond more spontaneously, behave less compulsively, and appear less guilt ridden.

One of the hallmarks of dementia is the client's ease of recovery from expressing strong or dramatic feelings. Sobbing or convulsive laughter is often not the expression of felt emotion but the result of the individual's inability to modulate his emotional expression. Instead of being able to express sadness, anger, anxiety, or pleasure in degrees of more or less, the person characteristically expresses these feeling states in terms of all or nothing. The more severe the organic impairment, the more likely the individual is to experience euphoria, rage, morose depression, or panic. Once removed from the offending environmental or interpersonal situation, the individual almost immediately stops crying or laughing, but is slow to recover his usual level of energy. Seldom does he exhibit residual happiness, anger, sadness, or anxiety; he tends to become more or less unresponsive, failing at otherwise easy tasks and avoiding or resisting people, activities, or situations that elicit the response.[22]

When dementia progresses to a moderate or severe stage, emotional expression is increasingly characterized by the absence of spontaneous emotion and subsequently by lability of emotional expressions. To the casual observer, the client may appear depressed; facial expressions may be absent, and he may appear to have a blank, empty gaze directed purposelessly into space. If asked about sadness or depression, he is most often mystified by the suggestion. Some clients report that they do not feel anything, and the nurse, physician, or family members often conjecture that the individual is engaging in the protective mechanism of denial.

However, once a feeling state is elicited, its expression tends to be overwhelming. Even a client who is moderately impaired may progress suddenly from a rather normal verbal expression of sadness to a state of uncontrolled sobbing. The observer usually notices that the individual is overreacting, but frequently tries to rationalize the response. The nurse may underestimate the importance of a particular issue, or the client's response may be out of proportion. This determination is not an easy one to make; however, significant insight can be obtained by asking the following questions:

1. How would I expect someone of the same sex, age, and sociocultural background to react to the same or similar comment or situation? What is an expected and appropriate response?
2. Are there any data to suggest that the client may have a primary or secondary OMD? Is he or has he been sick?
3. How has this client responded to similar situations or comments in the past? Do family members or close friends find his emotional responses unusual, exaggerated, or disturbing?
4. How quickly and under what circumstances does the client recover from apparent dramatic expressions of emotions? Does he cry easily, but once distracted, does he seem as if he had not cried at all? Does the individual seem mystified or confused when asked later about feeling so sad?

As the OMD worsens, the client has more trouble handling anxiety. In the unimpaired individual, moderate levels of anxiety tend to improve motivation and performance; clients with OMD are further impaired by even low levels of anxiety. To the degree that these clients have lost the capacity for abstract thought, they are confined to the eternal present and, like infants, unable to react selectively or sequentially to particular aspects of an experience. A common example of this total undifferentiated response in an adult is catastrophic anxiety. Individuals with this response show signs of incipient physical collapse as well as overwhelming emotional distress.[52]

Anxiety is inherent in many routine aspects of living, therefore *catastrophic reactions* are common in the organically impaired. Diminished physical and intellectual capabilities increase the probability of catastrophic anxiety. The individual may initially appear calm, pleasant, cooperative, and competent. However, when confronted with a task (such as putting on a shirt or shoes, cutting meat, or answering a question) that he cannot accomplish, mood and behavior change drastically. He may appear dazed, become agitated, fumble, and become hostile, assaultive, or evasive. His reactions are not only inadequate but disordered and inconsistent.

Because the conditions that produce catastrophic reactions are neither fully predictable nor consistent, those who work or live with the predisposed individual need to be aware of the possibility and signs of an impending catastrophic reaction. Common indicators include sudden and profound deterioration in mood, resistance or stubbornness, and increased agitation. After a catastrophic reaction, the individual is even more vulnerable and less competent; therefore caregivers need to assess for transient deficits and attend to more basic needs so that the exhausted individual is not neglected or unduly endangered.

✳ *Intellectual dimension.* The intellectual symptoms of delirium are deficits in attention, memory impairment, and misperception or misinterpretation of stimuli. These deficits lead to secondary symptoms such as poor recall of recent information, incoherent communication, lack of judgment, misunderstandings, inability to make commonplace associations, and diminished ability to organize personal possessions or behaviors. Often it is the client's noncompliance with medical regimens or hospital policy or his blatantly poor decisions that attract professional attention to his condition.[24,50]

Deeper assessment of the intellectual deficits associated with delirium usually reveals additional deficits that parallel the client's premorbid compulsive habits and cognitive vulnerabilities. Impaired clients who have smoked habitually, eaten compulsively, or shopped indiscriminately are more likely than ever to engage in these activities even if it clearly jeopardized their immediate health, safety, and security. More marginal areas of intellectual functioning, such as calculations, are likely to show the obvious signs of deterioration and incompetency. Learning, especially in strange environments or of new material, is likely to be significantly impaired, because it depends on the ability to attend to a situation selectively and commit relevant aspects of new information to memory.

Agnosia, apraxia, and aphasia usually result from disruption in any of the cerebral lobes; the location of the lesion determines the specific deficit or impairment. Lesions in the left frontal lobe are most likely to interfere with the expression of speech, whereas a similar lesion in the right lobe is more likely to interfere with the understanding of speech. Following is a listing of right- and left-brain activities[42]:

LEFT BRAIN	RIGHT BRAIN
Logic	Intuition
Symbols	Experience
Scheduling	Free
Language	Simultaneous
Structuring	Pictures
Planning	Timeless
Numbers	Imaginative
Specifics	Patterns
	Whole

Agnosia, aproxia, and aphasia are not always pathological. For the most part, they are exaggerations of common interruptions of thought, movement, or expression. Everyone occasionally has difficulty finding the right words, naming an object, or understanding how pieces of a pattern fit together. Measurable differences in performance occur when one is anxious, distracted, frightened, or confident. These deficits usually become pathological when they are consistently more severe or more frequent. The frequency and severity of these symptoms are often best assessed individually. The distinction between normal and abnormal is not absolute; consequently change in the frequency and severity of symptomatic behaviors may be more significant than the behaviors themselves. For some individuals, something so subtle as hesitancy or erratic performance may be more significant than consistent, overt errors; therefore it is usually important to know about an individual's past performance and to observe the individual in many situations to determine the significance or implications of a particular behavior or symptom.

Dementia is characterized by deterioration in intellectual functioning with no obvious clouding of consciousness. The confusion associated with dementia arises more from diminished understanding of stimuli than diminished perception. The two functions are intimately associated, so dysfunction in one area creates problems in the other. As dementia progresses, the individual is only able to understand objects and events in the most concrete, personalized way.

Differentiating between delirium and dementia is difficult among the aged. Delirium that masquerades as dementia is often referred to as *pseudodementia*[28] or pseudodelirium.[23] In the elderly, the onset of delirium is more likely to be insidious or superimposed on an existing (and possibly unrecognized) dementia. In either case the more typical, florid symptoms of delirium are often muted or absent and the delirium overlooked.[34]

The brain becomes more sensitive to its internal environment with aging. Consequently almost any disorder or substance that alters the body's homeostasis may mimic dementia. In the elderly, common causes of pseudodementia (reversible impaired intellectual functioning) include diuretics, digitalis, oral antidiabetic drugs, analgesics, antiinflammatory agents, sedatives, and psychopharmacological agents. Pseudodementia may also be present in clients who develop cardiac, pulmonary, renal, or hepatic failure; endocrine disorders; fluid and electrolyte disturbances; depression, anoxia, anemia; disruption of circadian rhythms; infections; nutritional deficiencies; hypothermia or hyperthermia; and increased intracranial pressure or intercranial lesion.[23,34]

Alzheimer's disease, hardening of the arteries, and multiple cerebral infarcts account for well over 80% of the dementia associated with advancing age.[34,52] These diseases cause the gradual intellectual and functional deterioration commonly associated with dementia. These changes are qualitatively different than those normally associated with aging. Eslinger and others[11] found that individuals known to be suffering from dementia were significantly more likely than control subjects to have deficits in activities requiring temporal orientation, logical memory, and retention of visual stimuli.

These types of deficits reflect more fundamental impairment in abstract reasoning. Such deficits make it increasingly difficult for the client to use ideas and concepts (for example, clock time, or sequencing of tasks) to order his life or to employ bureaucratic hierarchies to order his social relationships. The individual becomes increasingly dependent on experience and sensation (for example, hunger, tiredness, and darkness) to know how to behave, even when to eat or sleep. This supports the empirical observation that highly educated and intellectually oriented individuals are more likely to be impaired and be impaired sooner by brain damage or deterioration than those who are illiterate and rely on less conceptual means for knowing and relating to the world.[47] Ultimately the individual's entire personality and life-style are altered.

Aberrations in short-term memory and disorientation to time and place are the most obvious intellectual symptoms. The client may appear to comprehend and may accurately repeat requests or instructions. However, a short time later the behavior is contradictory. Behavior tends to be an automatic response to need, and conscious thought is diminished if not obliterated. Judgment and discrimination are impaired, and the meanings of all events and phenomena are personalized.

Impairment in the individual's recent memory can approximate the time of disease onset. Memory disturbances that involve past memories, particularly the remote past, indicate an extensive disease process and an unfavorable prognosis.[18,33] In addition, the nature and extent of memory loss infrequently provide clues to both the origin and the location of a lesion or tumor.

Assessment of memory loss is seldom as straightforward as is often believed. Past and present memories are highly variable categories; the individual's observable behavior and responses are seldom if ever a reflection of only one category of memory. The more mundane aspects of day-to-day living are essentially automatic and based on remote memories. Not until familiar ways of doing things become impossible is there evidence to suggest that an individual is not incorporating new experiences, stimuli, or information. As may be expected, an individual who lives in a stable, predictable, secure environment may have significant memory deterioration before he is unable to cope and others notice his impairment.

The client is likely to automatically compensate for the failure of his recent memory. He is increasingly likely to use generic terms and generalizations to deal with specific incidences, situations, or individuals.

Clues of memory loss are initially subtle and are frequently undetected. Nurses need to control their desire to fill in the details. Careful observation of the individual in novel situations, and his responses to new people and to familiar people in new social roles, are particularly revealing. Besides the usual memory-related questions on the mental status examination, the nurse may ask some of the following questions or make some of the following observations:

1. Does the client resist going to new places or resist new activities? Is this characteristic, or is there any indication of increased resistance?
2. Does he have difficulty accepting a new individual or role? Difficulties are commonly related to issues of authority and responsibility. Those which are frequently problematic involve a transfer of authority or responsibility from the client to a previous subordinate.
3. Is the individual using a known title, such as nurse, doctor, lawyer, pastor, or Father, to address recently introduced individuals rather than their names?
4. Is the conversation of the individual becoming increasingly historical? Does the client talk about current affectual states by recounting previous situations that elicited the current feelings and conflicts?
5. Is the individual's conversation decreasing in both spontaneity and elaboration? Does he fall asleep

when others are discussing immediate, but ordinary matters and concerns?

6. Is the individual's speech increasingly characterized by cliches?
7. Does the individual have trouble telling a story or putting thoughts together?
8. Is the individual's ability to engage in either oral or written discourse impaired? Are his responses to letters or memos essentially restatements of the originals?

Individuals with OMD have decreased capacity for learning and therefore are considered to have lost intelligence. However, unlike the lack of intellectual endowment in the mentally retarded individual, the problem focuses around the loss of intellectual capacities. Recent observations of those suffering from dementia, especially Alzheimer's disease,[36,41] suggest that performance in intellectually demanding tasks or judgment in socially sensitive situations is initially compromised. In most instances the individual can successfully hide his cognitive impairment.

In the early phases of dementia, the impaired individual is still capable of learning and to some degree can compensate for deteriorating skills.[48] This is particularly true if the new learning involves less complex strategies and the use of preexisting social or psychomotor skills. However, the ability to learn is closely associated with the individual's memory capacity or impairment.

Because judgment is such a complex intellectual phenomenon, it is also the most susceptible to impairment in OMD, especially those which result from a general toxic condition or generalized deterioration of cortical tissue. In fact, deterioration in judgment is often one of the first indications of OMD. Once an individual's memory is impaired, he is less able to learn from his current experiences. The meanings of all events and phenomena are personalized. The degree to which his past memory is impaired provides a crude measure of the individual's ability to use previous knowledge and experience as the basis for guiding his behavior.

As the individual's capacity for abstract thinking deteriorates, he is less able to see similarity or likeness in present and past experiences. Consequently the individual's responses become increasingly situation specific; every situation is increasingly isolated. Although the client's learning is not totally impaired, he may be unable to transfer learning from one situation to another.

The inability to recognize new forms of old stimuli is also a common manifestation of a decreased ability to think abstractly. If magazines or newspapers change their covers, they are likely to be left unread or discarded. The impaired individual is even likely to make vehement protests that he did not get the goods or services he ordered or wonder why he is receiving this junk.

Language disorders are particularly common manifestations of OMD. Dementia is characterized by a *poverty of speech.* The vocabularies for speaking, reading, or writing become progressively restricted. The client in the early stages of dementia may preserve a facade of normalcy. However, this is possible only as long as the individual is not under emotional, physiological, or social stress. The individual relies on stock words and phrases, especially for conversational purposes, and may start sentences and allow the listener to finish them. He may have difficulty with finding words; although he does not always hesitate to apply a term to an object, the term may be inappropriately applied or the term may be a neologism. If asked for examples of a generic class such as dogs, cats, cheeses, or wines, he may be unable to respond or give only singular or limited examples. The examples he gives are likely to be those of special relevance to him. The capacity for symbolic language, one measure of the ability to think abstractly, is impaired. This impairment may range from mild to severe.

Telegraphic speech patterns are another language disturbance commonly experienced by individuals with OMD, especially those with dementia. Replies to questions may be relevant, but with little elaboration. Speech is less spontaneous, characterized by the use of less descriptive words and fewer examples. As the individual's capacity for language decreases, he is less likely to be able or willing to make declarations or propositions unless there is some immediate bodily need.[5] Even then, the individual is likely to resort to exclamations and demands. Perseveration is also common.

The individual's ability to appreciate and engage in humor is also severely affected. Inappropriate and sexually explicit jokes often seem to make up the clients total humorous repertoire. He may tell ethnic, racial, and sexual stories to anyone at any time. The organically impaired individual is less able to conform his behavior to societal norms because he is less able to make the necessary discriminations. He tells jokes for their immediate effect, his immediate pleasure, or even as a way of reducing his anxiety. Also jokes are an effective way of distracting another person and avoiding confrontation with one's own disabilities.

Poor judgment is evident in the individual's apparent need for immediate gratification. Bodily needs become paramount and tend to increasingly dominate the individual's relations with the environment and other people. The body needs may be primary, such as hunger, thirst, sex, rest, or elimination, but they may also include addictions or cravings, such as for alcohol, sugar or tobacco.

Behavior in relation to these needs is characterized by an increasing sense of urgency. The request is frequently voiced as a demand; the client's sensitivity to where or when, as well as how requests are made, is decreased. The client may demand to return to his room to rest in the middle of a meal or church service. If cigarettes are not immediately available, the markedly impaired individual is likely to prowl the halls looking for cigarettes.

The impaired individual is frequently thought to be rude, inconsiderate, dangerous, or a thief, particularly when he does not comply with requests to cease such behaviors. However, the client perceives most strongly his immediate needs and has little capacity for insight into how his behavior effects others. He does not necessarily realize that he is functioning less appropriately or less effectively. Consequently, as the OMD progresses, the client can be expected to have progressively more interpersonal and social difficulty unless his environment and relationships are appropriately limited and structured.

Personality changes are commonly associated with OMD. However, the individual's personality does not become so much different as it does increasingly rigid. Existing personality traits or characteristics are exaggerated. If the individual was prone to suspiciousness, compulsivity, passivity, or frankness, these traits would become less amenable to modification.

The maturation process perfects and adds to an individual's repertoire of adaptive skills; cerebral dementia depletes it. The client has only the coping skills that he knows best. Loss of flexibility often causes innappropriate responses, especially in novel or stressful situations. Defense mechanisms such as sublimation, repression, and denial give way to regression and projection. The markedly impaired client often assumes a paranoid or passive attitude that makes it increasingly difficult for him to exploit or cooperate with others or his environment. The use of projection also tends to increase the angry responses the client elicits from others.

In advanced dementia the client has virtually no ability to communicate with his environment or control his bodily functions. Once stupor or coma develops, death usually follows shortly.

Along with observation and interviewing, the mental status examination and psychometric testing are frequently used to assess a client's intellectual capacities (Chapter 7).

Social dimension. Increased dependence is common in organically impaired individuals. The nature of this change is determined by the severity and nature of the cortical impairments and the usual responsibilities and expectations of the client. An individual can suffer significant cortical damage while living much as before. Other family members may routinely have cooked, cleaned, or shopped for the client, so inability or difficulty in performing these tasks may go unnoticed. On the other hand, if the individual is unable to competently perform in an expected manner, the other family members will feel the burden of increased responsibilities and duties.

The burden that families assume varies a great deal and their perceptions of the manageability of this burden depend on many factors. Following are some factors that play a part in determining whether a family can successfully cope without additional input or assistance:

1. The ability and willingness of the family to identify its own needs and those which the impaired individual met but can no longer or only partially meet
2. The ability and willingness of another family member to assume the functions of the impaired individual
3. The number and ages of family members available for sharing the additional tasks and responsibilities
4. The extent of the family members' existing responsibilities and commitments
5. The care or direct supervision that the impaired family member requires

As indicated in the Research Highlight on p. 623, the decision to institutionalize the client also depends on the family's perception of the client's condition as irreversible.

Every family member has different responsibilities, whether financial or housekeeping or a combination of these; indeed, the loss of the family organizer may be more devastating than loss of the breadwinner.

The amount and nature of care and supervision required often determines whether clients can remain in their own homes or be cared for adequately in the home of an adult child. Dangerous or socially disruptive individuals are difficult to care for at home. When the individual does not perceive his limitations, ordinary activities such as cooking or taking a walk can become problems. Forgetting the stove is on not only results in burnt food but fires; forgetting where one was going and how to get home can result in the individual's becoming lost. If the behavior of the impaired individual endangers others, the need to supervise him can become the predominant factor for organizing the family's relationships and activities.

Care-related responsibilities and hardships are especially dramatic if only a few members can share or are willing to assume these additional responsibilities. If the family can obtain assistance from the community or extended family and friends, an otherwise intolerable situation may be made manageable. Financial, personal, and interpersonal resources available to care for the client are important factors in the decision as to where the client will stay. Neglected clients and sick or exhausted family members are the consequences and clues of overtaxed, overwhelmed families.

The amount of physical care required by an impaired individual is another important consideration. Infirm or paralyzed clients require frequent care or assistance to meet such basic needs as toileting, eating, bathing, moving, and socializing. When these needs are substantial, meeting them is time consuming; the client needs the constant presence of another person. Planning more than a few minutes or hours ahead may be impossible, because the demands for toileting or comfort are largely unpredictable.

Interpersonal conflict is another problem that tends to become exacerbated, particularly in the case of progressive generalized deterioration. Unable to perceive errors in reason or judgment, some individuals will insist on performing their usual activities and making their usual decisions. Attempts to frustrate these behaviors, particularly in a previously aggressive or determined personality, can lead to physical resistance and angry outbursts. If the individual's premorbid personality was dependent, passive, or congenial, he is less likely to oppose increased supervision and control. For these individuals, the increased attention is likely to be perceived as love and caring; they are more likely to be comfortable in a dependent position. However, if his independent domains of functioning, such as driving, cooking, cleaning, enjoying hobbies, and caring for himself are limited, he too is likely to become resistive and defensive.

Other family members often receive a disproportionate

Research Highlight

A Microanalysis of "Senility": The Response of the Family and Health Professionals

C. Johnson & F. Johnson

PURPOSE

This study was designed to investigate and account for the increased incidence of institutionalization among the behaviorally impaired elderly. The study evolved from the investigators' observation that families were less willing or less able to continue to care for members with behavioral symptoms (particularly incontinence and sleep disturbances) than those with debilitating impairments.

SAMPLE

Clients and families were randomly selected from client lists of two San Francisco Bay–area hospitals.

METHODOLOGY

Interviews were conducted with the clients and their families. These interviews were then analyzed for recurrent attitudes and responses to professional interaction.

FINDINGS

The investigators found that the decision to institutionalize a cognitively or behaviorally impaired elderly family member could not be clearly associated with progressive cognitive deterioration. Instead, the issue of institutionalization most frequently arose when the individual had to be hospitalized for a medical or surgical problem. Hospitalization tends to both accentuate cognitive or behavioral disorganization and make the problem a public rather than a private affair.

As symptoms become more public, past events and actions are officially reinterpreted. The professional's suggestion of nursing home placement offers a ready solution and allows the family to rationalize the acceptability of their decision. If the physician confirms and certifies the client's condition or behavior as irreversible, the family often concludes that they have done all they can and have no other alternative.

IMPLICATIONS

Health professionals' tendency to view chronic conditions with therapeutic nihilism has no doubt contributed to their failure to differentiate between clients with mental deterioration and those with recent deterioration of social status. Failure to make this differentiation has no doubt contributed to uncritical recommendations for institutionalization. Because the client's "bad behavior" is so clearly associated with family intolerance and the individual's subsequent institutionalization, systematic physical and emotional assessments need to be conducted to determine whether the behavior problems are symptoms of a treatable condition or disease. Even if there are no clearly treatable diseases, many of the behavior problems associated with dementia can be effectively managed through social, emotional, and environmental manipulation. Institutionalization remains an alternative, but other alternatives need to be offered to the family.

Based on data from Culture, Medicine, and Psychiatry 7:77, 1983.

---

share of the client's paranoid attitude and defensive behavior. Children who assume responsibilities for a parent can be particularly problematic if they have never established an adult relationship with the parent. In such a relationship, the signficantly impaired parent is unlikely to see the child as more competent than he or be willing to be supervised or controlled by his offspring. This is especially true if the parent is physically unimpaired and unable to perceive his increasing deficits.

Attempts by the family or significant others to point out the client's disabilities to him may change the nature of the relationship and be of limited or no success. The family's inexperience and ineptness with their new tasks and roles may only compound the problem. Even to a skilled observer it may appear that the client is being victimized, that he is being displaced, and that he can, in fact, perform his role better than those who are overtaking it. Consequently the client may succeed in gaining outsiders' support, therefore validating his suspicions about his family and co-workers. Conflict can subsequently escalate, and open verbal battles frequently occur between opposing factions; the issue of the client's incompetence or ill-

ness becomes secondary. People who need to work together and share their information and efforts on the client's behalf may be irrevocably split. Anger, hostility, and hurt feelings are common and may be reflected in behaviors that sever the troublesome relationships; friendships are terminated, wills are changed, family members may be ostracized, and the client may ultimately be abandoned.

Sometimes attempts to displace or redelegate the individual's authority, responsibilities, and duties are threatening to the client. In dramatic cases he may become certain that others are out to get him or take his job, money, or even family. Not unexpectedly, the client may use his resources to prevent this perceived assault. Verbal assaults, physical defenses, employment of detectives to scout out the culprits, reports to the police, and repeated changes in phone numbers or complaints about tapped lines are among the more common defensive moves. Less common, but potentially disastrous, is the growing tendency of clients to arm themselves or booby-trap their home and property as a means of warding off the expected threat.

Often what begins as social or interpersonal conflict ends in familial conflict, as family members either try to control the aberrant behavior or are embarrassed, disgusted, or even ostracized because of it.

Consequently, by the time a family seeks professional help, they are discouraged and tired. They have tried everything they could imagine and judged all to have failed. The medical help they seek is often some combination of a rest and a miracle. If neither is forthcoming, family members may become angry, overly hostile, or withdrawn into their own obligations and activities.

The behavior of tired, discouraged families and that of uncaring, uninterested, unsupportive families often look similar to the observer. Professional efforts to care and plan for the client can impose additional burdens if the nature and needs of the particular family are not considered. This almost certainly causes resistance, and even the most skillfully designed arrangements may be destined to fail for the client, the family, or both. Careful attention to and assessment of the condition of both the family and the client enable the family to remain supportive. The ongoing assessment of the family's ability to cope with stress is facilitated if the nurse regularly asks the following questions:

1. What types of trouble or embarrassment has the client caused his family and individual members of his family? Is the family exhausted, discouraged, angry, and depressed?
2. What was the nature and quality of the relationships before the recent problem? What new interpersonal problems have developed? What problems have been exacerbated?
3. When did the famiy become suspicious that the client was having problems? When and how did they become involved? What is different? What happens now or does not happen that used to happen?
4. What has the family tried to do? What were the results of their efforts? What was the final incident or observation that made them seek help?
5. What does the family want and expect to happen? Are these expectations realistic in regard to (a) the client's condition and prognosis, (b) the client's financial resources, (c) community resources and services, and (d) available technology?
6. Is the family able to mourn the loss of their previous relationships with the client?
7. Can family members assume the roles and responsibilities that the client can no longer fill?
8. Can the family allow the client a new, still valuable role within the family, one based on being rather than doing?
9. Does the family have resources to help them learn and assume new tasks and roles? Are there untapped resources, neighbors, friends, extended family or community agencies? Do people need help finding the resources and learning how to appropriately use them?

Spiritual dimension. Variation in the expression of symptoms and in how these symptoms affect the process of life and living continually make assessment and

treatment for clients with OMD difficult. Generally, understanding how organic impairment affects an individual's sense of himself and his purpose for living depends on the interaction of numerous factors, including the following:

1. The individual's philosophy of life, his beliefs and values, and what life and living have meant to him and his significant others
2. The nature and extent of cortical impairment, the individual's perception of that impairment, and the personal meaning ascribed to his particular disabilities
3. The socially and culturally ascribed meaning of personhood: How are personal and social competence defined and judged? What social or cultural meanings are ascribed to the individual's deficits?

The organically impaired individual is less able to participate in the activities he values. The more his deficits conflict with his values, the more dramatic the impact. If a person is no longer able to engage in the activities and relationships that were central to his social acceptability, feelings of hopelessness and despair may be anticipated. In addition, the individual's ability to receive another's caring gestures may be diminished by feelings of unworthiness and failure or loss of ability to perceive the symbolic expressions of others.

As an individual becomes increasingly impaired, particularly by processes that diminish intellectual capacity, he is unable to successfully engage in the activities or maintain the attitudes prescribed by his values. Unlike persons whose incapacities are predominantly physical, those who have significant intellectual deficits also have diminished capacity to adapt and change. Thus they are less likely to learn new things and to engage in alternative but valued activities.

The maintenance of self-worth becomes particularly problematic when the individual's worth is determined by the values of progress, achievement, individualism, and activism. Investing time, energy, and love in the care of a person who may never again be independent, achieve goals, or show progress may seem unproductive. Rational reasoning provides little support or motivation; values of kinship, loyalty, obligation, belonging, and mutual dependence effectively convey unconditional acceptance of the client. The degree to which families and caregivers can accept the impaired individual provides important clues to their ability to make necessary adjustments in their expectations and attitudes and to meet and to sustain the client's spiritual needs.

Measurement tools. Psychological tests, usually performed by a psychologist, are useful not only in confirming the existence of an OMD but also in describing the nature and extent of the intellectual deficits. The tests selected depend on the client's history, the results of neurological examination, and the examiner's current neuropsychological knowledge. General examination, and the examiner's current neuropsychological knowledge. General examination of an individual's intelligence, memory, and comprehension is often assessed by the Wechsler Adult Intelligence Scale (WAIS). The WAIS is divided into a series of subtests, which measure of the individual's ver-

MEMORY DEFICIT

DEFINITION

Progressive deterioration in the individual's ability to recall information. Usually begins with recent or new information and skills. In time, may progress to interfere with long-term memories and behavioral patterns.

DEFINING CHARACTERISTICS

Physical Dimension
Presence of any one or combination of the following:
1. Infection
2. Drug toxicity
3. Chronic metabolic or hemolytic condition
4. Neurological disease or cerebral injury

Neglect of hygiene
Forgotten or inappropriate use of medications
Forgets to eat

Emotional Dimension
Increasingly prone to severe anxiety
Affect flat when not engaged in a specific activity
Increasingly fearful of new situations

Intellectual Dimension
Increased difficulty learning/remembering new information/skills
Inability to generalize or apply old skills in new situations
Incomplete recall, but rarely total forgetting
Perseveration
Diminished IQ, diminished academic ability
Poor attention to detail, unable to perceive/correct mistakes
Forgets appointments, social obligations
Forgets visits, gifts, phone calls

Social Dimension
Avoids unfamiliar social and geographical settings

Spiritual Dimension
More obsessive about religious obligations or neglect of religious/church activities

Adapted from North American Nursing Diagnosis Association Classification of Nursing Diagnosis: Proceedings of the seventh conference, St. Louis, 1987, The C.V. Mosby Co.

bal and performance abilities and give an overall assessment of his intellectual capacity.

Other neuropsychological tests are constructed to assess more specific intellectual functions associated with specific areas of the cortex. These tests are usually given when an individual is having difficulty coping with a specific type of task or when neurological tests indicate the probability of specific dysfunction.

Analysis

Nursing diagnosis. The NANDA nursing diagnosis related to organic mental syndromes is memory deficit. The nursing diagnosis of generalized disorientation at night is not yet accept by NANDA. The defining characteristics of these two diagnoses are summarized in the boxes above.

GENERALIZED DISORIENTATION AT NIGHT

DEFINITION

Increasing disorientation as evening hours approach, often followed by marked confusion and agitation during night hours.

DEFINING CHARACTERISTICS

Physical Dimension
Increasing restlessness
Markedly combative
Elevations in temperature, pulse, respiration
Prone to remove irritating appliances and to refuse food or medication

Emotional Dimension
Increased fearfulness
Increased anxiety
Marked paranoia
Overt hostility
Catastrophic anxiety

Intellectual Dimension
Progressive disorientation
Progressive memory impairment
Inability to reason rationally

Social Dimension
By nighttime may no longer recognize caregivers as nurses and be unable to cooperate
May report caregivers as imprisoning or trying to harm him
May attempt to call relatives or authorities for assistance

Spiritual Dimension
Praying or cursing may reflect anxiety or fear

The following Case Example demonstrates the characteristics of the nursing diagnosis of memory deficit.

Case Example

Mr. Johnson was a 59-year-old accountant. Some years ago he was diagnosed as having multiple sclerosis. Although he had some changes in his gait, there was little obvious physical deterioration. At this time, his wife sought consultation for him because he had made several errors in clients' tax returns and was irregular about keeping appointments. These changes were evident because he had always been very compulsive about being prompt and accurate. On admission to the neurological unit, Mr. Johnson had trouble remembering his room number, although he could remember numerous other, more complex numbers. While in the hospital his home phone number changed. He was unable to call home until the new number was written down and attached to his phone. He distinguished the nurses from other types of caregivers, but he could not remember the names of the four or five nurses who usually cared for him. Psychological testing revealed a "normal" IQ of 108, but this was significantly lower than his previous IQ of 125. Although he could still perform many complex intellectual tasks, he no longer knew how he did them, nor was he able to identify and correct an error if it occurred. It was determined that Mr. Johnson's multiple sclerosis had progressed and that he was no longer able to assume the responsibilities of his job.

The following Case Example demonstrates the characteristics of the nursing diagnosis of generalized disorientation at night.

Case Example

Mrs. Toczko, an 81-year-old widow, was admitted to the psychiatric unit with a diagnosis of mild dementia. Laboratory reports revealed an elevated WBC and bacteria in her urine. Mrs. Toczko, however, never had a temperature elevation over 99.2° F, although her pulse rate usually went from 78 in the morning to over 100 by evening. Although she was cooperative and only disoriented to time during the daytime hours, by late afternoon she no longer knew she was in the hospital and often attempted to go home. By 10 PM she was markedly disoriented, hallucinating and accusing the nurses of attacking her and stealing her clothes. She was combative and cried loudly until she fell asleep, exhausted, about 2 AM. In the mornings she would rationally complain about how she had been treated the night before. This pattern of orientation and disorientation continued until a bladder infection was diagnosed and treated. Subsequently she resumed her previous level of functioning, returning to her own apartment and receiving assistance from her son and Meals On Wheels.

The following list provides examples of NANDA-accepted nursing diagnoses with causative statements:
1. Social isolation related to poverty of speech
2. Alteration in thought processes related to dementia
3. Self-care deficit related to physical impairments
4. Fear related to memory loss
5. Sensory perceptual alterations related to delirium
6. Alteration in nutrition: less than body requirements related to inability to feed self.

DSM-III-R diagnoses. The DSM-III-R diagnoses related to organic mental disorders are listed in the left box below.

The essential features and manifestations of the features of delirium, dementia, and organic personality disorder according to the DSM-III-R are listed in the boxes below and on p. 627.

Planning

Table 33-2 provides some long-term and short-term goals and outcome criteria related to OMD. These serve as examples of the planning stage in the nursing process.

Implementation

✦ ***Physical dimension.*** Professionals or family members often need to supervise the administration of medication and take measures that decrease the risk of physically or socially complicating conditions and events.

Even if the ultimate outlook is favorable, the physical

DSM-III-R CLASSIFICATIONS RELATED TO ORGANIC MENTAL DISORDERS

DEMENTIAS ARISING IN THE SENIUM AND PRESENIUM

	Primary degenerative dementia of the Alzheimer type, senile onset
290.30	with delirium
290.20	with delusions
290.21	with depression
290.00	uncomplicated
290.1x	Primary degenerative dementia, presenile onset
290.4x	Multi-infarct dementia
290.00	Senile dementia not otherwise specified
290.10	Presenile dementia not otherwise specified

Organic Mental Disorders associated with Axis III physical disorders or conditions, or whose etiology is unknown.

293.00	Delirium
294.10	Dementia
294.00	Amnestic syndrome
293.81	Organic delusional syndrome
293.82	Organic hallucinosis
293.83	Organic mood disorder
	Specify: manic
	depressed
	mixed
294.80	Organic anxiety disorder
310.10	Organic personality disorder
	Specify if explosive type
294.80	Organic mental disorder not otherwise specified

From American Psychiatric Association: Diagnostic and statistical manual of mental disorders (DSM-III-R), Washington, D.C., 1987, The Association.

293.00 DELIRIUM

ESSENTIAL FEATURES

Clouding of consciousness with reduced ability to focus on and sustain attention to environmental stimuli and to shift attention from one stimulus to another.

MANIFESTATIONS

Physical Dimension

Disturbance of sleep-wake cycle with insomnia or daytime sleepiness

Evidence from history, physical examination or laboratory tests of a specific organic factor that is judged to be etiologically related to the disturbance

In the absence of such evidence, an organic factor necessary for the development of the syndrome can be presumed if the behavioral change represents clouding of consciousness of relatively abrupt onset and if conditions other than OMD have been reasonably excluded.

Increased or decreased psychomotor activity

Intellectual Dimension

Perceptual disturbances such as misinterpretations, illusions or hallucinations

Thinking, as reflected in speech content, is disorganized, or at times incoherent

Disorientation and memory impairment, such as inability to learn new material

Adapted from American Psychiatric Association: Diagnostic and statistical manual of mental disorders (DSM-III-R), Washington, D.C., 1987, The Association.

symptoms can be expected to clear unevenly and often slowly. Even clients with favorable prognoses need to be treated symptomatically. Continual reassessment facilitates changes in the care plan. In addition, health care providers and family members need to adjust their expectations of the client to be consistent with the individual's capacity to function intellectually and socially. This helps ensure that the client is neither unduly restricted nor pushed to assume tasks and responsibilities before he is physically able.

Responsibilities and control can be gradually returned to the client. Responsibility for hygiene and grooming usually return first, followed by the more mundane household, family, and job responsibilities. Physical endurance may determine whether the individual is able to resume a particular task. Activities and responsibilities that involve discrimination, motivation, planning, and judgment are the most problematic and therefore the most difficult to resume competently. This is why a client's inability to comply with a regimen of medication and treatment does not necessarily contradict his ability to drive a car, operate sophisticated machinery, or do bookkeeping.

Generally the more ordinary and routine the activity has been for the client, the less judgment and discrimination he needs to perform it competently. Therefore when a client does not comply satisfactorily with treatment, does not meet the expectations of his family, or appears to be socially insensitive or inept, his higher intellectual functions need to be reassessed and treatment and expectations realigned accordingly. Accusing the client of being disgusting or unmotivated are rarely helpful strategies for changing unacceptable behaviors. Since the offending observable behaviors are more often a result of the client being unable to do something (rather than unwilling), it is often more effective to simplify or change the task than try to alter the client's attitude.

As the impairment worsens, the individual becomes less able to attend to his physical needs without direct supervision or intervention. Interventions that reduce demands on the individual's energies often are most helpful. Providing Meals-on-Wheels, housekeeping services, shopping help, laundry services, and occasional haircutting or grooming facilitate the client's doing a few things more adequately. Secondarily these direct services help prevent complications. The individual is less likely to have anemia from not eating, accidents from cluttered or poorly repaired homes, and loneliness from unacceptable personal and environmental odors and appearances.

294.10 DEMENTIA

ESSENTIAL FEATURES

General deterioration in intellectual abilities due to the structural deterioration of nervous tissue.

MANIFESTATIONS
Physical Dimension

Existing evidence from the history, physical examination or laboratory tests, of a specific organic factor that is judged to be etiologically related to the disturbance. In the absence of such evidence, an organic factor necessary for the development of the syndrome can be presumed if the behavioral change represents cognitive impairment in a variety of areas, and conditions other than OMD have been reasonably excluded.

Intellectual Dimension

Objective evidence of impairment in long-term
    memory inability
Impairment of abstract thinking
Impaired judgment
Aphasia
Apraxia
Agnosia
Constructional apraxia

Social Dimension

Loss of intellectual abilities interferes with occupational functioning or with usual social activities or relationships with others

Adapted from American Psychiatric Association: Diagnostic and statistical manual of mental disorders (DSM-III-R), Washington, D.C., 1987, The Association.

310.10 ORGANIC PERSONALITY DISORDER

ESSENTIAL FEATURES

Diminished ability to mobilize available organic energy and to use available intellectual functions because of damage to the frontal lobes.

MANIFESTATAIONS
Physical Dimension

Evidence from the history, physical examination, or
    laboratory or neuropsychological tests of an abnor-
    mality in brain function or structure

Emotional Dimension

Affective Instability
Irritability
Anxiety
Recurrent outbursts of aggression or rage are grossly
    out of proportion to any precipitating psychosocial
    stressors
Marked apathy and indifference

Intellectual Dimension

Paranoid ideation

Social Dimension

Markedly impaired social judgment

Adapted from American Psychiatric Association: Diagnostic and statistical manual of mental disorders (DSM-III-R), Washington, D.C., 1987, The Association.

TABLE 33-2 Long-term and short-term goals and outcome criteria related to OMD

Goals	Outcome Criteria

NURSING DIAGNOSIS: DISORIENTATION AT NIGHT RELATED TO CONFUSION

Long-term goal

To become oriented to person, place, and time	Knows location of clocks and calendars.
	Follows daily routine.
	Finds the bathroom at night.
	Calls appropriate person for assistance.
	Knows own nurse.
	Knows address and phone number and carries identification.
	Distinguishes between day and night.

Short-term goals

To become less upset about confusion	Performs requested tasks without increased anxiety.
	Maintains emotional control.
	Thinks about the consequences of the action (indicated by statements).
	Stays relatively calm and noncombative when upset or fearful.
To feel safe and secure in the environment	Responds to being called by name.
	Knows daily schedule of activities.
	Wears own clothes.
	Uses own furniture and possessions.
	Is physically comfortable (indicated by statements).
	Does not smoke in bed.

NURSING DIAGNOSIS: INABILITY TO CARE FOR SELF DUE TO PHYSICAL IMPAIRMENT (POOR VISION AND UNCOORDINATION)

Long-term goal

To maintain optimal level of functioning	Lives in own home or in least restrictive environment possible.
	Uses supportive community services.
	Maintains hobbies, interests, or employment.
	Asks family for assistance with responsibilities (bill paying, taxes).
	Wears glasses, dentures, hearing aid, or mobility aids as necessary.
	Maintains health by avoiding infections, constipation, and undue stress.

Short-term goals

To meet physical needs at highest level of functioning	Eats three balanced meals per day or several small meals per day.
	Wears clothes that are clean and appropriate.
	Bathes twice weekly or more often if necessary.
	Moves bowels regularly without undue concern.
	Drinks adequate fluids.
	Wears glasses as necessary.
To meet emotional needs at highest level of functioning	Enjoys diversional activities such as television and hobbies.
	Has emotional outbursts less frequently or is less labile.
	Accepts own irritability and frustrations as part of illness.
To meet intellectual needs at highest level of functioning	Reads paper, books, and magazines or looks at pictures, as appropriate.
	Discusses news topics.
	Works at puzzles and word games.
	Remembers significant events and talks about them.
	Learns new ways to deal with problems of eating and mobility.
To meet social needs at highest level of functioning	Joins others in group activities, such as watching television or sitting on porch.
	Writes to family members or has nurse write for him to family member.
	Communicates verbally with others.
To meet spiritual needs at highest level of functioning	Goes to church, synagogue, or other place of worship.
	States that he feels accepted, cared about, and esteemed.
	States that he feels a sense of belonging and importance within the family.
	Shows some creativity in thoughts and actions.
	Includes some humor in day-to-day events.

Once an individual becomes markedly or severely demented, his ability to perceive and to meet his own physical needs is minimal. In fact, the ability to cooperate or interact constructively with one's environment is severely decreased. At this time, the individual needs to have others take the responsibility for physical care, which may include washing, dressing, toileting, and feeding. On the other hand, a client who is physically capable of feeding or dressing himself may need step-by-step direction about what to do and how to do it. If left alone to eat the client will not eat or will wander off, or will report that he is not hungry and does not like the food. The nurse or caretaker needs to remember that the client cannot, rather than will not, do these things for himself.

Measures to stabilize the client's internal and external environment are important, because of his diminished tolerance for either internal or external physical stress. Maintaining a stable temperature, a familiar environment, adequate nutrition, preventing infections, and preventing injuries, particularly immobilizing injury, are important nursing interventions.

With markedly severe dementia, physical safety for the client and those around him becomes more of a problem. The client needs continual supervision, which means that he is not left alone for even brief periods. Locked doors and windows may be necessary. Even then, disoriented clients seem to somehow slip away. Authorities, coworkers, and neighbors need to be alerted about the client's disappearance immediately. One never assumes that the impaired individual will or can return on his own. A search needs to begin immediately. The subject matter of the client's most recent conversations and fondly remembered places often provide clues for the search. However, the impaired individual may become easily distracted and forget his destination. Consequently, he is likely to become frightened and wander randomly trying to find a familiar place; he could go anywhere. Radio and television announcements and distributing a description are sometimes necessary and helpful for finding the lost individual.

Modern appliances become hazardous when used inappropriately or when they are abandoned without being turned off or disconnected. Because even the moderately organically impaired individual is easily distracted, coffeepots, stove burners, and heating pads are often left operating unattended. Setting a bag of groceries or the mail on a hot stove burner can quickly cause a fire, potentially a tragic situation and one that the individual cannot be expected to respond to appropriately.

Enforcing common safety regulations frequently involves the removal of problematic appliances or supervising their use. Requests for cigarettes and matches and requests to borrow small or personal appliances are often accommodated almost automatically. However, the danger such common objects pose needs to be explained to some clients. Involving family or other responsible adults in the supervision of the client while he smokes, shaves, or makes coffee often provides a satisfactory alternative way for maintaining social contact and expressing interpersonal caring.

Other problems include the use of flammables such as cleaning fluids, cigarettes, gasoline, or firewood. The client's inability to identify dangerous environmental factors and to anticipate the consequences of his method of handling dangerous materials make some situations potentially explosive.

Cigarette smoking is no doubt the most common source of fire. Dangerous smoking habits such as indiscriminately flicking the hot ash, forgetting and abandoning half-smoked cigarettes, and smoking in bed or while dealing with gasoline are responsible for innumerable fires and injuries.

Because smoking is often a response to physiological and emotional urges, the client often needs to meet this immediate urge more than to comply with social norms. Once the urge is satisfied, the client may abandon the cigarette without further concern about it. Consequently smoking often needs to be controlled or supervised. Control may include removing the cigarettes from the client or restricting cigarette smoking to specific supervised situations and environments.

Emotional dimension. Because the client is increasingly unable to manage his own emotional expression, someone may have to assist him. To do so, the assisting person needs to understand that the degree of expression is not an accurate assessment of the initial feeling. The intensity of the feeling may better be judged by the situation within which it originates. Unless the caregiver can establish an accurate sense of proportion, either of two responses is likely to occur: (1) the caregiver does not take any part of the individual's expression as valid and withdraws, ignoring the client as well as the disturbing behavior, or (2) the caregiver overevaluates the seriousness of the emotion and begins to consider ways to provide extraordinary support instead of trying to understand and manage the individual's behavior.

Generally, interventions seek to control the expression of the emotion. Being aware of the client's escalating behavior may allow both time and opportunity to withdraw the client either emotionally (change the subject, distract him) or physically (remove him to another location) before the response is totally out of control.

Once it is clear that certain types of situations or subjects are prone to elicit either catastrophic anxiety or severe emotional lability, it is often helpful to avoid these situations. By keeping the environment stimulating but calm and routine, avoiding conflict, and avoiding confrontation, many catastrophic responses can be prevented.

The client's lack of control of emotional expression does not imply that he does not experience emotions. Although their expression may become distorted, their emotions can be interpreted. Again, attention to context, to theme, and particularly to action is often more revealing than verbalizations or facial expressions. Clients who are only mildly or moderately impaired often use biographical stories as a means of dealing with a particular emotion. If the client is experiencing personal loss, the stories often focus on other incidences of personal loss. Concern about abandonment may be expressed by talking about people leaving or dying. All the nurse may have to do is listen, state simply that she understands, or just stay quietly until the end of the story. At this point the client may begin to relax and move on to other things.

In the early stages of OMD, some clients are partly aware of losing control. Emotional support, treatment, antidepressants or electroconvulsive therapy, and even limited psychotherapy may be immensely helpful. If these clients focus on what they can still do and recruit old skills,[39] they can find alternative ways to express themselves and gain recognition. As indicated in the Research Highlight below, exercise and activities are also helpful in decreasing anxiety and fear.

Grieving the loss of the previous self may be necessary before reduction and rehabilitation efforts are beneficial and readaptation possible. Depression in conjunction with OMD often makes the individual look and act far more impaired than he really is. Recognizing and treating depression may facilitate independence and productivity for several months or years.

Intellectual dimension. Organically impaired individuals depend particularly on external cues for knowing what to do, how to behave, or what others ex-

pect from them. Simple things such as familiar tablecloths and table settings remind the client to eat in a socially acceptable manner. Wearing his own pajamas and robe can help the client to stay in bed or at least rest, curtailing the urge to wander. Familiar furnishings and possessions often help remind the individual that he is at home, he belongs here, and this is his room. These surroundings and routines are reassuring and also facilitate the maximal level of independent function.

The following strategies compensate for the individual's decreased intellectual capacities:

1. Give the client specific, personalized written and verbal instructions for such things as diet, medication, and treatment.
2. Minimize the complexity of new information.
3. Adapt diet, care, and medication schedules to existing patterns and schedules.
4. Plan for additional time and instruction to accomplish new learning; learning is facilitated by teaching in the client's usual environment and with the equipment that the client is expected to use.

Research Highlight

Relieving the Anxiety and Fear in Dementia

H. Schwab, J. Rader & J. Doan

PURPOSE

To deal more effectively with the nursing problems of cognitively impaired individuals and to help these clients function more effectively, these investigators designed a special intervention program called SERVE. SERVE is an acronym for self-esteem, relaxation, vitality, and exercise. The guiding concept for the SERVE program was that reversible aspects of dementia existed. The study was to determine whether the SERVE program could be an effective means for increasing clients' functional capacity. Unlike reality orientation programs, this intervention program focused on participation in concrete simple activities rather than orientation to abstract concepts of time and space.

SAMPLE

The sample was drawn from a 127-bed intermediate to long-term care facility associated with a university-based nursing school. Participants included several severely disoriented ambulatory residents who had been admitted to one unit within a few weeks. Four components comprised the SERVE program: simple stretching and range of motion exercises, a "fun" activity, walking, and a massage/relaxation period. The group leaders focused their attention not so much on the activity but the response of the participants.

METHODOLOGY

Group leaders made individual assessments of the participants' cognitive abilities and emotional responses. Changes in a participant's behavior were evaluated and encouraged if

they represented progress, discouraged if they were disruptive. The object of each session was to create an atmosphere of safety, predictability, and acceptance. Success was expected to be observed indirectly as reduced fear, anxiety, or excess disability both within the group and on the unit.

FINDINGS

This program had dramatic results for some, more modest improvements for others. Generally the authors reported less noisy disruptive behavior, increased interactions between participants outside of the group sessions, and less wandering away from the facility. Most seemed to have gained some relief from symptoms of fear and anxiety.

In addition, the program seemed to have positively influenced the attitudes of the staff. These changes included encouraging clients to go to group sessions, facilitating their timely arrival, coping with the interactions of the group leaders, placing clients together for meals, walking with restless clients and seeking alternatives to using restraints.

IMPLICATIONS

Although it is unclear why some clients respond better than others, the activities and interpersonal contact facilitated by the SERVE program were beneficial. The results also indicate that the medical prognosis of irreversibility did not preclude measures that offered symptom relief and quality life experiences. Also, such programs appear to affect nursing staffs positively and facilitate a more understanding and personalized approach to care.

Based on data from Journal of Gerontological Nursing 11:8, 1985.

5. Use more than one sense to help the client see changes in his environment and relationships.
6. Use many sensory approaches to assist the individual with learning; for example, taste, feel, and look at new medication.
7. Use visual cues such as picture charts to help the individual make necessary associations.
8. Encourage the simplifying and structuring of the client's interpersonal relationships, financial responsibilities, and occupational obligations and tasks.
9. Use existing knowledge, old learning, and habitual strategies to deal with new situations and expectations.
10. Elicit desired behaviors and responses by evoking them rather than requesting them
    a. Begin the activity (for example, hum or sing a few bars of a familiar song or gently put the spoon or toothbrush to the client's mouth) and then let the client take over; remain close by in case the client forgets or is distracted.

Because problems with intellectual function are all interrelated, management takes into consideration all deficits that the individual is experiencing. The interventions in Table 33-3 are often helpful in assisting the client and family to cope. Success in working with the severely impaired individual often involves changes in the caregivers' own attitude and expectations.

As the client becomes more intellectually impaired, verbal communication becomes more limited and self-centered. Frustration, a common consequence of the client's attempts to communicate verbally, leads to acting-out behaviors. The client's concrete thinking and impaired memory make it difficult if not impossible for the client to think of alternative ways to say things to obtain attention or fulfill needs.

Throwing things, yelling, cursing, pushing, soiling, or spitting are often the means of communication the client thinks of. Such socially aberrant behavior often indicates that the client's immediate needs are not being met or that he has been confronted by his deficits. These outbursts are often avoidable if nurses can anticipate the client's needs and control the physical and social environment. Careful attention to the theme, environmental context, and emotional tone of the client's story often provides more information than the actual words he speaks. Standing in the bathroom may mean the client needs help to toilet himself. Recounts of previous incidences of being left alone or expressions of anger at those who left may mean that the individual is lonely or concerned that the nurse will not stay with him.

Clients with significant disturbances in verbal communication have trouble not only expressing themselves but also understanding what others mean. Simplifying communication is an important strategy for communicating effectively with the severely impaired client. Ideally only one idea is communicated at a time.

Verbal communications are best understood when they are kept simple and direct. Single words and short sentences facilitate understanding. However, verbal communication often needs to be supplemented with visual clues, pictures, or pointing. The client who has difficulty finding the right word also has difficulty remembering the meaning of words. Although the word may sound familiar, association with the object can be problematic. Even more difficult for the severely impaired client is remembering how to use objects and tools. Pictures of the needed object or desired activity help the client remember to perform a task.

If telling a client what to do next does not elicit the desired behavior, the behavior may be demonstrated or initiated. Physically guiding a client's movements often helps him understand more effectively than verbal directions. Touch is a concrete, direct way to express care and concern, and it is often understood long after verbal or written comprehension has deteriorated. A hug, firm grip, or guiding arm communicates presence and attentiveness; sitting quietly beside an individual often provides more security and relief than words could.

These strategies may allow some effective communication with a severely aphasic client. Those with limited disorders often benefit from intensive therapy, either relearning speech skills or learning alternative symbolic methods of communication such as sign language. For those who have more generalized disease, more iconic methods, particularly the use of pictures and gestures, are often successful. Singing and listening to music rather than talking may still be possible and provide an avenue for communication as well as an alternative source of pleasure. It is also important to remember that clients who are no longer able to readily comprehend verbal communications often become more attuned to the nonverbal aspects of others' communication, enabling them to comprehend some or all of messages. The inability to effectively comprehend words paradoxically makes the aphasic individual more sensitive to falsehood, malice, or equivocal intention.

Social dimension. New physical and social environments are often disorienting, because it is difficult for the marginally oriented to adapt their knowledge and skills to new environments. When the client is confronted with the impersonal and unfamiliar routines of a hospital or a nursing home, his behavior often deteriorates quickly. New environments and unfamiliar routines render him more dependent, often on strangers. Since these changes often create the potential for hazardous situations, every attempt needs to be made to support the efforts of customary caregivers and to maintain the client in a familiar environment.

As OMD becomes more severe, the individual's sense of self becomes more restricted and his needs more self-centered. This does not mean that these clients need less social contact, only that they can no longer gain approval through their achievements. They can only receive unqualified acceptance. Social acceptability is often fundamental to meeting the client's needs for human contact and support. Families, friends, and even professional caregivers are more likely to care for, visit, or just sit with the client if they are not overwhelmed by offensive behaviors, appearances, or odors.

Successful maintenance or reestablishment of family relationships is particularly important to the client's well-being. If the family is unable to cope with the client or renegotiate their own roles and relationships, the family not only becomes less cohesive but also may be in danger of disintegration. This significantly increases the likelihood that the client will be abandoned or neglected either physically or emotionally. Providing for necessary and timely help to the family is often the most significant way to ensure immediate and future support for the client. Some families may need assistance in identifying the meaning of their loss and in redefining their roles and responsibilities. These are appropriate issues and problems for short-term family therapy.

In addition, most families benefit from professional interventions that help them maintain a physically and emotionally safe environment. Fundamental to the achievement of this goal is support for the primary caregiver(s). Zarit and Zarit[44] suggest the following interventions for maintaining continuity of caregivers and of the physical and social environment:

1. Provide caregivers information that helps them understand what is happening to the client; support their efforts to anticipate and plan for present and future needs.

2. Assist caregivers to understand the effects of cognitive deterioration on the individual's behavior. Sometimes health care professionals can help by acknowledging the caregivers' frustrations and explaining that the client with severe memory loss cannot remember that he cannot remember.

3. Encourage caregivers to slow down, to make only one request or give one instruction at a time. This facilitates maximum independent performance by the client and minimizes the emotional and physical demands of the responsible caregiver.

4. Caregivers need to be encouraged and assisted in their efforts to solve problems as the individual's cognitive status deteriorates and/or new dilemmas arise. Health care professionals can often help by reminding caregivers that there is no "right" approach and encouraging them to try different attitudes, approaches, and responses and use the most successful.

5. Caregivers need to be encouraged to attend to their own needs and to plan for periods of relief from their caretaking responsibilities. Caregivers may schedule intermittent breaks before tensions get too emotionally or physically exhausting. This often involves helping family members, particularly spouses, to accept help for some of their ongoing responsibilities. Before these alternatives can be explored, however, primary caregivers may need an opportunity to share their pain, frustration, conflicts, and grief with someone.

6. Alternative ways of getting help need to be presented. For the professional health care provider this means not only knowing about and suggesting available community resources (respite care, Meals on Wheels, homemaker services, home care by nurses or physicians, day care centers, activity programs, sitters) but serving as an advocate for the development of relevant support services.

Generally environmental disruptions are best avoided; however, if they become unavoidable the event needs to be treated as having the potential for immense emotional crisis. If the client's increased dependence is unrecognized and no additional support is provided, he typically becomes more anxious and his behavior more intolerable and unmanageable. When home management is no longer feasible, special consideration is given to admitting a cognitively impaired person to an institution. Clients can be expected to become less anxious and less confused in circumstances that require them to make the fewest changes in their routines. It is particularly helpful if institutional care is individualized to accommodate the client's habits and capitalize on existing memories.

New social norms can also be confusing and provoke anxiety for clients. When old memories are inadequate or provide inappropriate prescriptions for behavior, the individual is likely to become withdrawn, disoriented, or dependent or to behave inappropriately. Interactions with those who hold differing personal, social, ethnic, and religious beliefs can be as confusing and disorienting to a severely impaired client as moving him to a totally new neighborhood or city. Confrontations and challenges can occur when such interactions are forced.

Provisions for social and environmental stability also enhance the individual's perception of being cared for, as well as the nurse's ability to care about the clients. Caring is probably the most culturally determined aspect of human expression. Teasing, arguing, embracing, or closeness is understood differently depending on one's social and cultural background. Teasing can be an expression of affection in one case and an expression of hostility in another. Food, gifts, and visitors also have their cultural specificity; favorite foods or the giving of food is, for some, essential to the expression of love and concern. Rules or conditions that inhibit such usual exchanges effectively restrict both the expression and reception of human caring. The client needs to be successful in his social interactions, and sensitive, perceptive nursing interventions can ensure that success.

Spiritual dimension. Despite significant cognitive deterioration, an individual is still capable of having religious feelings and beliefs. Because of their diminished intellectual capacities, however, organically impaired clients depend on their families and caregivers to evoke spiritual or religious memories and to communicate associated attitudes of love, dignity, peace, and belonging. Attitudes of peace and belonging are often communicated through the caregivers' own sense of accountability to a high spirituality or deep sense of commitment to their fellow humans. The presence of the client's supreme being, the integration of the universe, and the meaning of life are often evoked through continued participation in familiar religious rituals and ceremonies.

Given the present lack of scientific understanding of most OMD and the limited technological resources for intervention, interpersonal relations that communicate love and acceptance are the nurse's primary means for imparting hope to these clients. Hope may be generated when-

TABLE 33-3 Interventions for clients with OMD

Problem	Interventions
Significant impairment of immediate memory	Simplify and adapt new procedures and treatment regimens to established habits and preferences. Stress only the essential. Expect less frequent and more erratic compliance.
Concrete thinking and impaired judgment	Use recognized authority rather than rationale and explanations for gaining compliance. Supervise the client's administration of medication, treatments, and activities of daily living by way of a family member or a community agency (for example, a visiting nurse). Avoid confronting the client with decisions and judgments he is unable to make. Begin to structure the physical and social environment so that the client is not confronted with choices or situations he cannot make. Limit the client's choices. Alternative ways of accomplishing the same goal can be unnecessarily confusing. Make expectations clear; give simple, clear directions in simple, short sentences. Avoid the use of inferences, allegories, or metaphors.
Intensification of premorbid personality and increased use of projection	Anticipate less flexibility of attitude and more stereotyped reactions. Expect the client to assume less responsibility for the consequences of his behaviors; avoid punishing and scolding. Structure activities and situations to ensure successful participation. Do not ask the client to do what he cannot. Explain to the family and significant others the implications of the deterioration. Help them avoid overpersonalizing what the client either does or says. Avoid conflict and threatening behavior that could increase the client's paranoia.
Increased disorientation	Expect increased confusion at night; avoid shadows and total darkness. Observe activity more closely; be alert for wandering. Provide lighting, especially to the bathroom. Avoid use of central nervous system depressants as sleep aids; use instead a warm bath, warm milk, or low dosages of phenothiazines; increase activity during the day. Help the client clearly identify environmental stimuli. Avoid physical discomfort (for example, cold, constipation, hunger, tight clothes). Minimize disorientation to sequence and time; provide clear verbal and visual indication as to time of day (clock, open curtains); date (calendar, talk about seasonably appropriate activities), and year (calendar, talk about major news events and public personalities). State how long it has been between one event and another. Identify tangible changes over a specified period. Avoid activities that follow a detailed rigid sequence (for example, games in which players take turns, large group activities, group tasks). Encourage small-group activities characterized by parallel activity and simple physical responses. Encourage activity, modify exercise to client's capabilities. Encourage activity in which previous memories and skills might be evoked (for example, dancing, singing familiar songs). Minimize disorientation to place; avoid moving the client from a familiar environment if possible, or provide accompaniment by a familar person. If possible, use personal belongings of the client as integral parts of any new environment (for example, clothes, bedspread, blanket, pictures, appropriate furnishings). Use color rather than numbers to help the client identify his room; put his name on important personal objects, if possible. Allow him to establish as his a chair at the dinner table or community area. Encourage and facilitate regular visits from family and friends. Limit the number of professionals who care for the client. Facilitate the client's recall by immediately and matter-of-factly stating your name and your relationship to the client. Remind the client matter-of-factly what you want from him or expect of him. Encourage the client to use his own clothes and possessions; clearly identify them as his and reserve them for his exclusive use.

ever people realize that other people care about them and will rally to their needs when they are afflicted.

Religious rituals are usually a part of one's lifelong experiences. Imbedded in these rituals are prescriptions for attitudes, behaviors, and relationships. Participation in familiar religious services is often most beneficial, because the service remains familiar and recognizable. In Catholic and orthodox denominations, regular attendance is often sufficient, because the services have been ritualized, and are forever familiar. In Protestant and other heterodox religious traditions that are not highly structured, it may be more important that the individual attend a familiar church or join in the singing of familiar hymns to recognize and to meaningfully participate in the service. To the degree that the religious service remains familiar, the experience is capable of evoking the associated attitudes and behaviors. The totality of the experience may give the client a sense of wholeness or completeness, which has become increasingly rare in his incomprehensibly fragmented everyday life.

The former director of a Jewish nursing and retirement home described marked changes in behavior in clients with some of the home's most severely regressive cases of Alzheimer's disease during Passover services.[23] Many of these clients were able to participate in the Seder; many others sat quietly and responded appropriately throughout the entire pre-Seder service. With some amazement, the director noted that these same residents were incapable of attending to even their most basic personal needs and had been wandering the halls aimlessly just before the services.

Although nurses rarely have a direct role in the organization or conduct of religious or spiritual services, they may facilitate these activities and experiences by following some of the measures listed here:

1. Alter institutional routines and schedules to facilitate conduct and attendance at services.
2. Welcome clergy and religious leaders in the care facilities and help them understand the problems of the impaired clients so they can adapt their care and services accordingly.
3. Encourage families to continue to include even the more impaired member in important religious occasions, (holy days and religious rituals and ceremonies—marriages, communion, bar or bas mitzvahs, and so on).
4. Participate with clients in spiritual activities held in the institution if able to do so sincerely and comfortably.

A summary of interventions for clients with OMD is presented in Table 33-3.

Evaluation

Evaluating the care of a client with an OMD is highly individual but generally revolves around identification of the organic impairment and management of the resulting symptoms. It is essential to preserve the client's maximal level of functioning and independence, while ensuring that his basic physical, emotional, intellectual, social, and spiritual needs are met. Success is not particularly objective or measurable, nor does it necessarily involve a cure. Rather, successful nursing care sustains individuals and their families. Salient parameters of evaluation include the provision of quality relationships and meaningful experiences for the clients and the personal and professional growth of caregivers. Care can generally be considered effective if secondary complications do not occur or, in the case of the more severely impaired individual, an optimal level of functioning is maintained.

BRIEF REVIEW

Organic mental disorders include a broad spectrum of conditions and symptoms caused by trauma, disease, or physical impairment to the brain. Delirium and dementia, two of the most common forms of OMD, involve disturbances in every dimension of the person. Disturbances in the physical dimension include the client's inability to care for himself, illness and trauma, and a possible genetic basis. Disruptions in the emotional dimension are seen in the client's emotional lability and inappropriateness of emotional expression. Impairments within the intellectual dimension include false perceptions such as delusions and difficulty communicating, understanding, remembering, and making judgments. In the social dimension, disruptions in relationships with family members and other caregivers are seen. Because of the numerous disruptions clients with OMD frequently are unable to accept and understand their illness or to develop a philosophy about life that promotes hope and spiritual contentment.

Relating to clients with OMD requires patience, tolerance, and a belief that the care given makes a difference in the quality of the client's life. Those who successfully care for the organically impaired client often come to appreciate the less objective and less material aspects of life and come to better appreciate their own humanity and that of others. The warmth, patience, tolerance, and understanding acquired through caring for clients with OMD are often transferred to other aspects of the caregivers' lives.

The nursing process provides a systematic way of caring for clients with OMD by assessing disturbances and impairments within the five dimensions and analyzing the data to form nursing diagnoses. Planning and interventions are focused on maintaining the client at his highest level of functioning. Evaluation is based on the successful management of symptoms.

REFERENCES AND SUGGESTED READINGS

1. Beam, I.: Helping families survive, American Journal of Nursing **84:**229, 1984.
2. Burnside, I.: Working with the elderly, ed. 2, Monterey, Calif., 1984, Wadsworth, Inc.
3. Cahel, C., and Arana, G.: Navigating neuroleptic malignant syndrome, American Journal of Nursing **86:**671, 1986.
4. Colston, L.: The handicapped. In Wicks, R., Parson, R., and Capps, D., editors: Clinical handbook of pastoral counseling, New York, 1985, Paulist Press.
5. Coyle, M.K.: Organic illness mimicking psychiatric episodes, Journal of Gerontological Nursing **13**(1):, 1987.
6. Critchley, M.: The divine banquet of the brain, New York, 1979, Raven Press.

7. Cummings, J.: Dementia: neuropathological correlates of intellectual deterioration in the elderly. In Vlatowska, H., editor: The aging brain: communication in the elderly, San Diego, 1985, College Hill Press, Inc.

8. Davidhegar, R., Gunden, E., Wehlage, D.: Recognizing and caring for the delirious patient, Journal of Psychiatric Nursing and Mental Health Services, **16**:38, 1978.

9. Detmer, W., and Lu, F.: Neuropsychiatric complications of AIDS: a literature review, International Journal of Psychiatry in Medicine, **16**:21, 1986.

10. Devaul, R., and Hall, R.: Hallucinations. In Hall, R., editor: Psychiatric presentations of medical illness, Jamaica, N.Y., 1980, Spectrum Publications, Inc.

11. Donahue, E.: Reality orientation: a review of the literature. In Burnside, I., editor: Working with the elderly, Monterey, Calif., 1984, Wadsworth, Inc.

12. Ellenberger, H.: Psychiatry from ancient to modern times. In Arieti, S., editor: American handbook of psychiatry, vol. 1, New York, 1984, Basic Books, Inc., Publishers.

13. Eslinger, P., Damasio, A., Benton, A., and VanAllen, M.: Neuropsychologic detection of abnormal mental decline in older persons, Journal of American Medical Association **253**:670, 1985.

14. Freeman, A.: Delusions, depersonalization and unusual psychopathological symptoms. In Hall, R., editor: Psychiatric presentations of medical illness, Jamaica, N.Y., 1980, Spectrum Publications, Inc.

15. Goldstein, K.: The effects of brain damage on the personality, Psychiatry, **15**:245, 1952.

16. Guynn, R.: Psychiatric presentations of cardiovascular disease. In Hall, R., editor: Psychiatric presentations of medical illness, Jamaica, N.Y., 1980, Spectrum Publications, Inc.

17. Gwyther, L., and Matteson, M.: Care for the caregivers, Journal of Gerontological Nursing **9**:92, 1983.

18. Hall, R.: Anxiety. In Hall, R., editor: Psychiatric presentations of medical illness, Jamaica, N.Y., 1980, Spectrum Publications, Inc.

19. Jeste, D.V., editor: Neuropsychiatric dementias: current perspectives, Washington, D.C., 1986, American Psychiatric Press, Inc.

20. Johnson, C., and Johnson, F.: A micro-analysis of senility: the response of the family and the health professionals, Culture, Medicine and Psychiatry **7**:77, 1983.

21. Katzman, R.: Dementia in the context of the teaching nursing home. In Schneider and others, editors: The teaching nursing home, New York, 1985, The Beverly Foundation Raven Press.

22. Lezak, M.: Neuropsychological assessment, New York, 1976, Oxford University Press, Inc.

23. Lipowski, J.: A new look at organic brain syndromes, American Journal of Psychiatry **137**:674, 1980.

24. Lipowski, Z.: Transient cognitive disorders (delirium, acute confusional states) in the elderly, American Journal of Psychiatry **140**:1426, 1983.

25. Lucus, M., Steele, C., and Bognanni, A.: Recognition of psychiatric symptoms in dementia, Journal of Gerontological Nursing **12**:11, 1986.

26. Luria, A.R.: The man with a shattered world, New York, 1972, Basic Books, Inc., Publishers.

27. Luria, A.: The working brain, New York, 1973, Basic Books, Inc., Publishers.

28. Luria, A.: Higher cortical functions in man, ed. 2, New York, 1980, Basic Books, Inc., Publishers.

29. MacDonald, E.: Personal communication, 1986.

30. Mackey, A.: OBS and nursing care, Journal of Gerontological Nursing **9**:74, 1983.

31. McKean, K.: Memory, Discover **4**:10, 1983.

32. Mesulan, M.: Dementia: its definition, differential diagnosis and subtypes (editorial), Journal of the American Medical Association **253**:2559, 1985.

33. Morgan, A., and Morgan, M.: Manual of primary mental health care, Philadelphia, 1980, J.B. Lippincott Co.

34. National Institute on Aging Task Force: Senility reconsidered, Journal of the American Medical Association **244**:259, 1980.

35. National Interfaith Coalition on Aging, Inc.: Spiritual well-being: a definition, Washington, D.C., 1985, National Retired Teachers Association–American Association of Retired Persons.

36. Pajik, M.: Alzheimer's disease inpatient care, American Journal of Nursing **84**:216, 1984.

37. Palmateer, L., and McCartney, J.: Do nurses know when patients have cognitive deficits? Journal of Gerontological Nursing **11**:6, 1985.

38. Palmer, M.: Alzheimer's disease and critical care, Journal of Gerontological Nursing **9**:86, 1983.

39. Pincus, J., and Tucker, G.: Behavioral neurology, ed. 2, New York, 1978, Oxford University Press, Inc.

40. Price, W., Forejt, J.: Neuropsychiatric aspects of AIDS: a case report, General Hospital Psychiatry **8**:7, 1986.

41. Reisberg, B.: Stages of cognitive decline, American Journal of Nursing, **84**:225, 1984.

42. Richerson, K.: Right brain—left brain: the nurse consultant and behavior change following stroke, Journal of Psychiatric Nursing and Mental Health Services **20**(5):37, 1980.

43. Richardson, K.: Hope and flexibility: your keys to helping OBS patients, Nursing 82, **12**:64, 1982.

44. Roach, M.: Reflections in a fatal mirror, Discover **6**:76, 1985.

45. Sacks, O.: The man who mistook his wife for a hat, New York, 1985, Summit Books.

46. Schuster, M.: Psychiatric manifestations of gastrointestinal disorders. In Hall, R., editor: Psychiatric presentations of medical illness, Jamaica, N.Y., 1980, Spectrum Publications, Inc.

47. Schwab, M., Radar, J., and Doan, J.: Relieving the anxiety and fear in dementia, Journal of Gerontological Nursing **11**:8, 1985.

48. Shamoian, C.A., editor: Biology and treatment of dementia in the elderly, Washington, D.C., 1984, American Psychiatric Press, Inc.

49. Shapira, J., Schlesinger, R., and Cummings, J.: Distinguishing dementias, American Journal of Nursing **86**:698, 1986.

50. Trzepacz, P., Teague, G., and Lipowski, Z.: Delirium and other organic mental disorders in a general hospital, General Hospital Psychiatry **7**:101, 1985.

51. Walsh, K.: Neuropsychology: a clinical approach, Edinburgh, 1978, Churchill Livingstone.

52. Weddington, W., Jr.: The mortality of delirium: an underappreciated problem? Psychosomatics **23**:1232, 1982.

53. Wolanin, M.: Physiologic aspects of confusion, Journal of Gerontological Nursing **7**:236, 1981.

54. Wood, F., Novack, T., and Long, C.: Post-concussion symptoms: cognitive, emotional and environmental aspects, International Journal of Psychiatry in Medicine **14**:277, 1984.

55. Zarit, S., Cole, K., and Guider, R.: Memory training strategies and subjective complaints of memory in the aged, The Gerontologist **21**:1981, 1981.

56. Zarit, S., Miller, N., and Kahn, R.: Brain function, intellectual impairment and education in the aged, Journal of the American Geriatrics Society **26**:58, 1978.

57. Zarit, S., and Zarit, J.: Cognitive impairment. In Lewinsohn, P., and Teri, L., editors: Clinical geropsychology, New York, 1983, Pergamon Press.

ANNOTATED BIBLIOGRAPHY

Hall, R.C.W., editor: Psychiatric presentations of medical illness: somatopsychic disorders, Jamaica, N.Y., 1980, Spectrum Publications, Inc.

This text provides a perspective on the interrelatedness of psychiatric and somatic diseases and symptoms. Special attention is given to anxiety, depression, delusions, hallucinations, and hysteria. The psychological manifestations of infections, endocrine disorders, cardiovascular disease, pulmonary disorders, gastrointestinal disorders, and hematological disorders are singled out for specific discussion. This is a valuable reference not only for those interested in psychological illness, but also for those interested in illnesses traditionally classified as physical or medical.

Luria, A.R.: The man with a shattered world, New York, 1972, Basic Books, Inc.

This book is based on the life experiences of a Russian soldier who received a bullet wound that destroyed part of his brain. It incorporates material from his journals, which provide first-person memories. Particularly interesting are the descriptions of his attempt to use these memories to participate in the more mundane activities of living. How a brain injury makes the familiar strange and the simple complicated is conveyed through this soldier's accounts of determining right from left, taking a train home, and attempting to repair a barn door. The soldier's accounts are supplemented by Luria's discussion of neurophysiology and neuroanatomy.

Sacks, O.: The man who mistook his wife for a hat, New York, 1985, Summit Books.

Currently available in the popular press, this collection of clinical cases for the professional and layman provides numerous, sometimes amusing examples of what it might mean to have a neurological disease. The author describes the problems of neurological disease and how individuals consciously and unconsciously attempt to adapt to their altered circumstances. The star of this book is not the physician but his patients; from each one he learns something more about human determination and capability.

C H A P T E R

34

THERAPY FOR CLIENTS WITH PSYCHOPHYSIO-LOGICAL ILLNESSES

Sharon Holmberg

After studying this chapter the learner will be able to:

Discuss the historical development of psychophysiological disorders.

Define and describe the most common psychophysiological disorders.

Discuss the significant aspects of theory related to understanding psychophysiological disorders.

Apply the nursing process in the care of clients with psychophysiological disorders.

Psychophysiological disorders are health problems that result from influences of both the mind and the body. The term "psychophysiological disorders" expresses the notion of emotional influence on various organ functions. Another term, "psychosomatic," meaning mind and body, is used to describe emotional symptoms such as phobias, obsessions, and insomnia.[21] Sometimes these terms may be used interchangeably. Closely related is the term "psychobiologic," which suggests that specific psychological conflicts from early life, mobilized by later life experiences, produce certain diseases such as peptic ulcer, rheumatoid arthritis, bronchial asthma, migraine, essential hypertension, ulcerative colitis, and dermatitis.

Understanding how the body and the mind function together in health and illness is a relatively new and rapidly expanding field. The idea that "it is impossible for the mind to suffer without the body becoming sick"[4] is at least 2 centuries old, but the complex, synergistic action of biological, psychological, social, and environmental interactions is just beginning to be understood. Basic research, especially in neuroendocrinology, immunology, and neurobiology, accompanied by the study of psychological adaptation processes has developed an expanding scientific base for analysis and treatment of psychophysiological illnesses.

Anxiety and stress can affect most body systems or the organism as a whole. Some of the systems and physical conditions in which psychological factors are considered significant are the gastrointestinal tract (peptic ulcer, nausea and vomiting, ulcerative colitis, irritable bowel syndrome), the cardiovascular system (hypertension, arrhythmia, tachycardia, angina pectoris), musculoskeletal system (tension headaches, rheumatoid arthritis), genitourinary tract (painful menstruation, urinary frequency, impotence), and the respiratory system (asthma). A number of other illnesses, such as obesity, anorexia nervosa, some skin conditions, and migraine headaches, are also referred to as psychophysiological. As scientific knowledge expands, evidence is being accumulated to support theories about the probable impact of stress in the development or exacerbation of "biological" diseases such as diabetes, hyperthyroidism, hypothyroidism, cancer, myocardial infarction, and kidney disease.

Because psychophysiological conditions can become serious and even life threatening, appropriate medical treatment is essential. Control of life-threatening symptoms may be the first phase of a comprehensive treatment program. Such treatment usually occurs in the general hospital. Increasingly, psychiatric-medical units are emerging in general hospitals.[25, 41] The psychiatric liaison nurse may also contribute significantly to the care of these clients in a general hospital setting, either by providing direct services or through consultation to the nursing staff. Psychotherapy and pharmacotherapy extend beyond the phase of acute illness to treatment in psychiatric hospitals, outpatient clinics, and private offices. Approaches to therapy need to be client specific since the illness reflects the individual's particular difficulty coping with his own life situation in a style tolerable to the physiological system.

DATE	EVENT
Ancient Times	Hippocrates described the unity of the individual in his environment, recognizing how health is affected. The Greek philosopher, Aristotle, observed that afflictions of the soul such as passion, pity, joy, loving, and hating have corresponding afflictions of the body.
1600s	Descartes reasoned that the human is divided conceptually into body and mind, a description of Western, dualistic thought.
1700s	Some writings suggest the interaction of the mind and the body by describing verbal suggestions that can produce physiological changes.
1800s	The term "psychosomatic" was introduced, which referred to emotional symptoms such as phobias, obsessions, and insomnia.
1900s	Freud published his first papers describing the psychodynamics of anxiety and conversion hysteria.
1920s	Psychoanalytic formulations were further developed. Somatic symptoms were interpreted as hysterical and viewed as symbolic expressions of unconscious instinctual urges.
1930s	Cannon's[12] research in physiology led to the concept of homeostasis. Pavlov's[47] research with dogs, which demonstrated stimulus-response feedback mechanisms, was published. Von Bertalanffy[82] described new approaches to biological research, which were later developed into general systems theory.
1940s	Constructs were developed by Wolf and Wolf[84] and Dunbar[22] that attempted to link a specific personality pattern or conflict situation to specific diseases such as migraine, diarrhea, or ulcerative colitis. Specificity theory developed by Alexander[2] suggested that every emotion has a somatic concomitant; certain kinds of conflicts have affinities for certain organ systems.
1950s	Psychosomatic research included the cause of duodenal ulcer, the relationship of separation and depression to illness, and the psychological stress of surgical patients. Selye[73] published a seminal work defining stresss as the nonspecific response of the body to any demand made on it that leads to increased wear and tear in the organism, predisposing the individual to disease. Friedman and Rosenman[30] identified a cluster of behavior traits (type A personality) that is correlated with coronary atherosclerosis.
1960s	Sources of environmental stress were identified and described, including noise, job stress, environmental hazards, and sensory deprivation. Holmes and Rahe[42] developed a stress scale in an effort to standardize the extent of stress experienced by a person and relate it to the disease process. Lazarus[50] published the first phases of research emphasizing cognitive processes and adaptive mechanisms in stress. The role of major life changes and disruption in social networks was related to increased episodes of physical illness. Type A and B behaviors were further related to the predisposition to coronary heart disease.
1970s	Newly discovered hypothalamic factors and hormones demonstrated the connection between the brain and neuroendocrine axis. Complex models of stress and illness were proposed and tested. These examined stimulus characteristics, response characteristics, and attempts to describe a "lack of fit" between person and environment. Psychiatric, mental health nursing programs that integrated biological and psychological studies in the curriculum were developed. Roy[70] and Rogers[68] proposed theories of nursing based on an integrated, holistic concept of humans.
1980s	Links between anxiety and the immunological system are established in animal research. The discovery of hormones secreted by the brain such as endorphins opens new avenues for research and demonstrates the complexity of biochemistry associated with behavior. Psychiatric-medical units are developed in general hospitals that recognize the need for a holistic nursing approach.
Future	With emphasis on the biological bases of illness, nurses will be more active in managing psychophysiological disorders in direct and indirect roles.

THEORETICAL APPROACHES

General Systems

The basic constructs of general systems theory are outlined in Chapter 3. Systems theory was an outcome of new scientific doctrines of wholeness, dynamic interaction, and organization. As such, it was important for providing the possibility of an integrated concept of mental disorder. The relative nature of biological factors (physical appearance, endocrine balance, intellectual endowment, sex, age, and so on) and life experiences (family relationships, interpersonal relationships, education, social status, cultural factors, and so on) could be conceptualized together with the nature of the environment.

In this framework *mental health* was viewed as "that state in the interrelationship of the individual and his environment in which the personality structure is relatively stable and the environment stresses are within an absorptive capacity."[50] Mental illness then is viewed as existing on a continuum that extends from the well-integrated (healthy) personality structure to the poorly balanced personality structure that can tolerate few internal or external demands. Constitutional factors function as a dynamic substrate, molding and being molded by environmental influences. Disturbances in any of the systems influence the individual. For example, an overlying stressful job that produces prolonged emotional disequilibrium is likely to produce physical symptoms or changes.

Psychosomatic disorders clearly exemplify the interactions between biological traits, life experiences, and the environment. This group of disorders represents an exaggerated physiological response to prolonged stress and can occur in all human beings. Reasons for the psychosomatic reaction as opposed to other neurotic reactions are specific to the individual, probably based on previous life experiences or learned behavior. Systems theory, as an interactional theory, also addresses the nature of the multiple interactions and reactions taking place.

Stress

The basic concepts of stress described by Selye can be found in Chapter 3. Selye's original use of the term "stress" was limited to "an orchestrated set of bodily defenses against any form of noxious stimuli. . . . a universal physiological set of reactions and processes,"[52] created by an environmental demand. In this framework, stress is the individual's physiological response and the stressor is an environmental condition. A variety of environmental conditions, such as natural disasters, war, imprisonment, and forced relocation, would produce a stress response for almost anyone. Psychological stress occurs when a particular relationship between the person and his environment occurs that is viewed by the individual as threatening or exceeding personal resources. For example, depending on an individual's relationship with a particular family member, the death of that family member may be a stressor.

If the individual perceives the death of a family member as a stressor, his stress response may lead to illness. Levi and Kagan[55] suggest that psychosocial stimuli can cause physical disease. Their thesis is that most life changes evoke physiological stress responses intended for the physical activity of coping. The nature and extent of the stressor interacting with the individual's genetic and psychosocial response set may provoke precursors to disease that can lead to disease itself. The stress-illness response for psychological stress that leads to physical illness is complex. Consideration needs to be given to the following factors: (1) the nature and extent of environmental stressors; (2) the characteristics, usually genetic and physical, of the individual; (3) the perception of the individual or the meaning given to the event, commonly called cognitive appraisal; and (4) the coping abilities of the person.

Environmental stressors. Both quantitative and qualitative differences affect psychological stress. For instance, in the preceeding example, the death of a family member, how could a quantitative difference in stress be evaluated? If the death were that of a mother who was the primary source of financial and emotional support for two preadolescent children and thus resulted in the children being moved to foster homes, changing schools, giving up friendships and adapting to different expectations, the adjustment is extensive compared to, for example, a married man in his 50s whose mother dies while living in a nursing home where she has been for the past 3 years. This addresses quantitative demand for change presented to an individual from an environmental stressor. The qualitative demand may vary depending on the individual's ability to anticipate or control an environmental stressor or the relative valence of emotion involved. As an example, the man who can anticipate his mother's death because of an extended illness is likely to experience it differently than he might have had she died suddenly in his home from a heart attack.

Another suggested way to categorize stressors is based on duration. Four broad and somewhat overlapping categories have been defined[23]:

1. Acute, time-limited stressors, such as arriving late to work or falling out of a canoe
2. Stressor sequences, which involve a series of events over time but which occur as the result of one event, such as losing a job
3. Chronic, intermittent stressors, such as having disliked in-laws to dinner, which may occur on a regular but not constant basis
4. Chronic stressors, such as coping with a long-term physical illlness or long-term job stress, in which there is no clear precipitant but the stress is continuous and long lasting

These are only general categories intended to facilitate ways to think about stressors. The crucial test is how the individual responds. For example, having in-laws to dinner could be a chronic stressor for the individual who is very frequently preoccupied by the problem relationships.

Stressors can also include environmental characteristics such as heat, humidity, cold, altitude, noise, and amount of light. Overexposure or underexposure to any of these may cause serious physical illness or minor changes in physiological functions or mood. For example, studies have shown two effects of noise: (1) it damages hearing; and (2) it has a "stress" effect, changing mood, intellectual and motor performance, general behavior, and general body state. Some people exposed to high noise levels for several years develop hypertension. Environmental pollutants are another, increasingly commonly recognized source of stress. Some of these, when severe enough, will produce immediate illness, such as ionizing radiation, whereas others are a source of chronic stress that gradually changes physiological functioning.

Characteristics of the individual. The obvious traits of the individual (for example, sex, age, and physical appearance) and the less obvious traits (for example, endocrine balance, genetic makeup, and functioning of the immune and autonomic nervous systems), taken together, help to determine available coping abilities and techniques.

The physical properties and chemical composition of body tissues tend to be reasonably constant. When there is too much variation (for example, elevated body temperature), the individual is considered ill. However, more understanding of physical systems has led to new theories about the importance of subtle variations and the extent of system interdependence. Stress can ultimately produce physiologically observable changes in various body systems. Reactions of physical systems, that is, the internal environment, are contingent on the emotional and social responses of the person as well as activity and influence from the external environment. Some of the physical systems associated with stress responses are summarized in Table 34-1.

Cognitive appraisal. Cognitive appraisal is the process that probably takes place in the cerebral cortex and intervenes between the environmental stimulus and the reaction. It is the mental activity of judgment, discrimination, and choice before action, an analysis based on past experience. Thus the degree and kind of reaction to the same event can vary considerably from person to person. Consider, for example, two women, each of whom is sitting alone in her house late at night. Woman A has a recent history of being assaulted and robbed. Both hear a weird, indiscriminate noise from the upstairs bedroom. Woman A's response is immediate panic; her pulse rate and respirations increase, and her pupils dilate; she jumps from the chair to telephone a friend, fearing grave danger. Woman B feels a slight chill run up her spine but rapidly concludes that it is a windy evening and the shifting atmospheric pressure has caused the bedroom door to swing shut. When a crisis or threatening situation occurs, these physical and mental processes seem to take place instantaneously and intuitively. Clearly there is an instant arousal response in which the autonomic nervous system responds, but this can be rapidly modified by cognitive appraisal. Usually the appraisal process takes into consideration (1) risks and consequences (that is, "What will happen if I don't change?"), (2) resources (that is, "Am I strong enough to tolerate this? Who [or what] would help?"), and (3) imminence (that is, "Do I have time to search, to think more?").

Lazarus and Folkman[52] describe three types of stress appraisals, namely, those that include harm/loss, threat, or challenge. When some damage has already been done to the individual, harm/loss appraisals take place essentially to evaluate the degree of loss. Threat appraisals concern the anticipation of harm/loss and include anticipation of future problems as a consequence of the harm/loss already incurred. Both have primarily negative emotional implications such as fear, grief, or anger. Challenge appraisals involve the potential for harm/loss or for gain or growth. Thus pleasurable emotions of eagerness or excitement are associated with challenge appraisals.

Intrinsic to the notion of cognitive appraisal is that it is subjective. How a specific environmental event (especially an ambiguous one) is perceived does not necessarily have much to do with objective reality. Personality factors can influence or distort perceptions. For example, a new situation will be judged on past similar experiences. Timing of the event may also influence perception. Those events that occur at an unexpected life phase (for example, a teenager whose parents die) or several stressful events together may influence the person's overall interpretation of those events. It has been suggested that the individual who tends to perceive things negatively or who

---

TABLE 34-1 Summary of physical systems and their role in stress responses

Physical System	Role in Stress Response
Brain	Interprets and evaluates stressors
	Provides memories of past emotional experiences
	Controls feelings, emotions, and behaviors that ensure survival, and perhaps sociability and sexuality.
Autonomic nervous system	
Sympathetic	Reacts to acute demands made on the body, such as in acute anxiety or fight-flight response.
Parasympathetic	Directs functioning of physiological processes such as digestion and body fluids.
Endocrine System	Stressful environmental events change neurochemical and hormonal levels in the body. This function prevents illness and facilitates adaptation, but can also cause illness.
Immune System	Stress has an immunosuppressant effect that can increase vulnerability to certain diseases.
	Major life changes, such as bereavement, increase the risk of illness, probably by suppression of the immune system.

Psychological Changes Accompany Aerobic Exercise in Healthy Middle-Aged Adults

J.A. Blumenthal, R.S. Williams, T.L. Needles & A.G. Wallace

PURPOSE

This study was conducted to assess the psychological effects of physical exercise on a sample of healthy, physically deconditioned, middle-aged adults. A matched control group for comparison was included in the design.

SAMPLE

Experimental subjects were 16 men and women between the ages of 21 and 61 years who registered for a 10-week adult fitness program. They were given a physical examination and determined to be free from overt cardiovascular disease based on medical history and treadmill exercise testing. The control subjects consisted of community volunteers who were matched to the subjects on the basis of age, education, sex, and health status.

METHODOLOGY

Experimental and control subjects were individually given psychological tests before and shortly after completion of a 10-week physical conditioning program. Only the experimental subjects participated in the exercise program, which consisted of 10 minutes of stretching exercise followed by 45 minutes of walking or jogging to reach 70% to 85% of maximum heart rate. Psychological tests consisted of a profile of mood states, assessment of state and trait anxiety, and a retro-

spective change questionnaire. Experimental subjects were also given a physical examination but the control group was not.

FINDINGS

The major finding in this study was a significant improvement in the overall psychological functioning of experimental subjects after a brief structured exercise program. The exercise group experienced reductions in state and trait anxiety, felt more vigorous, and had less tension, depression, fatigue, and confusion.

IMPLICATIONS

This study is consistent with other studies which suggest that improved physical health is associated with improved psychological health. It also supports the notion that basically healthy, well-adjusted people can increase their sense of well-being through exercise. The study group had volunteered for the exercise program, which implies their desire for self-improvement, but this effect on the results was not measured. The study supports the potential utility of regular physical exercise as a means to promoting psychological and physical health.

Based on data from Psychosomatic Medicine 44(6):529, 1982.

expects fear, harm, or danger will be more likely to interpret new situations from that perspective. Cognitive responses can probably be changed or influenced by a variety of factors such as psychotherapy, advice from family or friends, or a change in one's health (see the Research Highlight above). The individual's philosophy, beliefs, and sense of control also influence cognitive appraisals.

Coping. Coping addresses the active process of using personal, social, and environmental resources to manage stress. One model views coping as a stress and control mechanism by which arousal is minimized through learned behaviors. The ego psychology model considers coping to be the most effective approach to managing person-environment relationships. A third model suggests that coping does not necessarily imply control over noxious stimuli but implies making an effort to minimize their effects.

The first model suggests that once an individual has developed a particular set of psychological adaptive mechanisms they will remain relatively constant throughout life. Type A personality represents one coping style; type A coping traits are a strong desire to control situations, receiving personal gratification from achievements, setting very demanding work standards, and having a great sense

of urgency. Failure in any of these leads to despair and to a redoubled effort to achieve, creating coronary-prone behavior. An individual's coping style can presumably be described and future responses predicted from studying his reactions in a few specific situations. If specific sets of coping styles can be developed, then relationships between these and the development of specific illnesses can be studied.

An alternative, the second model, considers coping as a process between the individual and a constantly changing environment and relies on the notion of cognitive appraisal as essential to the determination of a behavioral response. Research by Shontz[75] that examined individuals' responses to being told of a serious physical illness suggests that there may be various stages in the coping response: the first is shock, followed by encounter, then retreat, and gradually reality testing. These cycles repeat as the coping process continues, leading eventually to psychological growth. Lazarus and Folkman[52] describe a third model of the coping process that includes *emotion-focused coping,* a process by which the meaning of the stressful transaction is changed, and *problem-focused coping,* which means intellectually evaluating a situation and then selecting one or more alternative actions. The se-

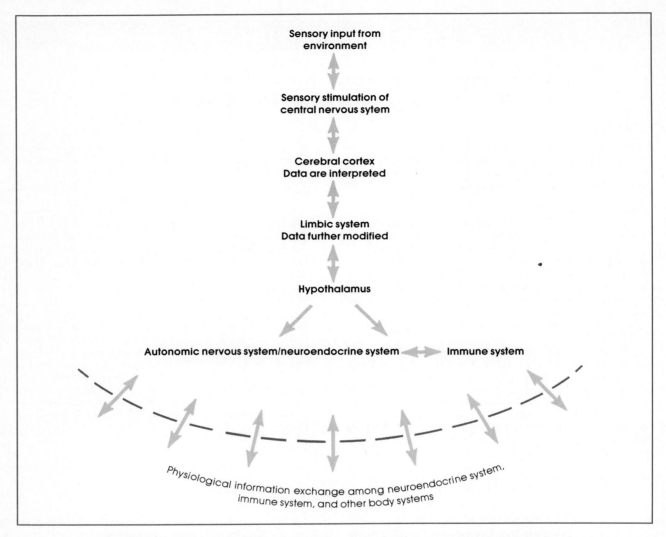

FIGURE 34-1 The path of information exchange between sensory inputs and body organs.

lected action is taken and the situation reevaluated to determine effectiveness of the coping actions and what, if any, further action is necessary. The way in which an individual responds depends on how the stressor is evaluated as well as the availability and access to resources. To understand behavior one must understand the individual's process of analysis (Figure 34-2).

Table 34-2 provides a summary of theoretical approaches.

CHARACTERISTICS OF THE THERAPIST
Qualifications

Clients with psychophysiological disorders are likely to be treated in a variety of settings such as general hospital inpatient units, psychiatric hospital inpatient units, medical and psychiatric outpatient clinics, and private offices.

TABLE 34-2 Summary of theoretical approaches

Theory	Theorist	Dynamics
General Systems		There is dynamic interaction between various parts of the individual's systems. Any disturbance in any system influences the individual as a whole.
Stress	Selye	Psychological stress occurs when a particular relationship between the person and his environment occurs that is viewed by the individual as a threat. The nature and extent of the stressor interacting with the individual's genetic and psychosocial responses may lead to disease.

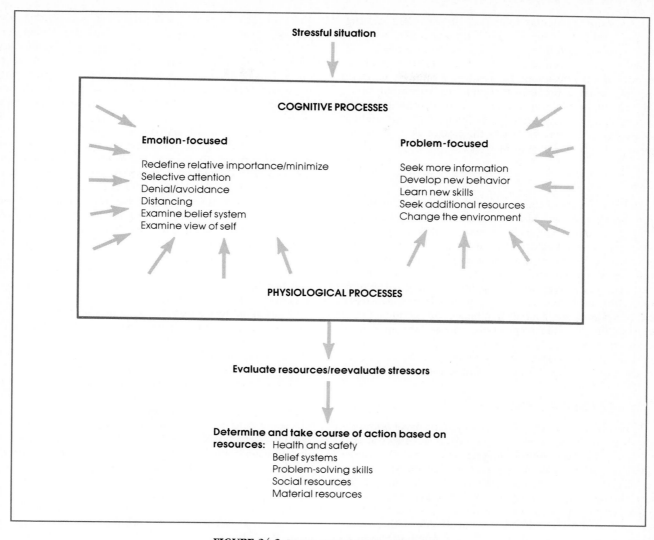

Stressful situation

COGNITIVE PROCESSES

Emotion-focused

Redefine relative importance/minimize
Selective attention
Denial/avoidance
Distancing
Examine belief system
Examine view of self

Problem-focused

Seek more information
Develop new behavior
Learn new skills
Seek additional resources
Change the environment

PHYSIOLOGICAL PROCESSES

Evaluate resources/reevaluate stressors

**Determine and take course of action based on
resources:** Health and safety
Belief systems
Problem-solving skills
Social resources
Material resources

FIGURE 34-2 Interactional mode of coping.

Each setting provides a different emphasis so it is not unusual for the client to move from one setting to another depending on the phase of the illness. The client's health problems often require a medical specialist as well as persons who have learned one or more techniques of psychotherapy.

Persons with academic preparation in nursing, medicine, psychology, and social work may be involved in the treatment process. Most of these disciplines require at least a master's degree. The multidisciplinary approach common to inpatient units will involve all of these professional groups. Some clients have specific needs for therapists skilled in other therapy techniques such as physical, nutrition, or respiratory therapy.

Special knowledge and skills required of the nurse are a thorough understanding of pathological mechanisms underlying the specific disease processes combined with the knowledge and techniques required for psychotherapy. She may need to be well versed in medical crisis intervention techniques and surgical procedures involved in the management of acute physical health problems. The nurse's knowledge of psychodynamics, physiological processes, and drug effects and interactions combined with knowledge of the client as an individual will facilitate the integration of various treatments.

Role

The role of the nurse may vary depending on the type of treatment facility and the theoretical framework underlying the treatment regimen. The nurse has a significant role on inpatient medical and psychiatric treatment units as one of the providers of direct care and a member of the multidisciplinary team. In addition to utilizing her skills as a nurse, an important task of the nurse treating clients in outpatient clinics and private practice is to ensure the coordination of care received from medical and rehabilitation personnel. There are roles for the psychiatric nurse as a consultant to medical treatment units in hospitals, nursing homes, or community treatment facilities. Prior experience in direct care roles helping clients learn to manage activities of daily living while integrating psychological aspects of care is the pragmatic knowledge most needed by these care providers.

Goals

The major goal of the nurse is to reestablish, maintain, or improve the individual's physical health status. Frequently the client has little awareness of how stress can influence physical health. A key task of the nurse is to help the client develop an understanding of the relationship between increased stress and increased physical symptoms. The client may need considerable help to identify environmental demands or relationships that cause stress. Another significant goal is to change or modify coping skills so the individual can more successfully manage a variety of roles (for example, employee, parent, spouse, student). Accomplishing such changes usually means increasing the client's self-esteem and self-direction.

CHARACTERISTICS AND TYPES OF THERAPY

Implementing therapy for persons with psychophysiological disorders has some unique characteristics but also calls on general psychiatric nursing skills. One of the most significant differences in treatment is that individuals are very likely to be initially seen in an acute, life-threatening state. Medical crisis intervention techniques need to be employed first. In addition, the physical health problems may persist throughout the individual's life with periods of remission and exacerbation so continued attention to the client's physical state is required. Another significant difference is that management or succcessful control of symptoms, both physical and psychological, is likely to require more than one therapeutic approach at any given time. For instance, medical management of the physical disease process might be accompanied by biofeedback training and long-term psychotherapy.

Most clients with mild or well-controlled physical symptoms and few overt behavioral symptoms of psychiatric disorder are treated by family physicians or medical clinics rather than in a psychiatric setting. Those clients referred to and treated in psychiatric settings are likely to be persons who have experienced repeated, severe episodes of physical illness that are likely to be accompanied by clear behavioral manifestations of psychological stress.

It is important to consider the interrelationship between physical and psychological conditions. For example, the two conditions may coexist, without any clear evidence of a causal relationship; a person with a diagnosis of schizophrenia and varicose veins of the legs is an example. The medical and psychiatric conditions may interact, which is the case in psychophysiological disorders

and can occur in many other instances; for example, the first sign that an elderly person with organic brain syndrome has developed a mild infection may be a marked decline in mental status. In a causal relationship one condition caused the other. Some examples of this are acute depression caused by hypothyroidism and kidney disease secondary to the use of lithium. Understanding the interrelationship of physical and psychological symptoms is essential for determining appropriate treatment.

Therapeutic approaches to psychophysiological disorders can vary greatly depending on the philosophy of the professsional; the attitudes, expectations, and resources of the client; and the availability of specific types of treatment. Somatic treatment of the medical condition is usually required on a regular basis or at least an episodic basis to maintain physiological balance. This may be the extent of treatment, particularly if the physical symptoms are well controlled and the client is not interested in psychotherapy or fails to see a connection between somatic state and psychic state. Psychotherapy may be provided in conjunction with somatic treatment.

Traditional forms of psychotherapy, such as individual, group, and family therapy, may be effective in helping the client to resolve many of the relationship problems that produce stress. Determining which of these therapies to implement is based on the particular client's conflicts.

Increasingly more utilized in the treatment of psychophysiological disorders are behavioral therapy approaches. Behavioral therapies combine multiple treatment approaches and can encompass dietary modification, biofeedback, hypnosis, autogenic training such as learning relaxation techniques, and exercise. Usually the behavioral therapies require active interest, emotional involvement, and participation from the client. Some clients wish to actively participate in their treatment and seek out the necessary information to do so. The nurse can respond by teaching the client sspecific techniques or providing specific data about medications, diet, exercise, and the like. Another important task of the nurse involves motivating clients who are particularly passive or dependent and tend to be less active in their treatment.

Behavioral therapy may be short term or long term, but it usually requires consistent effort by the client. For example, teaching the client relaxation techniques may take only a few sessions. However, the client needs to practice such techniques over a longer period of time to gain full benefit and to eventually change his behavior. In such cases the nurse is available to reinforce the practice of techniques and discuss benefits as well as potential problems with the client.

Certain other alternative treatments are useful in the treatment of psychophysiological disorders. These therapies are often directed toward the spiritual dimension of the person and include various forms of meditation such as yoga or transcendental meditation. Another alternative treatment that is gaining acceptance is acupuncture. In general, these treatments are viewed with skepticism by professionals since there is not yet conclusive research evidence of their efficacy and the physiological mechanisms contributing to the response are poorly understood.

However, the constructive potential of religious beliefs and practices should not be disregarded. Recent research by Lilliston and others[56] indicates that for some problems, such as life-threatening illnesses, religious practices such as churchgoing or prayer are considered valuable in learning about the illness.

NURSING PROCESS
Assessment

Physical dimension. Assessment of an individual with a psychophysiological disorder may reveal symptoms in only one body system, symptoms in several systems, or responses that include the whole organism. Consequently, this discussion presents a general overview of physical assessment and then focuses on the assessment of specific body systems influenced by the stress response.

Assessment generally includes a complete physical examination and general laboratory tests. A health history, including family history of disorders such as diabetes, cancer, hypertension, various cardiovascular disorders, and genetic diseases, gives an overall picture of the client. Specific information about use of prescription and nonprescription drugs is obtained. The health inventory also assesses risk factors such as smoking, use of illegal drugs or alcohol, caffeine intake, and exposure to environmental contaminants such as chemicals, pesticides, radiation, and automotive exhaust. It may be relevant to explore with the client the nature of contaminants in the workplace such as frequent contact with specific chemicals, high levels of noise, or extremely demanding physical activity. Another relevant arena to be explored is the client's lifestyle, including general activity level, diet, and eating patterns. It is important to inquire about the use of dietary supplements such as vitamins, which are known to cause health problems if ingested in insufficient or excessive quantities.

Cardiovascular system. Distinctly pleasant or unpleasant stimuli are likely to evoke cardiovascular responses such as changes in heart rate, heart rhythm, blood pressure, and stroke volume. Research has indicated that cognitive work such as mental arithmetic or public speaking and psychological stresses or intrapsychic conflicts can produce tachycardia and increase levels of noradrenalin and free fatty acids in the blood. The atherosclerotic process, which can be found in children as young as 15 years of age, is thought to be due to a number of interacting variables including exercise, diet, genetics, obesity, and the functioning of the central nervous system.

Physical assessment includes checking pulse, respirations, weight, and blood pressure as well as specific tests (see Table 34-3) that can be diagnostic if any one condition is suspected. The client is asked specific questions about episodes of tachycardia and any other related physical symptoms. Most diseases of the cardiovascular system develop subtly and slowly and are likely not to be discovered except serendipitously until there is episodic recurrent chest pain or a dramatic presentation of acute illness such as myocardial infarction. In addition to those ill-nesses presented in Table 34-3, other conditions, such as cardiac dysrhythmias or sudden death (see the Case Example below), may also be partially attributed to psychological factors.

Case Example

Sam V., 27 years old and single, walked into the psychiatric emergency room one morning and asked to be seen. He complained of severe anxiety and a sense of impending doom. During the examination Sam stated that he was now living in a somewhat unhappy situation with his mother after having broken up with his girlfriend approximately 4 months ago. He also acknowledged that he occasionally used some drugs, primarily marijuana and cocaine, and had from time to time sold drugs to get money, because he did not have a steady job. The mental status examination revealed an acutely paranoid, very guarded, and highly anxious man. All other cognitive and mental functions were normal. His blood pressure was 170/90. Sam reported that he had been seen in a local health clinic about 2 weeks earlier where he had been told that he had mild hypertension. He remained in the emergency room for several hours for observation, during which time the paranoid and anxious symptoms abated and he requested to leave, stating that he felt much better. He was released after signing permission for medical records to be obtained and accepting an appointment at the mental health clinic for the next day. That evening's local news reported a "crackdown" on local drug dealers; seven people had been arrested in Sam's neighborhood. The following morning it was reported to the emergency room staff that Sam had been found dead at home at approximately 9 PM the night before. Several weeks later the coroner's report indicated that the most probable cause of death was cardiac arrest.

Severe cardiovascular disease may also produce sufficient circulatory difficulty that other organic conditions occur. One of the most serious of these is delirium and other organic mental disorders associated with cerebral anoxia (see Chapter 33). Another psychogenic cardiovascular disorder is that in which the person experiences and describes symptoms of cardiac conditions with no physiologically measurable changes such as in ECG or serum enzymes.

Gastrointestinal system. An emotional response is accompanied by a variety of gastrointestinal changes, some of which are clearly physiological and many of which have been individually learned from repeated training. Consider, for example, the learning process established by a mother who always feeds her crying infant, regardless of the cause for the crying.

Not everyone responds to stress with serious or life-threatening conditions involving massive changes in gastrointestinal mucosa. These changes occur in conditions such as ulcerative colitis, irritable bowel syndrome, Crohn's disease, and peptic or duodenal ulcers. In addition to psychological factors, persons who develop these conditions are thought to have a genetic predisposition, or perhaps a propensity to develop the illness because of some other cause, such as a change in neuroendocrine function, a metabolic dysfunction, an immunological disorder, or a slow virus.

Respiratory system. A multitude of factors influence the normal functioning of the respiratory system: exercise

Text continued on p. 651

TABLE 34-3 Common psychophysiological disorders

Body System Affected	Illness	Significant Physical Signs and Symptoms	Associated Emotional Components	Associated Social or Environmental Conditions
Cardiovascular system	Coronary artery disease	Episodic chest pain usually on exertion, in cold weather, or in emotionally loaded situations Characterized by dull, aching sensation in middle sternum Pain may radiate to left shoulder or arm and lasts approximately 5 minutes Diagnosed by ECG; cardiac catheterization May be accompanied by complaints of fatigue, irritability, insomnia	May be accompanied by depression, anxiety, chronic poor self-image, decreased energy, lowered ambition May exhibit overt anxiety, emotional lability in response to stress Elation, excitement, or frightening dreams can precipitate attacks	Smoking Employment demands related to deadlines, intense desire for achievement, work overload, job conflicts Frustration and discontent of persons with little education and low economic status; hard work not associated with success Diet rich in saturated fats or calories
	Myocardial infarction	Damage and death of cardiac muscles Characterized by severe, prolonged chest pain described as crushing and radiating to left arm and shoulder Frequently occurs during rest Accompanied by ashen color; cold sweats; tachycardia or arrhythmias; nausea and vomiting; rapid, shallow breathing Diagnosed by ECG, elevated serum enzymes	Initial response of fear and apprehension then followed by minimization or denial During hospitalization, feelings of anxiety and depression Severe emotional response possibly leading to inability to return to work Generally repression of emotions	As above Also increased work responsibility, loss of spouse by death or divorce, social isolation Increased anxiety or depression, business or domestic problems possibly preceding myocardial infarction
	Essential hypertension	Blood pressure over 140/90 can indicate development of disease; may increase with age Occurs more commonly in black population May be accompanied by morning headaches, shortness of breath, chest pain, intermittent claudication in legs, and vascular changes in retina Hypertensive encephalopathy: serious risk of death	Theory of personality or intrapsychic conflicts between passive-dependent and aggressive impulses with repressed anger, resentment, or hostility not proven Positive association between anxiety, anger, and elevated blood pressure Stress from broad environmental conditions leading to fear, anger, or frustration Elevated blood pressure: noted after disasters or loss of job and in air traffic controllers	Rapid sociocultural change, urbanization, migration, socioeconomic mobility, high-stress job, natural disasters contributing factors to elevated blood pressure
	Headaches	Mild to severe, bilateral, throbbing or nonthrobbing; pain lasting a few hours to several days May be accompanied by nausea and vomiting or neurological symptoms No organic cause such as brain tumor May be associated with trigger factors, such as premenses, or allergic response	Emotional conflicts dealt with ineffectively Response to anxiety or worry	Trigger factors possibly environmental, such as specific foods, glare, weather changes, alcohol, odors, or hunger

System	Disorder	Description	Psychological factors	Precipitating factors
Gastrointestinal system	Irritable bowel syndrome	Motility disorder that can affect both large and small bowel Episodic abdominal pain and change in bowel habits, including diarrhea, constipation, and passing of mucus No abnormal physical or laboratory findings Symptoms: possible nausea, vomiting, abdominal distention, headaches, insomnia, dizziness, appetite and weight loss	Conscious reports of a distressing event, nervous symptoms Possibly represents struggle over controlling and letting go of aggressive impulses Alternative suggestion: constipation associated with stubborn active striving and diarrhea associated with inadequate and helpless feelings	Precipitated by obviously stressful life events such as illness of family member, financial loss, job loss, increase in work hours
	Ulcerative colitis	Inflammation of colon mucosa primarily in rectum and sigmoid colon Can occur in ileum Onset may be acute and can be lethal in severe cases Symptoms: rectal bleeding, diarrhea, weight loss, fever, abdominal tenderness Diagnosis by proctoscope examination or biopsy More common in whites and Jews May be genetic predisposition or autoimmune disorder Anal fissures, fistules, perirectal abscesses possible Associated with high incidence of colon cancer	Personality type described as "primitive personality organization," characterized by neatness, oversensitivity, egocentrism, grandiose self-concept, and excessive need for love, sympathy, affection Naive concept of love and overattachment to mother Inability to be aware of or express feelings and fantasy Exceedingly sensitive to interpersonal loss but also maintains ambivalent object attachments	May be precipitated by separation, bereavement, or situations in which individual feels unable to cope or has failed
	Crohn's disease	Inflammation of small bowel and sometimes colon Similar to above except abscess, fissures, ulceration, and perforation of bowel more common Cause thought to be genetic, immunological, or slow virus	Very similar to above Early ego deficits resulting in compulsive or paranoid traits, excessive dependence, demanding or explosive manipulation Regression, helplessness, and hopelessness possible No reliable personality factors	Symptoms may be precipitated by object loss, loss of self-esteem, interpersonal struggles
	Peptic and duodenal ulcer	Chronic ulceration of digestive mucosa in esophagus, stomach, or duodenum Onset acute, possibly accompanied by tarry stools, depressed hemoglobin and erythrocyte counts, vomiting, and epigastric pain Hemorrhage or perforation: medical emergency Less acutely, pain may be relieved by food or antacids Diagnosed by x-ray examination or endoscopy May be genetic predisposition since members of blood group O more likely to develop the illness	May be associated with oral conflict and frustration, accompanied by constitutional predisposition Personality factors in men described as assertively independent and in women as overly dependent	Situations where personal defeat is imminent but individual does not allow himself to be aware of it May be associated with being single or alcoholic Higher frequency of ulcers in concentration camp survivors Associated with high-stress jobs

Continued

TABLE 34-3 Common psychophysiological disorders—cont'd

Body System Affected	Illness	Significant Physical Signs and Symptoms	Associated Emotional Components	Associated Social or Environmental Conditions
Respiratory system	Bronchial asthma	Recurrent bronchoconstriction, edema, and excessive secretions in response to varied stimuli Wheezing that is mild or severe, episodic or paroxysmal Respirations may increase in frequency, accompanied by coughing and increased perspiration More common in boys than girls in childhood but approximately equal frequency in adults	Psychological profile confounded by inability to determine if certain factors cause disease or develop in response to it Relevant psychological factors: strong wish for protection, especially by mother Separation may precipitate attack, or intense conflict associated with separation may be relieved by being apart and symptoms decrease Other precipitants: sexual excitement, fear, angry outbursts, disappointment, or jealousy May be poorly attuned to environment, with immature coping mechanisms, dependence, tendency to become depressed and helpless unless given much support from others	Allergens, cold air, odors, physical exercise can precipitate attacks Increased frequency of attacks at night and during weather changes
	Hyperventilation syndrome	Breathing rapidly and deeply for a few minutes; produces vertigo, giddiness, buzzing in the ears, fainting, blurred vision, dry mouth, uncontrolled laughter or crying May be followed by apnea Can include increased heart rate, lowered blood pressure, nausea, increased perspiration	Responses to fear, anxiety, pain, anger, or situations with special meaning to person	Exercise such as climbing stairs or running
Dermatological conditions	Generalized pruritus	Abnormal sensation of itching not caused by insect bites, dermatitis, diabetes, nephritiss, liver disease, leukemia, and other diseases associated with itching May also be localized to specific areas of the body such as the anus or vulvae May lead to an itch/scratch such that individual produces severe, self-inflicted wounds	Anxiety and tension possibly producing a misinterpretation of cutaneous sensations May be a means to express repressed anger Possible exceptional need for affection	Lacks sexual partner or sexual outlets
	Atopic dermatitis	Also known as neurodermatitis Dry, flaky skin with redness, papules, scaly hyperkeratosis, exudation of clear serum, crusting Commonly on the face, knees, elbows Occurs intermittently May be allergic response	Related to lack of physical contact early in life Precipitated by emotionally disturbing situations, loss of or longing for love	Reaction to loss of significant person

	Psoriasis	Large red plaques covered with thick white scales usually on elbows and knees May involve deformity of nails May be genetic predisposition	Response to worry or stress Person with symptoms likely to feel he is repulsive May reflect desire for security	Systemic infection, excess or deficiency of sunlight, dampness, cold weather
	Acne vulgaris	Common at puberty; related to androgen-estrogen imbalance and overproduction of androgens Sebaceous glands overactive	Emotional stress or sexual difficulty may aggravate condition Sebaceous secretions may increase with anger	Diets rich in fats and carbohydrates may aggravate condition
Musculoskeletal system	Rheumatoid arthritis	Symmetrical joint swelling and deformity accompanied by morning stiffness, and tenderness or pain on motion of joint Other systemic symptoms: fatigue, loss of appetite and weight, occasional fever Most frequently involves joints in knees, hands, feet Subcutaneous nodules and ocular lesions possible Diagnosed by x-ray examination of joints Rheumatoid factor and anemia may be found in laboratory reports	Personality: self-sacrificing, conforming, inhibited or shy, perfectionistic, and masochistic Varied patterns of controlling anger, hostility, and aggression but tendency for experiencing conflict over expression of anger Personality traits possibly caused by pain, distress, and treatment of illness rather than premorbid traits May be chronic depression	Numerous life changes in year preceding onset of symptoms; major life conflicts, sexual difficulty, marital problems likely High incidence of family members with psychiatric disturbance
Endocrine system	Thyrotoxicosis	Excess thyroid hormone Symptoms: palpitations, heat intolerance, increase in appetite with weight loss, increased sweating, generalized weakness, insomnia, fine tremor of hands, elevated temperature, tachycardia, exophthalmous Diagnosed by protein-bound iodine, basal metabolic rate, and iodine-131 uptake	Tension, excitability, and possible emotional lability, temper outbursts, crying spells, distractability, short attention span, impaired recent memory; severe symptoms may include overt psychosis Disease possibly precipitated by acute emotional trauma or extreme fright	
	Hypothyroidism	Insufficient thyroid hormone Symptoms: peripheral neuropathy; hearing loss; headaches; skin pale, yellow, thickened; hysky voice Accompanied by cold intolerance, aching muscles, irregular menstrual periods, weight gain, lowered body temperature Diagnosed by thyroid hormone level and iodine-131 uptake	Predominant depression, sometimes dementia, complaints of fatigue, lethargy, decreased initiative, impaired recent memory May include paranoid suspicions and auditory hallucinations	
	Addison's disease	Decrease in corticosteroids caused by adrenal insufficiency Symptoms: weakness, fatigability, anorexia, weight loss, hypotension	Poverty of thought, apathy, fatigue, psychomotor retardation, depression May be frank psychosis, stupor, coma	

Continued.

TABLE 34-3 Common psychophysiological disorders—cont'd

Body System Affected	Illness	Significant Physical Signs and Symptoms	Associated Emotional Components	Associated Social or Environmental Conditions
	Cushing's syndrome	Excess of circulatory cortisol leading to increased appetite, truncal and facial obesity, frail skin, weakness, hypertension, muscle wasting, lowered glucose tolerance, impotence, amenorrhea	Depression with high risk of suicide, acute anxiety, emotional lability, irritability, insomnia Confusion and disorientation similar to organic mental disorders	
	Diabetes mellitus	Disordered glucose metabolism caused by insufficient insulin Genetically transmitted Symptoms: polydipsia, polyuria, increased appetite with weight loss, fatigue	Produces psychological stress and may provide means to meet needs for attention, caring, affection	Need for insulin possibly altered by life changes such as loss of interpersonal relationships
	Hypopituitarism	Lack of pituitary hormone caused by lesions in gland such as infections, head injury, tumors, myxedema, loss of pigmentation of breast areolae, inability to tan in the sun, loss of body hair, weight loss In children: dwarfism Severe symptoms: hypothermia, delirium, hypertension, stupor, coma, ultimately death	Mental disturbance common and includes apathy, indifference, fatigue, drowsiness, depression, dependence, cognitive deficits, delusions, loss of libido	

increases rate and depth of breathing; severely obese people may have shallow breathing because of restricted movement of the diaphragm; and drugs such as morphine and codeine suppress respirations while others such as salicylates are likely to increase them. The respiratory system can also be controlled voluntarily. Physical disorders that affect the respiratory system and result in difficult breathing, such as lung cancer, emphysema, congestive heart failure, or tuberculosis, are likely to produce psychological responses, primarily fear and anxiety, that will further increase respiratory difficulty.

Bronchial asthma has multiple predisposing, interacting factors, including: (1) possible genetic factors, (2) exposure to viruses or bacteria that results in infection, (3) exposure to allergens, (4) a tendency to bronchoconstriction, (5) a family history of allergy, and (6) psychological components. Physical symptoms are produced by a combination of events that lead to partial obstruction of bronchial passages because of constriction and edema. Acute asthma attacks are obvious by audible wheezing, diaphoresis, increased respirations, and the use of accessory muscles to aid ventilation and forced expiration.

Hyperventilation may be noted in persons who report repeated episodes of losing consciousness but who do not have epilepsy or other physical disorders that can produce loss of consciousness. Rapid breathing can be observed when the individual is under emotional stress.

Dermatological conditions. An itch, a tickle, and a pain are all conducted by the same nerve fibers, and the same sensation may be interpreted differently by the individual. The skin and sensations from it are a major source of environmental stimuli. Responses to pain, temperature, and touch are essential for maintaining body integrity, protecting the body, and providing one mode of interaction with the environment. The sexual function of skin has been demonstrated by Freud's descriptions of libidinal erogenous zones. Touch has also been shown to be important to normal physical and psychological development.

Abnormal skin sensations and manifestations can occur as a result of allergies, damage (for example, burns, nerve trauma), infections, and emotions. Exaggerated responses such as blushing with embarrassment or pallor with fear are relatively common. In addition to those disorders listed in Table 34-3 there are several other primarily physical skin responses to emotional states: (1) hyperhidrosis: excessive sweat secretion, especially of the palms, soles of feet, and axillae, which may lead to rashes, blisters, or infections; (2) rosacea: a vascularity with papule formation commonly occurring on the face or upper chest; (3) alopecia areata: sudden patchy hair loss more common in children and young adults, which usually occurs about 2 weeks after a significant emotional event.

Musculoskeletal system. Rheumatoid arthritis affects primarily the musculoskeletal system, but it is considered a systemic disorder with an unknown cause. Onset of the disease most commonly occurs in the fourth decade but can occur at any age, including childhood. Several causes have been suggested, but most data point to multifactorial influences including genetic predisposition; disordered immune, especially cell-mediated, mechanisms; a slow virus; and psychosomatic mechanisms that influence several hormones such as growth hormones, thyroxin, androgens, estrogens, and andrenocorticosteroids. Hypothalamic regulation of the immune response, especially in relation to corticosteroid production, may ultimately implicate an autoimmune response as responsible for rheumatoid arthritis symptoms.

The illness is usually not life-threatening but can lead to chronic pain and disability. An acute onset is characterized by high fever, extensive polyarticular inflammation, and rapid development of joint deformities. See Table 34-3 for other symptoms. After the initial onset of the disease most persons will improve, and about one fifth will recover completely. In spite of remissions and exacerbations, the majority continue to work and function to some degree in daily life activities.

Endocrine system. The endocrine system is ultimately involved in mediating mind-body interactions although the exact mechanisms of hormonal influence on mood, cognitive functions, and response to psychological and social factors is poorly understood. Disorders of the endocrine system, just as the disorders described above, may result from psychosocial stress and therefore be considered psychosomatic. However, it is important to realize that endocrine disorders may also be somatopsychic. That is, the hormonal imbalance caused by glandular dysfunction may produce mental symptoms, sometimes very severe and difficult to differentiate from depression or psychosis.

The major endocrine disorders are listed in Table 34-3. In addition, gonadal dysfunctions such as decreased androgen production in men and decreased estrogen secretion in women are known to result both normally and from psychological causes. For instance, acute physical or psychological stress may lead to decreased testosterone production in men, which leads to decreased beard growth. Menopause is a normal reduction in estrogen secretion for women. It may produce significant changes in calcium and lipid metabolism in the body that are associated with coronary atherosclerosis and osteoporosis as well as changes in skin and mucosal surfaces, hot flashes, and insomnia. Amenorrhea may occur in premenopausal women as a result of certain drugs, such as reserpine and phenothiazines, or massive obesity.

Multiple systems responses. There are several disorders that involve the whole body's response to combined physical and psychological factors. Eating disorders, for example, are very common, complex, and serious (see Chapter 35). Pain responses can also be considered partly psychosomatic. Headaches are a common cause of pain that may be transitory or severe and disabling. "Tension" headaches, usually mild and self-limiting, represent one end of the scale, whereas migraine headaches can be severe, lasting for days and accompanied by other symptoms such as flashes of color or wavy lines in the visual field. Migraine headaches are usually thought to be caused by increased vasomotor activity and tension headaches by contraction of skeletal muscles. Both causes coexist in some persons with headaches (see Table 34-3).

✳ *Emotional dimension.* The range of emotional expression in persons with psychophysiological disorders is very broad. The nurse works with those persons who have the ability to be consciously aware of their feelings and emotional responses as well as those persons who are far removed from realizing, understanding, or accurately expressing their feelings. With this in mind, it is important to both listen to the client's description of feelings as well as observe the expression of feelings. Conflicting data may give important clues to appropriate intervention.

One of the most significant problems for the client is to learn how to identify and develop more effective modes of coping with generalized anxiety. Generalized anxiety is reflected by such physiological measures as elevated blood pressure, tense muscles, exaggerated reflex responses to environmental stimuli, and many other physiological symptoms. Anxiety can also be expressed indirectly through anger, irritability, and frustration. Other common responses of persons with significant disabling symptoms over a period of time are depression, grief, and despair. (See Chapter 14).

The major emotions associated with most psychophysiological disorders are negative, for example, anger and anxiety. Observation of the client in a variety of situations helps to determine what precipitates these feelings. Listening to descriptions of the client's daily activities and relationships is another source of data. The person may be overcommitted, be responsible for too many others, not feel that others care, or long for more attention or affection. These feelings may be expressed through hostile or sarcastic humor rather than directly.

Table 34-1 lists some of the common feelings and personality traits associated with specific psychophysiological disorders. Much of the data available regarding emotional expressions related to any one disorder indicates that they can range from seriously distorted to quite normal emotional expression. Psychophysiological disorders may be chronic, painful, debilitating, and socially restricting. These factors themselves can contribute to distorted emotional responses. Therefore, if a client has been ill for an extended period of time, it may be useful to consider and even discuss with the client the emotional impact and changes since the first onset of symptoms.

Self-expectations may be high. The individual may experience jealousy or anger but consider it a failure to express such feelings, and if expressed there is an accompanying sense of guilt. Another manifestation of high self-expectations is excessive competitiveness. Friends and family members may describe the individual as a perfectionist. The usual forms of emotional expression such as angry outbursts, crying, or admitting disappointment are thought to be not only irrational but also personal failures.

One of the common emotional responses to chronic psychophysiological illness is depression. The client may discuss feelings of sadness, helplessness, and an inability to cope directly or indirectly through self-derogatory comments. Assessment of the degree of depression and potential for suicide is essential (see Chapter 14).

✳ *Intellectual dimension.* Ordinarily the psychophysiological disorders do not have a direct impact on the individual's intellectual capacity or cognitive abilities. Occasionally, cognitive functions are compromised by an acute medical crisis or a chronic degenerative process. Symptoms then are similar to organic mental disorders (see Chapter 33), or the person may develop psychotic symptoms and sometimes coma. In addition to determining the medical and organic processes, the most significant aspects of the person's intellectual dimension to be assessed are as follows:

1. Understanding of the disorder
2. Knowledge about the disorder
3. Decision-making processes
4. Cognitive processes used in coping

Understanding of the disorder is meant to address what the client believes to be the cause or causes. Typically the client has some basic knowledge about the effect of the disease process on the body. Assessment needs to be made regarding the advisability of providing more information to the client. For some persons, this increases their anxiety and use of defense mechanisms while for others it facilitates their interest in managing the disease and contributes to self-care practices.

Knowledge about the disorder refers to the client's information about the illness, that is, what changes may occur or have already taken place in the body and the potential or real limitations these impose.

The individual's understanding of his disorder is influenced by the usual decision-making style employed and the cognitive processes of coping. Clients with psychosomatic disorders typically are constant worriers. This may mean putting off significant life-style changes, or it may mean selectively excluding data that do not fit into the client's coping plan (rationalization and denial). For example, the client is very likely to ignore, minimize, or dispute data suggesting that emotional responses are in any way related to physical symptoms, especially if admitting such means drastically altering one's self-concept or learning a new way to relate to one's environment. Understanding the client's intellectual style and cognitive processes helps the nurse develop a more effective teaching plan.

Denial is common, especially if the psychophysiological condition is not obvious yet requires making major life changes or influences the person's view of self. For instance, the person who has had a myocardial infarction may not follow the prescribed treatment and act as if nothing has changed. Other clients are directly confronted with the physical realities of an illness such as immobility of joints or having to learn to manage a colostomy.

✳ *Social dimension.* Assessing the social dimension with the client establishes what aspects of work life, family life, friends, and community involvement are creating stress sufficient to cause illness. Interpersonal relationships are likely to be the most significant both for creating stress and as a source of healing. Establishing what life-style changes are necessary is also an important goal.

The way in which an individual's personality interacts

with employment demands can be an essential element in stress. Significant aspects to assess are (1) Are the demands, expectations, and work load considered reasonable by the client? (2) Is there a possibility of loss of the job? (3) Are job responsibilities and expectations in keeping with the individual's skills and intellectual capacity? (4) Are there conflicts with a supervisor or manager that prove difficult for the client? (5) What, if any, satisfaction is obtained from employment? and (6) Are financial rewards reasonable, and do they meet the needs and expectations of the client? Other sources of interpersonal stress in the workplace may come from sexual harrassment, ridicule, or other forms of abusive behavior. Support, understanding, and friendship from coworkers may be essential to job satisfaction for some individuals. For instance, one young woman began to complain that her job in a factory had become "too stressful," ostensibly because a procedure on the assembly line had been changed. Further exploration revealed that an older employee had resigned. She had been a significant buffer and protector of the young woman from intimidation by other coworkers. Without her, the job was no longer satisfying.

Disturbed interpersonal relationships may contribute to the maintenance of symptoms once they are established. Assessment of these relationships can be done by discussions with the client but are likely to also involve discussions with family members and close friends. A family evaluation, during which the client and family members are interviewed together, may be necessary to determine troublesome patterns of interaction. Marital and family assessment as described in Chapters 29 and 30 is applicable to this client group.

Finding a satisfying balance of interdependence with others can be a source of unconscious conflict. Striving for independence accompanied by the wish to be dependent can be "acted out" through the development of illness. Being sick allows the grown-up person to be cared for in a socially acceptable way but even so may be accompanied by anger and resentment for needing the care.

Table 34-3 describes social and environmental conditions relevant for specific diseases. One of the more common themes is the impact of losses, especially the loss of significant others in the year preceding illness. The assessment of loss includes exploring the meaning of losing intimacy such as affection, concern, touching, and sexual intercourse as well as practical supports such as fixing the car, paying the bills, doing the dishes, or cooking the meals.

The amount of community involvement can be stressful because it is too much or too little. Some persons become so overinvolved in church, civic, and social clubs that those things, intended as a source of pleasure, become liabilities. Other clients are totally isolated from developing friends or participating in community life. This may be a personality style or a consequence of debilitating symptoms. Determining the cause will provide data about possible solutions.

The nature of the community may be a significant factor. Neighborhoods with a high incidence of crime or a lot of traffic or noise can be stressful. The nurse also examines factors such as the frequency of moves from community to community, a change in socioeconomic status, or the need for the individual to modify his life-style. These factors may influence the stability of the client's social network, create unexpected problems with adaptation, and require making new friends.

The life-style and habits of the individual arising from his interests and social network may contribute to a psychophysiological illness. Excessive use of alcohol, smoking, or use of illicit drugs negatively influence health. Assessing the client's use of leisure time will give important data regarding the degree of physical activity, the need for competitive interactions, and the ease of accommodating to new environmental demands and making new friends.

Spiritual dimension. Personal beliefs and values contribute to the individual's understanding of his environment and give it meaning. They contribute in conscious and unconscious ways to establishing a life-style, determining a hierarchy of importance to life demands, and providing the guiding principles on which choices are made. Existential beliefs, such as faith in God, fate, or some other higher authority, contribute to maintaining hope and giving meaning to life. Generally these personal beliefs are helpful, but they can become a source of stress when the individual cannot accommodate his modes of behaving to his own belief system or when expectations and demands from others are contrary to his interpretation of right and wrong.

Assessment of the individual's values and value conflicts is probably best done indirectly. Often the person is aware of feeling stressed but does not relate that directly to his belief system. Having acted in a way contrary to the belief system may lead to feelings of guilt, personal condemnation, or even hopelessness. Sometimes careful listening to details of a client's problem with strategically placed questions from the nurse helps the client to understand his own conflicts. He may realize that he is questioning the validity of beliefs and values that he had previously taken for granted.

When expectations and demands from others do not fit with the client's view of proper behavior and actions he may be faced with giving up long-held beliefs, learning to live with the conflicts, or modifying the source of unacceptable expectations and demands (for example, changing jobs, moving to another community, divorce). Sometimes the client is unaware of the source of the conflict or ways to resolve it and responds with hopelessness, powerlessness, and despair.

These situations can precipitate a spiritual crisis. An assessment of these confllicts as well as determining how the client usually meets his spiritual needs can be valuable to planning his care.

Analysis

Nursing diagnosis. Ineffective individual coping is an example of a nursing diagnosis approved by NANDA that applies to clients with psychophysiological disorders. The

INEFFECTIVE INDIVIDUAL COPING

DEFINITION

The impairment of adaptive behaviors and problem-solving abilities of a person in meeting life's demands and roles.

DEFINING CHARACTERISTICS

Physical Dimension
Destructive, self-mutilating behavior
High rate of accidents
*Broad range of physical symptoms
*Sleep pattern disturbance
*Appetite disturbance; excessive or too little food intake
*Excessive alcohol intake; smoking

Emotional Dimension
*Anxiety
*Fear
*Anger
*Irritability

Intellectual Dimension
Inability to make decisions
Verbalization of inability to cope
*Impaired problem solving
Ineffective or inappropriate use of defense mechanisms
*Knowledge deficits

Social Dimension
*Life stress
*Not meeting role expectations
*Decreased social participation
*Low self-esteem
*Altered self-image

Spiritual Dimension
*Confusion about values and beliefs
*Conflict between values and behavior

Adapted from North American Nursing Diagnosis Association Classification of Nursing Diagnosis: Proceedings of the seventh conference, St. Louis, 1987, The C.V. Mosby Co.
*Indicates characteristics in addition to those defined by NANDA.

defining characteristics of the nursing diagnosis are listed in the box above.

The following Case Example demonstrates the characteristics of the nursing diagnosis of ineffective individual coping.

Case Example

Elaine, a 31-year-old single woman, was brought to the emergency room yesterday via ambulance. She had severe epigastric pain, vomited "a brown liquid," and had been having "black, soft stools for several days." Endoscopy revealed a gastric ulcer, and she was admitted for further treatment.

Elaine had lost her job as a typist about 5 months ago after missing many days because of severe headache, allergies, and "premenstrual tension" that involved irritability, crying, abdominal cramps and swelling, fatigue, and back pain. She had been to see three physicians in the past year and had multiple tests to determine what causes the allergic reaction and if there is an explanation for "premenstrual tension." Outcomes of the tests

revealed that she was allergic to house dust. The results of a 24-hour urine test showed mildly elevated corticosteroid levels, consistent with ovarian cysts. Oral estrogens were prescribed, but according to Alaine, "they did not help." Elaine is angry with the physicians for not helping her feel better.

In addition, Elaine's 73-year-old mother had fallen and broken a hip about 2 months ago and was recently placed in a nursing home. Elaine and her mother cannot afford the nursing home, but Elaine is unable to decide if she can care for her mother at home. Today she said to the nurse, "I can't cope with all of these problems, I don't know what to do."

The following list provides examples of NANDA-accepted nursing diagnoses with causative statements.
1. Potential disturbances in self-concept related to role change
2. Grieving: pathological pattern related to denial of cardiac condition
3. Anxiety related to fear of suffocation
4. Impaired physical mobility related to limited motion of limb
5. Ineffective individual coping related to excessive uncontrolled internal anger

DSM-III-R diagnoses. The diagnostic category in the DSM-III-R is 316.00 Psychological factors affecting physical condition. No essential features are listed in the DSM-III-R for this condition. This category is used when psychological factors contribute to the physical condition. Examples of physical conditions for this diagnoses are vomiting, obesity, and migraine headaches.

Planning

Table 34-4 provides examples of long-term and short-term goals and outcome criteria related to psychophysiological illnesses. These serve as examples of the planning stage in the nursing process.

Implementation

Physical dimension. The first task in the case of persons with psychophysiological disorders is to evaluate and treat the physical symptoms. Many clients are seen in an acute or even life-threatening state so that diagnosis and determining an initial plan of care are done quickly. A thorough physical examination with routine laboratory studies provides the initial basis for decisions. Specific procedures such as x-ray films, cardiac catheterizations, endoscopy, and proctoscopy may be necessary. It is essential for the nurse to explain these procedures to the client, telling him what to anticipate, the purpose of the test, and what may be learned from it. Such explanations facilitate the client's understanding and decrease anxiety and fear. The nurse needs to be available to respond to questions from the client and uses these opportunities to discover how much the client knows about his condition.

Some psychophysiological conditions require surgical procedures. There are conditions that require urgent surgery, but more often it is anticipated and planned in advance. This time with the client can be used for preoper-

TABLE 34-4 Long-term and short-term goals and outcome criteria related to psychophysiological illness

Goals	Outcome Criteria

NURSING DIAGNOSIS: INEFFECTIVE INDIVIDUAL COPING: EPIGASTRIC PAIN, NAUSEA, VOMITING, AND TARRY STOOLS RELATED TO LOSS OF JOB, MOTHER'S ILLNESS, AND FINANCIAL DIFFICULTIES

Long-term goals

To resolve problem of how to meet mother's need for care	Investigates community resources available for assisting with home care
	Assists with applications for financial assistance for mother
	Discusses personal resources and mother's needs with appropriate personnel
To demonstrate ability to tolerate unavoidable stress situations without reactivation of ulcer symptoms	Subjectively states she feels better
	Is able to renew search for another job without developing symptoms
	Utilizes social support systems and friends to discuss problems

Short-term goals

To maintain a diet that reduces epigastric distress	Eats frequent small meals
	Uses antacids as prescribed
To learn relaxation techniques	Meets with nurse at prearranged time
	Expresses interest in lowering anxiety
	Attempts relaxation exercises

NURSING DIAGNOSIS: INEFFECTIVE INDIVIDUAL COPING DEMONSTRATED BY HYPERTENSION AND CHRONIC RESTLESSNESS RELATED TO STRESS OR POOR DIETARY HABITS

Long-term goal

To modify life-style to one more conducive to health	Stops smoking
	Loses 50 pounds in 1 year
	Makes adjustments in work schedule
	Maintains blood pressure below 130/90

Short-term goals

To modify diet to reduce calories and salt intake	Participates with wife in discussion of eating habits
	Accepts dietary counseling
	Eats low-calorie, low-salt diet
To establish plan for stopping smoking	Calls local hospital and lung association for advice
	Evalutes available programs to determine which might be most effective
	States desire to stop smoking
	Begins a stop smoking program
To implement regular exercise program	Determines time to be set aside for exercise
	Seeks out friends involved in physical activities
	Begins participation in exercise program
To establish plan for regular checkups	Obtains equipment and learns technique of taking blood pressure
	Agrees to checkup every 3 months at local health clinic

ative teaching and to prepare the client physically and psychologically. This aspect of care usually occurs in the general hospital where the psychiatric nurse may be consulting although it is common for the inpatient or outpatient psychiatric nurse to discuss these issues with the client before general hospital admission.

Either because of the surgical procedure or as a consequence of the disease process itself, the client needs assistance to cope with changes in body image. For example, the client with rheumatoid arthritis notes changes in body size and shape accompanied by pain and loss of function. The nurse assists clients to realistically examine the meaning and impact of such changes. Some clients prefer to deny their existence and persist with attempts to do tasks that can cause further harm. A gentle approach aimed at helping the client gradually understand the reality of the limitations allows the client to make a psychological adjustment while learning new behaviors. At the other extreme and also an indication of inadequate adjustment to a change in self-image is the client who refuses to participate in any aspects of self-care. Such persons need assistance to discuss their reactions. A behavioral approach that reinforces the client's taking over a self-care activities in a step-wise fashion may be effective.

An added concern for the client is how significant others will react to the physical changes. This may be particularly profound if the client's body has become obviously distorted. It is also a significant concern for clients with alterations in particularly sensitive areas of the body that may not be readily observable, such as colostomies and ileostomies. Not only must the client adapt to these changes and learn new procedures to manage elimination but also those persons intimately involved with the client need to adapt to the changes.

Sexual problems may develop as a consequence of body changes. These may take the form of embarrassment and shame because the person or significant others cannot adapt to body alterations. Other reasons for sexual problems may be related to a lack of desire because of generalized pain and discomfort or restriction of flexibility and movement. Treatment of the underlying cause such as the use of analgesics for pain is a helpful first step, but if problems are not resolved further evaluation may lead to referral to sex therapy or couples' counseling.

The majority of persons with psychophysiological disorders receive one or more medications specific to their symptoms. The nurse needs to be familiar with the medication regimen and sufficiently knowledgeable about those medications so that the expected effects can be assessed. Equally important is the knowledge necessary for identifying side effects, allergic or other untoward effects, medication and food interactions, or the synergistic effects of several medications, alcohol, and food. Teaching the client about his medication regimen, including the schedule, effects, and precautions, is an important responsibility of the nurse. This is an opportunity to educate the client, perhaps improve compliance, and obtain data for other interventions. Some physical interventions will have little immediate impact but require an extended period before observable changes are apparent. The nurse informs the client that this is the case and encourages him to stay with the treatment.

Certain physiological problems such as insomnia or discomfort may not be related to the specific disease process but may be responses to a variety of factors such as the physical environment, generalized anxiety, or fear of the unknown. The client is encouraged to discuss the responses before alternative measures are implemented since this may be sufficient to resolve the problem. Behavioral approaches to the management of insomnia have been described by Pawlick and Heitkemper[56]; these include keeping a diary of sleep patterns, eliminating sleep outside of normal nocturnal patterns, going to bed and getting up at the same time each day, increasing physical exercise, and reducing caffeine intake.

Emotional dimension. The client needs help to identify his unique emotional responses. The nurse can facilitate this by careful listening and reflection. Identification of sensitive issues and exploring them in depth with the client may facilitate considerations of the interrelationships between feeling states and physical symptoms by the client. Until the client has grasped the notion of a temporal relationship between stress and physical symptoms, he will probably give little credence to important techniques of stress management.

The nurse can teach the client a number of stress management techniques that will help to control severe anxiety. Among the most common are relaxation techniques and guided imagery, which are intended to encourage positive thinking, support the client's use of self-control measures, and modify the neuroendocrine response system. These techniques, once learned, are readily available to the client in any environment. Other relaxation techniques such as various forms of meditation and biofeedback have been found to be helpful for some persons. The nurse can explain the essential elements of these tech-

niques and help interested clients seek the necessary resources. Special training or the use of specialized equipment may mean that these resources are not universally available.

Attempts to study the personality profile of persons with specific psychophysiological disorders have led to the suggestion that certain emotional responses may be responses to extended periods of disabling symptoms rather than preexisting character traits. Nevertheless, responses such as depression, guilt, and despair interfere with adequate coping and may become severe enough to be identified as primary problems requiring specific interventions. Very often the treatment involves long-term exploratory, individual, group, or family therapy depending on the expression of problematic behaviors. Supportive group interventions that encourage the expression of troublesome emotions in an accepting, tolerant environment can be valuable for clients who fear rejection or lack of understanding from their family and friends.

Intellectual dimension. Since the intellectual and cognitive functions of the client are essentially intact, the nurse's attention is usually directed toward assessing knowledge deficits and implementing teaching plans to address these. Exceptions to this may occur if the client experiences an organic mental syndrome, which can occur with certain endocrine disorders or cerebral anoxia. These are almost always completely reversible providing appropriate physical interventions are implemented.

Teaching plans are developed to address the specific needs of the client. Consideration needs to be given not only to the intellectual capacity of the client but also to the physical and emotional state of the individual. High levels of anxiety, for example, are known to minimize retention of information. The most effective teaching plans are those that support the individual's active involvement in the recovery and rehabilitation process. The nurse provides specific factual information and at the same time attends to the emotional and social components related to the factual data.

Given that the etiology of most psychophysiological disorders is exceedingly complex and the specific mechanisms leading to a particular group of symptoms are often poorly understood, it is important not to overwhelm the client with too much information. The nurse can develop unique and interesting ways to raise the client's interest in the health and illness process and then gradually present information as the client's knowledge base expands. The ultimate aim is to help the client grasp the relative importance of heredity, diet, life-style, stressful events, emotional responses, and social interactions on states of health. With this knowledge, clients may begin to formulate their own care plan and strategies to reduce or resolve stressors.

Understanding the need for medical regimens such as exercise programs, dietary restrictions, or medication-taking schedules makes more sense to the client if the disease process is understood. Since the client may view some medical regimens (for example, mediations that reduce blood pressure) as having more problems associated with them than obvious positive gains, understanding the rationale may enhance compliance.

A broad range of behavioral and educational approaches that complement physical interventions are considered. Some techniques of stress management can be effectively taught as didactic courses with positive benefits, as indicated in the Research Highlight below. Others, such as relaxation techniques, can be taught by the nurse on an individual basis or specific referrals can be made for the client interested in biofeedback, meditation, or acupuncture. The nurse explains to the individual that these techniques can be helpful but are not always effective nor can every individual fit them into daily activities. However, effectiveness may depend on the client's attitude and willingness to try different approaches. The nurse may need to assist the client to develop a plan to modify certain aspects of his life-style.

Understanding the client's use of defense mechanisms in coping with emotional responses facilitates reinforcing those that are effective and modifying unhelpful ones. The nurse considers how she can modify the client's cognitive appraisal (subjective interpretation) of situations and events. She may be able to offer alternative interpretations to a sequence of events described by the client, which, when framed differently, may not be as anxiety producing. Offering alternatives helps the client develop new patterns of assessing situations without directly confronting ineffective coping behavior. Directly confronting the client's style of coping can further escalate the client's anxiety responses by leaving him vulnerable and psychologically unable to defend himself.

Social dimension. Interpersonal relationships can provide personal fulfillment, or they may be a source of great stress. Becoming familiar with the person's social network and identifying the significant positive or troublesome relationships establish the groundwork for the nurse and client to begin to evaluate what changes need to take place. Whenever possible, the nurse encourages the client to make decisions regarding his treatment.

Conflicts from interpersonal relationships may evolve

Research Highlight

A Stress Management Program for Inflammatory Bowel Disease Patients

B. Milne, G. Joachim & J. Neidhardt

PURPOSE

In spite of aggressive medical treatment, it is common for inflammatory bowel disease patients to suffer chronic or recurrent symptoms. Psychological therapy may help to minimize these symptoms. Therefore this study was implemented to investigate whether or not practicing stress management techniques would decrease disease activity in this group of clients and if psychosocial functioning would show any improvement.

SAMPLE

Eighty subjects, including both men and women between 18 and 55 years of age, with inflammatory bowel disease were recruited from interested gastroenterologists. They could not have concomitant physical or psychiatric disorders requiring daily drugs or injections. Subjects were randomly assigned to either the treatment or control group after a baseline assessment interview.

METHODOLOGY

Six 3-hour classes were held for the treatment group to provide information about stress management. The classes included (1) personal planning skills, covering techniques such as time management, worry control, goal setting, problem solving, and mental clearing; (2) communication skills, including clear verbal and nonverbal communication, feedback, active listening, and assertive communication; and (3) autogenic training, meaning repetition of autogenic phrases that describe desired body condition, such as heaviness, warmth, and breathing. All subjects were administered the following data collection instruments at 4 months, 8 months, and 1 year: Crohn's Disease Activity Index, Inflammatory Bowel Disease Stress Index, and Individual Stress Assessment Questionnaire. Demographic data, length of illness, current medications, surgical interventions, and family history were collected initially. Follow-up interviews asked about increase or decrease in medication.

FINDINGS

At baseline, the treatment group, as opposed to the control group, was significantly older, had been symptomatic for a longer period of time, and scored higher (indicating more symptoms) on the objective and subjective measures of disease activity and psychosocial dysfunction. At the first assessment point and throughout, the treatment group demonstrated significant improvement while the control group showed no change from baseline. Over a 1-year period stress management techniques had significant benefit for this group both for reducing disease activity and improving psychosocial functioning.

IMPLICATIONS

The finding that stress management techniques decrease disease activity and improve psychosocial functioning indicates that nurses need to consider treatment of the whole client and not just focus on managing the diarrhea or abdominal pain; nurses need to deal with the symptoms and psychosocial considerations. Managing stress may help clients adapt to and cope with the chronic problem of inflammatory bowel disease.

Based on data from Journal of Advanced Nursing **11**:561, 1986.

from the person's view of self. To relate well to others, the person needs to have a sense of self-worth and to know he has positive traits and personal characteristics. Clients, particularly those who have had disabling symptoms for an extended period, may have a very low sense of self-worth. The nurse can work with the client to identify the particular positive interpersonal traits and styles of relating, such as a sense of humor, thoughtfulness, or interest in another's ideas. Observation of the client with significant others followed by discussion with the client can help the nurse identify ways in which the client distorts or misperceives the relationship. Comments from the nurse that describe the positive qualities observed can be the beginning of the client's redefinition of self. Often a negative sense of self arises from problems in very early childhood relationships. In-depth exploration of these is probably best managed by long-term individual psychotherapy.

If the locus of control remains with the client, it provides some independence even while the client is dependent in other respects. It is also relevant for the nurse and the client to discuss the realistic aspects of dependence. For instance, the person who is severely crippled by rheumatoid arthritis realistically may not be able to get to the bathroom alone, but angry and resentful feelings about that only increase tension in relationships and the stress level. Behavioral approaches that help the client intellectually determine which dependence issues are "worthy" of the response and which are not and then supporting and rewarding the client's implementation of these may prove useful. (See Chapter 16.)

Symptoms of physical illness tend to result in gradually narrowing or changing the client's cultural roles and network of social supports. A slow shift can take place that moves the client's central support network and role identity away from work and family into illness roles and relying on health professionals for support. The nurse is actively involved with the client and family to help them maintain normal role behavior. There may be serious interpersonal problems in the client's family life requiring resolution, which may involve termination of significant relationships or major shifts in interpersonal dynamics. In addition to family or couples therapy, the nurse can encourage the client to develop new support systems when necessary by joining church groups, adult education classes, community activity groups, or special interest groups.

Sources of stress in the workplace may come from environmental factors, difficult interpersonal relationships, or the nature of the work itself. Once the sources of stress and anxiety have been identified, the client may want assistance in determining a plan of action. For example, if the stress comes from environmental pollutants that cannot be avoided, the client may need to decide about continuing to suffer the health risks or finding another job. Encouraging the client to resolve these questions through discussion is important. The client's central support network of family and friends is often the most important source of assistance in alleviating stress arising from the nature of the work itself. Teaching the client that certain life-style changes can also help with stress is important.

Maintaining social contacts away from work, developing hobbies or learning new skills, and maintaining a program of regular, vigorous physical exercise provides diversion from preoccupation with work problems. Assertiveness training may help the client better cope with difficult interpersonal relationships at the workplace, especially if this is the only significant arena where problems occur. More generalized interpersonal problems usually indicate the need for psychotherapy.

Self-help groups and a variety of other supportive group approaches have evolved over the past 2 decades. Specific support groups such as ostomy clubs give members the opportunity to share feelings, exchange advice, and share practical and realistic ways of coping. Discovering that others share similar problems reduces loneliness and the feeling of differentness while providing emotional support to cope with the unique problems arising from the illness. For example, Levitt and others[54] described a support group for persons with premenstrual syndrome that is intended to give participants a sense of increased self-control. Sometimes self-help or support groups are available in the community or at local mental health treatment facilities or hospitals. The nurse who identifies a need but cannot find a specific group for a specific client may consider developing one.

✂ *Spiritual dimension.* Determining the stress arising from the client's confusion over his belief system or inconsistency between behavior, beliefs, or values may be a key in determining an overall treatment program. Discussion of the client's beliefs and values can be completely separate from knowing the client's religious affiliation. Existential questions about the meaning of life or the degree of responsibility for one's own behaviors, actions, and condition are particularly likely to arise with sick persons. These questions become even more profound if the individual begins to integrate the notion that there may be some degree of personal control over body responses.

Troublesome spiritual conflicts are likely to be unconscious and not readily available for discussion primarily because many of the beliefs and values held by the person developed early in life from social and cultural influences that went unquestioned. Additional life experience can expose the person to other, unfamiliar ways of thinking and behaving that challenge previously learned ideas. Sometimes clarifying the conflict is sufficient to resolve it.

Illness as punishment for misbehavior is a common theme. Beyond the notion of guilt for known or unknown misbehaviors may be questions related to "why me, why now, what value is my life" that reflect confusion about the validity of long-held beliefs and values and may imply the person's readiness for changing his basic approach to life. Patterns such as constant striving for power or control may be modified by examining the "expense" of these wishes when compared to satisfying needs through less demanding alternatives. The nurse provides a stable, open-minded approach to the client's pursual of these questions and provides feedback that helps the individual draw his own conclusions and make decisions along what is significant and valuable. The major task of the nurse is to assist the person to attain peace of mind.

BRIEF REVIEW

Psychophysiological disorders are manifestations of physical illness in one or more major organ systems. A significant component to the development of the symptoms is the client's response to stress. How the illness manifests itself is contingent on genetic traits, the personality characteristics of the individual, and the particular pattern of environmental stressors to which the person is exposed. The concept of stress-related disorders has been considered valid for centuries. However, exploration into the possible physiological and psychological mechanisms of these disorders has taken place during the past 60 years.

Initial theories were proposed which suggested that a specific personality profile resulted in the development of specific psychophysiological disorders. New approaches to science as represented by general systems theories brought specific theories into question. The explosion of knowledge based on basic science research into the complexities of the neuroendocrine system and its interaction with cognitive mechanisms in the cerebral cortex has led to the development of complex theories about person-environment interactions.

These theoretical constructs fit well with nursing's holistic approach to the person. The nurse uses these theoretical ideas as the basis for assessment and management of persons with stress-related disorders. In addition to assessing the symptoms of illness, the nurse evaluates the emotional, social, intellectual, and spiritual components of the person with regard to conflicts and demands from those sources that contribute to illness. External environmental factors that may not be controllable are also relevant to the development of illness. Interventions are developed from the assessment of unique patterns of the individual and are directed toward maximizing the effective coping potential of the person. Establishing new coping patterns may require interventions such as psychotherapy, behavioral techniques, education, and change in external environmental conditions.

The overall goals of the work with clients are directed toward modifications in the environment and within the individual that minimize the stress response. Environmental modifications may include changes in the actual physical environment or the interpersonal dynamics of the person in relationships so that there is less conflict. The individual can learn new ways of thinking, new approaches to problems, and techniques that influence biological responses to stress-producing events.

REFERENCES AND SUGGESTED READINGS

1. American Psychiatric Association: Diagnostic and statistical manual of mental disorders (DSM-III-R), Washington, D.C., 1987, The Association.
2. Alexander, F., French, T.M., and Pollock, G.: Psychosomatic Specificity, vol. I, Experimental study and results, Chicago, 1968, University of Chicago Press.
3. Andreasen, N.C.: The broken brain, New York, 1984, Harper & Row, Publishers.
4. Axen, D.M.: Chronic factitious disorders: helping those who hurt themselves, Journal of Psychosocial Nursing 23(3):19, 1986.
5. Baker, G.: On the affections of the mind and the diseases arising from them. In Hunter, R., and MacAlpine, I., editors: Three hundred years of psychiatry: 1535-1860, New York, 1963, Oxford University Press.
6. Baker, G.H.B.: Life events before the onset of rheumatoid arthritis, Psychotherapy and Psychosomatics 38:173, 1982.
7. Beland, I.L., and Passos, J.Y.: Clinical nursing pathophysiology and psychosocial approaches, New York, 1975, Macmillan Publishing Co.
8. Besedovsky, H., and others: Hypothalamic changes during the immune response, European Journal of Immunology 7:323, 1977.
9. Blumenthal, J.A., and others: Psychological changes accompanying aerobic exercise in health of middle-aged adults, Psychosomatic Medicine 44(6):529, 1982.
10. Burchfield, S.R., editor: Stress: psychological and physiological interactions, Washington, D.C., 1985, Hemisphere Publishing Corp.
11. Campbell, C.: Nursing diagnosis and intervention in nursing practice, New York, 1978, John Wiley & Sons, Inc.
12. Cannon, W.B.: Bodily changes in pain, hunger, fear and rage, ed. 2, Boston, 1953, Charles T. Branford Co.
13. Chess, S., and Thomas, A.: Origins and evolution of behavior disorders, New York, 1984, Brunner/Mazel Publishers.
14. Chess, S., and Thomas, A.: Temperament in clinical practice, New York, 1986, The Guilford Press.
15. Choi, M., and Steptoe, A.: Instructed heartrate control in the presence and absence of a distracting task: the effects of biofeedback training, Biofeedback and Self-Regulation 7(3):257, 1982.
16. Cohen, S.: Benzodiazepines in therapy, Current Psychiatric Therapy 22:111, 1983.
17. Cox, T.: Stress, Baltimore, 1979, University Park Press.
18. Daines, B., and Holdsworth, A.V.: Impotence, Nursing Times, 78(18):763, 1982.
19. D'Arcy, C.: Unemployment and health: data and implications, Canadian Journal of Public Health 77(suppl. 1):124, 1986.
20. Doenges, M.E., Jeffries, M.F., and Moorhouse, M.F.: Nursing care plans: nursing diagnoses in planning patient care, Philadelphia, 1984, F.A. Davis Co.
21. Dorfman, W., and Cristofar, L., editors: Psychosomatic illness review, New York, 1985, Macmillan Publishing Co.
22. Dunbar, F.: Emotions and bodily changes, ed. 4, New York, 1954, Columbia University Press.
23. Elliott, G.R., and Ensdorfer, C.: Stress and human health, New York, 1982, Springer Publishing Co.
24. Field, H.: Psychosomatic illness: semantic and theoretical evolution. In Gallon, R.L., editor: The psychosomatic approach to illness, New York, 1982, Elsevier Biomedical Publications.
25. Fogel, B.: A psychiatric unit becomes a psychiatric-medical unit, General Hospital Psychiatry 7(1):26, 1985.
26. Fontaine, R., and Roisvert, D.: Psychophysiological disorders in anxious patients: hypertension and hypotension, Psychotherapy and Psychosomatics 38:165, 1982.
27. Ford, C.V.: The somatizing disorders: illness as a way of life, New York, 1983, Elsevier Biomedical Publications.
28. Ford M.R., and others: Quieting response training: treatment of psychophysiological disorders in psychiatric in-patients, Biofeedback and Self-Regulation 7(3):331, 1982.
29. Frederickson, R.C.A., and others: Neuroregulation of autonomic, endocrine and immune systems, Boston, 1986, Martinus Nijhoff Publishing.
30. Friedman, M., and Rosenman, R.H.: Type A behavior and your heart, New York, 1974, Alfred A. Knopf, Inc.
31. Frese, M.: Stress at work and psychosomatic complaints: a causal interpretation, Journal of Applied Psychology 70(2):314, 1985.

32. Gadlin, W.: Psychiatric consultation to the medical ward: a group analytic and general systems theory point of view, International Journal of Group Psychotherapy **35**(2):263, 1985.

33. Gagan, J.M.: Imagery: an overview with suggested application for nursing, Perspectives in Psychiatric Care **22**(1):20, 1984.

34. Gallon, R.L., editor: The psychosomatic approach to illness, New York, 1982, Elsevier Biomedical Publications.

35. Ganong, W.F.: The neuroendocrine system. In Frederickson, R.C.A., and others, editors: Neuroregulation of autonomic, endocrine and immune systems, Boston, 1986, Martinus Nijhoff Publishing.

36. Goldsmith, S.: Strategic psychotherapy in psychiatric consultations, American Journal of Psychotherapy **37**(2):279, 1983.

37. Gordon, M.: Nursing diagnosis: process and application, New York, 1982, McGraw-Hill Book Co.

38. Gould, D.: The myth of menopause, Nursing Mirror **160**(23):25, 1985.

39. Gunderson, E.K.E., and Rahe, R.H., editors: Life stress and illness, Springfield, Ill., 1974, Charles C Thomas, Publisher.

40. Hebert, D.J.: Psychophysiological reactions as a function of life stress and behavioral rigidity, Journal of Psychiatric Nursing and Mental Health Services **14**(5):23, 1976.

41. Hoffman, R.S.: Operation of a medical-psychiatric unit in a general hospital setting, General Hospital Psychiatry **6**(2):93, 1984.

42. Holmes, T.H., and Rahe, R.H.: The social readjustment scale, Journal of Psychosomatic Research **11**:213, 1967.

43. Hopping, M.: Psychic seizures, Bulletin of the Menninger Clinic **48**(5):401, 1984.

44. Iyer, P.W., Taptich, B.J., and Bernocchi-Losey, D.: Nursing process and nursing diagnosis, Philadelphia, 1986, W.B. Saunders Co.

45. Jokinen, K., Koskinen, T., and Selonen, R.: Flupenthixal versus diazepam in the treatment of psychosomatic disorders: a double-blind, multi-centre trial in general practice, Pharmatherapeutica **3**(9):573, 1984.

46. Kaplan, H.I., Freedman, A.M., and Sadock, B.J., editors: Comprehensive textbook of psychiatry, vols. 1 to 3, ed. 3, Baltimore, 1980, The Williams & Wilkins Co.

47. Kaplan, M.: Essential Works of Pavlov, New York, 1966, Bantam Books.

48. Kim, M.J., and Moritz, D.A., editors: Classification of nursing diagnoses: proceedings of the third and fourth national conferences, New York, 1982, McGraw-Hill Book Co.

49. Krupp, M.A., and Chatton, M.J.: Current medical diagnosis and treatment, Los Altos, Calif., 1980, Lange Medical Publications.

50. Lazarus, R.S.: Psychological stress and the coping process, New York, 1966, McGraw-Hill Book Co.

51. Lazarus, R.S., and Monat, A., editors: Stress and coping, ed. 2, New York, 1985, Columbia University Press.

52. Lazarus, R.S., and Folkman, S.: Stress, appraisal and coping, New York, 1984, Springer Publishing Co.

53. Lesse, S.: Masked depression, Current Psychiatric Therapies **22**:81, 1983.

54. Levitt, D.B., and others: Group support in the treatment of P.M.S., Journal of Psychosocial Nursing **26**(1):23, 1986.

55. Levi, L., and Kagan, A.: Adaptations of the psychosocial environment to man's abilities and needs. In Levi, L., editor: Society, stress and disease, vol. 1, London, 1971, Oxford University Press.

56. Lilliston, L., Brown, P., and Schliebe, H.P.: Perceptions of religious solutions to personal problems, Journal of Clinical Psychology **39**(3):546, 1982.

57. Marmor, J., and Pumpian-Mindlin, E.: Towards an integrative conception of mental disorder. In Gray, W., Duhl, F.J., and Rizzo, N.D., editors: General systems theory and psychiatry, Boston, 1969, Little, Brown & Co.

58. Meichenbaum, D., and Jaremko, M.E., editors: Stress reduction and prevention, New York, 1983, Plenum Press.

59. Mendelson, G.: Psychosocial factors and the management of physical illness: a contribution to the cost-containment of medical care, Australian and New Zealand Journal of Psychiatry **18**:211, 1984.

60. Miller, D., and others: A pseudo-AIDS syndrome following from fear of AIDS, British Journal of Psychiatry **146**:550, 1985.

61. Mitchell, W.D., and Thompson, T.L.: Some methodological issues in consultation-liaison psychiatry research, General Hospital Psychiatry **7**:66, 1985.

62. Pasnau, R.O.: Psychiatric considerations in coronary artery disease, Bulletin of the Menninger Clinic **48**(3):209, 1984.

63. Pawlick, R.E., and Heitkemper, T.: Behavioral management of insomnia, Journal of Psychosocial Nursing **23**(7):14, 1985.

64. Peplan, H.: Interpersonal relations in nursing, New York, 1952, G.P. Putnam's Sons.

65. Philippopoulos, G.S., and Lucas, X.: Dynamics in art group psychotherapy with psychosomatic patients, Psychotherapy and Psychosomatics **40**(1/4):74, 1983.

66. Purilo, D.T., Hallgren, H.M., and Yuris, E.J.: Depressed maternal lymphocyte response to phytohaemagglutinin in human pregnancy, Lancet **I**:769, 1972.

67. Redd, W.H.: Behavioral analysis and control of psychosomatic symptoms of patients receiving intensive cancer treatment, British Journal of Clinical Psychology **21**:351, 1982.

68. Rogers, M.: An introduction to the theoretical basis of nursing, Philadelphia, 1970, F.A. Davis Co.

69. Rogers, M.P., Dubey, D., and Reich, P.: The influence of the psyche and the brain on immunity and disease susceptibility: a critical review, Psychosomatic Medicine **41**:147, 1979.

70. Roy, Sister Callista: Adaptation: a conceptual framework for nursing, Nursing Outlook **18**(3):43, 1970.

71. Sarti, M.G., and Cossidente, A.: Therapy in psychosomatic dermatology, Clinical Dermatology **2**(4):255, 1984.

72. Schwartz, G.E.: Testing the biopsychosocial model: the ultime challenge facing behavioral medicine? Journal of Consulting and Clinical Psychology **50**(6):1040, 1982.

73. Selye, H.: The stress of life, New York, 1976, McGraw-Hill Book Co.

74. Selye, H., and Neufeld, R.W.J.: Psychological stress and psychopathology, New York, 1982, McGraw-Hill Book Co.

75. Shontz, F.C.: The psychological aspects of physical illness and disability, New York, 1975, Macmillan Publishing Co.

76. Sifness, P.E.: Short-term dynamic psychotherapy for patients with physical symptomatology, Psychotherapy and Psychosomatics **42**(1/4):48, 1984.

77. Stefanek, M.E., and Hodes, R.L.: Expectancy effects on relaxation instructions: physiological and self-report indices, Biofeedback and Self-Regulation **11**(1):21, 1986.

78. Svedlund, J., and Sjodin, I.: A psychosomatic approach to treatment in the irritable bowel syndrome and peptic ulcer disease with aspects of the design of clinical trials, Scandinavian Journal of Gastroenterology (Suppl.) **109**:147, 1985.

79. Takashima, H.: Humanistic psychosomatic medicine, Berkeley, Calif., 1984, Institute of Logotherapy Press.

80. Throll, D.A.: Transcendental meditation and progressive relaxation: their physiological effects, Journal of Clinical Psychology **38**(3):522, 1982.

81. Viney, L.L., and others: The effect of hospital-based counseling service on the physical recovery of surgical and medical patients, General Hospital Psychiatry **7**(4):294, 1985.

82. von Bertalanffy, L.: General systems theory, New York, 1968, George Braziller, Inc.

83. Weiner, H., Hoffer, M.A., and Stunkard, A.J.: Brain, behavior and bodily disease, New York, 1981, Raven Press.

84. Wolf, G.A., Jr., and Wolff, H.G.: Studies on the nature of certain symptoms associated with cardiovascular disorders, Psychosomatic Medicine **8:**293, 1946.

85. Wong, L.D.: The interface between medicine and psychiatry, Bulletin of the Menninger Clinic, **48**(3):193, 1984.

86. Young, L.D., and Harsch, H.H.: An inpatient unit for combined physical and psychiatric disorders, Psychosomatics **27**(1):53, 1986.

87. Zales, M.R., editor: Stress in health and disease, New York, 1985, Brunner/Mazel Publishers.

88. Zenmore, R.: Systematic desensitization as a method of teaching a general anxiety-reducing skill. Journal of Consulting and Clinical Psychology **43:**157, 1975.

ANNOTATED BIBLIOGRAPHY

Gallon, R.L., editor: The psychosomatic approach to illness, New York, 1982, Elsevier Biomedical.

This book provides an overview and straightforward approach to understanding the psychosomatic concepts of illness. There is a comprehensive approach to psychosomatic disorders that includes description of and treatment for "typical" psychophysiological disorders as well as consideration of the psychophysiological components of cancer, chronic medical illness, and pain. One chapter addresses the role of the family. Current research data are included as well as some case examples. While written for physicians with emphasis on medical treatment, this book provides a good overview of medically focused treatment for all professionals treating clients with these disorders.

Lazarus, R.S., and Folkman, S.: Stress and appraisal and coping, New York, 1984, Springer Publishing Co.

This book, written by two psychologists, presents a major theory of stress emphasizing the cognitive and cognitive and emotional aspects of human coping. Current research trends and directions are described in an interesting and comprehensive manner. The effort is to develop ideas and raise questions about how individuals adapt and cope to life situations from a psychological perspective. The physiology of stress mechanisms is not included. The book is directed toward a multidisciplinary audience and succeeds in providing thought-provoking ideas about how persons make decisions that influence their behavior and consequently modify stress responses.

Neufeld, R.W.J., editor: Psychological stress and pathology, New York, 1982, McGraw-Hill Book Co.

There is a body of evidence that supports the idea that major psychiatric disorders are responses to psychogenic stress. This book brings together many of the current ideas and evaluates some of the work that has been done on the associations between stressing agents and psychiatric symptomatology. This is a rapidly expanding area of research and clinical practice.

CHAPTER 35

THERAPY WITH CLIENTS WITH EATING DISORDERS

Rauda Salkauskas Gelazis   Alice Kempe

After studying this chapter the learner will be able to:

Define obesity, anorexia nervosa, and bulimia nervosa.

Discuss historical perspectives of eating disorders.

Describe theoretical bases for eating disorders

Apply the nursing process to clients with eating disorders.

Discuss special issues related to eating.

Identify current research findings on eating disorders.

Nutrition is crucial to growth and development throughout the life cycle. Food and the fulfillment of needs are linked in infancy. As a person matures, eating behaviors take on new meaning and significance. Meanings that stem from family and culture influence the individual's self-concept. When problems exist in family relationships and interaction patterns and in one's self-concept, *eating disorders* can result.

Eating disorders are gross disturbances in eating behaviors. Three types are discussed in this chapter: obesity, anorexia nervosa, and bulimia nervosa. Also included are brief discussions of fasting, low-calorie diets, drug and hormone use, and the effects of vitamin deficiencies on mental health.

Obesity

Obesity, a major health problem in the United States, is defined as weight 15% to 20% more than one's ideal body weight, determined by the Metropolitan Life Insurance Standards. Also, there is an excessive proportion of fat or adipose tissue in the body mass. About 60 million Americans (one in five) may be considered obese. Many emotional factors are associated with obesity, but studies fail to clearly differentiate between those related to the development of obesity and those caused by being obese.[54]

THEORETICAL APPROACHES
Biological

Obesity often begins early in life. The infant's body generally is 10% to 15% adipose tissue. In the first year of life there is a definite increase in adipose cell size but not in cell number. In puberty and late adolescence the number of adult adipose cells stabilizes. There is evidence that adipose tissue usually does not decrease during the life cycle.

Cellular hypertrophy results from increased food intake and decreased energy expenditure, suggesting that obesity is not a disease but a symptom of an imbalance between caloric ingestion and energy use. Obese individuals tend to be less active than nonobese people. One study concludes that heredity is involved in obesity but that environmental factors may have a greater influence.[4] Genetic studies indicate that 60% of obese subjects have one or both obese parent(s). Studies of environmental factors affecting obesity suggest that infants' eating habits are a result of caregivers' feeding behaviors. If the caregiver ignores the child's cues, feeds him when the caregiver thinks he is hungry, and insists that he eat everyting on his plate, the child learns to ignore physical cues of hunger as a basis for eating or not eating.

Other biological theories suggest that endocrine disease, altered metabolism, and thyroid dysfunction may contribute to obesity (see Figure 35-1).

🍇 *Historical Overview* 🍇

DATE	EVENT
1800s	Being overweight was considered healthier than being thin, which was associated with malnutrition. Excess weight was valued and considered beautiful.
1850	Florence Nightingale documented the importance of a sound diet for health in *Notes for Nursing,* with recommendations for foods and fluids to be included in one's daily diet.
1873	Anorexia nervosa was first described in the literature by two physicians, Sir William Gull and Dr. E. Laseque.
1890s	Freud observed that nutrition affected neuroses by influencing energy levels and promoting healthier brain cell functioning.
1900s	Worldwide interest in health and nutrition grew in the early twentieth century. Chemists and physiologists in Europe and the United States identified the need for proteins, minerals, vitamins, hormones, enzymes, and fatty acids to ensure digestion and metabolism for maximal health.
1930s	The League of Nations established standards for adequate nutrition.
1950s	The National Nutritional Conference set up committees in every state to promote better nutrition. Recommended dietary allowances for various age and sex categories were established.
1960s	Studies to look at the effects of food intake on behavior and emotions showed that schizophrenia and depression are affected by chemical imbalances and nutritional deficits.
1980s	Today the American public, especially women, value thinness. Billions of dollars are spent on diets and the pursuit of thinness. However, current treatment strategies have had only limited success.
Future	Professional nurses will be challenged to educate the public about nutrition and to treat individuals with eating disorders to improve quality of life and longevity.

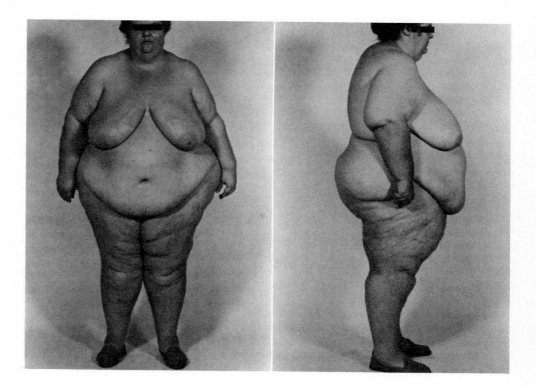

FIGURE 35-1 Obese client.

Psychoanalytic

Psychoanalytical theorists view obesity as an expression of some intrapsychic conflict that occurred during the oral stage of psychosexual development. Obesity is seen as a regression to the infant oral stage to fill unmet needs. Overeating is explained as a way to:

1. Decrease anxiety, insecurity, worry, frustration, or monotony
2. Express hostility or rebellion against authority or assert independence
3. Express anger at oneself
4. Punish oneself
5. Avoid competition in life
6. Compensate for lack of love, affection, and friends
7. Justify interpersonal or career failures
8. Achieve greatness by becoming bigger and stronger than others
9. Modify a depression
10. Destroy oneself

Cognitive

Ellis[19] stated that irrational thinking may contribute to continued obesity. The obese person may describe himself as fat and unable to do anything about it. Because he may have unsuccessfully tried to lose weight in the past, he may fear failure again. The irrational assumption that there is nothing to do about it prevents people from altering their eating behaviors.

Sociocultural

Eating is a socializing experience. Through the family the child learns the social customs, values, and mores of eating behaviors. Eating experiences in adulthood can symbolize childhood. In each eating experience there is a relationship of giving and receiving. For example, the mother makes a meal for the family, who in turn receives the food. Rejection of the food may be seen as rejection of the mother. Mealtimes can becomes arenas where the give and take of relationships have lifelong effects.

Orbach,[43] in studying family influence on obesity, relates obesity to the parent-child relationship. Ambivalence and conflicts are played out in feeding and eating behavior. For example, a child in a hostile environment of marital conflict who is used as a scapegoat for one or both parents may become obese.

Culture also strongly influences the development of feelings, attitudes, and preferences about food and eating that are built into the personality. Every culture has food preferences, habits, taboos, and variations in methods of eating. In some cultures everything revolves around food; in others food is deemphasized. The United States encompasses many cultural food value systems and many foods that represent or symbolize a person's "roots."

Investigations of social influences on eating patterns indicate differences between obese persons and persons of normal weight. Both groups are influenced by the eating habits of the people with whom they eat. Some families spend considerable time conversing while eating, prolong-

TABLE 35-1 Summary of theories of obesity

Theory	Dynamics
Biological	There is an imbalance between caloric ingestion and energy use. There is a genetic tendency toward obesity. Endocrine disease, altered metabolism, or thyroid deficiency may cause obesity.
Psychoanalytic	Obesity is an expression of an intrapsychic conflict that occurred in the oral stage of psychosexual development.
Cognitive	Irrational assumptions about food, weight, and body contribute to continued obesity.
Sociocultural	Family and cultural values, customs, and mores strongly influence the development of feelings, attitudes, and preferences about food and eating behaviors. Ambivalence and conflicts in family relationships contribute to obesity.
Learning	Overeating is a learned behavior related to environmental cues and emotional states.

ing the meal and discussing events of the day. Others eat quickly with little or no interaction.

Learning

Learning theory focuses on overeating as learned behavior resulting from environmental cues and states of emotional arousal. An obese individual learns to respond to various emotional states, such as anger, loneliness, boredom, or stress by eating. Parents' use of food to deal with these emotions teaches the child that eating is a way of receiving attention or reward and that feelings do not have to be dealt with directly and appropriately. Food becomes associated with feelings; later those feelings elicit eating.

Table 35-1 summarizes the theories of obesity.

NURSING PROCESS

Assessment

Physical dimension. The physical dimension encompasses all the effects and ramifications of obesity on the physiological functioning of the body, particularly the cardiovascular and respiratory systems. Symptoms include elevated blood pressure, shortness of breath, heart palpitations on exertion, and feeling warm even on cold days or with minimal activity. The nurse assesses the client's activity level, physical limitations, and exercise program. The nurse compares the client's weight to his ideal weight according to Metropolitan Life Insurance standards (Tables 35-2 and 35-3).

TABLE 35-2 Desirable weights for men 25 years of age and over (in indoor clothing)

Height		Small Frame	Medium Frame	Large Frame
Feet	Inches			
5	2	128-134	131-141	138-150
5	3	130-136	133-143	140-153
5	4	132-138	135-145	142-156
5	5	134-140	137-148	144-160
5	6	136-142	139-151	146-164
5	7	138-145	142-154	149-168
5	8	140-148	145-157	152-172
5	9	142-151	148-160	155-176
5	10	144-154	151-163	158-180
5	11	146-157	154-166	161-184
6	0	149-160	157-170	164-188
6	1	152-164	160-174	168-192
6	2	155-168	164-178	172-197
6	3	158-172	167-182	176-202
6	4	162-176	171-187	181-207

Courtesy Metropolitan Life Insurance Co., New York; revised 1983.

TABLE 35-3 Desirable weight for women 25 years of age and over (in indoor clothing)

Height		Small Frame	Medium Frame	Large Frame
Feet	Inches			
4	10	102-111	109-121	118-131
4	11	103-113	111-123	120-134
5	0	104-115	113-126	122-137
5	1	106-118	115-129	125-140
5	2	108-121	118-132	128-143
5	3	111-124	121-135	131-147
5	4	114-127	124-138	134-151
5	5	117-130	127-141	137-155
5	6	120-133	130-144	140-159
5	7	123-136	133-147	143-163
5	8	126-139	136-150	146-167
5	9	129-142	139-153	149-170
5	10	132-145	142-156	152-173
5	11	135-148	145-159	155-176
6	0	135-151	148-162	158-179

Courtesy Metropolitan Life Insurance Co., New York; revised 1983.

Research Highlight

Effects of Being Overweight

A.L. Stewart & R.H. Brook

PURPOSE

This study was designed to determine the effects of being overweight. The relationship of perceived overweight to objective overweight was studied. Also studied was the relationship between being overweight and functional status; general health perceptions; mental health; the extent of pain, worry, and restricted activities that overweight persons ascribe to their weight; and what they are doing to lose weight.

SAMPLE

Data were gathered from a cross section of a general population of 5,817, ages 14 to 61 years.

METHODOLOGY

Analyses were based on measures of weight and overweight (obtained by a self-administered medical questionnaire, attempts to lose weight (measured by the number of approaches taken to lose weight), functional status (measured by an index of personal functioning and an indicator of role functioning), general health perceptions (measured by the General Health Index), and mental health (measured by a Mental Health Index). Regression analyses were performed with ordinary least squares regression.

FINDINGS

Forty-one percent perceived that they were overweight. A higher percentage of women than men said they were severely overweight, whereas a higher percentage of men than women said they were moderately overweight. Of those who perceived they were overweight, only four out of 10 were classified objectively as overweight. Being overweight was given as a main reason for limitations in personal functioning and role functioning by 13% of people in the sample aged 14 to 61, and by 18% of people aged 30 to 49. Mean mental health scores were nearly identical, 74 for those of normal weight and 75 for those overweight. Of those who perceived they were overweight, 54% were taking no steps to reduce, 32% were dieting, 24% were exercising, and 72% were in a physician's care.

IMPLICATIONS

Nurses can use these findings to promote weight loss that improves personal functioning and mental health and lessens restricted activities attributed to being overweight. Findings can also be used to legitimize being moderately overweight in a society that values thinness.

Based on data from the American Journal of Public Health **73** (2):171, 1983.

A thorough nutritional assessment is needed. Obtaining a dietary intake for several days to identify eating patterns is helpful. Because the client may skip meals or eat several meals a day with numerous snacks, he may have trouble accurately describing usual dietary intake and daily food requirements. Obese clients often underestimate the amount of food they eat and the size of the portions. A person of normal weight eats when hungry; an obese client eats if food is available.

It is important to obtain information about the client's perception of his body image and sexuality (see the Research Highlight, p. 665). The nurse questions the client's views of his physical self, his thoughts and feelings about his body (its functioning and size), and perception of his body. Obese clients typically do not like their body. They avoid looking in mirrors and may try to mask their size by wearing loose clothing.

The nurse also assesses clients medications that may influence weight. Birth control pills and antipsychotics such as Thorazine are known to cause weight gain.

Emotional dimension. Feelings of anxiety, anger, guilt, boredome, hopelessness, loneliness, frustration, unattractiveness, and depression induce overeating. Many obese clients feel hopeless about changing their weight. Guilt frequently follows a deviation from a weight loss diet. Depression is common in obese clients. They have chosen to cope with their emotions by eating. See Chapters 12, 13, 14, and 19 for further information on assessment techniques.

Intellectual dimension. The nurse determines whether the client's thoughts about being obese are rational. Statements such as, "I can't control my eating," demonstrate irrational thinking. The client's self-control and motivation for changing eating habits are assessed. It is important to determine the client's use of defense mechanisms. Rationalization is common. The client may excuse his overeating with statements such as, "It's Christmas, everyone eats too much." Knowledge of nutrition and healthy eating behaviors are determined; many obese clients do not have an adequate knowledge of basic nutrition.

Social dimension. Cultural background and ethnicity strongly influence dietary intake and the value placed on food. This influence is so strong that changes are slow and difficult to maintain over time. Patterns of eating are developed early in life based on family traditions and beliefs. The nurse therefore considers cultural and ethnic background.

The client's support system is assessed. If family relationships are disturbed, the client may eat to compensate for it. Studies show that clients who have the cooperation of a partner lost significantly more weight than those with an uncooperative partner.[5] A partner who is critical and negative toward the client's eating behavior may even sabotage a weight loss program. Fearing that the client's loss of weight may create a loss of bargaining power in arguments or promote infidelity, the partner may offer or talk about food. After a successful weight loss program clients may have more control and independence in relationships.

For some persons food takes on more significance than their relationships. Obese clients see food as an important part of social activities. Sometimes a client's report of a social event focuses on what food is served rather than time spent relating to others.

The obese client's self-esteem is generally lowered. He is self-conscious and may lack confidence in himself and his achievements.

Spiritual dimension. The nurse assesses the meaning and significance of food in the client's life. Ingesting food has many purposes: to socialize, to meet a basic need, to cope with stress and disturbed relationships, to adhere to religious and cultural values, to demonstrate economic status and personal achievement, and to reward himself. Obesity is also a self-destructive behav-

---

ALTERATIONS IN NUTRITION: MORE THAN BODY REQUIREMENTS

DEFINITION

The individual experiences an intake of nutrients that exceeds metabolic needs.

DEFINING CHARACTERISTICS

Physical Dimension
Overweight (10% over ideal weight for height and frame)
†Obese (20% over ideal weight for height and frame)
Undesirable eating patterns
Intake in excess of body requirements
*Low activity and exercise level
Pairing food with other activities
Eating in response to external cues (time of day)
Eating in response to internal cues other than hunger (anxiety)
*Pregnancy

Emotional Dimension
Anxiety
Depression
Boredom
Guilt

Intellectual Dimension
*Lack of basic nutritional knowledge
*Irrational thoughts about food and eating

Social Dimension
Sedentary life-style or work
Ethnic or cultural expectations that emphasize hearty eating and a hefty body
Negative self-concept
Loneliness

Spiritual Dimension
*Conflicts with religious beliefs and values about food
*Devaluing self
*Hopelessness
*Lack of faith in self

Adapted from North American Nursing Diagnosis Association Classification of Nursing Diagnosis: Proceedings of the seventh conference, St. Louis, 1987, The C.V. Mosby Co.
*Indicates characteristics in addition to those defined by NANDA.
†Indicates a critical characteristic for the diagnosis.

ior; the client's continued overeating may be hastening his own death. He is generally unaware of this.

Clients may devalue themselves, believing that they are weak willed for being obese. Such a belief system increases guilt and anxiety and leads to further overeating and hopelessness. The nurse determines the client's beliefs about his personal worth and his ability to change his eating habits.

Analysis

Nursing diagnosis. Alterations in nutrition: more than body requirements is a diagnosis approved by NANDA that applies to an obese person. The defining characteristics of this diagnosis are listed in the box on p. 666.

The following Case Example illustrates the characteristics of this nursing diagnosis.

Case Example

Jane, a 58-year-old housewife of Italian heritage, has been overweight since age 40. Her husband is a successful businessman of normal weight. He is the decision maker for the family. Jane reports that her three children are all independent. In the last few years she has noticed that she is less active and lacks interest in exercise or new experiences. She states that she feels "bored and useless" much of the time. Her husband has begun to frequently remind her of her 25-pound weight gain this past year. She has attempted to lose weight by various fad diets but becomes easily frustrated and does not stay with them for more than a few days. Most recently she has begun to use diet pills to suppress her appetite. At her last physical examination her blood pressure was elevated. She was instructed to stop her diet pills, and her physician advised her to lose weight.

DSM-III-R diagnoses. Obesity is not generally associated with any distinct emotional or behavioral syndrome. However, when there is evidence that emotional factors are important in the cause or course of obesity, it is discussed under the DSM-III-R category *psychological factors affecting physical condition.*

Planning

See Table 35-4 for examples of long-term and short-term goals and outcome criteria related to obesity. These serve as examples of the planning stage in the nursing process.

Implementation

Physical dimension. The nurse helps the client plan and incorporate a realistic weight loss program to reach ideal weight based on height and body frame. The client can monitor his weight and food intake by keeping a diary of all foods eaten daily for a time to help him more accurately describe the amount, types, and portions of food eaten at what times. The client can modify rate and amount of food eaten by putting utensils down between bites, talking between bites to increase the social pleasure of eating, chewing food more thoroughly, and designating only one place for eating.

The nurse establishes an exercise program compatible with the client's interests. The information in the box on p. 668 can be used to help clients change their activity and exercise routines.

Emotional dimension. The nurse helps the client identify feelings and how they relate to eating be-

---

TABLE 35-4 Long-term and short-term goals and outcome criteria related to obesity

Goals	Outcome Criteria
NURSING DIAGNOSIS: ALTERATION IN NUTRITION: MORE THAN BODY REQUIREMENTS RELATED TO SEDENTARY LIFE-STYLE	
Long-term goals	
To control eating behaviors	Stays within daily intake
To identify a variety of measures to change eating habits	States at least 10 techniques for decreasing food intake, such as eating more slowly, chewing each mouthful 20 times, and putting utensils down between each bite
To establish and maintain a desirable weight	States desirable weight for age and height
	Establishes a pattern of exercise that assists to maintain the desired weight
	Monitors own weight daily
	Reinstitutes weight reduction diet at an increase of more than 3 pounds
Short-term goals	
To discuss habitual eating patterns	Identifies daily eating habits
	Identifies problem foods and times
	Identifies uncontrollable, irrational eating behaviors
To identify desirable changes in eating behaviors	States planned change with established timetable
To establish a nutritionally balanced daily diet including the basic food groups	Recognizes necessary daily nutrients and foods that contain them
To participate in planned exercise for 30 minutes three times per week	Exercises for 30 minutes three times per week

ENERGY EXPENDITURE FOR SELECTED ACTIVITIES*

Walking		Football (while active)	11	Running		
3 mph (leisurely)	5	Gardening	6	5 mph (jogging)	10	
4 mph (fast)	7	Golf (carrying clubs)	6	7 mph (moderately fast)	15	
5 mph (very fast)	8	Handball (competitive)	11	10 mph (very fast)	21	
Downstairs	7	Horseback riding		Upstairs	17	
Upstairs	14	Slow	4	Sawing hardwood	10	
Downhill (2.5 mph)	4	Trot	6	Shoveling snow	9	
Uphill (3.5 mph)	11	Hunting	8	Shuffleboard	4	
Hiking (with 40-pound pack)	7	Karate or judo	12	Skating (ice or roller)		
Badminton (singles)	6	Mountain climbing	10	Leisurely	7	
Baseball or softball	5	Mowing		Rapidly	12	
Basketball	6	Riding	3	Skiing		
Boating		Pushing power mower	5	Snow downhill	8	
Rowing	8	Pushing hand mower	8	Cross country		
Sailing	5	Paddleball	10	4 mph	10	
Bowling	4	Painting	6	8 mph	17	
Calisthenics		Ping-pong	6	Water	8	
Light	6	Playing musical instrument	4	Snowshoeing	10	
Heavy	10	Raking leaves	6	Soccer	13	
Cycling		Rope skipping		Squash (competitive)	11	
5 mph	4	Leisurely	5	Swimming (crawl)	9	
10 mph	7	Vigorously	13	Tennis		
13 mph	11			Doubles	6	
Croquet	4			Singles	8	
Dancing				Volleyball (competitive)	7	
Slow foxtrot	6					
Fast step	9					
Square dancing	9					
Modern	5					
Fishing (from pier or boat)	4					

*Numbers indicate calories burned per minute.

haviors, particularly those that trigger overeating. Facilitating the expression of anger, guilt, anxiety, depression, and hopelessness is an initial step in becoming aware of the relationship between feelings and eating. Relaxation, exercise, sports, art (including writing and music), and assertive behaviors are appropriate ways to express feelings. Developing new strategies for dealing with feelings may help eliminate the need to overeat. See Chapters 12 through 15 for further interventions.

❋ ***Intellectual dimension.*** Many irrational beliefs are held by the obese client. The nurse may first confront the client with the irrational thought, then work out a more rational response with him. For example, if the client thinks, "I can't control my eating," he tends to act on this belief and will not try to stay with his eating regime. By helping the client recognize that he has control over his own behavior in numerous ways throughout each day, the nurse can help him use this control in eating behaviors. The client then begins to feel more confident that he has a certain amount of control in his life.

Cognitive restructuring is essential for the client to begin to think about himself in a new way. As he becomes aware of some of the negative ways he views himself, he can begin to change to more positive thinking and move toward positive self-regard. The nurse facilitates change in thoughts and feelings from negative to positive by:

1. Explaining the overall change desired
2. Identifying client's typical thoughts about being fat
3. Introducing new, rational thoughts
4. Helping the client practice positive thinking and self-talk
5. Encouraging rational thinking in daily life and following up with discussions of its effectiveness

❀ ***Social dimension.*** Mobilizing social support for the obese client is an important aspect of care. A partner can assist by pointing out the positive aspects of change. A social network of significant others reinforces support through the weight loss process. It also discourages eating when lonely or bored, since others can be called on to fill the void. Support groups, such as Weight Watchers, Overeaters Anonymous, and Take Off Pounds Sensibly (TOPS), are useful for weight loss and maintenance. They decrease feelings of helplessness and hopelessness; increase feelings of confidence, power, esteem, and sexual attractiveness; and offer rewards for positive change. To maintain ideal weight, the client uses a variety of environmental supports, such as co-workers, who can be a powerful adjunct to treatment.

It helps to generouly praise any amount of weight loss and ignore slight deviations from the prescribed diet. Nagging and criticism are detrimental. The nurse assist the client to develop a system that provides rewards for a successful week, such as a special movie or weekend activity. The nurse promotes the client's participating in pleasurable activities other than those involved in eating.

When family relationships are disturbed, the client may be referred to family or marital therapy (see Chapters 29 and 30).

The nurse assists the client to accept responsibility for his eating behaviors. He alone can change his eating habits. He cannot change others' behaviors toward his weight problem, and others may not be helpful or tolerate his continued emphasis on dieting.

The nurse is careful to promote activities in accordance with the client's family, culture, and ethnic traditions. New behaviors for special holidays can be established.

Spiritual dimension. The nurse helps the client to value himself as a unique and special person of worth, even though he is large. Focusing on positive attributes, skills, and personal strengths counteracts the client's devaluing and negative belief system. Promoting better communication through assertiveness skills helps the client establish meaningful relationships with others and experience the give and take of loving, caring relationships.

The nurse offers hope to counteract depression and hopelessness by accepting lack of progress in weight reduction and by continuing to work with the client when he chooses not to accept treatment.

The client is assisted to describe the meaning and significance of food and eating in his life and to integrate those meanings into a life-style that balances gratification from eating with gratification from other sources.

Evaluation

Nursing intervention is successful when the client eats a balanced diet composed of the four basic food groups; maintains optimal physical functioning; exercises adequately; and has increased self-esteem, feelings of control, and awareness of feelings that trigger eating.

Anorexia Nervosa and Bulimia Nervosa

Anorexia nervosa is the life-threatening eating disorder of self-induced starvation. The most obvious symptom is extreme weight loss, up to as much as 15% of the client's body weight. An exaggerated interest in food is coupled with refusal to eat and denial of hunger.

Anorectic persons eat little, exercise vigorously, and have excessive fears of being fat or gaining weight, even though they are abnormally thin. Anorectic clients are predominantly female (95%). As many as one in 250 girls between 12 and 18 years of age develop the disorder (see the following Case Example).

Case Example

Sharon, a 17-year-old high school senior, has become increasingly secretive about her eating for the past 2 months. Her parents are concerned about her recent loss of 20 pounds and her preoccupation with thinness and diets. After school, rather than doing her homework, she focuses on food. She frequently cooks the family dinners but eats only salads, carrot sticks, and celery. Sharon reads about nutrition and preparation of foods. She cooks many deserts and high-calorie foods but does not eat them.

She is an excellent student but feels she has not done well enough. She is interested in sports and exercises at least 2 hours a day. It is not unusual to find her jogging early in the morning and again in the evening.

Sharon is the second of three siblings. She strives to be better than her older sister and tries to mother her younger brother. She has a very strong attachment to her father but is often ignored by him. Her mother tries to compensate for his lack of interest in the family.

At the beginning of the school year, when the school annual physical was required, the physician was unable to obtain blood for routine laboratory work. Extreme emaciation and anemia were noted, and her parents were advised to seek further medical help for Sharon. Her mother wanted to handle this on her own by insisting that Sharon begin to eat more, which resulted in continual struggles for control. By the time Sharon came to the nurse's attention she weighed only 80 pounds (she is 5′6″ tall) and had fainted during gym. She was hospitalized on the recommendation of the school nurse. At the hospital Sharon refused to eat and did not communicate with anyone.

Bulimia nervosa is characterized by an uncontrollable craving for food that results in binges—the rapid, surreptitious consumption of high-calorie food in a short time. The bulimic person may consume two to three times the amount of an average meal. The binge is followed by vomiting and/or use of laxatives, diuretics, and enemas. The disorder usually occurs in females and begins in adolescence. It is six times more common than anorexia nervosa.

After a period of *binging* and *purging* the client becomes "hooked" on its tranquilizing effects. Many learn to vomit by reflex action. The bulimic client usually falls into a cycle of guilt, self-loathing, and devastating isolation (see the Case Example below).

Case Example

Jean, a 19-year-old college freshman, came to the hospital after taking 30 Dulcolax tablets with reported abdominal pain. Jean gave a history of having tried many diets for weight loss without success. She began to respond to stress by compulsive binge-purge behaviors. She talked readily about herself and described the development of her eating disorder in great detail. She was fixated on achieving thinness at any cost and became more and more frustrated, guilty, and depressed with each binge. She used induced vomiting when she was alone but turned to laxative use to enhance weight loss. Many times this made her very weak; it was almost impossible for her to function at school, despite past scholastic success. The last binge episode convinced her to increase her laxative use, which resulted in a fluid-electrolyte imbalance requiring hospitalization. Her physical condition was quickly stablized, but Jean continued to show signs of depression and guilt about the cost of the hospitalization and the exposure of her eating disorder to her family.

THEORETICAL APPROACHES

The theoretical approaches for anorexia nervosa and bulimia nervosa are presented together because of the similarity of their dynamics.

Biological

The disease process of anorexia nervosa usually begins with the client deciding to lose weight. As she loses weight, she feels a great deal of satisfaction from the suppression of hunger. She fears regaining the weight and becomes preoccupied with remaining thin, although she looks emaciated (see Figure 35-2). The need for exercise becomes exaggerated, at times obsessional. Physical activity, frequently to the point of collapse, is used to distract attention from hunger. The bulimic client, instead of getting satisfaction from the suppression of hunger, satisfies her hunger by binging, followed by self-induced vomiting.

Psychoanalytic

Theorists with a psychoanalytical orientation view eating disorders as regression to prepuberty. Generally persons who develop eating disorders are experiencing difficulties in coping with life, their feelings, or the transition into adolescence. They feel anxious and out of control. There seems to be a resistance to growing up and maturing. The fact that anorexia nervosa and bulimia nervosa most often appear at puberty and are accompanied by amenorrhea leads theorists to believe that the disorder is related to sexual problems or to repudiation of sexuality.

Cognitive

Cognitive theorists see perceptual disturbances as contributing to anorexia nervosa and bulimia nervosa. The client with a distorted body image may perceive herself as too fat. She may draw her body as large and depict others' in correct proportion. The client may have irrational beliefs and thoughts; she may be obsessed with the idea that she needs to exercise after eating or drinking even small amounts. She may spend all day thinking about and preparing food, while preoccupied with thinness.

Sociocultural

Bruch[5] believes the central factor in anorexia is the overly rigid parental expectations of the anorectic child. She described families who are educated and happy but who implicitly or explicitly burden their children with living up to their ideal. These children are usually described as exceptionally "good" but seem to lack the ability to set their own goals. Without clear goals of their own they become overly compliant. Bruch suggests these children may have skipped the period of resistance in early childhood or adolescent development. Anorectic clients seem to remain convinced of the perfection of their parents and feel an obligation to obey them. Thus Bruch suggests anorexia nervosa is an internal conflict between feeling enslaved and exploited and wanting to lead an independent life.

Parental concern is often expressed in overprotection and hypervigilance. The anorectic client is enmeshed in a family system with inordinately close family relationships.

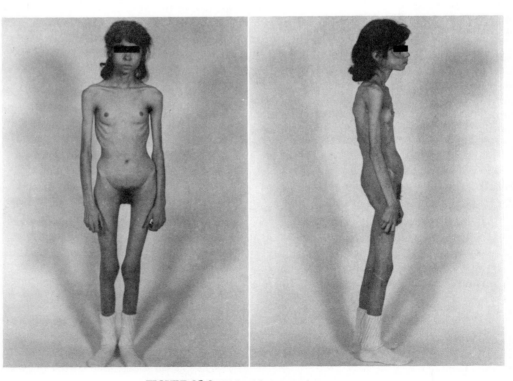

FIGURE 35-2 Girl with anorexia nervosa.

TABLE 35-5 Summary of theories of anorexia nervosa and bulimia nervosa

Theory	Dynamics
Biological	The disease process begins with attempts to lose weight and an intense fear of gaining weight.
Psychoanalytic	Eating disorders result from difficulties in coping with life, feelings, or the transition to adulthood with regression to the prepubertal stage.
Cognitive	Irrational thoughts and beliefs and distorted body image contribute to eating disorders.
Sociocultural	Family conflicts involving high parental expectations, controlling parents, and a resistant, dependent daughter contribute to eating disorders. The cultural overemphasis and value on thinness contributes to eating disorders.

Parents and others find it more and more difficult to empathize with the anorectic person, who seem to focus only on weight and eating.

The family places a high value on appearance, conformity, and obedience. The typical anorectic client is intelligent and performs well in school. The client's accomplishments are not for herself, however, but an effort to gain family approval. The client is fearful of embarrassing the family in any way. She is generally very dependent on them; any independent activity is difficult for her. Feeling she has little control in her environment, she finds that her body is something she can control and use to manipulate her family. The struggle over food intake is an emotional struggle for autonomy and self-control.

The anorectic client is also handicapped in developing relations with peers. The client can put on a facade of normalcy, but her difficulty with independent self-expression makes peer relationships hard to achieve.

The cultural overemphasis on thinness may be seen as a contributing factor in eating disorders. The disorder may start as a diet, common with adolescent girls, and continue as a weight maintenance technique until it becomes life threatening. Table 35-5 summarizes the theories of anorexia nervosa and bulimia nervosa.

NURSING PROCESS

Assessment: Anorexia Nervosa

Physical dimension. The client's physical appearance is notable. Usually she appears emaciated, with a hollow face and sunken eyes. There may be a yellow tinge to the skin from eating large numbers of carrots. The hair is usually dry and may fall out excessively. *Lanugo* (fine body hair), a possible reaction to prolonged malnutrition, is seen. There is deterioration of mucous membranes and teeth; brittle nails and hair; amenorrhea; and loss of muscle mass. To attempt to make weight loss less apparent, the anorectic client often wears loose clothing.

The anorectic client avoids high-carbohydrate foods but may allow herself substantial amounts of bulky low-calorie foods, such as celery, crisp breads, or cottage cheese. She usually avoids eating with others at conventional mealtimes to keep up abstinence in the face of hunger.

After collecting data on physical appearance and eating patterns, the nurse notes the client's activity level; daily caloric intake, physical signs and symptoms of malnutrition; and results of diagnostic studies, such as serum electrolyte studies, urinalysis, and hormone studies.

Emotional dimension. Anorectic clients are often cold, indifferent, stubborn, angry, depressed, anxious, and withdrawn. Their fear of loss of control results in a hostile, overcontrolled affect. They may be out of touch with their emotions, reporting feeling good when they are physically ill or feeling angry when there seems to be no justification for it. The client fears sexual maturity; her emotional development may not have kept up with her physical development. The adolescent stage of development requires skills or strengths she may not have, and she feels incompetent, helpless, and ineffective in dealing with a changing body and new social and emotional requirements.

Intellectual dimension. The anorectic client is often negative about herself and her achievements and describes her body critically. The nurse needs to explore irrational beliefs, such as: it is important to be perfect in everything; it is necessary to have love and approval at all times; and happiness is achieved by being thin.

The client's preoccupation with food, eating, thinness, and exercise is obsessional and needs to be discussed. The client has usually been a high achiever in school, with grades gradually declining as she placed increasing emphasis on weight loss and control. The nurse needs to assess the client's usual coping mechanisms (other than food and starvation). Because the client tries to be controlled in all aspects of her life, she may resist the nurse, who is an authority figure.

Social dimension. Most anorectic clients demonstrate low self-esteem. The nurse therefore determines issues that are important to the anorectic client that can be used to build success into the plan of care to increase self-esteem.

The nurse looks for signs of overly close, enmeshed family dynamics. Clues to this include: a parent speaking for the client; one parent sitting extremely close to the client while the other is detached and further away; and communication patterns that do not include all members. Focus of attention and blame may be placed on the anorectic client. Seen as a model child, the client shows evidence of trying to conform to parental demands, goals, and expectations. Frequently the client drives herself mercilessly to meet the high expectations of herself and her family. She may in some cases withdraw from family and peers.

✴ *Spiritual dimension.* Since the client and family may not come for treatment until much trauma has been experienced, the nurse may find considerable hopelessness about altering behaviors. The nurse assesses the meaning of life for the client and family, especially if there has been suicidal thoughts or suicide attempt.

Because of the client's poor physical condition, her motivation for emotional health and growth is constricted. Her preoccupation with food and thinness leaves little time to reflect on a purpose or direction of her life. Isolation and alienation from significant others further reduces her ability to receive pleasure. Assessment of the client's beliefs about health and illness reveals erroneous ideas about thinness based on distorted perceptions. She is unable to accept herself as she is with strengths and weaknesses; she sees herself with mostly weaknesses and little value.

Assessment: Bulimia Nervosa

✴ *Physical dimension.* The bulimic client reports frequent, recurrent episodes of binge eating, an awareness of abnormal eating patterns, frequent fluctuations in weight of more than 10 pounds because of alternating binges and fasts, self-induced vomiting after binging, abdominal pain, and use of cathartics or diuretics. The nurse further assesses this client for the more severe physical signs and symptoms of malnutrition and pathophysiological changes.

Often the bulimic client has a history of attempting to adhere to fad diets with little success in controlling eating behaviors. The client continues to eat large amounts of food, even though she is attempting to follow a restricted diet. When the client acknowledges her lack of success with low-calorie diets, she resorts to vomiting and/or use of cathartics to maintain her weight. The vomiting and amount of cathartics used is increased gradually as the client fails to lose weight.

The nurse questions the client about weight gain and loss patterns. The bulimic client may report weight gain (20 to 30 pounds) or weight loss in a short time span. When vomiting or laxative use help her lose weight, the bulimic client tries to regulate her binges so that her actual weight at the time of the nurse's assessment may be within 10 to 15 pounds of normal ranges, thus giving her a falsely normal appearance.

Only after the binge-purge pattern has been used for a long time does the client begin to show physical signs and symptoms other than abdominal aches and feelings of fullness. Other symptoms include severe constipation; vitamin and mineral deficiencies from lack of absorption (as a result of vomiting); and ulcerations and/or possible perforation of the gastrointestinal tract from frequent irritation from vomiting and laxative abuse. Binging may also result in acute dilation of the stomach, menstrual disturbance, and salivary gland disturbance. Self-induced vomiting may produce metabolic disturbance (especially hypokalemia), cardiac dysrhythmias, renal damage, tetany and peripheral parasthesias, dehydration, epileptic seizures, erosion of dental enamel (perimolysis), chronic hoarseness, and gas-

trointestinal reflux. The purgative abuse may lead to steatorrhea and finger clubbing from rebound water retention.[52]

The bulimic client is commonly overweight, usually within 10 pounds of ideal weight. Laboratory and radiological studies, such as blood work, urinalysis, and barium studies, usually reveal few abnormal findings, although the client often describes abnormal bowel patterns and many other physical symptoms in great detail.

✴ *Emotional dimension.* When the nurse assesses the emotional status of the bulimic client, she needs to keep in mind that this client often has strong feelings and emotions associated with the binge-purge pattern. The nurse observes the client's verbal and nonverbal responses carefully for signs of anxiety; helplessness; anger; depression; frustration; and feelings of futility, inability to meet the expectations of others, or even elation or joy. These feelings typically are experienced before binging. Feelings often reported during and after the binge-purge behaviors are guilt, repulsion, self-disgust, or the opposite extremes—excitement, increased energy, and stimulation. Frequently bulimic clients report that tension drives them to food and that the binging and purging relieves it, producing a high or release similar to an orgasm, followed by calmness and a sense of relaxation. Often the bulimic client hides binge-purge behaviors from family and significant others; the clandestine element adds to the excitement of it. The excitement and frenzy of binging is frequently reported. Often the binge-purge behaviors end in sleep.

✴ *Intellectual dimension.* Manipulating body size and food intake may be an attempt to hide inner stress or adjustment difficulties. In making her assessment of the bulimic client, the nurse is alert to clues that lead to uncovering the sources of the stress. This may be difficult, because the client (and family) may be locked into a pattern of denying underlying emotional causes of the eating disorder. The client attempts to appear normal, except for the binge-purge behaviors. The nurse's attempts to identify problems can be met with hostility and anger, since the client's anxiety is increased by any remote hint of breaking through the denial system.

✴ *Social dimension.* Weight loss from techniques such as vomiting and laxative and diuretic abuse tends to decrease an already low self-esteem. Assessing the client's current level of self-esteem assists the nurse to identify ways to aid the client in building positive feelings about herself. Self-esteem tends to grow as relationships with significant others improve.

It is essential that the nurse assess the client's support system. The family may include overweight members, and the client may have identified with the family's established pattern of overeating. The client may describe a dominating, controlling mother and a distant, powerful father. Few clients describe good relationships with their fathers. The nurse observes the family dynamics, watching for signs of power struggles, dominance, dependence, and enmeshment.

Bulimic clients may also have other impulsive behaviors. It is not unusual for her to have a history of shoplifting, alcohol or drug abuse, suicide attempts, and self-mutilation. The nurse is alert to signs of the pathological behaviors and considers them in her assessment.

Spiritual dimension. The interaction of all the dimensions affects the client's spiritual dimension. Her generally poor physical health, guilt, depression, self-disgust, self-criticism, irrational fears, and preoccupation with weight constrict the quality of her life and prevent her from giving and receiving many pleasures. Although the disorder is not as life threatening as anorexia nervosa, the condition may become chronic; without treatment the client feels a sense of hopelessness about herself and her life.

Analysis

Nursing diagnosis. The defining characteristics of the nursing diagnosis alteration in nutrition: less than body requirements are listed in the box below.

ALTERATIONS IN NUTRITION: LESS THAN BODY REQUIREMENTS

DEFINITION

The state in which an individual experiences an intake of nutrients insufficient to meet metabolic needs.

DEFINING CHARACTERISTICS

Physical Dimension

Loss of weight with adequate food intake
Body weight 20% or more under ideal
Weakness of muscles required for swallowing or mastication
Evidence of lack of food
Aversion to eating
Satiety immediately after eating
Abdominal pain
Sore, inflamed buccal cavity
Capillary fragility
Abdominal cramping
Diarrhea
Hyperactive bowel sounds
Lack of interest in food
Poor muscle tone
Excessive loss of hair

Emotional Dimension

Inability to ingest or digest food because of emotional factors

Intellectual Dimension

Reported inadequate food intake less than RDA (recommended daily allowance)
Reported altered taste sensation
Perceived inability to ingest food
Lack of information
Misinformation
Misconceptions

Adapted from North American Nursing Diagnosis Association Classification of Nursing Diagnosis: Proceedings of the seventh conference, St. Louis, 1987, The C.V. Mosby Co.

DSM-III-R CLASSIFICATIONS RELATED TO EATING DISORDERS OF ADOLESCENCE AND ADULTHOOD

307.10	Anorexia nervosa
307.51	Bulimia nervosa
307.50	Eating disorder not otherwise specified

From American Psychiatric Association: Diagnostic and statistical manual of mental disorders (DSM-III-R), Washington, D.C., 1987, The Association.

The following list provides examples of NANDA-accepted nursing diagnoses with causative statements:

1. Alteration in nutrition: less than body requirements related to self-induced vomiting
2. Alteration in bowel elimination related to insufficient food and fluid intake
3. Fluid volume deficit related to self-induced vomiting
4. Ineffective individual coping related to denial of hunger
5. Fear related to maturing sexuality

DSM-III-R diagnoses. The DSM-III-R classifications related to anorexia nervosa and bulimia nervosa are listed in the box above.

The essential features and manifestations of the features of anorexia nervosa and bulimia nervosa according to the DSM-III-R are listed in the following boxes.

307.10 ANOREXIA NERVOSA

ESSENTIAL FEATURES

The individual is intensely fearful of becoming obese and has a disturbed body image, significant weight loss, and amenorrhea (in females). The disturbance cannot be accounted for by a known physical disorder.

MANIFESTATIONS

Physical Dimension

Disturbed body image
Weight loss of at least 15% of original weight
No known physical illness
Absence of three consecutive menstrual cycles

Emotional Dimension

Feels fat even when emaciated
Intense fear of becoming obese

Intellectual Dimension

Refuses to maintain body weight above a minimal weight for age and height

Adapted from American Psychiatric Association: Diagnostic and statistical manual of mental disorders (DSM-III-R), Washington, D.C., 1987, The Association.

307.51 BULIMIA NERVOSA

ESSENTIAL FEATURES

The individual indulges in binge eating without awareness that the eating pattern is abnormal and fears not being able to stop eating voluntarily.

MANIFESTATIONS

Physical Dimension

Recurring episodes of rapid consumption of large amounts of food in a discrete period (usually less than 2 hours)

Consumption of high-calorie foods

Inconspicuous eating

Termination of eating episodes by abdominal pain, sleep, social interruption, or self-induced vomiting

Repeated attempts to lose weight by severely restricted diets, self-induced vomiting, or use of cathartics or diuretics

Frequent weight fluctuations greater than 10 pounds from alternating binges and fasts

No known physical disorder

Emotional Dimension

Fears not being able to stop eating voluntarily

Depression

Intellectual Dimension

Self-deprecating thoughts following eating binges

Adapted from American Psychiatric Association: Diagnostic and statistical manual of mental disorders (DSM-III-R), Washington, D.C., 1987, The Association.

Planning

See Table 35-6 for examples of long-term and short-term goals and outcome criteria related to anorexia nervosa. These serve as examples of the planning stage in the nursing process.

Implementation: Anorexia Nervosa

✦ *Physical dimension.* The immediate goal of nursing intervention is to restore the anorectic client's nutritional state to normal. Nutritional rehabilitation occurs most efficiently and rapidly in the hospital. The severely ill client requires daily monitoring of weight, fluid, calorie intake, and urine output. Clients are usually fearful of various types of foods, especially high-calorie foods, so the nutritional formula of vitamins, minerals, fatty acids, and carbohydrates given may be blended so the client cannot discard any item. If the client still fails to eat, lifesaving physical interventions, such as a gastrostomy tube, can be used.

The nurse defines a target weight for the client based on average weight tables. If the client has been ill for years, it may be appropriate to agree on a weight that is lighter than average.

Initially the nurse monitors the client 24 hours a day and provides one-to-one supervision. It may be helpful to encourage the client to weigh herself daily and set a realistic goal for weight maintenance. This helps reduce the client's anxiety and fear about weight gain. Gradually the nurse moves the client away from the preoccupation with weight. As the client gains weight, the staff can relax the controls. During the weight restoration period the client may be allowed to select her own foods, which allows a smoother transition to normal eating patterns, and to practice maintaining her target weight with less aid from the nursing staff. Daily exercise is included in the client's activities. The type and amount is clearly specified to discourage overactivity (see the Research Highlight, p. 675).

✳ *Emotional dimension.* When the client seems unconcerned about the seriousness of her eating problem, the nurse attempts to help the client understand it and gain insight into its effect on her physical health. The client needs some awareness of her need to control the environment with her maladaptive eating patterns. It is also important to help the client deal with the many fears she may have: fear of getting fat, of losing control, of maturing sexually, of failure, of becoming independent from her family, and of accepting adult responsibilities.

✳ *Intellectual dimension.* Cognitive restructuring is useful to help the client replace irrational thinking and distorted perceptions about her body and eating. Cognitive restructuring revolves around ways to challenge and change the irrational belief system that the client uses to maintain the eating disorder.

The nurse helps the client substitute her preoccupation with being a perfect person with a more realistic perception of herself by being a role model of an adult, rational thinker. The nurse shows that she is human, capable of making mistakes and accepting responsibility for them. The nurse also helps the client value her abilities and be more accepting of her limitations.

A difficult task facing the nurse is helping the client who does not see that she has an eating problem. The nurse is aware of the client's defenses (denial) and helps reduce the client's anxiety by discussing and exploring possible causes of her anxiety, thus lessening the need for the strong defenses.

❀ *Social dimension.* Behavior modification is the treatment of choice for anorectic clients. Reinforcers include physical activity, visiting privileges, and social activities, contingent on weight gain. Negative reinforcements, such as bed rest, isolation, and tube feeding, are also used at times, especially if the client is severely ill physically.

Most eating disorder programs include family therapy in the treatment regime. The nurse needs to help both the client and family recognize the importance of whole family involvement in treatment. Often family members feel it is the client who has "the problem" and resist coming to therapy sessions. The client, who is usually searching for approval from family and peers, is helped toward less dependence on others. The nurse can help the client move toward more mature, independent, and interdependent actions by exploring the client's perceptions about her current status and can help her become more assertive by allowing her to try out more independent actions

TABLE 35-6 Long-term and short-term goals and outcome criteria related to alteration in nutrition: less than body requirements

Goals	Outcome Criteria

NURSING DIAGNOSIS: ALTERATION IN NUTRITION: LESS THAN BODY REQUIREMENTS RELATED TO FEAR OF GAINING WEIGHT

Long-term goals

Goals	Outcome Criteria
To eat normally and gain weight	Establishes a pattern of eating that promotes weight gain
	Discovers there is nothing to fear in food
	Understands that past food preferences are self-serving to maintain anorexia nervosa
	Sets a reasonable ideal weight and stays in the desired range
To have a positive and realistic self-concept	Statements indicate a positive and realistic view of self

Short-term goals

Goals	Outcome Criteria
To experiment with new and increased amounts of food	Tries new foods with an open mind
	Keeps a diary of when hunger is felt; writes times and what satisfies the hunger
To change perfectionist attitude	Decides that everyone cannot like or love you all the time
	Expects less from self and others
	Learns that communication is necessary
To mature sexually	Verbalizes fear of sexual development
	Realizes that sexual development is not an affront to mother
	Increases intimacy with boyfriend
	Sees that sexual behavior is under self-control
To admit that a problem exists	Admits she is underweight
	Admits fear of weight
	Understands her choice of foods is a compulsion
To examine family relationships	Explores relationship with parents
	Discusses how parents dominate her life
	Recognizes that anorexia nervosa is an expression of family problems
To accept self as a person of value	Statements indicate self-value

Research Highlight

Activity Measures in Anorexia Nervosa

J. Falk, K. Halmi & W. Tryon

PURPOSE

This study was designed to measure the relationship between weight gain and motor activity in anorectic clients.

SAMPLE

The sample consisted of 20 hospitalized anorectic females in their first 2 weeks of hospitalization. Ages ranged from 13 to 21.1 years.

METHODOLOGY

Measurement of wrist and ankle kinetic energy was obtained every 24 hours for 2 weeks. Measures of weight and depression and Minnesota Multiphasic Personality Inventory scores were also examined.

FINDINGS

Results challenge the commonly held notion that activity decreases in anorectic clients as their condition improves: motor activity increased in the first 2 weeks of hospitalization. Increased motor activity is associated with weight gain as treatment progresses.

IMPLICATIONS

Because anorectic clients may have been hyperactive before hospitalization, the emaciated condition that precipitated their hospitalization may have lowered their activity level. Hospitalization also curtails movement to some extent. As clients improve medically, they are able to participate in more activities both inside and outside the hospital. Nurses can be alert to the fact that no increases in motor activity may correspond to an unsuccessful treatment response.

Based on data from Archives of General Psychiatry 42:811, 1985.

(see Chapter 16). The family also needs help in understanding the changes in the client's behavior and in allowing the client to separate from the family.

Some clients are withdrawn and want to spend considerable time alone in their rooms. The nurse helps this individual by establishing a one-to-one relationship and gradually encouraging her to tolerate and eventually enjoy other people. This type of client isolates herself particularly at mealtime. The nurse intervenes by helping the client gradually increase her tolerance of another person's presence at mealtimes. Diversional or recreational social activities are therapeutic. The nurse encourages the client's full participation in activities and recreational therapies, such as occupational therapy and school-related activities (if appropriate).

Therapy is most successful when a multidisciplinary approach is used. Usually a combination of group, individual, behavioral, pharmacotherapy, family, hypnotherapy, and nutritional therapy is required. Self-help groups and eating disorder clinics are growing in popularity. A complete list of self-help organizations for persons with eating disorders may be obtained from the National Anorexic Aid Society, P.O. Box 29461, Columbus, Ohio 43229, 614-895-2009.

Spiritual dimension. A primary goal in treating the spiritual dimension is to offer the client hope, thereby decreasing her feelings of despair. The nurse's confidence that the client can control her pathological eating patterns and her acceptance of the client as a worthwhile and valuable person are ways of offering hope. Promoting meaningful relationships with others and pleasurable activities can increase the client's feelings of worth and value. In addition, it is important to help the client accept herself as a person with potential for achievements and with some limitations.

It is essential to help the client examine reasons for her existence, since eating disorders are seen as self-destructive behavior (see Chapter 14 for specific interventions for suicide and self-destructive behavior).

Implementation: Bulimia Nervosa

Physical dimension. Because the client may attempt to vomit clandestinely, limits and close observation are needed, especially following meals. A contract is made with the client to stop laxative and diuretic use and vomiting. The bulimic client usually feels desperate at this point and is open to a new approach. Reinforcement that it is possible to learn controls is important. The nurse also emphasizes dental and mouth care (since frequent vomiting erodes dental enamel and may ulcerate the mucous membrane of the mouth), checks electrolyte studies, and monitors weight.

Emotional dimension. The nurse recognizes the client's feelings of helplessness, anxiety, anger, frustration, guilt, and depression associated with her eating problem. In addition, she fears that she will not be able to stop eating voluntarily. The nurse helps the client get in touch with these feelings by observing and acknowledging them. Helping the client identify feelings as she experiences them, discussing their possible causes, and exploring other ways of responding to situations that evoke these feelings are important. For example, because stress and tension often precipitate a binge, the nurse explores with the client the cause of the stress and tension and discusses alternative ways to cope with them.

Intellectual dimension. The client is aware that her eating is abnormal yet lacks control of her eating habits. The nurse explores with the client impulses, needs, and feelings that originate in herself. This learning about herself helps repair some of her perceptual difficulties and promotes more realistic thinking. Examining her preceptions about her body and weight also assists in promoting realistic thinking and lessens self-criticism and self-disgust. The nurse does not argue or set unrealistic limits in response to the client's lack of progress.

A cognitive-behavioral approach works well with bulimic clients. Keeping a record of meals and binge episodes helps them become aware of their eating behavior. Self-monitoring is followed by a contract to restrict the client's eating to three or four planned meals a day. Self-control is emphasized. Gradually the client learns to identify circumstances leading to the loss of control and to explore more adaptive ways of coping.

Social dimension. It is essential that the nurse help the client improve her self-concept. Participating in activities that are pleasant for the client, achieving success in tasks or projects, learning new skills, having meaningful relationships with others, giving positive statements to herself, and receiving positive statements from others enhance the self-concept.

Since the bulimic client may be involved in impulsive, acting-out behaviors, such as sexual promiscuity, stealing, lying, or drug abuse, the nurse needs to intervene in these behaviors also. Setting and adhering to agreed-on limits for the client's behavior is an important part of helping the client who exhibits these behaviors. The nurse also needs to help this client face and recognize her feelings and express these feelings in a socially acceptable way. The need to act on feelings is eventually replaced by appropriate ventilation and expression.

It is useful for the nurse to examine the sociocultural influences on binge-purge behaviors. The client needs to know that although society places great value on thinness and the mass media bombards the public with more and more foods to consume, the client can learn to ignore the temptations and control her impulse to eat.

The client may attend groups with other bulimic clients to receive peer support and to begin to reach out to others, which lessens her preoccupation with her own problem. She may also enjoy the humor and lightheartedness often found in groups of young people and begin to experience satisfaction in relationships with others.

Spiritual dimension. The nurse helps the client deal with feelings of hopelessness by displaying confidence and encouragement. By offering hope that the client can control her impulse to binge, the nurse helps the client view life less pessimistically. The nurse helps her find pleasures, either in activities involving others or in those that are satisfying to do alone. A sense of humor is encouraged, as bulimic clients tend to be serious na-

TABLE 35-7 Comparison of anorexia nervosa and bulimia

Features	Anorexia Nervosa	Bulimia Nervosa
Similar	Fear of fatness	
	Pursuit of weight loss	
	Fear of loss of control of eating	
	Distortion of body image	
Contrasting	Severely restricted food intake	Loss of control of intake leading to binges
	Diuretic laxative abuse	Abuse of laxatives, diuretics, or both
	No vomiting	Vomiting
	Younger	Older
	Obsessional, perfectionistic	Histrionic, antisocial, with loss of impulse control
	Denies hunger	Experiences hunger
	Severe weight loss	Variable weight loss
	Introverted	More extroverted
	Eating behavior source of pride	Eating behavior source of shame
	Less sexually active	Sexually active
	Amenorrhea, loss of sex drive	Variable amenorrhea and change in sex drive
	Death from starvation or suicide	Death from hypokalemia or suicide
	"Model" child	May have behavioral problems

tured. New activities, meaningful relationships, and decreased depressive symptoms increase the client's feelings of value and worth, restore a healthy balance to her life, and help to decrease obsession with food and weight.

See Table 35-7 for a comparison of features of anorexia nervosa and bulimia nervosa.

Evaluation

The nurse uses the outcome criteria for each goal that she and the client have established to evaluate the nursing care plan's effectiveness. Treatment for clients with eating disorders is seen as effective when the client maintains an appropriate weight over time according to her height and frame. The client's overall general health is improved. She is in touch with her feelings and uses new adaptive skills to meet her needs rather than relying on food (or the lack of food). She has a realistic perception of herself and her body, and irrational beliefs are replaced with more authentic ones. Her self-concept is positive. Family relationships are improved, and the client moves toward greater independence. In general the client experiences more satisfaction and pleasure when there is less focus on thinness and more emphasis on relationships and activities that lead to a balanced and productive life.

SPECIAL ISSUES
Fasting

Fasting is complete abstinence from food for 24 hours to several weeks. It results in protein loss and severe nitrogen imbalance. Persons fasting show progressive reduction of intestinal activity, which changes the overall physiological and biochemical activities of the gastrointestinal tract. Potassium, sodium bicarbonate, and multivitamin and mineral supplements are important. Therefore, per-

sons should only fast when under close medical supervision. Complications associated with fasting are muscle wasting, severe postural hypotension, hyperuricemia, acidosis, mineral loss, hepatic and renal impairment, nausea and dizziness, increased uric acid levels, and dehydration. About one third of the weight lost in a 24-day fast is fluid and body mass.

Low-Calorie Diets

One popular low-calorie diet consists of liquid mixtures of protein, carbohydrates, and minimal fat and powdered minerals and vitamins. The powder is mixed with water, club soda, or other noncaloric beverage or with fruit juice. The daily calorie content of such a diet ranges from 300 to 800 calories. Serious, sometimes fatal complications have been attributed to these diets. Potential complications are headache, nausea and vomiting, diarrhea or constipation, lethargy and lack of stamina, exacerbation of gout, mineral and electrolyte deficiencies, gum disease from lack of chewing, and cardiac dysrhythmias. Very low-calorie diets administered under careful medical supervision, however, can be effective, particularly for the moderately obese (41% to 100% overweight) and the severely obese (100% overweight). Such programs typically last up to 3 months and can be repeated if needed. An adequate diet provides at least 45 g of protein and 50 mEq of potassium per day. Persons on the diet are examined by health care professionals at least every 2 weeks so that health parameters can be monitored, including EKG and blood tests.

Other popular diets also have dangerous complications, or at best do not meet their claims. The grapefruit diet, for example, is said to help burn off excess calories. On this diet a grapefruit is eaten with each meal to allegedly increase metabolism of the other foods eaten. None of the claims can be substantiated. Resulting weight loss is due not to the grapefruit, but to the reduced calories consumed by the dieter. Another diet, the Zen Macrobiotic diet, is a semistarvation regimen that can lead to nutrient (such as Vitamin C) deficiencies, anemia, hypocalcemia, hypoproteinemia, and decreased renal function.[50]

Human Chorionic Gonadotropin Hormone

Injections of human chorionic gonadotropin hormone (HCG) obtained from the urine of pregnant women have been used to treat obesity. The mechanism of weight reduction is unknown. The claim by its proponents that HCG oxidizes fatty acids and melts fat from the waist and hips is not supported by sound evidence. The American Medical Association warns against this method of weight control.

Appetite Suppressants and Thyroid Hormone Use

Many people turn to pills and injections to lose weight. Anorectic agents help an individual lose only a small amount of weight (about 0.23 kg per week), and efforts at weight loss using appetite suppressants may last only 6 weeks.[3] Appetite suppressants are generally amphetamine derivatives. Appetite suppressants and thyroid hormones have different modes of action, but both increase thermogenesis or depress appetite.

The common belief that obese persons have a hypothyroid or other thyroid problem is not true. Less than 1% of overweight persons actually have abnormal thyroid function. The use of thyroid hormones has complications, including palpitations, sweating, and increased heart rate, systolic blood pressure, and urine calcium excretion.[3]

Vitamin and Mineral Deficiencies

A lack of vitamins and minerals affects a person's total health. Behavioral changes can result from deficiencies in required nutrients. There is much controversy today about the biochemical effect of various nutrients on the brain and thereby on behavior and emotions. Some symptoms of vitamin and mineral deficiences mimic mental illness. Table 35-8 lists some of the behavioral effects of some vitamin deficiencies.[39]

BRIEF REVIEW

Obesity is a severe eating disorder affecting not only the client but also the family and society at large. Millions of dollars are spent annually by overweight individuals trying new methods for weight loss. Anorexia nervosa and bulimia nervosa are reaching epidemic proportions as young people seek to lose weight and severely impair their physical health by self-induced starvation and binging and purging.

Theoretical explanations for eating disorders are excessive dieting and exercising, rejection of female sexual development, a learned response to emotional arousal, irrational beliefs about thinness, a negative self-concept, family conflicts (especially between mother and daughter), and family and cultural influences about food and eating.

The components of the nursing process are described as they relate specifically to obesity, anorexia nervosa, and bulimia nervosa. Fasting, low-calorie diets, and the effects of vitamin and mineral deficiencies on behavior are also discussed.

Research findings indicate that many people perceive themselves as overweight when objective measures do not substantiate it. Findings also indicate that obese persons are clearly at risk for impaired physical health.

TABLE 35-8 Behavioral effects of vitamin deficiencies

Vitamin	Behavioral Effect
Thiamine (B$_1$)	Wernicke's encephalopathy
	Memory loss
	Depression
	Apathy
	Irritability
	Korsakoff's psychosis
Riboflavin (B$_2$)	Change in body perception with severe physical symptoms
Niacin, niancinamide (B$_3$)	Organic dementia
	Delirium
	Memory deficits
	Apathy
	Depression
	Anxiety
	Hyperirritability
	Mania
Pyridoxine, pyridoxal, pyridoxamine (B$_6$)	Poor concentration
	Memory impairment
	Depression
	Nervous irritability
	Hyperacousia
Pantothenic acid	Poor concentration
	Restlessness
	Irritability
	Fatigue
	Depression
Biotin (H)	Lassitude
	Depression
Cyanocobalamin (B$_{12}$)	Confusion
	Irritability
	Memory loss
	Hallucinations
	Delusions
	Paranoia
Folic acid (B$_c$)	Forgetfulness
	Apathy
	Irritability
	Depression
	Psychosis
	Delirium
	Dementia
Ascorbic acid (C)	Lassitude
	Hypochondriasis
	Depression
	Hysteria

Adapted from Mahan, L., and Rees, J.: Nutrition in adolescence, St. Louis, 1984, The C.V. Mosby Co.

REFERENCES AND SUGGESTED READINGS

1. American Psychiatric Association: Diagnostic and statistical manual of mental disorders (DSM-III-R), Washington, D.C., 1987, American Psychiatric Association.
2. Anderson, A.: Anorexia nervosa and bulimia, Journal of Adolescent Health Care 4:15, 1983.
3. Blackburn, G., and Pavlov, K.: Fad reducing diets: separating fads from facts, Journal of Dentistry for Children 84:382, 1984.
4. Bray, G.A.: The obese patient, Philadelphia, 1976, W.B. Saunders Co.
5. Brownell, K.: Obesity: understanding and treating a serious, prevalent, and refractory disorder, Journal of Consulting and Clinical Psychology 50:820, 1982.
6. Bruch, H.: The golden cage: the enigma of anorexia nervosa, 1978, Harvard University Press.
7. Carpenito, L.: Handbook of nursing diagnoses, Philadelphia, 1984, J.B. Lippincott Co.
8. Casper, R., and others: Bulimia: its incidence and clinical importance in patients with anorexia nervosa, Archives of General Psychiatry 37:1030, 1980.
9. Cauwells, J.: Bulimia, New York, 1983, Doubleday & Co., Inc.
10. Chapian, M., and Coyle, N.: Free to be thin, Minneapolis, 1979, Bethany House Publishers.
11. Ciseaux, A.: Anorexia nervosa: a view from the mirror, American Journal of Nursing, 80:1468, 1980.
12. Colliver, J., Frank, S., and Frank, A.: Similarity of obesity indices in clinical studies of obese adults: a factor analytic study, American Journal of Clinical Nutrition 38:640, 1983.
13. Cosens, R.: Obesity in the aged, Nursing Clinics of North America 17:227, 1982.
14. Court, J.: Energy expenditure of obese children: techniques for measuring energy expenditures over periods of up to 24 hours, Archives of Diseases in Childhood 47:153, 1972.
15. Crisp, A.H.: Anorexia nervosa: let me be, Orlando, Fla., 1980, Grune & Stratton, Inc.
16. Crocker, K., Gerber, F., and Shearer, J.: Metabolism of carbohydrate, protein, and fat, Nursing Clinics of North America 18:3, 1983.
17. Daniels, A.: Obesity in adolescence. In Wolman, B., editor: Psychological aspects of obesity, New York, 1982, Van Nostrand Reinhold Co.
17a. Deering, C.: Developing a therapeutic alliance with an anorexia nervosa client, Journal of Psychosocial Nursing and Mental Health Services 25(3):10, 1987.
18. DeJong, W.: The stigma of obesity: the consequences of naive assumptions concerning the causes of physical deviance, Journal of Health and Social Behavior 21:75, 1980.
19. Ellis, R., and Harper, R.: A new guide to rational living, North Hollywood, Calif., 1975, Wilshire Book Co.
20. Falk, J., Halmi, K., and Tryon, W.: Activity measures in anorexia nervosa, Archives of General Psychiatry 42:811, 1985.
21. Fisher, J., Nadler, A., and Whitcher-Alagna, S.: Recipient reactions to aid, Psychological Bulletin 91:27, 1982.
22. Garfinkel, P.: Some recent observations on the pathogenesis of anorexia nervosa, Canadian Journal of Psychiatry 37:1036, 1980.
23. Garner, D., and Garfinkel, P., editors: Handbook of psychotherapy for anorexia nervosa and bulimia, New York, 1985, The Guilford Press.
24. Gierszewski, S.: The relationship of weight loss, locus of control, and social support, Nursing Research 32:43, 1983.
25. Grosniklaus, D.: Nursing interventions in anorexia nervosa, Perspectives in Psychiatric Care 18:1, 1980.
26. Hagenbuch, V.: Obesity and the school-age child, Nursing Clinics of North America 17:207, 1982.

27. Halmi, K.A.: Pragmatic information on the eating disorders, Psychiatric Clinics of North America 5:371, 1982.
28. Hawkins, R., Fremoow, W., and Clement, P.: The binge-purge syndrome, New York, 1984, Springer Publishing Co., Inc.
29. Herzog, D.: Bulimia in the adolescent, American Journal of Diseases of Children 136:985, 1982.
30. Hudson, J., Laffer, P., and Pope, H.: Bulimia related to affective disorder by family history and response to the dexamethasone suppression test, American Journal of Psychiatry 139:685, 1982.
31. Jarvis, W.: Food fads, fallacies, and frauds, CDA Journal 12:24, 1984.
32. Johnson, P.: Getting enough to grow on, American Journal of Nursing 84:336, 1984.
32a. Kaye, W., and Gwirtsman, H.: A comprehensive approach to the treatment of normal weight bulimia, Washington, D.C., 1985, American Psychiatric Association.
33. Keltner, N.: Bulimia: controlling compulsive eating, Journal of Psychosocial Nursing and Mental Health Services 22:24, 1984.
34. Kempe, A., and Gelazis, R.: Rational emotive techniques for overweight adults: a cognitive-behavioral group approach. In Abstracts of Research Day, Little Rock, Ark., 1984, The University of Arkansas for Medical Sciences.
35. Kruse, M., and Mahan, L.: Food, nutrition and diet therapy, Philadelphia, 1984, W.B. Saunders Co.
36. Lasky, P., and Eichelberger, K.: Implications, considerations, and nursing interventions of obesity in neonatal and preschool patients, Nursing Clinics of North America 17:199, 1982.
37. Leon, G.R.: Personality and behavioral correlates of obesity. In Wolman, B., editor: Psychological aspects of obesity: a handbook, New York, 1982, Van Nostrand Reinhold Co.
38. Lukert, B.: Biology of obesity. In Wolman, B., editor: Psychological aspects of obesity: a handbook, New York, 1982, Van Nostrand Reinhold Co.
39. Mahan, L., and Rees, J.: Nutrition in adolescence, St. Louis, 1984, The C.V. Mosby Co.
40. Marks, R.: Anorexia and bulimia: eating habits that can kill, R.N. 84:44, 1984.
41. Minuchin, S., Rosman, B.L., and Baker, L.: Psychosomatic families: anorexia nervosa in context, Washington, D.C., 1978, Harvard University Press.
42. Myers, K., and Smith, M.: Psychogenic polydypsia in a patient with anorexia nervosa, Journal of Adolescent Health Care 6:404, 1985.
43. Nightingale, F.: Notes on nursing: what it is and what it is not, Mineola, N.Y., 1960, Dover Publications, Inc.
44. Orbach, S.: Fat is a feminist issue: the anti-diet guide to permanent weight loss, New York, 1982, Jason Aronson, Inc.
45. Pope, H., and Hudson, J.: New hope for binge eaters, New York, 1984, Harper & Row, Publishers, Inc.
46. Phillott, W., and Kalita, D.: Brain allergies: the psychonutrient connection, New Canaan, Conn., 1980, Keats Publishing, Inc.
47. Popkess-Vawter, S.: Reducing cardiac risk factors in the obese patient, Nursing Clinics of North America 17:233, 1982.
48. Rand, C., and Stunkard, A.: Obesity and psychoanalysis: treatment and four-year follow-up, American Journal of Psychiatry 140:1140, 1983.
49. Reed, G., and Sech, E.: Bulimia: a conceptual model for group treatment, Journal of Psychosocial Nursing and Mental Health Services 23:16, 1985.

50. Richardson, T.: Anorexia nervosa: an overview, American Journal of Nursing **80**:1470, 1980.

51. Russ, C.: Fat diets for the treatment of obesity, CDA Journal **12**:60, 1984.

52. Stewart, A., and Brook, R.: Effects of being overweight, American Journal of Public Health **73**:171, 1983.

53. Stunkard, A., and Stellar, E.: Eating and its disorders, New York, 1984, Raven Press.

54. White, J.: An overview of obesity: its significance to nursing, Nursing Clinics of North America **17**:191, 1982.

55. Williams, S.: Mowry's basic nutrition and diet therapy, St. Louis, 1984, The C.V. Mosby Co.

56. Wilson, G.T., and Brownell, K.: Behavior therapy for obesity: an evaluation of treatment outcome, Advances in Behavioral Research and Therapy **3**:49, 1980.

57. Wilson, P., editor: Fear of being fat, New York, 1983, Jason Aronson, Inc.

58. Wolman, B., editor: Psychological aspects of obesity: a handbook, New York, 1982, Van Nostrand Reinhold Co.

ANNOTATED BIBLIOGRAPHY

American Journal of Nursing **80**(8), 1980.

Several articles in this issue discuss anorexia nervosa from a nursing perspective: Ciseaux, A.: Anorexia nervosa: a view from the mirror, p. 1468; Clagett, M.: Anorexia nervosa: a behavioral approach, p. 1471; Richardson, T.: Anorexia nervosa: an overview, p. 1470.

Carino, C., and Chmelko, P.: Disorders of eating in adolescence: anorexia nervosa and bulimia, Nursing Clinics of North America **18**:343, 1983.

This article suggests a holistic approach to nursing care for the anorectic or bulimic client. It provides helpful suggestions for therapy, including ways to involve not only the client but also significant others. Definition of the disorders and underlying theoretical premises are clearly stated.

White J.: An overview of obesity: its significance to nursing, Nursing Clinics of North America **17**:191, 1982.

This article gives a thorough overview of obesity and discusses appropriate nursing care. The multiple causes of and treatment approaches to obesity are explored.

CHAPTER 36

THERAPY WITH VICTIMS OF ABUSE

Virginia Koch Drake

After studying this chapter the learner will be able to:

Define and identify major types of abuse and neglect.

Discuss theoretical approaches to abusive situations.

Describe characteristics of individuals at risk for being a victim or perpetrator of abuse.

Review common myths and beliefs about victims and perpetrators of abuse.

Implement the nursing process to provide care for clients at risk for or involved in abusive situations.

Types of abuse include child abuse, sexual abuse, consort abuse, elder abuse, and rape. These types of abuse occur irrespective of age, race, religious, socioeconomic, occupational, educational, cultural, or other boundaries. Experts agree that each of these forms of violence needs to be of serious concern to society and to health care professionals.

For the purpose of this chapter the following definitions are given of the forms of abuse:

Physical abuse is an intentional injury, harmful deed, or destructive act inflicted by a parent, spouse, guardian, mature child, or caregiver on another person with whom an interpersonal or advocacy relationship is shared.

Physical neglect is the volitional deprivation of essential care necessary to sustain life, growth, and development. Neglect may ensue from acts of omission in securing the essential physical care or through failure to provide a safe environment.

Emotional abuse is the use of implicit or explicit threats, verbal assaults, or acts of degradation that are injurious or damaging to an individual's sense of self-worth. Verbal or nonverbal actions intended to provoke suffering or disrupt another's psychological equilibrium constitute emotional abuse.

Emotional neglect is the lack of maintaining an interpersonal atmosphere conducive for psychosocial growth and development of a sense of personal worth and well-being. Healthy psychological maturation is stifled and thwarted, resulting in varying degrees of emotional crippling.

Material abuse, primarily perpetrated on the elderly, is the theft or misuse of an individual's property or money.

Violation of rights is a form of elderly abuse occurring when an individual is forced from his home or coerced into a nursing home unnecessarily.

Definitions of child abuse, sexual abuse, consort abuse, elderly abuse, and rape are provided as these specific topics are discussed in this chapter.

THEORETICAL APPROACHES
Social Learning Theory

General agreement exists among social learning theorists that violence in the family begets violence. Children learn behavior by imitating or modeling the behavior of family and friends. Physical punishment by a parent can teach a child some unintended lessons. They learn that the persons who love them the most are the same ones who strike them. They also learn that violence may be used to obtain a desirable result, which implicitly sanctions the use of violence as a means to an end. Because most parents do not use physical punishment until all else has failed, the child may learn violence as a solution when other methods have been unsuccessful. Children become

Historical Overview

DATE	EVENT
1800s	British common law permitted husbands to discipline their wives as long as the "rod" was no thicker than the husband's thumb.
Mid-1800s	The Society for the Prevention of Cruelty to Animals interceded on behalf of a child discovered in New York City who was suffering from malnutrition and severe beatings inflicted by her adoptive parents.
Late 1800s	U.S. laws gave men implicit and explicit permission to beat their wives.
1871	The Society for the Prevention of Cruelty to Children was established in New York City.
1886	A bill proposed in Pennsylvania to make wife beating a crime failed.
1962	The phrase *battered child syndrome* was originated by Kempe[35] to emphasize the malevolent actions perpetrated on children by their parents or other adults.
1968	All states had developed legal mandates to report child abuse.
1973	The Child Abuse Prevention and Treatment Act advanced the legal responsibilities of nurses and other health care providers encountering child abuse or neglect.
1975	The label *battered child syndrome* was replaced by the term *child abuse and neglect.*
Late 1970s to Early 1980s	Recognition of elderly abuse expanded, and nurses began to write about their role in responding to the problem.
1980s	Legislation affording women protection from their husbands' physical assaults emerged; at least 43 states enable abused spouses to obtain civil protection orders without initiating divorce proceedings, as was previously required.
1985	Approximately half of the states recognized marital rape as a criminal offense.
	A U.S. Surgeon General's report stated that health care professionals must take the lead in preventing and protecting individuals against family violence.
	Only eight states had legally abolished corporal punishment in schools.
Future	With the number of elderly people expected to double in the next 50 years, it is highly probable that the incidence of elder abuse will increase. Other types of family violence will probably be affected by a refocusing of family values brought about by the AIDS epidemic.

violence-prone adults or potentially vulnerable victims of violence.

Mounting evidence suggests that the dynamics of abuse within a family are essentially the same whether a child or adult is the object of the attack. The perpetrator of the assault responds to a perceived threat from the victim with aggressive behavior. At the time of the assault one individual is subordinated by the other's use of force. Exposure to violence within a family affects every member of the household, even those not directly involved.

Straus, Gelles, and Steinmetz[34] found a positive correlation between the amount of physical punishment experienced by a child and the rate of spouse abuse. Each form of abuse increases in relation to the other: "The people who experienced the most punishment as teen-agers have a rate of wife-beating and husband-beating that is four times greater than those whose parents did not hit them." The lowest rate of conjugal violence is among individuals who were not struck by their parents when teenagers.

Stress management is a skill lacking in abusive families. Their inability to handle stress contributes to problems of abuse or neglect. Increased stress generates greater frustrations. Poor impulse control, a characteristic of abusers, causes them to react without benefit of problem solving. Victims tend to blame themselves for the chaos the family is experiencing. No one in the family feels good, each member feels pulled in many directions, and support for one another is minimal or nonexistent.

The Cycle of Violence

Similarities in the cyclical nature of family violence exist regardless of the age, sex, or role status of the victim. Walker[38] has identified three phases in the cycle of violence: the tension building phase, the explosion phase, and the honeymoon phase (Figure 36-1).

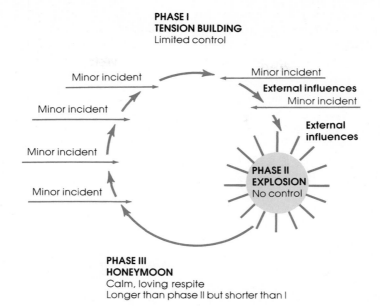

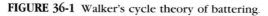

FIGURE 36-1 Walker's cycle theory of battering.

Phase I of the cycle of violence is labeled the tension building phase. During this time of minor assaults, perpetrators may push or throw things at their victims, inflict contusions, subject them to verbal assaults and threats, or humiliate and harm them in other ways. Initially victims may attempt to comply with demands of their mates in an effort to squelch their anger and hostility. In so doing the victims become unwitting accomplices, in effect implicitly accepting partial responsibility for the abusive situation. Batterers become increasingly oppressive and possessive to maintain control over their victims. This approach is usually effective. Women take extraordinary measures to maintain the precarious equilibrium. Fearing that the aggression may be unleashed on others close to them, battered women distance the couple from supportive persons such as grown children, parents, siblings, and close friends. This isolation provides batterers with even greater leverage and control, further jeopardizing the women's safety. As the delicate balance becomes more difficult to maintain because of escalating tension, coping mechanisms begin to disintegrate. Mounting tension can no longer be contained, and phase II erupts.

Phase II is ushered in by an incident of major trauma. It is characterized by a volatile discharge of aggression by the offender, lack of control, and destructiveness. During this time some batterers are so consumed by rage that they lose conscious control of their behavior.

Lack of predictability and total lack of control characterize phase II, which lasts approximately 2 to 24 hours. Only the batterers are able to interrupt this stage. Victims can do little more than try to protect themselves or find a safe place to hide. Acute battering ceases when perpetrators become so physically and emotionally drained they collapse.

Shock and disbelief follow these attacks. To minimize their fear, victims attempt to ignore or understate the se-

verity of their injuries. The gravity of the injuries usually determines whether and when battered women will seek medical care.

The cycle concludes with phase III, the honeymoon phase, a period of tenderness, love, contrition, or truce, which is a respite for the couple from the viciousness of Phase II. The calm characteristic of phase III, follows almost immediately on the heels of the storm of phase II. Victims yearn to believe that love will prevail and that the last attack will be the final one. Phase III lasts longer than phase II but is briefer than phase I when the cycle begins again.

Chronic cycles of violence are often shortened into two phases: tension buildup and violent eruption. Periods of respite become shorter and the truce more uneasy.

Characteristics of Victims

Victims of abuse share common characteristics regardless of age or sex. They are dependent, helpless, and powerless or suffer crippling feelings of dependence, helplessness, or powerlessness. Feelings of terror, anger, and heightened anxiety, numerous physical complaints, and health problems characterize the victim profile. These individuals feel responsible for the abuse or neglect inflicted on them, accepting blame or blaming themselves for the perpetrator's actions. The victims are unclear about their reasons for feeling guilty; they assume they must cause the offender to behave the way he does. Victims will recite a litany of specious explanations for the perpetrator's actions.

The victims also exhibit low self-esteem and depression. They question that they are worthy to be loved and treated with respect. If they are worthy, victims wonder, why then do they suffer at the hands of those who profess to love them? When blamed by perpetrators for their malevolent behavior, victims readily accept the idea. In addition to the physical injuries sustained, emotional damage persists long after physical health is restored. Permanent scars from physical trauma are not uncommon to victims of abuse.

In both child and consort abuse, the response of victims is to "try harder." They believe that if they can only do better in the future, the abuse will cease. Batterers readily support this fallacious logic and are more than willing to shift the blame for their offenses. Victims are doomed to fail, because they can never fulfill the unrealistic needs and expectations of the offenders.

Characteristics of Persons Who Abuse

Perpetrators of abuse exhibit a frightening lack of control over aggressive impulses which are discharged through explosive behavior. Many similarities exist among consort, child, and elder abusers. The offenders explain their assaultive behavior as attempts at disciplinary action that "got out of hand." They protest their innocence as abusers with spurious explanations.

Abusers experience low self-esteem and project the blame for their shortcomings on others. They are easily frustrated and unable to channel their feelings of frustration in a constructive fashion.

Emotional immaturity is characteristic of perpetrators of violence. They find themselves unable to process reality favorably. As their levels of tension and anxiety escalate, these individuals finally erupt, striking out at the most accessible, vulnerable person in their environment.

The deficit in their level of emotional maturity is characterized by narcissism. The self-centeredness of those who abuse prevents them from engaging in meaningful adult relationships. Abusers are too preoccupied with self-gain to invest any substantial quality of themselves in others. Their egocentricity interferes with their ability to recognize needs of others. Narcissistic, emotionally immature adults perceive others as objects responsible for meeting their needs.

Persons who abuse have a tendency to be suspicious of everyone—family, friends, business associates, and strangers. An obvious explanation for their suspicion is fear of being exposed. The fact that individuals who batter usually become violent within the confines of their own homes lends credibility to the speculation that they are aware of their trangressions against the norms of western society.

Distrust of others compels persons who abuse to isolate their families. The spouse and children are discouraged from having friends and attending activities unaccompanied by the one who abuses. The omnipresent fear is that someone will discover the abuse situation. Children are urged not to answer questions or talk to persons outside the nuclear family. Even the nuclear family becomes distanced from the extended family to preclude discovery of the abusive pattern. The one who abuses often goes to extraordinary lengths to protect the cover-up. The social network of the family becomes minimal.

Ordinarily the person who abuses possesses greater physical strength than the victim, which may be one reason more women than men are abused during cohabitation. In elder abuse, gender may not be a dominant factor.

Physical size, strength, and power do not play as important a role in child abuse. Clearly both parents are stronger, larger, and more powerful than their children until adolescence.

Persons not familiar with characteristics of abusive situations are misled if they expect the participants in violence to appear abnormal, mentally ill, or mentally incompetent. Individuals who abuse are difficult to detect in a social or business setting. Some may exhibit overt symptoms of emotional dysfunction; however, the nurse cannot rely on overt psychopathological features to identify perpetrators of abuse and neglect.

Nursing Process

One individual needs to be responsible for conducting the in-depth interview in each treatment setting so that detailed interviews are not conducted repetitiously by every person requiring information in each setting.

The victim's interview needs to be private. Someone remains with the victim at all times to provide emotional support and ensure the client's safety. In general, each victim needs to be interviewed separately from other individuals providing data. This arrangement provides an opportunity to evaluate the reliability and consistency of interview data. If abuse has occurred, this separate arrangement may meet with resistance from the perpetrator. In some agencies, one staff member interviews the victim while others interview the people who accompanied the victim to the treatment setting.

Interviews are approached with a matter-of-fact, nonthreatening demeanor. Tones and inflections in the voice are carefully controlled. A nonjudgmental attitude is crucial to the process, and establishing trust is essential. Histories of assault are accepted as being truthful unless concrete evidence to the contrary is uncovered. Victims will err more often by not admitting to assault than persons will fabricate an assault.

The interview is best structured by asking general, less-threatening questions initially. For example, the nurse may begin with, "What can I do to help you today?" rather than focusing immediately on obvious injuries. This communicates the nurse's personal willingness to assist the client and indicates her readiness to listen to the client. Some victims experience a sense of urgency to discuss their abuse or crisis as if waiting will prevent them from admitting the truth. Other victims may test the nurse before revealing intimate information they think will reflect on them unfavorably.

When abuse is suspected, the nurse needs to question the client about it directly. For example, the nurse may say, "Your injuries are like those of another woman (or child) I cared for. That person had been beaten (assaulted, attacked, or raped). I am wondering if the same thing happened to you. We are prepared to help people in those circumstances here." The victim needs to be reassured that if abuse is revealed she will be afforded some protection. Frequently the victim's assailant is the person who accompanies her to the health care agency! Offers for assistance that cannot be provided must never be extended to the victim.

The nurse needs to exercise extreme caution in contact with suspected batterers. They expect to encounter hostility and skepticism and to have their statements impugned. If so, their expectations that no one understands or will help them are confirmed. They are then lost as allies in the nursing process. Cooperation from the alleged batterer will benefit the victim's treatment. A stalemate or negative relationship between the nurse and suspected batterer is destructive to the treatment process. Although it is difficult for others to understand, the nurse needs to remain mindful that most victims continue to love their abuser.

Abusers and victims may choose alternate treatment settings to avoid arousing suspicion. They do not want to become known or familiar to any specific caregivers. In this way they avoid establishing an obvious or traceable pattern of repetitious injuries.

The nurse involved in cases of abuse may be called to testify in court. The nurse's assessment is recorded carefully, comprehensively, and explicitly. Verbatim statements are used whenever possible. A tape recorded statement or interview is more useful. Clear, precise statements about observations, supplemented by examples when possible, are necessary. The nurse's notes need to be decisive. Terminology such as "Client *appears* to have a contusion on left upper arm" is avoided. Either a contusion is present or it is not. When the nurse cannot be certain about an observation, clarity is provided by noting what was observed or heard that contributed to the conclusions.

Basic psychiatric nursing principles are required to provide optimal care for victims of abuse, even though these individuals are not usually seen by psychiatric nurses. Commonly, victims are assessed for their physical injuries in emergency rooms, private physicians' offices, and other facilities. When hospitalization is required, the client is usually admitted to a unit specializing in care for the victim's type of physical injuries. Whenever possible a psychiatric nurse is consulted for input to the care plan, even when she will not be the primary care provider. Keen observation of the interactions and behavior of the individuals being interviewed can yield a wealth of information. The box below left outlines some general guidelines for the assessment interview with the abused client.

CHILD ABUSE

Child abuse or neglect is the physical or mental injury, sexual abuse, negligent treatment or maltreatment of the child under the age of 18 years by a person who is responsible for the child's welfare under circumstances which indicate that the child's health or welfare is harmed or threatened thereby.

Because all states have mandatory reporting laws for confirmed or suspected child abuse, failure to report these cases puts the nurse in direct violation of the law.

Assessment

Physical dimension. Their essentially total dependence on caregivers places infants, toddlers, and preschool children at particularly high risk for abuse. Unrefined cognitive, motor, and verbal skills preclude children from comprehending their predicament, defending themselves, or articulating their plight. Still more vulnerable are children with handicaps and special needs or problems. Although the probability of physical abuse decreases with age, incest and sexual abuse become more likely.

An important feature of child abuse is the cyclical, repetitious nature of the act. Previous trauma may have left the child with permanent physical impairment or other telltale signs, such as scarring.

A detailed history focusing on the injury is obtained from the parents. The child is interviewed in a manner suitable to his age and physical and emotional status. The interviewer proceeds with extreme caution to mitigate defensiveness in the parents and child. Age-appropriate explanations are given to the child as the examination proceeds.

All external signs of trauma are observed and precisely recorded for appearance, size, location, color, and shape. Evidence of scarring is recorded. Head injury is the major cause of death and permanent disability in children under 2 years of age; therefore special attention is given to internal ear and ophthalmoscopic examinations. All body orifices are inspected carefully for indications of trauma. Bones and joints are manipulated for tenderness and range of motion.

Sleep patterns are explored with child and parent. Evidence of *night terrors, somnambulism, somniloquy,* en-

---

ASSESSMENT GUIDELINES FOR ABUSED VICTIMS

Nonverbal communication between client and parent, partner, or caregiver

Verbal communication between client and partner or parent

Nonverbal communication between client and nurse and parent, partner, or caregiver

Body language of client and parent, partner, or caregiver

Balance of communication among interviewer, client, and parent, partner, or caregiver

Dominant or submissive behavior of client and parent, partner, or caregiver

Affectual responses to interview material

Ability to answer directly versus subject changes and evasive, tangential, or irrelevant answers

Comfort levels of individuals during interview

uresis, insomnia, excessive sleeping, chronic fatigue, or any change is probed. Eating patterns are investigated. Failure to thrive and malnourishment are common manifestations of child abuse. The child's height, weight, and head circumference are graphed for comparison to the norm. Excessive weight gain or loss may signify interpersonal problems. Difficulty swallowing or chewing may result from head or neck trauma. Because head injuries are so prevalent among battered children, neurological function is carefully evaluated. Mastery of age-appropriate developmental tasks is assessed and deficiencies recorded. The current status of immunizations and dental care is evaluated. These health needs are usually unmet in children suffering from abuse or neglect.

Individuals unfamiliar with child abuse find it difficult to comprehend the severity and atrocity of trauma inflicted. No form of torture can be ruled out. Health care providers need to avoid appearing shocked and disbelieving when hearing histories of abused children. Those who work with child abuse are familiar with cases of infants being placed in hot frying pans on the stove, submerged in scalding water, or burned with cigarettes, electric cords, or electric cattle prods. Common injuries resulting from battering of children are listed below.

Any delay in obtaining medical attention alerts the nurse to consider child abuse. Parents who inflict injury on a child postpone seeking treatment for the victim. Victims of child abuse are often dead on arrival at the health care agency.

Radiological studies need to be conducted in every case of suspected abuse of children under age 5. Decisions on older children about such studies are made consistent with initial signs and symptoms. Frequently, multiple bone injuries in various stages of healing are demonstrated in abused children.

If death results from an assault, the case automatically becomes a police matter. The nurse needs to scrupulously avoid disturbing any possible evidence. The body is not to be handled without permission. Nothing is discarded or cleaned until clearance has been granted.

Identification or suspicion of child abuse immediately evokes the question of sexual abuse. If a vaginal examination is required, all persons involved need specific knowledge about proper protocol. Evidence that meets legal criteria is collected during the course of the examination. Specimens for sexually transmitted diseases need to be collected if there is evidence of genitourinary trauma.

Emotional dimension. The emotional sequelae of abuse may be expressed through a myriad of behaviors. A child who has been maltreated by persons who should love him the most finds it difficult, if not impossible, to trust. Efforts to "give to" the child undoubtedly will precipitate suspicious feelings. The child will find it difficult to accept that strangers want to give him what his parents will not. Emotional responses to note are fear, sadness, hopelessness, helplessness, depression, suspicion, withdrawal, flat or blunted affect, unusual aggressiveness, hostility, mood swings, inappropriate affect, or other erratic behavior. Any child may experience any of these responses for other reasons. It is the responsibility of the nurse to make some sense out of the child's emotional response or consult with someone about the meaning of the child's behavior.

Fear in the presence of parents is an especially revealing clue to child abuse. The child may avoid looking at his parents or his eyes may dart back and forth nervously. The youngster may appear to shrink away from his parents or to hide from one parent behind the other. In strange or otherwise frightening situations, most children look to their parents for comfort and reassurance—this may not be so in the abused child.

Inappropriate interaction between parents and child warrants exploration by the nurse. The parents may hover too closely about the child or may be preoccupied with themselves. Some adults and children demonstrate unusual affects in times of stress. Unusual affect is not prima facie evidence of child abuse; however, its significance to the total assessment needs to be noted.

Intellectual dimension. Delayed speech and limited vocabulary are not uncommon in abused children. Academic achievement may decline or classroom performance may be poor from the onset for no reason obvious to educators. The cognitive skills usually present in children who are of like age, developmental stage, and intellect may be lacking in young victims of abuse. These youngsters can manifest decreased attention spans or memory impairments.

Social dimension. Observation of parent-child interaction is a fertile area for cues that may indicate difficulty. Do the parents appear overly solicitous or protective of the child? Will the parents allow the child to answer questions directed toward him, or do they interrupt and try to answer instead? Are the parents unwilling or reluctant to leave the child alone with the nurse or other health care providers? The parents may be afraid of what the child will say if asked how the injury occurred.

COMMON INJURIES OF BATTERED CHILDREN

Head injuries
Internal injuries
Multiple fractures
Soft tissue trauma
Facial trauma (for example, black eyes, gag burns, nose injuries, damaged or missing teeth)
Contusions over entire body
Marks on neck suggestive of strangulation
Burn marks from cigarettes, stove burners, or radiators
Rope burns on wrists and ankles
Lacerations from belt buckles or coat hangers, especially on back or buttocks
Hematomas
Blisters or burns from scalding water
Human bite marks
Bald spots on head from which hair has been pulled
Trauma to genitalia
Injuries in various stages of healing
Evidence of scarring and healed fractures

They want to control or "interpret" anything the child says. If the parents demand to be in the room when the nurse is talking to the child, the nurse firmly reminds the parents that the question or comment was directed to the child for his response. Is the parents' behavior appropriate to the situation? The Case Example below illustrates inappropriate parental behavior.

Case Example

A 9-year-old girl was admitted to an emergency room on an extremely hot day in July after having sustained third-degree burns over 60% of her body. The mother explained that the girl had been playing with matches and "caught on fire." The girl corroborated the mother's explanation of the fire. This mother demonstrated behaviors characteristic of an abusive parent. The nurse noticed the mother was wearing a coat and chain smoking. When the nurse suggested that the mother remove her coat, she became very defensive, verbally assaulting the nurse. The mother maintained she was extremely cold. Later, when it became necessary for the mother to remove her coat, her clothes beneath reeked of gasoline. The mother had drenched her daughter in gasoline and set her afire. The girl was unable to admit the truth until she had established a trusting relationship with one of the nurses after being hospitalized for several weeks.

Lack of age-appropriate anxiety in the presence of strangers is characteristic of abused infants; instead of experiencing the separation anxiety normally seen in infants 9 to 12 months of age, abused babies may relate to anyone. Decreased discrimination may continue for several years and may be misinterpreted as evidence of a well-adjusted baby.

Older children may be too intimidated and frightened of adults to interact comfortably with anyone. The environment of victimized youngsters is perceived as a terrifying place.

The child's school attendance record is explored in cases of suspected abuse. School nurses and teachers are potentially good sources of information. Their observations about classroom attendance and behavior may provide useful input to the assessment. Abused children may have a pattern of visits to the school health clinic with vague complaints or problems from their injuries. Recurrent physical illnesses caused by inadequate health care or physical trauma may keep the child out of school. The child may lack adequate clothing or supplies, and it is not uncommon for parents to keep older children out of school to care for younger siblings or perform household chores. Distancing the child from school is another way to socially isolate the youngster from inquisitive people. The child may not grasp the implications of not going to school.

Abused children may not be allowed to establish relationships with peers, or in view of their circumstances, they may be reluctant to do so. Being a "loner" provides some protection from questions about visible injuries. Deficient social skills may interfere with the victim's ability to establish or maintain peer relationships. The more isolated the victim's social network, the less likely it is that the abuse will be uncovered.

Spiritual dimension. The child may question the existence of a benevolent superior being who allows his life to be so miserable and painful. The child might decide on the basis of the maltreatment he receives that he is unloveable or bad. Parents may tell the child he is being beaten to ward off or drive out evil spirits. Some parents view this form of "discipline" as their religious duty. These practices are more common in strict, fundamentalist religions.

Analysis

Nursing diagnosis. The following list provides examples of NANDA-accepted nursing diagnoses with causative statements:
1. Alterations in parenting related to having been abused as a child
2. Ineffective family coping related to secrecy about abusive situation
3. Fear related to child abuse
4. Anxiety related to parent's abusive behavior
5. Disturbance in self-concept related to repeated abuse by mother
6. Sleep pattern disturbance related to fear of being abused

Planning

Table 36-1 provides some long-term and short-term goals and outcome criteria related to child abuse. These serve as examples of the planning stage in the nursing process.

Implementation

Physical dimension. When abuse is suspected or confirmed, immediate intervention is directed toward protecting the child from additional trauma and treating his current injuries. Hospitalization may be indicated for temporary protection and an in-depth diagnostic workup to gain time to outline long-term treatment strategies.

The laboratory and x-ray procedures ordered by the physician are carefully explained to the parent by the nurse, who remains with the child for support. Depending on the injuries, a tetanus booster may be indicated and other immunizations updated. Special diets are provided for nutritional deficiencies or excesses. Classes in nutrition can be offered for parents who lack the essential knowledge to provide adequate nourishment. Subsidized meal programs may be available at school to provide for children nutritionally neglected at home because of low income.

If a child experiences sleep disturbances, the nurse plans extra time with the youngster at bedtime for a story, back rub, or another activity to promote sleep. Medications for rest or pain can be administered when ordered. The nurse anticipates the needs of battered children, who, unaccustomed to having their needs met by others, are unlikely to make requests.

TABLE 36-1 Long-term and short-term goals and outcome criteria related to fear secondary to child abuse.

Goals	Outcome Criteria
NURSING DIAGNOSIS: FEAR RELATED TO CHILD ABUSE	
Long-term goals	
To eliminate fear of interaction with adults	The child demonstrates ability to be with adults without feeling fearful.
To trust adults in interpersonal relationships	The child experiences positive feelings about interpersonal contact.
To evaluate adult relationships on a safe/unsafe continuum	The child differentiates between safe and unsafe relationships.
To report any threats or abuse to authorities	The child initiates appropriate interpersonal interaction with adults.
	The child demonstrates ability to report abuse.
Short-term goals	
To interact with adults with less fear	The child discusses feelings of fear related to interpersonal relationships.
	The child discusses feelings of fear related to the abuser.
	The child identifies one adult with whom he feels safe.
To feel safe in the present environment	The child reports feeling safe in present environment.
To understand that all adults are not harmful	The child accepts safe touch and closeness from an adult.

✳ *Emotional dimension.* Therapeutic experiences for the abused child permit him to explore his feelings about his family and a society that allows him to be mistreated. Intensive psychotherapy is critical for resolution of the conflicts and negative feelings experienced by battered children. Lifelong emotional sequelae are not uncommon for victims of child abuse, because their ability to form trusting, interpersonal relationships is damaged.

The nurse can encourage the abused youngster to express his feelings by reassuring him that he is safe in the health care environment and will not be punished for verbalizations of anger and hostility. Abused children need to be taught acceptable ways of expressing their feelings. Most find it difficult to modify behaviors they have adopted for protection. The nurse explains when, where, how, and with whom it is safe to express negative feelings.

Caregiver behaviors useful for decreasing victims' fears and anxiety include the following:

1. Moving slowly around the child
2. Using night lights, avoiding loud noises
3. Giving frequent explanations and reality orientation
4. Administering oral medication instead of injections whenever possible
5. Keeping the child near the center of activity
6. Placing oneself at eye level to the child instead of above him

To reduce feelings of helplessness, the child is encouraged to participate as much as possible in decisions about his care.

Few if any demands are placed on the victim. The nurse invites him to share feelings and thoughts or participate in activities, but does not insist. Victims often think that nonvictims do not have these negative thoughts and feelings. The nurse may stimulate discussion by sharing a comment; for example, the nurse can say, "I really get scared (or angry) when people do mean things to me, " or "My feelings are hurt when I try hard to do things right and someone yells at me or calls me stupid," or "I've been punished for things that were not my fault, and I remem-

ber feeling confused because I didn't understand why I was punished." Responding to a child's mood swings, withdrawal, apathy, slow progress, and erratic behaviors requires abundant patience.

✳ *Intellectual dimension.* Interventions in the intellectual dimension focus on reeducating the child and family to alternate methods of expressing hostility and frustration. If rage behavior is learned from punitive parents, as many theorists believe, abusive families can be taught nonviolent coping mechanisms. The cycle of abuse and violence is broken only by teaching victims and offenders healthy behavior to substitute for unhealthy behavior. Parent Effectiveness Training (PET) is offered in most communities to teach effective parenting. Nurses teach problem-solving skills that enable parents to identify healthy alternatives to violence and expand their repertoire of coping mechanisms.

Maltreatment resulting from parental ignorance can be resolved through plans designed to eliminate specific knowledge deficits. In cases of educational neglect, efforts are made to secure appropriate educational opportunities for the child. For the child absent from school for a long time as a result of his injuries, a home tutor is arranged for. The public school system is mandated to provide appropriate educational opportunities for children unable to attend school. This is paid for by the taxpayers out of the school budget. One secures these teachers by consulting the child's school, following the policy prescribed by the school system. Preschool-age children who are educationally disadvantaged in the home can be referred to an educational program to compensate for deficiencies. The abusive family may be too disorganized or unaware of available resources to implement useful suggestions; therefore the nurse provides specific information and assistance to effect the plans. Battered children may lack certain skills for daily living because they have not been taught. Lessons for managing the activities of daily living can bolster the child's self-confidence.

Even young children can be taught basic survival tactics. They can learn to get out of the house until the crisis fades if they sense a battering may be imminent. Some victims are very perceptive in identifying warning signs of violence. For example, if the parent is intoxicated and usually batters when in that state, victims can be instructed to leave the home. They are reminded frequently to tell someone if they are being battered or neglected. They can be taught who the appropriate people are to contact about their situation. Some children who may be inclined to tell someone about their abuse fail to do so because they do not know how to find assistance. The nurse can teach them how to dial the emergency telephone number for child protective services, a health care provider, police, or 911 if available. Used selectively, this strategy can save a youngster's life. However, it needs to be very carefully planned on an individual basis. The nurse needs to explore the responsiveness and attention given to a call from a child in her community before suggesting that the child call a particular number for help. She can have practice help sessions with her client, in which she teaches him how to call and what to say. The primary message to the child is to tell someone as quickly as possible when abuse occurs.

Social dimension. The role of the nurse is not to "rescue" the child from his parents. The nurse is hopeful that, with adequate treatment for the child and his family, they may be reunited and violence ended. Nurses are careful not to criticize the parents. As difficult as it is for others to understand, victims and perpetrators of child abuse generally do love each other. The battered child is given reassurance that he is loved and loveable and is not responsible for his parents' behavior. Unquestionably, the nurse is the child's advocate, but a working relationship with the parents is essential to treatment.

Recognition that the child's input is important may help him begin to build or renew a positive sense of self-esteem. Activities to encourage positive feelings about himself are planned according to the child's interests and preferences. Initially, the activities need to be short term to provide immediate gratification. Occupational therapy can assist the child's success with selected projects. Self-esteem can be enhanced by acknowledging behaviors that would be effortless for others but are taxing for battered children. For example, attending or participating actively or passively in group activity, initiating or responding to conversation, requesting something for himself, or saying no can represent major advances for the maltreated child.

Nursing interventions also include assisting abusive family members to expand their interactions with society. Families are encouraged to develop support systems and social networks.

Battering parents are referred to Parents Anonymous, a group similar to Alcoholics Anonymous. Interaction with other perpetrators of abuse allows parents to learn that their abusive behavior is not unique. Another parent who has learned not to abuse is assigned as an advocate for the batterer to contact when feeling stressed. Reformed abusers can serve as role models for active batterers. Parents Anonymous groups provide a perspective that abusers cannot find elsewhere.

Parents are referred to all applicable social and community service programs. The nurse gives written numbers of these programs to the offenders during their first contact. Trained volunteers working 24-hour hotlines are available to talk with offenders. Crisis hotlines provide immediate and continuous availability. It is useful for the nurse to assist the batterer in establishing this contact before he leaves the treatment setting.

Poverty is not a prerequisite for child abuse; however, socioeconomic conditions contribute to the problem. Subsidized programs to alleviate hardships caused by these stressors may decrease the incidence of battering in a family. Housing assistance, food programs, temporary child care, unemployment compensation, employment counseling, and medical care programs are useful services for many abusive families. Battered women who abuse their children can find themselves economically strained and in need of temporary assistance during times of separation or divorce.

Intervention with the parents is necessary for the child's welfare. Both parents need treatment if the family is to stay together. Siblings need to have the opportunity for therapy as well. The nurse decides the most appropriate treatment modality; for example, individual or family therapy. The role conflicts, guilt, and frustrations of parenting are explored. As parents learn to meet their own needs, they become better able to meet the needs of their children.

The nurse assists maltreated children to develop peer relationships. This can be done in the hospital if other children are there. Otherwise the nurse can role-play meeting other children and practice communication skills with the child. Interactions with sensitive, empathetic adults allow the youthful victim to experience healthy, nontraumatic relationships. Gradually, these experiences may allow the abused child to begin to trust.

Spiritual dimension. When a child has been told by his parents that his beatings are punishment from God because he is not a good child, the nurse is cautious in disagreeing. The nurse comments in a matter-of-fact tone that some people have different beliefs and do not believe God punishes children. However, the nurse does not criticize the parents' belief. Reassuring responses are given to the child that he is not a bad person. The nurse assists the child to strengthen his inner resources by emphasizing his self-worth and inherent value as a human being.

Pastoral counseling is available in many health care agencies. A member of that discipline needs to be included on the family violence interdisciplinary team. For hospitals without a task force, the nurse may find a member of pastoral counseling a willing ally to lobby for the formation of a task force.

Nurses can facilitate the requests of children who request clergy. The nurse can offer to listen to a child's prayers or may say one with him. A child accustomed to attending church or Sunday school may profit from a visit to the hospital chapel. The pastoral counseling member of the family violence team can be enlisted for input to meet the spiritual needs of the child.

SEXUAL ABUSE AND INCEST

Sexual abuse is the engagement of dependent children or developmentally immature individuals in exploitative or physically intimate sexual activity. Activities include fondling, masturbation, unclothing, oral and/or genital contact, and the use of objects for the purpose of physical stimulation. Sexual abuse may be violent or nonviolent. In nonabusive situations sexual partners have the ability to comprehend the significance of the intimate activity and grant informed consent. In abusive situations comprehension and consent are not part of the sexual activity.

Incest is a particular form of sexual abuse. The National Center on Child Abuse and Neglect views incest as sexual activity performed "on a child by a member of the child's family group," not limited to sexual intercourse but including any action performed to sexually stimulate the child or use the child to stimulate other persons.

Assessment

Physical dimension. Children or adolescents of either sex discovered with injuries of the perineum and/or genitourinary system are probable victims of some type of sexual assault. Health care providers are obligated to vigorously pursue this possibility until a diagnosis has been established beyond any reasonable doubt. Trauma of this type rarely results from other causes. Contusions, hematomas, genital edema, vaginal or rectal bleeding, genitourinary infections, or burns on the genitalia are strongly suggestive of sexual abuse. Venereal disease in children is almost conclusive evidence of sexual abuse. Incestuous relationships may be limited to being forced to fondle, fondling, exhibitionism, or other forms of sexual interaction not including intercourse.

Pregnant adolescents are questioned about a history of incest or sexual abuse especially if they are vague about boyfriends or other voluntary sexual activity. Pregnant teenagers are often defensive, evasive, fearful, or anxious when questioned about the paternity of the fetus. Their verbal and nonverbal responses to inquiries about incest or sexual assault need to be carefully evaluated. Younger pregnant girls may heighten suspicions of incest, though age is not the major clue to the presence of these crimes.

Emotional dimension. Despite the absence of conspicuous evidence of emotional trauma, child sexual abuse has the potential to completely shatter the victim's existence in later life. Sexual molestation without intercourse can be as emotionally destructive as assault including intercourse.

Most victims display symptoms of emotional distress, though the cause may be unclear or concealed. The omnipresent need to keep their molestation secret generates substantial fear for victims. Molesters use intimidation, threats, bribes, and manipulation. They endear themselves to the victim and use their dominant positions to secure the victims' cooperation for the sexual activity and silence. Victims are convinced by the perpetrator that no one will believe them if they tell. Some victims may be persuaded to think that these sexual activities are acceptable.

Responses to child sexual abuse include immobilizing anxiety, depression, guilt, shame, substance abuse, suicide attempts, and other forms of self-destructive behavior. Young victims, especially females, who show these behaviors alert health care providers to consider incest or sexual abuse. A history of sexual exploitation may be uncovered for the first time in adult women initially seen with symptoms of emotional disequilibrium. Cases of child molestation or incest may be repressed for many years.

Intellectual dimension. Adolescents victimized by incest or sexual abuse can find themselves so emotionally drained and preoccupied with concealing the secret that their academic performance suffers. These youngsters may respond with increased absences from school or by quitting school.

Young children describe their symptoms in rudimentary language. For example, during a physical examination the child may say, "It hurts down there," or "He hurt me down there," or "He put something inside of me." The child may use sexually explicit terminology too advanced for his age. Such comments must never be ignored! Children do not fabricate sexual experiences. They lack the information and background to articulate such events unless they occurred. Children whose attempts to tell their mothers have been rejected are unlikely to tell others. If a mother expresses disbelief, victims presume strangers will not believe them either.

Social dimension. The burden of keeping the secret of incest prevents sexually exploited youngsters from forming close peer relationships. As these children mature, they are fearful of physical and emotional intimacy with others. Superficial relationships and social isolation are characteristic of these victims.

Role confusion and ambivalence are major factors of the father-daughter incest victim profile. The victims experience intense rage toward the offender from whom they expected nurturing, guidance, and love. Many children risk parental rejection if they attempt to reveal their secret. The mother may respond with hostility, disbelief, and punishment. She may blame the victim for initiating the intimacy, leaving the victim without an advocate or protector in the family.

Commonly, missing children or runaways are victims of sexual abuse. The parents may profess not to know why their child would leave. Rarely does an incestuous relationship exist without the mother's knowledge. Mothers may remain passive and uninvolved for reasons that meet their own needs.

Some teenagers will remain in their abusive situation to "save" younger siblings from the same fate. It is not unusual for fathers to victimize all of their daughters when the girls reach a certain age. Some fathers claim they believe it their duty to teach their daughters about sex through incestuous relations.

Spiritual dimension. Victims may feel spiritually unclean after they have been sexually violated. They may distance themselves from their spiritual support system as a result of these feelings or a perceived need for secrecy. Older victims may feel they have been unfaithful to religious teachings, promoting a greater sense of isolation. Sexually exploited youngsters may emerge with a developmentally distorted sense of values and morality.

Analysis and Planning

Since sexual abuse and incest are types of child abuse, the reader is referred to p. 687 for a list of nursing diagnoses and to p. 688 for examples of long-term and short-term goals and outcome criteria related to child abuse.

Implementation

Physical dimension. Prenatal care for the pregnant adolescent addresses the higher risks incurred by the younger obstetrical client. Venereal diseases must be reported, and the client needs to be questioned about her sexual partners. The nurse remains with the client during the interview to provide support.

Emotional dimension. The most significant contribution to the victim's emotional well-being is early case-finding to interrupt patterns of chronic sexual abuse. The earlier the incest victim is treated the greater the chance to prevent or resolve major emotional trauma. The prognosis for full emotional recovery without permanent emotional scarring becomes more grave the longer the abuse continues.

Nurses assist victims by responding to them in a nonjudgmental, supportive manner. Victims are repeatedly reassured that they are not to blame for the sexual offenses. Opportunities to experience a safe closeness, with the potential for interpersonal trust, are provided. The nurse recognizes that a pregnancy conceived under these circumstances may generate ambivalent or hostile feelings. The nurse encourages expression of these feelings and makes herself available to listen. Assistance is provided so the victim can make a mutually beneficial, informed decision about her baby.

Victims are encouraged to join groups specific for incest and sexual abuse. These groups allow victims to confront their fears and rage with support from other victims. They begin to conceptualize themselves as survivors rather than helpless victims. Individual therapy also promotes emotional healing.

Intellectual dimension. Children are taught that their bodies are private. They need to understand that it is permissible to say "no" to any adult urging intimate contact. Activities which involve close body contact and cause youngsters to feel uncomfortable probably have incestuous overtones. Numerous booklets addressing sexual abuse of children are available.

Sex education that includes a discussion of healthy sexual attitudes and age-appropriate sexual activities is provided for victims. Negative feelings and confusion about sexual function are resolved. These topics are taught by individuals who are comfortable with their own sexuality and can facilitate candid discussion about sexual concerns.

Youngsters are instructed to inform their parents or another responsible adult if they are sexually exploited. They are urged to keep telling until they find someone who believes them and agrees to help. The child's dilemma is identifying a safe person with whom to communicate. This task requires children to be assertive in a difficult situation. Role-playing can be used to give children practice in telling.

Social dimension. Suspected or confirmed cases of incest or sexual exploitation are reported to authorities in accordance with state laws. Health care providers are in violation of the law if they do not report these cases.

Interventions are designed to assist victims to develop peer relationships and expand social networks. The nurse helps them identify activities that may lead to meeting people their own age with similar interests (for example, church groups, scouting, special interest groups at school, YWCA programs, community education programs, or volunteer programs). Nursing intervention can help the victim understand that everyone has events in their lives they prefer not to reveal. Positive interpersonal interactions promote self-confidence and decrease fear of intimacy with other persons.

Child protective services (CPS) are notified to assist in protecting the victim. The nurse collaborates with CPS in the youngster's care. CPS attends to the family, including other siblings at risk in the home. This relieves the victim of the burden to protect and care for her siblings while she is struggling to maintain her own equilibrium. Public health nurses may be assigned to follow a pregnant adolescent through her pregnancy and provide postpartum care.

Teenagers are encouraged to remain in or return to school. The nurse collaborates with the school nurse to discuss a general treatment plan. She promotes understanding among school personnel about the feelings and problems experienced by victims of sexual exploitation. Adult dropouts are given information about obtaining a high school equivalency diploma, which may improve their feelings of accomplishment and self-worth.

Spiritual dimension. The nurse can locate clergy of various religions in the community who are particularly sensitive to counseling victims with spiritual problems resulting from sexual abuse. Many hospitals have nurses who are pastoral counselors on staff. These people are good resources for the nurse who needs assistance in this area of nursing care.

CONSORT ABUSE

Consort abuse is the battery of an emancipated minor or female aged 18 years or older who is the victim of an intentional act of physical violence occurring during the course of an intimate, interpersonal relationship with a spouse or male partner.

There are no uniform laws to mandate reporting of suspected or confirmed consort battery.

Assessment

Physical dimension. Consort abuse is seriously considered as a problem for any woman who has injuries that appear to be trauma induced. Frequently, the first incident of battering will occur during a pregnancy. Caregivers need to consider the possibility of battering in pregnant women with any type of injury.

Common injuries incurred by battered women are listed in the box below.

Women are pushed down the stairs and thrown out of moving cars and have their hands purposely slammed in doors. The cruelty of these acts can strain the boundaries of believability.

Battered women are reluctant to reveal the cause of their injuries, preferring spurious explanations such as falling down the stairs, automobile accidents, stumbling over objects, or bumping into things. When the victim's statement about the cause of her trauma is incongruent with her injuries, abuse is likely. Consort abuse is suggested by the manner in which the victim responds to the history taking and physical examination. If the woman fails to acknowledge her situation, the nurse who suspects abuse directly asks her if she was battered.

The unrelenting emotional trauma caused by battering precipitates many alterations in victims' health. Women who reside in an atmosphere of escalating tension before the acute battering episode are afraid to go to sleep, fearing they will be attacked in bed. These women may spend weeks unable to obtain proper rest. When they do get sleep, it is fitful and restless. They may experience eating disturbances (especially anorexia), insomnia, fatigue, unremitting headaches, gastrointestinal disorders, hypertension, palpitations, hyperventilation, and dermatitis.

Emotional dimension. Emotional problems often follow an acute battering episode. Other responses include depression, malaise, withdrawal, feelings of despair and helplessness, suicidal thoughts, guilt, shame, blunted or inappropriate affect, increased anxiety, and hostility.

COMMON INJURIES OF BATTERED WOMEN

Facial injuries (such as black eyes, missing, chipped, or loose teeth, fractures of the nose or jaw, and hematomas or lacerations of the lips and mouth)

Head injuries (such as concussions, bald spots from which hair has been pulled and blurred vision or tinnitus)

Fractures of the upper extremities incurred by raising the arms to ward off blows

Joint tenderness from the perpetrator grabbing or twisting the arms

Contusions or other strangulation marks on the neck

Contusions and hematomas of the abdomen in pregnant women

Cigarette burns

Spontaneous abortion

Damage to the fetus

Human bite marks, especially on the breasts

Trauma to the genitalia

Fear permeates the existence of battered women. Rarely do they feel safe from the impulsive rage of their abuser, even when they are not together. They are afraid the batterer will return or find them wherever they may be and beat them again.

Intellectual dimension. The intellectual abilities of abused women may be compromised because of the adversity they face. Physical and emotional impairments interfere with ego functioning. The victim may stutter, exhibit halting speech or grope for words. Memory may be impaired by physical or emotional difficulties. Many different coping mechanisms are employed by battered women. Rationalization, projection, displacement, denial, suppression, repression, and regression are common. Battered women may try to minimize or deny the event by understating its severity. Some women experience periods of dissociation.

Not uncommonly, victims can articulate intellectual comprehension of their plight, yet experience behavioral immobilization. Battered women characteristically report feeling "trapped" or being "under mind control." External locus of control is characteristic of battered women, as indicated in the Research Highlight on p. 693. Furthermore, there is no relationship between level of intelligence and the ability to think and act rationally while being abused or evaluating the abusive situation. The victim's terror is so extensive and denial so pervasive that rational assessment eludes them.

The nurse gathers data about the couple's behavior during times of disagreement and methods they use to solve arguments. A high correlation exists between verbal aggression and physical violence. Recurrent verbal disputes within a relationship increases a couple's risk for physical abuse.

Social dimension. Abused women are also victimized by a society that tolerates comments implying lack of intelligence or placing the blame on battered women. "She should have sense enough to leave," "You'd think she'd be smart enough to get out," "She must like it to put up with it," and "I'd never let someone do that to me" are recurring themes.

Social isolation prevails among abused women for several reasons. Societal attitudes contribute to their perceived need to isolate themselves. The perpetrators use social isolation to increase their control over the victims' lives and reduce threats of exposure. Support systems are weak or absent because of the victims' withdrawal. Fearing the batterer will vent his rage on others, victims distance themselves from extended family members and friends. Some women remain in their homes for days following a severe beating to avoid embarrassing questions and detection. Tinted glasses may be worn to cover eye injuries. The nurse evaluates patterns of socialization in victims of trauma and looks for changes in patterns of social activity that denote increasing isolation.

The less the victim interacts with others, the less opportunity she has to develop support systems and maintain social skills. Isolation contributes to self-doubt and thwarts efforts to validate behaviors in the relationships of her peers. Many women are genuinely surprised to learn

Research Highlight

An Investigation of the Relationships Among Locus of Control, Self-Concept, Duration of the Intimate Relationship, and Severity of Physical and Nonphysical Abuse in Battered Women

V.K. Drake

PURPOSE

The purpose of this study was to determine whether specific variables were significantly related to severity of physical and nonphysical abuse in battered women.

SAMPLE

The sample consisted of 51 battered women from three counties near greater metropolitan Washington, D.C. The women had requested assistance from four agencies in the area. Demographically, the sample was closely representative of the general population as to socioeconomic status, education, marital status, race, and religion. The mean length of cohabitation was 9.36 years, with a median duration of 19.42 years. The range of cohabitation was 10 months to 38 years with the abusive partner. The mean age of the women was 33.16 years.

METHODOLOGY

Four tools were used for this descriptive, correlational study: (1) a demographic data questionnaire, (2) the Nowicki-Strickland Internal-External Scale, (3) the Tennessee Self-Concept Scale, and (4) the Index of Spouse Abuse, which gave two separate scores for physical and nonphysical abuse.

FINDINGS

No significant relationships were found between self-concept and physical or nonphysical abuse. Statistical analysis revealed a significantly lower sample mean self-concept than the norm group mean self-concept. Premorbid self-concept scores were not available; therefore it could not be determined whether low self-concept scores existed before the abusive relationship. External locus of control scores were associated with greater severity of physical and nonphysical abuse scores. Frequency and severity of physical abuse increased with the length of the relationship. Statistical analyses of demographic variables indicated no differences in the sample for the major variables of the study with one exception—higher self-concept scores correlated positively with length of cohabitation.

IMPLICATIONS

The association of external locus of control with greater severity of physical and nonphysical abuse in battered women suggests that interventions leading toward internal control, by assuming more responsibility for life events and outcomes, may be beneficial in reducing the severity of physical and nonphysical abuse in battered women.

Battered women need to be apprised of the greater propensity for more severe and frequent abuse as cohabitation continues. Low self-concept is a characteristic of battered women. Interventions to strengthen self-concept may be generally useful for battered women; however, the benefit for reducing severity of physical and nonphysical abuse is questionable.

Based on data from Dissertation Abstracts International 46(7)B, 1986.

that all women are not battered on occasion during the course of marriage or an intense relationship, especially if violence existed in their family as children. Victims are commonly blamed by their extended families for the conjugal violence. Family members pressure the victim to resolve the conflicts. The nurse assesses the potential availability of support from extended family members.

Spiritual dimension. Although no religious denomination escapes consort battering, lack of religious affiliation in both partners correlates with the highest rate of conjugal violence.

The woman's value system and religious beliefs influence her responses to the abusive situation. Religion may be a dominant factor in determining the victim's alternatives to an abusive marriage. She may feel it would be morally reprehensible to expose the father of her children. Her commitment to keep her family together at any cost may be an extension of her religious beliefs. Also, religious commitment can support victims who are wrestling with thoughts of committing suicide or killing their attacker.

To a battered woman, religion may be viewed as a support or cause for punishment. The battered woman may think she has been victimized for not adhering to her faith or attending church regularly. She may see the abuse as her punishment for failure as a wife, infidelity, or other indiscretions. Unmarried women may link abuse to involvement in a legally unsanctioned intimate relationship.

Analysis

Nursing diagnosis. The following list provides examples of NANDA-accepted nursing diagnoses with causative statements:

1. Anxiety related to anticipation of next abusive episode
2. Alteration in comfort related to trauma of physical abuse
3. Ineffective family coping related to poor utilization of support system to bring relief from abuse
4. Ineffective individual coping related to inability to leave abusive situation

TABLE 36-2 Long-term and short-term goals and outcome criteria related to consort abuse

Goals	Outcome Criteria
NURSING DIAGNOSIS: FEAR RELATED TO CONJUGAL VIOLENCE	
Long-term goals	
To establish a safe environment.	Client resides with her family without being assaulted.
	Family does not participate in family violence.
To use appropriate support systems to alleviate stress	Client identifies potential stressful situations.
	Client uses support systems before violence erupts.
	Client identifies alternate approaches to avoid being victimized.
Short-term goals	
To find a safe shelter for temporary residence.	Client resides in a safe setting.
	Client makes decisions about future living arrangements to ensure her safety.
To make decisions that promote safety.	Client participates in treatment sessions.

5. Disturbance in self-concept related to continual derogatory statements by spouse
6. Social isolation related to embarrassment about physical scars from abuse
7. Alteration in thought processes related to extreme fear of being beaten
8. Sleep pattern disturbance related to fear of abuse

Planning

Table 36-2 provides some long-term and short-term goals and outcome criteria related to consort abuse. These serve as examples of the planning stage of the nursing process.

Implementation

Physical dimension. Women are most likely to seek care for their battering during the brief interval at the termination of the explosion phase in the cycle of violence. Their vulnerability at this time makes them particularly receptive to intervention. Trauma has been inflicted, and the victims are in pain or worried about their injuries. Caregivers who fail to identify abuse at this time usually have to wait until the cycle of violence repeats itself to get another opportunity to help.

Commonly victims are in a state of shock following the assault and may be unaware of the severity of their injuries. Intervention may include hospitalization for observation and full evaluation. Nursing care appropriate to specific injuries is implemented.

A signed permit is obtained from the victim allowing photographs of her injuries at the time of treatment. The client's name; the time, date, and place; and the name of person taking the photos are noted on the film. If the client decides to prosecute, these photos are valuable evidence. The nurse reminds the client to get additional color photos in the next few days if possible, because soft tissue injuries become more apparent with time.

Care for victims' other health problems, such as sleep and nutritional deficits, is also planned. Warm soaks, heating pads, extra pillows for support, massages, and muscle relaxants or pain medication as ordered are therapeutic interventions for general body soreness and pain. Pain reduction promotes restful sleep. Many muscle relaxants produce drowsiness. Creative approaches to oral hygiene may be needed as a result of trauma to the jaw, mouth, or teeth. These injuries may also necessitate a special diet.

If the victim is pregnant, interventions are planned to protect the fetus. Possible pregnancy is ruled out before completing orders for x-ray studies. Head injuries may preclude the use of medication until a definitive medical diagnosis has been established. Medications are used cautiously in pregnant victims. A tetanus booster may be required for women with bites, burns, puncture wounds, or lacerations.

Emotional dimension. The nurse may find crisis intervention techniques useful during initial contact to reduce the client's anxiety level (see Chapter 26).

Following an acute episode of battering, the victim needs to reconstitute emotionally and physically. During the initial 24 to 72 hours after the battering, victims are helped to rest and reduce stress levels. The nurse acts as a facilitator to locate sources to relieve the victim of child care and housekeeping chores.

The strong relationship between external locus of control and greater severity of physical and nonphysical abuse indicates that victims may profit by learning to be responsible for controlling or influencing the outcome of events in their lives.

Battered women are encouraged to verbalize their feelings of ambivalence, hostility, and guilt. The nurse facilitates communication by her attitudes. Victims find it difficult to understand why they love a man who treats them so cruelly. Although most interventions in the emotional dimension require extended nurse-client contact, therapeutic principles of basic psychiatric nursing are equally essential in short-term encounters. Each positive interaction has the potential to demonstrate to the victim that she deserves to be treated with dignity and respect.

✳ *Intellectual dimension.* Women with injuries suggestive of battering are given written information about available health, social, and legal services. For victims who feel their safety may be jeopardized if found with the material by their abuser, instructions on how to conceal the information are given. The victim may tape the phone number of a shelter or crisis hotline to the bottom of a drawer. A preferable alternative for some women is to show them where the numbers are listed in the telephone book; however, in times of crisis it is more difficult to find the numbers.

The client learns to accept that she cannot control the batterer, only her responses to the batterer and to her situation. Battered women are informed that the frequency and severity of abuse increase the longer the abusive relationship lasts, which puts them in greater danger the longer they stay with an untreated abuser. Interventions are focused on emotional difficulties contributing to inability to disengage from a destructive relationship. The nurse helps the client identify her options in response to the abuse. Problem-solving skills are taught to the client who demonstrates these skills by assessing and discussing alternatives related to one of her problems.

The victim needs to make her own decision regarding the abuse. If she chooses to leave the abusive situation, books that focus on learning to leave are available. Victims who leave precipitously usually leave with only the clothes they are wearing. By the time they get assistance, the batterer has cleared any mutual bank accounts of all funds, terminated the woman's access to charge accounts, changed the door locks, and prevented the victim from getting her belongings. Victims are encouraged to plan leaving to their own advantage and not to leave abruptly except to protect themselves and their children. Once the client has made a decision, the nurse supports her in that decision whether or not the nurse agrees.

✳ *Social dimension.* Efforts are aimed toward assisting the victim to increase her self-concept. A trusting relationship between the nurse and client is the foundation for the client to be more receptive to positive statements about her. Groups are valuable resources and can provide support and feedback. Consistent positive responses from other persons can slowly reduce negative feelings.

The victim is assisted to identify her strengths and capitalize on them. Realistic awareness of liabilities and ways to overcome them are developed by the victim with the caregiver's help.

Legal options such as protective orders and prosecution are discussed with the woman. Sources to contact include the League of Women Voters, the state bar association, and the state central office for domestic violence. Community services are now available to battered women. There are shelters for battered women and their children in or near almost every community.

Crisis hotlines offer a wide variety of services to abused women. They are good resources for women or caregivers needing information about available services. The nurse

may want to coordinate her care plan with the services offered through the hotline. Many communities provide support for the woman choosing to prosecute.

Lack of education and job skills narrows some victims' options. Women wanting to leave find themselves in a financial dilemma. They may be unable to secure employment to support themselves and their children. These clients can be referred to vocational rehabilitation or employment counseling programs.

✳ *Spiritual dimension.* Interventions are personal and are guided by the clients' values and beliefs. The nurse can function as a facilitator in arranging spiritual counseling if the client desires. Victims contemplating divorce or other actions resulting in separation of the family unit may profit from pastoral counseling. It is best if the clergyman has had specialized training in working with the problems of family violence.

ELDER ABUSE

Elder abuse is any willful or negligent act that results in malnutrition, physical assault or battery, or physical or psychological injury of an elderly person by other than accidental means, including failure to provide necessary treatment, rehabilitation, care, sustenance, clothing, shelter, supervision, or medical services.

In 1985 there were laws mandating reporting of elderly abuse in every state with the exception of Colorado, Wisconsin, Iowa, and Wyoming, which had voluntary reporting laws.

Assessment

✦ *Physical dimension.* As with other types of abuse, a thorough history and physical examination needs to be performed in the case of elder abuse. The client is observed for signs of striking, shoving, beating, or restraining injuries like those described for physically abused women and children. The client is asked if he has been shaken, shoved, hit, restrained, burned, locked up, or left unattended inappropriately.

Medication abuses include excessive, missed, or withheld medicines. The nurse explores the possibility of these types of abuse by questioning the client and caregiver. Some older persons require assistance with their personal hygiene. Omitting or refusing required assistance can lead to multiple physical problems. Clients inappropriately dressed for the environment also evoke concern.

Malnutrition is one of the most common forms of elder abuse. Clients are carefully questioned when weight loss occurs. They may not be receiving an adequate amount of food or their diet may be grossly unbalanced. Some older people need assistance to eat. Inattention to oral hygiene and dental care impact on abilities to eat properly.

Contusions, hematomas, and fractures can be attributed to conditions such as circulatory impairments, osteoporosis, failing vision, or skin changes caused by aging. Similarly, changes that interfere with the perception of extremes of hot or cold could delay reflex responses and result in injury. Thus the nurse is cautious in assessing the origins of the injuries and in interpreting the explanation provided by the caregiver and client. Adequate consideration is given to possiblities of injuries occurring in nonabusive situations in the aged client.

Emotional dimension. Abused elderly individuals share many responses to abuse common to those of other victims. They fear retaliation from the perpetrator if they complain or reveal their plight. Their fear may be reflected in vigilant attention to the caregiver's actions, distancing themselves from the caregiver, and dodging or ducking when their caregiver moves. This fear needs to be distinguished from paranoid behavior or confusion.

The older person may experience guilt and shame for raising children who abuse him. Shame can be as powerful as fear of retaliation in keeping the client from revealing his abuse situation. The control the caregiver exercises may promote feelings of helplessness and hopelessness, which can lead to depression and withdrawal.

The caregiver is observed for hostile, secretive, insulting, threatening, destructive, or aggressive behavior. The caregiver may also show little concern for the elderly person and appear withdrawn, passive, or disinterested in suggestions offered by the nurse. On the other hand the caregiver may demonstrate exaggerated concern or defensiveness, indicative of guilt or an effort at disguise.

Caregivers' feelings about maintaining or losing control of their own behavior and the older person's are important because those who abuse are often obsessed with their fear of losing control.

Intellectual dimension. Because of the stereotype of elderly individuals as "forgetful" or "confused," their credibility may be questioned when they attempt to act in their own behalf by reporting abuse. Thus it is crucial to assess the elderly person's clarity of thinking and memory. Nurses need to know that loss of recent memory and focus on remote events can be within normal limits for an elderly person. Ample time is allowed to respond to questions during assessment. A client who feels pressured to respond quickly may experience increased anxiety, which impairs cognition.

The caregiver's knowledge of the client's medical condition and necessary care is assessed. What looks like neglect or abuse may be the caregiver's inadequate knowledge about providing care.

Social dimension. Elderly abuse is more likely to be committed by those who have been victims of or witnesses to familial abuse as children.

The client is questioned about theft or misuse of finances, property, or possessions. He may believe that his caregivers are entitled to make all decisions about disposition of his material goods. He may be forced to forfeit control of his material possessions to others.

The roles and relationships, past and present, of all family members are evaluated for their actual or potential contribution to an abusive situation. For example, if an adult child has unresolved negative feelings toward his parents, he may consciously or unconsciously use reverse roles with the elderly parent to enact some of these negative feelings through abuse.

The family's cohesiveness, its social isolation or alienation, and its available support system are other important considerations. The amount of contact away from home gives an indication of the client's level of social isolation and the caregiver's role in facilitating or controlling this contact. Such control is common when there is a need to keep others out of the home to maintain the secrecy of the abuse.

The degree of the client's dependence on caregivers for financial and physical support is assessed. Knowing who assists the client with daily living needs provides data about the degree of stress the family may be experiencing. It is important to assess whether the caregiver's own dependent needs have been met, since it is more difficult to accept the dependent needs of the aged person if the caregiver's own needs for dependence have not been met.

The elderly person's role expectations of himself and the caregiver, as well as the caregiver's expectations of his own role and the aged person's role, need to be explored. Data from this assessment can assist the nurse in determining whether these sets of experiences are realistic or unrealistic and in identifying areas of role conflict or role reversal.

Spiritual dimension. The values of both the aged person and the caregiver affect their reactions in situations in which there is a potential for abuse. If the spiritual values of the elderly person and the caregiver include a deep respect for another person's life and a sense of caring that transcends problems imposed by the losses of aging and the resulting responsibilities incurred by the caregivers, there is a strong force against potential abuse. On the other hand, if the spiritual values of the individuals in the situation do not support them in their acceptance of the losses experienced in aging and the necessity of the caregiver's role in support of the elderly person, those involved may more readily accept an abusive situation as justifiable.

Other aspects of the assessment of the spiritual dimension are the resources for support of both the elderly person and the caregivers from the religious affiliations and activities.

Analysis

Nursing diagnosis. The following list provides examples of NANDA-accepted nursing diagnoses with causative statements:

1. Alterations in health maintenance related to caregiving responsibilities
2. Fear related to maltreatment by caregiver
3. Alterations in family processes related to grandparent moving into home
4. Ineffective family coping related to acting-out behavior of older adult

Planning

Table 36-3 provides some long-term and short-term goals and outcome criteria related to elderly abuse. These serve as examples of the planning stage of the nursing process.

TABLE 36-3 Long-term and short-term goals and outcome criteria related to elderly abuse

Goals	Outcome Criteria
NURSING DIAGNOSIS: INEFFECTIVE INDIVIDUAL COPING RELATED TO CAREGIVER'S INCREASED RESPONSIBILITIES	
Long-term goals	
To establish a caring, cooperative relationship between the caregiver and the elderly person.	Elderly person experiences satisfaction with the care given him.
	Caregiver experiences satisfaction with her role as caregiver.
To use adequate support systems for the caregiver when responsibilities become unmanageable.	Caregiver can identify family and community resources available for assistance in caregiving responsibilities.
	Caregiver uses support systems.
Short-term goals	
To stop the occurrence of medication abuse	Elderly person shows no signs of overmedication.
	Elderly person states that he is receiving proper medication doses.
	Behavior indicates that medication is given appropriately.
To realistically balance job and caregiver responsibilities.	Caregiver sets realistic limits on her responsibilities.
	Caregiver recognizes her needs and responsibility for her own health.

Implementation

Physical dimension. Adequate physical care to meet the victim's health needs is provided. This includes a diet tailored to the individual's requirements. The client is given foods that he can manage. To promote his independence, the client is encouraged to do as much as possible for himself. Caregivers supplement care as warranted by the person's condition.

Emotional dimension. Frequently a feeling of helplessness discourages older people from making efforts to stop their abuse. They may need assistance in restoring feelings of control and hopefulness about their situation. Fear of retaliation by the caregiver or fear of losing a preferred living situation may also be present. The nurse can assist the older person in exploring and working through the fear by providing a relationship in which the older person feels comfortable enough to express his fear.

The caregiver's feelings of guilt and frustration can be examined on an individual basis with the mental health–psychiatric nurse. Group therapy, such as Children Anonymous groups, can be formed in which middle-aged children explore together their feelings and difficulties in caring for an elderly parent and use each other's experiences in identifying ways to cope.

Intellectual dimension. The client is provided with as much information about his care as he can understand. Apprising clients of realistic care expectations enables them to recognize abuse or neglect when it occurs.

Preventive interventions include teaching nonviolent behavior early in life and educating the family about the normal aging process. Managers of senior centers or nutrition sites, as well as community "gatekeepers," such as postal workers or grocery clerks, may suspect abuse and neglect but not know what to do. Training can be provided that focuses on signs of abuse, available services, and reporting procedures. Health care professionals need to convey to gatekeepers that it is all right to be suspicious and also to reinforce their reporting and other forms of involvement. Programs such as the Gatekeeper Project in Philadelphia have been successful in promoting the detection of abuse.[10] Nurses can also teach self-care to elderly clients or appropriate care to caregivers.

Social dimension. Most interventions involve ways of providing relief from the often continual caregiving responsibilities. This may include the use of a home health aide for personal care or an adult day care center. Selecting an alternate living arrangement, such as a nursing home or an adult foster home, may be necessary. Hospitals have begun to form Adult Protection Teams (APT). These teams employ an interdisciplinary group of professionals to implement care for families involved in elderly abuse.

Family counseling to clarify role expectations is a useful intervention within the social dimension. When role conflicts are identified, expectations about the needed roles can be clarified, the family member's ability to enact the new roles can be strengthened, and families can be assisted in performing the new roles.

Families need to be encouraged to develop extended kinship networks. Because older people are often more likely to bring their problems to friends in the neighborhood than to formal agencies, nurses need to encourage a mutual help model in communities that emphasizes a reciprocal exchange of services and "watching out for each other." For example, a neighborhood block home for the elderly can be identified as a place to which families turn for assistance, or a neighborhood elderly sitting pool could be established. Shelters for battered women can also develop support groups for aged women who have left abusive situations.

❈ *Spiritual dimension.* Actions by the nurse that display a valuing of older people and a concern for the quality of their existence serve as an example for families who may be discouraged in their caregiving efforts. At the same time, the degree of love and concern displayed by many families caring for older people in the most difficult of situations is often an inspiration to the nurse and serves to extend the knowledge of the nurse about ways to assist families who are not able to cope successfully in similar situations.

Frequently church or synagogue members provide a variety of supports to families of the elderly, including actual participation in the care and an affirmation of the family's spiritual beliefs regarding their important role in providing for the older family member. Counseling may also be given as a part of the church's or synagogue's ministry to its members.

RAPE

Rape is the legal term for an act of engaging another person in unlawful sexual intercourse through the use of force and without valid consent of the sexual partner.

Statutory rape is a legal term for the act of sexual intercourse with a female under the age of consent determined by state law. Sexual intercourse with a minor female is considered unlawful even with consent of the minor to the sexual act.

Acquaintance rapes are committed by men known to the victim. Nurses and other health care providers are not required to report rape or sexual assault to authorities in most states. In the absence of a legal mandate, health care providers must have permission from the client before notifying the authorities.

Assessment

∴ *Physical dimension.* Physical assessment of sexual assault victims includes the standard history and physical examination outlined in professional protocols. For sexual assault victims, special attention is given to menstrual, sexual, and obstetric history. Date of the last menstrual period, present form of birth control, current use of medications, and last act of coitus before the assault are recorded. Explanations are given to the victim to emphasize the necessity for candid disclosure of this information. The assault needs to be described and recorded in minute detail.

Specific data is obtained about penile penetration, orifices violated, duration of intercourse, use of a condom, occurrence and/or site of assailant's orgasm, and physical activities since the assault. The victim is asked whether she has bathed, showered, douched, urinated, defecated, vomited, cleansed her mouth, or changed clothes.

The total body is examined for any contusions, abrasions, lacerations, hemotomas, burns, scars, or other anomalies. The victim's clothing is examined and retained, with her approval, for use as evidence. All body orifices are carefully inspected for signs of trauma. Swabs of body cavities are taken as deemed necessary. The pelvic examination includes appropriate procedures to detect sexually transmitted diseases and the presence of semen. The woman's pregnancy status is determined with appropriate laboratory tests. Pubic hair samples and fingernail scrapings are obtained. With consent of the victim, photographs are taken for additional documentation of injuries. Evidence is sealed, labeled, dated, and signed by the collector and the receiver. Nurses need to be aware of the importance of adhering to strict protocol for evidence collection. A breach of protocol could result in evidence being inadmissible in court if the woman prosecutes.

A variety of somatic responses follow forced sexual contact. Sleep disturbances, increased motor activity, sobbing, crying, headaches, oropharyngeal trauma from oral sex, disrupted eating patterns, musculoskeletal discomfort, gastrointestinal difficulties, genitourinary problems, sexual dysfunction, nausea, vomiting, and malaise are examples of the more common problems.

❈ *Emotional dimension.* Rape victims display a vast array of emotional responses. Personality structure, previous coping strategies, and life circumstances at the time of the attack are contributing factors to the victim's reaction.

The prevailing initial response to sexual assault is extreme fear. The unexpectedness of the attack, coupled with loss of control and threats from the assailant explain the overwhelming fear experienced by victims. Some women feel grateful to have escaped with their lives, and others feel guilty for having survived. Victims report being frightened of physical injury, mutilation, and death during the attack. Fear prevents them from leaving their homes or being alone.

Other emotional responses to sexual assault are feelings of acute stress, persistent uncleanliness, guilt, shame, embarrassment, humiliation, shock, disbelief, phobias, night terrors, anxiety, vulnerability, and depression. These feelings may be intermittent or prolonged. Alcohol or drug use is not uncommon following a sexual attack; it is used in an effort to numb the pain.

❈ *Intellectual dimension.* The psychic energy required by the victim to prevent further emotional decompensation is depleted leaving little energy for cognitive tasks. Disorientation and disorganized thought processes are common immediately following sexual assault and may continue for some time. Decision-making and problem-solving skills may be weakened or disrupted. Some sexual acts are so repulsive to the victim that she may suppress or repress their occurrence or feel too ashamed to report them. Some victims perseverate about the experience and are preoccupied with thinking about what they could have done differently to prevent or change the outcome of the assault. Other victims may focus on their work to avoid thinking about the rape.

The victim has to make many decisions during this time, when she is least prepared to make them—decisions about seeking health care, preserving physical evidence, notifying the police, securing any breach of the living premises, telling the family, caring for children, and other practical matters of daily living. The victim's basic intellectual capacity affects her ability to comprehend the significance of the event and make decisions about necessary arrangements.

✿ *Social dimension.* One major problem confronting victims of sexual assault is what, when, and how to inform the family or significant others. These persons are usually viewed as the frontline support system for loved ones in crisis. In cases of sexual assault family members are, in a sense, victimized as well. Reports have indicated that husbands and significant others often respond to the victim's rape with divorce, terminating the relationship, or blaming the victims. Such reactions further intensify the victim's trauma.

Husbands, fathers, or significant others, usual sources of support for victims during crises, may find themselves unable to meet the victim's needs because they are dealing with their own feelings and needs. Men may distance themselves sexually and emotionally from their mates. For others, the implicit or explicit question is whether the victim provoked her attack. Family members may pressure the victim not to prosecute or notify authorities because they do not want to risk publicity. This lack of support is another way the family communicates its shame or embarrassment to the victim. Victims may express reluctance to reveal their attack because they are concerned about the impact on their family. Relationships are also threatened if the assailant is an employer, family friend, relative, or neighbor.

Social isolation is common following a rape. Victims are uncomfortable being with other people, even close friends. Fear, suspicion, and other emotional responses prevent victims from wanting to leave their homes.

✿ *Spiritual dimension.* Religious beliefs, faith, and moral values may be highly significant for the rape victim. She may be confronted with very difficult decisions if she becomes pregnant. Some women are unable to cope with a pregnancy resulting from rape yet would experience extraordinary guilt consenting to an abortion. Pregnancy prevention therapy may conflict with the victim's religious beliefs. Children conceived as a result of rape may not be accepted by the victim, husband, or other family members. Relinquishing a child, even though fathered by a rapist, may provoke guilt for the victim. The victim may find herself forced to choose from a list of undesirable alternatives.

Rape victims who believe in God may question their faith, feel angry at God, or feel they have been punished by God. Victims may experience guilt if they are unable to forgive their assailant. Religious faith may be a victim's greatest source of comfort during times of stress.

Analysis

Nursing diagnosis. The defining characteristics of the NANDA-accepted nursing diagnosis of rape trauma syndrome are presented in the box at right. This syndrome includes three subcomponents: rape trauma, compound reaction, and silent reaction. Those characteristics unique to the compound reaction and the silent reaction are indicated in parentheses.

RAPE TRAUMA SYNDROME

DEFINITION

Forced, violent sexual penetration against the victim's will and consent. The trauma syndrome that develops from this attack or attempted attack includes an acute phase of disorganization of the victim's life-style and a long-term process of reorganization of life-style.

DEFINING CHARACTERISTICS

Physical Dimension
Gastrointestinal irritability
Genitourinary discomfort
Muscle tension
Sleep pattern disturbance
Reactivated symptoms of previous physical illnesses or psychiatric illnesses (compound reaction)
Reliance on alcohol and/or drugs (compound reaction)
Increase in nightmares (silent reaction)
Pronounced changes in sexual behavior (silent reaction)

Emotional Dimension
Anger
Embarrassment
Fear of physical violence and death
Humiliation
Dealing with repetitive nightmares and phobias
Increased anxiety during interview (silent reaction)
Sudden onset of phobic reactions (silent rection)

Intellectual Dimension
No verbalization of the occurrence of rape (silent reaction)
*Short attention span
*Difficulty understanding communications
*Difficulty making decisions
*Increased attention to irrelevant matters
*Selective impaired memory

Social Dimension
Revenge
Changes in residence
Seeking family support
Seeking social network support
Abrupt changes in relationships with men (silent reaction)

Spiritual Dimension
Self-blame
*Angry at God
*Feels punished or abandoned by God
*Struggles with abortion decision
*Unable to accept offers of spiritual support

Adapted from North American Nursing Diagnosis Association Classification of Nursing Diagnosis: Proceedings of the seventh conference, St. Louis, 1987, The C.V. Mosby Co.
*Indicates characteristics in addition to those defined by NANDA.

The following Case Example illustrates characteristics of the nursing diagnosis of rape trauma syndrome.

Case Example

Beth, a 34-year-old divorced mother of two, was brought to the emergency room by her neighbor. The neighbor found Beth, clothed in a nightgown, rocking back and forth in a chair and crying. Her children, a daughter age 12 and a son age 10, reported their mother was "acting funny." Beth reported she had been raped by a man wearing a ski mask who surprised her on the way to her car the previous evening after work. Although Beth had several contusions on her face and arms and signs of perineal trauma, she expressed concern that perhaps she had not fought off her attacker vigorously enough. "I was afraid he would kill me if I screamed or fought him anymore. At least, that's what he told me he would do." Beth had stayed home from work because she did not want anyone to see how bad she looked. She had not notified the police because she feared her fiance would learn she had been attacked. He had cautioned her not to go to her car alone after dark. She believed he would break their engagement because she had been assaulted. Beth worried she could not be a "real wife" to her prospective husband.

Planning

Table 36-4 provides some long-term and short-term goals and outcome criteria related to rape. These serve as examples of the planning stage of the nursing process.

Implementation

✦ *Physical dimension.* Ideally, the client is treated initially in a designated sexual assault treatment center. These facilities are best equipped to provide comprehensive care for rape victims, because they follow a detailed protocol to maximize treatment. If the victim makes telephone contact before being seen by a professional caregiver, she is encouraged not to shower, bathe, douche, or change clothing and to seek health care as soon as possible.

Evidence is collected according to strict legal guidelines, even if the client has not decided whether to notify the police. Initially, the victim may feel overwhelmed and unable to make that decision. Properly collected evidence preserves the victim's option to press charges.

The manner in which the victim's needs are met during initial contact has major implications for her prognosis and recovery. Many facilities provide female nurse practitioners or female physicians to take the history and perform the physical examination of the rape victim. A detailed, verbatim account of the sexual attack is included in the client's record. The examination proceeds slowly, with clear explanations provided before every procedure. The victim is not touched without being told first and asked for her permission. Careful attention is given to make the victim as physically comfortable as possible, because she is likely to be in great pain from her ordeal. Short rests may be necessary if the victim expresses fatigue or undue discomfort. The victim may appreciate being offered a beverage at some point during the treatment process unless contraindicated by incomplete laboratory work or specific injury. The victim will welcome an opportunity to wash out her mouth as soon as possible if she had oral contact with her assailant. Anything that can be done to help the victim clean up will benefit her physically and emotionally.

Pregnancy prevention measures are discussed with the client if the rape occurred within the previous 72 hours. All options are explained, including the strengths and weaknesses of each alternative. The possibility of sexually transmitted diseases is addressed. Some agencies implement prophylactic antibiotic therapy, appropriate for specific venereal diseases, during the initial visit. Other agencies administer treatment only after a sexually transmitted disease is diagnosed. A third alternative is to treat only

---

TABLE 36-5 Long-term and short-term goals and outcome criteria related to rape trauma syndrome

Goals	Outcome Criteria
NURSING DIAGNOSIS: RAPE TRAUMA SYNDROME RELATED TO RECENT RAPE EXPERIENCE	
Long-term goals	
To resume prerape activities	Demonstrates ability to resume full range of activities of daily living.
To resume prerape level of functioning	Feels comfortable without antianxiety medication.
	Demonstrates understanding of her role as a victim by discussing the incident calmly and rationally.
Short-term goals	
To decrease anxiety level	Identifies and discusses factors that increase her anxiety level.
	Sleeps at least 6 hours per night.
	Showers only once each day.
To identify members of her support system and accept their assistance	Informs fiance of sexual assault.
	Accepts assistance from friends and others trained to provide post-rape interventions.
	Contacts rape crisis unit.
To obtain necessary medical care	Permits physical examination.
	Complies with medical treatment recommendations.

those victims deemed to be high risks to not receive follow-up care.

Victims are given medication for sleep or pain if needed. They are encouraged to contact the health care provider if pain or sleep disturbances continue.

Emotional dimension.
The priority for intervention in the emotional dimension is to establish trust with the victim. Ideally, the client is seen as quickly as possible by a rape counselor. Initial contact with the rape counselor may occur by telephone or in an emergency room, outpatient unit of a hospital, counseling center, crisis center, physician's office, victim's home, or police station.

Nursing intervention focuses on reducing the victim's fear. The nurse understands that her client's temporary fear about a repeat attack is real, and not immediately amenable to logic. Repetitive reassurance of the victim's safety is offered. The client is urged to focus on measures enacted for her protection. The nurse assists the client to concentrate on increased security measures such as new window and door locks, police intervention, someone to stay with her, or someone to accompany her outside her home. If the fear continues after a few weeks and shows no signs of abating, psychotherapy is considered. Crisis intervention techniques are also useful following sexual assault. (See Chapter 26).

Sexual assault is an experience during which the victim is controlled. She has been degraded and humiliated. It is important for the victim to regain control. Well-intentioned persons may try to take charge of the victim's life and do everything for her. However, she needs to be given as many opportunities as possible to make decisions for herself. Consulting the victim about who she prefers to be with her, her daily schedule, and her follow-up treatment are examples of giving her control.

Treatment choices are the victim's decision. Once the victim makes a decision, that decision is supported. Others may not agree with her decisions; however, it is important that their values are not imposed on her.

The nurse assists the victim to resolve feelings of self-blame. Victims are not responsible for their assaults. They are urged not to accept the responsibility for another's behavior or the projections of others' feelings onto them.

Intellectual dimension.
Intellectual disorganization and disorientation may mean the victim needs assistance with problem solving and decision making during the period immediately following the rape. The nurse helps the client identify options for situations about which decisions need to be made.

Finding the assailant, preserving evidence, and successful prosecution are issues that hinge on prompt notification of the authorities. The victim is not pressured into the decision during a period of vulnerability, but needs to be aware of the reasons for a quick decision. The victim or family members need to be reminded not to clean the scene of the crime if police involvement is anticipated. As the shock, disbelief, fear and anxiety levels subside, the victim will have more energy for cognitive functions.

Information about available treatments and services is given in language the victim understands. Medical and anatomical jargon is avoided. Communication is on the client's level, with statements such as, "I am going to have to ask you some difficult questions," or "Some things may be difficult for you to discuss. We can take it slowly, but there are things which need to be discussed as soon as possible."

Apparent reluctance to discuss the sexual assault may not be directly related to the attack, but to other information that would be revealed. For example, girls whose parents don't know they are sexually active or women using birth control without their husband's knowledge may be hesitant to report the incident to the police, knowing that their secret may surface during an investigation. Victims are not questioned in front of family members unless they ask that the family member be present for support.

Written instructions for home care, signs and symptoms necessary to report, follow-up care, appointments and medication information are given to the client. Clients are unlikely to remember verbal instructions under stressful circumstances. Classes in self-defense for women, often taught by local police departments, may help decrease a woman's feelings of vulnerability.

Social dimension.
Rape victims are afforded privacy in a quiet room. An individual trained to handle rape crisis stays with the victim. The number of personnel attending to the victim is kept to a minimum. Required tasks may be shared to keep personnel involved with the victim to a minimum; for example, the nurse or physician may collect blood samples rather than an unfamiliar laboratory technician.

National registers are available to provide callers with information about the nearest victim assistance program. Services are listed in telephone directories under terms such as rape, abuse, or battering. Some provide transportation services, accompany the victim to court, bring clothes to the hospital if the victim's are held as evidence, or see the victim in her home to provide support. The victim is given information about rape support groups and services. She is urged to avail herself of those services, which are usually free.

Many geographic areas have support groups for husbands, fathers, or significant others. These groups help the men resolve their feelings about the assault and teach them ways to provide support for the victim. The nurse can implement a referral to a treatment service for these persons.

The nurse assists the victim to identify ways to inform others about the assault. Role-playing is a useful technique to practice telling others. The victim may decide not to tell others, but plans are made in case the need arises.

Spiritual dimension.
Pastoral counseling is appropriate for the victim suffering from a sexual assault. Issues about which a victim may desire pastoral counseling are pregnancy prevention, abortion, prosecuting her assailant, disclosing the rape to her fiance or husband, and the implications of her hatred, vindictiveness, and rage toward the rapist. The nurse offers to contact clergy of the victim's choice.

Evaluation

Progress in the prevention of family violence and in helping families and health care providers in dealing with abusive situations is extrinsically tied to society's attitudes toward abuse and rape, and its willingness to recognize and give attention to the problem. When society can better accept that abuse and rape respect no boundaries, it is more likely that additional resources will be allocated to find solutions.

The success of the nursing process with abused clients and their families is measured by the cessation of the abuse through interruption of the cycle of violence, and on a more long-term basis, by the ability of the victim to come to an intraphysic resolution of the abuse. Other indicators of goal attainment are the learning of impulse control and problem solving by the abuser and the ability of the family to learn less destructive methods of handling their negative emotions.

BRIEF REVIEW

Abuse is a dynamic, interactive process involving two or more persons. Clients seeking treatment for physical injuries are asked directly if they are victims of abuse unless there is concrete evidence to the contrary. Every health history contains questions designed to elicit information about possible abuse. Case-finding of any victim enters an entire family into the health care system.

Failure to identify abused clients remains an important issue in prevention and treatment of health problems resulting from abuse. Informed nurses increase the probability of identifying abusive situations. Their knowledge, skills, and expertise can be used to raise the consciousness of and educate other health care providers about the problems experienced by victims of abuse.

All nurses will encounter victims of abuse. Early diagnosis and treatment provide the best opportunity for rehabilitation and improved prognosis.

REFERENCES AND SUGGESTED READINGS

1. Anderson, C.L.: Abuse and neglect among the elderly, Journal of Gerontological Nursing 7(2):77, 1981.
2. Attorney General's Task Force: Family violence, Washington, D.C., 1984, Department of Justice.
3. Bahr, R.T., Sr: The battered elderly: physical and psychological abuse, Family and Community Health 4(2):61, 1981.
4. Beck, C.M., and Ferguson, D.: Aged abuse, Journal of Gerontological Nursing 7:333, 1981.
5. Beck, C.M., and Phillips, L.R.: Abuse of the elderly, Journal of Gerontological Nursing 9(2):97, 1983.
6. Bergman, A.B., Larsen, R.M., and Mueller, B.A.: Changing spectrum of serious child abuse, Pediatrics 77:113-116, 1986.
7. Bragg, D.F., Kimsey, L.R., and Tarbox, A.R.: Abuse of the elderly: the hidden agenda. II. Future research and remediation, Journal of the American Geriatrics Society 29:503, 1981.
8. Burgess, A.W., and Holmstrom, L.L.: Rape crisis and recovery, Bowie, Md., 1979, Robert J. Brady Co.
9. Champlin, L.: The battered elderly, Geriatrics 37(7):115, 1982.
10. Collins, A., and Pancoast, D.: Natural helping networks: a strategy for prevention, New York, 1976, National Association of Social Workers.
11. Drake, V.K.: Battered women: a health care problem in disguise, Image 14(2):40, 1982.
12. Drake, V.K.: An investigation of the relationships among locus of control, self-concept, duration of the intimate relationship, and severity of physical and nonphysical abuse of battered women, Ann Arbor, Mich., 1985, University Microfilms International.
13. Drake, V.K., and Steinmetz, C.: Spouse abuse: dynamics and intervention strategies—Training Key No. 352, Gaithersburg, Md., 1985, International Association of Chiefs of Police.
14. Elder abuse in the home found widespread by congressional inquiry, Geriatric Nursing 1(5):153, 1980.
15. The elderly: newest victims of familial abuse, Journal of the American Medical Association 243:1221, 1980.
16. Falcioni, D.: Assessing the abused elderly, Journal of Gerontological Nursing 8:208, 1982.
17. Federal Bureau of Investigation: Crime in the United States, Washington, D.C., 1984, Department of Justice.
18. Fulmer, T.: The hidden victim, Aging and Leisure Living 3(5):9, 1980.
18a. Giarretto, H.: Humanistic treatment of father-daughter incest. In Helfer, R.E., and Kempe, C.H., editors: Child abuse and neglect: the family and the community, Cambridge, Mass., 1976, Ballinger Publishing Co.
19. Hickey, T., and Douglas, R.L.: Mistreatment of the elderly in the domestic setting: an exploratory study, American Journal of Public Health 71:500, 1981.
20. Hickey, T., and Douglas, R.L.: Neglect and abuse of older family members: professionals' perspectives and case experiences, Gerontologist 21(2):171, 1981.
21. Jacobs, M.: More than a million older Americans abused physically and mentally each year, Perspective on Aging 9:46, 1973.
22. Katz, K.D.: Elder abuse, Journal of Family Law 18:695, 1979-1980.
23. Kimsey, L.R., Tarbox, A.R., and Bragg, D.F.: Abuse of the elderly: the hidden agenda. I. The caretakers and the categories of abuse, Journal of the American Geriatrics Society 29:465, 1981.
24. Koop, C.E.: Introduction to workshop on violence and public health, National Organization For Victim Assistance Newsletter: 9:11, November, 1985.
25. Long, C.M.: Geriatric abuse, Issues in Mental Health Nursing 3:123, 1981.
26. Mancini, M.: Adult abuse laws, American Journal of Nursing 80:739, 1980.
27. Newman, G.: Understanding violence, New York, 1979, J.B. Lippincott Co.
28. O'Reilly, J.: Wife beating: the silent crime, Time, p. 23, September 1983.
29. Rubinelli, J.: Incest: its' time we face reality, Journal of Psychiatric Nursing and Mental Health Services 18(4):17, 1980.
30. Salholz, E., and others: Beware of child molesters, Newsweek, p. 45, August 9, 1984.
31. Select Committee on Aging: Elder abuse: an examination of a hidden problem, U.S. House of Representatives, Comm. Publ. No. 97-277, Washington, D.C., 1981 U.S. Government Printing Office.
32. Steinmetz, S.: Elder Abuse, Aging 135-136:6, January-February 1981.
33. Steuer, J., and Austin, E.: Family abuse of the elderly, Journal of the American Geriatrics Society 28:372, 1980.

34. Straus, M.A., Gelles, R.J., and Steinmetz, S.K.: Behind closed doors: violence in the American family, Garden City, N.Y., 1980, Anchor Books.
35. Thobaben, M., and Anderson, L.: Reporting elder abuse: it's the law, American Journal of Nursing 85(4):371-374, 1985.
36. U.S. Department of Health and Human Services: Elder abuse, Washington, D.C., Administration on Aging, DHHS Publ. No. (OHDS) 81-20152, Washington, D.C., 1980, U.S. Government Printing Office.
37. U.S. Department of Health and Human Services: Executive summary: National study of the incidence and severity of child abuse and neglect, DHHS Publ. No. (OHDS) 81-30329, Washington, D.C., 1982, U.S. Government Printing Office.
38. Walker, L.E.: The battered woman, New York, 1979, Harper & Row, Publishers.

ANNOTATED BIBLIOGRAPHY

Campbell, J., and Humphreys, J.: Nursing care of victims of family violence, Reston, Va., 1984, Reston Publishing Co.

This comprehensive text discusses theories of violence, theoretical frameworks for clinical practice and implications for research, and organizes interventions according to the nursing process. Nursing care is described in detail from primary to tertiary prevention. This book is essential for interdisciplinary students, clinicians, educators, and researchers engaged with topics related to family violence.

Deschner, J.P.: The hitting habit: anger control for battering couples, New York, 1984, The Free Press.

This book provides in-depth information on social, personal, cognitive, and physiological factors related to battering and violence among family members. Alternatives to violent behavior and treatment models are presented. A practical book for interdisciplinary professionals seeking additional in-depth knowledge.

Finkelher, D.: Child sexual abuse, new theory and research, New York, 1984, Free Press.

This book offers information for parents about ways to inform their children about sexual abuse. It provides a section on professional responses to sexual abuse, long-term effects of this crime, and more data about boys as victims and women as perpetrators. A unique chapter addresses the triad of implications for theory, research, and practice.

Psychiatric Annals 17:4, 1987.

This issue contains six articles on child abuse, including the family's role in the abuse of children; sexual abuse of children; current research reviewed; psychodynamics of exaggerated accusations; child abuse aspects of child pornography; psychological damage associated with extreme eroticism in young children; and evaluating suspected child sexual abuse cases. It has excellent current information and useful assessment tools.

Sonkin, D.J., Martin, D., and Walker, L.: The male batterer, a treatment approach, New York, 1985, Springer Publishing Co., Inc.

An innovative text with a singular focus on the male batterer. In depth information and special issues for treatment of this population are addressed. Suggestions are provided for the development of counseling programs for male batterers.

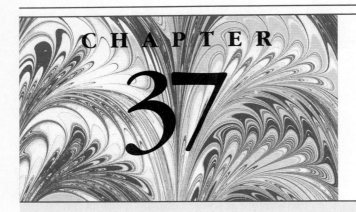

THERAPY WITH DYING CLIENTS

Linda Hannawalt Rickel   Barbara G. Williams

Judith Eberle Seidenschnur   Malinda Garner Pappas

After studying this chapter the learner will be able to:

Trace the historical changes in attitudes toward caring for the dying client.

Differentiate among acute grief, delayed grief, and pathological grief.

Identify appropriate developmental tasks of the dying process.

Describe the major theorists' approaches to dying and death.

Discuss characteristics of therapy with the dying client.

Discuss characteristics of the nurse working with the dying client.

Implement the nursing process in caring for the dying client.

Describe how current research enhances care of the dying client.

Dying is the final stage of human growth and development. Like birth, death is a naturally occurring, normal process. As the process of birth can be eased through the timely intervention of a knowledgeable, caring nurse, so can the process of dying.

The care of the dying client and his family, while an integral part of the continuum of health care, can be one of the most challenging roles for health care providers. Because of the strong emphasis in health care on the cure of disease and promotion of optimal health, a client's death can and often does represent failure to health care professionals. When dealing with dying clients and grieving families, health care professionals are confronted with their own mortality and other discomforting issues. These factors can influence the quantity and quality of care. The American Nurses' Association[1] addresses nursing care for the dying client in its *Code for Nurses.*

THEORETICAL APPROACHES
Grief

Dying and death result in multiple losses for the client and family: loss of job, goal fulfillment, roles, and ultimately life itself. Emotional responses to these losses, known as *grief,* are experienced by client, family, and sig-

nificant others. *Acute* or *functional* grief, the process of acknowledging and expressing feelings associated with loss, is a syndrome with psychological and somatic symptoms, which appear in each dimension of the person.

Grief reactions. Lindemann[29] divides the symptoms of normal grief into five categories:
1. Somatic distress
2. Preoccupation with the image of the deceased person
3. Feelings of guilt
4. Hostile reactions
5. Loss of patterns of conduct

Anticipatory grief is the range of feelings experienced by both client and family in anticipation of a loss. If the family's anticipatory grief results in grief resolution before the client's death, the client may feel abandoned, and family members may feel guilty and frustrated.

Distortions of normal grieving patterns are sometimes encountered. Failure to experience or express grief at the time of loss may result in a *delayed* or *dysfunctional* grief reaction. Reaction to the loss may occur weeks, months, or years later. Grief may also be expressed as *pathological* or *morbid* grief—an excessive response resulting in health problems, such as impotence, eating disorders, delusions, drug or alcohol abuse, or paranoia.

Historical Overview

DATE	EVENT
Early 1900s	The role of professionals who worked with dying clients, other than clergy, became prominent with the proliferation of hospitals, increased legal concerns over wills and inheritance, the development of the nursing and medical professions, and the establishment of the funeral director and licensed mortician.
1950	Before this date death usually occurred at home with loved ones. After 1950 the majority of people died in hospitals or institutions.
1960s	Dying and death became topics of research and seminars. Glaser and Strauss developed the awareness context. Kübler-Ross identified the stages of death and dying.
1970s	Hospices in the United States became recognized as a care delivery system.
1976	The American Nurses' Association addressed nursing care for the dying client in its Code for Nurses.
1980s	Today client and family involvement in determining the setting, circumstances, and management of the dying process is encouraged. Grief therapy and therapists are used. Life quality issues are openly discussed, and client choice of treatment options is encouraged.
Future	Living wills will be upheld as legal documents. More individuals will be dying at home because of the cost of hospitalization and the improvement in home health care. Nurses will be increasingly viewed as primary caregivers.

Table 37-1 summarizes acute, delayed, and pathological responses to grief.

Grief outcomes. Bugen's model[8] of human grief with empirically validated concepts has contributed significantly to grief theory. The model defines grief outcome as mild or intense, brief or prolonged, based on the significance of the relationship of the bereaved to the deceased and whether the death was perceived as preventable. The relationship is identified as either central or peripheral. When the relationship is central the grieving process is most intense, and the survivor feels that life can no longer be significant and feels helpless and unable to cope. If the relationship is peripheral, the grief response is less intense, and the grief work is likely to progress more rapidly to resolution. When the death is viewed as preventable, survivors feel direct or indirect responsibility for it. Working through this belief increases the intensity and prolongs the grieving process. If the survivors view the death as unpreventable, they are less likely to feel responsible and guilty, and the grief response will be milder and briefer.

Grief stages. Kübler-Ross[28] proposed five stages or series of reactions to dying. The stages apply to both bereaved and dying individuals. Although not scientifically supported by quantitative research, Kübler-Ross's theory has received considerable support from professional and lay communities.

Stage I—denial and isolation. An initial state of shock and numbness typically follows a terminal diagnosis. Some degree of denial is used by all clients, not only during the first stages of illness or confrontation but also later as the disease progresses. Denial and isolation serve as buffers permitting the client to pull himself together and mobilize alternative defenses.

Stage II—anger. Anger replaces denial and is frequently displaced to loved ones or health care providers. Anger is difficult to understand and may result in the family and others rejecting the client.

Stage III—bargaining. The client attempts to formulate an agreement to postpone death. He thinks if he behaves well, he may be granted an extension of life, the removal of pain, or the opportunity to reconcile with a loved one. Most bargains are secretly made with God.

Stage IV—depression. No longer able to deny his illness because of his deteriorating physical condition and need for more treatment, the client feels a sense of great loss. This sense of loss is intensified as financial burdens increase because of required medical treatment. Job and family roles are altered, and dreams and future plans are recognized as futile. Preparatory grief, the process by which the client prepares himself for separation and impending losses, occurs at this stage. The client struggles with the painful realities of his life as he prepares himself for death.

Stage V—acceptance. When a client has sufficient time and support to work through the previous stages, he may reach the stage of acceptance. Acceptance is almost void of emotion, because emotional pain is gone, and the struggle is past. When the dying client has reached peaceful acceptance, the silent presence of the nurse becomes the

TABLE 37-1 Responses to grief

Acute or Functional Grief	Delayed or Dysfunctional Grief	Pathological or Morbid Grief
PHYSICAL DIMENSION		
Crying	Absence of acute symptoms	Anorexia or gluttony
Sobbing	Hyperactivity or hypoactivity	Insomnia or excessive sleeping
Wailing or silence	Muscle tension	Uncontrolled screaming or mutism
Lump or tightness in throat		Running
Shortness of breath		Exhaustion
Sighing respirations		Pounding heart
Empty feeling in abdomen		Diarrhea
Lack of muscle power		Vomiting
Loss of appetite		Fainting
Insomnia		Impotence
Altered libido		Homicidal or suicidal attempts
Pain		
EMOTIONAL DIMENSION		
Anger	Apathy	Hysteria
Guilt	Sense of emotional numbness	Hostility
Hostility	Denial	Lack of feeling
Fear of losing control		Torment
		Lability
		Preoccupation with grief
		Depression
INTELLECTUAL DIMENSION		
Focusing attention on the loss	Preoccupation with image of deceased	Paranoia
Lack of contact with here and now	Concrete thinking	Delusions
Decreased concentration	Indecision	Hallucinations
Sense of unreality	Increased effort with decreased productivity	Confusion or disorientation
		Lack of concentration
SOCIAL DIMENSION		
Closeness with significant others	Avoidance of reminders of the loss	Isolation or clinging behavior
Lack of warmth in casual relationships	Uninhibited seeking of people	Sexual acting out
Stiff social manner	Habitual activity	Encounters with the law
Seclusion	Drug and alcohol use	Drug and alcohol abuse
SPIRITUAL DIMENSION		
Feeling presence of deceased	Ambivalence	Religiosity or atheism
Search for meaning	Sense of void	Helplessness
		Hopelessness
		Powerlessness or omnipotence

most meaningful communication. The client may experience fatigue and weakness and need extended hours of sleep.

Not all dying clients go through each of these stages, nor do they necessarily go through them in the order described. A client may move back and forth among them or may accept death without experiencing each of them. Some clients never accept death, but live with hope until the end. People are unique in the manner they choose to cope with death.

Overlapping phases of grief. Weisman[53] viewed the emotional responses of the dying process as overlapping phases, not distinct stages. He described an initial acute crisis phase in which client is faced with the insoluble problem of a potentially fatal disease. Typical reactions are shock, anger, and tension as the client attempts to cope with this problem for which he has no previous experience. His ability to cope positively is strongly influenced by his self-concept and how he has learned to deal with past crises. The client then gradually moves into the chronic living-dying phase, which is accompanied by multiple fears of dying and death. Eventually the client enters the terminal phase of dying, characterized by acceptance of death.

TABLE 37-2 Summary of theoretical approaches

Theory	Theorist	Dynamics
Grief reactions	Lindemann	Grief and bereavement in response to death will lead to a crisis in most individuals.
Grief outcome	Bugen	The degree of the bereaved's grief is related to the significance of the relationship and whether the death was perceived as preventable.
Grief stages	Kübler-Ross	There are five probable stages of the dying client and the family's emotional and intellectual reactions: denial, anger, bargaining, depression, and acceptance.
Overlapping phases	Weisman	The overlapping phases of the dying process are: initial acute crisis phase, chronic living-dying phase, and terminal phase.
Awareness context	Glaser and Strauss	The dying client and his significant others can have different levels of awareness of the client's condition and each other's awareness.
Intentionality	Shneidman	The client who is willing to accept life and take responsibility for choices is more likely to live longer.

Awareness Context

Awareness context describes what the client and family know of the client's condition. Following are several types of awareness contexts as described by Glaser and Strauss:[21]

1. *Closed awareness.* Attempts are made to prevent the client from knowing of his possible death.
2. *Suspicion awareness.* The client becomes suspicious, usually because of personal physical clues, that information about his condition is being withheld.
3. *Mutual pretense.* The client and others know that he is dying but pretend otherwise.
4. *Open awareness.* The client and others know that he is dying and relate to each other openly.

In an open awareness context the client feels more trust toward those around him, because they afford him the information he needs about himself.

Intentionality

Shneidman[45] saw an element of *intentionality* in most deaths. The holistic health concept, in which the client is given responsibility for his wellness or illness, is in accor-dance with this idea. The client who is willing to accept life and take responsibility for his life choices is more likely to live longer. This same individual, when death approaches, will die peacefully and with a sense of accomplishment. According to Shneidman, life has multiple phases and closings that involve mourning and grief as intense as the mourning produced by death.

Table 37-2 summarizes the various theoretical approaches.

Transitions and Loss in the Life Cycle

The stage of dying involves many struggles and tasks. The dying client continues to live fully aware that soon he will have to give up life and be separated from loved ones. Thus it is often the emotional pain that makes dying problematic and difficult. The problems in living caused by a loved one's dying are also experienced by the family and significant others. They need to find a way to cope with the dying process and death while retaining enough energy to manage the pain of surviving.

Age groups, because of their particular stage of development and probable personal experience with death, have common characteristics in their view of death (Table

TABLE 37-3 Views of death of various age groups

Age (Years)	Characteristics of View
3	Fears separations; unable to comprehend permanent separation
3-5	Generally reacts as parents do; views death as temporary and reversible; curious about death and what happens to body; may feel guilty if previously had wished harm to the deceased
6-10	More aware of permanence of death, but views it as avoidable; possible morbid ideas about body after death; fears pain and mutilation of body
11-12	Recognizes inevitability and irreversibility of death; attitude and beliefs influenced greatly by parents
13-21	Usually has developed personal philosophy of life and death; views own death as distant; often views it as a challenge and takes risks with own safety
22-45	Tends not to think about death unless confronted, then philosophizes and emotionally distances self from it
46-65	Usually experiences the death of parents or friends; may be preoccupied with death as he adjusts to aging; may put life in order to prepare for own death
66+	Usually fears lingering, incapacitating illness; views death as inevitable in near future

Research Highlight

Home Care for Children Dying of Cancer

Ida M. Martinson, D. Gay Moldow, Gordon D. Armstrong, William F. Henry, Mark E. Nesbit & John H. Kersey

PURPOSE

This nonexperimental study was designed to explore the provision and process of home care for the dying child and to specifically examine (1) the family's ability to provide good care at home until the child's death; (2) the family's willingness to provide such care; (3) the degree of nurse and physician involvement in such care; and (4) the nurse and family's abilities to procure adequate medication, medical equipment, and supplies.

SAMPLE

Fifty-eight children diagnosed as dying from cancer were cared for at home during the 2-year project. The children were 17 years of age or younger.

METHODOLOGY

Data were obtained from questionnaires and interview schedules developed during a pilot study, including health records, records completed by home care nurses, questionnaires on standard demographic and personal characteristics, grief support lists, care ratings, and progress recordings. The interviews were semistructured and conducted by trained individuals. Interviews were also conducted with the family 1 month and 1 year after the child's death. Home care was nurse directed with a consultant physician and did not entail extensive participation by other health care professionals; the option of readmitting the child to the hospital was always open.

FINDINGS

Forty-six of the 58 children (79%) died at home; 11 died in the hospital, and one died en route to the hospital. One month after the child's death, only two of the 73 parents whose children died at home expressed uncertainty about choosing home care again. Six (37.5%) of the 16 parents whose children did not die at home said they would choose home care again; six (31.5%) expressed uncertainty; and four (25%) said they would definitely choose hospital care. One year after their child's death, 56 families stated they would definitely choose home care again.

IMPLICATIONS

Home care was found to be a feasible alternative for a wide age range of children with a variety of special needs and was satisfactory for families of diverse backgrounds. Additional studies need to examine economic aspects of home care and develop and test criteria for children and parents who can or cannot benefit from the home care alternative.

Based on Data From Research in Nursing and Health **9**:11, 1986.

37-3). Of course, individual differences occur in each age group; a precise reaction depends on religion, illness, quality of life, relationships with others, age, growth, and development. The Research Highlight above presents the results of a current developmental investigation of children dying at home.

CHARACTERISTICS OF THERAPY WITH DYING CLIENTS

The implementation of therapy with dying clients differs from general psychiatric nursing psychotherapy. The type of illness and the process of dying limits the time available for therapy, and the goals, characteristics, and phases of the therapeutic process are different.

The nurse may have little time for intervention with clients facing sudden or unexpected death and longer periods with other clients. When a client dies suddenly and unexpectedly or is rushed to the hospital and dies soon after admission, crisis intervention techniques are appropriate for both the client and family. On the other hand, clients with short-term fatal illnesses may have weeks or months to prepare for death. The nurse has time to develop rapport with the client and family and to assist them in coping with the impending death.

Clients with long-term fatal illnesses have more time to develop a close relationship with the nurse and to resolve conflicts associated with their impending death. Clients diagnosed with a potentially fatal illness, such as cancer, live with both the possibility of survival after treatment and the possibility of death. The nurse supports these clients as they cope with potential death and possible alterations in body image resulting from the illness and treatment.

The overall goal of therapy with dying clients is to help them die comfortably and appropriately. The alleviation of as much pain as possible is also of primary concern. Issues causing conflict are handled in ways that promote emotional comfort.

The dying client sets the pace for the therapy. The nurse does not force issues or confront him with unresolved business. In-depth insight therapy is not usually appropriate. Very few people die with all their complexes and neuroses completely worked through; this is not a goal of psychotherapy with the dying client. Any type of therapy that damages the client's defenses against unbearable anxiety is avoided. The nurse reinforces and strengthens all of the client's intact coping mechanisms.

The termination phase of therapy differs from other forms of psychotherapy because of its finality. The nurse usually works with the client at least intermittently throughout the dying process. This commitment to support the client until death is an important aspect of therapy.

Another characteristic of therapy with the dying client is the relationship between the nurse and the client's survivors. The client and significant others will grieve throughout the dying process. The nurse usually develops rapport and works with significant others. She may see them intermittently for up to a year after the death, during which her primary task is supporting their efforts to free themselves from emotional bondage to the deceased and to find new patterns of rewarding interaction.

CHARACTERISTICS OF THE NURSE

Effective nurses have specific knowledge of the dying process, the needs of dying clients and their significant others, and expected patterns of behavior of dying and grieving clients. These nurses possess therapeutic interpersonal skills and quickly develop an open, honest relationship with both the dying clients and their families.

The nurse's ability to therapeutically intervene with the client and family is also related to personal characteristics and experiences. The nurse needs to examine her own feelings and attitudes about dying and death, since these are reflected in her care. The value the nurse places on health, productivity, independence, religious faith, and the meaning of life and death influences the way she interacts with dying clients. The nurse accepts the client's attitudes and responses to death, even if they are very different from her own. If the nurse feels conflict or fear when dealing with dying clients, she may inadvertently avoid them. Thus failure to assess and acknowledge her own feelings, beliefs, and values about dying and death may result in inadequate emotional care and minimal physical care.

Additional education is necessary for nurses who work with dying clients and their survivors and may be obtained by taking courses in death and dying, attending workshops, working with other therapists who deal with dying clients, and reading independently.

Nurses who work continuously with dying clients also have to deal with their personal feelings of grief and loss when their clients die. A client's death can and does affect the nurse and puts her at risk for depression. The nurse needs support from loved ones, other professionals, and sometimes a psychotherapist to work through her feelings from her involvement with death, grief, and loss.

NURSING PROCESS
Assessment

Physical dimension. During history taking the nurse asks questions about sleeping patterns, body image, activities of daily living, mobility, general health status, medications, and pain. The basic needs of nutrition, fluid and elimination, adequate oxygenation, and safety are also addressed.

Interruptions in previous sleeping patterns suggest possible causes of additional physical stress. Dying clients of-ten resist sleep because they worry about dying while asleep. The early morning hours are especially frightening because others are asleep and the client is alone.

Body image can be a major concern for the dying clients and those around them. The dying client's perceptions of his appearance may be assaulted by physical alterations from the illness or treatment, such as weight changes and hair loss; inability to maintain appearance because of weakness; and mutilations from surgical procedures or trauma. Illness and other factors that distort body image can make it difficult for the client to accept his appearance, causing changes in the responses of others to him.

Dying clients, especially those with cancer and other diseases that produce pain, often fear incapacitating pain and are concerned about whether it can be controlled. The nurse's assessment needs to be grounded in a working knowledge of pain assessment. The severity and duration of pain may change as manifestations of the disease increase. When death is imminent, clients usually become severely weak, with decreased sensations and reflexes and impaired circulation. These changes may decrease the need for pain medication (see Chapter 19).

Emotional dimension. Preparation for one's death is a personal endeavor in which anxiety and fear are often predominant emotions. Anxiety can be intense and is a threat to the client's well-being, self-esteem, and identity. Helping clients identify their fears is an integral part of the nurse's emotional assessment. Dying clients commonly fear:

1. The unknown
2. Loneliness
3. Sorrow
4. Loss of family and friends
5. Pain and suffering
6. Loss of self-control
7. Loss of body
8. Loss of identity

Often clients do not fear the fact of death itself as much as the feelings they experience as they proceed through the dying process. The fear of losing self-control is common, because illness may alter clients' life-styles, making them more dependent on others and altering role responsibilities in relationships. Losing control of body functioning can produce strong feelings of losing identity. The impending losses and changes in identity can be a serious threat to the client's self-esteem, leading to depression and regression.

Assessment of grief responses in the dying client and significant others is based on the identification and recognition of behaviors associated with the various types of grieving (discussed earlier in Theoretical Approaches). The nurse explores all family members' previous experiences and responses to loss. Based on the behaviors assessed and the definitions of acute or functional grief, delayed or dysfunctional grief, and pathological or morbid grief, the nurse is able to determine the grieving pattern of the client and family members. Anger, depression, and acceptance are expressed by both the family and client, and seldom is the group in unison. While one member is experiencing anger or denial, another may be depressed or attempting to bargain, and a third may have accepted the death and begun to grieve.

Assessing the guilt feelings of the client and family is also important. Dying clients frequently blame themselves for what is happening. Family members often feel guilty about their actions. They may say they are "not doing enough" for the client or feel they have contributed to the illness by actual or perceived offenses. Guilt may be manifested in destructive punishment. A client might not follow therapeutic plans because he believes he does not deserve to feel better. A spouse might quit work because she believes her job took her away from her husband and now she is being punished. Direct questions about guilt (such as "Do you feel your illness is a result of something you did or failed to do?") can help determine the extent of the guilt.

Anger is often exhibited by dying clients and is assessed by examining manifestation, extent, time of occurrence in the grieving process, response of others to it, and its effects on the client. Clients' expressions of anger can have either a positive or negative effect on their response to dying. Constructive anger is a mild resistance to the events occurring. It can be helpful as the client seeks ways of maintaining greater control over his remaining life. Constructive anger is also characterized by the client's setting of concrete goals and use of the anger to guard against depression and to maintain identity.[22] For example, a hospitalized client may insist on wearing his own clothes and maintaining his usual evening routine of watching television and taking a shower. Anger that is destructive to the client or others has a negative overall effect. Violence or hostility toward family members can further increase the client's isolation and perpetuate his anger.

The nurse assesses indications of depression, such as discontinuance of the use of denial and an abatement of anger. Denial and anger are often replaced by decreased physical activity. Talking or other activities may appear to be difficult for the depressed client; withdrawal from others also often occurs.

Careful assessment of depression is needed, because what appears to be depression may actually be introspection, in which the client sorts out and orders priorities. During introspection the client's external boundaries are limited, and he usually takes in only one significant other. For example, he may be unresponsive to most visitors, yet request that his son be with him. Because the client seems withdrawn and unapproachable, nurses often mislabel introspection as depression. Following are direct questions that can help to distinguish depression from introspection:

1. "What do you do with your spare time?"
2. "What are you thinking about?"
3. "Who do you need at this time?"

The depressed client may respond, "It's hopeless," "I'm useless," or "What's the use?" The introspective client may say, "I'm figuring some things out" or "I'm sorting through some stuff."

To determine if a client has reached the acceptance stage, the nurse assesses his freedom from strong emo-

tional components and the resolution of anger and denial. At this time the client makes no more commitments to life and deals with dying in a manner he can accept.

Intellectual dimension. All aspects of the intellectual dimension can be altered in the process of grieving and dying. Changes in sensory processes and perceptions of stimulation result from physiological changes from the disease process, medications, or the client's emotional state. Hearing and sight are sometimes diminished near death, as indicated by the client's turning toward light and listening intently. Although decreased sensation is most common, heightened sensory perception is also possible. A client may be overly sensitive to stimulation and find normal levels annoying. Because responses are highly individual, the nurse carefully watches the client's responses to sensory stimulation and asks him what level of stimulation he thinks is comfortable.

If the dying client is withdrawing from his immediate world, his short-term memory may diminish. This may be due to decreased motivation to remember as he attempts to detach himself from his immediate environment. Some dying clients seem to have an increased ability to remember events from the distant past as they engage in life review. They think about their childhood, young adulthood, career choices, and so forth.

It is widely accepted that a person knows that he is dying even when not told. It is also not uncommon for clients to know their time of death more precisely than the most sophisticated health care providers. The nurse needs to recognize that dying clients can possess this knowledge.

The nurse also assesses symbolic language. Dying clients often speak of one thing that represents another either by association or resemblance. If a client describes his illness as a "loss of freedom," he is most likely describing loss of control or a feeling of being trapped. Exploring these language symbols can reveal additional data about the client, his feelings, and his fears.

Another way to assess the intellectual dimension is through the use of imagery—calling up mental pictures to symbolize or typify something not present. Imagery can be described verbally or through art. For example, dying children often reveal knowledge of their impending death through drawings. Imagery arising from memories or internal representations of external stimuli allows clients to view something not present. It permits a client to convey what he may be unable to state directly to the nurse through descriptions of images or art; thus additional data is garnered. Individual clients may reveal a polarity of expressions about death from morbid fear to peaceful acceptance. When exploring these extremes and any area in between, imagery can be used to interpret the client's expressions. The fearful person frequently imagines death as dark, painful, and lonely. Peaceful clients picture it as bright, comfortable, and a place for reunion with lost friends, and family.

When the client discusses his death, the nurse ascertains his ideas of an appropriate and meaningful manner of dying. Questions to elicit this information are the following:

1. "What would be the ideal way in which you would like to die?"
2. "Who would you like to be with you when you are dying?"
3. "Where would you like to die?"
4. "What would you like to do before your death?"

The awareness contexts identified by Glaser and Strauss[21] provide some parameters for the assessment of the client's and others' knowledge about his dying process; their desire for this knowledge; and the family's beliefs and feelings about how much and what information needs to be shared with them and the client. Although it is commonly assumed that the open awareness context is best, clients and their families may prefer to be in closed awareness or mutual pretense. Thus a careful assessment of the level of the client and family's knowledge of the impending death is needed.

The dying client's perception of time needs to be evaluated. Living in the present is very important, but other realms of time perception are also to be recognized. The client's view of the past, present, and future can offer clues to how he may cope with death and the challenges faced in the process. Time seems to fly during periods of interest, commitment, or creativity and to drag during periods of waiting, boredom, or unpleasant emotions.[31] Dying clients who feel time is moving rapidly are usually committed to living their last days to the fullest as creative human beings, either by accomplishing tasks or making final plans. The client who feels time is dragging may be bored and simply waiting.

The nurse assesses the extent to which defense mechanisms are employed and their usefulness. Defense mechanisms can be beneficial if they do not interfere with relationships or distort reality. Sometimes, however, distorting reality may help dying clients to cope or preserve hope. Assessment of denial, the most common defense mechanism, includes the type and degree of use by the client. He may use denial for a few minutes to help cope or for a long period, refusing all help because "nothing is wrong." The prolonged use of denial can result in ignored medical treatment orders and exacerbated symptoms, can disrupt family interactions, and can prevent the client from making decisions that affect the family's future well-being.

Clients may also intellectualize as a defense mechanism. For example, a client may talk openly about impending death; relate all the statistics, facts, and figures on the particular illness; have read all the latest death and dying books; and express appropriate insights. This client may be coping on a cognitive level only, not on an emotional one. Clients who intellectualize use few emotional words (such as "sad," "happy," "angry," and "hurt") to express their reactions to dying; instead they use mostly cognitive words (such as "understand," "know," and "recognize").

Social dimension. If the client is not able to care for himself completely, the nurse assesses which activities are most important to his self-image and self-esteem and facilitates his participation in these. The family may desire to perform some of the activities involved in the client's care. This can be therapeutic for both parties.

Most clients' needs for social interaction remain similar to patterns established earlier in life. The nurse assesses previous styles and frequency of social interactions and who is in the client's network of family members and significant others. Family members who have previously played a minor role in the client's life may appear to assume a major role. The nurse determines whether this has a negative or positive effect on the client.

During the dying process clients are afforded a last chance to include significant people in their life. Clients and their families need to feel free to identify individuals who will contribute to the desired support in this crisis. A good friend at work, the occasional tennis partner, or the person they work out with at the gym may be part of the support system. Often people from important past social systems, such as old school friends, army pals, or childhood chums, may be called on. The nurse ascertains who the client views as significant, including any health care providers. The nurse can then call on these people when the client is near death and unable to call them himself.

The functional level of the family is assessed. After the initial shock a well-functioning family usually adapts to stressful situations by being able to shift roles, levels of responsibility, and patterns of interaction. The following information is necessary for asssessment:

1. Family structure, developmental state, and roles
2. Norms, values, and attitudes, especially toward illness and death
3. Extended family and outside supports, such as church, work, friends, and community resources

As the family faces and works through their grief, some behavior patterns will alert the nurse to growing distortions in the grieving process. Examples are changes in relationships with friends and other family members; loss of customary patterns of social interaction; and behavior that is detrimental to physical, social, or financial existence. If the grief becomes pathological, family members may begin missing work or school, getting in trouble with law officials, or abusing alcohol or drugs. Instead of drawing closer to loved ones, they may strike out destructively or maliciously. In extreme cases individuals can become homicidal or suicidal.

An assessment of the trust among client, family, and nurse is also essential in dealing with dying clients and their families. Learning to trust is no less important during the dying process than during life. The dying client who has a basic mistrust suffers more anxiety and fears than the who is trusting. Mistrusting behaviors include the client's asking the same questions of several health care professionals and being unwilling to share information with family members.

Spiritual dimension. The nurse assesses the spiritual dimension by asking questions such as: What are the spiritual aspects of the client's philosophy of life? Which religious resources and rituals of his faith group have significance for him in dealing with death? How are the client's values and beliefs about life, death, and the afterlife compatible or incompatible with those held by

Research Highlight

Religiousness Among Terminally Ill and Healthy Adults

Pamela G. Reed

PURPOSE

This study compares terminally ill and healthy adults' religiousness and sense of well-being.

SAMPLE

Fifty-seven terminally ill, unhospitalized adults and fifty-seven healthy adults were matched on four variables found to influence religiousness: age, gender, education, and religious affiliation. The terminally ill subjects were all diagnosed with incurable forms of cancer and were cognizant of their illness.

METHODOLOGY

Subjects were asked to complete demographic and health status questionnaires, two scales to determine religious perspective, and an index of well-being.

FINDINGS

The terminally ill subjects rated themselves considerably poorer in health status with a shorter life span and indicated significantly greater religiousness than the healthy group. The two groups did not differ significantly in their sense of well-being. There was a significant correlation between age and well-being in the terminally ill group only and between well-being and religiousness in the well group only. Women in both groups indicated greater religiousness than men, although only significantly in the terminally ill group.

IMPLICATIONS

The results of the study support that a person's age may influence how he views terminal illness. Further study is needed to assess the characterisitcs and needs of terminally ill people of various age groups. Although the client's spiritual dimension is considered relevant to nursing, there is little research on religion and health.

Based on data from Research in Nursing and Health 9:35, 1986.

individuals important to him? Incompatible beliefs among family members may increase distance and produce added stress. An exploration of these beliefs is less traumatic for the survivors if dealt with early than if discrepancies surface at the deathbed.

The spiritually healthy client has inner resources to assist him in coping with the stresses of the dying process. Inner resources may include faith and trust in God or a superior being, belief in the immortality of the soul, or belief in an overall purpose of life. Church or synagogue affiliation and its significance to the client, family, and significant others is explored to help identify spiritual support systems.

Clients who would not have considered themselves religious before their illness often turn to religion at this time (see the Research Highlight above). The particular religion may be the faith of their childhood, their family, or a friend.

The client may feel a sense of spiritual unrest if he feels he has not been faithful to his religion or that his disease is a punishment. Recognizing these feelings during the initial assessment allows more time to explore them.

Analysis

Nursing diagnosis. The major nursing diagnoses approved by the North American Nursing Diagnosis Association (NANDA) pertaining to the dying client are grieving, anticipatory grieving, and dysfunctional grieving. The de-

fining characteristics of these three diagnoses are presented in the boxes on the opposite page.

The following Case Example illustrates some of the defining characteristics of the nursing diagnosis of grieving.

Case Example

Mr. Caver was diagnosed 6 months ago with adrenal carcinoma. Because of pain and lethargy he gave up his position as a successful car salesman; he and his wife and son now depend on his wife's income.

Mr. Caver has trouble sleeping at night and has become increasingly withdrawn. He sometimes has difficulty concentrating on a topic in a conversation. His wife is concerned because he often becomes silent when his friends come to visit and wants to spend more and more time alone.

The following Case Example illustrates the defining characteristics of anticipatory grieving.

Case Example

Mrs. Piercy's 18-year-old son Mark suffered a serious head injury in an automobile accident. The doctor has informed the family that he will probably not come out of his coma. After seeing her son once, Mrs. Piercy refuses to visit him again. She expresses guilt to her family for letting him drive the night of his accident and talks as if Mark had already died.

The Case Example on p. 713 illustrates the defining characteristics of dysfunctional grieving.

GRIEVING

DEFINITION

Grieving is a state in which an individual or family experiences an actual or a perceived loss (person, object, function, status, relationship) or the state in which an individual or family responds to the realization of a future loss (anticipatory grieving).

DEFINING CHARACTERISTICS

Physical Dimension
Crying
*Altered appetitie or gastointestinal or elimination pattern
*Altered sleeping patterns
Emotional Dimension
Guilt
Sorrow
*Fears of losing control
Intellectual Dimension
Anticipates loss
Reports an actual or perceived loss
Denial
*Decreased concentration
Social Dimension
*Lack of warmth in casual relationships
Spiritual dimension
*Search for meaning

Adapted from North American Nursing Diagnosis classification of Nursing Diagnoses: Proceedings of the seventh conference, St. Louis, 1987, The C.V. Mosby Co.
*Indicates characteristics in addition to those defined by NANDA.

ANTICIPATORY GRIEVING

DEFINITION

Grief that occurs before the actual loss of an object or person. (NANDA definition not yet developed)

DEFINING CHARACTERISTICS

Physical Dimension
Changes in eating patterns
Alterations in activity level
Altered libido
Emotional Dimension
Potential loss of significant object
Expression of distress at potential loss
Guilt
Anger
Sorrow
Choked feelings
Intellectual Dimension
Denial of potential loss
Altered communication patterns

Adapted from North American Nursing Diagnosis Classification of Nursing Diagnoses: Proceedings of the seventh conference, St. Louis, 1987, The C.V. Mosby Co.

DYSFUNCTIONAL GRIEVING

DEFINITION

The grief reaction is delayed, excessive or leads to excess symptomology. (NANDA definition not yet developed)

DEFINING CHARACTERISTICS

Physical Dimension
Alterations in eating habits
Alterations in sleep patterns
Alterations in dream patterns
Alterations in activity level
Alterations in libido
Interference with life functioning
Emotional Dimension
Expression of guilt
Anger
Sadness
Crying
Developmental regression
Labile affect
Difficulty in expressing loss
Intellectual Dimension
Verbal expression of distress at loss
Denial of loss
Expression of unresolved issues
Idealization of lost object
Reliving of past experienices
Alterations in concentration and/or pursuit of tasks
Social Dimension
*Alterations in social relationships
Spiritual Dimension
*Questioning meaning of existence

Adapted from North American Nursing Diagnosis Association Classification of Nursing Diagnosis: Proceedings of the seventh conference, St. Louis, 1987, The C.V. Mosby Co.
*Indicates characteristics in addition to those defined by NANDA.

Case Example

Marilyn is a 42-year-old woman whose 87-year-old mother recently died from a heart attack following lengthy hospitalization for cancer. Since Marilyn's father is also deceased, her two brothers are involved in making the arrangements to settle the family estate and need Marilyn's cooperation in these efforts. However since the funeral two weeks ago, Marilyn has been unable to sleep and has not stayed at work for an entire day because she cannot concentrate on her job. When her brothers approach her about the need to settle some financial matters she begins to cry and expresses guilt over not spending enough time with her mother over the last 20 years.

The following list provides examples of NANDA-accepted nursing diagnoses with causative statements:
1. Alteration in comfort related to pain
2. Impaired physical mobility related to disease process
3. Severe anxiety related to impending death
4. Grieving related to loss of significant other
5. Powerlessness related to loss of independence

6. Ineffective coping related to awareness of impending death
7. Dysfunctional grieving related to hostility
8. Noncompliance related to feeling of separation from care providers
9. Knowledge deficit related to disease process
10. Disturbance in self-concept related to changes in body image
11. Spiritual distress related to guilt about one's life
12. Social isolation related to separation from family
13. Social isolation related to abandonment of friends
14. Ineffective family coping related to role changes

DSM-III-R diagnoses. The DSM-III-R diagnosis for dying clients and their significant others is *uncomplicated bereavement* (see the box at right).

Planning

Table 37-4 contains long-term and short-term goals and outcome criteria related to death and dying. These serve as examples of the planning stage in the nursing process.

Implementation

✦ *Physical dimension.* The client's energy level can fluctuate daily or even hourly. He is often weak and fatigued; thus his physical care is scheduled to allow rest periods between activities, and the nurse assumes physical care activities the client is unable to perform. Since the client's physical condition can change rapidly, the nurse needs to be prepared to modify nursing care.

The nurse ensures that adequate rest is provided and promotes activity by maintaining the client's regular

---

V62.82 UNCOMPLICATED BEREAVEMENT

ESSENTIAL FEATURES

This category can be used when a focus of attention or treatment is a normal reaction to the death of a loved one.

MANIFESTATIONS
Physical Dimension

Poor appetite
Weight loss
Insomnia

Emotional Dimension

Full depressive syndrome
Guilt, if present, is chiefly about things done or not done by the survivor at time of death

Intellectual Dimension

Regards depression as "normal"
Thoughts of death usually limited to individual's thinking he would be better off dead or he should have died with the client

Social Dimension

May seek professional help for relief of associated symptoms (duration of "normal" bereavement varies considerably among different subcultural groups)

Adapted from American Psychiatric Association: Diagnostic and statistical manual of mental disorders (DSM-III-R), Washington, D.C., 1987, The Association.

---

sleeping patterns as much as possible. Restful sleep is promoted when the client maintains his usual evening rou-

---

TABLE 37-4 Long-term and short-term goals and outcome criteria related to the dying client

Goals	Outcome Criteria
NURSING DIAGNOSIS: ANTICIPATORY GRIEVING RELATED TO THE KNOWLEDGE OF IMPENDING DEATH	
Long-term goal	
To express grief appropriately to family and significant others.	Expresses feelings of grief to family members and others in appropriate and meaningful way Shares feelings and fears about death
Short-term goal	
To identify problems in the grieving process.	Shares concerns of grieving with appropriate others
NURSING DIAGNOSIS: FEAR OF LONELINESS RELATED TO ABANDONMENT BY FAMILY AND OTHERS	
Long-term goal	
To maintain interaction with significant others throughout the dying process.	Requests visits from significant others Initiates relationships with staff and clergy
Short-term goals	
To express fear of loneliness to nurse.	Expresses feelings of fear to appropriate other(s) Identifies behaviors related to fear of loneliness
To initiate methods of reducing loneliness.	Requests personal items to be included in environment Uses telephone and letters to maintain contact with others Asks to spend time with other clients in unit

tines and bedtime. Placing the client near others is often helpful, because dying clients may fear being alone, especially at night. The view that the dying client needs to be in a quiet, subdued, softly lit area may be incorrect. If the client is at home, he may rest better with someone else in the room or even in bed with him. Placing hospitalized clients near activity areas is often advisable. A semiprivate room may be more comforting than a private room. A nightlight can be helpful to keep the client oriented to familiar places and objects in the room.

The dying client needs to be kept as comfortable as possible. Nursing measures are instituted to enhance proper functioning of the body systems, to maintain comfort, and to prevent further disability. The client's skin condition needs to be frequently monitored because of his inactivity, the possibility of edema, and the fragility of the tissues. The skin is maintained and skin breakdown is treated. Although the client is dying, the nurse is still responsible for assisting him to maintain correct body alignment and flexibility of joints through proper positioning, turning, and range-of-motion exercises. These activities increase comfort for the client with decreased sensations, reflexes, and circulation. Even if the dying client looks comfortable, positioning change at least every 2 hours is essential. Writing a nursing order to turn the client each even hour promotes physical comfort and staff contact with him, decreasing feelings of isolation.

Families who want to assist in client care can be instructed in massage. This allows the family to be helpful and increases comfort, amount of touching, and feelings of togetherness. Family members or friends who do not feel comfortable massaging the upper body or trunk can massage the feet. If heightened sensation causes a massage to be painful for the client, the foot is usually relatively free of pain, and the results are similar to those of body massage.

Pain management is essential in promoting comfort for the dying client. All clients do not experience pain, but most fear it. Open communication in the early stages of therapy allows the client to discuss his ideas of pain and the nurse to explain ways it can be controlled. The nurse reassures the client that all possible ways of managing pain will be used. The nurse addresses the client's fears of addiction by explaining that addicts use medications for emotional highs; not to relieve pain. One medication's gradual ineffectiveness does not mean that addiction has occurred; switching to other medications may be beneficial to clear the body of those chemicals. The same drugs can often be used effectively again later.

The dying client's body image is assaulted by the effects of illness and treatment. The nurse encourages clients to wear their own clothes, put on their makeup, comb their hair, or purchase a wig to enhance their self-image. Because many clients lose a great deal of weight, it is helpful for them to wear clothing that fits properly and does not accentuate the change.

Emotional dimension. The nurse accepts the client's feelings, attitudes, values, and means of coping. When the client does not want to talk, sitting quietly with him expresses an understanding and acceptance of him. Nonverbal expressions of acceptance, such as touch, can be meaningful. However, the nurse needs to verify that touch is acceptable to the client. His stiffening or pulling away may indicate that touching makes him feel uncomfortable. This client may be comfortable with the nurse sitting close to the bedside. Spending time with the client other than when physical care is being performed communicates that the nurse is interested in him as a person. The nurse shows commitment to continued work with the client by following through on agreements and by being consistent in actions and time spent with the client.

The nurse assists the grieving client through encouragement and support. She does not interfere with the client's own pattern of grief. Grief work can be physically and emotionally exhausting. The client needs rest periods and may wish to be alone to restore himself and grieve privately.

The dying client commonly feels low, anxious, or depressed on some days and peaceful on others. The nurse can help prepare the client for this cycle by explaining its possiblity.

When a person is first diagnosed with a potentially fatal illness, fear surfaces in many forms. A goal of therapy at this stage is to reduce fears and anxieties. Verbalizing the fears is helpful. Forcing the client to talk about it may increase his discomfort rather than give peace. Allowing dying clients to verbalize when they choose provides sensitive comfort.

Anxiety can occur throughout the dying process. The nurse assists the client in identifying anxiety and exploring its origins. She can ask, "When you begin to feel nervous about a particular event, what was it that may have caused the anxiety?" Being able to identify the cause transforms the nameless into a known fear. Once the problem has been named, it can be assessed and diagnosed, and appropriate plans and interventions can be developed.

Anger needs to be accepted by the nurse undefensively. Responding defensively tells the client that he is only accepted if he is "good" and frequently intensifies the anger and hostility. The nurse validates that the client's anger is a normal response and encourages him to vent his feelings about his impending death, providing positive reinforcement for openness and honesty. If the client still has pent-up emotions, the nurse provides alternative ways of expressing the anger, such as physical exercise and games of skill, that are not harmful to others or to himself. Attempts to make light of or to criticize the client's anger are unsupportive. For example, the statement "You ought to be glad you're alive" is telling the client he is ungrateful.

The nurse assists the client in expressing his guilt, examining it realistically, considering what his alternatives may have been, and determining if they were realistic. The following is an example:

Client: *I should have gone to the doctor earlier.*
Nurse: *Did you have earlier warning signals?*
Client: *No.*
Nurse: *Then how would you have known to go to the doctor earlier?*

Even if symptoms were disregarded or health habits neglected, the nurse can help the client realize that it is normal to ignore symptoms, to think they are insignificant and will go away. Statements such as "Well, you smoked long enough, didn't you?" will only add to his guilt.

When the client is ready, the nurse can provide assistance as he says good-bye to his family and friends and to her. The nurse provides time and privacy for the good-byes. She may engage him in role-playing before he actually says good-bye. The nurse provides acceptance and support by allowing the client to lead her through his dying process.

✳ *Intellectual dimension.* Information about the illness and dying process is given to the client as he requests it. Most clients wish to know the illness' extent and the prognosis. The client and family frequently benefit from a description of and the rationale for the treatment and plan of care. Withholding information in the name of "protecting the client" may be more for the comfort of staff members and family. Information about the prognosis, however, is never to be forced on the client; it is only given when he is ready for it.

No specific guidelines exist for precisely what information is to be given, when to disclose the information, or whom can best present the information to the client. The client needs to be allowed to set the pace. The nurse uses terminology that the client can easily understand. Frequently the information needs to be repeated because of distracting pain, effects of disease and medications, shortened attention span, interference from emotional responses, and other factors. Verifying that the information is understood allows for clarification and ensures that it is understood. The nurse asks the client to repeat the information in his own words and what the information means to him. The nurse can also ask the client to relay the information to a family member in her presence.

Clients are always allowed to ask questions. The nurse is truthful but refrains from destroying all hope, positively reinforcing realistic hopes. For example, a common question of dying clients is, "Am I going to die?" An appropriate response is reflective, such as "Do you feel you are dying?" This allows the client to express his thoughts and fears and allows the nurse to ascertain the real meaning of the client's question. Answering, "Yes, you know you have about a month to live," destroys all hope. Examples of realistic hopes are that a loved one will arrive before the client dies or that he will be in less pain or more alert.

The nurse can ask the client to imagine his own death and use his images to help him die comfortably and appropriately. For example, if the client imagines that he is dying pleasantly and comfortably at home with his wife and child present and relatively free of pain, the nurse works with the family to meet that goal. If moving the client home is not a suitable option for the family or client because of his physical condition, the nurse helps him amend the previous image. For this particular client, dying in the hospital can be cushioned by bringing familiar articles from home, such as his favorite pictures, music, and pillow, to his room.

If the dying client imagines his death very fearfully and negatively, the nurse encourages him to alter the picture to gain control over the fearful aspects. The client who fears death's darkness can begin to imagine lights and soft music in the room. Imagery can be used to explore fears and concerns and to alleviate those fears by altering the image and ultimately reality.

The nurse needs to allow and accept the client's intermittent use of denial. She is truthful with him but does not force him to accept information or discuss subjects that he resists. The following is an example:

Nurse: Did they tell you what the biopsy report said?
Client: No.
Nurse: Do you want to know?
Client: No.
Nurse: Okay. I'll be back tomorrow, and we can talk about it then if you're ready.

If the client's denial interferes with therapy and is destructive, the nurse simply confirms that the information he has received is true, rather than confronting him with his unwillingness to openly deal with death. She tells the client that the choice of whether or not to accept and respond to the information is his but that she wants him to have it. The nurse's manner is matter-of-fact and not judgmental.

If the client's denial is manifested by going from one physician, hospital, or form of therapy to another, the nurse helps him examine the purpose of his behavior rather than criticizing him or trying to talk him out of his plans. She might ask him how he thinks this behavior will help him, what he expects to be told, and what he will do if he hears the same thing again.

If the client decides to return home, additional teaching may be necessary for him and family members. The nurse teaches the family skills to enable them to care for the client at home. The physical environment is considered when developing plans for home care. The nurse also explains the signs and symptoms of deteriorating health and when and how to seek professional help when needed. Positive and negative aspects of the client's return home are explored to ascertain the support needs of the family. It is often helpful to assist the family in identifying additional means of support, such as hospice nurses, health care personnel from home health care agency services, public health nurses, friends, and other family members who can help either routinely or occasionally.

Often the client requests information about will preparation, organ doanation, and financial assistance. Information that the nurse cannot provide is obtained, or the client is referred to the appropriate person.

Because a client near death may have decreased hearing and sight, the nurse stands close to the bed, speaks loudly and clearly, and informs the client of procedures initiated for him and what is occurring elsewhere in the room. If the client has heightened sensations, environmental stimuli are decreased (for example, the room is darkened).

❈ *Social dimension.* To promote the client's independence and maintain self-esteem, the nurse allows him to perform as much hygienic care as he can. If he cannot perform complete self-care, the nurse allows him to do what is most important for his self-image and self-esteem.

Often the family wants to participate in the physical care of their loved one, which can be therapeutic for both parties. It is still important, however, that the client's independence be maintained as much as possible. The client may feel belittled or babied if the family performs care that he is capable of doing himself. Also, the nursing staff does not rely on the family to perform this care. Inappropriate use of the family in the provision of nursing care can result in hostility and mistrust of the nursing staff.

Pointing out the client's positive attributes is helpful in increasing self-esteem. Sincere comments such as "You sure have pretty eyes," "I like how you fixed your hair," or "That color shirt is really right for you" can help a client focus on positive rather than negative attributes.

The nurse supports the client's realistic adaptation to loss and assists him in restructuring his life-style to promote a meaningful existence. This is accomplished through the client's continued involvement in established relationships, particularly the most significant ones. Another method is to promote renewal of former meaningful interests. Resuming a hobby can be a therapeutic outlet and contribute to a sense of accomplishment.

The client and family may need encouragement to maintain current roles, personal interests, and life-style for as long as possible. There is a tendency to prematurely abandon jobs, hobbies, vacations, and social interests; the nurse can intervene to prevent this. The celebration of special events, such as birthdays, anniversaries, and other holidays, is encouraged.

The nurse also assists the client and significant others in exploring the impact the client's death may have on the survivors. The client may identify specific actions that he can take to help the family readjust after his death, such as making a will, updating insurance policies, paying bills, providing instruction for handling of family financial responsibilities, or completing professional or business obligations. It also may be necessary to provide opportunities to discuss personal preferences about funeral and burial arrangements, such as place and type of funeral, clothing to be worn, pallbearers, and burial site.

As the client's condition deteriorates, the family will require assistance and support to shift roles and assume new behaviors. If the client has previously handled all the business matters, this task may now fall to a family member unfamiliar with such transactions. The nurse may suggest resources available to assist in solving problems and to help family members feel less overwhelmed.

Dying clients frequently enjoy talking about the past. Life review enables them to talk about past accomplishments, pleasures, and hardships and gives them pride. How they succeeded in their job, dealt with adversity, or overcame setbacks is reminiscent of happy, healthier times. The past represents control that dying clients may feel they are losing. Past recollections offer affirmation of self. The past is something known and cannot be taken away like the future. Discussing subjects that span the past, present, and future allows clients to make a statement about their being.

Nurses and family members often do not allude to present events, since the client is possibly unable to fully engage in them. The past is avoided for fear of upsetting the dying client and making him yearn for what "used to be." Discussions of future holidays, vacations, or special events are avoided, since the client may not be there to enjoy them. Dying persons are often afraid to mention future plans for fear of being labeled as unrealistic. These beliefs contribute to the client's feelings of aloneness, isolation, and abandonment. The opportunity for real communication and sharing is lost if health care personnel and significant others assume that talking about the past or future makes the dying person uncomfortable. Exploring and validating the degree of comfort in these topics can greatly enhance communication and afford a vast repertoire for conversation.

Framing memories is a specific, effective tool for encouraging clients and family members to review the past and envision the future. The client and family reminisce about happy experiences. The nurse can urge the client to give family members meaningful information to pass on to future generations. In return family members can tell the client what he means to them and tell him of their future aspirations; this way the client is able to share in their future.

As death approaches, family, friends, and staff members may avoid the dying client because of their own discomfort. The nurse encourages involved individuals to express their feelings and supports their efforts to cope with their fears. Support groups for clients, families, or nursing staff can reduce the probability of client abandonment as death approaches.

The client needs the opportunity to say good-bye to others. The nurse encourages and supports the client and significant others as they terminate relationships in a healthy, appropriate, and positive manner. The nurse acknowledges the painful feelings of termination and reinforces the importance of the client's completion of this task.

After the death the family is allowed to vent their feelings and encouraged to accept the pain of the loss. Avoidance of the pain of loss and bereavement can produce destructive delayed responses. Reviewing a family member's relationship with the deceased and helping him express feelings of sorrow, anger, or guilt can facilitate healthy resolution of grief.

Spiritual dimension. To help meet the spiritual needs of the client, the nurse supports and accepts him and his spiritual beliefs, even though they may differ from her own. If the client finds comfort in prayers, the nurse ensures time and privacy for praying. If he expresses comfort in the concepts of grace and faith, the nurse explores them with him.

The clergy can be a valuable resource. Some clients are comfortable only with clergy from their own faith; visits from the clergy of their home congregation are often very important.

Some clients may ask the nurse to participate in religious activities with him, such as praying or communion. In such instances a meaningful relationship has usually developed between this nurse and client. If the activity is acceptable to her personal values, it is appropriate for the nurse to join the client. If the nurse is uncomfortable with the request and declines, she explains the reason in a manner that is not critical of his beliefs. To demonstrate continued acceptance of the client and the client's beliefs, the nurse may offer to find another person to participate with him.

Evaluation

The therapeutic process is considered successful if the client's death was meaningful and appropriate to him. The family may be included in the evaluation, but the fact that the care culminates in the client's death has an impact on their feelings and responses. Whether the death was sudden or long anticipated, the family and care providers experience a loss. The immediate reaction can include questions about the adequacy of the health care provided. The family may express a variety of feelings, ranging from appreciation to anger and hostility toward the nurse and other health care providers. Evaluating these feelings openly and honestly can facilitate the healing process and generate new ideas for care delivery.

A nursing process summary for the dying and grieving client is presented in the box below.

NURSING PROCESS SUMMARY: GRIEF

ASSESSMENT

Responses characteristic of the different types of grief are given in Table 37-4.

ANALYSIS

See the nursing diagnoses list on pp. 713-714.

PLANNING AND IMPLEMENTATION

Physical Dimension

Promote the client's physical comfort.
Meet nutritional, fluid, and elimination needs.
Promote the highest level of functioning possible.
Provide for rest and activity.
Provide for hygienic and skin needs.
Administer pain medication.
Provide assistance in mobility.
Provide a safe environment.

Emotional Dimension

Spend time with the client, family, and client and family together at times other than when administering physical care.
Provide appropriate support to the client according to his current grieving; change support as required as he moves through the grieving process.
Help the client and family express reactions to previous losses, to the current loss, and to responses of family and others to the current loss.
Ensure and respect the client's privacy.
Use touch and other nonverbal communication appropriately to provide support and acceptance.
Encourage meaningful activities.
Provide emotional support to significant others so they will be able to support the client.

Intellectual Dimension

Explore the client's and significant others' level of knowledge about the diagnosis, illness, and dying process.
Provide information as requested.
Support useful coping mechanisms.
Allow time for the client and significant others to talk.
Discuss the therapeutic regimen—its components, purposes, options.
Use imagery to assist the client in exploring the meaning of the dying process and death.
Assist the client in reviewing his life.
Allow the client to make as many choices as possible.
Allow the client to set the pace for grief work.

Reduce demands placed on the client, but refrain from performing nonessential procedures for him.
Allow the client to speak openly about dying and death.

Social Dimension

Explore with the client and significant others the cultural significance of dying and death.
Identify and plan for customs related to dying and death that are important to the client and significant others.
Allow client to perform as much self-care as he is capable of to enhance self-esteem and self-image.
Allow family members to perform mutually satisfactory and beneficial client care.
Incorporate important social events, such as birthdays, anniversaries, holidays, and graduations, into care as much as possible.
Educate the client and family members about shifts in role behaviors.
Assist the client and family in maintaining previous roles and life-style to the degree possible.
Identify and offer options and resources for environmental changes and ways of coping with physical, financial, and role changes resulting from or concomitant with illness.
Identify and explore alternative environments for care, their advantages, disadvantages, and locations.
Refer client to appropriate agencies and health care professionals to meet needs not met by nursing.

Spiritual Dimension

Explore with the client and significant others the meaning and significance of dying and death in their religion.
Identify and plan for religious activities related to dying and death that are important to the client and significant others.
Encourage and provide for religious observances.
Encourage and provide for use of spiritual resources.
Determine the client's conditions for a meaningful death.

EVALUATION

Answering the following questions will reveal whether the client's death was meaningful and appropriate to him:
Did the client die where he wanted to?
Were the people he wanted present at his death?
Was he comfortable?
Had he been able to express thoughts to family and friends?
Had he experienced desired religious activities, such as communion?

BRIEF REVIEW

Individuals differ in their responses to death. Dying as the final stage of life is an important aspect in holistic health care. The nurse is often a key person in providing care to dying clients and their families.

Death and responses to death are beginning to be explored in all aspects of American culture. The roles of professionals in caring for the dying have expanded rapidly since the early 1900s with the recent interest in death education programs, hospice care, and holistic approaches.

The nurse who therapeutically intervenes with dying clients and their families uses her knowledge of the dying process and the needs of the client and family and effective interpersonal skills to facilitate the client's open expression of feelings.

The nurse thoroughly assesses all areas of the client's life. Goals are the mutual objectives determined by the client and nurse. Goals remain realistic and constitute a form of hope that is essential during the dying process. Planning and implementation change as the dying process changes. Through the nursing process the nurse assists the client in meeting his death in a way that is comfortable and acceptable to him.

REFERENCES AND SUGGESTED READINGS

1. American Nurses' Association; Code for nurses, Kansas City, 1976, American Nurses' Association.
1a. American Psychiatric Association; Diagnostic and statistical manual of mental disorders (DSM-III-R), Washington, D.C., 1987, The Association.
2. Barton, D., editor: Dying and death: a clinical guide for caregivers, Baltimore, 1977, The Williams & Wilkins Co.
3. Berry, J.O., and others: The stage model revisited, Rehabilitation Literature 44(9-10):275, 1983.
4. Bowlby, J.: Attachment theory, separation anxiety, and mourning. In Arieti, S., editor: American handbook of psychiatry, ed. 2, New York, 1975, Basic Books, Inc., Publishers.
5. Brice, C.W.: Mourning throughout the life cycle, American Journal of Psychoanalysis 42(4):315, 1982.
6. Brown, J.T. and Stoudemire, G.A. Normal and pathological grief, Journal of the American Medical Association 250(3):378, 1983.
7. Browning, M.H., and Lewis, E.P., editors: The dying patient: a nursing perspective, New York, 1972, American Journal of Nursing Co.
8. Bugen, L.A.: Human grief: a model for prediction and intervention, American Journal of Orthopsychiatry 47(2):196, 1977.
9. Castles, M.R., and Murray, R.B.: Dying in an institution: nurse/patient perspectives, New York, 1979, Appleton-Century-Crofts.
10. Collison, C., and Miller, S.: Using images of the future in grief work, Image 19(1):9, 1987.
11. deBeauvoir, S.: A very easy death, New York, 1973, Warner Paperback Library.
12. Dobson, C.C., and others: Unresolved grief in the family, American Family Physician 27(1):207, 1983.
13. Dracup, K.A., and others: Using nursing research findings to meet the needs of grieving spouses, Nursing Research 27:212, 1978.
14. Elbirlik, K.: The mourning process in group therapy, International Journal of Group Psychotherapy 33(12):215, 1983.
15. Epstein, C.: Nursing the dying patient, Reston, Va., 1975, Reston Publishing Co.
16. Feifel, H., editor: The meaning of death, New York, 1959, McGraw-Hill Book Co.
17. Franks, J.: Toward understanding understanding. In Weimer, Wand Palermo, D: Cognition and the symbolic processes, New York, 1974, John Wiley & Sons, Inc.
18. Granstrom, S.L.: Spiritual nursing care for oncology patients, Topics in Clinical Nursing 7(1):39, 1985.
19. Furman, E.: Children's patterns in mourning the death of a loved one, Issues in Comprehensive Pediatric Nursing 8(6):185, 1985.
20. Garfield, C.A., editor: Psychosocial care of the dying patient, New York, 1978, McGraw-Hill Book Co.
21. Glaser, B.G., and Strauss, A.L.: Awareness of dying, Chicago, 1965, Aldine Publishing Co.
22. Grollman, E.A., editor: Concerning death: a practical guide for the living, Boston, 1974, Beacon Press.
23. Horowitz, M.J., and others: Brief psychotherapy of bereavement reactions: the relationship of process to outcome, Archives of General Psychiatry 41(5):438, 1984.
24. Johnson, J.: Call me healthy, Oncology Nursing Forum 9:73, 1982.
25. Kalish, R.A.: Death, grief, and caring relationships, Monterey, Calif., 1981, Brooks/Cole Publishing Co.
26. Kavanaugh, R.E.: Facing death, Kingsport, Tenn., 1972, Kingsport Press, Inc.
27. Kübler-Ross, E.: On death and dying, New York, 1969, Macmillan Publishing Co., Inc.
28. Kübler-Ross, E.: To live until we say good-bye, Englewood Cliffs, N.J., 1978, Prentice-Hall, Inc.
29. Lindemann, E.: Symptomatology and management of acute grief, American Journal of Psychiatry 101:141, 1944.
30. Lunden, T.: Long-term outcome of bereavement, British Journal of Psychiatry 145:424, 1984.
31. Maguire, D.C.: Death by choice, New York, 1975, Schocken Paperbacks.
32. Megerle, J.S.: Surviving, American Journal of Nursing 83(6):892, 1983.
33. Melges, F.T.: Time and the inner future, New York, 1982, John Wiley & Sons, Inc.
34. Mitford, J.: The American way of death, Greenwich, Conn., 1963, Fawcett Books.
35. Oberfield, R.A., Terminal illness, death and bereavement: toward an understanding of its nature, Perspectives in Biology and Medicine 28(1):140, 1984.
36. Peterson, J.A.: Social-psychological aspects of death and dying and mental health. In Birren, J.E., and Sloane, R.B., editors: Handbook of mental health and aging, Englewood Cliffs, N.J., 1980, Prentice-Hall, Inc.
37. Ptalum, M.C., and others: Understanding the final message of the dying, Nursing 16(6):26, 1986.
38. Pinker, S., and Kosslyn, S.M.: Theories of mental imagery. In Sheikk, A. A., editor: Imagery, New York, 1983, John Wiley & Sons, Inc.
39. Polanyi, M.: The tacit dimension, Garden City, N.Y., 1967, Anchor Books, Doubleday.
40. Putnam, S.T., and others: Home as a place to die, American Journal of Nursing 80:1451, 1980.
41. Roy, P.F., and others: Group support for the recently bereaved, Health and Social work 8(3):230, 1983.
42. Rubin, S.S., Mourning distinct from melancholia, the resolution of bereavement, British Journal of Medical Psychology 7:339, 1984.
43. Sahler, O.J., editor: The child and death, St. Louis, 1978, The C.V. Mosby Co.

44. Shneidman, E.S., editor: Death: current perspectives, Palo Alto, Calif., 1976, Mayfield Publishing Co.

45. Shneidman, E.S.: Deaths of man, Baltimore, 1974, Penguin Books.

46. Shneidman, E.S.: Some thoughts on grief and mourning, Suicide and Life-Threatening Behavior **15**(1):51, 1985.

47. Shanfield, S.B., and others: Death of adult children in traffic accidents, Journal of Nervous and Mental Disease **172**(9)533, 1984.

48. Shapiro, E.T.: Death and dying, Journal of the Medical Society of New Jersey **80**(2):110, 1983.

49. Schulman, J.L., and Rehm, J.L.: Assisting the bereaved, Journal of Pediatrics **102**(6):1008, 1983.

50. Spradley, J.P.: The ethnographic interview, New York, 1979, Holt, Rinehart & Winston General Book.

51. State Historian: Ecclesiastical records, State of New York, Albany, 1901, State Press.

52. Toynbee, A.: Various ways in which human beings have sought to reconcile themselves to the fact of death. In Shneidman, E.S., editor: Death: current perspectives, Palo Alto, Calif., 1976, Mayfield Publishing Co.

53. Weisman, A.D.: The realization of death: a guide for the psychological autopsy, New York, 1974, Jason Aronson, Inc.

54. Wilcox, S., and Sutton, M.: Understanding death and dying: a multidisciplinary approach, Port Washington, N.Y., 1977, Alfred Publishing Co., Inc.

55. Wilkes, E.: Quality of life: effects of the knowledge of diagnosis in terminal illness, Nursing Times **73**:1506, 1977.

56. Zlsook, S., editor: Biophysical aspects of bereavement, Washington, D.C., 1987, American Psychiatric Press, Inc.

ANNOTATED BIBLIOGRAPHY

Collison, C. and Miller, S.: Using images of the future in grief work, Image **19**(1):9, 1987.

Encouraging dying clients and family members to imagine future events is presented as a supportive nursing therapy. Imaging allows the dying individual to preserve his identity and facilitates a mutual redefinition of relationships with significant others. The authors promote imaging as a mechanism to address the existential crisis facing the dying client and his family.

Corr, C.A. and McNeil, J.N., editors: Adolescence and death, New York, 1986, Springer Publishing Co., Inc.

This book explores the issues of death, dying, and bereavement in the lives of adolescents. It identifies ways in which adults can assist teenagers to cope with death-related issues.

Kalish,R.A.: Death, grief, and caring relationships, Monterey, Calif., 1981, Brooks/Cole Publishing Co.

Personal observations, research, and theory are integrated in this thorough and highly readable book. The four major sections are the meaning of death, the process of dying, grief and bereavement, and caring relationships. Each section begins with an allegory or personal story.

Worden, J.W.: Grief counseling and grief therapy: a handbook for the mental health practitioner, New York, 1982, Springer Publishing Co., Inc.

The phenomenon of grief is developed in a concrete, well-organized manner. The book provides many useful suggestions for helping clients work through grief reactions in a meaningful and healthy way.

CHAPTER 38

ALTERNATIVE TREATMENT MODALITIES

Elizabeth Jane Martin

After studying this chapter the learner will be able to:

Identify assumptions underlying alternative treatment modalities.

Discuss the historical development of the human potential movement.

Compare and contrast body-focused, mind/psyche-focused, spirit/consciousness-focused, and holistic alternative treatment approaches.

Identify a typical alternative treatment approach in each of the four types, giving characteristics of the therapist, therapy, and therapeutic process.

Mental health–psychiatric nurses today have a wider range of treatment modalities available than ever before. The more traditional modalities discussed in preceding chapters continue to be important and useful. However, in the last few decades alternative treatment therapies, sometimes called *the new therapies,* have emerged to challenge conventional modalities.

Alternative treatment modalities differ widely in focus and method. However, in general all of them rest on the following assumptions:

1. People are fine as they are (not sick) but could be better.
2. People all have unrealized (some say limitless) potential.
3. Individual change is best accomplished through self-responsibility and self-help.

Some alternative treatment modalities, like conventional therapy, have stringent qualifications for their practitioners, rigidly structured sessions, and legal and social sanctions. However, conventional psychotherapy assumes that its major task is to work on the mind. Its proponents believe that when the mental problem is corrected, clients automatically do things that enrich their lives in other ways. In the alternative forms of therapy the mind is only one dimension addressed. Of equal or greater importance, depending on the particular therapy, is the body, spirit, and environment. Conventional psychotherapists conduct their sessions in offices and have regular

meetings; alternative therapists may meet for extended periods at irregular intervals, at retreats, in public meeting rooms, or even in forests. Whereas conventional psychotherapists emphasize exploring the past, human potential practitioners emphasize the present and value feelings more than ideas. They borrow heavily from the wisdom of ancient societies, particularly Eastern religions and philosophies. They emphasize the body in all its beauty and grace and advocate using its fullest capacity for movement and pleasure, believing that it also provides a means of feeling better emotionally.

The new therapies discussed in this chapter are those which have emerged as significant treatment approaches. They have either attracted large numbers of followers or have had a recognized impact on health care in the United States.

BODY-FOCUSED THERAPIES

The body-focused treatment approaches are based on the premise that the client's problem is housed in the body and that relief from symptoms will occur if the body is properly treated. These therapies focus on the physical dimension and use manipulative techniques to alter some component of the body structure. Although corresponding changes often take place in other dimensions of the client—intellectual, emotional, social, and spiritual—they are coincidental to the treatment of the body and are not

🍇 *Historical Overview* 🍇

DATE	EVENT
1960s	New, alternative forms of therapy emerged in response to the development of the holistic view of the person, which emerged from the human potential movement. Astrology, meditation, body manipulation, exercise, nutrition, control of involuntary physiological states, and psychic phenomena were included in the expanding human potential movement and were reflected in the development of alternative therapies.
1970s-1980s	People became fascinated by the human potential movement and explored the new forms of therapy to determine for themselves the advantages and disadvantages of each. Adam Smith[64] wrote about his 3-year journey in *Powers of the Mind.* Steven Applebaum,[4] a psychoanalyst from the Menninger Clinic, recorded the adventures of his odyssey in *Out in Inner Space.* Richard Alpert, a wealthy, well-educated social scientist and psychotherapist, journeyed to India, emerged as Ram Dass,[49] and wrote about his adventures in *The Only Dance There Is* (which is life).
	Some of the far-reaching effects of the human potential movement and the new types of therapy are an increased sense of community and acceptance of responsibility, a decreased emphasis on competition with a shift from aggression to gentleness, a renewed appreciation of nature and awareness of ecological responsibility, and a commitment to a holistic approach to all of life in development of the fullest human potential in body, mind, and spirit.
Future	Practitioners of the new types of therapy, dissatisfied with society as it exists, are optimistic that with their diversity of interests and plurality of approaches they can make a difference in the quality of their clients' lives.

emphasized. However, neither are they denied. All of these alternative treatment approaches are said to be holistic and as such are expected to affect all five human dimensions.

Alexander Technique

The *Alexander technique* is one of the oldest treatment approaches to be considered here. A precursor of the human potential movement, this body-focused technique has gained wide respectability. Frederick Alexander[3] (1869-1955) was an Austrian actor whose career was threatened by repeated loss of his voice during performances. From self-observation he concluded that the cause of his voice loss was his tendency to pull his head backward and downward during every movement. He trained himself not to do this, and his difficulty disappeared. Alexander continued his observations and created a system that encouraged people to "unlearn" harmful or habitual movements that cause tension, stress, and even dysfunction. He gave up acting and devoted the remainder of his long life to teaching his technique to medical and lay groups in England and the United States.

The Alexander technique, a method of reintegrating the body by relearning positive habits, is a self-reeducation process encouraged and led by an expert. The client is considered a student, and the therapist a teacher. The assessment process is limited to the physical dimension. The teacher first observes the student's misuse of the body as revealed in posture and musculature. This technique stresses that each person has a unique body and implements the prinicples of coordination and adjustment in a unique way. The teacher determines each student's ideal configuration. During treatment the student lies flat on a waist-high table, and the teacher begins the manipulation designed to correct the specific misuses of the body. The student is actively involved in the process, learning first how to inhibit and prevent faulty use of physical mechanisms and then how to move properly while being physically manipulated. The student's responsibility continues between sessions; moves are to be practiced regularly. The therapy is over when the student can move freely with well-coordinated muscles, breathe deeply and rhythmically without tension, and use the body to optimal efficiency in all endeavors in daily living. The number of sessions required to complete the work of reintegrating the body may be equal to the number of years the student has lived. Although not emphasized by Alexander, his followers say that this treatment results not only in improved physical function but also in release from emotional stress.

Rolfing

Rolfing, or *structural integration,* was developed by Ida P. Rolf.[55] Her belief that a human is basically an energy field operating in the gravitational field of the earth is the cornerstone of this treatment. The purpose is to change the client's energy field so that it is supported and enhanced by the greater energy field of the earth (gravity). The client's field is altered by the therapist's use of massage to better vertically align the head, shoulders, thorax, pelvis, and legs. Usually requiring 10 hour-long sessions, therapy consists of a carefully formulated sequence of *manipulations*. The therapist's energies are directed at the deviant myofascial connective tissues; the force necessary to free them may be applied by using fingers, elbows, clenched fist, and open hands. Once the tissues are freed, the body realigns itself with the gravitational field of the earth, resulting in increased energy.

Rolfing is limited to the physical dimension. The client strips to his underwear, and the therapist carefully inspects the body. Posture and knots of tense muscles are observed. The client is photographed from the front, back, and side. He then lies flat on a mat, and the therapist continues the assessment with palpation and percussion. The therapist analyzes the findings, carefully formulates and implements a sequential plan of manipulations, and notes any changes. Rolfing requires the active willingness and conscious cooperation of the client. It demands responsibility and awareness of personal goals and purposes and results in feelings of autonomous accomplishment. Evaluation of the effectiveness of the treatment by the therapist is based on observable changes in posture and musculature. Successful rolfing results in a relaxed upright posture in natural alignment with the forces of gravity.

Although symptom relief, often dramatic, is a result of rolfing, Rolf's primary interest is the potential of humans. She believes that rolfing is one of the most basic and reliable means of developing this potential, whether emotional or physical. She has argued that emotional pain and anger are often repressed and held in the musculature, which requires energy. During rolfing it is not unusual for the client to experience painful blockages in areas that contain residues of repressed, painful emotional experiences. After rolfing the anger and pain seem to disappear, and the energy that has been tied up within the musculature is available.

Bioenergetic Therapy

Bioenergetic therapy, developed by Lowen,[34] also focuses on the body. Lowen believes that the observable "body armor" of chronic muscular rigidity expresses a person's constricting early life experiences. The purpose is to free the client from the chronic constrictions that limit breathing and from the muscular tensions that block the flow of energy so that energy pulsations can fill deadened areas of the body with a new consciousness of life. The constrictions and tensions are released through stressor and "releaser" exercises, usually beginning with deep breathing. The exercises that follow emphasize stretching and loosen the particular body areas that correspond to particular emotions. For example, Lowen says that inhibitions to reaching out for love and affection are manifested by shoulder muscle tension. In addition to stretching, the exercises may include kicking a sofa or punching a pillow while yelling to help clients let go of their usual controls

and release the great amounts of energy that have been tied up with negative emotions.

The therapeutic process focuses on observing the client's posture and physique. The therapist frequently asks him to assume a stress position, such as arching the body over a chair and touching the feet and head to the floor, which reveals chronic muscular tension and rigidity. After assessment the therapist directs each client through warm-up exercises and increasingly difficult stretching exercises based on the assessment findings. Kicking, punching, and yelling are also tailored to each client's needs.

Bioenergetic therapy requires client cooperation and responsibility. The underlying premise is that the body's movements are reflections of the body's feelings and thus are a key to the client's emotional status. Improved body movement can be interpreted as reflecting improved body feelings and attainment of a higher level of emotional functioning. Lowen and his followers believe that people do not simply have bodies; people *are* their bodies.

Feldenkrais Therapy

Feldenkrais therapy, or *functional integration therapy,* developed by Moshe Feldenkrais,[23] is based on the belief that humans are unique in their capacity to learn. Feldenkrais sees the therapist-client relationship as one of teaching and learning. The client's physical and emotional complaints are not viewed as diseases to be cured but as the results of faulty learned modes of doing. The therapist's job is to reeducate the client, emotionally and physically.

A basic goal is the establishment of a positive self-image. According to Feldenkrais, three factors contribute to this process: heredity, education, and self-education. Heredity is the physical structure with which the client is born. Education provides the means by which the client acquires concepts and socialization. It also determines the direction of self-education that begins in childhood with the development of individual characteristics. Self-education is the component with which the therapist is working when the client is charged with the responsibility for self-help and self-improvement.

Awareness, the central component of self-improvement, is characterized as a waking state with four interacting characteristics: sensation, feeling, thinking, and movement. Correction of movement is the most viable means of self-improvement for many reasons: its quality is easier to judge, people have a greater capacity for movement than for thinking and feeling, moving well enhances self-esteem, and most important it is a means of changing the pattern-directing function of the motor cortex of the brain, which, by influencing thought and feeling, changes patterns of existing.

Feldenkrais corrects movement through exercise. His elaborate schema of exercises—all deliberate, slow, and mild—are based on the reversibility of the relationship of the muscular and nervous system. This means that clients' muscle movements, of which they are unaware, are brought into awareness by a reversed pattern. Most exercises are performed lying down to help break the habitual motion of the muscle in gravity. For example, the client might have to work 40 minutes to relax one shoulder so that it touches the floor, but may need only a few minutes to do the same with the other shoulder. The brain has learned the muscular arrangements that allow what was first seen as impossible. When the client has learned the exercises and realizes the importance of practicing them daily, therapy is over, and the client is ready to assume responsibility for self.

Biofeedback

Biofeedback uses equipment to reveal internal physiological events as visual or auditory signals. The purpose is to teach clients to manipulate these otherwise involuntary or unfelt events.[7] Biofeedback is a type of training because it involves teaching the body to modify specific activities based on experience. In its simplest form the therapist uses an electronic instrument to monitor a particular output, then displays it so that the client can be aware of changes (Figure 38-1). For example, a woman with migraine headaches can be trained to ward off the headache before it starts by dealing with its classic onset signal, the cold hands that indicate that blood vessels in the extremities are narrowing. The client learns to increase the blood flow to her hands in the laboratory, where she is wired to machines that register and indicate with a pointer the temperature of her hands as measured by the thermistor she holds. She is instructed to keep the pointer moving upward; nothing is said about increasing the blood flow to her hands, although clearly it is the desired outcome. Once the client is trained in the laboratory, she is given autogenic training (discussed next) and a regular home practice schedule. Numerous research studies have validated this treatment approach as effective for migraine headaches as long as the client continues to practice the techniques at home. Tension headaches have also been relieved (see the Research Highlight on p. 725). Biofeedback has additionally been found to be useful in treating high blood pressure, insomnia, Raynaud's disease, and a variety of psysiological disorders.

As a technique, biofeedback training is used by many different health caregivers. It is generally used as an aid or auxiliary to other approaches. Evaluation of the training's effectiveness is based on assessment of the client's ability to control the desired body function. Clearly the client's responsibility is great. In very successful cases the client assumes full responsibility for the biofeedback and monitors body function at home.

Autogenic Therapy

Autogenic therapy was developed from research on sleep and hypnosis by Jonathan Schultz,[60] who identified the physiologically oriented steps that became the core of this training: heaviness and warmth in the extremities, regulation of cardiac activity and respiration, abdominal warmth, and cooling of the forehead. Autogenic therapy is based on a belief that the brain mechanisms know what to do to remove disturbing interferences. It gives the natural forces in the brain the opportunity to reestablish functional harmony in a homeostatic or autogenic way. The effects of autogenic therapy can be considered as diametrically opposed to changes caused by stress.

The client learns and practices to perfection the six autogenic standard exercises[60]:

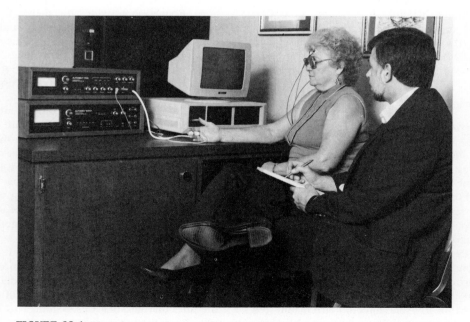

FIGURE 38-1 The client is being coached in biofeedback training. Changes are recorded on the computer and provide the client with feedback on changes that are occurring.

Research Highlight

Biofeedback Application to Migraine and Tension Headaches: A Double-Blinded Outcome Study

E.J. Daly, P.A. Donn, M.J. Galliher & J.S. Zimmerman

PURPOSE

This study was designed to determine the efficacy of progressive relaxation, fingertip temperature training, and electromyographic training of the frontalis muscles for relief of symptoms in clients with chronic migraine or tension headaches.

SAMPLE

Subjects were obtained through advertisements for chronic headache sufferers and by referral. Fifty-six subjects completed the training and submitted the required data for 2 years. They ranged in age from 18 to 61 years. Forty-five were female; 11, male. The mean duration of headache symptomatology was 15.9 years.

METHODOLOGY

Subjects were first seen by the team physician for a diagnostic work up and explanation of the headache record-keeping chart. All headache activity was to be noted and rated for level of intensity. Subjects were then assigned to one of three training condition groups. Treatments in each group consisted of 9½ hours of individual sessions for 5 weeks by the three psychologist authors in rotation. A tenth session was a reporting session with the physician. Each group's goal was for the subject to learn the procedure well enough to do it without assistance. All subjects were encouraged to practice twice a day on their own, without equipment, and at the completion of the training, they were to continue practicing at home for 3 months. The headache charts were used to assess the efficacy of the various treatments in alleviation of symptoms.

FINDINGS

Overall, a diminution of perceived severity of hours or months of headache was found for all treatment groups. Although both fingertip warming and training of the frontalis muscles produced more change by the end of treatment than the relaxation training, none of the treatment comparisons reached significance at either the end of the treatment or the 3 month follow-up. Also, the majority of subjects were able to reduce the strength of their medication and dosage level during the course of the study.

IMPLICATIONS

Any of the three treatments may work for some subjects; none of the treatments were effective for others, and both fingertip temperature and frontalis muscle training can be helpful for both types of headaches.

Based on data from Biofeedback and Self-Regulation 8(1):135, 1983.

---

1. My right arm (left arm, right leg, left leg) is heavy.
2. My right arm (left arm, right leg, left leg) is warm.
3. My heartbeat is calm and regular.
4. My breathing is calm and regular (or, "It breathes me").
5. My solar plexus is warm.
6. My forehead is cool.

Once the trainee can quickly (in 20 to 30 seconds) and effectively go through the standard exercises, the therapist determines if the client is ready to learn the meditative exercises, the special exercises developed specifically for each client to modify particular problem areas, or the neutralization exercises that promote *abreaction* (discharge of emotion) and verbalization. The decision is based on the client's condition.

An example of autogenic neutralization treatment follows. The client comes to the therapist's office for the scheduled appointment and lies on the couch. After quickly moving through the standard exercises, the client begins to abreact or verbalize. The entire session is tape-recorded. The therapist makes few if any comments. At the end of the session, she instructs the client to listen to the tape at home, transcribe it, and fill in details. The client rereads the transcript aloud and writes a step-by-step commentary to take with the transcript and read aloud at the next session, 7 to 10 days later. This requires 5 to 15 hours of work between sessions and considerable client motivation, but active participation and responsibility is seen as essential to success.

Autogenic therapists believe that the autogenic abreactive process originates from certain parts of the brain that have a need for unloading and is not influenced by insight-promoting interpretations from the therapist. Although greater self-understanding and self-realization are among the positive results of autogenic therapy, they are not accomplished by the therapist or client interfering in the brain-directed process of autogenic abreaction.

Rebirthing

Rebirthing, developed by Leonard Orr[40] in 1975, is based on the results of his experiments with the hot tub to induce altered states. Rebirthing involves submerging the client in a tub of water while he breathes through a snorkle reciprocally with the therapist. Rebirthing has two goals: to heal the breathing apparatus injured during birth

TABLE 38-1 Summary of body-focused therapies

Therapy	Founder(s)	Focus of Treatment	Therapist Activity	Client Activity	Goal of Treatment
Alexander technique	Frederick Alexander	Musculature, posture, breathing	Manipulation, teaching	Active practicing, learning	Reintegration of the body through reeducation
Rolfing, or structural integration	Ida Rolf	Posture, musculature	Manipulation, massage	Responsible, willing cooperation	Realignment of the body posture with the earth's gravity
Bioenergetic therapy	Alexander Lowen	Breathing, musculature	Teaching, leading stretching exercises	Responsible cooperating, practicing	Releasing the body armor to permit the flow of energy
Feldenkrais therapy	Moshe Feldenkrais	Awareness, body movements	Teaching exercises	Learning, practicing	Establishing a good self-image through correction of movement
Biofeedback	Neal Miller Joseph Kamiya	Involuntary internal events	Training to manipulate	Learning to manipulate	Being able to control the desired body function
Autogenic therapy	Wolfgang Luthe	Brain-directed processes	Listening, giving instructions	Analyzing therapy content	Establishing functional harmony by natural forces in the brain
Rebirthing	Leonard Orr	Breathing	Guiding, reassuring	Experiencing	Healing of birth-damaged breathing apparatus

and to help the client use breathing as a completely supportive and creative part of daily life.

Orr believes that when the umbilical cord is cut prematurely and the child is deprived of oxygen and forced to learn to breathe through fluid-filled lungs, panic and terror result. These feelings are reinforced subconsciously with every breath and, if not released, are stored in the body and subconscious, resulting in a generalized fear of life in adulthood. The initial stage of the rebirthing process may take place out of water to avoid overwhelming the client. Once the fear and panic associated with the initial breath have been reexperienced, the client is assisted to repeat the process in the hot tub.

Rebirthing therapists first go through rebirthing themselves to release their own birth traumas, so that clients can feel safe to experience and release theirs. Each therapist works with one client, communicating that the experience is safe and will be beneficial and offers suggestions that guide breathing. Healing the damaged breathing apparatus usually takes three to ten 2-hour sessions and is achieved when the client's breathing is relaxed and even, rhythmic and balanced, with pauses between exhaling and inhaling and no holding patterns that limit the movement of the ribs and diaphragm. The change is believed to be permanent. The client can then become his own rebirther and work independently on the long-term goal. This decreases dependence on the therapist and promotes self-responsibility.

The body-focused therapies are summarized in Table 38-1.

MIND/PSYCHE-FOCUSED THERAPIES

Mind/psyche-focused therapies, widely divergent in style and method, all share the underlying assumption that the client's problem is basically one of faulty thinking or feeling. Treatment is aimed at correcting the dysfunctional cognitive or emotional processes through learning better ways of thinking and releasing crippling emotions.

Primal Therapy

Primal therapy, developed in the late 1960s by Arthur Janov,[31] a psychologist who had become disenchanted with the Freudian approach to psychotherapy, is a psychotherapy in which clients reexperience intensely painful events of infancy and childhood. Janov believed that neurosis has only one cause, an integrated childhood pain, and only one cure, primal scream therapy. He explained that all people carry around great pain from their early years when their parents failed to meet their primal needs: to be fed when hungry, to be kept warm and dry, to be stimulated and held, and to be allowed to develop at their own natural pace. The pain is repressed, disconnected from awareness, and results in neurosis. The longer people live with this pain, the less "real" and the more neurotic they become. The goal of primal therapy is to be "real"; that is, to be free from neuroses. Anxiety, depression, addiction, and sexual dysfunction are all partial responses to primal pain. Janov further believes that when a neurotic response fails to relieve the pain, psychosis results.

Primal therapy lasts approximately 8 months. The first 3 weeks are intensive, with one therapist working with one client. The client is required to live at the treatment center and may not work or go to school. The weekend before beginning treatment, the client is instructed to stay alone. No alcohol, smoking, caffeine (for example, coffee, and colas), drugs, reading, or television is permitted. Treatment begins with discussion aimed at breaking down the client's defenses (already weakened by the stimulus deprivation of the past weekend). For as many consecutive hours as can be endured, the client is led back into the past and is assisted to reexperience the painful events of infancy and childhood. Such reexperiences are called *primal.* A primal event has two phases. First, there is a crescendo of involuntary panic during which the client cries or screams in agony. This peaks and is abruptly followed by a recovery phase, during which the client has a vivid memory of an earlier painful life event. At the end of a primal event the client feels slightly euphoric, very lucid, and profoundly calm. After 3 weeks of intensive therapy, the client returns to his life of work or school but joins a primal group that meets two or three times a week for 6 to 8 months. The client continues to experience primal events in the group. Many clients build a soundproof room in their homes so they can continue to practice this cathartic experience after the treatment is completed.

Since a primal therapist recognizes only one disorder, neurosis, and only one treatment, primal therapy, assessment may occur along any dimension. For example, a physical ailment such as peptic ulcer disease would be diagnosed as a neurotic response to primal pain and would be treated with primal therapy.(This would not exclude appropriate medical treatment by a physician if indicated.) Depression would be likewise diagnosed and treated, as would other neurotic manifestations in the other dimensions. It is strongly believed that a therapist must personally have primal therapy before being qualified to treat clients. Evaluation of the therapy's effectiveness is based on the client's surrendering of a neurotic defense and becoming "real."

Morita Therapy

Morita therapy, a Buddist-based treatment for neurosis, was developed in Japan in the early 1900s by psychiatrist Shoma Morita.[53] Verbal instruction and guided activities were used to teach clients to accept their symptoms as part of reality. Thus clients learned to live constructive lives despite various neurotic feelings, such as shyness, fear, and anxiety.

The therapist first listens to an account of the client's problems and symptoms. The therapist then teaches the client the basic principles of the treatment approach: recognize purpose, accept feelings, and control behavior. The client begins to keep a diary, usually writing at least a page a day. On one half of the page, divided lengthwise, the client records the time of day and his activities. On the other half, he records his thoughts and feelings during the activity. The therapist analyzes the diary at the weekly sessions. Through this analysis the client learns that many activities are performed because there is something that must be done and that feelings and desires about wanting to do the activity do not necessarily correspond to it. The diary becomes a record of what the client can do despite negative or fearful thoughts.

Morita therapy is particularly suited for treatment of a wide range of neurotic disorders. The goal is not symptom reduction; in fact symptoms may persist. The goal is to build character. Through application of the basic principles the client learns to live responsibly and constructively despite symptoms. Then, when success comes, it is the direct result of the client's efforts, and it forms a solid base for a lasting sense of self-worth. Treatment is usually brief (12 to 16 weekly 1-hour sessions), since the client quickly perceives what the therapist will typically say about the diary entries. When the client can independently respond to each life situation with the question "What needs to be done now?" and then do it, regardless of feelings that may accompany it, therapy can be ended.

Gestalt Therapy

Gestalt therapy is rooted in the early work of psychoanalyst Frederick (Fritz) Perls[46] in the 1940s. Perls was influenced by Reich[50] and Alexander[3] and used some of their ideas about body armor and bioenergetics. He also used ideas from Zen Buddism, Taoism, existential phenomenology, and general semantics. Phenomenological and existential, gestalt therapy explores the changing phenomena of life as they enter the individual's awareness in the here and now.

The word *gestalt* refers to the "whole." All the different parts of the whole (figure and ground) relate to each other in a functional way. Every aspect of functioning is part of a person's gestalt and has meaning only in relation to the whole. At any given time, one aspect of function is sharply in awareness (the figure) and said to be in the foreground, while all other aspects are less distinct (the ground) and said to be in the background. Gestaltists believe that a person who pays attention to and follows his awareness will discover his authentic interests and concerns. This often involves reversing the figure-ground relationship or becoming aware of a fuzzy, indistinct part of the background. Then the relatedness of each element to identity can be examined. Awareness is seen as curative in and of itself, because every bit of awareness strengthens and promotes growth.

The therapist helps the client overcome the barriers that block awareness, which is accomplished in several ways:

1. By feeding back the verbal and nonverbal experience and behavior of the client
2. By suggesting experiential here-and-now exercises for the client as a means of self-discovery
3. By explaining to the client the impact of a particular behavior on the therapist
4. By acting as a teacher to provide principles and strategies useful in deepening awareness

The client is responsible for following the ground rules, which create an atmosphere and attitude toward working in therapy that lead to greater awareness of the reality of self, how the self interacts with others, and how the self functions in the here and now. Some of the ground rules follow:

1. Clients are encouraged to be in touch with their flow of awareness, to tune in to what they are experiencing from moment to moment.
2. Clients are required to speak in the present tense. When it is necessary to bring in some memory from the past, such as a childhood episode with a parent, a gestalt technique may be used to bring it into the present, such as pretending that the parent is sitting in an empty chair and then talking to the parent as if the episode were happening at that moment.
3. Clients are expected to own everything they say and do by speaking in the first-person singular and avoiding abstractions and impersonal statement.
4. Interaction between clients is to be on a first-person basis, leading to meaningful dialogue in which what one person says to another is reflected in the response of the other.
5. There is no gossiping.
6. Questions are generally discouraged.
7. Clients are encouraged to get in touch with the *what's* and *how's* of behavior, not the *why's*.
8. Clients are to substitute "I won't" statements for "I can't."
9. Clients are to avoid pressuring anyone in the group.
10. Clients have the responsibility for and the freedom to take risks when they are ready.

The training of gestalt therapists focuses on the client-therapist relationship. It is expected that the trainees have already had training as psychotherapists. Thus they are free to create their own style of treatment while practicing gestalt therapy, which is consistent with the experiential and existential nature of the therapy. Gestalt therapy is most often implemented in a group format, but it is also suitable for individual psychotherapy. Regardless of how it is practiced, the goal remains authentic growth in the here and now, or, "Be here now and be truly yourself."

Encounter Therapy

Encounter therapy flourished in the United States in the late 1960s but is rooted in ancient Greece and the Delphic precept "Know thyself." William Schultz, a psychologist whose name is generally associated with the contemporary movement, described encounter as a method of relating based on openness and honesty, self-awareness and responsibility, awareness of the body, attention to feelings, and an emphasis on the here and now. Encounter is seen as a form of therapy because it removes blocks to better functioning. However, it is also seen as education, recreation, and religion in that it attempts to create conditions that lead to the most satisfying use of personal capabilities.[62]

Encounter therapy is almost always conducted in a group setting (8 to 15 people) and may take place in 3 to 5 days with frequent 2-hour meetings or on a weekend with all-day meetings *(marathon encounter)*. The basic principles are: group members focus on becoming aware of their feelings, expressing them honestly, and taking responsibility for them. A set of rules for group interaction implements the principles of encounter, which all members are expected to follow. The first group of rules establishes the open and honest communications; the second group focuses on the body, integrating it into group activity; and the third-group focuses on identity establishment and taking responsibility for self. Encounter principles have been widely applied in other areas such as education, industry, theater, parent-child relations, and daily life.

Reality Therapy

Reality therapy was developed in the late 1960s by William Glasser,[25] a psychiatrist disenchanted with the traditional psychodynamic approaches he had been learning in his residency. Glasser especially objected to labeling people with emotional and relational problems as sick, because it took the responsibility for changing behavior from them and gave them an excuse for continuing as they were.

At the core of Glasser's approach are the psychiatric three *Rs*—responsibility, reality, and right and wrong. Responsibility is the ability of the client to satisfy his needs without depriving others of the ability to do the same. Reality can be understood as the world that surrounds the client. Right and wrong concern the moral quality of behavior.

Glasser believed that all people are motivated by two main needs: to love and be loved and to achieve self-worth. The primary job of all clients in reality therapy is to accept the fact that they alone are responsible for their behavior and that no excuses for irresponsible behavior are acceptable. Then they are ready to learn to make appropriate choices, to develop a sense of responsibility, to learn how to interact constructively with others, and to understand and accept the reality of their existence. The therapist is essentially a teacher of need-satisfying living who follows a three-step process:

1. Gain the necessary emotional involvement with clients by being very responsible, tough, interested, humane, and sensitive.
2. Point out the unrealistic aspects of clients' irresponsible behaviors while still accepting and maintaining involvement with them.
3. Teach clients better ways of need fulfillment, praising their efforts and accomplishments as they try new ways while not accepting excuses for failure.

Reality therapists, who must themselves practice the principles of reality therapy, do not use conventional diagnostic labels and do not believe their clients are ill. They see any person who behaves irresponsibly as an acceptable client for their therapy. They assess clients in terms of their behaviors, which may be manifestations of irresponsibility in any of the five dimensions. Step 3, dependent on the achievement of steps of 1 and 2 occurs when the client participates in identifying immediate and long-term goals and negotiates a contract. During each session progress toward the goals is reported and evaluated objectively. The ways in which clients are blocking their progress are explored, and alternative approaches identified. The focus is always on the present. Past life events, no matter how terrible, are not accepted as excuses for failure. Therapy ends when goals have been met to the satisfaction of the therapist and client and the client can responsibly fulfill his own basic life need for love and self-worth. The length of treatment varies depending on the client's motivation and the therapist's skill but generally does not exceed a year. Reality therapy is both an individual and a group treatment. Its concepts have been shown to be of value in a number of diverse settings, such as schools, correctional institutions, mental hospitals, and private practice.

Rational-Emotive Therapy

Rational-emotive therapy (RET) was created in 1955 by Albert Ellis,[21] a psychoanalyst who found psychoanalysis "woefully inefficient." He also formulated a new theory of personality, the ABC theory (see Chapter 3).

Ellis believed that a therapist needs special training to practice RET, although many therapists have independently learned the theory and technique of RET through Ellis' writings and speeches and incorporated it into their practice. In addition, RET translates easily into self-help procedures that many lay people use (for example, *Help Yourself to Happiness* by Maultsby,[36] a colleague of Ellis). Teachers also have used RET principles in the classroom.

According to Ellis, RET is applicable and useful in treating all clinical problems, including neuroses, psychoses, sexual disorders, child-rearing problems, and even lack of assertiveness. It can be practiced in an individual, small group, or family format.

The goal of the therapy is to teach the client effective self-analysis so that after treatment, introspective analysis and correction of distortions of the world can continue. Therapy is usually brief (12 to 20 sessions). Evaluation is based on remission of the initial symptoms and the demonstrated ability of the client to carry out the ABCs of the therapy.

Radical Therapy

Radical therapy is more an attitude about the therapeutic process than a specific type of treatment. Its major premise is that all therapy is characterized by numerous social and political value choices. Since clients' values are influenced by the values of the therapist, the therapist is responsible for fully recognizing and understanding these values. Therapists who accept this premise and practice accordingly are radical therapists, regardless of their basic theoretical orientation.

The radical therapist knows well her theoretical orientation's system of bringing about emotional and behavioral change in the client. Some key techniques are suggestion, persuasion, emotional support for approved trends, information about alternatives, and approval-disapproval cues. Although these are necessary parts of the process, they are not value free. When the therapist recognizes the social meaning and impact of these techniques, she can use herself in a conscious way.

Divergent views about how to apply the basic insights of radical therapy have given rise to three categories: aggressive radical therapy, defensive radical therapy, and social radical therapy. Aggressive radical therapists propose that clients are radicalized through the therapeutic process. They believe that making all values explicit, sometimes through actual didactic input, results in the client's viewing the solution of emotional conflict and the raising of political and social consciousness as one and the same. The goal of this therapy is not to create pervasive radical consciousness as the norm for mental health but to create sufficient social awareness to assist in coping with an authoritarian social order. Defensive radical therapists view the therapeutic process as a survival tactic. They begin at the client's present state and encourage him to avoid self-defeating behaviors. The goal of this therapy is to create social awareness for clients to use in coping with their oppressive environments. Social radical therapists generally have given up on the notion of individual, group, or family therapy and instead see society as the client. Social radical therapists function by merging into the larger radical political movement and attempting to bring about change. Aggressive radical therapy is frequently useful for radical clients; defensive radical therapy is often useful for nonradical clients, and social radical therapy is an important aspect of the radical therapists' view of how to uproot the conditions that cause emotional oppression.[35]

Although the radical therapy movement has its own internal controversies, it is cohesive in its conviction that the social and political values of the therapist are a potent element in the therapeutic process and need to be recognized.

Feminist Therapy

Feminist therapy evolved from the second wave of feminism that began in the 1960s. Feminists report that it was partially a reaction to the chilling realization that many women were being harmed by traditional psychotherapy, which reinforced passivity, dependence, and helplessness in women seeking to change.

Feminist therapy incorporates a philosophical approach to the conduct of therapy or counseling. Feminist therapists may vary in their theoretical orientations and may incorporate a variety of techniques and methods. However, all treatment is based on the following assumptions:

1. The personal is political—all behaviors and experiences are viewed in the greater sociopolitical context in which they occur.
2. The options available to both men and women are limited by sexism and sex role stereotyping.
3. Therapists are responsible for developing new interventions based on the insights of political feminism.

4. Therapists are aware of and explicit about their own value system, particularly values regarding "gender-appropriate" behavior.

Feminist therapy demands the equalization of power between the client and therapist. Clients are assumed to be their own best experts; they define their own problems and set their own goals. Although practically any technique or approach can be used to achieve their goals, three are particularly helpful in feminist therapy: (1) assertiveness training, which helps women express their anger, develop autonomy, and accept self-nurturance; (2) life planning, which focuses on aiding clients in career planning; and (3) sex role analysis, which is used to help women become aware of the ways in which they are constrained by adherance to traditional sex roles.

Another form of feminist therapy, consciousness-raising (CR) groups, is advocated by feminists who believe that all other therapy is demeaning. They believe that CR groups are the appropriate treatment for women.

CR groups, popular since the late 1960s, often succeed in helping women after years of conventional therapy have failed. They have emerged as the primary educational vehicle of the women's movement. Some general characteristics of CR groups follow[13]:

1. The group is small (8 to 10 is optimal).
2. The group meets often enough and long enough to provide each member time for self-expression and group response (weekly for 2 to 3 hours is suggested).
3. All members participate.
4. There is no formal leader.
5. Meetings are held on a rotating basis at each member's home or a neutral place.
6. All other members listen respectfully when one member speaks and accept what is said without criticism.
7. Regular attendance is expected.
8. What is said in the group is kept confidential.
9. A topic for the meeting may be introduced to organize and focus the discussion.
10. The discussion moves from the personal to the political.

Common denominators of personal experiences are identified and related to the political, including the concept of power in society—who has it, how it is used, how it can be obtained. Unless the political point is made for each topic, the participants may not have their consciousness raised. Unless they see the connection between what happens to them as individuals and what happens to all women in a sexist society, they are not experiencing real feminist consciousness raising.

Erhard Seminar Training

Erhard seminar training (est) was founded in 1971 by Werner Erhard, a layman who studied and participated in a wide variety of therapies (including yoga, gestalt, encounter, and Zen). Erhard reported that he had a catalytic experience—a transformation—after which things began to work for him in an incredibly simple yet powerful way. He developed est so that he could share his experience with others and provide an opportunity for them to experience a similar transformation.

Est is a practically oriented philosophical educational experience lasting 4 days, usually 9 AM to midnight, Saturday and Sunday, on two successive weekends. Included in the tuition are three 3½-hour seminars, one the week before the training weekends, one during the week between, and one the week after. Approximately 250 people participate, usually seated on hard chairs arranged theater style in a hotel ballroom. One trainer, located at the front of the room, conducts the workshops.

Four principal topics are addressed in the training: belief, experience, reality, and self. Trainees examine their experience of each of these topics in three ways:

1. Lectures by the trainer
2. "Processes," or guided experiences
3. Sharing, or communications from individual trainees to the trainer or seminar group

Each day one of the four principal topics is examined. On the first day the participants observe the role of belief in defining their experience of living. The trainer teaches that people live lies because they live according to belief systems that cannot be proved. Also, there are no absolutes other than people's individual experiences. After the lecture, participants move into the process component, during which they are asked to close their eyes and "take what comes up for them" as the trainer leads them through body sensation awareness exercises. Then participants are invited to say whatever they would like about the process or their own experiences. The other principal topics are dealt with similarly.

On the fourth day the trainees should experience the transformation—the shift in the nature of experiencing—that allows them to experience life not as a victim but as a whole, responsible person. Suddenly they get the point: they are who they are, and the world is what it is.

Although est is one of the most popular of the alternative treatment modalities, its proponents emphasize that it is not a psychology or therapy. Current estimates of the number of people who have attended the 60-hour training seminars exceed 200,000. Trainees have often learned about est from friends and co-workers who have already experienced it and enthusiastically recommend it to all who will listen. Trainers are elicited from the graduates who continue to be involved in est through attendance at graduate seminars on special topics such as communication, money, the body, and sex.

Several scientific investigations have been done to explore the effectiveness of est. One major survey study of 1,400 randomly selected graduates of est states that "respondents reported strong positive health and well-being changes since taking the est standard training, especially in the areas of emotional health and well-being and those illnesses with a large physiological component."[41] Ornstein, a highly respected researcher and clinician at Langley Porter Neuro-Psychiatric Institute in San Francisco, concluded that the findings were powerful enough to warrant further research in the areas in which change occurred for the better.

Assertiveness Training

Assertiveness training (AT) is rooted in behavioral therapy, but a considerable humanistic gestalt influence is also evident. Since the early 1970s, when the two frameworks were integrated, the technique has been popularized and its application extended to a wide range of nonclinical situations.

According to Robert Alberti,[2] a recognized expert in the technique, AT (also known as *assertive behavior therapy, assertion training,* or *social skills training*) is a procedure that trains the person in socially appropriate behaviors for self-expression of feelings, attitudes, wishes, opinions, and rights. Three components follow:

1. *Skills training.* Specific verbal and nonverbal behaviors are taught to and practiced by the client.
2. *Anxiety reduction.* Anxiety is reduced as a direct result of specific techniques (desensitization) or as an indirect result of the skills training.
3. *Cognitive restructuring.* Attitudes, values, or beliefs that limit the client's self-expression are changed as a result of insight or behavioral achievement.

AT may be used as the sole intervention in some situations (for example, in a CR group), used as an adjunct to other treatments (for example, with behavioral therapy for a client with acute dysphonia), or used independently as a self-help technique. AT is used in management training, children's programs, and minority rights groups.

AT is frequently conducted in a group format to provide an adequate social environment. The skills training component emphasizes rehearsal and role playing in the group; clients then try the new behaviors in real-life situations and report back to the group. Cognitive restructuring procedures may include didactic presentations by group members on issues of individual human rights and values. Barriers to individual expression may be examined and challenged. At all times the emphasis is on standing up for one's rights without denying the rights of others. A basic tenet of AT is that people have the right to be, to express themselves, and to feel good (not guilty) about doing so as long as they do not hurt others in the process. When these criteria have been met, AT is terminated.

A summary of mind/psyche-focused therapies is presented in Table 38-2.

SPIRIT/CONSCIOUSNESS-FOCUSED THERAPIES

Spirt/consciousness-focused approaches address the spirit or consciousness. All of these therapies employ techniques to enable clients to achieve higher levels of consciousness, meditation being the most common. These forms of therapy have come to the United States from other countries and very different cultures. Some have been practiced for thousands of years in their countries of origin, but all have only recently gained acceptance and become popular in the United States.

Yoga

Yoga, an ancient Indian meditational discipline rooted in the teachings of Buddha, has many forms today. *Hatha yoga,* one of the most common and the focus of this discussion, strives for the attainment of physical and mental well-being through mastery of the body. Other common types are *karma yoga,* its path being service to others, and *bhakti yoga,* its path being devotion and love.

Hatha yoga is a step-by-step system of physical training that involves the entire body in stretching exercises *(asanas),* holding postures, breathing control, and meditation. The rhythm of the exercises is slow and precise. There is no exertion or strain. The holding postures affect every major system of the body and can be used therapeutically for relief of a variety of disorders, including nervousness, tension, high blood pressure, ulcers, and obesity.

Proper breathing control is also necessary. Yogis maintain that breathing is the center of life not only because it supplies oxygen but also because it vitalizes the autonomic nervous system. Exercises in breathing are designed to rid the body of harmful emotions and promote relaxation[28] (see the Research Highlight on p. 734). Even more important, correct breathing is a stimulus for achieving higher levels of consciousness. Subjects are taught to use the diaphragm for slow, controlled respiration. Inhaling to a count of 16 and exhaling to the same count are optimal.

When incorporated with physical training and proper breathing control, the practice of meditation takes its place as the key to the consciousness toward which all yogis strive. Yoga meditation is a way of turning off the stimulation from the senses. It is aided by a life-style of relative isolation and a select but sparse diet primarily of fruit, nuts, seeds, raw and cooked vegetables, brown rice, and herbal tea. This life-style better enables the subject to perform the meditative technique of centering the mind on one simple thought. A specific word or sound is used to develop the "one-pointed" concentration and keep out intruding thoughts. Intruding thoughts are triggered by unfulfilled wishes; maintaining focus allows the mind to transcend such wishes and their interfering stimulation.

For hundreds of years there have been reports of the unbelievable feats of Indian yogis such as being buried alive, walking on hot coals, and stopping the heart. In modern times, with the aid of technology, these feats have been recorded and validated. Yogis can drop their metabolic rate to half the normal rate and survive well in a freshly dug grave. They can turn off pain signals and increase vagus nerve firing while blocking the action of the sinoatrial nerve.[69] The implications for health care and self-care are immense. Unfortunately, yoga originates from a culture so alien that its major beliefs may need to be translated into concepts the Western mind can grasp.

Zen

Zen, also an ancient meditational discipline rooted in the teachings of Budda, originated in Japan and is similar to yoga. The major difference is the meditational style. The goal of Zen is to achieve mindfulness. The meditator makes no effort to regulate flow of consciousness; instead he aims for full awareness of any and all thoughts of the

TABLE 38-2 Summary of mind/psyche-focused therapies

Therapy	Founder(s)	Focus of Treatment	Therapist Activity
Primal scream therapy	Arthur Janov	Repressed childhood pain	Listening and interpreting
Morita therapy	Shoma Morita	Neurotic symptoms	Listening and teaching
Gestalt therapy	Frederick Perls	Barriers that block awareness	Giving feedback, suggesting, and teaching
Encounter therapy	William Schultz	Blocks to better function	Participating, relating and leading
Reality therapy	William Glasser	Three Rs: responsibility, reality, and right and wrong	Teaching, relating, and leading
Rational-emotive therapy	Albert Ellis	Irrational belief systems	Teaching
Radical therapy	Many contributors	Social and politcal value systems of therapist, client, and society	Recognizing and verbalizing own values and using self
Feminist therapy	Many contributors	Sexism and sex role stereotyping	Developing new interventions and recognizing and verbalizing own values
Erhard seminar training	Werner Erhard	Belief, experience, reality, and self	Lecturing, teaching, leading, and supporting
Assertiveness training	Robert Alberti, Michael Emmons, and others	Behaviors for self-expression of feelings, attitudes, wishes, opinions, and rights	Skills training, teaching and confronting

mind. The meditator is a neutral witness, barely noticing each successive thought as it passes through the mind. He neither rejects nor pursues the thought but drops it from awareness after it has been noticed. The meditator gives each and every object of awareness equal value.

The hierarchy of altered states in Zen meditation moves from the initial stage of noting each object and dropping it from awareness to noting the random and discrete units from which the mind builds reality. When this has been accomplished, a second phase in the process of meditating is achieved. The final stage, when mental processes cease, is the *nirvanic state.* It is believed that radical and lasting alteration of the personality can occur when the meditator has reached nirvana.

All of the feats of the Indian yogis have also been reported and validated for Zen meditators.[28] The effects of both practices on the human mind and body are similar.

Transcendental Meditation

Transcendental meditation (TM) is a simple, natural, mental technique that produces deep rest for the body and clarity for the mind. The goal is to achieve a state of enlightenment and full human potential. TM is easily learned, but it must be taught by a qualified instructor because of the *mantra,* a unique secret sound selected by the instructor specifically for each participant. The mantra is matched to the participant's personality and is used during meditation.

TM is taught in two brief lectures, a weekend initiation ceremony (during which the mantra is given), another lecture, and one more weekend. The participant is required to meditate for 20 minutes twice a day, using the secret mantra. During meditation the individual sits quietly, usually with eyes closed, and repeats the sound silently over and over. Thoughts are allowed to come and go. The entire process is meant to be easy and pleasant. It does not involve trying or concentrating. It simply allows an innate ability of the nervous system to unfold. Meditators report brief periods of pure awareness, or transcendence.

Numerous beneficial effects of TM have been reported, from stress reduction to increased energy and creativity. TM proponents cite research studies that support these claims, but critics question the quality of the research (for example, some studies had no control groups). Herbert Benson,[8] a cardiologist and professor at the Harvard Medical College, was initially impressed by research that identified various physiological effects, such as decreased blood pressure and decreased lactate concentrations in the blood. However, he continued to explore and found that many techniques in addition to TM produce altered states of consciousness, which in turn produce a response of relaxation and the same physiological effects.

Client Activity	Goal of Treatment
Obeying rules, practicing, and abreacting	Surrendering neurotic defense and becoming real
Diary keeping and learning	Character building, enabling client to live responsibly and constructively
Obeying the ground rules	Authenic growth in the here and now
Communicating, using the body, and taking responsibility for self	Making the most satisying use of personal capabilities
Accepting responsibility for self and learning	Fulfilling basic needs for love and self-worth
Learning and analyzing	Acquiring effective self-analysis skills
Understanding own values, recognizing therapist's values, and deciding	Coping with society and becoming active for change
Defining problems and setting goals	Consciousness raising
Listening, experiencing, and sharing	Transformation in the nature of experiencing
Practicing, learning, and role-playing	Being, expressing self, and feeling good without hurting others in the process

Psychosynthesis

Psychosynthesis, a therapeutic process of combining individual components of the mind to achieve a whole personality, was developed by Roberto Assagioli,[5] an Italian psychoanalyst dissatisfied with the Freudian emphasis on the unconscious. Assagioli described three levels of the unconscious, somewhat analogous to the id, ego, and superego, called the lower, middle, and higher, or superconscious. The true self, or the creative center, is found in the superconscious. Assagioli's therapy was designed to synthesize all areas of the personality and to affirm the natural drive of humans to grow by integrating their lives at higher levels. Psychosynthesis emphasizes the following:

1. The function of the will as integral to all choices and decisions
2. The direct experience of the self as manifested by self-awareness
3. The phenomenologically lived experiences that are positive, creative, and joyous

The process of psychosynthesis concentrates on the transforming and redirecting of psychological (sexual and aggressive) energies toward creative goals, the development of weaknesses into strengths, and the activation of energies. It is a conscious and carefully worked out process of re-creation, or integration, of the personality.

Clients go through four stages in the integration process:

1. Learning about the various elements of the personality
2. Controlling the various elements of the personality
3. Discovering the psychological center of the personality
4. Integrating the parts, or psychosynthesis

The task of the therapist in psychosynthesis is complex and requires systematic use of many active psychological techniques. For example, in the first stage of integration the therapist may use psychoanalytic techniques to reach the depth of the unconscious where images of early fears and conflicts reside. Assagioli recommended that all therapists interested in practicing psychosynthesis should first experience it, in much the same way that candidates for psychoanalysis go through a training analysis first.

Arica Therapy

Arica therapy was developed by Bolivian Oscar Ichazo,[30] in 1964, who brought it to the United States in 1971 when he founded the Arica Institute in New York City. Ichazo's goals were to train as many teachers of Arica as quickly as possible to bring about a spiritual awakening and to save Western civilization from decline. Aricans believe that if enough people learn the theory and system, a metasociety can be created—one in which relations between people are based on a recognition of unity rather than competition.

Arica is a mystical approach that offers a message for spiritual development and the attainment of full enlightenment and freedom. The theory explains the unity of the whole; it provides tools to systematize and describe the human psyche—to draw a "map" and make the territory known.

There are nine levels of training in the Arica system. Many training exercises can be done independently with the proper manuals obtainable from Arica centers, but guidance from certified Arica trainers greatly accelerates the process. It is said that anyone who is exposed to the training will benefit from it and that the 40-day training program (a combination of physical body work and meditation) will produce permanent altered states of consciousness for most people. The final portion of the training program is "the desert," 40 hours to be entirely alone, without books, television, radio, or telephone, to practice self-observation.

Most Arica therapy experiences are conducted in groups led by certified Arica trainers who aim at breaking down the overdeveloped intellect common in Western society. If the client can be led back to his original self or essence, he can then experience the unity of the whole.

Silva Mind Control

Silva mind control, a method for increasing the powers of the mind, was developed by José Silve[27] a self-taught electronics engineer, to teach individuals how to voluntarily enter into and control various states of consciousness.

Research Highlight

The Effect of Yogic Breathing Exercises on Mood

J.R. Harvey

PURPOSE

This study was designed to evaluate the effects of yogic breathing exercises on a self-report measure of six separate dimensions of mood and a total mood disturbance measure. The literature supports the importance of breathing control as a therapeutic modality and maintains that there is a critical link between breathing pattern and emotional functioning. Further, respiration is very closely related to the activation of the autonomic nervous system and thereby to affective states.

SAMPLE

The volunteer sample included 20 subjects: six in the experimental yogic breathing group (three men, three women); six in a meditation control group (three men, three women); and eight in a psychology class control group (three men, five women). The age range was 20 to 55 years.

METHODOLOGY

Mood was measured by the Profile of Mood States (POMS), which has six affective dimensions: tension-anxiety, depression-dejection, anger-hostility, vigor-activity, fatigue-inertia, and confusion-bewilderment. A total mood disturbance (TMD) score is obtained by summing the scale scores (vigor-activity is weighted negatively). The experimental group subjects participated in a 4-week class in yogic breathing techniques, the first control group in a 6-week class on the philosophy and psychology of meditation, and the second control group in an introductory course in abnormal psychology. The POMS was administered before and after the third meeting of both the yogic breathing and the meditation control group and at the beginning and midpoint of the fourth session of the

psychology class. The third class in the yogic breathing group contained a lecture on the psychology of breathing and 45 minutes of practice on diaphragmatic breathing and other breathing techniques known to cleanse and energize and to soothe and calm.

FINDINGS

No significant differences were found on the pretest scores on all scales. Examination of mean gain scores on posttests showed that all three groups changed somewhat in the desired direction. However, t-test results showed that the yogic breathing group's total mood improvement score was significantly higher than the meditation control group's score. (p ≤ .05) and the psychology class control group's score (p ≤ .01).

IMPLICATIONS

The results suggest that the practice of yogic breathing exercises may be effective in creating immediate improvement in some parameters of mood as measured by the POMS, specifically, increased vigor and decreased tension, fatigue, and depression. Replication of the study with a larger number of subjects randomly assigned to groups is recommended. Also, future studies can include physiological- and behavioral-dependent variables in addition to self-report.

The study offers evidence that yogic breathing exercises may produce beneficial changes in mood and emotional state and thus may have clinical potential as a nonpharmacological, self-control technique. Because the exercises involve specific physical actions, they can be taught in a skill-building approach.

Based on data from Journal of the American Society of Psychosomatic Dentistry and Medicine 30(2):39, 1983.

Silva's earliest efforts in the 1940s involved the use of lower brain wave frequencies to increase retention and recall of information and thus raise the IQ. Silva also found that when individuals attained the alpha range, they could sense information beyond themselves and even solve problems that had not yet been posed. Silva then turned his attention to discovering the full powers of the mind at the alpha-theta range and in 1956 began teaching his newly formulated mind control method. Since then more than 450,000 people in the United States have learned the method.

Silva mind control is taught on two successive weekends from 9 AM to midnight each day by a specially trained leader. The meetings are held in small hotel rooms; participation is limited. Each day a basic lecture is given, and the content is applied through various exercises and other experiential learning.

The four lectures deal with the development of two forms of communication, objective and subjective. Les-

sons in objective communication focus on controlled relaxation and general improvement, such as learning muscle relaxation, falling asleep and awakening at will, and relieving a headache. Also, memory can be improved, problem-solving capability increased, and undesirable habits such as smoking or overeating controlled. Lessons in subjective communication focus on increasing effective sensory perception and learning how to apply it. Participants learn how to project their minds into inanimate objects, animate objects, and then animals. Participants also have the opportunity to project themselves into other humans, to diagnose and possibly heal the pathological condition they identify.

The prevailing philosophy of Silva mind control seems to lie in the belief in positive thinking. Throughout the training program participants are frequently exhorted to think and act in uplifting ways. For example, they are taught to silently repeat to themselves during quiet moments of the day, "Everyday, in every way, I am getting

TABLE 38-3 Summary of spirit/consciousness-focused therapies

Therapy	Founder	Focus of Treatment	Therapist Activity	Client Activity	Goal of Treatment
Yoga	Unknown	Musculature, posture, breathing, and consciousness	Teaching	Exercising, holding postures, practicing proper breathing, and meditating	Attainment of physical and mental well-being through mastery of the body and "one-pointedness" meditation
Zen	Unknown	Musculature, posture, breathing, and consciousness	Teaching	Exercising, holding postures, practicing proper breathing, and meditating	Attainment of physical and mental well-being through mastery of the body and "mindful" meditation
Transcendental meditation	Maharishi Mahesh Yogi	Consciousness	Teaching	Meditating	Achievement of a state of enlightenment and full human potential
Psychosynthesis	Roberto Assagioli	Three levels of the unconscious; lower, middle, and higher, or superconscious	Interpreting, supporting, teaching, and guiding	Free-associating, learning, forming goals, and practicing	Re-creation or integration of the personality
Arica	Oscar Ichazo	Human psyche with its overdeveloped intellect	Training and guiding	Practicing, body work, and meditating	Attainment of full enlightenment and freedom
Silva mind control	José Silva	Consciousness	Lecturing and training	Learning, practicing, and experiencing	Increase in powers of the mind

better and better." They are advised to look people in the eye, to smile at them, to joke, and to ask them how they are doing. Thinking positively and treating others with respect result in increased self-esteem and improved interpersonal relations.

Silva mind control is very popular in the United States. As with est, those who receive the training frequently suggest to friends and family members that they too could benefit from it.

A summary of spirit/consciousness-focused therapies is presented in Table 38-3.

HOLISTIC APPROACHES

Although all alternative treatment modalities claim to be holistic, only a few focus their interventions on all five human dimensions.

Wholistic Therapy

Wholistic therapy was developed by Herbert Otto in the early 1970s.[41,42] His interest in the concept of a wholistic treatment program stems from his work as part of the Human Potentialities Research Project at the University of Utah. Wholistic therapy is an approach to treatment that

may be used by all therapists, regardless of their basic theoretical orientations.

Following are the seven components of Wholistic therapy:

1. *The health model perspective of the person seeking treatment.* All people seek health. Symptoms are an expression of need and motivate the person to seek help.
2. *Combined group and individual treatment.* Most of the treatment occurs in groups because of the numerous advantages of group therapy. Individual sessions are scheduled as needed.
3. *The use of body work as an integral part of treatment.* Mind and body are treated simultaneously. Body work ranges from supportive touching to full use of body work modalities (rolfing, bioenergetics, dance).
4. *Optimal use of life space in treatment.* The total interpersonal and physical environment of the person is used to support and foster therapeutic aims and goals.
5. *Working with the belief system.* Emphasis is on assessing life-style and life goals and exploring the meaning of life as seen by the person, including spiritual resources or religious beliefs.

6. *Self-concept, self-image, and human sexuality as major factors in treatment.* A clear focus is on enhancement of the self-concept and self-image. Treatment also includes exploration of sexual attitudes and sexual self-image.

7. *The new eclecticism and the expanded therapeutic team.* The therapist is familiar with and willing to try diverse treatment methods drawn from a variety of schools of treatment. If the therapist does not have the knowledge or skill to implement a different appropriate treatment technique, the therapeutic team is expanded to include a therapist who is qualified to do so.

Wholistic therapy is appropriate for many disorders. Therapists simply incorporate this program into their theoretical orientation. This treatment addresses all dimensions of the person and yields maximal treatment benefits.

Holistic Counseling

Holistic counseling began in 1975 with William Woodson's introduction of Arica techniques into his more traditional practice of counseling and psychotherapy. He first added relaxation techniques, physical conditioning, and *Chua K'a* (a system of muscle tension release) to his counseling, which emphasized clarification and cleansing of both mind and emotions. Later he expanded the sessions to include meditation, visualization, nutrition, and other techniques.

Holistic counseling is a comprehensive approach to mental health that fosters growth of the whole person. It is concerned with health, not illness. The role of the holistic counselor is to clarify and educate the total person. Through clarification, clients obtain a new perspective on their behavior, recognizing that their activities are manifestations of the universal laws of human behavior. Clients are taught how to cleanse their minds and bodies, balance their emotions, and gain more energy. Self-responsibility is an important dimension to holistic counseling. Clients agree to practice exercises and carry out agreed on routines between sessions, with the goal of making the new techniques an integral part of their lives.

Currently there are six groups of techniques used in holistic counseling[62]:

1. *Clarification process.* This helps clients understand the effect of their assumptions, unresolved emotional conflicts, and expectations. By clearly isolating and examining their belief systems, clients begin to see patterns of behavior and the effects these patterns have on their lives. Clients are taught how to release distress associated with past traumatic events (psychological cleansing). They are also given information about Ichazo's[30] "maps of consciousness," which helps them see their behavior more clearly, understand it, and change it.

2. *Chua K'a, muscle tension release.* This is used to release tension stored in the body, cleanse the body of toxins, and restore maximal flexibility of thought and action. A manipulation and massage technique is used in which pressure is applied along the bones.

3. *Exercise.* This is used to increase the flexibility and elasticity of the body, restore and maintain the balance of body and psyche, increase the flow of vital energy, and elicit a sense of inner calm.

4. *Relaxation.* Additional exercises are taught that have deep relaxation as their primary benefit.

5. *Meditation.* To activate the healing energies in the body, three types of meditation are used:
   a. Those using repeated words or phrases (mantra) to quiet the constant clatter in the head
   b. Those using precise body positions to make the body receptive to positive emotions
   c. Those using visualization to awaken the body's natural healing energies

6. *Nutrition.* Clients are taught the significance of food selection, preparation, and combination; the dangers of food additives, preservatives, and supplements; and the importance of periodic cleansing diets or fasts.

Holistic counseling can be used in individual and group work with adults and adolescents who are facing stressful life situations. It is also applicable for persons suffering from psychophysiological disorders. Business and professional people have found it helpful for stress reduction

TABLE 38-4 Summary of holistic approaches

Therapy	Founder	Focus of Treatment	Therapist Activity	Client Activity	Goal of Treatment
Wholistic therapy	Herbert Otto	Psyche and soma, environment, and belief system	Leading, teaching, and supporting	Experiencing, learning, practicing, body work	Addressing all dimensions of the person and achieving optimal health
Holistic counseling	William Woodson	Mind, body, spirit, and health	Clarifying, teaching, guiding, and massaging	Examining belief systems, relaxing, exercising, meditating, altering dietary habits, and accepting self-responsibility	Growth of the total person

and career planning. It is equally applicable for use in corporate or educational settings.

The two holistic approaches are summarized in Table 38-4.

BRIEF REVIEW

Alternative treatment modalities emerged in response to a holistic view of the person—a view that people have physical, emotional, intellectual, social, and spiritual dimensions.

The holistic view grew out of the human potential movement in the 1960s. Dissatisfaction with society and its limitations sparked the movement, and it spread rapidly. As barriers between mind and body—limited self and limitless self—were broken down, new therapies were developed in unexpectedly large numbers.

Because so many different alternative treatment modalities emerged and because they varied so widely in focus and method, one precise definition is not possible. However, certain common assumptions underlie all: people are fine as they are (not sick), and all have unrealized potential that is best developed through self-responsibility and self-help.

Although almost all of the new treatments identify their approach as holistic, each tends to focus primarily on one component. Thus each therapy is classified as body, mind/psyche, or spirit/consciousness-focused or holistic.

Body-focused therapies assume that the client's problem is physical. All of these therapies focus on the body and use body manipulation techniques to change the body structure. Included in this group are the Alexander technique, rolfing, bioenergetic therapy, Feldenkrais therapy, biofeedback, autogenic therapy, and rebirthing.

Mind/psyche-focused therapies view the client's problem as faulty thinking or feeling. Treatment aims to correct the dysfunctional cognitive or emotional processes by teaching clients better ways of thinking, releasing emotions, or both. Primal therapy, Morita therapy, gestalt therapy, encounter therapy, reality therapy, rational-emotive therapy, radical therapy, feminist therapy, Erhard seminar training, and assertiveness training are included in this group.

Spiritual/consciousness-focused approaches employ techniques to enable their participants to achieve higher levels of consciousness. Included here are some of the oldest therapies, but all have been introduced fairly recently to the United States. Yoga, Zen, transcendental meditation, psychosynthesis, Arica therapy, and Silva mind control comprise this group.

The two truly holistic alternative treatment approaches (which focus on all five dimensions of the person) are wholistic therapy and holistic counseling. They are recent and perhaps indicate a trend toward a more integrated, holistic approach.

REFERENCES AND SUGGESTED READINGS

1. Agel, J.: The radical therapist, New York, 1971, Ballantine Books, Inc.
2. Alberti, R.E., and Emmons, M.L.: Your perfect right, San Luis Obispo, Calif., 1978, Impact Publishers, Inc.
3. Alexander, F.M.: The use of the self, New York, 1932, E.P. Dutton, Inc.
4. Appelbaum, S.: Out in inner space: a psychoanalyst explores the new therapies, New York, 1979, Anchor Books.
5. Assagioli, R.: Psychosynthesis: a manual of principles and techniques, New York, 1971, The Viking Press.
6. Barlow, W.: The Alexander technique, New York, 1973, Alfred A. Knopf, Inc.
7. Basmajian, J., editor: Biofeedback: principles and practice for clinicians, ed. 2, Baltimore, 1983, The Williams & Wilkins, Co.
8. Benson, H.: The relaxation response, New York, 1975, William Morrow & Co., Inc.
9. Blanchard, E., and Epstein, L.: A biofeedback primer, Reading, Mass., 1978, Addison-Wesley Publishing Co., Inc.
10. Bloomfield, H., and Kory, R.: Happiness: the TM program, psychiatry and enlightenment, New York, 1976, Simon & Schuster, Inc.
11. Brandon, J., and others: Training meditation and behavioral relaxation techniques, Health Values, **10**(2):3, 1986.
12. Brier, B., Schneidler, G., and Savits, B.: Three experiments in clairvoyant diagnosis with Silva mind control graduates, Journal of the American Society of Psychical Research **69**:263, 1975.
13. Brodsky, A.: The consciousness-raising group as a model for therapy with women, Psychotherapy: Theory, Practice and Research **10**(11):24, 1975.
14. Browne, L., and Ritter, J.: Reality therapy for the geriatric psychiatric patient, Perspectives in Psychiatric Care **10**(3):135, 1972.
15. Bruner, L.: The spiritual dimension of holistic care, Imprint **31**(4):44, 1984.
16. Chang, S.C.: Morita therapy, American Journal of Psychotherapy **28**:208, 1974.
17. Cox, S.: Female psychology and the emerging self, ed. 2, New York, 1981, St. Martin's Press.
18. Daly, E., and others: Biofeedback applications to migraine headaches: a double-blinded outcome study, Biofeedback and Self-Regulation **8**(1):135, 1983.
19. DiGiuseppe, R.A., Miller, N.J., and Trexler, L.D.: A review of rational emotive psychotherapy outcome studies, Counseling Psychologist **7**(2):64, 1977.
20. Ellis, A.: Rational-emotional therapy: research data that supports the clinical and personality hypotheses of RET and other modes of cognitive behavior therapy, Counseling Psychologist **7**(1):2, 1977.
21. Ellis, A., and Grieger, R.: Handbook of rational-emotive therapy, New York, 1977, Springer Publishing Co., Inc.
22. Erhard, W., and Gioscia, V.: est standard training, Biosciences Communication **3**:104, 1977.
23. Feldenkrais, M.: Awareness through movement, New York, 1972, Harper & Row, Publishers, Inc.
24. Foss, R.: Nontraditional approaches to mental health and their relation to counseling psychology, Counseling Psychologist **7**(2):21, 1977.
25. Glasser, W.: Reality therapy, New York, 1965, Harper & Row, Publishers, Inc.
26. Greenwald, J.: The ground rules in Gestalt therapy. In Stephenson, F.D., editor: Gestalt therapy primer, Springfield, Ill., 1975, Charles C Thomas, Publisher.
27. Guzman, E.: Mind control: new dimensions of human thought, Laredo, Tex., 1976, Institute of Psychorientology, Inc.
28. Harvey, J.R.: The effect of yogic breathing exercises on mood, Journal of the American Society of Psychosomatic Dentistry and Medicine **30**(2):39, 1983.

29. Hirai, T.: The psychophysiology of Zen, Tokyo, 1974, Igaku Shoin.

30. Ichazo, O.: The human process for enlightenment and freedom, New York, 1976, Arica Institute.

31. Janov, A.: The primal scream, New York, 1970, G.P. Putnam's Sons.

32. Kamiya, J.: Conscious control of brain waves, Psychology Today 1(11):56, 1968.

33. Kerr, N.: I believe in primal therapy, Perspectives in Psychiatric Care 12(1):32, 1974.

34. Lowen, A.: Bioenergetics, New York, 1975, Coward, McCann & Geoghegan.

35. Maglin, A.: The role of radical therapy, Monthly Review 28:51, 1977.

36. Maultsby, M.C., Jr.: Help yourself to happiness, New York, 1975, Institute for Rational Living.

37. Nelson, P.: Involvement with Betty: an experience in reality therapy, American Journal of Nursing 74:1440, 1974.

38. Ornstein, R., editor: The nature of human consciousness, New York, 1974, The Viking Press.

39. Ornstein, R.: A self-report survey: preliminary study of participants in Erhard training seminar, San Francisco, 1975, est Foundation.

40. Orr, L., and Ray, S.: Rebirthing in the new age, Mallbrae, Calif., 1977, Celestial Arts.

41. Otto, H.: Wholistic therapy. In Harper, R., editor: The new psychotherapies, Englewood Cliffs, N.J., 1975, Prentice-Hall, Inc.

42. Otto, H., and Knight, J., editors: New dimensions in wholistic healing, Chicago, 1978, Nelson-Hall Publishers.

43. Owen, P.: Stress tag: you're it—walking meditation, American Journal of Nursing 86(1):52, 1986.

44. Perls, F.: Gestalt therapy verbatim, Lafayette, Calif., 1969, Real People Press.

45. Pownall, M.: Holistic nursing: all in the mind's eye, Nursing Times 82(8):26, 1986.

46. Rachin, R.L.: Reality therapy: helping people to help themselves, Crime and Delinquency 20:45, 1974.

47. Randolph, and others: Stress: meditation versus the rat race, Nursing Management 16(2):30, 1985.

48. Rahula, W.: What the Buddha taught, New York, 1974, Evergreen-Grove.

49. Ram Dass: The only dance there is, New York, 1976, Jason Aronson, Inc.

50. Reich, W.: Character analysis, New York, 1972, Farrar, Straus & Giroux, Inc.

51. Reisser, P.: Holistic health and psychic healers, Journal of Christian Nursing 3(3):30, 1986.

52. Rew, L.: Exercises for spiritual growth, Journal of Holistic Nursing 4(1):20, 1986.

53. Reynolds, D.K.: Morita psychotherapy, Berkeley, 1976, University of California Press.

54. Rolf, I.P.: Rolfing: the integration of human structures, Boulder, Colo., 1977, Rolf Institute.

55. Rolf, I.P.: The vertical: an experiential side to human potential, Journal of Humanistic Psychology 18(2):37, 1978.

56. Rosen, R.D.: Psychobabble, New York, 1977, Atneneum Publishers.

57. Roszak, T.: The making of a counterculture, New York, 1969, Doubleday & Co., Inc.

58. Sargent, J.: A follow-up evaluation of the Menninger pilot migraine study using thermal training, Headache 17:198, 1977.

59. Sayre, J.: Radical therapeutic techniques, Current Psychiatric Therapies 17: 103, 1977.

60. Schultz, J., and Luthe, W.: Autogenic therapy: autogenic methods, New York, 1969, Grune & Stratton, Inc.

61. Schultz, W.: Joy, New York 1967, Grove Press, Inc.

62. Schultz, W.: Elements of encounter, New York, 1975, Bantam Books, Inc.

63. Severtson, B., and others: Effects of meditation and aerobic exercise on EEG patterns: stress level of student nurses, Journal of Neuroscience Nursing 18(4):206, 1986.

64. Smith, A.: Powers of the mind, New York, 1982, Summit Books, Inc.

65. Tien, H.: Pattern recognition and psychosynthesis, American Journal of Psychotherapy 23:53, 1969.

66. Valentine, K.: Massage in psychological medicine, New Zealand Journal of Physiotherapy 12(3):15, 1984.

67. Watts, A.: The way of Zen, New York, 1967, Pantheon Books, Inc.

68. Weinberg, R., and Hunt, V.: Effects of structural integration on state-trait anxiety, Journal of Clinical Psychology 35:319, 1979.

69. Wenger, M.A., and Bagchi, B.K.: Studies of autonomic functions in practitioners of yoga in India, Behavioral Science 6:312, 1961.

70. Woodson, W.: Holistic counseling. In Harper, R., editor: The new psychotherapies, Englewood Cliffs, N.J., 1975, Prentice-Hall, Inc.

71. Yates, A.: Biofeedback and the modification of behavior, New York, 1980, Plenum Press.

ANNOTATED BIBLIOGRAPHY

Applebaum, S.: Out in inner space: a psychoanalyst explores the new therapies, New York, 1979, Anchor Books.

A variety of new psychotherapeutic and holistic approaches to treatment of mental health problems are described and evaluated based on actual experiences of the author. Some of those therapies included are gestalt, primal, psychosynthesis, rolfing, Feldenkrais, Alexander, biofeedback, est, Silva mind control, TM, and yoga.

Ram Dass: The only dance there is, New York, 1976, Jason Aronson, Inc.

Based on two lectures Ram Dass gave to health professionals in the United States, this book explores the nature of consciousness. It represents an amalgamation of Western training (received when he was Richard Alpert, Ph.D., Psychology, Stanford University) and Eastern experiences (as Ram Dass in India).

Smith, A.: Powers of the mind, New York, 1982, Summit Books, Inc.

A research article on health grew to a book based on a 3-year exploration of the new therapies. All therapies described were personally experienced and include biofeedback, Zen, yoga, TM, rolfing, Feldenkrais, Arica, and est.

Van Dyke, C., Temoshok, L., and Zegans, L.: Emotions in health and illness, Orlando, Fla., 1984, Grune & Stratton, Inc.

The authors build on theoretical and research foundations to explain ways the knowledge of emotions enhances the understanding of health problems and how they apply to clinical interventions. The focus is on biological correlates of emotions that may mediate the relationship of emotions to disease promotion.

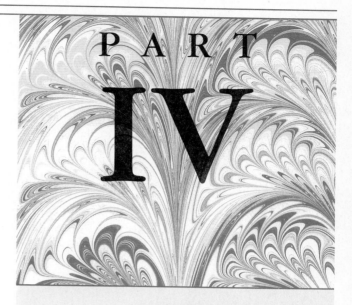

PART
IV

Life-Cycle Phases

From conception to death, each person continues to evolve and change while undergoing a series of alternating periods of stability and transition. At each stage in the life cycle, individuals have distinct developmental tasks to achieve, and they encounter stressors that are specific to the stage. To enhance understanding of the discrete stages in the life cycle, the following artificial age delineations were chosen for this text: the prenatal period (conception to birth), the infant (birth to 1 year), the child (1 to 12 years), the adolescent (12 to 21 years), the young adult (21 to 45 years), the middle-aged adult (45 to 65 years), and the aged adult (over 65). Although the dissection of the life cycle into discrete stages is necessary for purposes of discussion, the mental health–psychiatric nurse best applies the knowledge gained from this discussion by looking at all ages and stages as they intermingle.

Each chapter in Part IV discusses the process of mental health–psychiatric nursing with clients at a specific stage in the life cycle. Theories that explain the individual's physical, emotional, intellectual, social, and spiritual development are examined. The process of mental health–psychiatric nursing with individuals at each stage in the life cycle is presented with emphasis on the developmental tasks and stressors unique to each age. A holistic assessment tool in each chapter contains assessment information specific to each stage in the life cycle. Treatment modalities that are commonly used with individuals of each age conclude each chapter.

Chapter 39 begins by discussing life before birth and the influence of the mother's experience during pregnancy on the newborn. Development during the first year of life is then presented. In Chapter 40 the childhood years are divided into several stages and the unique patterns of growth within each are discussed. During the adolescent years, the individual is growing out of childhood into adulthood. This transition stage is the subject of Chapter 41. The three adult phases of the life cycle are presented in Chapters 42 to 44.

CHAPTER 39

THE INFANT

Eva Hester Lin

After studying this chapter the learner will be able to:

Discuss significant historical contributions to the development of infant psychiatry.

Describe the major developmental theories of infant mental health and illness.

Describe the unique nature of the therapeutic relationship with the infant.

Apply the nursing process to the mental health care of infants.

Describe current research findings on infant mental health and illness.

Infancy, beginning with birth and ending with the emergence of language and ambulation, is the most dependent phase of human development. For many years the infant was considered a totally passive organism, little more than a bundle of undifferentiated reactions and responses. Healthy physical and mental development of the infant was believed to depend almost completely on the mother's nurturing. The evolving relationship between the infant and caregiver is still viewed as a basic determinant of mental health, but the focus now is on its reciprocal nature and includes the prenatal period (see the Research Highlight on p. 743). The infant today is seen as an active, striving individual, who not only seeks and elicits stimulation from the environment, but also influences parental attitudes and behaviors.[54]

Knowledge of normal mental health development in infancy has expanded rapidly in the past decade and continues to grow. Researchers are working to integrate theoretical frameworks, from genetics to psychology, to address the complexity of infant development. Equipped with new insights, health care professionals are able to identify and treat infants at risk for mental health problems at increasingly earlier ages. Early intervention is therapeutic and preventative. Behaviors and relationships are easier to redirect during infancy than in later life, when maladaptive coping strategies may have become more entrenched.

Nurses, currently active in settings for the newborn, well-baby clinics, and pediatric units that emphasize primary prevention, are also taking on expanded roles as educators and counselors to those at risk. A clear understanding of the dynamic nature of the first 18 months and an appreciation of this phase's challenging tasks are requisite for examining infant mental health. Awareness of general developmental trends allows for early intervention and prevention of long-term problems. The main objectives of infant mental health are prevention of maladaptive behavior and promotion of normal development.

THEORETICAL APPROACHES

The infant development theories of Gesell, Greenspan, Erikson, and Piaget share some basic assumptions: that there is a reciprocal relationship between the infant's biological makeup and social environment and experiences (nature and nurture); that the gradual emergence of the personality occurs in an orderly, sequential, and progressive pattern; and that infant personality is linked to a consideration of the physical self and the caregiver. The merging of the self with the world, of body with mind, is the bedrock of infant experience. Holistic and family frameworks are particularly crucial in accurately evaluating an infant's mental health.

Historical Overview

DATE	EVENT
1905	Publication of Freud's *Three Essays on the Theory of Sexuality* highlighted the significance of infantile sexuality in personality development and adult mental health.
1940	Arnold Gesell's publication of *The First Five Years of Life* presented new observational data on early behavior patterns of infants.
1943	Article on *Infantile Autism* by Leo Kanner was a milestone in identifying early psychopathological conditions.
1945	Rene Spitz published his findings on the profoundly pathogenic effect of institutionalization and hospitalization on infants.
1951	John Bowlby in *Maternal Care and Mental Health* identified mother-child attachment as the core of the infant's emotional life.
1954	Graduate nursing programs in child psychiatry were created, providing a professional psychiatric nursing corps for infants and children.
1972	Advocates for Child Psychiatric Nursing formed a nationwide professional nursing organization to promote research in this field. Annual scientific meetings were initiated.
1974	American Academy of Child Psychiatry established a Committee on the Psychiatric Dimensions of Infancy that meets annually.
1976	*Infant Psychiatry* (Rexford, Sanders, and Shapiro), a book of articles by experts in child psychiatry and child development synthesizing research and clinical observations was published.
1977	National Center for Clinical Infant Programs was formed to improve and support professional work in infant mental health and development.
1981	National Institute of Mental Health established a Center for Study of Child and Adolescent Psychopathology.
1985	*Guidelines for Health Supervision,* which identifies emotional milestones to help pediatricians assess the emotional (as well as physical) well-being of infants, was published by the American Academy of Pediatrics.
Future	More psychiatric nurses are needed to identify infants at risk for psychiatric problems, work with problem infants, and to help families alter unhealthy childrearing practices.

Biological

Gesell's studies of infant behavior were linked to a careful, detailed analysis of physical maturation. He believed that behavior is a function of structure; that is, the body one inherits determines the way one behaves. In the first year of life the rapid development of the infant's central nervous system (CNS) provides the organic pathway for personality development. The sequence of development, with increasingly complete behavior emerging, is continuous and the same for all, although the rate varies. Thus all infants sit before they walk, but they sit and walk at different ages.[20] Infant development is closely tied to the maturation of the nervous system: no amount of encouragment can make an infant sit without support until the nervous system is ready for it.

Gesell and Amatruda focused on four major behavioral areas: motor, adaptive, language, and personal-social. Using data from extensive observational studies, they identified norms of behavior in these areas at successive stages in infancy. They perceived infancy as a dynamic period of progressive development in all spheres of behavior, based on increasing neuromuscular maturity. In the earliest phase basic physiological regulation is achieved. Most of the infant's energy is then consumed by growth. The physical aspects of nurturing are primary; the infant can survive only under carefully controlled conditions. As physiological homeostasis is achieved, social interaction between infant and caregiver increases as the infant, with growing initiative and power, assumes an increasingly active role in the family life. Sensory stimulation and social

Research Highlight

An Exploration of Paternal-Fetal Attachment Behavior

R.H. Weaver & M.S. Cranley

PURPOSE

This study was designed to explore whether men prepare for fathering by developing a relationship with their unborn infants. It was predicted that there would be a positive relationship between the strength of the marital relationship as perceived by the expectant father during gestation and the father's attachment to the fetus. Also, the incidence of paternal physical symptoms mimicking pregnancy was predicted to be positively associated with the father's attachment to the fetus.

SAMPLE

One hundred expectant fathers attending childbirth classes at a midwestern university were studied. All had a pregnant spouse in her third trimester. Ninety were expecting their first child.

METHODOLOGY

Subjects were given the Paternal-Fetal Attachment Scale (PFA), the Marital Relationship Scale (MRS), and the Health and Physical History Scale (HPH). The PFA measured attachment behaviors, the MRS assessed feelings and attitudes about the marital relationship, and the HPH scale assessed the presence of paternal symptoms resembling pregnancy symptoms or discomforts.

FINDINGS

The results supported the hypotheses that expectant fathers demonstrate attachment behaviors toward the fetus during gestation and that the strength of the marital relationship as perceived by the father is positively associated with paternal-fetal attachment. Although the correlation between the expectant father's physical symptoms and paternal attachment to the fetus was positive, it was not significant.

IMPLICATIONS

The findings support the existence of paternal-fetal attachment behaviors. However, because of the homogeneity of the sample and the convenient sampling technique, generalizations are not possible.

Based on data from Nursing Research **32**:2, 1983.

experience then become important "nutrients" for further development.[29]

Psychoanalytic

Erikson emphasized how the personality develops within the web of its particular social fabric in a sequence of psychosocial critical tasks. The challenge of infancy is to establish a capacity for basic trust.[13,14] The caregiver's responsiveness to the completely helpless infant, dominated by body needs and impulses, determines the outcome of this task. Earliest needs are physiological but satisfied in a social context. If babies can eat, sleep, and achieve a sense of physical comfort with relative ease during the period in which they need others to manage these functions, they learn to feel that life is sufficiently consistent and reliable and develop a sense of security. Because the boundary between the self and the outer world is not clear in infancy, the infant's feelings about the environment and self are one and the same. If the world is perceived as predictable, caring, and responsive, infants also establish a basic trust in themselves, their physiological processes, and their self-image. These intricately enmeshed physiological and psychological experiences are also the prototype of the social world gradually unfolding. The sense of inner certainty and outer predictability, which forms basic trust by the end of infancy, also pro-

vides the hope that is necessary if the next developmental step is to be attained. The infant can then reach out for new experiences with the prerequisite confidence. With a firm foundation of basic trust, the child's energy can be used in the acceptance of new challenges. Once achieved, this basic trust remains throughout life as the core of self-confidence and trust in others; this crucial task affects the whole of emotional life and all social relations.

Interactional

Greenspan[22] described the sequential stages of emotional development of infants and young children. To him, emotions play a critical role in the infant's development of a self-concept. Through sensations and feelings the infant gradually learns to discriminate, differentiate, and organize experiences. Intellectual and emotional functions merge in this process, and consequently their respective development cannot be separated. The child's capacity for organizing experiences depends on the infant's social experiences and CNS maturity. Thus emotions are the result of the interaction among the child's neurological, cognitive, social, and expressive functions. Each infant has a unique constitution and temperament, but each passes through predictable stages of emotional growth. Greenspan[20] identified six stages in emotional development, four in the first 18 months of life (Table 39-1).

TABLE 39-1 Summary of Greenspan's stages of emotional development

Stage	Stage-Specific Task	Stage-Specific Behaviors and Accomplishments
Achievement of homeostasis (birth to 3 months)	Self-regulation and interest in the world	The infant begins to control or regulate attentional states by focusing on sensory experiences.
Attachment (2 to 7 months)	"Falls in love" with primary caregiver	The infant's interest in external environment progresses and becomes more selective. Vocalizations for the primary caregiver induce a response.
Intentional communication (3 to 10 months)	Purposeful signaling	The infant's communications become more interactive; emotions are expressed in response to specific situations. Through the process of affecting others by emotional reactions, the infant learns cause and effect.
Behavioral organization (9 to 18 months)	Development of conceptual philosophy about world	The infant begins to reason about the world, as newly developed physical abilities (crawling, standing, walking) are integrated with previously acquired emotional skills (self as causal agent, intentional communication). The infant becomes a unique person, demonstrating complex and innovative behaviors.

Cognitive

Piaget focused on intellectual development in infants and children. He emphasized the role of adaptation in the organism-environment relationship. Piaget noted that development occurs in invariant stages, each building on previous ones. All infants pass through the same sequence of development but at different rates. Intelligence evolves from the interplay between infant and environment. Thus environmental understimulation slows the rate and hinders the complexity of learning.

Piaget viewed intellectual development as one aspect of general adaptation to the world. His four stages of intellectual development encompass only the sensorimotor stage in infancy. Babies are born with reflexes and reflexlike behavior that enable them to interact with and make discoveries in the environment. Through their senses—mouth, eyes, ears, nose, and skin—infants incorporate experiences of their motor activities, from objects with which they have contact—mother's body, bottle, crib. Behaviors such as sucking, biting, touching, grasping, and kicking provide bits of experience that gradually assume meaning. Thus mental functions are ultimately derived from the infant's motor actions on concrete objects. The growth of intelligence can be seen as the progressive transformation of these motor patterns into thought patterns.[37, 38]

The original reflexlike behavior of the newborn is gradually modified by contact with the world into more complex motor coordinations. They become aware of occasional discrepancies between previous experience and new stimuli. This tension creates curiosity, which leads to further extension of behavior beyond the body to the perception of the effect of personal actions on objects. The beginning of intentional behavior lies in this increasing exploration, which displaces earlier random activity. Purposeful behavior enables infants to accommodate their actions to real circumstances. They reach out toward an increasingly interesting and ever-expanding world. Increasing cognitive development occurs with the development of memory and object constancy (the ability to represent an object internally, which enables infants to perceive the object as externally existent). Babies learn that other people exist independently of themselves and their actions. The magical omnipotence of infancy is gradually reduced, leading to the beginning of a more objective and accurate appraisal of reality.

At the end of the sensorimotor stage, infants are far more competent in getting what they want through their actions. The emergence of goal-directed behavior, which signals the end of infancy and the beginning of the preconceptual stage of development, is the hallmark of intelligence and a landmark achievement. The infant's simple need to repeat inborn reflexes has evolved into the complex, purposeful activity characteristic of all intelligent action.[37, 38]

Social Learning Theory

Ainsworth[1] believed that social attachment is achieved in four stages, three of which occur in the first 18 months of life. In the first 3 months the infant learns to identify the individual characteristics of the primary caregiver. Through reflexes (sucking, rooting, grasping, cuddling, smiling) and sensory experiences (visual tracking, gazing, vocalization) the infant is able to seek closeness with the caregiver. In the second stage at 3 to 6 months of age) the infant begins to show preference for familiar people by smiling more and showing more excitement (see the Research Highlight on p. 745). In the third stage (at 7 to 18 months) large motor competencies (crawling and walking) emerge and enable babies to seek physical closeness with the object of attachment. Such behavior is purposeful, with the intent to maintain or prolong physical contact. Two behaviors in this stage signify the development of *attachment: stranger anxiety* (at 6 to 9 months) and *separation anxiety* (at about 9 months). Stranger anxiety is an infant's wariness or discomfort with unfamiliar adults. Generally infants demonstrate stranger anxiety

Research Highlight

The Perception of Facial Expressions by the 3-Month-Old

M.E. Barrera & D. Maurer

PURPOSE

This study was designed to investigate the abilities of 3-month-old infants to discriminate and recognize smiling and frowning expressions posed by the mother and a female stranger.

SAMPLE

Experiment 1 (using mother's picture) involved 24 full-term, healthy, 3-month-old infants (12 girls, 12 boys). Experiment 2 (using stranger's picture) involved 28 full-term, healthy, 3-month-old infants (14 girls, 14 boys).

METHODOLOGY

Each subject was placed in an infant seat in front of a projection screen. Observers watched the infant's eyes through 1 cm holes on both sides of the screen. Each observer independently timed the infant's visual involvement with the projected picture. Half of the infant's were habituated to the smiling expression, and the other half to the frowning expression. Specifically, the expression was presented repeatedly until the infant looked less than half as long as on the first three trials. After reaching habituation, the infant was tested twice with the habituated (H) and twice with the novel (N) expression. Infants were tested in two different experiments, the first using their mother's faces and expressions, the second using a female stranger's face and expressions.

FINDINGS

Infants in both experiments discriminated smiling and frowning expressions. However, a greater number (23 of 24) showed the discrimination with the mother's picture than with the picture of the stranger (21 of 28). The infants did not demonstrate a preference for the smiling face, although there was a higher attrition rate (two in experiment 1, six in experiment 2) because of uncontrollable crying and inconsolability in the groups habituated to the frowning face.

The findings also indicate that boys and girls differ in their perception of the mother's photographed face. In experiment 1 boys looked at the pictures significantly longer than girls (an average of 91 seconds compared with 56 seconds). There was no difference between the sexes in experiment 2, which used the stranger's picture.

IMPLICATIONS

This study demonstrates that 3-month-old babies can discriminate between smiling and frowning faces posed by both the mother and a stranger. Previously, such discrimination had only been demonstrated in older infants. The fact that sex differences were found in the responses in experiment 1 but not experiment 2 suggests that boys and girls differ in their perception of photographed faces only when the mother's face is used.

Based on data from Child Development **56**:203, 1981.

through a variety of avoidance behaviors, including gaze aversion, tensing at a stranger's touch, or refusing to be held by anyone but the primary caregiver.[26] Observable stranger anxiety is a good indication that the infant has developed an attachment to the primary caregiver. The ability to discriminate between familiar and strange adults emerges from the infant's secure and intimate association with a familiar adult.

Separation anxiety is the term used to describe the fear and loss infants feel when separated from their primary attachment figure. Separation anxiety is believed to be a normal corollary of attachment[2,6]; the infant must have an investment in another person to notice his absence. The infant usually responds to separation in one of two ways. Separation may either stimulate attachment behaviors (the infant seeks to find the attachment figure and regain physical proximity) or evoke protest, despair, or detachment, depending on the duration of the separation. Initially, the anxiety occurs at the time of actual separation, but gradually the infant may experience it when separation is anticipated. The emergence of separation anxiety parallels the infant's development of object permanence (since

now the infant is able to include the attachment figure in the imagination), at 8 to 10 months of age. In time infants become more adaptable and tolerant of separation, and eventually the anxiety diminishes almost totally.

Table 39-2 summarizes the major theories discussed.

RELATING TO THE CLIENT

In the past an infant's mental health problem was addressed by treating the mother's emotional problems. Although individual therapy with the infant's primary caregiver is often an appropriate intervention, it is no longer the only available approach. Perhaps the most popular and effective method for promoting infant mental health now is by treating both the infant and primary caregiver together.[17,22]

Therapy is usually sought by the infant's primary caregiver. Except for in crises involving legal intervention, direct therapeutic care of infants cannot be initiated without the consent and cooperation of their legal guardians. In cases of profound physical or social impairment from abuse or neglect, the nurse may become responsible for a

TABLE 39-2 Summary of theoretical approaches

Theory	Theorist	Dynamics
Biological	Gesell	Infant development is closely tied to CNS maturation. The sequence of development is similar for all; the rate varies.
Psychoanalytic	Erikson	The caregiver's response to the helpless infant determines capacity for basic trust.
Interactional	Greenspan	Emotions result from the interaction among individual neurological, cognitive, social, and expressive functions and develop in sequential stages.
Cognitive	Piaget	Evolvement of intelligence occurs in stages as the result of the interplay between infant and environment.
Social learning	Ainsworth	The ability to discriminate between familiar and strange adults emerges from secure and intimate associations with a familiar adult.

direct therapeutic relationship with an infant. Similarly, primary nurses in chronic care settings often establish direct relationships as surrogate parents.

In joint therapeutic relationships the nurse has two main objectives: to make a thorough assessment of both the infant and the primary caregiver and to develop a specialized plan to foster competent functioning by both caregiver and infant. The following is an example of this process.

Case Example

Elizabeth, age 3 weeks, is described by her parents as "a terrible baby! She's irritable, cranky, and cries all the time, no matter what we do!" Elizabeth's parents are becoming increasingly frustrated and beginning to verbalize feelings of inadequacy. After interviewing the parents, observing the interaction between Elizabeth and her parents, and direct observation and examination of Elizabeth, the nurse is able to tell the parents that their infant has visual hypersensitivity: bright lights hurt her eyes and make her fussy. Together the nurse and parents devise a simple solution of limiting Elizabeth's exposure to bright lights and plan other ways to stimulate Elizabeth's interest in the world that will not be painful.

Often problems that prompt parents to seek professional help are more complex than this. Many times, how-

ever, a simple problem is complicated by the parents. An "inconsolable" infant in a different setting might trigger a parent's underlying feelings of helplessness and rage and become a convenient target for these emotions. The focus of a therapeutic relationship in such a case would be to help the caregiver achieve the emotional equilibrium necessary for optimal infant mental health. Frequently, unsatisfied parental needs affect the quality of parenting and therefore infant well-being. When parental needs are great, the therapeutic course has a parallel thrust: (1) direct intervention with the infant when necessary to supply unsatisfied nurturance and (2) creation of models of responses and behaviors for the caregiver to emulate.

The therapeutic relationship begins with the primary caregiver's acknowledgment of need and acceptance of the nurse. It is crucial during this contracting phase that the nurse accept the caregiver as the primary client. Often the first step is the fulfillment of the caregiver's own dependence needs. Emphasis on the infant at this time can increase competition with the baby in emotionally immature parents and between a parent and the nurse, who may be viewed as a competitor for the role of the "good parent." When a helping relationship is accepted as useful and there is a willingness to meet regularly, the first stage of contracting is completed.

In the working phase of the relationship problems are identified, and alternative responses are explored together. The mutual effect of the caregiver and infant's emotional states, needs, and behavior is gradually recognized. The nurse maintains a supportive approach when working with the caregiver, fostering the development of a therapeutic alliance based on trust. Problem areas are carefully assessed to plan appropriate therapeutic approaches.

Specific suggestions and new information coupled with appropriate feedback are often sufficient to assist some caregivers to develop new patterns of interaction with their infants. In other situations the nurse may need to function as a role model for alternative behaviors. In these cases the nurse recognizes the caregiver's dependence need and supports this need long enough to permit the caregiver to internalize a sense of personal competence. The caregiver may feel threatened and defensive as new behaviors are demonstrated and encouraged and may test the strength of the therapeutic relationship through noncompliant and provocative behavior. The nurse is prepared for such behavior, remaining consistent and supportive while helping the caregiver to explore the meaning of the behavior. The nurse needs to recognize this behavior as part of the therapeutic process and not react emotionally to the caregiver's seemingly hostile attitude.

A wide variety of interventions are used in the helping relationship, depending on individual need. The duration, pattern, and modalities of treatment employed depend on the parents' background, readiness, and insight. An eclectic approach is helpful in determining individual plans. The ultimate goal is the same: to promote mental health in infants through improved reciprocal caregiver-infant interactions.

The caregiver's improved responsiveness, self-confidence, and competence and the achievement of normal developmental tasks indicates a readiness for termination. Termination of the helping relationship with an infant has a unique and paradoxical feature: absolute termination is not desirable. Instead, it is often restricted and relative. With the consent of the caregiver(s) frequent and regular meetings cease gradually, as weaning. It is also advisable to include auxillary care and availability in the termination agreement. An explicit plan for reentry into treatment at times of extra stress, whether developmental, personal, or social, is essential. Predetermined, periodic meetings for careful, caring monitoring of child rearing are imperative. These meetings, which constitute primary preventive care, are particularly useful at transitional stages of child development, when reassessment and anticipatory guidance can be provided.

NURSING PROCESS
Assessment

✦ *Physical dimension.* The integrity of the sensorimotor functions are critical to the optimal development of the infant. Physical maturity at birth varies widely. Several factors influence it: sex (on the average girls are about 2 weeks more mature in CNS and bone development), gestational age, and birth weight. Premature infants (weighing less than 2500 g, or 5½ pounds) often have serious physical problems that interfere with the early functions of breathing, digestion, sleeping, and waking. These difficulties often impair the infant's ability to adjust and adapt to the environment in ways that promote mental health.

Assessment of the physical status of the newborn begins immediately after delivery. The Apgar score is commonly used in the delivery room to evaluate cardiopulmonary and neurological integrity.[3] The Apgar scale also identifies gross CNS abnormalities.

In the first 28 days of extrauterine life the infant makes a number of physiological adjustments to the world and begins to respond to internal and external stimulation. Life outside the protective environment of the womb requires dramatic adjustments. For example, before delivery infants live in a state of nutritional equilibrium supported by the maternal environment. Once born, infants' survival depends in part on their ability to recognize and convey feelings of hunger to their caregivers. Successful nourishment, then, depends in part on the integrity of an infant's physiological and sensory capacities (sensing hunger) and his expressive and motor capabilities (crying and sucking).

Neonates' voluntary muscles are poorly controlled, but they come equipped with a variety of reflexes, including sucking, grasping, rooting, coughing, and stepping (the prancing movements of the legs when the infant is held upright with feet touching a table or crib). Many of these reflexes are used by the infant as protection against noxious stimuli. Additionally, the sensory system of the newborn functions at a much higher level than the motor functions. Optimal mental health development during the first year of life is seen as the result of successful melding of sensory experiences with motor activities,[20] as the following Case Example illustrates.

Case Example

Maureen, age 3 months, one of a set of identical twins, was referred to an infant mental health specialist by her pediatrician, who could find no physiological cause for her recent weight loss, poor muscle tone, and withdrawn appearance. Her mother described Maureen as "the good one, she hardly ever cries, and is content to sit for hours, just playing with her hands. She always goes right to sleep—sometimes I think she'd sleep all day if I didn't wake her up." Christine, Maureen's twin, was smaller at birth, and had developed respiratory distress syndrome after delivery. She was described by the mother as "very difficult, very fussy. She's so demanding, just the opposite of Maureen."

Maureen's inability to elicit a response from her environment has placed her at both a physical and mental health risk. She shows signs of hypoarousal and appears sleepy, subdued, and shuts out sensory stimulation by ignoring it or falling asleep. She fails to recognize sensory experiences in the world and has a limited ability to communicate her needs to her mother. Her mother, stressed from attempting to nurture the difficult and possibly hyperaroused twin, believes that Maureen does not demand attention because she does not need attention. Thus a potentially dangerous pattern of mother-infant interaction is under way.

Other areas the nurse considers when assessing the physical dimension are the infant's state of arousal or attention; the consolability of the baby; and feeding, elimination, and sleeping patterns. Before looking for problems in behavior or activities, however, the nurse needs a basic understanding of what is considered "normal." Pediatric texts will validate normal physical development. Ideally, an infant is able to use sensory experiences as a means of prolonging interest in the world. Thus the infant's level of attention is enhanced by the ability to taste, feel, smell, see, and hear. These experiences in turn provide a means of self-consolation. An infant who is relaxed and attentive while awake will also eat and sleep better than one who is tense and overwhelmed by sensations.

The infant's digestive processes (including feeding and elimination patterns) provide information about sensorimotor and expressive abilities. The caregiver's reciprocal behavior can provide valuable insight into his or her ability to read the baby's cues and signals of hunger and satiation. Feeding and elimination change with age.

Sleeping difficulties are distressing for parents and may produce long-lasting maladaptive patterns of interaction. Sleeping problems also often accompany attentional or arousal problems, in which the infant is unable to "turn off" exciting environmental stimuli. In the opposite extreme the infant uses sleep to escape from the world.

✳ *Emotional dimension.* Infants' emotional development evolves from the unique and highly individual blend of at least three basic ingredients: (1) the integrity of their cognitive and physical (sensorimotor) structures, (2) their basic behavioral style (temperament), and (3) the type and amount of social feedback they receive. Infants' ability to notice and react to the environment is crucial to their emotional development. Sensorimotor functions, discussed previously, enable the infant to experience the environment. Cognitive abilities, discussed in the next section, change with time. The gradual development of full emotional capability parallels the emergence of intellectual abilities, which enable the infant to organize and make sense of experiences and respond differentially.

An assessment of the infant's temperament provides important data. As any parent of more than one child knows, no two babies act alike. Some infants are born with a zest for life, a happy-go-lucky attitude that allows them to adapt gleefully to the world. Others respond to the world with behavioral intensity and chaos. Research by Thomas and Chess[48,49,50] identified three specific constellations of behavioral traits in neonates: the easy child, the difficult child, and the slow-to-warm-up child.

Temperamental individuality is well established by the time a baby is 2 to 3 months old and is thought to be influenced by genetic makeup and prenatal and early postnatal experiences. Studies by Plomin and others[41,42,43] indicate that individual differences of emotionality (reactiveness), activity (including tempo and vigor), and sociability are influenced by heredity.

Social feedback is the third element necessary for infant emotional development and an essential assessment factor. Emotions are critical to infant-caregiver communication. Through feelings, expressions, and reactions babies become actively involved with others. Infants depend on others to stimulate and encourage their emotional behavior. Consider the following Case Example.

Case Example

Sammy, 10 months old, is playing by himself. He is having a good time banging two wooden blocks together. His mother dislikes the noise and comes toward him to take the blocks away. When Sammy sees his mother, his excitement builds and he squeals loudly and throws one of the blocks toward her, his way of "sharing" his joy, attempting to involve his mother in his play. However, his mother sees this behavior as disrespectful and mean; the block struck her painfully on the shin, and she is angry with Sammy. She reaches down, grabs the other block from him, shakes him by the shoulders and yells, "*No! You bad boy! Don't you ever hit me again!*"

Sammy's mother has misinterpreted her son's intentions. She has projected her own ideas (that he was intentionally trying to hurt her) onto his behavior. She responded to his feeling of joy with anger and outrage, and he is left with new feelings of pain, fear, and anger. His feelings of joy and delight were neither reciprocated nor enhanced. If this pattern of interaction is repeated often, Sammy may begin to think that his feelings of joy and desire for his mother's company are bad and that he needs to be punished. Similarly, Sammy's mother (observing her son with a look of obvious delight on his face before throwing something at her) might begin to think that Sammy was happy because he was about to do something he knew she would not like. This type of emotional mis-

reading or miscommunication is detrimental to the development of optimal emotional health.

A gradual differentiation of emotions occurs during the first 12 months. Early emotional responses tend to involve the entire body. The hungry infant, for example, communicates this feeling by crying, stiffening the body, and clenching the fists. As infants mature, emotions are not tied as closely to their internal state, and they begin to react to things and events in the environment. Later emotional expression (between 6 and 12 months) is related to increasing awareness of the social context of events.[36] Feelings of hunger are expressed differently by the 6-month-old baby, who stops fussing and smiles at the parent who has arrived with the bottle. Older infants (who have a better idea of where and when hunger is relieved) may become upset and cry when hungry but will also crawl toward the high chair and become ecstatic when the parent opens the refrigerator to begin meal preparations. A wide range of emotional responses emerge in a regular pattern. Specific emotions appear with age and depend on both cognitive and social development.[47]

An assessment tool to uncover specific infant behavior patterns is shown in Figure 39-1.

✳ ***Intellectual dimension.*** An evaluation of mental health begins with an assessment of sensorimotor capabilities. Infants with serious sensory or motor problems often do not develop optimal intellectual functions. The nurse also assesses the infant's environment, which needs to allow safe and stimulating exploration and produce consistent, dependable responses. The nurse then examines the infant's patterns of vocalizations and (later) verbalizations, since language development is closely tied to cognition.

Infants' intellectual development depends on active experiences with the environment during the first year of life. This environmental involvement takes two forms: first, an organizing of basic rhythms, such as crying, sucking, breathing, and resting; second, an active and voluntary participation in environmental experience. Both provide opportunities for the infant to associate patterns of movement and sensation with specific environmental events and signal the beginning of intellectual development.[12] Each facet of environmental involvement needs to be assessed.

During the first 12 months intellectual abilities emerge sequentially. Through repetition of simple reflex activities the infant begins to differentiate between self and environment. In the beginning "self" is the cause of everything in the world. When the hungry baby cries, milk arrives. Eventually, with repetition, different stimuli become associated. The hungry baby learns to stop crying when the caregiver's voice is heard (since now the arrival of milk is anticipated). The infant begins to recognize objects in the environment as separate from self as well as the self's effect on these objects.[39]

This early notion of cause and effect is directly related to a beginning self-conception. Through repeated experiences, the infant begins to sense relationships between action and the stimulation of action. This awakening awareness of the part the infant plays in the action helps to

I. SELF-REGULATION AND INTEREST IN THE WORLD
Birth to 3 months

Increasingly (but still only sometimes):   YES   NO
—able to calm down
—sleeps regularly
—brightens to sights (by alerting and focusing
 on object)
—brightens to sounds (by alerting and focusing
 on your voice)
—enjoys touch
—enjoys movement in space (up and down,
 side to side)

II. FALLING IN LOVE
2 to 7 months

When wooed, increasingly (but still only
sometimes):   YES   NO
—looks at you with a special, joyful smile
—gazes at you with great interest
—joyfully smiles at you in response to your
 vocalizations
—joyfully smiles at you in response to your
 interesting facial expressions
—vocalizes back as you vocalize

III. DEVELOPING INTENTIONAL COMMUNICATION
3 to 10 months

Increasingly (but still only sometimes)
responds to: YES   NO
—your gestures with gestures in return
 (you hand her a rattle and she takes it)
—your vocalizations with vocalizations
—your emotional expressions with an emotional
 response (a smile begets a smile)
—pleasure or joy with pleasure
—encouragement to explore with curiosity
 (reaches for interesting toy)

III. DEVELOPING INTENTIONAL COMMUNICATION—cont'd
3 to 10 months

Increasingly (but still only sometimes) initiates: YES   NO
—interactions (expectantly looks for you to
 respond)
—joy and pleasure (woos you spontaneously)
—comforting (reaches up to be held)
—exploration and assertiveness (explores your
 face or examines a new toy)

IV. THE EMERGENCE OF AN ORGANIZED SENSE OF SELF
9 to 18 months

Increasingly (but still only sometimes):   YES   NO
—initiates a complex behavior pattern such as
 going to refrigerator and pointing to desired
 food, playing a chase game, rolling a ball
 back and forth with you
—uses complex behavior in order to establish
 closeness (pulls on your leg and reaches up
 to be picked up)
—uses complex behavior to explore and be
 assertive (reaches for toys, finds you in
 another room)
—plays in a focused, organized manner
 on own
—examines toys or other objects to see how
 they work
—responds to limits that you set with your voice
 or gestures
—recovers from anger after a few minutes
—able to use objects like a comb or telephone
 in semirealistic manner
—seems to know how to get you to react (which
 actions make you laugh, which make
 you mad)

FIGURE 39-1 Assessment of specific behavior patterns in the infant. (From First feelings—milestones in the emotional development of your baby and child, by Stanley Greenspan, M.D., and Nancy Thorndike Greenspan. Copyright © Stanley Greenspan, M.D., and Nancy Throndike Greenspan, 1985. Reprinted by permission of Viking Penguin, Inc.)

further differentiate self from environment. The nurse, then, assesses the infant's ability to separate self from others and the effect the separation has on the infant.

❀ ***Social dimension.*** The infant, dependent on the social environment for optimal development, has a repertoire of capacities and characteristics designed to attract the caregiver. For example, from birth infants are drawn to the human voice and face. Their physical appearance (large eyes in proportion to the face; large head in proportion to the body; fuzzy hair; soft, smooth skin; and baby fat) entices most adults into some form of nurturing. Furthermore, infants are able to shape interactions by their abilities to communicate, or signal, their feelings.

Infants' signals and responses enable them to become involved in reciprocal interactions with their caregivers. This interaction helps ensure survival during the long period of physical and emotional dependence.

Two important areas of social assessment are attachment and development of a sense of trust. Trust emerges from a strong primary attachment to the caregiver. Attachment is the specific positive emotional relationship that forms between infant and primary caregiver (Figure 39-2). Newman and Newman[36] list three indicators of formed social attachment: (1) the infant tries to maintain contact with the object of attachment, (2) the infant shows distress when the object of attachment is absent, and (3) the

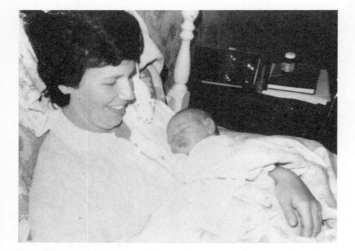

FIGURE 39-2 Attachment has begun between this mother and her 1-hour-old newborn.

infant is more relaxed and comfortable with the object of attachment than with others.

Development of a sense of trust is the main task of infancy, according to Erikson.[14] The infant's trust evolves from repeated experiences with a consistent and responsive caregiver. Caregiver responsivity, however, is influenced in part by the infant's ability to successfully communicate. Ideally, the caregiver learns to interpret the infant's behavior appropriately. The infant begins to feel confident of the caregiver's ability to understand his needs, and mutual trust is established. The infant's ability to trust is critical for becoming a successful member of a larger social network later.

When assessing the strength of the social dimension of the infant, the nurse looks for signs of attachment and trust, such as separation and stranger anxieties.

✳ *Spiritual dimension.* Human spirituality may begin to develop at birth. There is no literature on infant spirituality; but one logical assumption is that the basis of spirituality is derived from the infant's earliest role models of nurturing authorities; consequently, it is rooted in family experiences and closely related to the development of trust. The spiritual aspect, related to an understanding of the ultimate meaning and purpose of life, is linked to later cognitive and moral development. However, cognitive and emotional structures (which permit moral reasoning) begin to develop in infancy and at the very least serve as a foundation for full spiritual capabilities in later life. The ultimate development of an individual's spiritual dimension, then, at least partially depends on the integrity of the underlying intellectual, emotional, and social dimensions. Assessment of the infant's spirituality involves consideration of these three areas.

The following holistic assessment tool contains assessment information specific to infants. It is to be used in conjunction with the assessment tool in Chapter 8.

PHYSICAL DIMENSION

Genetic History

Are there any family members with mental or emotional illnesses, such as depression, schizophrenia, or alcohol or drug addiction?

Are there any genetically linked conditions in the family that could affect the infant's growth and development (such as metabolic or neurological disorders)?

Prenatal History

Did the mother receive prenatal care?

Did the mother use alcohol or drugs or smoke during pregnancy?

Was there any maternal illness, unusual stress, or injury during pregnancy?

Neonatal History

Is this a high-risk infant (for example, premature, small for gestational age, one of a multiple birth, offspring of an adolescent mother)?

Were there any problems at birth that required medical treatment (for example, respiratory distress, jaundice)?

What were the infant's Apgar scores?

PHYSICAL EXAMINATION

Has the infant had a complete physical examination by a physician or a certified pediatric nurse practitioner?

Have arrangements been made to obtain well-baby health supervision?

Have routine immunizations been started?

Is the infant in good physical condition?

Is growth and development progressing normally?

Does the infant have any health deficits?

Are all sensorimotor capabilities present?

Does the infant have any congenital anomalies?

Level of Arousal

How does the primary caregiver describe the infant's temperament?

What does the primary caregiver think about the infant's sleeping and waking cycle?

Is the baby sleepier or more awake than expected?

How does the baby react to new situations and people?

How does the baby react to a sudden loud noise, such as a door slamming nearby?

Does the baby ever seem upset for no reason at all?

Consolability

Does the baby enjoy being held and cuddled?

How does the primary caregiver get the baby to stop crying?

Does the same method always work?

Does the baby ever stop crying without intervention?

Does the baby ever suck his thumb or fingers?

How does the baby fall asleep (for example, only while being held, while nursing or being fed, in crib alone)?

Is it hard for the baby to calm down once upset?

HOLISTIC ASSESSMENT TOOL: THE INFANT

Feeding and Elimination

How does the baby convey feelings of hunger?

Does the baby have any problems with feeding?

How does the baby respond to new foods and new textures when eating?

Does the baby have problems making bowel movements?

Sleeping

How many hours (in 24) does the baby sleep?

Does the baby ever have trouble falling asleep?

Does the baby wake up frequently in the night?

Are there any specific positions the baby cannot tolerate (for example, on the back, tummy)?

Does the baby need help to fall asleep (for example, being swaddled, rocked, or walked)?

Does the baby ever engage in self-induced rhythmic activities, such as rocking or head banging?

Does the baby require a bottle to go to sleep?

Where does the baby sleep (for example, parents' bed, own crib)?

EMOTIONAL DIMENSION

How does the primary caregiver characterize the infant's predominant style of behavior (for example, easy going, slow to warm up, irritable)?

Does the primary caregiver find the infant's temperament difficult to deal with?

How regular is the infant's schedule?

Does the infant seem to mind a lot if this schedule is altered?

How would the infant react to delayed or interrupted feeding or naps?

Is the infant easily distracted during feeding?

How does the infant react to other people?

How does the infant react to being bathed?

INTELLECTUAL DIMENSION
Intellectual Activities

0 to 4 months of age

Does the infant show special interest in some sights and sounds?

Does the infant enjoy being moved up and down, side to side, through space?

Will the infant follow a slowly moving object or person a full 180 degrees?

Is the infant able to hold and briefly mouth two objects?

4 to 8 months of age

Does the baby enjoy playing with rattles?

Does the baby shake the toy to produce the rattling sound?

Will the baby reach out to the primary caregiver to be picked up (after caregiver initiates movement toward picking up the infant)?

Is the baby able to search for and find a partially hidden toy?

8 to 12 months of age

Does the baby engage in imaginative games, such as pat-a-cake and peekaboo?

Is the baby able to discriminate strangers?

Does the baby cry or attempt to retreat when strangers are present?

Can the baby anticipate events from signs, such as when the caregiver puts on a coat before leaving the house?

Does the baby drop or throw objects intentionally?

Does the baby ever use objects according to their social significance (for example, hugging a doll or wearing a hat)?

Language Skills

0 to 4 months of age

Does the baby coo and smile in response to another person's voice?

Does the baby cry in response to distress?

Is the baby able to repeat his or her own sounds?

4 to 8 months of age

Does the baby respond to his own name?

Does the baby ever babble repetitive syllables (for example, ba ba ba)?

Does the baby ever vocalize different emotional states, such as anger or happiness?

8 to 12 months of age

Is the baby able to initiate interactions through deliberate use of vocalizations?

Does the baby shake his head to show "no"?

Can the baby wave good-bye?

Can the baby say three or more words other than "mama" or "dada"?

"Does the baby respond to simple requests (for example, "come here," "sit down")?

Does the baby respond to "no, no"?

Does the baby vocalize in response to the presence of a familiar person?

SOCIAL DIMENSION
Social Skills

Does the infant exhibit prosocial behavior (for example, smiling, cooing, visual tracking, turning head to interesting sounds)?

Does the infant show a preference for the primary caregiver?

Does the infant imitate sounds or gestures?

Does the infant initiate interaction with the primary caregiver?

Does the infant engage in reciprocal social games, such as peekaboo?

Does the infant avoid new people? (If so, is it age appropriate?)

How does the infant react to separation from the primary caregiver? (Is this behavior age appropriate?)

Does the infant reach out for toys?

Does the infant initiate new behaviors by himself?

Can the primary caregiver generally figure out the infant's needs? For example, how does the caregiver determine whether the infant is crying from hunger as opposed to fatigue?

Does the infant ever engage in gaze aversion? If so, with whom and when?

TABLE 39-3 Instruments for assessing infant development

Instrument	Reference	Description
Bayley's Scale of Infant Development	Bayley	Intelligence test for children less than 3 years of age that evaluates cognitive and motor functioning and integration. Although measurements of infants are less reliable than those for older children, they can be predictive when scores are markedly subnormal or superior. This instrument is best used by developmental psychologists.
Brazelton Neonatal Assessment Scale	Brazelton	Assessment of such newborn behavior as motor maturity, alertness, and consolability. This focus on individual infant behavior can be used to prepare parents for their baby's individual temperament. Neonatal nurses and physicians can use this in promoting better mother-infant relations.
Developmental Diagnostic Profile	A. Freud	Comprehensive and dynamic evaluation of neuropsychiatric, intellectual, emotional, and social development, using psychoanalytic principles. For use by psychiatric professionals who work with infants and children.
Developmental Screening Inventory Scale	Knobloch and Pasamanick	Detailed questionnaire for use with caregiver of infant. Determines achievement level of infant in five areas: adaptive, gross motor, fine motor, language, and personal-social. Based on Gesell's findings, this instrument can be used by nurses and physicians with pediatric knowledge and interviewing skills.
Denver Developmental Screening Test	Frankenburg and Dodds	Objective screening test for development in four areas: personal-social, fine motor–adaptive, language, and gross motor. Based on Gesell's work establishing norms of development in these areas. Since this instrument is easy to administer and score and takes about 15-20 minutes to use, it is economical and widely used to screen for early abnormal development. Nonprofessionals and professionals can be trained to administer the test. It can be used in all settings that serve children's educational and health facilities.

Another simple screening tool, which provides a guide for data collection, was developed by Haslett.[24] It uses a mnemonic device, "SCREAM," to designate the six areas to address when assessing infant mental health:

S *Sensitivity.* Are there unusual sensitivities to sound, light, touch, smell, or taste? (To assess sensory integrity)

C *Cuddliness.* What is the infant's reaction to being cuddled? (To assess attentional state and consolability)

R *Reactivity.* What is the intensity of the infant's reaction? (To assess temperament)

E *Emotional maturity.* What level of emotional maturity has the infant reached? (To assess the progression of the infant's ability to relate to other human beings)

A *Automatic stability.* Is there any evidence of autonomic nervous system instability? (To assess early CNS vulnerability)

M *Motor maturity.* Is the infant progressing normally through the major motor phases? (To assess physical or motor development)

Other useful tools for assessment are growth charts and the instruments listed in Table 39-3.

Analysis

Nursing diagnosis. The following list provides examples of NANDA-accepted nursing diagnoses with causative statements.

1. Impaired physical mobility related to CNS dysfunction

2. Alteration in comfort related to colic
3. Alteration in comfort related to impaired sensory function
4. Alteration in nutrition related to feeding problems
5. Sleeping pattern disturbance related to colic
6. Sensory-perceptual alteration related to hearing impairment
7. Impaired communication related to alteration in sensory-perceptual state
8. Impaired communication related to caregiver's inability to adequately interpret infant cues or signals
9. Ineffective individual coping related to inconsolability
10. Anxiety related to stranger's presence
11. Anxiety related to separation from attachment figure

DSM-III-R diagnoses. Infant pathological conditions identified in the DSM-III-R are listed in the box below.

DSM-III-R CLASSIFICATIONS FOR INFANT PATHOLOGICAL CONDITIONS

313.89	Reactive attachment disorder of infancy
307.53	Rumination disorder of infancy
299.00	Autistic disorder

Adapted from American Psychiatric Association: Diagnostic and statistical manual of mental disorders (DSM-III-R), Washington, D.C., 1987, The Association.

The essential features and manifestations of the features of reactive attachment disorder, autistic disorder, and rumination disorder according to the DSM-III-R are listed in the following boxes.

313.89   REACTIVE ATTACHMENT DISORDER OF INFANCY AND EARLY CHILDHOOD

ESSENTIAL FEATURES

The essential feature of this disorder is markedly disturbed social relatedness that begins before the age of 5.

MANIFESTATIONS

Physical Dimension

Weight loss or failure to gain weight
Poor muscle tone
Hypomotility
Weak rooting and grasping in response to feeding attempts
Weak cry
Excessive sleep
Lack of visual tracking of eyes and face by 2 months of age
Lack of visual reciprocity by 2 months of age; lack of vocal reciprocity with caregiver by 5 months of age
Lack of alerting and turning toward caregiver's voice by 4 months of age

Emotional Dimension

Lack of smiling in response to faces by 2 months of age

Social Dimension

Lack of interest in the environment
Lack of spontaneous reaching for the caregiver by 4 months of age
Lack of participation in playful games with the caregiver by 5 months of age

---

Adapted from the American Psychiatric Association: Diagnostic and Statistical manual of mental disorders (DSM-III-R), Washington D.C., 1987, The Association.

Planning

Because the infant cannot be assessed or treated apart from the family and environment, plans include the entire family. Any plan that merely revolves around the baby is likely to fail, since the infant has no existence apart from the caregiver and environment.

Table 39-4 lists some examples of long-term and short-term goals and outcome criteria for two selected nursing diagnoses. They provide a model for the planning stage in the nursing process.

Implementation

The nurse's interventions are directed primarily toward the caregiver, with specific plans to alter infant behavior

---

299.00   AUTISTIC DISORDER

ESSENTIAL FEATURES

The child fails to respond to other people, and has grossly impaired communication skills and bizarre responses developing in the first 36 months of age.

MANIFESTATIONS

Physical Dimension

Bizarre environmental responses
Stereotyped body movements
Fascination with movement (staring at fans, spinning objects)

Emotional Dimension

Labile moods

Intellectual Dimension

Gross deficits in language development (echolalia, metaphorical language)
Preoccupation with parts of objects

Social Dimension

Lack of interest in other people
Pervasive lack of response to others
Failure to cuddle
Lack of eye contact and facial responsiveness
Indifference or aversion to affection or physical contact
Failure to develop normal attachment behavior
Abnormal social play

Adapted from the American Psychiatric Association: Diagnostic and Statistical manual of mental disorders, Washington D.C., 1987, The Association.

307.53   RUMINATION DISORDER OF INFANCY

ESSENTIAL FEATURES

The child repeatedly regurgitates food with weight loss or failure to gain expected weight, developing after a period of normal functioning.

MANIFESTATIONS

Physical Dimension

Repeated regurgitation of food without nausea or gastrointestinal illness
Weight loss
Malnutrition
Developmental delays

Emotional Dimension

Satisfaction from regurgitation
Irritability and hunger between episodes

Social Dimension

Discouraged caregiver by failure to feed child successfully
Alienation from caregiver
Avoidance caused by noxious odor
Understimulation caused by avoidance

Adapted from the American Psychiatric Association: Diagnostic and Statistical manual of mental disorders, Washington D.C., 1987, The Association.

TABLE 39-4 Long-term and short-term goals, and outcome criteria related to infants

Goals	Outcome Criteria

NURSING DIAGNOSIS: ANXIETY RELATED TO SEPARATION FROM ATTACHMENT FIGURE

Long-term goals

To develop normal human relationships with others	Infant demonstrates preferential response to attachment figure.
	Infant differentiates caregiver from strangers.
To develop trust in others.	Caregiver provides attachment: secure, consistent emotional base from which infant can explore.
	Caregiver demonstrates ability to allow infant to experience the environment and others (not overprotective).

Short-term goals

To reduce anxiety	Caregiver establishes methods to diminish infant's sense of abandonment: leaves doorways between rooms open so infant can see, caregiver responds verbally to infant when out of sight.
	Infant responds verbally to caregiver when out of sight.
To reduce attachment figure's anxiety	Caregiver accepts phase as normal and as a desired consequence of infant's ability for object permanence.
To foster ability to separate	Caregiver provides consistent alternative caregiver.
	Caregiver provides infant with transitional object, such as teddy bear or blanket.

NURSING DIAGNOSIS: SLEEP PATTERN DISTURBANCE RELATED TO COLIC

Long-term goals

To develop regular diurnal sleeping patterns consistent with age norms	Caregiver establishes consistent night sleep patterns
	Infant establishes day nap pattern.
	Infant falls asleep in crib instead of caregiver's arms.
To provide gratification in activities of daily living	Adequate caregiver-infant interaction during the day.
	Caregiver spends time each day in pleasure-producing play with infant.
	Infant can comfortably spend time alone.

Short-term goals

To reduce anxiety	Caregiver understands infant's physiological needs: has expectations, reads infant's signals and cues accurately (recognizes distress crying), recognizes own response to infant, seeks and receives support and encouragement from others.
To establish realistic, reasonable limits	Caregiver establishes regular bedtime, maintains regular routine; and responds to continued crying (after 15 minutes) by providing comforting measures (no feeding or playing).
	Caregiver eliminates excessive stimulation before bedtime and maintains quiet nighttime environment

or environmental factors. Consequently, the nurse will generally find the roles of consultant, role model, and teacher the most successful when implementing changes to foster infant mental health.

✦ Physical dimension. Infants at risk for serious physical problems (such as premature and low-weight babies, babies with birth defects, and those born to alcoholic and drug-abusing mothers) need to be referred to medical experts for thorough evaluation and treatment.

Feeding and sleeping problems are major concerns in young infants. Many such problems stem from the infants inability to regulate his state of arousal. Nurses can provide valuable assistance in teaching parents to facilitate their infant's self-regulating ability, which is often caused by CNS immaturity and usually outgrown by the age of 3 months. However, early intervention is important, since first experiences are critical in establishing healthy and mutually gratifying patterns of care.

Early self-regulatory problems can often be alleviated through interventions to increase the baby's attention and to help the baby learn self-consolation. Strategies include teaching the parents about the self-regulating capacities of the infant by stating that infants adapt to the world by using different attentional states and demonstrate distinct behavioral differences depending on their attentional state. For example, an actively crying and kicking baby is effectively shutting out other stimuli, whereas a quiet baby sucking on a thumb may be very attuned to visual and auditory events in the environment. Other strategies include encouraging self-consoling behaviors such as thumb sucking; providing simple sensory stimulation at an appropriate level for the baby; providing a consistent, calm atmosphere; and assisting the parents to accurately interpret the infant's signals.

Occasionally, self-regulation problems are related to specific sensory problems. In the case of sensory hyposensitivity or hypersensitivity the nurse can offer strategies to decrease or increase specific sensory stimulation. For example, some babies are extremely sensitive to high-pitched noises and will disorganize quickly when exposed to such sounds. Caregivers can be taught to moderate their own voices to a pitch that is not painful and to control environmental noises as much as possible. Severe sensory problems, such as visual or hearing impairments, require interventions that provide increased stimulation through other intact senses.

Generally an infant who is able to integrate sensory experiences and regulate attentional states will not develop major feeding or sleeping problems. Persistent feeding difficulties accompanied by vomiting, elimination problems, or weight loss may be due to a physical problem, and the nurse refers the parents and infant to a physician. Occasionally, a feeding problem may result from a temperamental mismatch between the infant and caregiver. An easily distracted, hyperalert baby will have difficulty settling down to nurse. Such behavior may cause the mother to feel tense and inadequate, which will further increase the infant's distraction. The nurse, through observation of the feeding process, is often able to suggest practical methods for promoting more rewarding feeding experiences. For example, a baby who feeds briefly, stops to look around frequently, and requires encouragement to return to the breast or bottle may need to be fed in a less stimulating environment, such as a darkened room. The caregivers distraction or tension can produce a reciprocal tension in the infant. Encouraging a relaxed attitude, which will enhance a mutual responsiveness, is accomplished by exploring the caregiver's feelings about and behavior during feeding and by teaching relaxation techniques.

Persistent sleeping problems require interventions to increase the infant's deep sleep period. When infants first fall asleep, they enter the rapid eye movement (REM) state. Later they enter the deep sleep stage, during which maturational processes occur in the body and CNS. The infant with a sleeping disturbance may be getting predominantly REM stage sleep and as a consequence may remain neurologically immature. This immaturity makes it difficult for the infant to self-regulate, which inhibits the infant's ability to fall asleeep without help. Thus, instead of arousing slightly when moving to deeper sleeping levels, the infant completely awakens and never gets to the deeper levels of sleep. Interventions that promote sleep include adequate feeding, being warm and dry, reducing environmental stimuli, and having a relaxed caregiver.

Emotional dimension.
An infant's emotional problems result either from his difficulty experiencing the environment (sensorimotor problems) or integrating and interpreting the experiences accurately (intellectual problems). As an example, consider the fretful, tense, and inconsolable infant, who cries easily and is often upset. The slightest change in the environment is enough to set this infant off; normal sights, sounds, and tactile stimulation are irritating. Interventions in this case increase the infant's self-regulatory capacities. Likewise, the depressed or apathetic infant requires stimulation that is interesting and enticing yet modulated to allow the baby to become involved gradually. Stimulation and affection with such babies is provided in a gentle and unobtrusive way, since these infants become easily overwhelmed and "tune out." Nurses working with withdrawn infants offer low-key stimulation, approaching them with one sensory experience at a time (lightly stroking the infant's limbs *or* talking in a quiet voice, not both at once).

When an infant appears to have an emotional impairment that is not due to a sensorimotor problem or is caused by intellectual deficits, the nurse considers the influence of social feedback. If the problem resulted from inappropriate or inadequate caregiver behavior, interventions are aimed at improving the emotional reciprocity between caregiver and infant. The nurse focuses on improving the quality of the caregiver's nurturing activities. First the nurse assesses the caregiver's level of child-rearing skills. When the caregiver is inexperienced and lacks knowledge of appropriate caregiving behaviors, the nurse intervenes by teaching the caregiver about the infant's individual emotional needs. Specifically, the nurse assists the caregiver in accurately interpreting and responding to the baby's cues, points out the infant's selective responses to the caregiver, and encourages the caregiver to remain consistent and available and to engage in pleasurable activities with the infant. In some instances the caregiver may not be able to provide adequate nurturance because of emotional problems; the nurse refers the infant and caregiver to an appropriate resource.

Intellectual dimension.
When a severe intellectual deficit is suspected, the nurse refers the infant appropriately to a neurologist, pediatrician, or an infant mental health center for further evaluation and treatment.

Several nursing interventions foster optimal intellectual developments. The nurse encourages caregivers to allow their infants to become actively engaged in the environment, to manipulate and explore as much of the world as safely possible. Many parents find developmental guidance helpful. The nurse interprets the infant's seemingly meaningless repetitive activities for the parents as desired and normal. For example, the infant who continuously drops dishes, food, and silverware from the high chair is developing early recognition of a sequence of events, which is necessary for attaining the concept of cause and effect. The nurse can also assist parents in understanding and facilitating the development of object permanence through simple games, such as peek-a-boo, "Where is it?," and waving bye-bye. The related concepts of stranger and separation anxiety are also explained. Specific strategies to decrease separation anxiety are teaching parents to increase the use of distal modes of communication; for example, calling to the infant from other rooms, keeping doors open to allow the infant to make visual contact with the parent; providing the infant with a transitional object, such as a teddy bear or security blanket; and maintaining consistent, sensitive responses that convey acceptance of the infant's feelings but do not reinforce the infant's fearfulness. For example, a quick hug of reassurance, coupled with a distraction to some other interesting toy or event is better than prolonged soothing and intense physical contact, which exaggerates the infant's dependence on the caregiver and ultimately makes separation more difficult.

Language development depends partly on the integrity of intellectual foundations that enable intentional, receptive, and expressive functions. Failure of the infant to meet age-expected vocalizations and verbalizations may necessitate referral for evaluation. Many community health centers and public school departments have speech evaluation services. The nurse may also refer the infant directly to a speech pathologist.

❋ ***Social dimension.*** The infant experiencing a problem in the social dimension, such as an attachment disorder, may demonstrate behavior such as gaze aversion and withdrawal from human contact or may demonstrate insecure attachments through clinging and intense fearfulness on separation from the attachment figure. Early interventions educate caregivers about the process of attachment. Parents can facilitate the development of a trusting relationship by learning to accurately interpret their baby's signals and providing a consistent and responsive environment.

Because attachment to a primary caregiver is one of the most important developmental tasks of infancy to ensure optimal mental health, the nurse encourages caregivers to form a rich and rewarding relationship with the infant. This can be facilitated by having parents observe their infants closely to get to know their individual behavioral style. Caregivers need to provide interesting experiences that allow the infant to experience multisensory stimuli. This can be as simple an activity as moving the infant gently through space, maintaining eye contact and offering warm expressions, and cooing or talking to the baby. Some infants require special wooing, a method to attract the infant's attention. Developing a sense of attachment requires first that a relationship exist between caregiver and infant, then the relationship is fostered by spending pleasurable time together at play. Some parents may need to learn *how* to play. The nurse provides valuable assistance through demonstration, role modeling, and observation and feedback sessions. Because the process of attachment is thought to be central to the optimal development of mental health, the nurse needs to refer parents and infants for further evaluation and treatment when serious attachment problems are suspected. Referral to an infant mental health specialist is critical when the infant's physical growth and development are affected by the attachment disorder.

When working with a caregiver-infant dyad, the nurse is sensitive to the needs of the caregiver and is careful to offer assistance in ways that are nonjudgmental and that will ultimately augment the caregiver's self-esteem. One useful technique is a method in which the nurse interprets the infant's behavior and speaks for the nonverbal infant. This can be done directly or indirectly. For example, in the direct approach the nurse who is enhancing the attachment process between caregiver and infant would point out the infant's preferential smile for the caregiver by saying, "See Mommy (or Daddy)? This is my special smile just for you. You make me feel so good, no one else is quite like you." In the indirect approach the nurse communicates the infant's needs and intentions by directing questions and comments to the infant in the presence of the listening caregiver. After observing and interpreting an infant's behavior, the nurse comments, "Are you sleepy? You always start to fuss and then you rub your eyes when you're tired. I think you're a sleepy baby." Both approaches are useful in helping the caregiver to accurately interpret the infant's behavior.

Many infant mental health centers have been established to provide programs that offer appropriate supportive environments for infants. Therapeutic daycare centers provide opportunities for caregivers to learn parenting skills in growth-enhancing environments. Other centers have therapeutic nurseries, which focus more on the direct care of infants who have special mental health care needs.

❋ ***Spiritual dimension.*** Interventions to ensure spiritual development in infancy are those that enhance optimal emotional, social, and intellectual development, since it is believed that spirituality encorporates all these dimensions.

Evaluation

Evaluation of the nurse's interventions is a judgment of the extent to which the treatment goals and outcome criteria have been met. Because care focuses on the caregiver-infant relationship, the behavior of both is evaluated. The caregiver's perception of the changes that have occurred and how goals for the infant have been met is important.

The promotion and maintenance of infant mental health necessitates an emphasis on continuing parent education, anticipatory guidance, and periodic evaluations.

BRIEF REVIEW

In mental health–psychiatric nursing the therapeutic relationship with the infant is unique. Parameters in the relationship are discovered through the nursing process, which includes data collection in all five dimensions during the prenatal, neonatal, and infancy period. Because the relationship between infant and caregiver is reciprocal, the nursing process is directed toward both.

Biological interactional, cognitive, psychoanalytic, and learning theories provide understanding of infant growth and direct clinical actions. Knowledge of normal emotional development provides the nurse with standards to assist in identifying deviations from the norm and high-risk factors.

A number of measurement tools are available for assessing infant development, such as "SCREAM," Brazelton's Neonatal Assessment Scale, and the Developmental Screening Inventory Scale. These tools aid in assessing the infant in each dimension. Referral to another professional or agency may be necessary for more serious conditions, such as reactive attachment disorder, rumination disorder, or infantile autism.

The ultimate goal is improved mental health in infants through improved caregiver-infant interactions. The nurse can be a change agent toward an improved climate for the promotion of infant mental health.

REFERENCES AND SUGGESTED READINGS

1. Ainsworth, M.D.S.: The development of infant-mother attachment. In Caldwell, B.M., and Ricciuti, H.N., editors: Review of child development research, vol. 3, Chicago, 1973, University of Chicago Press.

2. Ainsworth, M.D.S., and others: Patterns of attachment: a psychological study of the strange situation, New York, 1978, John Wiley & Sons, Inc.

2a. American Psychiatric Association: Diagnostic and statistical manual of mental disorders (DSM-III-R), Washington, D.C., 1987, The Association.

3. Apgar, V.: Proposal for a new method of evaluation of the newborn infant, Anesthesia and Analgesia **32**:260, 1953.

4. Barrera, M.E., and Maurer, D.: The perception of facial expression by the three-month-old, Child Development **52**:203, 1981.

5. Bayley, N.: The development of motor abilities during the first three years, Society for Research in Child Development Monograph 1, vol. 1, 1935.

6. Bowlby, J.: Attachment and loss, vol. 2, Anger, New York, 1973, Basic Books, Inc., Publishers.

7. Brazelton, T.B.: Neonatal assessment scale, Philadelphia, 1973, J.B. Lippincott Co.

8. Brazelton, T.B.: Precursors for the development of emotions in early infancy. In Plutchik, R., and Kellerman, H., editors: Emotions in early development, vol. 2, New York, 1983, Academic Press, Inc.

9. Bromwich, R.: Working with parents and infants, Baltimore, 1981, University Park Press.

10. Call, J.D., and Galenson, E.: Frontiers of infant psychiatry, New York, 1982, Basic Books, Inc., Publishers.

11. Children in hospitals: statement of policy, Washington D.C., 1981, The Association for the Care of Children in Hospitals.

12. Elkind, D.: Children and adolescents: interpretive essays on Jean Piaget, New York, 1981, Oxford University Press, Inc.

13. Erikson, E.: Childhood and society, ed. 2, New York, 1963, W.W. Norton & Co., Inc.

14. Erikson E.: Insight and responsibility, New York, 1964, W.W. Norton & Co., Inc.

15. Field, T.M.: High-risk infants and children: adult and peer interactions, New York, 1981, Academic Press, Inc.

16. Field, T.M.: Infants born at risk: behavior and development, New York, 1979, S.P. Medical & Scientific Books.

17. Fraiberg, S.: Clinical studies in infant mental health: the first year of life, New York, 1980, Basic Books, Inc., Publishers.

18. Freud, A.: Normality and pathology in children: assessments of development, New York, 1965, International Universities Press, Inc.

19. Gesell, A., and Amatruda, C.S.: Developmental diagnosis, ed. 2, New York, 1947, Paul B. Hoebner, Inc.

20. Greenspan, S.: Psychopathology and adaptation in infancy and early childhood, New York, 1981, International Universities Press, Inc.

21. Greenspan, S., and Porges, S.: Psychopathology in infancy and early childhood: clinical perspectives on the organization of sensory and affective-thematic experience, Child Development **55**: 49, 1984.

22. Greenspan, S., and Greenspan, N.: First feelings, New York, 1985, Viking Penguin, Inc.

23. Haslett, N.R.: Treatment planning for children: a complete child psychiatry evaluation outline, Journal of Continuing Education in Psychiatry **11**:21, 1977.

24. Howell, J.G.: Modern perspectives in the psychiatry of infancy, New York, 1979, Brunner/Mazel, Inc.

25. Kandzari, J.H., and Howard, J.R.: The well family: a developmental approach to assessment, Boston, 1981, Little, Brown & Co.

26. Kiltenbach, K., and others: Infant wariness toward strangers reconsidered: infants and mothers' reactions to unfamiliar persons, Child Development **51**:1197, 1980.

27. Klaus, M.H., and Kennell, J.H.: Parent-infant bonding, St. Louis, 1981, The C.V. Mosby Co.

28. Knobloch, H., and Pasamanick B.: Gesell and Amatruda's developmental diagnosis, ed. 3, New York, 1974, Harper & Row, Publishers, Inc.

29. Lidz, T.: The person, New York, 1968, Basic Books, Inc., Publishers.

30. Lipsitt, L.P., and Field, T.M.: Infant behavior and development, New York, 1982, S.P. Medical & Scientific Books.

31. Lugo, S.O., and Hershey, G.L.: Human development, New York, 1974, Macmillian Publishing Co.

32. Mack, J.E., and Ablon, S.L.: The development and sustenance of self-esteem in childhood, New York, 1983, International Universities Press, Inc.

33. Mahler, M.S., and others: The psychological birth of the human infant, New York, 1975, Basic Books, Inc., Publishers.

34. McCormick, L., and Schiefelbusch, R.: Early language intervention, Columbus, Ohio, 1984, Charles E. Merrill Publishing Co.

35. Maier, H.W.: Three theories of child development, New York, 1978, Harper & Row, Publishers, Inc.

36. Newman, B., and Newman, R.: Development through life, Homewood, Ill., 1984, The Dorsey Press.

37. Piaget, J.: The origins of intelligence in children, New York, 1952, International Universities Press, Inc.

38. Piaget, J.: The construction of reality in the child, New York, 1954, Basic Books, Inc., Publishers.

39. Piaget, J.: Psychology of the child, New York, 1969, Basic Books, Inc., Publishers.

40. Piaget, J.: The child's conception of time, New York, 1971, Random House, Inc.

41. Plomin, R., and Rowe, D.C.: Genetic and environmental etiology of social behavior in infancy, Developmental Psychology **15**: 62, 1979.

42. Plomin, R.: Developmental behavioral genetics, Child Development. **54**: 253, 1983.

43. Plomin, R., and DeFries, J.C.: Origins of individual differences in infancy, New York, 1985, The Colorado Adoption Project Academic Press.

44. Schaffer, R.: Mothering, Cambridge, Mass., 1977, Harvard University Press.

45. Steinhauer, P.D., and Rae-Grant, Q.: Psychological problems of the child in the family. 2, ed. New York, 1983, Basic Books, Inc., Publishers.

46. Stern, D.: The first relationship, mother and infant, Cambridge, Mass., 1977, Harvard University Press.

47. Stroufe, A.L.: Socioemotional development. In Osofsky, J.D., editor: The handbook of infant development, New York, 1979, John Wiley & Sons, Inc.

48. Thomas, A., and Chess, S.: Behavioral individuality in early childhood, New York, 1963, New York University Press.

49. Thomas, A., and Chess, S.: Temperament and behavior disorders in children, New York, 1968, New York University Press.

50. Thomas, A., and Chess, S.: Temperament and development, New York, 1977, Brunner/Maxel, Inc.

51. Weaver, R., and Cranley, M.: An exploration of paternal-fetal attachment behavior, Nursing Research **32**:2, 1983.

52. Winnicott, D.W.: Therapeutic consultations in child psychiatry, New York, 1971, Basic Books, Inc., Publishers.
53. Yarrow, L.J.: Historical perspectives and future directions in infant development, New York, 1979, John Wiley & Sons, Inc.

ANNOTATED BIBLIOGRAPHY

Ferber, R.: Solve your child's sleep problems, New York, 1985, Simon & Schuster, Inc.

This is an excellent and practical guide to understanding sleep mechanisms and requirements of infants and young children. Advice offered is based on sleep research done at the Center for Pediatric Sleep Disorders at the Children's Hospital in Boston (the only sleep center in the country devoted to children). It is easy to read and suitable as a parent resource.

Fraiberg, S.: Clinical studies in infant mental health: the first year of life, New York, 1980, Basic Books Inc., Publishers.

This easy-to-read collection of case studies of therapeutic relationships with infants and mothers reflects Fraiberg's sensitive and empathetic approach.

Greenspan, S.I., and Greenspan, N.T.: First feelings: milestones in the emotional development of your baby and child from birth to age 4, New York, 1985, Viking Penguin, Inc.

Written primarily for parents, this book is informative to health professionals as well. The emotional milestones are related to the different developmental stages that comprise Greenspan's developmental-structural framework, which emerged from research by Greenspan and his colleagues at the National Institute of Mental Health. The book is punctuated with interesting and illuminating vignettes from the original study.

Osofsky, J.: Handbook of infant development, New York, 1979, John Wiley & Sons, Inc.

This comprehensive collection of reviews on infant development covers cognitive, social, and emotional development and theoretical and clinical issues.

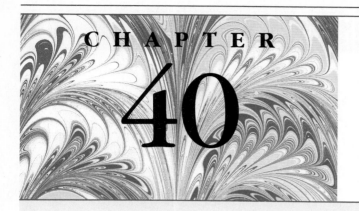

THE CHILD

Patricia Ann Clunn

After studying this chapter the learner will be able to:

Discuss historical developments related to psychiatric nursing care of the child.

Describe various theoretical approaches to explaining child development.

Identify important considerations in establishing a therapeutic relationship with children.

Apply the nursing process to the mental health needs of children.

Describe treatment modalities frequently used in caring for the mental health needs of children.

Of the 47.6 million children between the ages of 3 to 15 years reported in the 1980 U.S. census, it is generally estimated that about 15% are emotionally disturbed. An *emotionally disturbed child* is one whose personality development is arrested or interfered with so that the child shows impairment in reasonable and accurate perceptions of the world, impulse control, learning, and social relations with others. The following statistics summarize the magnitude and types of these problems[46]:

1. There are approximately 500,000 children with psychotic and borderline psychotic disorders, one million children with personality and character disorders, and one million children institutionalized for mental illness.
2. Drug abuse, including alcohol consumption, has increased markedly among children of elementary school age. One large metropolitan survey reported that 74% of children in grades 7 to 10 and 45% of the children from grades 4 to 6 were using drugs regularly.
3. Venereal disease is a major epidemic of childhood, with more than a million cases reported each year and the largest incidence (95%) in children between the ages of 10 and 14 years.
4. More than one million cases of child abuse are reported annually, with about 5,000 children under 5 years of age dying from abuses.
5. Between 1961 and 1975 suicide increased among

children over 10 years of age, with a 150% increase among children ages 5 to 14 years.

Population projections indicate that between 1980 and 2005 there will be an increase of approximately 11% in the number of children under 15 years old. Statistical data on disruptions in the family, the essence of the child's environment, are alarming[49]:

1. Eight to ten million children under age 6 are in child care centers, and about 5.2 million children 13 years or under have parents employed full time. These children are without supervision for significant periods of time.
2. Between 1970 and 1981 the proportion of children living with one parent increased from 11% to 19%, and the number of single-parent homes increased from 3.3 to 6.6 million.
3. Approximately 1 million children experience a marital breakup annually. Most children are 7 years of age or younger at the time of divorce.

Therefore the current emphasis in child psychiatry is on interventions for these many risk factors in the child's environment.

THEORETICAL APPROACHES
Psychoanalytic

The basic tenets of Anna Freud's[20] theory of developmental lines follow Sigmund Freud's psychoanalytic

Historical Overview

DATE	EVENT
Sixteenth Century and Before	No distinction was made between "little" and "big" people; the same social expectations were held for all beyond the age of infancy.[3]
Industrial Revolution	Childhood was recognized as a discrete stage of life as industry became the framework for organizing society. "The century of the child" began in France and took hold in America with the passage of child labor and compulsory education laws.
1850s	Compulsory school attendance brought large numbers of emotionally disturbed children in need of mental health services under the jurisdiction of public school officials. The child guidance movement began.
1900s	Clifford Beers founded the mental hygiene movement, predicting that direct methods of child treatment would provide for prophylactic interventions at the time of the onset of emotional problems.
1920s	Child's play was recognized as an accepted vehicle of research and treatment, fostered by the work of Darwin and other ethnologists. John Dewey introduced learning through play and discovery in the schools.
1930	White House Conference on Children proclaimed that "play was the work of children," giving educators and psychologists official support to use play to foster child development, learning, and socialization.
1933	American Psychiatric Association recognized child psychiatry as a unique subspecialty.
1954	The first graduate education program in child psychiatric nursing was started at Boston University.
1968	A resolution by the Child Psychiatric Nursing Educators Conference was passed supporting care of children in the community and outside custodial institutions.[46]
1971	President's Commission on the Mental Health of Children cited that the status of children's mental health had reached crisis proportions.
1976	American Nurses' Association developed a certification test for clinical specialists in child and adolescent psychiatric mental health nursing.
1979	The Year of the Child, sponsored by the United Nations, emphasized the increase in the number of children afflicted with emotional problems and the need for mental health–psychiatric services.
1984	American Nurses' Association published the standards on child and adolescent psychiatric and mental health nursing practice.[1]
1986	Nine graduate programs in child psychiatric nursing are available.
Future	The projected population increase in the number of children, combined with the disruptions in family life, indicate an ever-increasing need for child psychiatric services.

theory, stressing that ego defenses available to the child depend upon the child's maturational level. Her theory was unique, however, in conceptualizing the role of defense mechanisms in assisting the child's developing personality to adapt and to defend against stress and anxiety in the child's environment.

Klein[32] was one of the first theorists to describe attachment disorders in young children. She called the painful anxiety small children experience when they are first sep-

arated from their reassuring mothers a "depressive position," which she described as a normal developmental stage during which the child learned to modify ambivalence and sustain periodic loss of the "good mother." Klein expanded and refined descriptions of *anaclitic depressions* set forth by Rene Spitz[52] during the early 1940s. Spitz observed failure to thrive and *marasmus* among infants and young children prematurely separated from parents and in orphanages during World War II.

These theorists also described symbiotic reactions as the opposite behavioral manifestations of anaclitic depression. Symbiotic reactions occurred when children and their parents failed to negotiate the separation-individuation process. Since school attendance is the first enforced separation of mother and child, symbiotic reactions are usually first manifested in school phobias.

According to theories of separation anxiety and anaclitic depression, the child's behaviors were normal negotiations of the separation-individuation process, however, it was generally believed that the emotions of depression and grief are not possible during young children's developmental stages. Mourning includes the grieving process, which requires mature intellectual and emotional structures and the passage of time for emotional pain to be gradually experienced and resolved. Whereas the adult's developed personality structure and defenses provide for sustaining emotional pain and enable loss to be gradually experienced and resolved, children have a developmental unreadiness for grieving. Until adolescence, children are not able to employ the processes of introjection and identification with a lost love object.[16] Also, children function emotionally on an all-or-none principle; they cannot tolerate emotional pain, and they lack the ego defenses that regulate the gradual discharge of such pain.

In contrast to the five stages in the adult grief process identified by Kübler-Ross, Bowlby[5] posited a three-stage "loss" process for children: protest, despair, and detachment. Bowlby's theory held that when children lose a loved one, their initial feelings are ambivalent. This ambivalence is especially strong if the one lost is a parent or significant other who had disciplined or set limits on the child's behavior, thus angering the child by delaying immediate need gratification. The stronger the child's ambivalence, the less difficult the loss experience. Negative ambivalent feelings help the child to deny or delay grief through idealization and reaction formation. These defenses provide a mechanism for the child to resolve guilt aroused by negative (wish fulfillment) feelings. It was believed that if children felt sadness and unhappiness, these feelings were brief and manifested in transient grief behaviors of restlessness and hyperactivity. These behaviors were viewed as signs that the mechanism of reaction formation was being established in the child's intellectual structure.

Erikson's theory of child development[15] included stages that paralleled Anna Freud's theory and included play constructions, which he viewed as stages of ritualization of life. His theory emphasized that culture was the interplay of customs, and he stressed that children's play provides for resolution of the conflict or working through developmental crises.

In his classic work *Toys and Reasons*[15] Erikson described in detail the intrinsic reasons children use specific toys and games at various ages. For example, children ages 1 to 3 years are in the anal-muscular stage in which developmental tasks focus on resolving conflict that centers around the basic sense of autonomy versus shame and doubt. These children prefer parallel play. Children 3 to 6 years old are in the genital-locomotion stage, and the developmental tasks center on the basic sense of initiative versus guilt. They enjoy cooperative play, fantasy, and elaborate dramatic scenes and dramas through which they symbolically resolve many conflicts by imitating adults. Children ages 6 to 12 years are in the genital-locomotion stage in which the developmental task is one of resolving the conflict of a basic sense of industry versus inferiority. These children prefer games governed by complex rules and regulations, such as chess and checkers.

Cognitive

Piaget's[45] theories of the child's growth of intellect revolutionized traditional views of child development and established that children think differently from adults and that often children spontaneously learn on their own, without input from adults. He defined development as a process governed by the child's activities, resulting in increasingly complex cognitive structures. Stages are not caused by genetic predisposition but by the child's intrinsic growth. Piaget's definition of intelligence included a range of intellectual activities: reasoning, remembering, and perceptions. His cognitive theory focused on universals; his research verified that the first three stages of his cognitive theory applied to children of all cultures and changed at the stage of adolescence. It is only then, when the intellectual processes of formal operations mature, that thinking is less individualized and influenced more by environmental factors. In his research on how children understand their dreams, Piaget developed a six-stage developmental sequence showing that children progress from believing dreams are real-life occurrences to believing dreams exist outside themselves and are visible to others.

Piaget did not view the external environment as influencing intellectual development but as providing stimulating, interesting, conflicting information that in turn stimulates children's thinking and growth. Piaget posited that stimulation came from the child's peers during play and conversations. His theories of the child's growth of social thinking paralleled his theory of cognitive development. His study of moral reasoning verified that young children have a developmental inability to distinguish their perceptions from others'. Children cannot intellectually understand that rules can be changed until they reach adolescence.

Piaget's theory of moral development paralleled his theory of intellectual development and held that morality develops in age-specific, invariant sequences comparable to and dependent on the developing cognitive structure. He stated that the child is an active participant in the development of this cognitive structure and that the child's unique interpretations of experiences are part of the development of ethical precepts. Piaget believed that children learn morality and ethical behaviors from their interactions with peers, not from adults or established cultural norms. He attributed moral development to schemata within the child's cognitive structure that grow as the child interacts with others and from role-taking skills that result from participation in social activities.

Following many of Piaget's concepts, Chomsky[8] developed a theory of language development that was a major scientific contribution to understanding the developing child. His theory held that the child establishes internal rules (transformations) of grammar that help convey intended meanings. The child uses and interprets sentences he has not heard or used before through transformations (that is, reordering words into sentences to convey meaning). The child first develops use of noun phrases such as "I want" and then develops structure-dependent grammar spontaneously, as the result of an innate maturational process. Language growth is characterized by a fixed gross motor developmental schedule that follows universal sequences comparable to the cognitive developmental theory of Piaget.

Children learn an extensive language system on their own. They pick up language at home, at school, and from television. They then sort the "overload" of words into grammatical rules and structures to merge as language. There is a biological-maturational predisposition for the development of language and linguistic accomplishments are possible because of an innate *language acquisition device (LAD)*. The LAD helps the child establish rules and regularities in use of words. Whereas LAD is rudimentary at birth, it matures with the child's central nervous system, and the child's own activity and play foster the use of words.

Chomsky theorized that the innate LAD is sufficiently broad to accommodate the diverse languages of the world. Whereas they learn different languages, children from all cultures learn language in a standard sequence. Mastery proceeds from one word to two and progresses to working on syntactic rules of inflections, phrases, structures, and negatives in the same manner. Cognitive and linguistic structures have parallel development, exemplifying developmental progression along multiple lines. The development of speech, thoughts (ideation, cognition), and locomotion (walking) fosters the evolving of a self-concept separate from that of the mother. Balance among these developmental lines is essential for mental health, and a lag in any of these interdependent systems can result in serious mental health problems.

As children gain mastery in moving about independently, they begin to learn to control their emotions; perceptions, memory, and mobility combine to help distinguish self from the object world. First, children verbalize perceptions by naming or "labeling," and gradually verbalize feelings or emotions. The naming of objects and feelings reinforces the sense of control of feelings rooted in the child's emerging self-concept. It helps the child distinguish what is real, providing a vehicle for testing reality by verbally validating names of objects and feelings with others. The development of language facilitates the process of reality testing, is basic to self-identity and differentiation, and spans all dimensions of the developing child.

Mastery of language is a major developmental task of childhood and is a competency that emerges gradually. Most young children express their needs primitively through the use of primary process, nonverbal metacommunication, play, symbolic expressive activities, and games.

Theoretical approaches are summarized in Table 40-1.

RELATING TO THE CLIENT

Establishing a therapeutic relationship with children and their parents requires a helping attitude similar to a positive parent-child relationship. Children do not seek treatment on their own; they cannot define the problem, and often they are unaware that their parents or others perceive their behaviors as problematic.

Confidentiality is critical to the development of trust, because minor children are unable to give informed consent or grasp the implications of confidentiality. The parents' legal responsibility for social control of the child contributes to the parents' concerns about nursing interventions during the child-nurse relationship. It is essential for children to understand that their parents will be informed about their treatment progress and that potential changes in their behavior will be reviewed with the parents.

Very young children rely on nonverbal behaviors to evaluate the intent of others. The child, with fewer verbal

TABLE 40-1 Summary of theoretical approaches

Theory	Theorist	Dynamics
Psychoanalytic	Anna Freud	The defense mechanisms used by the child depend on the child's maturational level.
	Spitz and Klein	Separation anxiety and anaclitic depression result from the normal negotiation of the separation-individuation process.
	Bowlby	Children generally experience ambivalent feelings on initial loss of a loved one.
	Erikson	There are intrinsic reasons why children use specific toys and games at various ages; children's play provides for the resolution of conflict and developmental crises.
Cognitive	Piaget	The process of development is governed by the child's activities and results in increasingly complex cognitive structures.
	Chomsky	There is a biological-maturational predisposition for the development of language that occurs because of an innate language acquisition device.

and social skills than the adult has, moves slowly into relationships, and the necessity of third-person transitions needs to be acknowledged when initially relating to a child client. Just as children use transitional objects such as comfort blankets or toys to ease transitions, parents and significant others on whom the child relies serve as interpersonal transitional buffers or facilitators in the development of trust.

Often very small children who are depressed are "acting out" parental depression and come from disorganized homes. Therapeutic relationships may be difficult to establish and require time because the child's low self-esteem makes trusting difficult. Sometimes, after trust is established, the child may become overdependent on the nurse, especially if the parental anger continues. There is also the danger of the child finding safety with the nurse and continuing to be depressed so the relationship will continue.

Children in therapeutic relationships relate to the nurse in the same way as they relate to their parents. They bring the same expectations and reactions to the therapy session that they have come to expect and respond to with their parents. These response patterns are more fragile in children than in adults. The therapeutic alliance should expand and enhance the child's repertoire of expectations and responses.

The young child's values and conscience are in the process of development, and children are often in an intense stage of parental identification. Thus no matter how dysfunctional the parent-child relationship may be, children consciously and unconsciously identify with parental values and evaluations. Children seldom like, trust, or relate well to adults or to professionals that their parents distrust.

Parents provide important assessment data about the young child that the child cannot provide, such as the child's developmental history and family constellation. In all instances the goal of working with the child's parents is to engage them as collaborators, which requires parents to: report aspects of the child's behavior that occurs outside of treatment, not ask questions about the therapeutic relationship, support and bring the child for therapy when they do not wish to come, and develop tolerance of the child's behavioral changes.[27]

The child's level of cognitive development is a major consideration in the nurse-client relationship. The child's understanding of causality in terms of time, space, and numbers is dependent on developmental stages and affects understanding and interpretation of sequences of events. Developmental theories stress that the child's thinking is predominantly magical and that only through maturation do children develop adultlike reality testing and increasingly organized adaptive thoughts. The child's degree of egocentricity also limits his ability to understand and consider the other person's point of view.[23] The child's language development and nonverbal communication patterns provide rationale for the selection and ordering of language-appropriate data gathering and nurturing interventions (for instance, structure or unstructured play, symbolic play activities, games, group work with other children, or interviews with the individual child alone or with parents).

The working phase of the therapeutic relationship relies on nonverbal activities to compensate for the child's limited verbal abilities. No matter when the problem, interventions assist the child in maintaining developmental progression and enhance the young child's developing language skills.[2]

In addition to nonverbal communication, nurturing care within the nursing process is an important aspect of relating to the child. Children are physically small, and adults often touch, hug, or pick them up without considering the child's body personal space. Children relate touching to parenting and attachment bonding. Thus touching needs to be judicious, since transmission of feelings influences transference. Transference is less apparent in children than in adults, since parents and significant others, who are directly responsible for the child's wishes, fantasies, and feelings, are still present and are not past recollections. Nuances of transference occur when children express feelings toward the nurse that they feel for their parents. For example, children fearful of their parents may be fearful of the nurse. The nurse may unwittingly take over more of the parental role than appropriate, and the child's dependency needs and tendency to overidentify may stimulate countertransference, with the nurse's negative parental attitudes becoming competitive.

Unlike adults, the child has age-appropriate dependency needs. While the child's dependency needs on the nurse mature and change the nurse-child relationship, the child's appropriate dependence on the parent or significant adult is concurrently enhanced. This relationship facilitates termination of the nurse-child relationship, which than enhances the reestablishment of positive parent-child relationships. Children who overidentify with the nurse may become depressed after termination of the relationship, a major pitfall in child treatment.

NURSING PROCESS
Assessment

✦ *Physical dimension.* The child's age is important because of the developmental changes that occur with time. However, development is the outcome of intrinsic and extrinsic factors, and the child's capacity for continued progress from one age/stage to the next is often as important as the child "fitting" within the age/stage framework. A child's physical developmental patterns may differ from the norms of other children in that age range but be consistent with familial traits. For example, very short or very tall children may vary from the average yet be "normal" for their family genetic traits. Unusual developmental patterns may be due to genetically related disorders such as Down's syndrome.

There is an important relationship between neurological and both emotional and intellectual development. Therefore the neurological examination is an important part of the assessment of the emotionally disturbed child. This neurological play assessment[24] is a useful method to gather neurological data because it includes play activities that the child knows. These play adaptations of the neurological examination are less threatening and thus especially useful with children who are overly active, distractible, impulsive, and excitable. The following play assessment activities are suggested:

1. *Cerebral functions.* Games such as Hide-and-seek, Simon Says, Blindman's Buff, and naming games can be adapted to assess specific areas of cerebral functioning. Hide-and-seek can be used to assess the child's *stereogenesis* by having the child identify objects with eyes closed. Simon Says is a useful game for assessing the child's temporal sequence because it requires following a series of commands.
2. *Reflexes.* Games such as Let's Take Turns and You Play Nurse help eliminate the child's fear of reflex hammers and other instruments used in a physical examination.
3. *Cerebellar functions.* Games such as Follow the Leader and Pin the Tail on the Donkey can be adapted to evaluate the child's coordination and balance. The child's ability to hop or stand on one foot, rapidly touch various body parts, and balance with his eyes closed contributes to this evaluation.
4. *Sensory functions.* Body tapping and tickling games before the assessment of the child's responses to touch, pain, vibration, and temperature may alleviate this sensitive aspect of assessment that involves body contact. It is suggested that this part of the neurological examination be left to the final assessment because children often become uncooperative, which may affect the other data to be gathered.
5. *Cranial nerves.* Following lights, whispering games, and playing dentist assist in assessing the child's visual acuity, visual fields, movement of eyeballs, jaws, sensations of taste, corneal reflexes, hearing, movement of the mouth, throat, and tongue, facial expressions, and sensations in the forehead, jaw, and cheeks.

The normal, expected findings in the neurological-perceptual examination of a 5- to 6-year-old child are listed below:

1. *Alternating movements.* The child can turn hands over rapidly or tap thumb and index finger.
2. *Associated movements.* When wooden sticks are placed between the fingers of each hand, the child will not drop more than five extra sticks in six trials.
3. *Eye-hand coordination.* When the peripheral visual field is stimulated by a moving finger, the child can point to the moving finger without looking from side to side.
4. *Eye movements.* The child can visually pursue an object without head movement.
5. *Choreoid movements.* When arms are extended and eyes closed, no choreiform movements are noted.
6. *Copying ability.* The child can copy a circle, cross, square, and triangle.
7. *Perceptual reversals.* When asked to copy the letters *B, P, D, Q,* or other letters, the child reproduces the letters without reversals, inversions, rotations, or mirror images.

Freud believed that dreams require the use of repression and that children under 5 years cannot dream. Research on rapid eye movement (REM) sleep however, has led to a reevaluation of Freud's idea; it appears that infants and small children have some form of dream activity that is somewhat different than the REM (dream) activity experienced by children who can use symbols for recall.

Children's dreams are a product of the interactions of development, and thus their content contains the most pressing tasks that the child is experiencing at different developmental stages.

The child's body image is also assessed as part of the physical dimension. The body schema begins at birth and unfolds through the maturing child's gradual differentiation of self. The progressive inclusion of body imagery in the child's mind can be measured by children's drawings. A specific measurement, the Goodenough-Harris Draw-A-

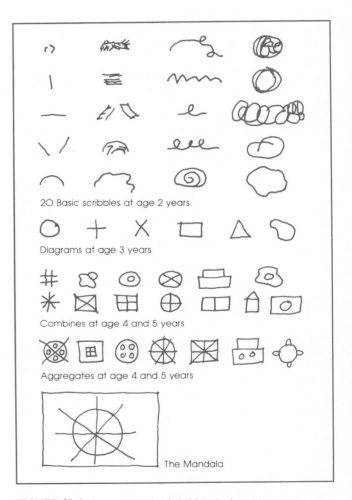

20 Basic scribbles at age 2 years

Diagrams at age 3 years

Combines at age 4 and 5 years

Aggregates at age 4 and 5 years

The Mandala

FIGURE 40-1 Components of children's drawing. (From Kellogg, R.: Stages of development of preschool art. In Lewis, H.P., editor: Child art: the beginning of self-affirmation, Berkeley, Calif., 1966, Diablo Press.)

Person (DAP) test, is based on the premise that a child's drawings are related to his developmental age. Norms for children's drawings have been established, and the child's neurological integrity, psychomotor skills, and graphomotor and fine motor development can be assessed through the DAP test. Figure 40-1 illustrates the progressive complexity of children's drawings. The *mandala* in children's art is of interest because it is a universal religious symbol spontaneously drawn by most children.

The child's drawings of human figures is an index of the child's body image and progresses in a predictable manner. Drawings of the 3- to 4-year-old child usually depict large heads and eyes, with arms and legs as appendages of the head. Gradually the trunk appears, with arms and legs as stick appendages. The child's overemphasis or omissions of body parts gives clues to the child's body image. Although the child's drawings are a rich source of assessment data, they are examined within the context of other assessment data for verification. For example, excessively large hands may indicate aggression, small arms and hands withdrawal and denial. Children's drawings are often used as evaluation data. For example, the child's drawings completed during assessment can be compared with drawings after the child has been in therapy to evaluate body image changes during the therapeutic process. Clearly defined body boundaries, a balance of body parts and appendages, and centering the person on the drawing paper are signs of a positive body image.

Generally, having children draw pictures of themselves and of their family provides important assessment data. When a child is asked to "draw a person" he tends to concentrate on objects and details.[14] When asked to draw a picture of himself and his family, the child projects specific fears, anxieties, and concerns, and the drawings tell more about how the child feels. In addition to viewing drawings within the child's developmental context, it is important to ask the child about the drawings because artwork can easily be misinterpreted. Winnicott[54] suggests that the therapist draw a "squiggly" mark on a piece of paper and encourage the child to add marks to it. Once the child starts to draw, the therapist can ask the child about the marks, and the relationship can begin.

Often children draw what they cannot say. "Drawing out" the child encourages the surfacing of problem areas that otherwise may not be disclosed. Because of cultural and family taboos, children are usually unable to discuss sexual issues and anxieties. Children's drawings rarely include genitals; these omissions are normal and reflect the child's internalization of taboo topics.[14] When the child draws genitals or stylized sexual figures, the nurse needs to be alert that the child's drawing may be in response to rape trauma or sexual abuse.

✳ ***Emotional dimension.*** Children's fears become more realistic, varied, and global as the child matures.[42] Normal fears of children between the ages of 2 and 7 years include fear of falling and fear of animals, such as dogs, snakes, or tigers. Children ages 7 to 11 years fear bodily injury, punishment, illness, death of a parent, and failure in social situations, such as at school. Between the ages of 11 and 12 years children express more global fears, such as natural hazards, accidents, and nuclear explosions. Many children have bedtime fears, which are often related to fears of dreaming and being alone in the dark. Since small children are unable to distinguish between dreams and reality, *night terrors* often occur in children under 5 years of age.

Theories of childhood anxiety hold that conflict is a normal and necessary component of growth, and most children negotiate developmental stage changes with a minimum of fear, anxiety, and crisis. Sources of anxiety in the preschool child are loss of parental love, anticipation of physical injury, loss of control, and expressions of dependency, aggression, and anger as the child develops independence. In the school-aged child major sources of anxiety are related to concerns about failing to master socially valued skills, such as inability to succeed in the classroom, and failure to demonstrate accepted sex role behaviors.

Overanxious behaviors concerning separation generally occurs in children between the ages of 3 and 6 years. These behaviors cannot be traced to a specific source and may result in phobic behavior in which the child overgeneralizes anxiety or fear of a specific object to all objects or situations similar to those in the initial fear-inducing encounter. For example, a child frightened by a dog may become afraid of all dogs. Childhood phobias are common and similar to phobias observed in adults (see Chapter 12).

Hospitalization for physical problems is a major source of anxiety during childhood with the potential residual effect of profound, debilitating anxiety reactions and phobias. The major fears during early childhood, cited earlier, are exaggerated when the child is physically in pain. In addition to observations, nurses can use various projective picture tests that depict specific hospital situations and use mutual story-telling techniques to assess the child's anxiety. These story-telling games include the nurse reading picture books and other illustrated child reading materials and the child "imagining" a story in response to these stimuli. Barton's[4] Hospital Picture Test, widely used in pediatric settings, assists the nurse in identifying misperceptions as well as anxiety and depression in young hospitalized clients.

Depression is often masked by acting-out behaviors, poor school performance, inability to study, isolation, somatic complaints, and accident proneness. The potential of suicide and suicide attempts by children are generally underestimated. Parents tend to deny their child's sad or depressed feelings. Depressed children often have low self-esteem and feelings of helplessness with resulting angry feelings toward parents or authority figures. The child may feel rejected and act out angry feelings toward the parents, who in turn become angry with the child, setting up a destructive cycle that may include child abuse. The cycle intensifies as parents become more determined to "straighten the child out" when their authority is challenged.

Temper tantrums are violent, unpredictable outbursts of anger during which the child is out of control and screams, kicks, and strikes out at others. Children often throw things and may lose bladder and bowel control. These violent outbursts have been related to power struggles between children and parents or significant others, such as teachers or caretakers.

Children with antisocial behaviors often lack the necessary ego strength to control overt expressions of anger and aggressive impulses. Impulsivity and hyperactivity can also be related to minimal brain damage when impulses are acted out. Deficits or limitations in language create situations for the child in which words fail and action seems the only resource. As the child develops language skills there is a decline in the hitting, shoving, and pushing of other children.

Expressions of anger and aggression in children also differ from those of adults. Through socialization children are expected to master impulse control and learn to delay gratification. Parental discipline provides external controls that the child gradually internalizes. As discussed earlier, small children are egocentric and tend to blame themselves for unpleasant happenings; thus they often have strong, unrealistic feelings of guilt and shame when they express their anger.

✳ *Intellectual dimension.* At the age of 18 months the child uses and understands a limited number of single-word utterances which are rooted in action, such as "run," "walk," and "give," and the child's first verbal activity is an extension of the sensorimotor structure.[45] By the age of 2 years the child begins to put two words together to express relationships. The two-word association phase is a universal characteristic of all human language development.

Between the ages of 2 and 3 years children begin using words in subject-verb-object order. In addition to adding the suffix -*ing* to words, children learn to use "no." Between 3 and 6 years of age children begin to use "where, what, and why" questions and tags, which are little questions at the end of a sentence, such as "isn't it—can't we—doesn't it." Tags result from complex transformation operations originating in the child's tendency to solidify new capacities by overuse.

Between 5 and 7 years children master verbal intricacies as operational thought evolves. As logical links are grasped in the manipulation of the external world, the thought processes include more than "surface" phenomena. Despite a growing command of grammar, words acquire meaning only in concrete life situations. Separation of speech from action does not occur in children until the ages of 11 to 13 years, when the human brain reaches physical maturation. At that time the neuroanatomical and neurophysiological framework necessary for hypothetical and deductive thinking replaces pragmatic "here and now" thinking. When the stage of formal thinking is achieved, children express thoughts independently of immediate experience and initiate language about past, present, and future events. Language becomes abstract and implements thought.

There are important distinctions to be made between normal dreaming and fantasy and the serious psychiatric disorders related to lack of contact with reality and reality orientation. Daydreams and fantasy are similar to the concepts of delusions, hallucinations, and loss of contact with reality, and the similarity of these behaviors concerns parents. Many parents become distressed about their child's daydreaming and fantasizing and consider them unacceptable, nonproductive activities. However, there is a great misunderstanding about the place of fantasy in the small child's life. The nurse needs to clarify the place of fantasy for overanxious parents. Most children use fantasy, play, dreams, and daydreams to strengthen their contacts with the real world and reduce stress. In contrast, emotionally disturbed children, like children with physical illnesses, do not use play to reduce their stress and anxieties. Usually the child's lack of play is the first sign parents perceive and report to clarify that "something" is wrong with the child. Conversely, parents usually report the child is improving when he resumes usual play behaviors.

✿ *Social dimension.* Collecting data from parents provides opportunities to assess the parent-child relationship and the parents' strengths and limitations. The parents' child-rearing behaviors are carefully evaluated as they affect the child's trust and dependence-independence needs. Information about the child's peer relationships, caretakers, and school activities is also assessed.

Assessment of the child's parents begins with the initial interview, a structured process during which roles, confidentiality, and rationale for family and individual interviews are clarified. The reasons for the visit (for instance, clarification of the problem, duration of symptoms, the parents' perceptions of the problem, their concerns and efforts to solve the problem) are initial topics. If the child is referred by a teacher or physician, the reason for the referral needs clarification. It is important to identify how the parents and others, such as teachers, may want the child to change and what role parents see for themselves in the change process.

Information about the child's family constellation is best gathered by developing a genogram. Genograms facilitate the establishment of the therapeutic relationship, may take several sessions to complete, and provide the parents with a concrete exercise that alleviates initial anxiety. By viewing themselves and their child within a broad intergenerational context, parents often feel less guilty and will more readily discuss their relationships.

During the data collection the nurse observes and records both content and process. Process includes behaviors such as seating arrangements, verbal and nonverbal patterns of communication, and who speaks and when. Verbal themes, such as assuming responsibility for others' behavior, are noted and clarified during the interview.

Family and social considerations in assessing the child have become increasingly important in recent years because the major mental health problems now confronting children are psychosocial. The effects of social change on the child and assessment of the changes discussed in this section represent a small segment of the many aspects of social changes affecting the child that the nurse assesses and integrates into the data analysis and treatment plan.

TABLE 40-2 Life event scale for preschool age group*

Life Event	Life Change Units
Beginning nursery school	42
Increase in number of arguments with parents	39
Change in parents' financial status	21
Birth of brother or sister	50
Decrease in number of arguments between parents	21
Change of father's occupation requiring increased absence from home	39
Death of grandparent	30
Outstanding personal achievement	23
Serious illness requiring hospitalization of parent	51
Brother or sister leaving home	39
Serious illness requiring hospitalization of brother or sister	37
Mother beginning to work outside home	47
Change to new nursery school	33
Change in child's acceptance by peers	38
Decrease in number of arguments with parents	22
Increase in number of arguments between parents	44
Serious illness requiring hospitalization of child	59
Loss of job by parent	23
Death of close friend	38
Having visible congenital deformity	39
Addition of third adult to family	39
Marital separation of parents	74
Discovery of being adopted child	33
Jail sentence of parent for 30 days or less	34
Death of parent	89
Divorce of parents	78
Acquiring visible deformity	52
Death of brother or sister	59
Marriage of parent to stepparent	62
Jail sentence of parent for 1 year or more	67

From Coddington, R.D. The significance of life events as etiological factors in the diseases of children: a study of normal populations, Journal of Psychosomatic Research **16**:205, Pergamon Press, 1972.

TABLE 40-3 Life event scale for ages 6 through 11 years*

Life Event	Life Change Units
Death of parent	109
Death of brother or sister	86
Divorce of parents	73
Marital separation of parents	66
Death of grandparent	56
Hospitalization of parent	52
Marriage of parent to stepparent	53
Birth of brother or sister	50
Hospitalization of brother or sister	47
Loss of job by parent	37
Major increase in parents' income	28
Major decrease in parents' income	29
Start of new problem between parents	44
End of problem between parents	27
Change of father's occupation requiring increased absence from home	39
New adult moving into home	41
Mother beginning to work outside home	40
Being told you are very attractive by friend	23
Beginning first grade	20
Move to new school district	35
Failing a grade in school	45
Suspension from school	30
Start of new problem between you and your parents	43
End of a problem between you and parents	34
Recognition for excelling in sport or other activity	21
Appearance in juvenile court	33
Failing to achieve something you really wanted	28
Becoming adult member of church	21
Being invited to join social organization	15
Death of pet	40
Being hospitalized for illness or injury	53
Death of close friend	52
Becoming involved with drugs	38
Stopping use of drugs	23
Finding an adult who really respects you	20
Outstanding personal achievement (special prize)	34

Courtesy R.D. Coddington, 1982.
*The purpose of this form is to record events that occurred in the child's life during a 3-month period.

The life event scales developed by Coddington[10] provide systematic assessment tools for evaluating the amount of stress the child is experiencing as a result of social factors. The life event scales presented in Tables 40-2 and 40-3 provide ranges of expectations for normal children. If the child is not progressing normally for his age the reaction is referred to as a *developmental crisis*.

The kinds of social changes children experience and the amount of stress that these changes cause in children are assigned life change units (LCUs). The standardized data on healthy children indicate that life stress increases with age; children in elementary school average 102.8 LCUs, and children in junior high school average 195.6 LCUs.[10] Also, as the assigned life change numerical values show, stress levels differ for children at different ages. For the preschooler the death of a parent has been assigned a weight of 89 LCUs, whereas the death of a parent of children ages 6 to 11 years has a higher life change value (109 LCUs).

The revised scale (Table 40-3) for children ages 6 to 11 years reflects changes in society since the life event scales were first developed. For example, on the 1972 life event scales a child becoming involved with drugs was assigned a weight of 38 LCUs; in 1983 stopping use of drugs was a new item and was assigned 23 LCUs. When the scale was developed most children ages 6 to 23 years did not have experiences of initiating and withdrawing from drug use. It is important that the nurse use the most recently available, updated editions of the life event scales because societal changes are reflected in the items. For example, the recession during the early 1980s and consequent parental unemployment affected children's stress and life change units.

Recently efforts have been made to examine stressful events from the child's perspective rather than from the adult's. The Research Highlight below discusses one of these efforts.

Because more of the child's time is spent in daycare centers and schools, assessments by the teacher or care provider are extremely important for a comprehensive data base of the child's social behaviors. Many problems during childhood, such as drug abuse, result in the child exhibiting some signs and symptoms at home and other symptoms in school or other social contexts.

Research Highlight

Feeling Bad: Exploring Sources of Distress Among Preadolescent Children

C.E. Lewis, J.M. Siegel & M.A. Lewis

PURPOSE

The purpose of this study was to begin to operationally define stress from the child's perspective.

SAMPLE

Two thousand four hundred fifth-graders were participants in this study. They were from communities selected for their diversity in terms of geographic location, size of community, and socioeconomic background of families. Boys and girls were equally represented in the sample.

METHODOLOGY

In preliminary interviews fifth- and sixth-graders were asked "What makes you feel bad, nervous, or worry?" From these interviews a 20-item list was developed of sources of distress. The 2,400 fifth-graders were presented with two lists of the same 20 items. On the first page the instructions read, "The following is a list of things that some kids say make them feel bad or nervous or make them worry. For each put an X showing how you would feel if this happened to you or, if this happened to you, how you felt." The children placed an X in one of five categories labeled: not bad, a little bad, pretty bad, real bad, and terrible. For the second list the instructions read, "Now please indicate if any of these things has happened to you in the past year and, if so, how often." The children placed an X in one of five categories labeled: never, one or two times, sometimes, often, and all the time. Subjects also self-rated their mental health status.

FINDINGS

There were significant associations between children's ratings of mental health and "feel bad" scores. Girls rated most items significantly higher (more bad) than boys. Factor analysis revealed that the items could be grouped into the following three dimensions: (1) anxieties surrounding conflict with parents, (2) self-image and peer group relationships, and (3) geographic mobility. The top two occurrences for the "badness" rating were having parents separate and being pressured to try something new. Children who had never been pressured to try something new or whose parents had never separated rated these occurrences as worse than did children who had experienced the event.

IMPLICATIONS

Based on the items identified it is possible that there are strains in childhood that may not be appreciated as such by adults—for example, having nothing to do and not spending enough time with parents. It is important that the child's perspective on the life events that influence his mental health be incorporated into nursing care of the child.

Based on data from American Journal of Public Health 74(2):117, 1984

Spiritual dimension. Moral development is one of the major tasks of the school-age child and includes development of the child's percepts of right and wrong, responsibilities in relation to others, and ability to understand the feelings of others. These data can be gained by assessing how the child relates to peers and adults.

Role taking, in Kohlberg's theory,[34] refers to understanding what situations mean to another person. Interpersonal perception includes the development of concepts of norms, social responsibility, and justice. As discussed earlier, there is a close relationship between intellectual and moral development. Children's verbalizations and actions, as well as teacher's and parents' reports of the child's social roles, provide guides to the child's level of moral development. Children who are socially popular and "leaders" generally have well-developed moral reasoning. Observation of the child playing with peers also provides data on the child's interpersonal awareness.

There are other opportunities for assessing the child's level of moral development in the nurse-child encounters. For example, as the assessment session begins the nurse carefully states the "rules" for behavior and confidentiality during the child-nurse relationship. School-age children will usually request rules if they are not volunteered, indicating their reliance on rules and structured situations.

The holistic assessment tool below contains assessment information specific to the child. It is to be used in conjunction with the assessment tool in Chapter 8.

See Table 40-4 for assessment norms for children.

Text continued on p. 774.

HOLISTIC ASSESSMENT TOOL: THE CHILD

PHYSICAL DIMENSION

Diet and Elimination
Are the child's food preferences, eating patterns, and elimination patterns appropriate for his age group?

Exercise and Activity
Are the child's play activities appropriate for his age group?

Sleep and Rest
Are the child's patterns of sleep and rest appropriate for his age group?

Body Image
What is the child's body image?

Sexuality
Is the child's curiosity in exploring his own sexuality appropriate?

EMOTIONAL DIMENSION

How appropriate is the child's mood to his experiences?

What is the child's ability to tolerate frustration, anger, sadness, and pleasure?

Has the child achieved the developmental tasks of his age group?

INTELLECTUAL DIMENSION

How appropriate is the child's attention span to his age group?

How appropriate is the child's memory capacity to his age group?

What, if any, difficulties does the child have in learning and in school performance?

Are the child's language skills and vocabulary appropriate to his developmental stage and chronological age?

What concerns does the child have?

What is the child's perception of his problems?

SOCIAL DIMENSION

What is the child's self-concept?

How age appropriate are the child's social interaction patterns?

How age appropriate is the child's attachment to and dependence on his parents?

How satisfied is the child with his friendships?

SPIRITUAL DIMENSION

What are the child's concepts of right and wrong, good and bad?

What importance does religion, God, or a supreme being play in the child's life?

TABLE 40-4 Assessment norms for children ages 2 to 11 years

	Dimension				
Physical	Emotional	Intellectual	Social	Spiritual	Characteristic Play

AGE 2 YEARS

Physical	Emotional	Intellectual	Social	Spiritual	Characteristic Play
Runs, balances, throws and kicks balls	Graduation from infancy with beginning of "me" and "I" concepts	With mastery of sensorimotor period, child has an efficient, well-organized mechanism for dealing with immediate environment	Presocial; masters object permanency, that is, that objects are separate from self, leads to sense of self as separate object, beginning of self-concept	Preconventional morality; knows "good" and "bad"	Sensorimotor play predominates
Opens doors, turns the pages of a book	Anal stage	Uses symbols, including images and words, requiring child to reorganize thinking; throughout preoperational period (2-7 years) child's thinking is unsystematic and illogical[45]	Enjoys looking and being looked at	Has unquestioning obedience to authority; rules are absolute, coming from higher authority	Enjoys solitary play or play with other children nearby (parallel play)
Can build a six-tower structure with play cubes	Tasks of autonomy vs. shame and guilt, yet still needs confirmation of trust, with mother within reach or within sight	Uses animism, attributes life to physical objects; egocentricism, thinks things function as he does; views things from one perspective; oriented toward present	Egocentric, views things only from own perspective	Begins to have self-judgment	Maternal, imitative play with dolls, relating to household things such as cleaning and cooking
Clumsy, falls often, ceaseless activity, curious	Volatile has suggestible feelings, imitates others, reflects their actions, attitudes, moods	Makes choices, uses projection and undoing as adaptive mechanisms	Requires constant supervision by adult	Pain and pleasure help child conform to rules	Repetition pervades with little risk, no plot, some fantasies
Explores body	Impulsive, functions on punishment-reward basis		Indicates wants other than by crying; talkative, chatters to self, enjoys songs, uses three-word sentences ("me do it" typical), uses "no"		
Establishes hand preference			Requires routines, upset by unpredictability; needs constant, firm, gentle discipline		
Scribbles, makes zig-zags and circles, holds crayons in fist guided by index fingers, copies horizontal stroke			Has egocentric perspective, knows others have thoughts and feelings, but cannot differentiate theirs from his; thoughts and feelings are responded to in physical terms or with egocentric wishes		
Muscular maturation for sphincter control; important for autonomy, independence			Tests limits of authority, resents help, may use toilet training as a battleground to assert self and self-control		
Needs 12 hours of sleep plus nap			Attention-seeking, self-assertive		
Dreams are considered real, external events					
Distractable, short attention span					

AGE 3 YEARS

Physical	Psychosocial	Cognitive/Language	Social	Conscience	Play
Nodal age in which previous processes of development culminate	Pre-oedipal stage	Represents thoughts through language, drawings, dreams, play	Interested in events outside immediate home	Uses rules to own advantage: "Don't get caught"; no longer totally dependent on external constraints, blames other people and things ("bad chair")	Recognizes others and otherness—takes turns
Domesticated; bladder and bowel training completed	Tasks of initiative vs. guilt	Continues to be preoperational, bases conclusions on what he feels or would like to believe	Has concept of "what's mine is mine" and is possessive; understands this by identification		Cooperative play is best with one or two others; plays with others in same activities with cross-references
Names pictures in books, knows action depicted in pictures, knows a few nursery rhymes by heart	Begins to use reality principle	Continues to think out loud, talk to himself but uses correct syntax; language deals with concrete situations but asks rhetorical questions	Status in family important		Dramatization and imagination enter into play; combines playthings such as dolls and cars
Holds a crayon with fingers, draws incomplete person, copies circles	Concepts of social and physical reality emerging	Dissociation of spoken word from associated body movements begins	Begins to understand social requirements, cultural norms, and expectations, wants to keep behaviors within family "norms" and acceptable bounds; often asks if behaviors are right; seeks approval; notices differences in home and others		Imitative, dramatic play, symbolic play to unburden guilt
Feeds and dresses himself	Can delay immediate gratification, is "in control," can stand alone, has impulse control	Uses gender words such as "he" and "she"; uses prepositions to denote a beginning of time concept formation			Rich fantasy life with difficulties telling what is real and what is pretend
Can walk a line, hand dominance established	Beginnings of initiative and self-control leading to self-esteem	Vocabulary of about 900 words, knows *up, down, over,* and action commands; uses three- to four-word sentences			Imaginary companions
Has eye-hand coordination; perceptual development includes size, colors; can make curved and straight lines with crayon	Needs things to be orderly and to have routines; will help pick up or clean up	Sound-symbol relationships begin			
Alternates feet when going upstairs, can stand on one foot and balance well	Self-protective stage				
Has body image and directionality					

AGE 4 TO 6 YEARS

Physical	Psychosocial	Cognitive/Language	Social	Conscience	Play
Fine visual motor organization with form and symbol discrimination	Continued phallic Oedipal stage	Continued preoperational level	Goes on errands outside home	Needs help with explanations of his behavior and conduct; time to talk to parents about ideas and value questions	Comparative, socialized, associative play; creative, uses props and infinite variety of roles, plots, family romance themes, settings; drama and risk involved
Ability to maintain balance (age 5)	Rivalry, jealous competition with parent of same sex	Thinking and reasoning begins replacing acting out	Friendships are strong, especially spurred on by rivalry, and competitive feelings evolve	Knows what is his but is willing to share, understands things can be used and returned	Plays in groups of two to five; likes to work on projects that are carried over, on and on
Right and left body orientation		Thinks in pairs, not wholes	Subjective perspective; sees people as interpreting social events—e.g., "a friend is someone you play with"	Begins a value judgment system, traits and ideals of role models now become part of self-ideal, an inner standard of behavior one strives for (superego)	Shares
Can copy cross, triangle, square, tie knots in string		Intuitive thought; thinking more complex and elaborate	Cooperative but interested in winning		Play helps dissolve Oedipal ties; development of followers, leaders; seeks adventure and accomplishment
Draws people with body parts		Egocentricism replaced by social signs			
Walks downstairs, one to step					

Continued.

TABLE 40-4 Assessment norms for children ages 2 to 11 years—cont'd

Dimension				
Physical	Emotional	Intellectual	Social	Spiritual	Characteristic Play
Can tell front from back Unilateral right-handed behavior predominates Draws square, stops at proper length to make a right angle		At age 4, formulates five-to six-word sentences; by age 5, 90% of language and words mastered (2,400 words); words used in thought Uses repression and identification; imitation very strong, especially as to behaviors, feelings, reactions More flexible in language use Begins to tell time by clock (6 to 7 years)	Self-ideal becomes the direction for behavior, providing more self-assurance and independence; "should" system evolves Conformist phase: begins to identify own welfare with that of family; obeys rules because they are family rules, not for fear of punishment; tradition-directed conformity	Concepts of God include notion that He is responsible for everything, yet good and bad continue to be what parents approve and forbid	

AGE 6 TO 8 YEARS

Physical	Emotional	Intellectual	Social	Spiritual	Characteristic Play
Continued neuromuscular growth Body image solidifies Prints name, defines concepts such as brave and nonsense Knows days of week Knows seasons Rides bicycle Muscles develop, energy and skill increase Practices to attain efficiency Learns value of money Orders, relates parts to whole	Latency stage Tasks of industry vs. inferiority Develops wholesome attitude about himself	Concrete operations Conceptual organization takes stability, coherence, and rationality Weight and volume viewed as consistent despite changes in size and shape (can conserve) Shift from inductive to deductive reasoning begins Uses reaction formation and rationalization to justify his behavior	Sibling relationships important; needs many exchanges with peers and adults Develops hobbies Seeks companionship Interested in community leaders, teachers; has many role models and ego models Self-reflective perspective in which child understands reciprocity, that is, not only can people have feelings but also they can react to one another—thus growth in self-awareness and clearer definition of self begins; acknowledges one can have several perspectives, thus the potential for inner conflict	Observes rules; develops conscience; conforms because conformity is itself a value Scale of values evolve.	Cooperative play with peers, prefers members of same sex; rules, programs, rituals, organized play, shared fantasy, gangs, group alliances and activities

AGE 9 TO 11 YEARS

Prelude to puberty; develops secondary sexual characteristics—breasts, pubic hair (girls about 1½ years ahead)	Continued tasks of identify vs. diffusion	Reaction formation and sublimation	Peer in-groups and out-groups	Superficial, but experiences sympathy for others	Rules can change by mutual agreement	Collaborates with groups in organized way
Boys voice deepens, he develops facial hair	Fantasies of romantic love	Intellectualization begins (11 to 12 years)	Emancipated from parents; makes inner-directed decisions, develops sexual identity, changes and experiments with roles, talks things over with peers	Other-directed conformity	Right and wrong are logically clear	Loyalty to "chum" may exceed loyalty to family
Period of steady growth, pause between childhood and adult		Formal operational thought begins at about age 11 years; can now deal with world effectively, not only with immediate but with possibilities, "as if" cognition is now of adult type, uses deductive reasoning, has ability to evaluate logic and quality of own thinking; ability for abstractions provides child with ability to deal with laws and principles	Needs "best" friend	Wins recognition through productivity	Follows peer group mores	
"Daring" years, most accident prone		Has capacity for insight	Third-person perspective leads to ability to take view of disinterested spectator or "generalized other",[39a] moves from reciprocity to mutual interest; people's attitudes become stereotyped because of limited discriminations		Conventional moral level oriented to authority, duty, law	
Absorbed interest in body changes—growth spurt		Can adapt to another opinion or point of view	Is self-aware			
Growth may seem disproportionate; may be clumsy, uncoordinated; increased interest in sports, athletics, "team" games		Makes decisions based on stored knowledge	Begins inner-directed conformity			
Heterosexual interests and experiences (some); concerned about appeal to opposite sex		Can define abstract terms	Has empathy for others			
			Uses slang, group "jargons," peer culture language			
			Prepares for vocational choice			

Analysis

Nursing diagnosis. The following list provides examples of NANDA-accepted diagnoses with causative statements.

1. Disturbance in self-concept related to disturbed relationships with peers
2. Sleep pattern disturbance related to anxiety over separation from parents
3. Impaired social interaction related to impulsive behavior
4. Dysfunctional grieving related to loss of sibling
5. Impaired adjustment related to academic problems
6. Altered growth and development related to chronic illness

DSM-III-R diagnoses. The DSM-III-R diagnoses related to infancy, childhood, or adolescent disorders are listed in the box below.

DSM-III-R DISORDERS USUALLY FIRST EVIDENT IN INFANCY, CHILDHOOD, OR ADOLESCENCE

Developmental disorders

(Note: These are coded on Axis II)

MENTAL RETARDATION

317.00	Mild mental retardation
318.00	Moderate mental retardation
318.10	Severe mental retardation
318.20	Profound mental retardation
319.00	Unspecified mental retardation

PERVASIVE DEVELOPMENTAL DISORDERS

299.00	Autistic disorder
299.80	Pervasive developmental disorder (not otherwise specified)

Specific developmental disorders

ACADEMIC SKILLS DISORDERS

315.10	Developmental arithmetic disorder
315.80	Developmental expressive writing disorder
315.00	Developmental reading disorder

LANGUAGE AND SPEECH DISORDERS

315.39	Developmental articulation disorder
315.31	Developmental expressive language disorder
315.31	Developmental receptive language disorder

MOTOR SKILLS DISORDERS

315.40	Developmental coordination disorder
315.90	Specific developmental disorder (not otherwise specified)

Other developmental disorders

315.90	Developmental disorder (not otherwise specified)

DISRUPTIVE BEHAVIOR DISORDERS

314.01	Attention deficit-hyperactivity disorder
312.20	Group type
312.00	Solitary aggressive type
313.90	Undifferentiated type
313.81	Oppositional-defiant disorder

ANXIETY DISORDERS OF CHILDHOOD OR ADOLESCENCE

309.21	Separation anxiety disorder
313.21	Avoidant disorder of childhood or adolescence
313.00	Overanxious disorder

TIC DISORDERS

307.23	Tourette's disorder
307.22	Chronic motor or vocal tic disorder
307.21	Transient tic disorder, specify; single episode or recurrent
307.20	Tic disorder (not otherwise specified)

ELIMINATION DISORDERS

307.70	Functional enuresis, specify; primary or secondary type
307.60	Functional encopresis, specify; primary or secondary type, specify; nocturnal only, diurnal only, nocturnal and diurnal

SPEECH DISORDERS NOT ELSEWHERE CLASSIFIED

307.00	Cluttering
307.00	Stuttering

OTHER DISORDERS OF INFANCY, CHILDHOOD, OR ADOLESCENCE

313.23	Elective mutism
313.32	Identity disorder
307.30	Sterotype/habit disorder
314.00	Undifferentiated attention deficit disorder

From American Psychiatric Association: Diagnostic and statistical manual of mental disorders (DSM-III-R), Washington, D.C., 1987, The Association.

The essential features and manifestations of the features of attention-deficit hyperactivity disorder, and separation anxiety disorder according to the DSM-III-R classification, are listed in the boxes below.

Planning

Table 40-5 provides some long-term and short-term goals and outcome criteria related to childhood. These serve as examples of the planning stage of the nursing process.

314.01 ATTENTION-DEFICIT HYPERACTIVITY DISORDER

ESSENTIAL FEATURES

A disorder in which there is disturbance in the areas of inattention, impulsiveness, and hyperactivity.

MANIFESTATIONS

Physical Dimension

Difficulty remaining seated
Excessive jumping about
Fidgeting
Manipulating objects
Twisting and wiggling in one's seat
Accident-prone behavior

Intellectual Dimension

Does not stick with tasks sufficiently to finish them
Difficulty organizing and completing work correctly
Gives the impression that he is not listening or has not heard what has been said
Work is often messy and is performed carelessly and impulsively
Makes comments out of turn
Failure to heed directions fully before beginning to respond to assignments
Failure to follow through on others' requests and instructions
Frequent shifts from one uncompleted activity to another
Excessively noisy activities
Failure to listen to other children
Interrupting
Excessive talking

Social Dimension

Failure to wait one's turn in group tasks
Interrupts the teacher during lessons
Interrupts other children during quiet work periods
Interrupts and intrudes on family members
Failure to follow the rules of structured games
Failure to wait one's turn in games

Adapted from American Psychiatric Association: Diagnostic and statistical manual of mental disorders (DSM-III-R), Washington, D.C., 1987, The Association.

309.21 SEPARATION ANXIETY DISORDER

ESSENTIAL FEATURES

The child, when separated from those to whom he is attached, experiences anxiety beyond that expected for the child's developmental level.

MANIFESTATIONS

Physical Dimension

Stomach aches, headaches, nausea, and vomiting when separation is anticipated or occurs
Has difficulty falling asleep
Insists that someone stay until he falls asleep
Nightmares

Emotional Dimension

Experiences anxiety to the point of panic
Fear of being lost and never being reunited with parents
Anticipatory anxiety when separation is threatened or impending
Fear of animals, monsters, and situations that are perceived as presenting danger to the integrity of the family or themselves
Exaggerated fears of muggers, burglars, kidnappers, car accidents, or plane travel
Concerns about death and dying
Extremely homesick when away from home

Intellectual Dimension

Preoccupation with morbid fears, accidents, or illnesses about themselves or significant others when separated
Preoccupation with reunion fantasies when away from home

Social Dimension

Uncomfortable when alone and away from the house or familiar surroundings
Refusal to visit or sleep at friends' homes, run errands, or attend camp or school
Unable to stay in a room by himself
Displays clinging behavior, staying close to the parent, or shadowing the parent
Exhibits recurrent instances of social withdrawal when without a major attachment figure
Becomes violent toward a person who is forcing separation

Adapted from American Psychiatric Association: Diagnostic and Statistical manual of mental disorders (DSM-III-R), Washington, D.C., 1987, The Association.

TABLE 40-5 Long-term and short-term goals and outcome criteria related to childhood

Goals	Outcome Criteria

NURSING DIAGNOSIS: DISTURBANCE IN SELF-CONCEPT RELATED TO INADEQUATE EMOTIONAL SUPPORT

Long-term goals

To develop trust	Interacts frequently with others
	Expresses feelings of others without hesitation, blockings, or fear response
To increase interpersonal perception	Makes positive statements about parents and peers
	Indicates improved self-esteem by spontaneously joining peers in play activities

Short-term goals

To express feelings without fear of punishment	Shares feelings in one-to-one relationship with nurse, expanding vocabulary to label feelings
	Relies on words rather than actions when expressing needs and wishes
To recognize effects of behaviors on others	Develops alternative ways of expressing needs that do not stimulate interpersonal anger
	Tests strategies for verbally expressing self in peer-group interactions and reviewing outcomes
To improve decision-making strategies	Explores alternative behaviors in situations requiring choices
	Completes a project successfully
	Initiates decision-making games with peers, expressing pleasure with these activities
To resolve dependence conflicts	Engages in activities that improve self-esteem
	Acknowledges successful experiences
	Cites behavioral changes in self
	Notes changes in behavior that enhance social relationships

NURSING DIAGNOSIS: INEFFECTIVE INDIVIDUAL COPING RELATED TO CHRONIC ILLNESS

Long-term goals

To develop strategies for coping with environmental stressors	Identifies potential environmental stressors and initiates activities to decrease stress responses
	Demonstrates alternative ways of decreasing stress, indicating a repertoire of coping techniques
	Collaborates with peers in constructive, goal-directed activities such as building projects
	Engages in competitive peer activities, demonstrating ability to win or lose without loss of self-esteem
To demonstrate age-appropriate self-care behaviors	Identifies early signs and symptoms of fatigue, frustration, and fear in self, initiating tactics to prevent escalation of these feelings
	Recognizes situations requiring assistance from others and seeks help appropriately
	Cooperates in medical regimens

Short-term goals

To identify frustrated and frustrating behaviors	Recognizes nonproductive responses to stressful environmental situations and identifies, with nurse's assistance, productive stress-reduction actions
	Expresses needs instead of expecting others to anticipate wishes
	Accepts taking turns and not having to be "first"
To increase self-competence	Identifies interest and initiates efforts toward mastery of skill, such as painting, macrame, woodworking, or model building
To increase social skills	Expands understanding of others' feelings through role taking and role playing and communications that facilitate peer interactions
	Learns a new competitive game (chess, checkers, Scrabble) and accepts losing and winning without offending partner
To participate in a health care regimen related to chronic illness	Knows rationale for dietary regimen and participates, with nurse, in planning and evaluating, gradually assuming more control of dietary regimen and himself
	Develops an exercise regimen, identifying early signs of fatigue
	Monitors sleep patterns and participates in activities that improve sleep
	Identifies situations related to medical regimen that incur frustration and feelings of lack of control, expanding self-help skills appropriate to age
	Recognizes anxieties and frustrations arising from dependence on others as a result of chronic illness, accepting others' role in treatment regimen

Implementation

✦ ***Physical dimension.*** Although most adults are watchful with small children, there is a need for increased vigilance with the child who has perceptual or neurological deficits. Rooms need to be uncluttered and well lit. Night-lights help control perceptual distortions that can stimulate fearful illusions.

Hyperactive children require environmental modifications. It is important that sensory stimulation such as noise, light, and colors be minimized. Arrangements are made for the child to receive additional rest and sleep, and plans need to be made for the hyperactive school-age child to rest during the day. Attention to the hyperactive child's diet is important because these children require a higher caloric intake than do less-active children. Parents need to monitor the child's diet and eliminate foods that seem to contribute to the child's overstimulation, such as sweets.

Most small children spontaneously establish a variety of rituals, and parental reinforcement of these rituals helps provide structure for the child. This is especially important for activities of daily living such as mealtimes, bedtime, and bathing and for other physical care activities.

Play activities can be used to help the child master the physical environment by strengthening integration of physical-neurological processes. When counseling parents of emotionally disturbed children, the nurse can prescribe specific, developmentally related play activities that use the child's energies constructively.[37] Activities that strengthen the emotionally disturbed child's control and mastery of the physical world and his self-control, such as games or sports, are major interventions. These interventions are critical in working with children who are hyperactive and distractible and who have short attention spans and reality distortions, regardless of the etiological factors underlying their psychopathology.

Physical activity is a prime aspect of child's play and a medium through which children develop physical skills and body confidence. The early explanations of play focused on its physical benefits such as expending "surplus energy." Gesell[22] stated that no one need teach a child how to play, that play is automatic and the result of intrinsic maturational forces that direct the child to "do what needs to be done" so that growth, maturation, and development are integrated and balanced. Most of children's spontaneous free play involves physical contact and closeness with one another; young children touch, hug, roll, and toss, whereas older children enjoy body contact sports and touching games.

Table 40-6 provides a schema for selecting age-appropriate developmental play activities developed by Florey.[19] In this schema the "self" refers to physical actions relevant to the physical dimension, not the self-concept. Type I objects are play materials that can change shape and form when manipulated, such as paints, clay, sand, water, and unstructured art media. Type II objects are those that change shape and form when combined with similar or dissimilar objects, such as blocks and tinker toys. Type III objects are toys that do not change shape or form, such as dolls and trucks.

❋ ***Emotional dimension*** The child's language and cognitive structures are not sufficiently developed to express concepts verbally. Developmentally children first express their feelings and desires through action, then through fantasy, and finally, through language. Therefore the therapeutic use of play assists children to resolve internal, emotional problems, such as stress, anxiety, depression and anger.

Interactions with a child 4 years of age or younger are limited to naming feelings, wishes, or fantasies relating to others and the child making simple requests of adults. The young child lacks the language and cognitive structures to discern relationships between events, and verbalizations need be limited to words to which the young child can respond. The nurse needs to make simple statements by "naming" feelings and objects, and through these identifications the nurse adds to the child's language repertoire and provides the child a new option of behavior.

Although the 5-year-old child has learned syntax and grammar, the child's ease in using language to express feelings is still limited. Play materials provide familiar concrete objects and materials that stimulate the child to symbolically express areas of concern. Engaging the child in ongoing dialogue while he plays helps clarify the child's thought organization. Conversation stimulated through play may be the most important part of the intervention. The child is assisted by verbal interactions and clarification to organize experiences and fill in missing data. The nurse has the opportunity to identify and clarify the child's misinterpretations.

Children 9 to 12 years of age are usually very verbal, and their language and communications skills can be expanded and refined during therapeutic dialogues. Although the older child's language and cognitive concepts may be sufficient for expressing feeling, the older child may be inexperienced or uncomfortable discussing feelings and interpersonal situations. Focusing on play materials may help alleviate uncomfortable barriers that eye-to-eye interaction may stimulate. Older children are extremely sensitive to social and adult-child size differences, and these perceptions may impede free and open verbal expression. Children ages 9 to 12 years spend much time talking with peers, and group therapies with children in this age range may be indicated.

Children often need parental help in mastery of impulse control and angry feelings. Most children have outbursts of anger and frustration while learning to delay gratification, and behavior modification interventions often enforce limits and help both child and parent to be consistent.

❋ ***Intellectual dimension.*** When nursing interventions include teaching, the child's learning capacity and style can be determined from conferences with nursery or school teachers. It is important that teaching interventions in the nursing care plan are consistent with the child's learning capacities and experiences. The child's language development, reviewed earlier, is an important consideration in teaching plans and interventions with the emotionally disturbed child. This is especially true with children with delayed speech or expressive language

TABLE 40-6 Play behaviors

	2-3 Years	3-4 Years	4-5 Years	5-6 Years
HUMAN OBJECTS				
Parents	Asking to listen to same story, over and over without any change in wording	Not asking to hear same story word for word	Bragging, e.g., "I can do _____; asking "why" questions, listening to stories—fairy tales	Asking "why" questions; wanting to know what to expect, wanting to listen to realistic stories as opposed to fairy tales
Peers	Parallel (playing alongside on same or different activity); fighting, pinching; defending play objects; taking objects from another	Parallel; beginning to take turns	Enjoys being with other children; sharing materials; bragging and name calling	Cooperative (two or more working on same project); wanting playmates; playing group games in which everyone has a turn—no competition; imaginative action—roles differentiated, e.g., one plays mother, one plays baby
Self	Practice of newly acquired motor skills, e.g., balancing, rolling	Identifying body with other people or things, e.g., I am a bear, I am a fireman—does not ask for costumes for such action, may have imaginary friends	May have imaginary friends	No play-specific information reported
NONHUMAN OBJECTS				
Type I	Emptying and filling containers, splashing (with water); making marks and using many sheets of paper (with paint or crayons); tasting, putting on self, squishing through fingers; patting; pulling apart; extending efforts beyond boundary of paper or surface; does not name product or ask to have it saved	Attending to results of efforts (e.g., "Look what I made," and naming of products); treating product as object itself and not a representation of object; likely to throw a clay ball	Intends to make something when begins although may end with different product; talking about what is being made; treating product as representation of object—not likely to throw clay ball—product does not have to be a realistic representation; wanting to put name on product and wanting it saved	Attempting to make realistic representation; definitely wanting products saved and displayed; putting name on products
Type II	Stringing beads, working puzzles, building vertically, placing in rows, building floorlike arrangement; making arch, transporting in containers	Working puzzles; building wall-like arrangement; floorlike arrangement, arch, or solid structure (a wall of several thicknesses), using the form built in; imaginative action	Naming what is being built although not intent on making product a realistic representation; wanting structures saved; collecting, e.g., variation of nature objects mainly	Constructing simple projects that can be completed within 20 minutes; projects must be useful (e.g., potholders)
Type III	Looking at and playing with same object, manipulating parts; taking simple things apart or off; placing pegs in board; pushing and propelling over obstacles; kicking, climbing, imaginative action—ascribing action (e.g., making dolly eat, sleep, cry, making truck "start")	Fine motor action—hitting nail with hammer, dropping buttons through small openings; propelling over obstacles; imaginative action—ascribing action; identifying one object as another by speech before using in action (e.g., paper as blanket, shell as cup)	Fine motor action—cutting, sewing on cards; gross motor action—arranging perilous feats for self, e.g., jumping, climbing jungle gym; imaginative action—identifying body with other people, wanting a few elements of costume; sequences more complex, e.g., more than one event (feeding, bathing dolly), or expansion of one event	Fine motor action—making mosaics; gross motor action—leaving earth with ropes in jumping; imaginative action—identifies body with other people and wanting whole costume; using miniature objects to represent real ones; attempting to imitate others

6-7 Years	7-8 Years	8-9 Years	9-11 Years
In listening to stories, has greater tolerance for fairy tales in the form of magic	Asking to listen to heroes own age in setting he can recognize; opinions of group more important than opinions of parents; boys want some individual time with father; girls want individual time with mother	Rebelling against parents especially when group opinions conflict with parental ones	No play-specific information reported
Wants to be with a group although there is little cooperation; important to obey customs of group—must act, look, talk like others; may tattle; game action—unable to put rules of game above need to win; learning to work as team in relay races; imaginative action—includes more than one or two children and often depends on leader; details in costume	Group is very important—a for or against age in which one is in or out of group; game action—rules apply to everyone except him; group games in which everyone has a chance to play; trading of objects; imaginative action—each group has organization and leader; imitation of reality; separation of sexes, e.g., girls—house, boys—war	Group is very important—must compete with others and conform to code; secrecy of gang important; game action—rules can still apply to everyone except him; imaginative action—done in group and reflects events outside of home and school; scouts or cubs important; trading of objects	Group is very important—joins many groups; game action—more conscious about rules and obeys them; competition is strong and plays for personal and team glory at the same time; imaginative action is rare
No play-specific information reported	No play-specific information reported	No play-specific information reported	No play-specific information reported
Attempting realistic representation	In a hurry for results—prefers crayons to paint as does not want to wait for paint to dry; concerned with realistic representation	Paints and uses casein; concerned with realistic representation	Making projects (for example, clay modeling)
Has trouble finishing any simple project—gets bogged down in middle; very critical of self in work	Sampling age—tries many different crafts and explores use of tools in relation to them; in a hurry for results so does not use best workmanship	Makes things that move and work; constantly overreaching self in projects—needs someone to help get materials and show procedures; exploring many processes in crafts (e.g., potato carving)	Exploring many crafts (e.g., model making, weaving, woodworking, metalworking, working with leather, carving, making baskets, sewing); projects made need to be useful
Collecting items—quantity important—taking objects apart (e.g., clocks); speed important in sport activities (e.g., roller skating)	Beginning to collect only certain items; gross muscle action—speed important; trying to improve physical skills and sampling new skills (e.g., swimming, archery, riding, skiing)	Reads and chooses fairy tales and legends—stories about everyday people in everyday situations; gross muscle action—gross muscle sports of hopscotch, roller skating, kite flying, wrestling, not ready for fine precision sports (e.g., tennis, golf); collecting according to individual interests	Exploring a variety of books (e.g., adventure, fantasy, biography, mysteries, westerns, sports, animal, scientific); exploring a variety of sports, trying many and concentrating on a few and practicing those skills

problems, such as blocking or stuttering. It is important that the child have a complete evaluation by a speech therapist to rule out the possibility of neurological or organic sensory problems. Many children with emotional problems fail to maintain the eye contact that is basic to learning the mouth movements necessary for clear enunciation. Thus many speech problems in children disappear when the underlying emotional stress has been alleviated. The resolution of the language problem symptoms is often an indication of effective intervention within the emotional dimension.

❀ *Social dimension.* The stressors on children can be addressed with many of the same stress management techniques that are used with adults. The effect of relaxation training on children is presented in the Research Highlight below. Because children and parents with mental health problems often withdraw from social relationships, it is important to encourage peer relationships for both child and parents. As part of the evaluation of the therapeutic process, social relationships need to provide the social support networks upon which families and children rely.

Implementation of the child's treatment plan depends on the therapeutic alliance with the child's parents. By the time parents seek professional help for the child, they usually have tried many techniques of their own and have followed advice of family and friends. Sometimes parents are troubled, deny the existence of a problem, and seek support to prove others wrong. Thus it is important that the nurse help parents regain confidence in the parenting role. Sufficient time needs to be taken to allow the parents to identify and discuss their feelings, successes, frustrations, and anxieties.

The therapeutic relationship with the child's parents begins with the initial assessment of their roles and relationships with the child and the child's problems and includes ongoing strengthening of the parents' potential to help the child. The treatment goal of working with emotionally disturbed children and their families is the reestablishment of the normal child-parent relationships appropriate for the child's developmental level. The problems identified by parents often have little or no relationship to the child's subjective feelings of distress. It is important, however, to learn parents' concerns and resolve them concurrently with intervention with the child. The nurse is nonjudgmental while gathering the information, allowing each parent to give his or her point of view. The parents' trust is gained, and the therapeutic alliance is established if positive feedback, information, and reinforcement are provided. For example, the mother of a hyperactive child can be asked how she provides for her own well-being and restoration of energies. The child's

Research Highlight

A Pilot Study of the Impact of Stress Management Techniques on the Classroom Behavior of Elementary School Students

R. Petrosa & D. Oldfield

PURPOSE

The purpose of this study was to assess the impact of stress management techniques on the ability of elementary school children to attend to teacher-assigned tasks.

SAMPLE

The sample contained 296 children 5 to 12 years of age. Based on school records the sample was composed of a higher percentage of high-mobility, low-income, single-parent families than the national average.

METHODOLOGY

Students were randomly assigned to a treatment or control group. Students in the treatment group received 8 days, approximately 25 minutes per day, of psychophysiological relaxation training in their classrooms. All students monitored and charted fingertip temperature changes 2 days each week while practicing the relaxation exercises. This self-monitoring was used both as a motivational technique to maintain student interest and to provide for some periodic feedback on their skill performance. Two weeks after the treatment group had completed the stress management curriculum, a trained examiner visited each of the treatment and control classes for a blind assessment of on-task behavior. On-task behavior was defined as student behavior that contributed to the completion of the teacher-prescribed activity.

FINDINGS

There was a significant difference between the posttreatment scores of the treatment and control groups. Thus teaching children psychophysiological relaxation skills was shown to promote on-task behavior.

IMPLICATIONS

Children's behavior improves with the use of stress management techniques, and the teaching of these techniques to both teachers and students is an appropriate role for the mental health–psychiatric nurse.

Based on data from Journal of School Health **54**(10):69, 1985.

and parents' strengths are emphasized to provide the parents with hope.

Therapeutic interventions with the child's parents are based on a parallel process that strengthens the parents' potential to help the child. The parents' and child's developmental tasks in progress are set forth in Table 40-7 (pp. 782-783) for the child under 5 years of age and 5 to 12 years of age. Table 40-8 (p. 784) gives psychopathological conditions of the child 18 months to 5 years and 5 to 12 years of age and related behaviors of the parents. Tasks in process, acceptable behavioral characteristics, minimal psychopathology, and extreme psychopathology are important guides to the nurse during implementation as well as during evaluation of behavioral change.

Spiritual dimension. Interventions in the spiritual dimension are so integrally related to the other dimensions for children that they are not addressed separately here.

Evaluation

Development is uneven, and not all children can be expected to change simultaneously. An important criterion is the child's developmental progress; Children with mental health problems often seem "fixed" at a developmental stage. Positive evaluation reflects the child's productive return to the expected developmental stage. Materials used in assessment often provide useful guidelines to evaluate therapeutic outcomes, such as children's drawings compared before and after interventions.

Evaluation takes into consideration the parents' perceptions of the child's progress and changes in parent-child relationships. Also, the Research Highlight on p. 768 indicates that the child's perceptions are of equal importance in the evaluation process. In many instances, parents are unaware of the child's worries and concerns.

SPECIFIC TREATMENT MODALITIES

Play Therapy

Children with neurotic problems usually have little insight and respond best to play therapies based on psychoanalytic theories. This approach uses play for working through or resolving conflicts through repetitive fantasy and make-believe. The therapist's role is active in that the toys used in therapy are purposefully selected for their therapeutic value. The therapeutic communication with the child during play helps him develop abilities in interpretation and insight.

Erikson[15] expanded Freud's psychoanalytic theory of play to include social mastery, stating that the purpose of children's play is to master the specific areas of conflict involved in developmental crisis. In Erikson's play therapy methods the therapist controls the play session by introducing toys and activities that facilitate the child's development and mastery, while recognizing at the same time that the child will spontaneously choose materials and activities to alleviate conflicts and developmental crises.

Theraplay

The technique of *theraplay* differs from traditional forms of child treatment. Theraplay uses active physical contact and control of the child. Theraplay grew from the work of DesLauriers and Carlson[13] with autistic children, in which they forced the child to acknowledge their presence by insisting on eye contact, speaking loudly when the child "tuned them out," and aggressively insisting on interactions. Their interventions involved physical contact that forced the autistic, self-absorbed child to acknowledge their presence in the here and now. The theraplay techniques have been adapted to interventions with children with less severe psychopathological conditions and are of benefit to children with psychosocial retardation and benefit children having difficulties in elementary school settings.

BRIEF REVIEW

Nursing care of children with emotional problems requires an understanding of the development of the five dimensions of the child and the interrelatedness of the dimensions in the developmental process. Assessment and interventions need to include the child's parents and significant others, for example, teachers and caretakers.

The developmental model holds that the child is an active participant in the developmental process and that direct treatment of the child is based on age/stage considerations. One of the specific treatment methods for children is the therapeutic use of play, which can be structured and focused on the content of the child's play or unstructured, providing a framework for learning, improving socialization, or setting limits.

Therapeutic communication with children focuses on communicating with the child at the appropriate age level of word usage and adding to the child's growing understanding of language. Therapeutic treatment of the child includes helping the child reach higher levels of development in all dimensions without overemphasizing one specific problem area.

The immediate goals of interventions with children are to alleviate the child's distress and help the child get back on the developmental tract. Long-range goals are to expand the child's coping strategies and alter his environment so the problems do not recur. The goals include working with families and significant others so that the individual child's uniqueness is understood, the developmental process and tasks are mastered, and changes are supported and facilitated.

Tables 40-7 and 40-8 follow.

TABLE 40-7 Developmental tasks and acceptable behavioral characteristics of the child and related tasks and behaviors of the parents

Tasks in Process		Acceptable Behavioral Characteristics	
Child	Parents	Child	Parents
18 months to 5 years of age			
To reach physiologic plateaus (motor action, toilet training)	To promote training, habits, and physiologic progress	Gratification from exercise of neuromotor skills	Is moderate and flexible in training
To differentiate self and secure sense of autonomy	To aid in family and group socialization of child	Investigative, imitative imaginative play	Shows pleasure and praise for child's advances
To tolerate separations from mother	To encourage speech and other learning	Actions somewhat modulated by thought, memory good; animistic and original thinking	Encourages and participates with child in learning and in play
To develop conceptual understandings and "ethical" values	To reinforce child's sense of autonomy and identity	Exercises autonomy with body (sphincter control, eating)	Sets reasonable standards and controls
To master instinctual impulses (Oedipal, sexual, guilt, shame)	To set a model for "ethical" conduct	Feelings of dependence on mother and separation fears	Paces herself to child's capacities at a given time
To assimilate and handle socialization and acculturation (aggression, relationships, activities, feelings)	To delineate male and female roles	Behavior identification with parents, siblings, peers	Consistent in own behavior, conduct, and ethics
To learn sex distinctions		Learns speech for communication	Provides emotional reassurance to child
		Awareness of own motives, beginnings of conscience	Promotes peer play and guided group activity
		Intense feelings of shame, guilt, joy, love, desire to please	Reinforces child's cognition of male and female roles
		Internalized standards of "bad," "good"; beginning of reality testing	
		Broader sex curiosity and differentiation	
		Ambivalence towards dependence and independence	
		Questions birth and death	

From Senn, M.J.E., and Solnit, A.J.: Problems in child behavior and development, Philadelphia, 1968, Lea & Febiger.

TABLE 40-7 Developmental tasks and acceptable behavioral characteristics of the child and related tasks and behaviors of the parents—cont'd

Tasks in Process		Acceptable Behavior Characteristics	
Child	Parents	Child	Parents
5 to 12 years of age			
To master greater physical prowess	To help child's emancipation from parents	General good health, greater body competence, acute sensory perception	Ambivalent towards child's separation but encourage independence
To further establish self-identity and sex role	To reinforce self-identification and independence	Pride and self-confidence, less dependence on parents	Mixed feelings about parent-surrogates but help child to accept them
To work towards greater independence from parents	To provide positive pattern of social and sex role behavior	Better impulse control	Encourage child to participate outside the home
To become aware of world-at-large	To facilitate learning, reasoning, communication, and experiencing	Ambivalence regarding dependency, separation and new experiences	Set appropriate model of social and ethical behavior and standards
To develop peer and other relationships	To promote wholesome moral and ethical values	Accepts own sex role: psychosexual expression in play and fantasy	Take pleasure in child's developing skills and abilities
To acquire learning, new skills, and a sense of industry		Equates parents with peers and other adults	Understand and cope with child's behavior
		Aware of natural world (life, death, birth, science); subjective but realistic about world	Find other gratifications in life (activity, employment)
		Competitive but well organized in play; enjoys peer interaction	Are supportive toward child as required
		Regard for collective obedience to social laws, rules, and fair play	
		Explores environment; school and neighborhood basic to social-learning experience	
		Cognition advancing; intuitive thinking advancing to concrete operational level; responds to learning	
		Speech becomes reasoning and expressive tool; thinking still egocentric	

TABLE 40-8 Minimal and extreme psychopathological conditions of the child and related behaviors of the parents

Minimal Psychopathology		Extreme Psychopathology	
Child	Parents	Child	Parents
18 months to 5 years of age			
Poor motor coordination	Premature, coercive, or censuring training	Extreme lethargy, passivity, or hypermotility	Severely coercive and punitive
Persistent speech problems (stammering, loss of words)	Exacting standards above child's ability to conform	Little or no speech, noncommunicative	Totally critical and rejecting
Timidity towards people and experiences	Transmits anxiety and apprehension	No response or relationship to people, symbiotic clinging to mother	Overidentification with or overly submissive to child
Fears and night terrors	Unaccepting of child's efforts; intolerant towards failures	Somatic ills; vomiting, constipation, diarrhea, megacolon, rash, tics	Inability to accept child's sex; fosters opposite
Problems with eating, sleeping, elimination, toileting, weaning	Overreacts, overprotective, overanxious	Autism, childhood psychosis	Substitutes child for spouse; sexual expression via child
Irritability, crying, temper tantrums	Despondent, apathetic	Excessive enuresis, soiling, fears	Severe repression of child's need for gratification
Partial return to infantile manners		Completely infantile behavior	Deprivation of all stimulations, freedoms, and pleasures
Inability to leave mother without panic		Play inhibited and nonconceptualized; absence or excess of autoerotic activity	Extreme anger and displeasure with child
Fear or strangers		Obsessive-compulsive behavior; "ritual" bound mannerisms	Child assault and brutality
Breathholding spells		Impulsive destructive behavior	Severe depressions and withdrawal
Lack of interest in other children			
5 to 12 years of age			
Anxiety and oversensitivity to new experiences (school, relationships, separation)	Disinclination to separate from child; or prematurely hastening separation	Extreme withdrawal, apathy, depression, grief, self-destructive tendencies	Extreme depression and withdrawal; rejection of child
Lack of attentiveness; learning difficulties; disinterest in learning	Signs of despondency, apathy, hostility	Complete failure to learn	Intense hostility; aggression toward child
Acting out; lying, stealing, temper outbursts, inappropriate social behavior	Foster fears, dependence, apprehension	Speech difficulty, especially stuttering	Uncontrollable fears, anxieties, guilts
Regressive behavior (wetting, soiling, crying, fears)	Disinterested in or rejecting of child	Extreme and uncontrollable antisocial behavior (aggression, destruction, chronic lying, stealing, intentional cruelty to animals)	Complete inability to function in family role
Appearance of compulsive mannerisms (tics, rituals)	Overly critical and censuring; undermine child's confidence	Severe obsessive-compulsive behavior (phobias, fantasies, rituals)	Severe moralistic prohibition of child's independent strivings
Somatic illness; eating and sleeping problems, aches, pains, digestive upsets	Inconsistent in discipline or control; erratic in behavior	Inability to distinguish reality from fantasy	
Fear of illness and body injury	Offer a restrictive, overly moralistic model	Excessive sexual exhibitionism, eroticism, sexual assaults on others	
Difficulties and rivalry with peers, siblings, adults; constant fighting		Extreme somatic illness: failure to thrive, anorexia, obesity, hypochondriasis, abnormal menses	
Destructive tendencies; strong temper tantrums		Complete absence or deterioration of personal and peer relationships	
Inability or unwillingness to do things for self			
Moodiness and withdrawal; few friends or personal relationships.			

From Senn, M.J.E., and Solnit, A.J.: Problems in child behavior and development, Philadelphia, 1968, Lea & Febiger.

REFERENCES AND SUGGESTED READINGS

1. American Nurses' Association: Standards of child and adolescent psychiatric and mental health nursing practice, Kansas City, Mo., 1985, The Association.
2. American Psychiatric Association: Diagnostic and statistical manual of mental disorders, ed. 3, Washington, D.C., 1987 The Association.
3. Aries, P.: From child king to child martyr: transformations of the attitude toward the child. In Anthony, E.J., and Chiland, C., editors: The child in his family: preventive child psychiatry in an age of transition, New York, 1980, John Wiley & Sons, Inc.
4. Barton, P.: The relationship between overt and fantasy stress reaction of children to hospitalization, Doctoral dissertation, Gainesville, 1964, University of Florida.
5. Bowlby, J.: Attachment and loss. II. Separation, New York, 1973, Basic Books,
6. Brody, V.: Developmental play: a relationship-focused program for children, Journal of Child Welfare **57**: 591, 1978.
7. Burgess, A., MrCausland, M.P., and Wolbert, W.: Children's drawings as indicators of sexual trauma, Perspectives in Psychiatric Care **19**:50, April 1981.
8. Chomsky, N.: Reflections on language, New York, 1975, Pantheon Books, Inc.
9. Clunn, P., and Payne, D.: Psychiatric–mental health nursing, ed. 4, New York, 1986, Medical Examination Publishing Co.
10. Coddington, R.D.: The significance of life events as etiological factors in the disease of children. II. A study of normal population, Journal of Psychosomatic Research **16**:205, 1972.
11. Coddington, R.D.: Personal communication, New Orleans, 1982.
12. Crain, W.: Theories of development, Englewood Cliffs, N.J., 1980, Prentice-Hall, Inc.
13. DesLauriers, A.M., and Carlson, C.F.: Your child's asleep: early infantile autism, Homewood, Ill., 1969, The Dorsey Press.
14. DiLeo, J.H.: Young children and their drawings, New York, 1970, Brunner/Mazel, Inc.
15. Erikson, E.: Toys and reasons, New York, 1977, W.W. Norton & Co. Inc.
16. Evans, D.L.: Explaining suicide among the young: an analytical review of the literature, Journal of Psychiatric Nursing and Mental Health Services **20**:9, 1982.
17. Feingold, B.: The Feingold book for hyperactive children, New York, 1979, Random House, Inc.
18. Fine, M.J., editor: Intervention with hyperactive children: a case study approach, Jamaica, N.Y., 1980, SP Medical Publishing Company.
19. Florey, L.: An approach to play and play development, American Journal of Occupational Therapy **25**(6):278, 1971.
20. Freud, A.: The concept of developmental lines, Psychoanalytic Study of the Child **8**:245, 1963.
21. Gardner, H.: The mind's new science, New York, 1985, Basic Books, Inc., Publishers.
22. Gesell, A., and Ilg, F.L., and Ames, L.B.: Infant and child in the culture of today, New York, 1974, Harper & Row, Publishers.
23. Goldman, J., Stein, C., and Guerry, S.: Psychological methods of child assessment, New York, 1983, Brunner/Mazel, Inc.
24. Goodman, J.D., and Sours, J.A.: The child mental status examination, New York, 1967, Basic Books, Inc., Publishers.
25. Greenspan, S., and Greenspan, N.: The clinical interview of the child, New York, 1981, Basic Books, Inc., Publishers.
26. Groos, K.: The play of man, New York, 1901, D. Appleton Co.
27. Group for the Advancement of Psychiatry, Committee on Child Psychiatry: The process of child therapy, New York, 1982, Brunner/Mazel, Inc.
28. Holmes, T.H., and Rabe, R.H.: The Social Readjustment Rating Scale, Journal of Psychosomatic Research **11**:213, 1967.
29. Jernberg, A.: Theraplay, San Francisco, 1979, Jossey-Bass, Inc., Publishers.
30. Kaplan, H., and Sadock, B.: Comprehensive textbook of psychiatry, IV, Baltimore, 1985, Williams & Wilkins.
31. Klaus, M.H., and Kennell, J.H.: Parent-infant bonding, ed. 2, St. Louis, 1982, The C.V. Mosby Co.
32. Klein, M.: The psychoanalysis of children, London, 1969, Hogarth Press.
33. Kohlberg, L.: Moral stages and moralization: the cognitive-developmental approach. In Lickona, T., editor: Moral development and behavior, New York, 1976, Holt, Rinehart & Winston.
34. Kübler-Ross, E.: On death and dying, New York, 1969, Macmillan Publishing Company.
35. Lawrence, J.A.: Moral judgement intervention studies using the defining issues test, Journal of Moral Education **9**:178. 1980.
36. Lazarus, A.: The practice of multimodal therapy, New York, 1981, Basic Books, Inc., Publishers.
37. Lee, J., and Fowler, M.: Merely child's play? Developmental work and playthings, Journal of Pediatric Nursing **4**:260, August 1986.
38. Light, N.: Counterpoint: family treatment for the disturbed child, Perspectives in Psychiatric Care **19**:79, 1981.
39. Mead, M.: Childhood in contemporary cultures, Chicago, 1955, University of Chicago Press.
39a. McFarland, G., and Wasli, E.: Nursing diagnoses and process in psychiatric mental health nursing. Philadelphia, 1986, J.B. Lippincott Co.
40. Mahler, M.: Notes on the development of basic moods: the depressive affect. In Loewenstein, R.M., and others, editors: Psychoanalysis: a general psychology, New York, 1966, International Universities Press, Inc.
41. Miles, M.: Playtherapy: a review of theories and comparison of some techniques, Issues in Mental Heath Nursing **3**:63, January-June 1981.
42. Miller, S.R.: Children's fears: a review of the literature with implications for nursing research and practice, Nursing Research **28**:217, 1979.
43. North American Nursing Diagnosis Association: Nursing Diagnosis I, St. Louis, 1986, NANDA.
44. Piaget, J.: The language and thought of the child, London, 1959, Routledge & Kegan Paul, Ltd. (Translated by M. Gabain.)
45. Piaget, J.: The construction of reality in the child, New York, 1964, Ballantine Books, Inc. (Translated by M. Cook.)
46. Pothier, P.C.: Child psychiatric nursing, Journal of Psychosocial Nursing **22**:11, 1984.
47. President's Commission on Mental Health: Report to the president's commission on mental health and mental illness in the United States, Washington, D.C., 1981, U.S. Government Printing Office.
48. Rapoport, J.L., and Ismond, D.: DSM-III training guide for diagnosis of childhood disorders, New York, 1984, Brunner/Mazel, Inc.
49. Sanoff, A.P., and Thornton, J.: Our neglected kids, U.S. News and World Report, p. 18, August 9, 1982.
50. Smith, P.K., and Vollstedt, R.: On defining play: an empirical study of the relationship between play and various play criteria, Child Development **56**:1042, 1985.

50a. Spitz, R.A.: Hospitalism: an inquiry into the genesis of psychiatric conditions in early childhood. In Psychoanalytic Study of the child, Independence, Mo., 1945. International University Press.

51. Wieczorek, R.R., and Natopoff, J.N.: A comprehensive approach to the nursing of children, Philadelphia, 1981, J.B. Lippincott Co.

52. Winnicott, D.W.: Playing and reality, New York, 1971, Basic Books, Inc., Publishers.

ANNOTATED BIBLIOGRAPHY

Adams, P.L., Milner, J.R., and Schrepf, N.A.: Fatherless children, New York, 1984, John Wiley & Sons.

This practical guide to working with fatherless children includes a review of research, specification of the major varieties of father-absence, conclusions about research methods, public policy, and psychotherapy of fatherless children. It discusses the effects of fatherlessness on the school and sex roles of children as well as on delinquency and mental disorders.

Erikson, E.H.: Toys and reasons, New York, 1977, W.W. Norton & Co., Inc.

In this book Erikson describes the stages in the ritualization of experience, from child's play to the adult's interplay. The space-time, visionary aspects of play for humans is reviewed, and the decline of ritualization is discussed as it relates to social disingegration. Erikson expands and refines the concepts presented in *Childhood and Society.*

Singer, D.E., and Revenson, T.A.: A Piaget primer: how a child thinks, New York, 1978, New American Library.

This primer provides a clear introduction and explanation of Piaget's theory of cognitive development. Topics include the stages of development, playing and imitating, discovering space, time, and numbers, and learning about right and wrong. Illustrations from *Alice in wonderland,* "Peanuts," and other child literature result in an easily understood presentation of this complex theory for parents and nonprofessionals, as well as a refreshing perspective for the professional nurse.

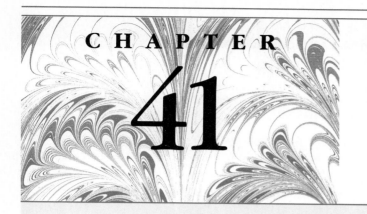

C H A P T E R
41

THE ADOLESCENT

Rae Sedgwick

After studying this chapter the learner will be able to:

Discuss the historical development of mental health–psychiatric nursing related to the adolescent.

Describe theoretical approaches to understanding adolescence as a unique phase of development.

Identify major considerations in establishing and maintaining a therapeutic relationship with the adolescent.

Apply the nursing process in the mental health–psychiatric care of the adolescent.

Describe specific treatment modalities that can be used in meeting the mental health–psychiatric needs of the adolescent.

Adolescent mental health–psychiatric nursing involves the care of adolescents, with particular emphasis on their emotional needs. Adolescence has been variously described but is generally agreed to be a phase of development during the years 12 to 20 when the individual experiences great surges of physical growth, engages in identity formation, and develops plans for the future.

Adolescence is an accelerated age in which a sense of balance is needed but rarely achieved until adulthood. In many ways adolescence is a unique period because during this time the physical and emotional characteristics of adulthood emerge and social, intellectual, and spiritual beginnings of the early years are sharpened, tested, and shaped for fuller use. Idealism, optimism, impatience, eagerness, and doubt characterize adolescence. Energies, once turned outward to explore the world, are now turned inward in introspection and self-analysis. It is a period when the mind becomes capable of deep thoughts, even able to think about the thoughts one is having. Perceptual abilities broaden, and intellectual capabilities expand.

Adolescence serves several functions. Structurally, adolescence links childhood with adulthood. Although factors such as environment and training can intervene or be disruptive, development is usually characterized by continu-

ity. Functionally, adolescence is a process within which physical, emotional, and intellectual growth prepares the individual for future roles: adult, sexual partner, parent, and responsible member of family, community, and society. As a process, adolescence unfolds systematically and, in spite of its chaotic appearance, occurs in an orderly sequential manner.

When this sense of order is violated, the individual may come to the attention of a health care professional whose task is to restore order and facilitate further growth and development of the disrupted process.

THEORETICAL APPROACHES
Biological

Hall,[22] who is generally regarded as the first psychologist to recognize adolescence as a unique developmental phase and to study it scientifically, expanded Darwin's concept of biological evolution into a theory that included a four-stage division of development. Adolescence was considered by Hall to be a period of "storm and stress," characterized by wide vacillation between contradictory tendencies such as idealism versus selfishness, solitude versus friendship, and cooperation versus rebellion. Hall's theory of adolescence postulated that adolescence

🍇 *Historical Overview* 🍇

DATE	EVENT
Pre-1700s	Children and adolescents were treated as chattel and often used as slave labor. Harsh treatment was based on the biblical idea of "spare the rod and spoil the child" and "children should be seen and not heard."
	The theological view of human nature encompassed ideas that humans had innate tendencies toward sinfulness, that people were basically bad, and that without severe discipline they would become worse during the developmental years.
1700s	Stern discipline and moral rigidity were prevalent. People believed that children and adolescents were miniature adults.
	John Locke challenged the notion that adolescents were miniature adults and suggested that social conditions and environment influenced the development of the adolescent's mind. He also saw adolescence as basically different from adulthood and as the period during which rational reasoning emerged.
	Rousseau emphasized the adolescent's need to be free from the unnatural, strict discipline of the adult world and advocated treatment and education of adolescents as adolescents rather than miniature adults.
1970s	Nurse leaders contributing to changes in attitudes and clinical practice that focus specifically on adolescents included Claire Fagan (*Readings in Child and Adolescent Psychiatric Nursing*, 1974), Shirley Smoyak (*The Psychiatric Nurse as a Family Therapist*, 1975), and Jeanne Howe (*Nursing Care of Adolescents*, 1980).
	Certification by the American Nurses' Association (ANA) now recognizes child and adolescent psychiatric–mental health nursing as a specialty area.
1977	The President's Commission on Mental Health identified adolescents as a high-risk group for mental health problems.
1980s	As society altered and expanded its view and care of adolescents, nursing altered and expanded its views of educational and clinical preparation of the professional nurse caring for adolescents.
1987	The increasing number of adolescent suicides today requires that nurses and other health professionals identify those adolescents at risk and that they intervene quickly with competence and confidence to prevent this tragic loss of life.
Future	It is estimated that problems associated with adolescence, such as alcoholism, drug abuse, pregnancy, sexuality, and bulemia, will increase in number and severity and require more nurses with special knowledge, skills, and attitudes to work with persons in this stage of development.
	Because the media exerts strong influence on adolescents it will be used in new, creative ways by interspersing rock music programs with health information or using live peer panel discussions on adolescent issues.

(1) is genetically determined and (2) occurs in a set pattern initiated by physiological factors. Hall underplayed the importance of cultural and environmental factors.

Psychoanalytic

Freud[18] postulated that psychosexual development occurs in genetically determined stages that are relatively independent of environmental factors. Sexual life begins not at puberty but earlier in life, with the first years being the most formative in terms of personality development and the later years being most formative in problem res-

olution. In this theory adolescence occurs between 13 and 18 years in the fifth, or genital, stage of development, during which sexual interest is reawakened because of physiological maturation, release of sex hormones, and sexual exploration. Two main developmental tasks are identified during this time: (1) the attainment of genital primacy, which includes detachment from the "incestuous object" (the parent) and forming an attachment with a nonincestuous object and (2) the establishment of a sense of balance between the self (ego), sexual drives (id), and parental and social mores (superego).

Erikson's[14] eight developmental stages were modifications of Freud's emphasis on instinct. According to Erikson, the main developmental task in the identity versus role diffusion phase is the acquisition of ego identity, during which the individual is faced with defining his ego identity. Self concept, body image, sexual identity, vocation or career, and independence from parents are all facets of the adolescent's identity. If the adolescent does not learn who he is, he may fail to develop ego identity resulting in role diffusion, and there is frequently trouble with sexual roles, social roles, choosing a career, separating from parents, and interpersonal relationships. If the adolescent enters young adulthood with a clear sense of identity, he is able to establish a mature relationship with a member of the opposite sex, choose a marital partner, and perform work and social roles.

Cognitive

Piaget[28] focused on qualitative changes in intellectual structure from birth to maturity, with each structure being built on the previous one. The integration of old into new provides continuity and development and leads to increasingly complex logical thought. During adolescence the individual is able to leave the objective world and enter into the world of ideas in which he is able to think abstract thoughts, to reflect, and to use symbols in a variety of ways. The ability to reason grows and matures, moral judgment is enhanced, and spiritual and religious beliefs are sought. As the adolescent increases his capacity of reasoning, new understandings are considered. Problem solving becomes possible at this time, as does the ability to see a situation from more than one viewpoint.

Sociocultural

Lewin envisioned that each person is surrounded by "life space," and the behavior within that life space is a function not only of the person within the space but also of the environment.[37] Biological, social, environmental, and emotional factors are seen as interdependently related within the life space. The life space begins somewhat simply and develops complexity as these factors change. Adolescence is a period of transition when the life space be-

comes further differentiated.[36] Lewin recognized that not only individual differences but also factors within the environment and within the social structure contribute to the life space changes. To understand the behavior of an adolescent, the nurse needs to have some knowledge of the environment in which the behavior occurs. In Lewin's field theory, the primary tasks of the adolescent include transition of membership from family group to peer group; transition of self-image as the body changes in unknown, unreliable, and unpredictable ways; and transition from the relatively structured world of the child to the unstructured world of the adult. The transition consists primarily of changing membership from the child world to the adult world. For a time the adolescent straddles the border between the two worlds. The adolescent experiences a conflict in values, life-styles, and ideologies between the two worlds; experiences emotional and social tension; and has a readiness to take extreme positions and to change behavior radically and quickly—all outgrowths of the differentiation and change within the life space.[36]

Table 41-1 summarizes theories of adolescence.

RELATING TO THE CLIENT

Establishing a relationship with an adolescent means initiating the relationship with a stated purpose, however tentative. It means recognizing that the adolescent is at a heightened physical and emotional phase of development in which intellectual capacity is increasing and the desire for change is nearly as great as the fear of it. It means remembering that the adolescent is struggling for a sense of identity and a sense of separateness from the family and may need to act out and practice the breaking away in the therapeutic relationship.

The nurse needs to resist the urge to rescue the adolescent, who often appears confused and vulnerable. The nurse encourages the adolescent from the beginning of the relationship to be actively involved in the process and to assume personal responsibility for his behavior.

With specific goals in mind, the nurse sets out to establish a relationship with and gain the trust of the adolescent.

Most adolescents, particularly those with adjustment

TABLE 41-1 Summary of theories of adolescence

Theory	Theorist	Dynamics
Biological	Hall	Adolescence is genetically determined and occurs in patterned, universal stages regardless of environment.
Psychoanalytic	Freud	Adolescence occurs in the genital (psychosexual; predominantly biological) stage of development during which sexual interest is reawakened because of physical maturity.
	Erikson	The developmental stages of identity versus role diffusion occurs.
Cognitive	Piaget	By adolescence there is an ability to reason, to think abstractly, to reflect, and to use symbols in logical ways.
Sociocultural	Lewin	The task of adolescence is the transition from family group to peer group, from the child world to the adult world. Changes occur as a result of biological development and environmental influences.

problems, believe that "no one cares and no one listens." Establishing trust involves listening and, in a sense, proving that one is hearing the message. One of the ways the nurse can do this is by reflecting to the adolescent the apparent message being conveyed.

Reflecting involves receiving what is heard and repeating it in an understandable way for the adolescent, for example:

Nurse: I notice that you grind your teeth when we talk about your father.
Nurse: When we talk about your failing the course, I feel like you pull away from me.
Nurse: You say that you look forward to leaving home, but you look so sad, I wonder how you really feel about going to college.

Reflecting gives the adolescent the opportunity to think about, change, and clarify what he is trying to say.

Clarifying means sharing with the teenager impressions, as well as conclusions drawn from them, in a way that encourages the adolescent to have input into the process:

Nurse: You look sad when you talk about leaving home.
Client: (Begins to cry quietly.) I was thinking about my brother who is away at school, and I miss him very much.

Failure to clarify the impressions that the nurse has drawn from facial appearance and body posture may lead the nurse to draw erroneous conclusions and act in ways that detract from the problem at hand. Sharing with adolescents lets them know that they are an important part of the relationship, that they are noticed, and that their opinions matter. This sets the stage for tentative conclusions to be drawn and indicates to the adolescent a sense of caring. The nurse says, "I care enough about you to share my impressions with you, and I want you to be able to do the same with me."

Caring and sharing means establishing a sense of give-and-take in the relationship. This may be a difficult aspect of the relationship in that the nurse is often dealing with an adolescent who has not learned to share, has not been rewarded for stating feelings, has perhaps been punished for expressing contradictory opinions, and in some cases may not be able to distinguish reality from fantasy. The nurse is often pulled in and becomes a part of the fantasy in the mind of the troubled adolescent. The adolescent who has not learned to share often needs to be coaxed.

Case Example

Hal is a 13-year-old who is asked to talk about the problems that brought him to the clinic.

Client: Why should I tell you? You'll only tell my father.
Nurse: No, I don't want to tell your father. I'm asking so that I can get to know you better. I want us to work together to help you get better.

The nurse has the opportunity and responsibility to model healthy ways of communicating and interacting, to demonstrate risk taking, and to provide limits that the adolescent is unable to provide. The more disturbed the adolescent, as in extreme depression accompanied by suicide attempts, the more structure and limit setting are needed.

Listening means hearing with all the faculties: sight and sound. One "listens to behavior" by paying close attention to *what* is said and *how* it is said. The nurse asks, "Do the adolescent's voice and body movement match the tone of the words?"

Case Example

Barbara, 14 years old, is asked to perform a sentence completion task during an evaluation visit. She slumps down in the chair, pulls her coat up around her ears, and looks down at the floor. In response to the statement, "Put words to your feelings," she replies, "There are days life just doesn't seem worth it."

Barbara's behavior and the words she uses to describe her feelings are congruent. In listening with the "third ear" one convinces the adolescent that he is being heard.

Remembering that adolescents are curious and eager to learn, especially about themselves, may help the nurse to get through times when the adolescent teases, tests, argues, and complains about the nursing care.

A contract can be drawn up in written form that spells out the purpose of the meeting and the specific goals that both hope to achieve by the end of the agreed upon number of visits. The contract is a vehicle through which the adolescent and the nurse can mutually agree upon needs and expectations. With the adolescent whose life space is rapidly changing and whose intellectual capabilities are increasing, the contract provides both a structured focus of attention and an avenue through which a relationship can be established that has built-in limits and expectations. Adolescents express a desire not only for structure but also for reliable information. Providing the structure, setting the limits, and supplying information can serve to reduce anxiety associated with whatever disruption has occurred in the healthy development of the adolescent.

The nurse helps the adolescent and the family plan for termination by setting goals, establishing a target date for the accomplishment of the goals, and ending the relationship when either the stated goals have been achieved or the target date has been reached. Like the adolescent, the nurse can expect to feel sadness or loss when the relationship is terminated. Such feelings help the nurse know that a relationship has been established in which an emotional closeness was achieved while specific goals were accomplished.

NURSING PROCESS
Assessment

✦ *Physical dimension.* The early phase of adolescent development is often referred to as *pubescence* and is marked by physical changes in the nurse such as skeletal growth, enlargement of the testes, appearance of straight pigmented pubic hair, and early voice changes. This stage is followed by ejaculation; kinky, pigmented pubic hair; maximal annual physical growth; the appearance of downy facial hair and axillary hair; and finally, voice changes, coarse, pigmented facial hair, and chest hair.[45] Although the age at which each of the body changes appears varies, the appearance of body changes is taken to represent the initial stages of adolescent development, and the sequential, orderly process of physical change is expected to be complete by the late teens or early twenties. Adolescent girls also undergo a similar orderly process of physical change: skeletal growth; breast development; and straight, pigmented pubic hair followed by maximal annual growth increment; kinky, pigmented pubic hair; menstruation; and the appearance of axillary hair.

Adolescents, particularly boys, express anxiety as well as curiosity about sexual development. For example, masturbation, a minor interest in latent years, now increases. Although masturbation appears to be more prevalent in boys than girls, such activity is normal unless it is excessive, prohibits physical and social relations with others, or results in excessive guilt. Curiosity, experimentation, tension reduction, and pleasure all contribute to the adolescent's enhanced interest in sexual development. Discussion of penis size or breast development is common, with attempts made to equate virility and attractiveness with physical size and appearance.

Although adolescents are prone to comparing, rigid norms for physical development are difficult to establish because of the wide range of individual differences in development. This variability makes it difficult for the adolescent who develops earlier or later than his peers.

Irrespective of the wide range of development, the nurse notes the adolescent's height, weight, system development, sexual development (breast buds, genital development, onset of menses), skin changes, and any anomalies that may have been previously undetected. Rapid growth may result in orthopedic problems, and absence of growth may signal endocrine deficits. A thorough family history of parents and siblings is needed to establish the family norm for growth and development. Conducting a physical examination provides the nurse an opportunity to explore adolescent concerns about sexuality, school problems, peer pressure, or family difficulties.

In addition to history taking and physical examination, the adolescent is asked to provide information regarding a typical day. The day is described in detail for a 24-hour cycle, including number of hours slept, soundness of sleep, time of rising, breakfast, morning activities, after-school activities, return home, supper, evening activities (family, school, church), friends visited, games attended, and bedtime and associated activities such as bathing. One may need to compile activities of several days before a representative day is profiled. This information gives the nurse an overall picture of the physical health practices in which the adolescent engages. Alterations in patterns from what the nurse considers normal need to be investigated more fully.

The patterns that emerge in the typical day of the adolescent are diagnostic in their deviation from the norm.

Sleep patterns differ from the norm in the depressed or anxious adolescent who reports uneasy sleep and early awakening. Eating patterns and meal habits often become bizarre, for example, in the girl with anorexia nervosa or bulimia (see Chapter 35). Activity patterns are useful in diagnosing the socially withdrawn, isolated, or shy adolescent and the adolescent who is abusing drugs or alcohol. The adolescent uses drugs and alcohol for reasons such as experimentation, boredom, curiosity, and most frequently peer pressure. The adolescent is often first introduced to drugs and alcohol by an older sibling, parent, or older peer. Many adolescents use drugs and alcohol infrequently as a form of relaxation, occasionally for experimentation, or at parties. When drugs are used in excess, school performance, social relations, and family life are often harmed. The adolescent engaging in substance abuse generally appears disinterested, lethargic, easily distracted, irritable, and moody. School performance and social relations hit highs and lows in relation to periods of substance abuse. Addiction to drugs or heavy reliance on alcohol may result in the adolescent's becoming abusive, hostile, and difficult to manage. The adolescent who abuses drugs and alcohol may engage in impulsive and self-destructive behavior and often draws attention to himself through such acts.

The nurse asks, "To what extent do the habits and patterns represented by this adolescent's typical day seem to promote health, and to what extent do these patterns seem to reflect deviations from health?" Patterns that reflect deviations often appear disorganized, are difficult to chart, and may vary widely. On the other hand, healthy patterns, although varying from day to day, present an overall consistent picture with a balance between sleep and exercise, eating, eliminating, and use of leisure time.

Therefore in assessing the physical dimension the nurse determines whether and to what extent the particular adolescent falls within the normal range of development; where the adolescent is within the sequential development of body changes; to what extent sexuality (masturbation, ejaculation, menstruation) is a concern; to what extent chronic health problems such as juvenile diabetes are affected by the onset of adolescence; to what extent physical changes or patterns are accompanied by alterations in mood; and to what extent overall patterns seem to promote and support healthy physical development.

Emotional dimension. Emotionally, adolescence is a time of highs and lows. One day the adolescent may be happy and outgoing. Within a matter of hours the adolescent may be crying and worried that he has no friends and is understood by no one. One moment the adolescent may feel good about himself and the next moment may express self-doubt and lack of self-confidence. The adolescent exists within a whirlwind of emotional change and unpredictability, particularly in the early phases of development from 12 to 15 years. After that time the emotions seem to even out, the adolescent can be more trusting of his feelings, and the periods of unpredictability are spaced farther apart.

The physical aspects of adolescent development are

difficult to fully separate from the emotional aspects because much of the emotional development is linked with physical and sexual changes. Body image, concern for physical appearance, ability to attract the opposite sex, and sensing oneself as appealing is integral to the adolescent's acceptance of himself as attractive (Figure 41-1). Skin blemishes, uncoordinated body movements, and physiological functions that are unpredictable and beyond conscious control, such as erections or menstruation, induce anxiety. While the adolescent is struggling with emotional control, the body's demands require energy; the adolescent responds to physical changes with fear and anxiety. Anxiety can take many forms ranging from an occasional sleepless night to excessive thinking and worrying about not only real problems but also fantasized ones. Anxiety often occurs around individual lags or extreme variations in growth and development. A year or two in the life of adults is a small segment of time; however, the same 2 years can seem much more important to adolescents, who may be worried and confused about their development. The adolescent often asks the question, "Am I normal?" Fears of not being normal, especially related to sexuality, can lead to feelings of anxiety and to acting out.

Emotional instability is indicated by a number of symptoms: inability to sleep; disrupted eating patterns (too much or too little); altered relations with friends and peers, especially withdrawal; increasing and unexplained conflict with family members; preoccupation with body functions; abrupt and unexplained mood swings; and inability to gain control over impulses. The degree to which such changes are present indicates the severity of the

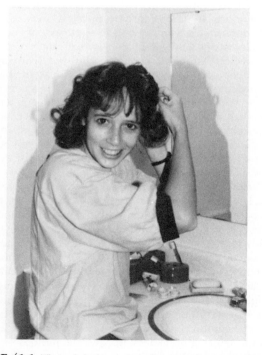

FIGURE 41-1 The adolescent spends many hours in front of the mirror making herself physically attractive.

emotional problem. For example, inability to sleep may indicate stress associated with an impending examination. When combined with other symptoms an underlying depression may be suspected.

Clinical depression in the adolescent can manifest itself in a number of ways:

1. Withdrawal
2. Acting out
3. Angry outbursts
4. School problems
5. Sexual difficulties
6. Running away
7. Inability to pay attention
8. Flat affect
9. Lack of hope
10. Poor self-regard
11. Negative attitude
12. Loss of interest in usual activities
13. Changes in physical appearance
14. Mood changes
15. Appetite changes
16. Marked decrease or sudden increase in physical or social activities
17. Unpredictable patterns of behavior

In cases in which depression is related to a specific event such as the death of a parent, it is generally considered a transitory adjustment problem in which the adolescent may experience unhappiness, tearfulness, nervousness, irritability, and perhaps even school problems. Such depression generally occurs from 3 to 9 months after the specific event and does not result in significant changes in family or social relationships.

Depression may also occur without any apparent link to a specific event, in which case a chronic pattern of low self-esteem, feelings of worthlessness, and a pervasive sense of failure may be triggered by some minor and unrelated situation. This type of depression manifests itself in sleeplessness, loss of appetite, lack of interest in physical appearance, decreased productivity at home and school, and feelings of hopelessness and may result in excessive use of alcohol or drugs or attempts at suicide.

An anxious adolescent may experience some of the same symptoms as the depressed adolescent, such as distractibility, fears about the future, and irritability. However, the anxious adolescent does not experience symptoms to the extent exhibited in depression, does not experience muted or blunted affect, has sleepless nights only occasionally, and generally overcomes the problem in a shorter time.

Like depression, anxiety can result from direct changes in the adolescent's life, such as frequent family moves or parental discord. Anxiety, self-doubt, and identity confusion can also occur unrelated to any specific event. In determining events that may be critical to the appearance of symptoms or changes in the emotional state of adolescents, a 5-year critical incident survey (see the box on p. 793) is helpful. The survey compiles a profile of information regarding critical incidents or events, such as death of a grandparent, divorce of parents, or severe physical illness, that may require emotional adaptation and coping and determines the extent to which these events preceded the onset of symptoms or problems. Symptoms and the onset of problems can occur anywhere from 3 months to 2 years after such events. The survey can be taken of the adolescent and of family members, since often the adolescent may not fully remember all events.

What differentiates the emotionally anxious from the more severely troubled adolescent is the degree of change in overall functioning, including perception of and reaction to reality. Adolescence has been described as a time of "natural craziness," when acting out and weirdness are accepted as typical teen behavior. However, when acting out occurs in more than transitory periods or when anxiety severely impedes the ability to function socially, academically, or in terms of personal care, the degree of disturbance is greater than typical teen behavior.

Assessment of the emotional dimension of the adolescent involves development of an overall profile of emotional development. In regard to suspected emotional problems such as anxiety, angry and hostile behavior, or depression accompanied by feelings of worthlessness and hopelessness, the nurse needs to determine the extent of the impairment and to assess the relationship between specific events that have occurred and the kinds of problems that the adolescent is experiencing.

✳ *Intellectual dimension.* Projection of one's own internal state onto others is probably never as prevalent as during adolescence. Adolescents find it difficult to trust others primarily because they do not trust or understand their own feelings. Because of this lack of trust and certainty, adolescents often project onto others a lack of understanding. "You don't understand me" is often a camouflaged way of saying that "I don't really understand myself; therefore how could you possibly understand me?" Just as uncertainty is associated with feeling states, actions that stem from these feelings are often considered by the adolescent to be unpredictable. The adolescent expressing his anger will say, "If I told my old man what I really thought, he'd knock my block off." Although the adolescent may be correctly predicting his father's response, a greater probability is that the adolescent fears that he himself will lose control, and he reads this possibility into his father's behavior. Intellectually, the adolescent is developing an increasing ability to think abstractly, to reason, and to understand at higher levels. Such heightened intellectual capabilities are competing with intense and distracting physical and emotional changes. The early years of adolescence are particularly troublesome in that the great surges of physical growth and sexual development and the increasing awareness of the self as a separate entity seem to develop simultaneously. The adolescent's energies are divided among the various facets of personality development. However, as adolescence progresses, the ability to think critically, to reason rationally, to probe into unknown areas, and to engage in intellectual and philosophical debates increases. The vigorous debates in which adolescents engage often seem pointless to the adult because of the adolescent's preoccupation with the debates themselves and overall lack of concern for any direct action based on the outcome of the debates. This is a time of asking, "Why doesn't someone do something about the poor . . . the disabled . . . the elderly . . . foreign countries?" while saying, "I don't know why we have to go to Grandmother's house every Sunday. There isn't anything to do there." The adolescent is usually better able to cope with personal inconsistencies in behavior and thinking than are adults, primarily because adolescents cope with such inconsistencies by ignoring them. When an adult focuses attention on these inconsistencies, heated arguments tend to occur.

The best gauge of intellectual functioning of the adolescent, despite the ups and downs in performance, is the overall academic record. One also needs to consider the home environment, the cultural background, and the role models available to the adolescent. However, despite individual differences, the adolescent's grade point average, motivation, achievement, and classroom performance are often indicators not only of intelligence but also of emotional states. The troubled adolescent often signals a need by altering his patterns of classroom behavior, acting out, picking fights, being tardy, demonstrating a loss of interest, and achieving lower grades.

Alterations in classroom behavior do not always signal acute or chronic episodes of mental illness; however, this is a critical time when previously undetected problems may become manifest. Classroom performance can signal a number of other problems, including use and abuse of alcohol or drugs; family problems; personal adjustment problems; fears or concerns about pregnancy, impotence, or venereal disease; unresolved grief process; or simply

---

FIVE-YEAR CRITICAL INCIDENT SURVEY

INSTRUCTIONS

Try to recall the important things that happened to you or your family at 5-year intervals. Which events stand out in your mind as being the most significant? What do you remember most about these incidents?

STAGES

Birth to 5 years:

6 to 10 years:

11 to 15 years:

16 to 20 years:

PROBLEM

What is the relationship between the events or series of events and emotional problems that have developed? Did emotional problems appear within 3 months to 2 years of any one event?

concerns about and uncertainty regarding the future. Whatever the source of the problem, classroom behavior is a critical signal that needs to be investigated further through observations and interviews with the adolescent, the family, and, when appropriate, school personnel and peers. Peers and peer group relations can provide valuable information about the adolescent. Changes in classroom behavior may be accompanied by changes in social relationships. Since the social clique often provides the adolescent with a sense of support and a testing ground for reality, any changes in these relationships need to be viewed with concern.

✼ *Social dimension.* One of the more prevalent problems encountered in adolescence is the inability to find an answer to the question, "Who am I?" The adolescent experiencing an identity crisis or conflict has not been able to find a sense of self and experiences much uncertainty about future goals, friendships, sexual orientation, and spiritual beliefs. This adolescent may express a desire to pursue goals but is unable to undertake direct actions to achieve those goals.

Following are questions nurses may use to confront adolescents experiencing identity problems:

What are your fantasies about yourself?

Where do you see yourself in 5 years?

If you could be anything or anyone, who would you be and what would you be doing?

Power struggles with parents and other authority figures are an outgrowth of the search for identity, a need to test and experiment with the limits of power. In an attempt to experience themselves as adults or nearly adults, adolescents often overstep the limits of their own ability. The obedient, cooperative adolescent may become a rebellious, argumentative, disobedient person who refuses to abide by curfews, insists on driving at breakneck speeds, and loses any and all interest in being part of the family, particularly refusing to engage in family activities. Family life and the interactions between the adolescent and family members play a significant part in the adolescent's development of autonomy, independence, self-esteem, and ability to communicate consistently and congruently outside the family. Disturbance in these relationships and inability to get along with or feel understood by parents can both contribute to and be factors in the adolescent's peer relations. Alterations in peer relations, running away, aggressive and hostile acts, and symptoms of anxiety and depression can be the outcome of parent-child conflict.

Parent-child conflict appears to be more prevalent in families with economic problems, marital discord, chronic physical health problems, inadequate sexual identities, and poor communication skills. Parent-child conflict can be minor (disagreements, irritability, and lack of communication) or more severe (angry outbursts, loud screaming matches, failure to communicate, unreasonable and restrictive discipline measures, and physical or emotional abuse).

Increasing conflict often erupts between the adolescent and younger siblings who are suddenly a source of embarrassment and a constant reminder of that which the adolescent has just experienced (childhood). Sibling rivalry during the adolescent years can be intense and severe. At the same time, the adolescent can be loyal and supportive. Many of the adolescent's feelings of uncertainty are vented on siblings, yet rarely with the awareness of or intent to do harm.

Adolescents are often ambivalent about intimacy, wanting to be close but fearing the loss of self. Adolescents frequently feel engulfed by their own emotional intensity but generally project the feeling of engulfment onto others, particularly close friends or members of the opposite sex. The need to nurture and be nurtured is strong in the adolescent; however, the fear of commitment and being "tied down" that accompany such feelings is also strong. Unable to work out a balance, the adolescent may engage in excessive sexual activity or may become socially withdrawn. Acting out or promiscuity is often evidence of strong, unmet emotional needs, just as shyness and social isolation can be evidence of the same unmet needs.

Acting out is usually characterized in the early stages by conflict at school, for example, minor and repeated infractions of rules that result in the student's being sent to the principal or having to serve detentions, and by conflict with parents, usually resulting in fights over curfews or minor scrapes with community authority figures. At this stage the adolescent is generally considered to be engaging in antisocial behavior by minor infractions of social and family norms. The adolescent may progress from the antisocial stage of acting out to repeated and more severe forms of rule breaking such as shoplifting, drinking excessively, driving at excessive speeds, street fights, or burglary.

Adolescents who engage in repeated patterns of breaking social and legal rules are often manipulative, distort the truth, run in gangs, create problems with peers, and become hostile and aggressive when confronted by authority figures. Without help, these adolescents become chronic rule breakers and difficult to reach. In later years they may engage in more serious rule breaking and criminal behavior.

In the early stages this behavior is often an attempt to signal the need for professional help either for the adolescent or for the family. More and more courts are assigning these adolescents and their families to therapy early in the process to prevent the acting-out, antisocial behavior from becoming a more severe conduct disorder.

The adolescent does not have a fully developed sense of consequences. Without life experiences to fall back on, the adolescent engages in behavior that often seems dangerous and self-defeating, for example, having sex without birth control, driving down a main highway with the lights of the car turned off, and refusing to take examinations because "tests are all stupid anyway." Most adolescents engage in some risky behavior, but the adolescent who consistently engages in such behaviors is not only experiencing the whirlwind of emotional turmoil but also losing control of it. The adolescent who is constantly engaging in dangerous and self-destructive behavior is asking for help to cope with changes that have gone beyond his ability to manage.

Case Example

Charlie is 15 years old. For his birthday his parents gave him a motor bike, which he has used to jump ditches and drive down railroad tracks.

Charlie is having trouble accepting the responsibility of the motorbike but is asking for help in controlling his behavior. In essence he says, "I'm a gambler. I'm out to see if I can beat life at its own game." Charlie has an unrealistic and self-destructive need to pit himself against powerful forces, probably hoping that someone will stop him and set the limits that he cannot set for himself.

Loneliness (see the Research Highlight below), fear of intimacy, and the strong need for comfort can lead to a number of problems, including obesity from oral attempts to be self-nurturing; sexual promiscuity in which sexual behavior is used to attain closeness; delinquency in a social attempt to gain recognition; and conflicts with authorities in an attempt to gain attention and even acceptance. Erikson says that a boy prefers to be a bad boy than no boy at all. By this he means that an adolescent seeks to establish an identity, even a negative identity, rather than having to think he is like no one at all, unnoticed and unrecognized. Lack of recognition and notice is often equated with lack of love by adolescents. Without recognition and the emotional support that comes with notice, the adolescent has a difficult time developing a positive, self-accepting identity.

The adolescent strives for a competent and stable sense of self. Through such development the adolescent experiences a wide range of feelings, on one hand, believing he is able, strong, and competent and, on the other hand, believing he is powerless, helpless, and vulnerable.

The adolescent strives to achieve balance among a number of competing forces, including physical change and emotional upheaval, identity development with internal fears of rejection, a need for autonomy, and a sense of closeness. When the balance is achievable and reachable, the adolescent often maneuvers successfully toward a competent sense of self. When this is not possible, emotional problems may result.

One of the tasks facing the adolescent is the transition from family group to peer group, during which the adolescent strives for autonomy and a sense of individual freedom. This striving for individuality is a concern on one level; on another level, adolescents want very much to be like their peers. An 18-year-old client expressed such concern by saying, "All my parents ever wanted for me was to be different. All I ever wanted was to be just like my friends." However, while striving for autonomy and associated freedom, the adolescent struggles with the need to be dependent on others. Following is a typical interview:

Client: My parents never give me any responsibility. I don't know how my parents expect me to make any decisions. I don't have any experience. (Pause.) *My parents don't trust me.*

Nurse: What have you done to make them feel that way?

Client: Nothing. (Pause.) *I got drunk and wrecked the family car, but that was 2 months ago.*

Research Highlight

Developmental Changes and Loneliness During Adolescence

N.E. Mahon

PURPOSE

The purpose of this study was to determine whether youngsters in the early adolescent phase of development have higher levels of loneliness than those in the middle or late phase.

SAMPLE

Subjects consisted of 470 volunteer students from three settings: 209 from an urban college, 179 from an urban high school, and 82 from an urban junior high school. Mean ages for students were 20.5 years for college students, 15.5 years for high school students, and 13.1 years for junior high school students.

METHODOLOGY

The revised UCLA Loneliness Scale and a general information sheet were used. Participants indicated on the general information sheet that they were free from anxiety and depression.

FINDINGS

Significant differences were found in mean loneliness scales, with early adolescents scoring higher in loneliness than middle or late adolescents. Thirteen-year-old girls were found lonelier than any other age group. This age group is thought to be particularly vulnerable because in this phase of development, detachment from parents is expected and identification with a peer group becomes important.

IMPLICATIONS

Since loneliness appears to be a significant problem among adolescents, nurses need an understanding of the behavioral and affective manifestations of loneliness in order to assess its presence. Knowledge of developmental trends and the experience of loneliness during adolescence can be used in planning nursing care for adolescents and parents.

Based on data from Topics in Clinical Nursing 5(1):66, 1983.

The nurse needs to ask the question, "How autonomous can an adolescent realistically hope to be, given the particular individual ability and set of circumstances in which the adolescent lives?" One observation the nurse needs to make is of the family atmosphere regarding individual independence.

Case Example

The Johnson family have brought their 16-year-old daughter, Jennifer, for counseling, expressing their concern that she is not demonstrating the "independence" required of her to go to college in 2 years. Jenny is the youngest of three children (two older brothers) of parents in their mid-fifties. The parents' expressed concern is that Jenny needs to gain and demonstrate independence at home and in her social life to show that she is dependable before she can earn privileges. However, observations of and sessions with the family reveal a conflict. When Jenny asks to date, her father refuses because the "boy is too old." When Jenny wants to go shopping to buy a dress for the school dance, her mother tells her she is "too young to be picking out her own clothes." When Jenny goes out after a football game on Friday night and doesn't come home until 1 AM (curfew is midnight), an older brother calls home from college the next day to ask Jenny how she could be so "inconsiderate" and "worry" their parents.

Although the parents express concern that Jenny lacks independence and that she cannot be trusted, their unexpressed fear is that she will become too independent, too self-sufficient. Their inconsistency acts as a barrier to her attaining independence. The parents say that they want Jenny to grow up; however, they are highly invested in keeping her a little girl. Both parents are indirectly threatened by Jenny's increasing independence and undermine her every attempt to successfully break away from their domination.

In assessing the adolescent's striving for independence, the nurse examines the emotional tenor in the family. She looks for warmth, authentic expression of feelings, honest exchange and communication, unconditional positive regard for one another, a physical expression of affection, expectations appropriate for age and experience, encouragement and support for individual aims, and support of conflict in allowing and providing for disagreement and argument. Especially important is the congruence of communication, that is, a consistent pattern in which what is said is congruent with what is done and in which underlying messages are brought out in talk and action.

Within the peer group the adolescent practices being independent and works to resolve the quest for freedom with the need for intimacy. The peer group serves as an important testing ground. In a sense the peer group becomes a subculture. Members of the peer group compete, tease, and test one another. But they also share their confusion and fear associated with breaking away. The adolescent is extremely loyal and expects a sense of justice in the peer group.

An adolescent reared in an open family will have a greater opportunity to seek and establish an individual identity than will an adolescent reared in a rule-dominated family. The warm, supportive, accepting family will tend to foster adolescent development that is outgoing, socially active, and independent, whereas the rule-dominated authoritarian family will tend to produce adolescents who lack self-confidence, experience low self-esteem, and express themselves in rebellious ways.[44] Rebellious behavior, social withdrawal, poor school performance, and overall lack of adjustment may be manifestations of a rigid family atmosphere.

At the other extreme is the family with no rules and little if any interest in the children. Adolescents from such homes may develop strong identities in spite of such indifference but more often are poorly motivated, indifferent to others, confused, and lacking in self-worth. The formation of a positive identity and a sense of autonomy is difficult at best in either a family that is excessively rule oriented or one in which emotional indifference is the norm.

The peer group is a safety net, above which the adolescent can play out the drama of fantasized relationships, can establish intimate and nonintimate relationships, is able to experience the social aspect of the personality, and practices the sexual aspects of personality development.

Adolescents seem to spend an inordinate amount of time with one another, which leads some authors to label this period a time of *pseudohomosexuality* in that adolescents often prefer the company of members of the same sex. The company of one another helps them avoid the anxiety of initiating contact with or having to establish a relationship with a member of the opposite sex. On the other hand, adolescents spend a great amount of time in mixed groups. The pressure is great among adolescents to be sexual partners to justify spending time together, to have a date on Friday night, and to avoid the anxiety of being alone and lonely.

Although a sense of loyalty is great within the peer group, intimate relationships can be transitory and brief; best friends may exchange best friends. Some adolescents can remain friends through such exchanges, others cannot. It is a learning experience in the building and maintaining of relationships.

How adolescents select the peer group within which to build relationships is not well known. Adolescents can be attracted to someone similar to them in terms of family background, religion, and social status, just as they can be attracted to someone from differing family, class, and religious backgrounds. The importance of peer-group relationships is that adolescents have a group with whom they can relate, be with someone they feel understands them, and have someone with whom they can practice testing reality. Without this source of support and reality testing, the adolescent may learn to rely on an untested, internal fantasy world.

Through peer relations, the adolescent is able to examine and explore topics that parents find embarrassing, repulsive, silly, or frightening, such as sex, war, death, and divorce. Whereas parents often assume that adolescents are unaware of and turned off by what goes on around them, adolescents are deeply affected by social and political issues in a way that often influences their outlook on life. No topic is taboo.

The adolescent is intrigued by life and death and may even fantasize what his own death may be like. An adolescent may say that "I'm sure I won't live past 20," and at the time he says it, he probably means it. It is perhaps a subconscious recognition that the person before the age of 20 is not the same person after his twentieth birthday; a certain amount of grief needs to be resolved when one leaves adolescence, just as when one leaves childhood. The peer group also helps in this transition.

The peer group helps establish acceptable norms of behavior, provides an arena for testing new behaviors and exploring old ones, and aids in the development of healthy coping skills in managing the struggle for independence. Of parent conflict around independence, adolescents often say that "It's only a stage your parents are going through. They'll get over it by the time you're a senior." In the "us against them" attitude of the adolescent against the parent, the adolescent when pushed will often choose the friend over the family member. The friend is an extension of the self—the good self and the bad self—and the adolescent will go to great lengths to protect and defend this fragile projection of self.

The adolescent who fails to make the transition in membership from the family group to the adolescent group will experience difficulty separating from family later and may exhibit signs of social isolation and lack so-cial interactive skills. The loner, the adolescent who rejects and is rejected by his peer group, may experience difficulty in later establishing long-term intimate relationships because the "practice time" was lost during the adolescent peer-group experimentation.

Suicide, as well as attempted suicide, is one of the more alarming problems that seems to occur with greater frequency among adolescents (see the Research Highlight below). Fear of failure, pressure to achieve, excessive concern for material gain, lack of acceptance among peers, and parent-child conflict are all factors related to teenage suicide. The three factors that seem to occur with the most frequency are family disorganization and marital discord between parents, family history of emotional disturbance with attempted suicides, and adolescent use and abuse of drugs and alcohol.

The suicidal adolescent may show previous symptoms of disturbance such as poor school performance; drunkenness; or incurring traffic fines, especially for excessive speed or reckless driving. The suicidal adolescent may make an apparently sudden and unexpected attempt at wrecking a car, drinking and driving, or physical recklessness with guns. Or the adolescent may engage in long-term self-destruction such as excessive use of drugs and alcohol, which borders on social suicide but may go undetected until a more drastic step is taken that brings the adolescent the professional help needed.

Research Highlight

Psychological Autopsy of Completed Suicide in Children and Adolescents

M. Shafii, S. Carrigan, J. Whittinghill & A. Derrick

PURPOSE

The purpose of this study was to develop methods for initiating contact and effective follow-up with bereaved family and friends, to explore the psychological factors contributing to completed suicide and to attempt to prevent future suicides in bereaved families and friends by being available for support, education, and referral.

SAMPLE

The sample consisted of families, relatives, friends, and significant others (teachers, counselors, ministers, physicians) of all children and adolescents 19 years of age or younger who committed suicide from January, 1980 to June, 1983 in Louisville, Kentucky. There were 24 cases of suicide during this period with 20 families agreeing to participate in the study.

METHODOLOGY

An initial interview was made after the death of the child or adolescent. The Psychological Profile of Suicide, the Louisville Behavior Checklist, and the Millon Multiaxial Clinical Inventory Questionnaire were administered to obtain data. A control group of friends was used as matched-pair control subjects because of the similarity in age, sex, race, eduction, socioeconomic status, and religious background. Contact was made with the family, friends, relatives, and significant others 1, 2, 3, 6, and 9 months following the suicide.

FINDINGS

There were no significant differences between victims and control regarding broken homes, overcrowded families, large number of children, parental dependence on drugs or alcohol, demanding parents, poor academic performance, being behind age-appropriate grade level, or being a school dropout.

IMPLICATIONS

A close relationship exists between suicidal wishes, threats, attempts, and completed suicide. This study suggests that the "talkers" become the "doers." Suicidal messages from children and adolescents need to be taken seriously to prevent the tragedy of childhood or adolescent suicide, which is rapidly reaching epidemic proportions.

Based on data from The American Journal of Psychiatry **142**:1061, 1985.

TABLE 41-2 Warning signs of suicide

Warning Sign	Example
Change in personality	From studious or withdrawn to the class clown; from an actively participating student to one who drops out of all activities
Sudden mood swings	Persistent ups and downs
Inability to concentrate, apathy	Declining grades, loss of interest in school
Loss of or dramatic change in friends	Dropping friends or becoming so obnoxious that friends drop him
Loss of important person or thing	Parents' divorce or death, remarriage of parent, loss of boyfriend or girlfriend, kicked off team
Feelings of hopelessness	Inability to get pleasure from any activity; loss of interest in appearance, in opposite sex; "what's the use?" attitude
Obsession with death	Suicidal threats, taking big risks, frequent accidents
Completing personal or business affairs	Unusual display of affection or generosity; giving away favorite records or tapes; making a will

Table 41-2 lists the warning signs that may alert the nurse to a possible suicide attempt by an adolescent.

In assessing the social aspect of development, the nurse needs to determine the people with whom the adolescent spends time, the groups to which he belongs, the kind of part-time job at which he works, and the kinds of relationships he has formed outside the family. The nurse is also interested in the following:

1. The extent to which relationships are enduring or transitory
2. The amount and quality of time spent with friends
3. The extent to which the adolescent is sexually active and, if active, the extent to which birth control and venereal disease protection are maintained
4. How active or passive a role the adolescent takes in making friends, keeping friends, and changing relationships
5. The amount of conflict between adolescent and parents regarding friends and social activities in which the adolescent participates
6. The amount of peer pressure that the adolescent feels in terms of social, sexual, and other activities

Spiritual dimension. Spiritually, the adolescent seeks to understand the meaning of life and to use this understanding to develop a framework for approaching present and future decisions. This searching takes many forms, for example, questioning parental beliefs, rejecting institutionalized religion, sampling differing religious beliefs, comparing religious and philosophical beliefs of peers, and examining one's own beliefs. Adolescents often ask the question, "What is life all about anyway?" This age is perhaps the first time in the life cycle that the individual comes to the realization that life is not forever, that humans are mortal, and that, in adolescence, life is beginning to take on a new seriousness.

Because of the fluid state of the adolescent, several opposing and contradictory beliefs can be held simultaneously. The adolescent often states a strong belief, for example, that all people (particularly oneself) should have the right to think and act in a unique and personal way. However, teachers and classroom instructors are often made fun of in a way that reflects intolerance and insensitivity, that is, they are imitated in walk, ridiculed because of outdated dress, and generally dismissed as "stupid" and "old-fashioned." The adolescent strives to develop a belief system by seeing the world in a "me" and "not me" framework. If the situation is one with which the adolescent can identify, then it makes sense. However, if the situation or individual within the situation is doing something with which the adolescent cannot identify, then the situation or person is viewed as irrelevant. This results from the adolescent's lack of life experience and underdeveloped ability to see any position other than his own. Empathy and a view of the world that includes the other person's perspective come after many years of life experiences.

The adolescent develops philosophical beliefs through trial and error as life experiences are collected. It is the age of the ideal, of heroes, and of perfection. The adolescent looks for the perfect parent, mate, class, friend, religion, and sense of self. It is a time of periodic disappointment when the perfect friend, parent, or hero is discovered to make mistakes, to not always agree with what the adolescent thinks or believes, or in some way to do something to make the adolescent feel let down. The adolescent may respond to such recognition of human fallibility with transitory disappointment, in which case other heros are found and other ideals sought. On the other hand, the adolescent may react with confusion, bitterness, despair, and caution about finding replacements.

The adolescent is often confused by the inconsistencies in the behavior of others, particularly when this behavior is an outgrowth of an underlying value, such as the parent who espouses honesty and intentionally fails to report income for tax purposes, the coach who instructs players in fairness and then pushes them to win at all costs, or the teacher who talks about equality but selects only a few favored students for recognition. The adolescent holds loyalty, fairness, and honesty as important and looks for examples of how to implement these qualities in daily practice.

Most adults in the adolescent's environment become fair game to use as examples. Parents' lifelong beliefs and practices are questioned and tested, as are the spiritual beliefs with which the adolescent has been reared. Part of the examination often results in temporary rejection of such beliefs, and the adolescent practices this rejection by attending services less often and questioning parental commitment to such practices. In later years the belief system of many adolescents will come to be very similar to that of their parents despite protests and early rejections.

At the same time that the adolescent is challenging, testing, and perhaps even rejecting social and religious norms, he holds firmly to a moral and peer-oriented code that guides behavior. This code can be identified as the nurse presents the adolescent with a set of hypothetical situations that are social, family, or peer oriented but that require a set of values and beliefs to arrive at a solution, as in the following examples:

1. Allen is a 13-year-old boy who has been caught shoplifting. Should he (a) be kicked out of school, (b) be grounded for 6 weeks, (c) be lectured by his parents, or (d) be turned over to the police to let them handle it? What is the most important aspect of this solution?
2. Tony is a 15-year-old boy who has been smoking marijuana on the school grounds. Would you (a) ignore his behavior, (b) report it to the principal or a teacher, (c) tell his older brother, (d) keep your mouth shut, or (3) smoke marijuana along with Tony? How did you make your decision?
3. Ann is 14 years old and is going steady with Butch, a senior in high school. He wants her to "go all the way" with him. If she refuses, Butch tells her he will find someone else. Should Ann (a) have sex with Butch, (b) tell Butch no and accept the consequences, (c) get Butch's best friend to reason with him, or (d) ignore the situation and hope that Butch forgets about it? Why?

In listening to the adolescent's response to situations involving shoplifting, substance abuse, and sexual behavior the nurse assesses the guiding belief or set of beliefs that compels the adolescent to select a particular option, the primary values that the adolescent is trying to uphold by acting in certain ways, and the compromises the adolescent is forced to make when the options are limited. An adolescent with strong religious beliefs about birth control and sex outside marriage may feel forced to choose between such beliefs and the strong need for intimacy and physical closeness. The same adolescent who later becomes pregnant may be forced to choose again between the value that says that life must be preserved and the value that is critical of the unwed mother.

The nurse assesses themes of fairness, honesty, loyalty, sanctity of family, authority of parents, and peer pressure (resistance or acceptance) that appear and reappear in the solutions that the adolescent chooses. An adolescent's ability to resist peer pressure is often based on a set of beliefs and convictions that operate despite such pressure. It is frequently a conviction that has been debated, argued, challenged, and perhaps once rejected but finally accepted as workable. An adolescent who believes in "a healthy mind in a healthy body" may be able to resist peer pressure to experiment with mind-altering drugs and alcohol not only to maintain good physical condition but also to remain consistent with beliefs.

Another mechanism for eliciting philosophical beliefs that guide the adolescent is to present the adolescent with a set of statements such as the following and ask the adolescent to agree or disagree:

1. People are primarily responsible for what happens to them.
2. People can achieve anything if they try hard enough.
3. A person's destiny is determined at birth, and nothing can be done about it.
4. Adolescents should be under the control and direction of their parents as long as they live in the parents' home.
5. Death is not a finality but a transformation of energy from one state to another.

Responses to such statements reveal underlying beliefs that guide the adolescent and give the nurse some indication of how much control the adolescent believes he has over life in general. Whereas adolescents experience a sense of uncertainty about the future and may even experience an occasional anxiety attack, the healthy adolescent maintains control over and believes he has some direction in his future, real or fantasized.

The nurse is interested in assessing that which the adolescent holds to be important, how the adolescent implements his belief system in setting priorities, how similar the adolescent's ideas and values are to those of the peer group, and how his beliefs contribute to overall functioning. Despite fluidity in thinking and expansion of personal and social space, the healthy adolescent works at developing consistent beliefs and practices. Regardless of his criticism of others, the adolescent maintains a sense of fairness, loyalty, honesty, and inner direction concerning present and future goals and is able to tolerate change in these goals. The unhealthy adolescent often cannot articulate a set of beliefs or has such a rigid set of beliefs that any change results in major emotional and social upsets.

The holistic assessment tool, pp. 800-801, contains assessment information specific for adolescents. It is to be used in conjunction with the assessment tool in Chapter 8.

Analysis

Nursing diagnosis. The following list provides examples of NANDA-accepted nursing diagnoses with causative statements.

1. Anxiety related to underdeveloped body
2. Ineffective coping related to abuse of alcohol
3. Ineffective coping related to depression associated with feelings of worthlessness
4. Grieving related to loss of grandmother

HOLISTIC ASSESSMENT TOOL FOR ADOLESCENTS

PHYSICAL DIMENSION

Genetic History

Who in your family has had any of the following mental or emotional illnesses?
Depression
Suicide
Drug addition
Schizophrenia

Health History

What illnesses, injuries, hospitalizations, or surgeries have you had?

Growth and Development History

Describe your physical growth.
Describe your sexual growth.
Tell me about your experiences in kindergarten, elementary school, high school, college or work.

Activities of Daily Living

Describe your typical day beginning with when you get up in the morning and moving through the day until you go to bed at night.

Diet and Elimination

What changes in your appetite and weight have occurred and over what period of time?
What problems are you having with elimination?

Exercise and Activity

What kinds of activities do you participate in? how often? for how long?
What kind of exercise do you participate in? how often? for how long?

Sleep and Rest

How many hours of sleep do you get? Is it adequate?
What difficulties do you have going to sleep or staying asleep?

Tobacco, Drugs, Alcohol

How much do you smoke?
What drugs or medications do you take?
How much alcohol do you drink? What kinds of alcohol?
In what ways do drugs or alcohol interfere with your daily activities?

Leisure Activities

What do you do for fun and recreation?

General Appearance

The nurse notes any unusual physical characteristics, the style of dress, grooming, gait and posture, and general behavior.

Body Image

Describe yourself physically.
What do you think about your body?
How do you feel about your body?
Do you see yourself as normal?
What would you change about your body if you could?

Sexuality

What are you worries, concerns about your sexual self?
What problems are you having with menstruation, birth control, erections, intercourse, or masturbation?
What is your sexual preference?

EMOTIONAL DIMENSION

Affect

What is the adolescent's affect?
How appropriate is his affect to the situation?

Mood

What is your predominant mood?
Does he have mood swings?
How well do you control your emotions?
How well does he express his feelings?
What are your fears and anxieties?
Are you depressed, suicidal, angry?
Do you feel hopeless?
What are your coping skills?

INTELLECTUAL DIMENSION

Sensation and Perception

Do you see, hear, feel, smell, or taste things that others do not?
Do you believe that your actions are outside your control?
How realistically does he perceive events and situations?

Memory

Immediate

Ask adolescent to repeat a question you asked

Recent

Ask for events leading up to the adolescent's seeking help.

Remote

Ask for descriptions of events in the adolescent's early childhood.

Cognition

Is the adolescent oriented to time, place, person?
What is his knowledge of current events?
How well is he functioning academically?

Judgment

How does the adolescent make decisions?

Insight

Does the adolescent recognize that he is ill and needs help?
How much does he blame others for his difficulties?
How much awareness does he have of the impact of his behavior on others?

Abstract Thinking

What is the adolescent's style of thinking, concrete or abstract?

Attention

What is the adolescent's ability to listen and concentrate?

Communication

What is the rate of speech?
What is the tone of speech?
Does the adolescent have any speech impediments?
Is he verbally active?
Does he respond freely to questions?
Are his responses relevant?

HOLISTIC ASSESSMENT TOOL FOR ADOLESCENTS—cont'd

How well are his thoughts organized?

Does he demonstrate blocking, circumstantially, tangentiality, flight of ideas, loose associations, neologisms?

Flexibility-Rigidity

How open to new ideas and alternatives is the adolescent?

How upset does he get when his routine is disrupted?

SOCIAL DIMENSION
Self-Concept

Describe yourself, including your strengths and limitations.

What kind of person would you like to be?

Interpersonal Relations

Who is your best friend?

How do you get along with your parents, your brothers and sisters, your peers, and people at school, at work, and in the community?

How much time do you spend with your family?

Who is supportive for you?

How do you get along with authority figures?

Cultural Factors

What traditions do you and your family observe?

What conflicts arise from these traditions?

Environmental Factors

What situations or events are stressful for you?

What risk-taking events do you participate in?

Level of Socialization

How conforming or nonconforming is the adolescent?

What evidence is there of legal difficulties?

How well does he accept responsibility?

Trust-Mistrust

How suspicious is the adolescent?

How naive is the adolescent?

Dependence-Independence

What evidence is there of dependence-independence conflicts?

In what areas does the adolescent demonstrate autonomy?

In what areas does he demonstrate dependence?

SPIRITUAL DIMENSION
Philosophy of Life

What is your purpose in life?

What is important about life to you?

Who is your hero?

Sense of Transcendence

Are you an optimist or a pessimist?

Do you think life can be better?

What can you do to make it better?

Concept of Deity

What is your view of God or a higher power?

How similar is it to your parents' or family's view?

How comforting is your relationship with God or a higher power?

Spiritual Fulfillment

What is beautiful to you?

What are your creative abilities?

What do you believe about life and death?

Are you preoccupied with religion?

What conflicts arise from your religious beliefs?

How much do you question or reject your parents' beliefs?

How do you implement your own belief system?

---

5. Potential for violence to self related to anger associated with alienation from parents and peers
6. Alteration in nutrition: more than body requirements related to feeling unloved
7. Alteration in thought processes related to unrealistic body perception
8. Disturbance in self-concept related to low self-esteem
9. Sensory-perceptual alteration related to hearing voices
10. Potential for harming one's self related to overdose of drugs

DSM-III-R diagnoses. The DSM-III-R diagnoses related to pathological conditions in adolescents are listed in the box at right.

The essential features and manifestations of the features of childhood and adolescent oppositional defiant disorders according to the DSM-III-R are listed in the box on p. 802.

DSM-III-R CLASSIFICATIONS RELATED TO ADOLESCENCE

V71.02	Childhood and adolescent antisocial behavior
V62.30	Academic problem
313.81	Oppositional-defiant disorder

From American Psychiatric Association: Diagnostic and statistical manual of mental disorders (DSM-III-R), Washington, D.C., 1987, the Association.

Planning

See Table 41-3 for examples of long-term and short-term goals and outcome criteria related to adolescents. These serve as examples of the planning stage in the nursing process.

313.81 OPPOSITIONAL-DEFIANT DISORDERS

ESSENTIAL FEATURES

The individual demonstrates a pattern of negativistic, hostile, and defiant behavior without the more serious violations of the basic rights of others seen in conduct disorders.

MANIFESTATIONS

Emotional Dimension

Temper outbursts
Anger
Resentfulness
Easily annoyed
Mood lability
Low frustration tolerance

Intellectual Dimension

Swearing
Blaming others

Social Dimension

Argumentative
Defies adult requests
Annoys other people
Low self-esteem
Heavy use of illegal psychoactive substances before the legal age, such as cannabis and alcohol

Adapted from American Psychiatric Association: Diagnostic and Statistical manual of mental disorders (DSM-III-R), Washington, D.C., 1987, The Association.

Implementation

✦ *Physical dimension.* Clinical intervention in the nursing care of the physical needs of adolescents occurs on two levels. One level is to focus on and intervene in the self-care habits of the adolescent that encompass eating, sleeping, exercise, and use of leisure time. The healthy adolescent is notoriously neglectful of self-care habits and often skips breakfasts, eats junk food for lunch, has nachos and soda for snacks, hurries through supper, runs to activities immediately after school, falls asleep late, and rises early. However, eventually the hectic pace catches up, and the adolescent makes adjustment to meet physical needs. The unhealthy adolescent may neglect self-care needs altogether.

On another level, the nurse is interested in physical needs as they relate to emotional factors. The adolescent does not quickly see or understand the relationship between emotional changes and physical responses. For example, in the obese adolescent, intervention strategies are geared toward the adolescent's developing insight into the relationship between emotional factors, such as disappointment, and physical responses, such as overeating and obesity or undereating and anorexia nervosa (see Chapter 35).

On both levels, the adolescent is instructed in specifics such as diet and dietary needs related to individual re-

quirements. When the nurse does not think she is adequately prepared to counsel the adolescent on dietary needs, a nutritionist can be consulted to assist in dietary instruction and planning. Adolescents are instructed in the relationship between physical activity and exercise and in the recognition of internal triggers such as fear, anger, or cravings and allergies that set off physical responses such as destructive eating habits.

Adolescents are also instructed in the recognition of external cues that set off patterns of self-neglect, self-abuse, or self-destructive tendencies. Overeating, going on food binges (bulimia), undereating (anorexia nervosa), anxiety attacks, substance abuse, or periods of depression may stem from externally triggered events or situations. Successful treatment of adolescents who are severely disturbed may include treatment of the family. Treatment for persons who abuse drugs and alcohol is discussed in Chapter 16.

To learn about the interrelationship of physical and external and internal cues, the adolescent is helped to develop self-monitoring skills. These skills include the recognition that stress, fatigue, and physical illness alter the body's need for nurturance and rest.

The adolescent's concern with body image may require help with physical appearance and establishing self-care habits that bolster self-esteem, for example, hair care, oral hygiene, or cleanliness. Discussing sexuality with the adolescent and instructing the adolescent about physical changes associated with development relieves anxiety.

✳ *Emotional dimension.* Through role modeling, the nurse demonstrates and supports attempts to put feelings into words. The nurse may ask the adolescent to "put words to your feelings so that I can understand what is going on inside you." The nurse accepts the adolescent's presentation of self, giving positive recognition for aspects that are appropriate and healthy and ignoring or confronting the adolescent on inconsistent, unhealthy, or inappropriate behavior. In giving positive recognition for healthy and appropriate actions, the nurse can say, "I like the way you stick up for yourself" (exhibiting self-confidence), "I appreciate your admitting that you made a mistake" (presenting self authentically), or "Thank you for coming. I learn something new about you each time you come" (saying by your coming that you think you are an important person).

The adolescent who is experiencing anxiety can be instructed in recognizing early symptoms such as rapid heart rate and in developing a self-monitoring program such as progressive relaxation, in which the adolescent gives himself quieting messages. The adolescent can be taught, after recognizing physical symptoms to find a quiet place and practice relaxing, saying, "I am in control of what happens to me. I can sit here and safely relax. As I breathe deeply, I will let tension and fear slip away from me. I experience calmness, relaxation, and serenity." As the adolescent gains an appreciation for the interplay between mind and body, he gains confidence in being able to control to some extent the interaction. Once physical control is mastered, the adolescent can proceed to gain new insight into underlying emotional factors, for exam-

TABLE 41-3 Long-term and short-term goals and outcome criteria related to the adolescent

Goals	Outcome Criteria

NURSING DIAGNOSIS: ALTERATION IN NUTRITION WITH LESS THAN BODY REQUIREMENTS RELATED TO INABILITY TO COPE WITH PROBLEMS

Long-term goals

To decrease family power struggle.	Alters focus from identified client to family problem.
To enhance individuality among family members.	Family tolerates individual expression of opinion.
	Members take individual actions.
To decrease hostile and dependent behavior by the adolescent.	Adolescent cooperates with the treatment team.
	Adolescent decreases victim role.
To establish healthy communication.	Family and adolescent cease to use adolescent's symptoms to communicate conflict.
To maintain adequate weight.	Adolescent's nutritional intake is sufficient to maintain adequate weight.

Short-term goals

To decrease rapid and destructive weight loss.	Maintains standard weight.
To decrease vomiting after meals.	Does not induce vomiting.

NURSING DIAGNOSIS: POTENTIAL FOR VIOLENCE TO SELF RELATED TO SUICIDE ATTEMPT SECONDARY TO LOSS OF GRANDMOTHER

Long-term goals

To develop positive self-attitude.	Makes positive "I" statements.
To resolve grief work.	Incorporates loss in daily living.
To develop hope for future.	Speaks in future terms with optimism.
To be self-directed.	Takes responsibility for acts.
	Exhibits initiative in decisions.
To accept loss of person as real person.	Does not speak of person in idealized terms.
To decrease apathy, hopelessness, and worthlessness.	Experiences feelings of happiness, joy, sorrow, and anger.
To accept self as separate from family and lost person.	Does not punish self for loss; views self as independent individual.

Short-term goals

To eliminate self-destructive acts.	Does not engage in self-destructive behavior.
To set limits.	Cooperates with regimen.
To convey attitude of acceptance.	Is receptive to approaches by staff members.
To accept feelings.	Expresses feelings to nurse.

ple, fear of death, loss, or separation that triggers anxiety attacks.

When the adolescent is depressed and a suicidal attempt is suspected, a few low-key questions such as "You haven't been yourself lately" or "You've been looking rather sad for the past few weeks. What is bothering you?" may help the adolescent to open up. Quite surprisingly, most suicidal adolescents honestly and openly discuss their thoughts about suicide once they are asked. Often the adolescent is relieved to have someone to talk to about his problems. Understanding and empathy are essential. Statements such as "You have had a lot of disappointments lately" or "Sometimes you wonder if it is worth it to keep struggling" are helpful and communicate understanding.

Hospitalization is necessary when there has been a suicidal attempt. Chapter 15 gives further information on interventions for suicidal clients.

Other interventions for specific emotional responses are found in Chapters 11 to 14.

✳ *Intellectual dimension.* The nurse provides for the intellectual needs of the adolescent who is experiencing a temporary crisis trhough maintaining conti-

nuity with formal learning settings. In cases in which the problem is more severe or extended, the nurse may be involved in providing for and assisting with learning needs.

Tutors, homebound teachers, and special education teachers are available for the hospitalized or homebound adolescent so that the student is able to continue his studies. These personnel are available from 1 or 2 weeks to an entire semester if necessary. Arrangements are made through the school system with either the school psychologist or the special education division at the district level. When the adolescent is hospitalized, the nurse needs to coordinate time for study, tutorial visits, and tests or examinations with the hospital routine to alleviate as much disorder and to promote as much cooperation as possible.

In preparing the tutor for the particular crisis with which the adolescent is coping, the nurse may arrange a conference time for mutual consultation. The nurse may need to educate the tutor about grief and its emotional requirements and impact on learning, about depression and its impact on attention spans, about anorexia nervosa and its effect, about divorce or parental separation and its impact on security and feelings about self, and about general emotional needs that detract from the ability to learn during periods of adolescent adjustment. The nurse may have to attend sessions with the tutor if the adolescent is severely depressed, suicidal, aggressive and hostile, or withdrawn.

Continuing with a program of study is important for the adolescent in terms of educational needs and the anchoring effect that school involvement has on the adolescent's overall adjustment and contact with reality. Attendance or continuing contact with these learning experiences is as important as accomplishing the work associated with such learning.

Length of educational sessions may vary depending on the adolescent's emotional and physical states. Intellectual stimulation needs to be geared to the adolescent's capacity at the given time to ensure some margin of success, especially for the adolescent experiencing an identity disorder. More difficult and complex material can be introduced as emotional problems or crises are resolved.

When the adolescent is seen exhibiting undesirable or inappropriate behavior, the nurse intervenes to alter the behavior. For example, when the adolescent is seen talking to himself, the nurse can say, "Jack, I see you talking to yourself. I'd be willing to listen if you'd like to talk to me." In giving a choice of whether to respond, the nurse not only lets the client know that she sees inappropriate behavior but also lets the adolescent know that he is not alone with his fears and fantasies. The relationship between the nurse and the troubled adolescent becomes an anchoring experience and provides contact with reality. Through the relationship, the adolescent may maintain control over fears and fantasies that contribute to confusion, disorientation, and impede learning.

For the less-disturbed adolescent, the nurse works to maintain previous patterns of learning and assists the adolescent in coping with problems that are contributing to the disruption in learning. The anxious adolescent may need help controlling fear and running-away reactions, the unhappy adolescent may benefit from an altered program of learning that includes insight into events causing the unhappiness, and the adolescent with low self-esteem needs small, achievable steps of success built into the learning program to bolster self-confidence and self-worth. Providing extensive work on developing coping skills enhances the adolescent's sense of self-control. Being able to recognize problems, engaging in work with other adolescents experiencing the same problem, talking about problems, and developing strategies for maintaining self-control are all intervention strategies aimed at bolstering the adolescent's problem-solving ability.

Following are interventions for an adolescent experiencing an academic problem:

1. Encourage and support school attendance.
2. Use positive statements regarding attempts to succeed.
3. Discuss events and situations that impede learning.
4. Recognize efforts to improve school work.
5. Explore with the adolescent thoughts and feelings about individual ability and parent-teacher expectations.

6. Coordinate health needs and goals of the learning environment.
7. Establish reasonable goals and priorities.

✿ *Social dimension.* Clinical intervention strategies that focus on the social needs of the adolescent include helping the adolescent find answers to the question, "Who am I?" The adolescent is encouraged to look for and identify options and to develop an internal sense of alternatives. The depressed or suicidal adolescent often replies to this question with "Nobody." Not only does the adolescent believe he is worthless, he also thinks his options are limited. Clinical strategies are geared toward restructuring the way the adolescent thinks about himself and the alternatives that grow from this restructuring.

In developing a sense of identity, the adolescent often needs assistance with developing a sense of ownership of behavior. For example, when the adolescent experiences anger, he needs to learn to discriminate his anger from the anger of others and to direct his anger in appropriate and productive ways. The adolescent is taught to recognize internal states of fear, sadness, and anger and to take responsibility for actions that stem from these feelings. The adolescent learns to share feelings with others but is often reluctant at first, particularly when the feelings are created by the person with whom the adolescent needs to share negative feelings. The adolescent is reluctant to reveal inner feelings primarily because of confusion in identifying these feelings and a lack of certainty about the outcomes of making the feelings known. Participation in group therapy and other planned peer groups helps the adolescent learn to share his feelings with others in a safe environment.

Confronting the adolescent on the aspects of the self that do not seem healthy or appropriate may include statements such as "I'm not going to let anyone push you around, but I'm not going to let you push anyone around either" (bullying), "We're not going to get anywhere if you just sit there and pout for the entire session" (withdrawing and controlling by silence), or "You say that you want to get better, but your behavior tells me that you would rather stay sick and be taken care of" (needing parenting and noncompliance).

Following are specific interventions for an adolescent experiencing an identity crisis:

1. Explore with the adolescent the question, "Who am I?"
2. Help the adolescent think in future terms:
   a. Where will you be in 5 years?
   b. What do you want to be like?
   c. Who is the ideal you?
   d. Who is the real you?
3. Explore intimacy needs and how best to appropriately meet them.
4. Instruct in recognizing emotional states and actions stemming from them.
5. Discuss sexuality.
6. Build self-esteem by recognizing the positive contribution of the adolescent to the therapy process.
7. Confront and eliminate inappropriate acts and self-degrading remarks.
8. Encourage positive "I" statements.

The adolescent is helped to gain a broadened perspective of himself and to be safe and confident in his abilities. For the adolescent to feel safe and engage in risk taking associated with self-examination, the nurse and staff provide a warm, accepting, and predictable environment. For example, when possible, appointments are made at a regular time on a regular basis with consistent personnel. The plan of care is shared with and made available to the adolescent, who can then know about and prepare for daily activities. As the adolescent explores more and more the internal dimensions of self, such environmental consistencies are internalized by the adolescent as his own.

The nurse promotes ongoing relationships with peers and assists the adolescent to gain independence and autonomy from the family. The nurse-adolescent relationship is often a bridge for the adolescent to maneuver from family to social and peer relationships. As the nurse builds a bridge through communicating with the adolescent, the adolescent observes and practices similar bridge building with peers. As the adolescent experiences himself as an individual and is encouraged by the nurse to experiment with autonomy by making decisions and being independent, he has a basis for moving away from the family system.

Clinical strategies with the adolescent provide social skills that the adolescent lacks. Long-range clinical intervention strategies are aimed at helping the adolescent develop successful and autonomous social relationships. The group exercises are geared toward teaching problem solving, sharing experiences, and developing networks to facilitate the transition from family to peer group relationships.

The adolescent who fails to develop these networks may exhibit acting-out behavior. Following are interventions for an adolescent who is acting out:

1. Encourage the client to elicit feedback from peers regarding the behavior.
2. Teach consequences (social and legal) of the behavior.
3. Instruct on interplay in social situations, internal triggers, and external triggers that prompt or support lack of impulse control.
4. Establish impulse control through a program that positively recognizes attempts and ignores, confronts, or penalizes loss of control.

The withdrawn adolescent may be experiencing a sense of worthlessness and abandonment because of perceived or fantasized losses. If the loss is real, clinical strategies aim toward the realistic interpretation of events and the incorporation of the lost person into the adolescent's life. The adolescent is helped to see the person as real and to avoid any idealization of the person. The adolescent is helped to express feelings of anger, resentment, and helplessness resulting from the person's leaving and from his inability to control life and death. When the loss is fantasized or potential, the adolescent is encouraged to view himself as independent from the other and capable of coping despite threats to integrity.

In addition to establishing a sense of options, encouraging the adolescent to experience and express feelings, and helping him to identify actions that stem from feeling

states, the nurse assists the adolescent in meeting and coping with intimacy needs. The adolescent who has been sexually abused may experience difficulty in establishing close relationships, especially in cases in which the perpetrator was a close family member or someone the adolescent trusted. The sexually or emotionally abused adolescent often thinks that he is to blame and lacks self-confidence in seeing himself as attractive, acceptable, and lovable. "If I am such a good person," one abused adolescent asked, "then why has this horrible thing been done to me?" Placing blame and seeking appropriate peers and adults for intimate relationships are actions the adolescent often learns by trial and error. (See Chapter 36.)

When the adolescent seeks to meet intimacy needs inappropriately, as with staff members, the nurse assumes responsibility for setting limits and letting the adolescent know that staff members are not to be included in the search for relationships even if they are the appropriate age or have the appropriate experience. The nurse may say, "It is important for you to make close friends with your peers. Staff members are here to help you and support you in making friends and in developing close relationships, but they are not here to become a part of an intimate relationship with clients." By so doing, the nurse sets limits and lets the adolescent know that he is safe within the environment and that the nurse is willing to support and assist but not engage in intimate relationships with the adolescent. As the nurse acts as a role model for behavior appropriate to age and sex, the adolescent may imitate and practice healthy ways of interacting.

Spiritual dimension. A crisis in beliefs occurs often in adolescence, and clinical intervention strategies promote normalizing these experiences as much as possible. The adolescent who experiences a crisis in beliefs because of the death of a friend or family member often challenges religion, doubts God, and strikes out at family and friends. The adolescent may say, "If there was a God, he would not let my brother die." Even the adolescent who does not experience severe loss may question religion and doubt God.

The adolescent who believes that family or friends have let him down or disappointed him often confronts and challenges not only deep-seated beliefs but also others' practices. Churchgoing parents who profess sanctity of family and then separate or divorce are often perceived by the adolescent as hypocritical. Inconsistency between professed and practiced beliefs often causes despair, disappointment, and unhappiness. These experiences can lead the adolescent through periods of doubt, skepticism, and lack of trust in institutionalized religion. The deeply disturbed adolescent may incorporate religious symbols into distortions of reality. Clinical strategies assist in separating reality from fantasy.

The nurse recognizes the normalcy of doubting, searching, and denial of belief and facilitates the adolescent's acceptance of questioning as essential to the development of personal values, beliefs, and practices. Adolescents can be philosophical and probing in their search for meaning and are able to raise doubts and questions in the mind of the unprepared adult or nurse. Just as the nurse accepts doubting and questioning on the part of the adolescent, the nurse needs to be prepared to accept similar episodes of doubting in herself.

The nurse encourages the examination of life, its meaning, and the meaning it has for the adolescent and supports the adolescent in doubting and critically examining beliefs without fearing punishment or loss of control. The nurse helps the parents accept such searching as normal and desirable adolescent behavior and not necessarily indicative of rebellion or parental disrespect. Clinical intervention strategies promote the development in the adolescent of a lifelong pattern of questioning that incorporates an acceptable and workable set of spiritual beliefs which meets the needs of the particular adolescent. If the nurse believes she is unprepared or in need of support, religious and spiritual personnel—priests, rabbis, ministers, and pastoral counselors—are available for consultation. Basically, clinical intervention strategies are geared toward assuring the client that thoughts which may be confusing and frightening are normal.

Following are interventions for the adolescent experiencing spiritual distress:

1. Encourage doubting and questioning.
2. Support examination of beliefs.
3. Encourage testing of values.
4. Involve the client in group sessions.
5. Pose questions such as "Why life?"
6. Read and share philosophical writers such as Fromm, Frankl, and Jourard.
7. Discuss relationship of values, beliefs, and practices.
8. Use resources of various religions to examine spiritual beliefs and practices.
9. Examine differences between doubting and having no faith.
10. Discuss the disappointment associated with inconsistencies between stated beliefs and practices of significant others and oneself.

Evaluation

Expected and observed changes in the behavior of the adolescent include demonstrating initiative; taking responsibility for actions; discussing thoughts and feelings without probing on the part of the nurse; identifying and rectifying inconsistencies in communication; taking risks and having positive regard for himself; accepting termination of the clinical relationship; using "I" statements that indicate a more positive self-esteem; participating in ongoing classroom work; being oriented to time, person, and place; being able to distinguish reality from fantasy; establishing contact with peers; being able to question life without undue anxiety; and being able to accept basic uncertainties in daily living and future plans.

The adolescent's progress and successful change reflect the extent to which a successful relationship of trust and collaboration has been established and reflect the appropriate use of intervention strategies.

SPECIFIC TREATMENT MODALITIES

Several treatment modalities can be used in treating the adolescent: (1) group therapy in which the adolescent

shares with other adolescents his concerns through discussions in sessions identified as YES and (2) group therapy in which the adolescent and his peers role-play setting up and solving a problem with feedback from peers (EDIT).

YES are group sessions in which adolescents are asked to think, talk, and exchange ideas and feelings in an atmosphere guided by an experienced and accepting therapist. The groups are designed to convey an attitude that is positive and accepting and to encourage the adolescents' active participation in a group that generally meets 1 to 3 hours a week for 8 to 10 weeks. Membership is open, with members joining along the way, to provide the experience of separation and termination of relationships within the framework of supportive peers. The meetings are held in homes, after school, or in a clinic but are designed to provide a format in which the adolescent can bring up issues, raise questions, seek support, and learn about the dynamics of interpersonal exchanges. The adolescent takes turns with other adolescents in leading the group, suggesting group activities, observing and making comments about the dynamics involved, and participating in exercises geared to teach decision making and conflict resolution. The group generally includes adolescents with a variety of backgrounds and experience, and in various stages of doubt, confusion, fear, and identity development. Positive sharing helps the adolescent experience others as helpful and experience himself as contributing positively toward the growth of others.

Basic rules that guide interaction in the YES groups are (1) each adolescent speaks for himself, (2) each adolescent listens to others and finds a way to let others know that listening is happening, (3) each adolescent gives at least one feedback comment per session, and (4) withdrawing, hostile, or destructive behavior is not accepted. Adolescents examine and discuss loneliness, depression, and divorce and experiment with new ideas. The adolescent learns to make connections between what happens at home and what happens at school and learns the value of peer support and feedback for handling conflict or disagreement. YES goups, named to develop an adolescent's saying YES to life, are uniquely prepared for, co-led by, and carried out by adolescents in various states of emotional and social development. It is one of several treatment modalities geared toward healthy adolescent development.

Another example of a structured learning experience for adolescents is EDIT, which involves the following steps: (1) finding an *e*xample of a situation that the adolescent would like to change or understand, (2) *d*escribing the situation to the group with the peer group asking clarifying questions, (3) having the peer group generate *i*deas about the problem, and (4) the adolescent, with peer help, *t*rying out suggested approaches and solutions through role playing. EDIT is essentially a semistructured role-playing situation in which the adolescent actively participates in describing a problem, seeking solutions, obtaining support from others, and practicing a variety of solutions with feedback from peers. Such activity promotes problem solving while enhancing social networking with peers. The success of the adolescent in the peer experience often ripples into family and school relationships.

BRIEF REVIEW

Adolescence is a time of change. The adolescent experiences great surges of physical development that are accompanied by emotional, social, intellectual, and spiritual changes. In Lewin's terms[37] the life space of the adolescent is expanding and becoming more complex. Throughout the changes, the adolescent experiences fluidity of ideas, attitudes, and emotions. When the changes and developing complexities result in imbalances in health, the adolescent may need the assistance of professional mental health-psychiatric personnel who establish treatment programs and intervention strategies to facilitate the resolution of problems and promote healthy development of the adolescent.

Throughout the treatment modalities, the nurse assists in establishing a warm, supportive, intellectually stimulating, and emotionally honest atmosphere so that the adolescent can question, doubt, rebel, and try out new behaviors while feeling safe and accepted. The nurse sets limits when necessary and encourages the adolescent to establish and maintain self-imposed limits when possible. The relationship the nurse establishes with the adolescent is temporary yet permanent; that is, the nurse conveys to the adolescent, "You belong here, but you may not stay forever." The nurse encourages the reengagement of the adolescent with his peers and supports the adolescent in seeking growth potential outside the therapy process.

Through the establishment of a positive, growth-inducing relationship, the mental health–psychiatric nurse encourages the adolescent to seek uniqueness. The adolescent learns to trust others and finally to rely on himself. The test of the success of the process comes in the adolescent's leaving the relationship; becoming a whole person in contact with and aware of the physical, emotional, intellectual, social, and spiritual dimensions of himself; and recognizing that the unfolding of those dimensions is a lifelong process.

REFERENCES AND SUGGESTED READINGS

1. American Nurses' Association, Division on Psychiatric and Mental Health Nursing Practice: Statement of psychiatric and mental health nursing practice, Kansas City, 1976, The Association.
2. American Psychiatric Association: Diagnostic and statistical manual of psychiatric disorders (DSM-III-R), Washington, D.C., 1987, The Association.
3. Arnold, E.: Preventing adolescent alienation: an interprofessional approach, Lexington, Mass., 1983, Lexington Books.
4. Aten, M., and McAnarney, E.: A behavioral approach to the care of adolescents, St. Louis, 1981, The C.V. Mosby Co.
5. Brooks-Gunn, J., and Peterson, A.: Girls at puberty: biological and psychosocial perspectives, New York, 1983, Plenum Press.
6. Carlson, J., Craft, C., and McGuire, A.: Nursing diagnosis, Philadelphia, 1982, W.B. Saunders Co.
7. Chambers, K.: Management of the child with severe anorexia nervosa: a multidisciplinary approach, Nursing 2:1198, November, 1985.
8. Chilman, C.: Adolescent sexuality in a changing American society: social and psychological perspectives for the human service professions, ed. 2, New York, 1983, John Wiley & Sons.
9. Cleveland, M.: Families and adolescent drug abuse: structural analysis of children's roles, Family Process 20:295, 1981.
9a. Corr, C., and McNeil, J.: Adolescence and death, New York, 1986, Springer Publishing Co.
10. Craft, M.: Preferences of adolescent for information providers, Nursing Research 30:205, 1981.
11. Crawshaw, J.: Anorexia and bulimia, the earliest clues, Patient Care, 19:80, October 1985.
12. DeLongis, A., and others: Relationship of daily hassles, uplifts, and major life events to health status, Health Psychology 1:119, 1982.
13. DiCroce, H.: The role of nursing diagnosis in the care of the hospitalized adolescent and his family. In Carlson, J., Craft, C., and McGuire, A.: Nursing diagnosis, Philadelphia, 1982, W.B. Saunders Co.
14. Erickson, E.H.: Childhood and society, ed. 2, New York, 1964, W.W. Norton & Co., Inc.
15. Evans, J.: Adolescent and preadolescent psychiatry, New York, 1982, Grune & Stratton, Inc.
16. Falley, G., Herbert, F., and Echardt, L.: Handbook of child and adolescent psychiatric emergencies and crises, New York, 1986, Medical Examiners Publishing Co.
17. Frankl, V.: Man's search for meaning, New York, 1969, Washington Square Press.
18. Freud, S.: A general introduction to psychoanalysis, New York, 1953, Permabooks. (Translated by J. Riviers.)
19. Fromm, E.: Man for himself, New York, 1967, Fawcett Publications, Inc.
20. Garfinkel, B.G.: Suicide attempts in children and adolescents, American Journal of Psychiatry 139:1257, 1982.
21. Gordon, M.: Nursing diagnosis process and application, New York, 1982, McGraw-Hill Book Co.
22. Hall, G.: Adolescence, vol. 2, New York, 1916, D. Appleton & Co.
23. Hamilton, J.: Development of interest and enjoyment in adolescence. II. Boredom and psychopathology, Journal of Youth and Adolescence 12(5):363, 1983.
24. Havighurst, R.J.: Developmental tasks and education, New York, 1951, Longmans, Green & Co., Inc.
25. Herskowitz, J., and Rosman, P.: Pediatrics, neurology, psychiatry: common ground, behavioral, cognitive, affective, and physical disorders in children and adolescents, New York, 1982, Macmillan Publishing Co., Inc.
26. Howe, C.: Developmental theory and adolescent sexual behavior, Nurse Practitioner 11:65, February 1986.
27. Howe, J., editor: Nursing care of adolescents, New York, 1980, McGraw-Hill Book Co.
28. Inhelder, B., and Piaget, J.: The growth of logical thinking, New York, 1958, Basic Books, Inc., Publishers. (Translated by A. Parsons and S. Milgram.)
29. Jourard, S.: The transparent self, New York, 1964, Van Nostrand Reinhold Co.
30. Kizziar, J., and Hagedon, J.: Search for acceptance: the adolescent and self-esteem, Chicago, 1979, Nelson-Hall Publishers.
31. Klerman, G.: Suicide and depression among adolescents and young adults, Washington, D.C., 1986, American Psychiatric Association.
32. Lambert, V., and Lambert, C.: The impact of physical illness, and related mental health concepts, Englewood Cliffs, N.J., 1979, Prentice-Hall, Inc.
33. Laufer, M., and Luafer, E.: Adolescence and developmental breakdown: a psychoanalytical view, New Haven, Conn., 1984, Yale University Press.

34. Levenkron, S.: The best little girl in the world, Chicago, 1978, Contemporary Books, Inc.

35. Leveton, E.: Adolescent crisis: family counseling approaches, New York, 1984, Springer Publishing Co.

36. Lewin, K.: Field theory and experiment in social psychology: concepts and methods, American Journal of Sociology **44**:868, 1939.

37. Lewin, K.: Field theory and social sciences, New York. 1951, Harper & Brothers.

38. Lynam, M.: Adolescent communication: understanding its dynamics and fostering its development, Nursing Papers **18**:67, Spring 1986.

39. Mahon, N.: Developmental changes and loneliness during adolescence, Topics in Clinical Nursing **5**(1):66, 1983.

40. Maslow, A.: Motivation and personality, New York, 1954, Harper & Brothers.

41 Mathai, J.: Staff perception of adolescent behavior problems, Journal of Adolescence **8**:243, September 1985.

42. Matteson, D.: Adolescence today: sex roles and search for identity, Homewood, Ill., 1975, Dorsey Press.

43. Miller, D.: Affective disorders and violence in adolescents, Hospital and Community Psychiatry **37**:591, June 1986.

44. Mussen, P., Conger, J., and Kagen, J.: Child development and personality, ed. 3, New York, 1969, Harper & Row, Publishers, Inc.

45. Muuss, R.: Theories of adolescence, ed. 2, New York, 1968, Random House, Inc.

46. Olderker, S.: Identity confusion: nursing diagnoses for adolescents, Nursing Clinics of North America **20**:763, December 1985.

47. Peck, M., Litman, R., and Farberow, N.: Youth suicide, New York, 1985, Springer Publishing Co., Inc.

48. Peplau, H.E.: Interpersonal relations in nursing, New York, 1952, G.P. Putnam's Sons.

49. Piersona, H.: Mom and dad: views on the relationship between direct care staff and therapists in residential treatment facilities, Adolescence **20**:975, 1985.

50. Rigg, A., and Shearin, R.: Adolescent medicine: present and future concepts, Chicago, 1980, Year Book Medical Publishers.

51. Rutter, M., and Hersav, L.: Child and adolescent psychiatry, ed. 2, Boston, 1985, Blackwell Scientific Publications.

52. Schwebel, M.: Effects of the nuclear war threat on children and teenagers: implications for professionals, American Journal of Orthopsychiatry **52**:608, 1982.

53. Sedgwick, R.: Family mental health: theory and practice, St. Louis, 1981, The C.V. Mosby Co.

54. Sedgwick, R., and Hildebrand, S.: The adolescent at risk: crisis, the delicate balance. In Howe, J., editor: Nursing care of adolescents, New York, 1980, McGraw-Hill Book Co.

55. Shafii, M., Carrigan, S., Whittinghill, J., and Derrick, A.: Psychological autopsy of completed suicide in children and adolescents, American Journal of Psychiatry **142**:1061, September 1985.

56. Silbert, T: Ethical issues in the treatment of children and adolescents, Thorofare, N.J., 1983, Slack, Inc., Publishers.

57. Sprinthall, N., and Collins, A.: Adolescent psychology: a developmental view, Reading, Mass., 1984, Addison-Wesley.

58. Stern, S., and others: Anorexia nervosa: the hospital's role in family treatment, Family Process **20**:395, 1981.

59. Storms, M.: Theories of sexual orientation, Journal of Personality and Social Psychology **38**:783, 1980.

60. Sullivan, H.S.: The interpersonal theory of psychiatry, New York, 1953, W.W. Norton & Co., Inc.

61. Tackett, J., and Hunsberger, M.: Family centered care of children and adolescents: nursing concepts in child health, Philadelphia, 1981, W.B. Saunders Co.

62. Tarter, R.: The child at psychiatric risk, New York, 1983, Oxford University Press.

63. Williams, E.: Adolescent loneliness, Adolescence **18**:51, Spring 1983.

ANNOTATED BIBLIOGRAPHY

Cleveland, M.: Families and adolescent drug abuse: structural analysis of chidlren's roles, Family Process **20**:295, 1981.

This article provides a structural analysis of sibling roles in families in which adolescents are involved in chemical drug abuse and suggests appropriate clinical interventions.

Hall, S., and Hall, R.: Clinical series in the behavioral treatment of obesity, Health Psychology **1**:359, 1982.

This article compares seven clinical treatment programs for obesity, noting one study (Robin) with college students in which a variety of treatment approaches were used with a high level of success.

Howe, J., editor: Nursing care of adolescents, New York, 1980, McGraw-Hill Book Co.

This text provides a comprehensive approach to nursing care of the adolescent in a variety of settings: school, home, and hospital.

Kizziar, J., and Hagedon, J.: Search for acceptance: the adolescent and self-esteem, Chicago, 1979, Nelson-Hall Publishers.

The authors address the issue of adolescent self-esteem and discuss ways in which environments can be created that are conducive to the development of healthy self-esteem.

CHAPTER 42

THE YOUNG ADULT

Sydney D. Krampitz

After studying this chapter the learner will be able to:

Discuss the historical developments in treating the young adult.

Discuss various theories of young adult development.

Identify issues of establishing a relationship with a young adult.

Apply the nursing process to the care of the young adult.

Young adult development encompasses maturation and socialization from age 20 to 44 years. Separating from the family of origin, establishing a viable career, developing an intimate adult relationship with an adult of the opposite sex, developing an individual life-style, and establishing and maintaining a social network are all critical tasks of the early adult years.[29] Since the largest component of the U.S. population will be between 25 and 44 years old until the year 2000,[28] health care providers need to recognize the complex and changing needs of young adults.

The basic stressors confronting today's young adult population are similar to those that confronted their parents as young adults. However, the rate of change of social values and the range of possible life-styles and family structures compound the decision-making process and may create confusion and anxiety for the young adult. Unemployment, relocation, and retraining will affect the life-style of the young adult and shape patterns of marriage, parenting, and relationships with the family of origin.

Young adulthood is a developmental period of rapid change. The young adult faces changes in perception of psychological self and body image, belief systems, values, expectations, and a wide range of environmental factors.[9] The adaptive response of the young adult is often challenged and confused by this rapidly changing scenerio. These changes demand fast assimilation and adaptation.

One of the most significant problems that affects the young adult population is the abuse of drugs and alcohol. Suicide risk from substance abuse is evident and increasing in this population. Depression may also be a significant factor in suicide in the young adult population. The de-

pressed young adult is approximately 30 times more likely to commit suicide than those in this age group who are not depressed.[25] Approximately three fourths of all suicides in the United States are associated with the use of drugs or alcohol, depression or both. Population projections predict that more than 100,000 adults between 18 and 44 years of age will commit suicide in the next decade.[28] These statistics clearly indicate the need for recognition of suicide potential in this high-risk population.

Successful mastery of milestones in previous developmental periods shape how later tasks are perceived and addressed. Young adulthood is an active period and requires the individual to make a number of significant choices with long-term implications. Previously learned behavior that enables good communication, effective interpersonal relationships, and an adequate support system influence how significant choices are made. These same factors are crucial in later coping behaviors and the individual's success as student, professional, spouse, and parent.

THEORETICAL APPROACHES
Psychoanalytic

Intrapsychic. Freud[14] identified unconscious conflict in early childhood as crucial to the development and use of defense mechanisms. The period of genital development, from 12 years to early adulthood, was seen to set the stage for the development of sexual maturity and *intimacy* in the adult. Relational problems with members of the opposite sex are thus demonstrated in subsequent problems,

🌿 *Historical Overview* 🌿

DATE	EVENT
1900	The initial focus on the development of young adults was the problems they experienced. Writings addressed specific areas of the young adult's development such as marriage and parenthood instead of a comprehensive approach.
1929	Oakland Growth and Development Study, conducted by the Institute of Human Development of the University of California at Berkeley, began as a longitudinal study that focused on the lives of 171 men and women from birth through age 40.
1938	Harvard University's Grant Study of Adult Development focused on adult men from the classes of 1942 and 1944 who were psychologically healthy.
1939	Valliant, a social psychiatrist from Harvard Medical School, conducted a longitudinal study on developmental issues of 260 male graduates of Harvard from ages 20 to 50.
1947	Cox conducted a longitudinal study of 65 young adult men and women who were considered mentally and physically healthy.
1950s	Erikson included the young adult in his writings about psychological development throughout the life cycle.
Late 1960s	Levinson, a Yale psychologist, conducted a 10-year study of the lives of 40 men, identifying two transitional periods and two stable periods. Gould, a psychiatrist at UCLA, conducted a 5-year cross-sectional study of issues and concerns of men and women.
	The establishment of community-based psychiatry and the emphasis on primary prevention and development of crisis intervention theory and technique greatly influenced the nursing management of the young adult in situational or transitional crises.
1970s	Sheehy described the predictable development of the young adult and compared the development of women and men.
1980s	Troll focused on the development of young adults in his writings. Baruch, Barnett, and Rivers studied the lives of young adult women; their findings highlighted the importance of the role of work in women's lives.
Future	As the young adult population grows and experiences stress in response to the effect that changing societal expectations have on their values, nurses will be more involved in interventions that prevent the development of chronic problems.

such as impotence, premature ejaculation, divorce, or serial marriages.

Erikson[11] identified intimacy as the major developmental task for young adults. Having dealt with issues of identity in adolescence, the individual now begins to develop an interest in an intimate heterosexual relationship. The movement toward commitment includes the development of the ethical strength needed to make sacrifices and compromises to maintain the relationship. The ability to develop a close affiliation with another necessitates a sense of trust and self-worth. Failure to achieve intimacy results in *isolation*, which can interfere with the development of the capacity to engage in a meaningful heterosexual relationship. Isolation may be a means to delay entry into the stage of generativity.

Interpersonal. Later work of Sullivan[32] focused on relationships between and among individuals as primary in

development. The late adolescent stage of Sullivan's theory of interpersonal growth and development extends from mid-adolescence to the establishment of a deep heterosexual love relationship in early adulthood.

According to Sullivan, the development of productive and effective adult relationships is critical in achieving maturity. Disparagement, or "putting others down," is a feeble prop for an inadequate self system. To Sullivan, mature adults have learned to satisfy important needs, to cooperate and compete with others, to develop and sustain intimate and sexually satisfying relationships, and to function effectively in the society in which they live.

Cognitive

Piaget's theory of development[30] recognizes four major stages in which biological change and maturation usher in new modes of responding. The successful resolution of the formal operations stage, or Piaget's final intellectual developmental stage, culminates in the refinement of higher order intellectual functioning of adulthood. The demands of professional education and career development require further refinement and expansion of intellectual operations. Cognitive functioning is seen to remain high during early young adulthood.

Sociocultural

Recent studies by Gould,[18] Levinson,[24] and Gilligan[16] focus on a sociocultural orientation, which appears to offer a helpful perspective to the health care provider in addressing conflict and ambiguity inherent in a rapidly changing society. Gould[18] identifies the 29- to 34-year period as critical, when young adults frequently commit to marriage, establish themselves as members of a new family, and assume the responsibility of parenting. This period is also stressful because of increased professional responsibilities.

The 35- to 43-year period is transitional, when values, work, and life-style may be seriously questioned. Gould[18] reported time during this period to be at a premium, the future looming ahead as an unknown. When the individual determines that professional or personal goals are unrealistic in light of previous experience or accomplishments, it becomes imperative to find other acceptable options to maintain self-esteem. Living with an adolescent family member during this transitional period was seen by many in the Gould study as stressful as the adolescent strives to become his own person and challenges his parents' values. Similar stress is encountered when the individual is confronted with increased responsibilities for an ill or aged parent.

Levinson[24] identified three distinct stages in a male's transition from adolscence to adulthood. They are the Early Adult Transition, or novice period, at 17 to 22 years; the Entering the Adult World period at 22 to 28 years; and the Age 30 Transition at 28 to 33 years. He identified several major developmental tasks as essential for the young man entering the first period. These include separating from the family of origin and forming a basis for living in the adult world, establishing more specific goals, making firmer choices, and articulating a clearer self-definition. Critical to mastering these tasks is separation from family and persons and groups in the world of adolescence. This separation results in a sense of loss, grief, and anxiety about the future. Thus internalizing adult behavior and the movement into the early adult period may prove stressful to the college student or newly employed worker. The individual begins to more clearly articulate future options and expectations, while continuing to develop personal and professional skills needed for entrance into the adult world.

Entry into the Adult World requires men to explore self and world, make and evaluate provisional choices, search for alternatives, and construct a more integrated life structure with increased personal and professional commmitment. The individual feels a sense of urgency about marrying, establishing a lifelong satisfying occupation, and developing a more organized life-style. He may opt for stability in marriage, while continuing to explore career opportunities, or he may focus on a professional career, while continuing to avoid closeness or commitment. This period is fraught with contradiction and inherent problems; mastery of these tasks significantly affects self-worth and adult identity.

Levinson[24] viewed the Age Thirty Transition as a period of opportunity, because the individual now has time for further refinement of the evolving life structure of the previous period. In this 5-year period men feel a sense of urgency, and that they have a second chance to create a more satisfactory life structure. However, this transition period may prove stressful if the individual feels unable to master its developmental tasks and reactivates unresolved conflicts of adolescence.

Each individual may identify his developmental prob-

TABLE 42-1 Summary of theoretical approaches

Theory	Theorist	Dynamics
Psychoanalytic	Freud	Genital development sets the stage for development of sexual maturity in young adulthood.
		Relationship problems with members of the opposite sex are seen in disorders such as impotence, and premature ejaculation and problems such as serial marriages and divorce.
	Erikson	The task is intimacy versus isolation. Failure to achieve intimacy interferes with capacity to engage in meaningful heterosexual relationships.
Interpersonal	Sullivan	The development of a productive and effective adult intimate relationship is critical to achieving maturity.
Cognitive	Piaget	Cognitive functioning is refined and remains high during young adulthood.
Sociocultural	Gould	Ages 22 to 28—commits to marriage, creation of a family, parenting and career advancement.
		Ages 29 to 34—reevaluates values, work, and life-style.
	Levinson	Ages 17 to 22 (Early Adult Transition)— separates from family, establishes specific goals, and makes firmer choices.
		Ages 22 to 28 (Entering Adult World)—explores self and world, makes conditional choices regarding career.
		Age Thirty Transition—the period of opportunity to create more satisfactory life.

lems as unique as values are challenged and larger social questions gain considerable attention. However, much remains to be learned about male and female development in this Transition and Settling Down period. The theoretical approaches are summarized in Table 42-1.

RELATING TO THE CLIENT

The nurse developing a relationship with the young adult client needs to be aware of the individual's striving for the development of an adult identity and the expectations inherent in a mature relationship. Rebellious and immature behavior from adolescence may be evident as the client confronts the myriad of demands of career or college. This behavior may have initiated the client's referral to the nurse for assessment and intervention and may continue throughout the nurse-client interaction.

The young adult entering a therapeutic relationship may express a high level of anxiety about the nurse's expectations and may test all facets of the relationship. The nurse needs to recognize the developmental needs of the client and to begin to establish clear parameters for the interaction with these needs in mind. The value of a verbal or written contract to facilitate trust in the relationship is well documented and essential if acting-out behavior is an initial problem. Establishing the treatment contract often provokes the client to test the contract's terms. Although this may be disruptive, the client's behavior frequently can be used effectively to address issues of trust and confidentiality in the relationship. Failure to keep an appointment or to arrive on time for an individual group or session provides an opportunity to discuss issues of trust, anger, or expectations inherent in responsible adult behavior. The nurse may perceive acting-out behavior as rejection or failure. This nurse needs adequate professional support and supervision to help clarify client behaviors and to assist her in processing the perceived rejection or failure.

The nurse's goal in the early treatment period is to develop a meaningful relationship with the client. The young adult client may appear fearful and move toward establishing a relationship only with considerable support and encouragement. Although the establishment of mutual openness and trust may be challenged, a consistent approach by the nurse provides the support essential for the relationship to progress.

The universal need to be loved and cared for is critical to the young adult, who is struggling with many stressful adjustments. The nurse who recognizes the client's need for acceptance, understanding, and individuality involves the client in all aspects of treatment planning.

The young adult may have an unrealistic perception of the nurse and lack insight into the role of the client in treatment. The inability to separate from strong family ties and the reluctance of family members to encourage independence may also delay engagement in treatment.

One of the first issues to address is a high level of anxiety or an obvious distrust in the initial nurse-client contact. A sense of failure or low self-esteem may have inhibited the client from seeking professional services before.

Thus it is imperative to be sensitive to the client's developmental needs. If the client has taken a risk and failed, he may appear very guarded. The nurse recognizes that this failure increases the client's reluctance to establish a relationship. A problem of this nature necessitates that the nurse plan for adequate time to begin to develop the relationship and establish priorities for working with the client on issues of trust. The young adult may also revert to earlier ways of coping with stress, including use of drugs and alcohol, and may drop out of therapy to return to an identified safer place. The nurse explores the acting-out behavior and the client begins to learn how to communicate his anger, fear, anxiety, and frustration, thus decreasing the need to act out.

During the working phase of the relationship, the client demonstrates increased trust and openness. The nurse has an opportunity to model open communication and to help the client explore and expand communication and other modes of adult behavior. As an authority figure in the client's life, the nurse has many opportunities to change his perception of authority and how one relates appropriately to other adults in authority. The insights gained and the opportunity to explore new behavior in a safe environment provide the client with new or refined skills critical for success in a myriad of social, employment, and school settings.

Resolution of issues not addressed in earlier developmental periods is a critical task of young adulthood. The nurse provides opportunities for the client to discuss how he learned to cope with stress during earlier periods and helps him identify how skills developed earlier can be refined to facilitate more mature expression and coping.

The termination phase provides many opportunities for resolving conflict and learning new behavior. The nurse recognizes the stress that the client may display at this time. Anger or rage directed at the nurse may be manifested in withdrawal or a range of disruptive behaviors. Exploration of this behavior may reveal that the client has had a number of unresolved traumatic losses or separations in childhood or adolescence. Loss of a parent or significant other by divorce, separation, or death or a real or perceived rejection by a significant other is addressed at this time if new patterns of coping with losses are to be explored. During termination the client may use defense mechanisms that foster continued immature behavior. The nurse explores the client's use of denial or repression, since a fear of loss or rejection may make the task of establishing an intimate adult relationship stressful, if not impossible. Other defense mechanisms and inappropriate behavior demonstrated during this period are also explored.

NURSING PROCESS
Assessment

✦ *Physical dimension.* Physical growth has been essentially completed in young adults. Aging and the maintenance of physical integrity is related to individual differences in nutrition, sleep, stress, and genetic variables. Physical signs of aging may be evident in the late

20s, with loss of skin elasticity and subsequent wrinkling. Signs of premature graying or balding may also be evident. These and other physical changes, seen as negative, may significantly affect the client's self-confidence.

Exploring the client's use of alcohol and drugs and routine dietary habits is helpful in assessing physical status. The young adult client may eat high-calorie foods at home and at fast food establishments. A rapid weight gain or loss may be a response to the caloric intake, a physical response to a high level of stress, or a sign of inadequate coping mechanisms for adaptation. Excessive weight gain or loss may contribute to a poor self-concept.

Assessing the client's physical symptoms is an integral part of the nurse's health history. Vague somatic complaints may mask underlying mental health problems and delay the client seeking early intervention for depression or anxiety related to school, work, or interpersonal relationships. Headaches, digestive complaints, and a lack of vigor may signal tension and stress or depression. A thorough assessment of onset of symptoms, duration, and other related or contributing factors helps the nurse differentiate between physiological stress or psychophysiological manifestations.

The nurse observes dietary and sleep patterns of the hospitalized client. She can explore the outpatient's dietary intake, and patterns of alcohol and drug use, sleep, and response to stress by asking him to record this information in a daily log or diary. These behaviors can then be explored in treatment, and new ways of coping with stress can be addressed. Some increase in depression or anxiety may be anticipated in therapy; the nurse identifies the impact of these changes on the client's health. When monitoring a client's response to drug therapy, the nurse is also acutely aware of possible physical changes in vital signs, bowel habits, and energy levels.

The depressed young adult may feel increased apprehension about body image and feel unacceptable as a sexual partner. Since Western culture places a high value on youth and beauty, shame about one's own body may greatly inhibit establishing an intimate relationship and thus delay the initiation or achievement of a key developmental task.

The value of peer acceptance in young adulthood has a number of implications for the *cachectic* or obese client. Both malnutrition and overnutrition may be psychogenic. The anorectic client may demonstrate self-starvation after a period of excess weight gain. This client may also eat excessively and exhibit a number of somatic complaints and irrational fears. The obese client may use ingestion of food to decrease anxiety and stress. This client may be warding off sexuality and subconsciously expressing fear of intimacy. The anorectic client may also fear the changes of young adulthood and thus demonstrate fears of rejection or of changing expectations of peers about intimacy and increased commitment.

Emotional dimension. The ability to function in a stressful environment is critical for the young adult to achieve success in work or school. Stress can serve a useful purpose in motivating the individual to strive for greater achievement. However, an inability to

cope effectively with the many stressors of this developmental stage may bring the young adult to seek help in learning new coping behaviors to decrease emotional outbursts. Assessment of the individual experiencing emotional stress includes his support systems and congruence in values and role expectations with spouse or significant other.

A number of emotions may contribute to the client's feeling stressed. Guilt, despair, anger, and loneliness contribute to depression or hopelessness. These feelings result from encounters on the campus, in the workplace, or at home. To assess the client's perception of emotions experienced, the nurse may ask him to identify a current stressful experience and the accompanying feelings or to explore behavior that seems inappropriate or troublesome, underlying feelings, and how these feelings are expressed.

The nurse assesses the client's perception of how control or lack of emotional control affects his ability to develop successful relationships or achieve professional goals. These experiences may be used to discuss individual responses to a wide range of economic, social, and intellectual demands. When conflicting demands are placed on the client, the nurse may observe responses ranging from inability to act and apathy to anger, rage, or destructive behavior.

During assessment, the client may become painfully aware of an inability to handle anger effectively. He may find expression of emotions or feelings threatening and thus may resort to using anger to distance others when stressed. The use of anger to ward off feelings of closeness may become an unhealthy defense mechanism. However, in assessing emotional response in the young adult, it is imperative to recognize that depression and guilt may be closely related to anger, manifested in angry ourbursts. Anger clearly involves the use of energy vitally needed for successful resolution of developmental tasks.

Assessment may help both client and nurse determine how the client uses defense mechanisms, such as repression, to alleviate the expression of anger or to deny feelings of loneliness or depression. Unfortunately, although repression often appears to alleviate the most pressing problem or immediate feelings, it fails to serve effectively to resolve the client's anger or depression.

Intellectual dimension. An assessment of the client's ability to handle cognitive and abstract problems and to process information in a timely and appropriate manner provides valuable information that can help the nurse structure interactions. The client may demonstrate an impulsive or irrational decision-making style or markedly vary in style when stressed. He may make decisions soundly by carefully weighing pros and cons or by using a trial-and-error approach.

Limitations identified in intellectual development may create major or minor adjustment problems for the client. Young adults are required to process large amounts of new information or rapidly develop skills for professional education or succeeding at work. Thus the capacity for a sustained effort and the intellectual ability to manipulate concrete data and comprehend abstract problems are crucial for success. The capacity to delay gratification and to demonstrate sound decision-making skills also is reflected in the client's ability to establish and maintain interpersonal relationships.

As the young adult is exposed to broader educational or work experiences, the ability to adapt to change becomes evident. Flexibility thus becomes an indicator of identity and self-esteem. Flexibility and risk taking greatly enhance the individual's response to opportunities available for new experiences and result in subsequent mastery in a broader intellectual or interpersonal arena.

Social dimension. Assessment of the client's social orientation focuses on interactions or relationships in living, working, or socializing with others. Interaction style has broad implications for success on the job, in an intimate relationship, or in other professional or social situations. Evidence of isolation or failure to develop interpersonal relationships may manifest itself in low self-esteem or alienation. The fear of an intimate adult relationship may inhibit the individual from dating or joining in group activities that involve close interpersonal relationships.

The expansion of high technology and increasing competition may force the individual to change employment or expand his educational background to continue to meet employment demands. This may be perceived as either a challenge or a threat. Underemployment or unemployment is often a stressor leading to feelings of inferiority, loss of confidence, and fear of economic insecurity. Underemployment often results in disruption or breakdown of social and family relationships. It may be further compounded if the individual has recently married or become a parent, thus appreciably increasing personal and fiscal responsibilities. The development of economic independence, however, goes beyond steady employment and an adequate income, it requires skill in money management.

For professionals the need to perform in many areas simultaneously and to accept additional responsibility to successfully compete may prove extremely stressful. Support of peers, spouse, and parents is crucial when time and energy are focused on educational or career goals. To deal with conflicting role demands, individuals may quickly find themselves confronted with the need to set priorities to succeed. Conflict occurs between individual needs and values and expectations of work, school, spouse, or others. Unfortunately, a failure to successfully establish priorities or disparity between expectation and external reality may create a climate that generates maladaptive coping—anger, anxiety, depression, or somatic complaints.

Although the capacity for establishing sexual intimacy begins in adolescence, the young adult needs to develop a sense of personal identity before merging with another in marriage or other long-term intimate relationship. Individuals with similar socioeconomic backgrounds, value systems, role expectations, and interests are most likely to establish a more lasting and secure intimate relationship.

During assessment, the client identifies individuals in his support sytstem and his usual interpersonal acitivity at work and in relationships. Assessment of how the client balances his role as an employee, a parent, a spouse, and as a part of other social situations, provide insight into his value system; personal adjustment is reflected in satisfaction with one's life-style.

Hoffman[19] found that although fathers' participation in child care has increased in the last 2 decades, the task of early child care is still viewed as primarily the mother's responsibility by both the mother and others. In light of the ambiguity inherent in the socialization of women, particularly the professional woman, this responsibility may create role strains not previously anticipated by the new mother.

Assessment of how young women perceive their roles as wage earner (or student), spouse, and parent will give useful clues to sources of stress on the job and in relationships. The assessment of young men, like young women, include a description of how they perceive their role as wage earner (or student), spouse, and parent. Financial pressures or career stressors compound the adjustment of young men and women to marriage and parenthood. Assessment of the importance of the workplace in meeting social needs of young men and women, is essential, as it identifies areas of ambivalence and stress related to relocation or upward mobility in the organization.

A lack of social support systems or financial resources may compound adjustment problems of new families. Relocating can cause additional strain. The importance of support of family members in parenting has been documented in a longitundinal study by Cronenwett,[7] who investigated the relationships among network structure, social support, and psychological outcomes of pregnancy (see the Research Highlight on p. 815).

Preparing for marriage is often more emotionally stressful than anticipated. The tasks of the premarital and early marriage period are disengaging from the family of origin and other exceptionally close relationships that may interfere with the spousal relationship, emotionally preparing oneself for the role of spouse and establishing a new life-style that provides gratification for both partners. A great deal of stress and dysfunctional behavior may be encountered in clients who are anticipating marriage or have entered a relationship with unrealistic expectations. An assessment of the social dimension addresses current experiences from the client's perspective.

Parenting is another major source of stress. Cohen, Cohler, and Weisman[6] and Lederman[23] identify potential regression as the predominant risk of parenthood. Previous loss of a parent or abandonment increases the new parent's level of vulnerability. The young adult may continue to be greatly influenced by earlier unresolved losses, thus experiencing a significant deficit in parenting ability. This deficit will increase anxiety and doubt about the individual's ability to succeed as a parent. Even in ideal conditions parenthood forces the individual to shift from focus on self to responsibility for another 24 hours a day. Child care demands may create a high level of anxiety and a sense of helplessness, which further compounds the emotional adjustment of the young adult.

The young married professional woman with home and

Research Highlight

Network Structure, Social Support, and Psychological Outcomes of Pregnancy

L.R. Cronenwett

PURPOSE

This longitudinal study investigated the relationships among network structure, social support, and psychological outcomes of pregnancy.

SAMPLE

A nonprobability sample of 50 primigravid couples was obtained through the private practices of local physicians and a Lamaze-sponsored film showing.

METHODOLOGY

The Social Network Inventory (SNI) was used to collect data on network structure and perceived social support. The four types of support described on the inventory were emotional, material, informational, and comparison. The postpartum outcome measures were obtained from subjects' response to the Postpartum Self-Evaluation Questionnaire (PSQ). The seven scales of the PSQ were designed to measure the quality of relationship with spouse, perception of spouse involvement in basic child care activities, gratification received from labor and delivery experience, general satisfaction with current life status, confidence in parenting tasks, satisfaction with parenting role, and perceived support in parenting role from parents, friends, and relatives.

FINDINGS

Men and women in the study had similar density and frequency of contacts with identified members of their network. They also perceived similar types of access to social support from identified social networks. However, the sources of social support differed significantly by gender, with men receiving more emotional support from family members and less from friends.

A significant relationship was identified for both men and women between network or support variables and the following PSQ items: ability to cope with tasks of parenting and satisfaction with parenting and satisfaction with parenting and infant care. Men's network or support variables also were significantly correlated with PSQ measures of quality of relationship with the spouse and support of parenting role.

IMPLICATIONS

The study further documents the need for emotional support of the new father in his parenting role. These needs can be determined by assessment during prenatal instruction and in the postpartum period. Interventions can strive to decrease conflict in the network ties needed to assist the father in his adjustment to parenting.

A plan can be established, if needed, to augment the natural network of the couple with personal contacts with peers, family members, or professional from whom they can receive the type of support needed.

Based on data from Nursing Research 34(2):93-99, 1985.

family responsibilities may find herself extremely stressed by the parenting role. Assessment of the client's response to the demands of her different roles is helpful in identifying stressors and planning intervention to decrease role conflict. The increased demands on the young father and the changing needs and expectations of his wife may be overwhelming, thus leading to increased anxiety, depression, and strained interpersonal relationships. These tensions may greatly affect the trust and intimacy needed to sustain the marriage relationship and lead to alienation, separation, or divorce.

For single or childless young adults between 20 and 30 years of age, the nurse assesses personal goals and established priorities, satisfaction with their quality of life, and their perceived need for increased social contacts or significant changes in life-style. The client may say that overcommitment has been a problem on the job or in social relationships, and failure to meet these commitments has lead to feelings of failure or loss of self-esteem. This sense of failure may also considerably affect clients' perception of their ability to marry or assume responsibility for a family.

Individuals with demanding educational or career goals may find little time for social activity and become increasingly isolated from family and peers. Young adults who have chosen a career over marriage and family or who have been too busy professionally to develop a social life or intimate adult relationship may become increasingly aware of a sense of "something missing" as the Age Thirty Transition approaches. The young adult may choose to make a significant change in life-style at this time to facilitate social contacts, may seek support in reaffirming the value of the current life-style, or may explore other options.

Married couples may reassess decisions to remain childless or to continue to defer childbearing during the Age Thirty Transition. If the couple fails to satisfactorily resolve conflict over this or other issues at this time, their relationship may become increasingly strained. The young couple is also faced with a growing need to broaden social contacts in this period. They may have been totally involved in careers, education, or the demands of children in the early years of marriage and now have a need to expand beyond the immediate family or work setting.

However, this broadening may be perceived by one spouse as a loss of interest in the relationship. This issue needs to be openly addressed to decrease conflict.

The nurse notes the social and emotional implications of separation or divorce when the client has a history of marital discord. The young adult frequently seeks counseling because of depression or feelings of failure from a recent divorce that may be further compounded by feelings of abandonment or rejection. Because divorce demands a major adjustment in life-style for both partners, support may be necessary for both. The stereotype that women have more difficulty coping with divorce may no longer be true. A woman's career may not only provide economic support but also peer support.

✂ ***Spiritual dimension.*** Conflict may be apparent as early values are challenged. (see the Research Highlight below). The young adult may have conflicts related to premarital sexual intercourse, abortion, or living with a person of the opposite sex. Some resolve these conflicts; however, others may need assistance. Some clients may experience a conflict because of failure to attend religious services as they were taught or a change of their religious affiliation.

As individuals establish themselves in a community and marry, time is spent reflecting on ethical and spiritual values. The responsibilities of a family may foster introspection on values and the sharing of philosophical and spiritual orientation with one's children. The focus of the young couple, however, is often primarily on the training of the young children, unless there is a major life crisis, such as divorce, loss of a parent or other family member, a life-threatening accident, or prolonged illness. The nurse may note that the client has begun to search for meaning in life or is actively reassessing spiritual values because of a loss. In today's society, reports of terrorism and destruction, war, and natural disaster confront the individual with many anxiety-producing sights and sounds, thus increasing one's sense of vulnerability. Vulnerability also provides impetus for young adults to assess their value system and reflect on spirituality.

Student, blue collar worker, and professional alike often face moral and ethical situations that demand an as-

---

Research Highlight

The Stressors of Nonmarital Sexual Intercourse

S. Snegroff

PURPOSE

This study was designed to survey male and female perception of psychosocial stressors that influence individual response to nonmarital sexual intercourse.

SAMPLE

The sample was 271 undergraduate students enrolled in an elective course entitled "Human Sexuality and the College Student." approximately 85% were junior or senior students, and 98% were age 23 or younger. There were 170 women and 101 men.

METHODOLOGY

The participants responded to a situation involving a couple with no commitments to each other by listing the concerns that a woman or man (depending on participant's gender) might have about sexual intercourse.

FINDINGS

Subject responses were arranged in seven categories: relationship, performance (general), performance (physical aspects), body image, reputation, communication, and morality. Statistics were reported on items with a 50% agreement after a group discussion of initial questionnaire response.

Women expressed more concern about relationship issues, especially involving respect and love. Conflict about morality and reputation were expressed only by the women.

Both women and men were concerned about sex performance and partner's satisfaction. However, general performance was more important to the men.

Men and women identified the physical aspects of intercourse as significant. The men, however, demonstrated greatest anxiety over the ability to achieve and maintain an erection and premature ejaculation. Women focused on reaching orgasm and the partner's gentleness. Both men and women expressed uneasiness about body image, with the size of breasts or penis of particular concern.

IMPLICATIONS

Among young adults, nonmarital sexual intercourse may become anxiety producing. This study documents how both sexes perceive the act of sexual intercourse in a nonmarital relationship. The male emphasis on sexual intercourse as a purely physical event and female emphasis on relationship and the commitment component clearly have potential for creating major stressors in communication, morality, and subsequent female guilt.

Nurses often have the opportunity to work with young adults who are in relationship crises, are unmarried, and pregnant, or feel inadequate or depressed because of negative self-concept. An understanding of the stressors of nonmarital sexual intercourse enhances management of the young adult experiencing anxiety, depression, or other psychosocial or physical developmental problems related to sexuality.

Based on data from Health Education 16(6): 21-23, 1985-1986.

sessment in light of individual values. A junior member of a management team or professional group may encounter interpersonal conflict as co-workers engage in business practices that fail to meet the young adult's ethical or moral standards. During the initial assessment, the client may be very confused or angry, having become aware of the value conflicts inherent in entering the adult society. These issues are often stressful to those who become acutely aware that they cannot continue to compromise

their values without loss of integrity. The nurse, however, is objective and provides opportunity for the client to explore options as they relate to his spiritual and moral values.

The assessment tool below, left contains assessment areas specific to the young adult. It is to be used in conjuction with the assessment tool in Chapter 8.

Analysis

Nursing diagnosis. Alteration in parenting is a nursing diagnosis approved by NANDA that applies to the young adult. The defining characteristics of this nursing diagnosis are listed in the box below.

The following list provides examples of other NANDA-accepted nursing diagnoses with causative statements for the young adult.

1. Powerlessness related to ineffectiveness in parental role
2. Impaired social interaction related to inability to maintain interpersonal relationships
3. Disturbance in self-concept related to obesity
4. Ineffective individual coping related to marital discord
5. Anxiety related to perceived threat to self-concept
6. Social isolation related to depressed mood

ASSESSMENT TOOL: THE YOUNG ADULT

PHYSICAL DIMENSION
   Describe your eating habits.
   What is your sleep pattern?
   What are your thoughts about your body image?
   How do you feel about your sexuality?

EMOTIONAL DIMENSION
   What do you think and feel when you experience stress?
   How does your spouse respond to you when you experience stress?
   What is a stressful experience you are now facing?
   How do you handle anger? guilt?
   What do you feel hopeful about?
   Describe your behavior the last time you were depressed.
   What is your response when faced with a conflict?

INTELLECTUAL DIMENSION
   What is your response to changes in your life?
   How do you make decisions about everyday situations? major situations?
   How do you feel about seeking professional assistance?

SOCIAL DIMENSION
   How many friends do you have at work?
   What type of social events do you participate in with your peers?
   How often do you invite friends to your home?
   What are your career goals?
   What do you think about your performance at your present job?
   Describe your marriage.
   Describe your parenting behavior.
   When faced with several tasks, how do you set priorities?
   How do you handle conflicts with your spouse?
   Describe the way you manage your finances.
   What do you consider your role in the family?
   What are your thoughts about assuming this role?

SPIRITUAL DIMENSION
   What are your thoughts about divorce? abortions? infidelity?
   How congruent is your value system with your spouse's?
   How do you behave when faced with a moral or ethical conflict?

ALTERATIONS IN PARENTING

DEFINITION
   The state in which one or more individuals experience a real or potential inability to provide a constructive environment that nurtures the growth and development of the individual's child or children.

DEFINING CHARACTERISTICS
Physical Dimension
   Growth and development lag in infant
   Evidence of abuse or neglect
Emotional Dimension
   Verbalization of perceived or actual inadequacy
Intellectual Dimension
   *Lack of knowledge of parenting
   Diminished or inappropriate visual, tactile, or auditory stimulation of infant
Social Dimension
   Verbalization of frustration of role
   Frequent verbalization of dissatisfaction or disappointment with the infant
   Lack of parental attachment behavior
   Inappropriate parenting behavior
Spiritual Dimension
   *Values conflict

Adapted from North American Nursing Diagnosis Association Classification of Nursing Diagnosis: Proceedings of the seventh conference, St. Louis, 1987, The C.V. Mosby Co.
*Indicates characteristics in addition to those defined by NANDA.

The following Case Example illustrates the defining characteristics of alterations in parenting.

Case Example

Joan's infant son has been seen repeatedly by the nurse, and a diagnosis of failure to thrive has been made. Joan is a single parent and unable to care for the child because of drug and alcohol abuse. The child lost 2 pounds since the previous clinic visit and appeared also to demonstrate signs of lack of sensory stimulation.

The child is placed in a temporary foster home at Joan's request, and she enters an outpatient rehabilitation program.

DSM-III-R diagnosis. The diagnoses for the young adult are listed in the box at right. There are no essential features in the DSM-III-R for these disorders.

An adjustment disorder is a maladaptive response to a psychosocial stressor. This response generally occurs within 3 months of the period of acute distress. Assessment will reveal an impairment in the client's ability to function in the social or work setting. The behavior manifested is not an isolated incident of overreaction but remits with decrease in stress or when a new level of adaptation is achieved.[3] Stressors such as divorce, separation, academic failure, or occupational failure are common for young adults.

Planning

Table 42-2 gives long-term and short-term goals and outcome criteria for the client with an adjustment disorder with depressed mood. These are examples of the planning stage in the nursing process.

DSM-III-R CLASSIFICATIONS OF ADJUSTMENT DISORDER

309.24	Adjustment disorder with anxious mood
309.00	Adjustment disorder with depressed mood
309.30	Adjustment disorder with disturbance of conduct
309.40	Adjustment disorder with mixed disturbance of emotions and conduct
309.28	Adjustment disorder with mixed emotional features
309.82	Adjustment disorder with physical complaints
309.83	Adjustment disorder with withdrawal
309.23	Adjustment disorder with work (or academic) inhibition
309.90	Adjustment disorder not otherwise specified
V71.01	Adult antisocial behavior
V62.20	Occupational problems
V62.20	Phase of life problem or other life circumstance problem

Adapted from American Psychiatric Association: Diagnostic and statistical manual of mental disorders, (DSM-III-R), Washington, D.C., 1987, The Association.

Implementation*

Physical dimension. Young adults are the healthiest people in the population, thus a major focus for meeting physical needs is health maintenance. Like other age groups, young adults need caloric intake based on ca-

*Some content in this section contributed by Malinda Garner Pappas.

TABLE 42-2 Long-term and short-term goals and outcome criteria related to the young adult

Goals	Outcome Criteria
NURSING DIAGNOSIS: ANXIETY RELATED TO PERCEIVED THREAT TO SELF-CONCEPT	
Long-term goal	
To develop increased awareness of anxiety	Identifies signs and symptoms of anxiety.
	Uses constructive strategies in coping with anxiety.
Short-term goals	
To assist in identifying anxiety-provoking situations	Increases awareness of precipitating factors
To explore individual indicators of increasing anxiety	Develops means to monitor increasing anxiety level
To develop skills in coping with anxiety	Develops adaptive coping skills and uses them in a high-stress situation
To demonstrate mastery in skill in work setting	Participates in new activity and successfully achieves new skill
NURSING DIAGNOSIS: SOCIAL ISOLATION RELATED TO DEPRESSED MOOD	
Long-term goals	
To increase interaction with others and environment	Establishes several significant relationships
	Returns to work and social environment with limited anxiety
Short-term goals	
To provide positive feedback when the client interacts with others	Participates in group activities
	Makes positive statements about self
To encourage group discussion of behavior that isolates client from others	Identifies behavior that fosters increased isolation
	Demonstrates skill in interacting with peer group members

loric need to avoid excessive weight gain or loss. Those in nonsedentary occupations and who actively exercise burn more calories than inactive young adults. Pregnant women require more calories than other young adults. Young adults can decrease the intake of salt and high cholesterol foods that may contribute to later diseases.

A young adult who feels worthless may think he is not worthy of food and may decrease food intake or avoid meals. This individual may require hospitalization. Careful observation of the client during hospitalization and follow-up to ensure that adequate food intake is maintained may be a short-term goal until the client has become involved in treatment and accepted increasing responsibility for maintainance of adequate nutrition.

Food may become the major means some young adults use to deal with stress. Some may overeat and become obese; others may become anorectic. The nurse monitors the amount of food eaten and the frequency of meals. These eating disorders need medical and psychiatric intervention (see Chapter 35).

Young adults who eat and exercise strenuously near bedtime may have decreased ability to sleep restfully. If an infant's needs during the night contribute to interrupted sleep, spouses can take turns getting up so that neither parent loses too much sleep. A young adult with chronic insomnia may need medical or psychiatric assistance.

The nurse makes sure that clients are aware of the hazards of excessive smoking and drinking. Young adulthood is an opportune time for attending a smoking clinic or Alcoholics Anonymous, if necessary. Individuals planning to have a baby need to be informed of the potential effects of smoking and drinking on the unborn child.

Genetic counseling is indicated for a couple with family histories of hereditary illness or a condition that is known or suspected to be inherited. Such counseling helps the couple determine their chances of having a normal child. The nurse or the genetic counselor to whom the nurse refers the couple can discuss alternative courses of action, such as adoption, artificial insemination, or sterilization. Some couples may benefit from counseling at Planned Parenthood as they decide to start a family.

The nurse informs young adults of the need for an annual physical examination to maintain their health status. Because breast cancer is increasing among women over 35 years of age, young women are taught to examine their breasts monthly, the week after menstruation. The nurse also informs women of the importance of a baseline mammogram between 35 and 40 years of age.

When the stresses of young adulthood cause somatic complaints, such as headaches and stomachaches, the individual needs to have a checkup and have any acute illness treated before the problem becomes chronic.

Interventions for the person who abuses substances focuses on maintenance of physical well-being. Sleep patterns, nutritional status, and degree of interest in maintaining personal hygiene are monitored. Interventions initially are directed toward assisting the client to attend to his physical needs by providing proper nutrition and encouraging personal cleanliness and grooming. The nurse assists the client in increasing awareness of the relationship between stress and physical symptoms.

A number of substance abuse programs provide lectures on the physiological effects of drugs, family dynamics in substance or co-dependent behavior, and other topics. Didactic groups can be extremely helpful to inform clients of the dangers of alcohol or drug ingestion, but these groups clearly focus on specific content and may fail to meet the immediate needs of some clients (see Chapter 16).

Emotional dimension. The young adult may fail to appropriately manage the stress of leaving home, establishing successful adult relationships, or achieving professional goals. The client may censor his own expression of feelings, leaving him angry and frustrated. When the client finds that his unexpressed anger is resulting in isolation from his peer group or co-workers, he may seek professional help. Sometimes a client is referred for counseling because of failure at school or work.

The nurse needs to provide an opportunity for the client to express his feelings about the current crisis. How the client identifies the current problem and how he has attempted to cope give valuable information. Once this has been accomplished, the nurse and client establish and set priorities for short-term and long-term goals. The nurse often finds that encouraging the client to identify alternative ways of coping is an effective means of increasing his awareness of the existing problem. The handling of emotional responses when stressed may require training in relaxation techniques or assertiveness.

A client's lack of experience in confronting adults may reflect social class differences or feelings of inferiority from previous negative experiences. Role playing, rehearsal, reframing, or other methods can be used to assist the young adult in learning new skills. The management of feelings of anger, fear, and conflict is a challenge to the young adult in a rapidly changing, complex society. Increased competence, cultural differences, and changing sex roles today often create frustration for young adults not experienced by previous generations.

The client is given an opportunity to verbalize feelings of failure or depression resulting from separation or divorce. Support and assistance often aid in the resolution of feelings of loss and guilt as the client adjusts to the change in life-style. Parents Without Partners and groups for divorcees at churches or community mental health centers allow young adults to express feelings of anger, abandonment, and rejection.

Intellectual dimension. Because young adults generally have a capacity to tolerate high levels of sensory stimulation, coping with multiple stimuli is not generally perceived as a stressor. However, if the client demonstrates low self-esteem or depression, it may be important to assist him in decreasing environmental stimuli until he feels a sense of control. These stimuli can be then increased as the client can tolerate them.

The student who has encountered academic stress or failure may need to reassess professional goals and to develop a realistic approach to achieving academic success. The nurse and client explore alternatives and establish long-term and short-term goals, which are structured to provide the opportunity for academic success and mastery of the developmental tasks of young adulthood. The involvement of the client in establishing goals allows success in independent decision making, which not only gives support in autonomous decision making but also provides the nurse with an opportunity to evaluate the client's decision-making process.

An ongoing evaluation of the client's ability to use various problem-solving operations and the client's level of intellectual functioning is essential if the nurse is to assist him in establishing realistic goals that will result in a sense of mastery, thus fostering self-esteem. It is important to recognize that the anxious or depressed client is often unable to perform intellectual functions at a level previously attained and may become angry and frustrated. Continued support from the nurse, family members, and significant others is critical in assisting the client to successfully achieve the level of intellectual functioning he is capable of reaching.

Ridigity in thinking and the inability to think abstractly may limit the client's ability to effectively participate in analytic therapy. This behavior may also create a management problem if the client interacts inappropriately with other clients and staff. Nursing intervention is directed at assisting the client to look at his current behavior and the limitations it places on his further development. The opportunity for the client to participate in a therapeutic milieu that necessitates group interaction enhances expressive functions and fosters intellectual responsibility.

Social dimension. Interventions for the failure to develop interpersonal relationships are directed toward increasing self-esteem and improving social interactions. The initial goal is to develop a trusting therapeutic relationship with the nurse. After a relationship has been established, the client is encouraged to talk about the problems he has encountered in his relationships and his feelings about them. The hospitalized client may be assisted to develop intimacy by initially participating in activities such as games and outings with the nurse that are noncompetitive and allow distance. The client is gradually encouraged to interact with peers, first with same-sex peers, then with those of the opposite sex. Then the client may be able to give of self in a relationship that demands intimacy.

The client is encouraged to develop a list of strengths and weaknesses. Much positive reinforcement is then given to build on the client's strengths to increase self-esteem. Assertiveness training, role playing, and the modeling of effective communication will assist the client in improving interpersonal skills. Group therapy can be especially helpful in providing young adults with feedback from peers on their behavior. Group members can also provide support and positive reinforcement as the client makes behavioral changes. Group therapy can also provide an opportunity to practice interpersonal skills and receive feedback.

When working with young adults having difficulty adapting to the parent role, open expression of feelings is encouraged. The nurse listens and responds nonjudgmentally as the client verbalizes disappointment and demonstrates lack of parental attachment. The client's expectations of fatherhood or motherhood are explored, and unrealistic expectations discussed. Information about the woman's acceptance of pregnancy and her relationship with her mother is often useful in assisting her to cope with stress after the delivery.

Clients can write a list of negative changes since the birth. The nurse assists clients in planning some activities on the list that have rarely been done since the child's birth. Child care, work schedules, and support from a spouse and other family members can critically affect solution of these problems. The client is also encouraged to seek out other young parents and share experiences and feelings.

Clients can also list positive aspects of being a parent, which the nurse emphasizes. The nurse may ask which friend or relative is most admired as a parent. The qualities of this parent are explored. Clients are encouraged to spend time with this admired friend or relative. As clients increase parental attachment, the nurse gives much positive reinforcement.

Some women may strive to be "super mom," succeeding at work and home, but allocating little time for personal interests or individual needs. Family demands on the young adult may add appreciably to stress on the job, at school, or as a member of the new family. Clients are assisted to realistically examine the basis of their expectations and to adjust their life-style accordingly. Sometimes family therapy is indicated as clients adapt to the parenting role.

Assisting the mother to develop parenting skills is most helpful when initiated before discharge from the hospital. However, this has become difficult, because women are discharged sooner than in previous years.

Interventions for young adults experiencing role conflicts attempt to reduce stress. The client describes the roles (parent, employee, spouse, boss) that contribute to the conflict. Expectations of self and others are explored, with attention to unrealistic expectations. The client is encouraged to make time for enjoyable activities. The nurse teaches the client relaxation exercises to reduce stress and encourages him to practice them. The nurse also emphasizes the importance of communicating with the person who is the source of the stress. Assertiveness training and role playing are useful approaches for intervention in role conflict.

The young adult may be faced with the challenge of relocation for educational or work opportunities. Some may question the value of leaving a close-knit family or community for such purposes. The nurse can often provide support by carefully listening and helping the client identify advantages and disadvantages of the opportunity and limitations or fears inherent in the proposed change. The opportunity to contact an individual who made a similar move often provides the client with a realistic perception of the adaptation needed to succeed in the new environment.

Young adults may seek treatment or are even hospitalized as a result of marital conflict, separation, or divorce.

Intervening with these clients usually requires couple or family therapy for effective conflict resolution. When these therapies are not possible, the nurse facilitates expression of feelings to increase self-esteem. The client is asked to describe situations or behaviors that precipitate conflict with the spouse. The client is encouraged to accept responsibility for hurtful or destructive behaviors and is asked to try new interaction techniques with the spouse and report the results. Specific measures for intervening in marital conflict are described in Chapter 30.

✴ *Spiritual dimension.* A young couple who experiences a significant loss, for example, loss of a newborn, may seek support and begin to explore their religious values, often for the first time, from an adult perspective. This shared experience either strengthens the relationship or creates tension that may inhibit communication and thus stress the relationship.

The nurse gains a critical client perspective by exploring his value system with him. The client's view of the meaning of life is helpful in assisting with feelings of depression or low self-esteem. The inclusion of the value system and religious orientation in the treatment plan can provide insight into areas of client conflict and outside resources or support systems that can be used to change the client's perspective and behavior.

A crisis precipitates a wide range of individual responses. The client with a strong religious orientation may become introspective and respond consistently with the goal of renewal. Thus the successful resolution of a crisis may provide a mechanism for continued growth.

The following Case Example demonstrates the role of the nurse in assisting the client to resolve an ethical and moral conflict.

Case Example

Mary, a 22-year-old newlywed, contacted the university mental health clinic to see a therapist because her high level of anxiety was interfering with her success in graduate school. The nurse interviewing Mary provided an opportunity for her to discuss the problem that initiated the contact and sought clues to other issues that may need to be addressed. Mary stated that she had only recently married and that both she and her husband had several more years of education. When questioned about her marriage, she became tearful and said all was going well until she found out she was pregnant a month ago. Her husband had become very angry, said that she was irresponsible, and accused her of tricking him. He refused to talk about the pregnancy and spent a great deal of time away from their apartment in the last month.

The nurse noted that Mary had been feeling a great deal of stress during this period and that her anxiety, sleeplessness, and failure to concentrate was caused by her pregnancy and her husband's reaction to it. Mary expressed a need to talk about options for the pregnancy. The nurse provided information and support as Mary began to deal with her husband's anger and ambivalence about abortion. The nurse also provided information on specific community agencies as requested and an oppor-

tunity for Mary and her husband to meet with her to discuss abortion, adoption, and ways to incorporate a baby into their life-style.

At the next appointment Mary told the nurse that confronting the problem had made it possible for her to continue school and that she and her husband had made plans to begin their family. They were looking into child care and other options so that they both could complete their education without delay. The nurse had assessed the scope of the problem and provided support during a stressful period when issues of values and morality had to be addressed by the young couple.

Evaluation

The involvement of the young adult in the evaluation phase of the nursing process is the culmination of the nurse-client relationship. Review of outcome criteria and achievement of short-term and long-term goals are the focus of the evaluation process. During the evaluation process, stress and current level of coping are also addressed. Since evaluation is an ongoing process, when the client progresses in treatment and new goals are established, the overall therapeutic plan is reevaluated and updated.

Positive growth is evident when the client is comfortable in intimate heterosexual relationships. This displays that the client has made some choices regarding his roles as an adult.

BRIEF REVIEW

Young adulthood (ages 20 to 44 years) encompasses a period of increasing societal expectations. Establishing financial independence from the family of origin, developing an intimate relationship, marrying, and parenting place demands on the individual that can produce stress. An individual unable to successfully cope with the demands of this period may experience high levels of stress, demonstrate substance abuse behaviors, or express feelings of unworthiness and depression.

The young adult is encountering a period of rapid emotional change. They are also faced with issues regarding the changing role of women and men in U.S. society. The adaptive response of the young adult is often challenged and confused by the wide range of life-styles to choose from.

Developmental tasks of this period are identified by a number of theorists. The individual's perception of his world greatly determines if he perceives himself as a success or failure. The demands of professional education and career development may prove extremely stressful, although cognitive functioning remains high during this period.

When working with the young adult, the nurse becomes acutely aware of the client's striving to meet the demands of school or work. The client's continued use of coping mechanisms that were successful in earlier developmental stages may interfere with more mature problem-solving activities. Resolution of issues not addressed in earlier developmental periods is a critical task.

REFERENCES AND SUGGESTED READINGS

1. Adams, C.G., and Macione, A., editors: Handbood of psychiatric mental health nursing, New York, 1983, John Wiley & Sons, Inc.
2. American Psychiatric Association: Quick references to the diagnostic criteria from DSM III, Washington, D.C., 1980, The Association.
3. Carpenito, L.J.: Handbook of nursing diagnosis, Philadelphia, 1984, J.B. Lippincott Co.
4. Chadrow, N.: Family structure and feminine personality. In Rosaldo, M.Z., and Lamphere, L., editors: Women, culture and society, Stanford, Calif. 1974, Stanford University Press.
5. Charlesworth E.A., and Nathan, R.G.: Stress management: a comprehensive guide to wellness, New York, 1984, Atheneum Publishers.
6. Cohen, R.S., and others: Parenthood: a psychodynamic perspective, New York, 1984, The Guilford Press.
7. Cronenwett, L.R.: Network structure, social support, and psychological outcomes of pregnancy, Nursing Research 34(2):93, 1985.
8. Delgaty, K.: Battered women: the issues for nursing, The Canadian Nurse 82(2):21, 1985.
9. Diekelman N.: Primary health care of the well adult, New York, 1977, McGraw-Hill, Inc.
10. Erikson, E.H.: Childhood and society, ed. 2, New York, 1964, W.W. Norton & Co., Inc.
11. Erikson, E.H.: Generativity and ego integrity. In Neugarten, B., editor: Middle age and aging, Chicago, 1968, The University of Chicago Press.
12. Freiberg, K.: Human development: a life span approach, Monterey, Calif., 1983, Wadsworth Publishing Co.
13. Freud A.: The concept of developmental lines: their diagnostic significance, Psychoanalytic Study of the Child 36:129, 1981.
14. Freud, S.: Three contributions to the theory of sex, ed 4, Washington D.C., 1930, Nervous and mental Disease Publishing Co.
15. Fromm E.: The sane society, New York, 1955, Rinehart.
16. Gilligan C.: In a different voice: psychological theory and women's development, Cambridge, Mass., 1982, Harvard University Press.
17. Gordon, M.: Nursing diagnosis: process and application, New York, 1982, McGraw-Hill, Inc.
18. Gould, R.: Transformations, New York, 1978, Simon & Schuster, Inc.
19. Hoffman, L.: Effects of the first child on the women's role, In Miller, W., and Newman, L., editors: The first child and family formation, Chapel Hill, 1978, University of North Carolina.
20. Horney, K.: The neurotic personality of our Time, New York, 1937, W.W. Norton.
21. Kaluger, G., and Kaluger, M.F.: Human development: the life span, St. Louis, 1974, The C.V. Mosby Co.
22. Keane, S.M.: Challenge within the community: crisis intervention for society's unemployed, Nursing Forum 21(3):138, 1984.
23. Lederman, R.P.: Psychosocial adaptation to pregnancy, Englewood Cliffs, N.J., 1984, Prentice-Hall, Inc.
24. Levinson, D., and others: The seasons of a man's life, New York, 1979, Alfred A. Knopf, Inc.
25. Lowenstein, S.R.: Suicidal behavior recognition and intervention, Hospital Practice 20:10A, Oct. 30, 1985.
26. McFarland, G., and Wasli, E.: Nursing diagnosis and process in psychiatric mental health nursing, Philadelphia, 1986, J.B. Lippincott Co.
27. Murray, R.B., and Zentner, J.P.: Nursing assessment and health promotion through the life span, Englewood Cliffs, N.J., 1979, Prentice-Hall, Inc.
28. National data book and guide to sources: statistical abstract of the U.S., ed. 105, Washington, D.C., 1985, U.S. Bureau of the Census.
29. Owen, B.D.: The young adult. In Hill, P.M., and Humphrey, P., editors: Human growth and development throughout life: a nursing perspective, New York, 1982, John Wiley & Sons, Inc.
30. Piaget, J.: The stages of the intellectual development of the child, Bulletin of Menninger Clinic 26:120, 1962.
31. Snegroff, S.: The stressors of non-marital sexual intercourse, Health Education 16(6):21, 1985-1986.
32. Sullivan, H.S.: The interpersonal theory of psychiatry, New York, 1953, Norton Publisher.
33. Toffler, A.: The third wave, New York, 1980, Bantam Books, Inc.
34. Valliant, G.: Adaptation to life, Boston, 1977, Little, Brown & Co.
35. Walster, E., and Walster, G.: A new look at love, Reading, Mass., 1978, Addison-Wesley Publishing Co., Inc.
36. Watson, J.: Nursing: human science and human caring—a thing of nursing, East Norwalk, Conn., 1985, Appleton-Century-Crofts.
37. Woods, N.F.: Human sexuality in health and illness, ed. 3, St. Louis, 1984, The C.V. Mosby Co.

ANNOTATED BIBLIOGRAPHY

Freeberg, K: Human development: a life span approach, Monterey, Calif., 1983, Wadsworth Publishing Co.

This book addresses the genetic, health, family, social network, and other determinants of development on persons of various age groups. Determinants of development are examined from the perspective of various research methodologies and theoretical viewpoints. Chapters on adulthood bring together valuable research and information needed by the nurse to address the needs of the adult client.

Hill, P.M., and Humphrey, P., editors: Human growth and development throughout life: a nursing perspective, New York, 1982, John Wiley & Sons, Inc.

This text gives an overview of psychosocial theories related to human growth and development. It addresses the dynamic, changing process experienced from infancy to senescence. Psychosocial, physical, and cognitive development of the young adult is explored and issues of career and job satisfaction explored. Tasks of the developing family and the crisis experienced in parenthood are seen to demand planning and timely preparation. A chapter focusing on common health and developmental problems of young adults provides a valuable perspective for the nurse.

Newman, B.M., and Newman, P.R.: Personality development through the life span, Monterey, Calif., 1983, Brooks/Cole Publishing Co.

An excellent overview of methods and measurements used to study personality development. Chapters on motivation, role, crises, and coping provide a theoretical basis for research related to the young adult period. The process of coping is identified as an interaction between personal resources and preferred coping strategies and the unique demands confronting the individual.

Schuster, C.S., and Ashburn, & S.S.: The process of human development: a holistic life-span approach, Boston, Mass., 1986, Little, Brown & Co.

Schuster and Ashburn provide several chapters of interest to those working in the area of young adults. Chapters on changing roles, initiating a family unit, and decision making regarding parenting provide an extensive overview of the issues encountered during the young adult period.

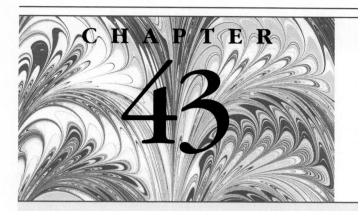

CHAPTER 43

THE MIDDLE-AGED ADULT

Sophronia R. Williams

After studying this chapter the learner will be able to:

Trace the history of interest in the middle-aged adult.

Discuss theories related to middle-aged adults.

Identify issues of a therpaeutic relationship with a middle-aged adult.

Apply the nursing process to the care of middle-aged clients.

Individuals of the post–World War II baby boom are now entering middle age. Middle-aged adults will compose 12% of the population by the year 2050. In addition to the number of "new"-middle-aged adults by virtue of birth rate, advances in health science contribute to the growth of this age group. The mental health–psychiatric nurse meets the mental health care needs of the middle-aged adult with special emphasis on prevention of problems.

Although there is no formal discipline for studying the middle years, there is noticeable interest in this stage. Some have tried to dispel some of the myths about middle age.[21] Fewer professionals now view middle-aged adults as "over the hill," although the stereotype of the middle-aged man who deserts his wife for a woman half his age still exists. Today the middle-aged woman whose children are grown may begin a second career instead of floundering in her "empty nest."

The middle years are viewed by some as the prime of life, when people change but are generally responsible and in control of their lives. Middle-aged persons are usually in fairly good physical and emotional health and financially secure. They have recognized their intellectual abilities, established themselves in the social world, and found ways to meet their spiritual needs. They also experience changes that result in satisfactions and stresses unique to this period of life.

The chronological definition of middle age varies, beginning at age 35 to 45 and ending at age 60 to 65. Levinson and others[51] define middle adulthood as five developmental periods:

40 to 45: Midlife transition
45 to 50: Entrance into middle adulthood
50 to 55: Age 50 transition
55 to 60: Culmination of middle adulthood
60 to 65: Late adulthood transition

Midlife transition begins when people become aware that life experiences such as reproductive and physical changes and children leaving home signify the beginning of another stage in life. The individual reappraises the meaning of his life and attempts to integrate past, present, and future. A goal of this period is to complete three major tasks: (1) to terminate the era of early adulthood by reappraising the life goals identified and achieved, (2) to initiate movement into middle adulthood by beginning to make necessary changes in unsuccessful aspects of the current life while trying out new choices, and (3) to deal with polarities that divide life.[28] The individual's ultimate goal is to rebuild his life structure. During introspection the middle-aged adult asks himself questions such as What have I done with my life? What do I really get from and give to my spouse, children, friends, work, community, and self? What are my strengths and liabilities? What have I done with my early dream and do I want it now? Based on the answers to these questions, the middle-aged adult in transition redefines his own individuality as a mature adult.

Some people make a smooth transition to middle adulthood. Others may experience a midlife crises. In either case what a middle-aged adult learns about himself during the transition may be experienced as a challenge to test his ability to learn to function as a middle-aged adult.

🍇 *Historical Overview* 🍇

DATE	EVENT
Pre-1900s	There was no systematic study of the developmental experiences of the middle-aged adult. Philosophers, prophets, and other writers emphasized either characteristic abilities or social and moral responsibilities of the middle-aged adult.
Early 1900s	Popular and professional writers portrayed the middle-aged adult as desolate, gloomy, and more despairing than hopeful. Much information used to describe middle-aged adults came from psychoanalysts' therapy with them. Psychoanalysts viewed the middle years as a series of crises that resulted in pathological behavior. Jung was the first to investigate the middle years while treating his clients.
1920s-1930s	Buhler and others conducted the first formal research on middle-aged adults and recognized them as relatively healthy with strengths. Although their lives were contracting, they could take stock and reassess their lives.
1940s-1950s	Attention was focused on the study of the relatively healthy middle-aged adult.
1960s	The Bethesda Conference on the Middle Years recommended that research be directed toward the potentials of the middle-aged adult instead of their problems. A federal conference on aging recognized that research on the problems of middle age was necessary to solve the problems of the older adult. Professionals became interested in maintaining the health of the middle-aged adult.
1975	The American Journal of Nursing discussed changes in the sexual, physical, and social needs of the middle-aged adult and later compared the middle years with other phases in the life cycle.
1977	The Schweppe Research and Education Fund Conference focused on the interaction between biomedical and social factors in the aging process, with emphasis on the middle-aged adult. Dissemination of information on realities of middle age to middle-aged adults, young adults, health care professionals, educators, and policy makers was emphasized. Nursing began demonstrating interest in all aspects of middle age. Stevenson,[75] a nurse, wrote a textbook devoted to issues and crises in the middle years.
1979	Burnside and other nurses comprehensively covered experiences of the middle-aged adult in their text.[14]
1980s	Articles on the middle years are included in journals, and nurses have included a discussion of this age group in textbooks.
Future	Interest in this age group will increase as the "new middle-aged adults" now begin their movement through the life span and greater emphasis is given to prevention of mental health problems.

Many theorists agree that age may not be the most significant determinant of entrance into the middle years. Individual differences, including cultural factors, mark transition to middle adulthood. Specific life events may also signal the beginning of middle age.[58] Social and positional cues show middle age as a period between young adulthood and retirement. A social position between these two generations increases middle-aged persons' awareness that they are in a separate class. Physical and biological cues indicate changes in the body. People may find they tire more readily. Psychological cues also mark entrance into middle years. These cues relate to the irreversible patterns established by people that determine their life goals. Parents realize their children have left home for good. The woman without children realizes she may never be a mother. Psychological cues may be used to assess career goals.

THEORETICAL APPROACHES
Psychoanalytic

Intrapsychic. Erikson's[21] seventh stage of life can be considered the middle years. The developmental task is generativity versus stagnation. *Generativity* is a commitment to care for and a willingness to counsel and guide others. Erickson believed no form of generativity is as meaningful as that with one's own children. Middle-aged persons who fail to achieve generativity may stagnate, which is manifested through a person's excessive concern with himself. Feelings of stagnation may also be manifested in destructive behavior toward one's children and the community. Although having children is itself no guarantee against stagnation, a person's concern for his own children and for the next generation can help prevent stagnation.

Jung's theories[45] about the middle years, based on a psychological model, addressed aspects of the spiritual dimension. He viewed life as contracting in middle age. The task for middle-aged people is to make a transition to their inner orientation, which may be threatening because it involves giving up the images of youth and recognizing one's mortality. The stresses that accompany this transition may motivate middle-aged adults to cling to behavior characteristic of youth. However, in the developmental process of self-individuation, they become more uniquely themselves. This process enables them to balance their four psychologial functions: thought, feeling, intuition, and sensation.

With this balance middle-aged people begin to feel more secure about their attitudes and feel they have discovered the right course in life and the right ideals.

Buhler's theories[10] about the middle years emphasized goal formulation. Like Jung, she viewed life as an expansion and contraction process. She proposed a critical assessment of life's goals, with acknowledgement of success or failure as the major task of middle age. The achievement of goals depends on (1) satisfaction of needs, (2) ability to expand creaatively, (3) adjustment to limitations, and (4) consistency of inner self. She believed that generally, by middle age, a person has either achieved his goals or has failed. Few people achieve all their life goals. Occasionally goals may not be identifed until late in life. The emotional responses to unfulfilled goals are depression, despair, and sometimes suicide.

Peck,[78] expanding Erikson's concepts, described four phases of psychological development for middle age.

1. Valuing wisdom versus valuing physical powers. Wisdom is the ability to make the best choices from the alternatives that are available to the person. The middle-aged person inevitably experiences decrease in physical strength, stamina and beauty. The person adjusts to declining physical stamina and health by investing more energy into mental activities. Peck recognized that a person's emotional status and intellectual ability affect his ability to achieve the task. Persons who value and define their lives in terms of physical power become increasingly depressed and bitter as that power inevitably declines.

2. Socializing versus sexualizing in human relationships. The sexual climacteric coincides with the general decline in physical powers. This change motivates middle-aged people to redefine men and women in their lives as individuals and companions rather than primarily as sexual objects.

3. Cathectic flexibility versus cathectic impoverishment. This task requires the ability to shift emotional investments from one person to another and from one activity to another. Peck believed the task is crucial in middle years, because people experience the loss of many relationships. Although middle-aged persons experience losses, they have a wide circle of acquaintances at work and in the community for reinvestment of emotions. People who are unsuccessful in replacing the lost relationships with new ones suffer increasingly impoverished emotional lives through the years.

4. Mental flexibility versus mental rigidity. This basic conflict affects all changes of middle age. Mental flexibility, meaning not being set in one's ways, is shown through openness to new ideas and acceptance of change in self and society. Flexible adults strive to master life experiences and use them as guides to solving new problems. Rigid middle-aged adults are set in their ways, inflexible in their opinions and actions, and closed-minded to new ideas. Peck believes that mental rigidity is most noticeable during middle age when people have a set of answers to life.

Sociocultural

Havighurst[40] also identified developmental tasks of middle age. The individual needs to assume a position of social responsibility and guidance in the following ways:

1. Achieve adult civic social responsibility
2. Establish and maintain an economic standard of living
3. Help teenage children become responsible and happy adults
4. Develop adult leisure activities
5. Relate to one's spouse as a person
6. Accept and adjust to the physiological changes of middle age
7. Adjust to aging parents

The literature since Havighurst first published his model in 1950 demonstrates its continuing validity. Some tasks, such as adjustment to aging parents, have only recently begun to receive attention.

Table 43-1 presents a summary of the theoretical approaches.

RELATING TO THE CLIENT

Most middle-aged persons cope effectively with the stresses of the middle years by themselves (see the Research Highlight on p. 827). Others contract for the services of a mental health–psychiatric nurse. Still others are motivated by acute and chronic problems to seek help. In general, middle-aged clients are able to participate in delineating the terms of the therapeutic relationship.

The nurse's attitude toward middle-aged clients and their attitudes toward themselves will influence the nature of the relationship. Because of previous pessimism about the possibilities for change in middle age, the nurse and client may share a fatalistic attitude. The nurse needs to accept the client's capacity for change to enhance the client's acceptance of potential for change. If, for example, the nurse thinks a woman who has symptoms of menopausal changes is merely a neurotic middle-aged woman, the development of basic trust is hindered.

Setting goals is based on the nurse's knowledge of events that normally occur in middle age. Equally essen-

TABLE 43-1 Summary of theoretical approaches

Theory	Theorist	Dynamics
Psychoanalytic	Erikson	Achievement of the developmental task generativity versus stagnation is evident in a commitment to care for and a willingness to counsel and guide the next generation. Failure to achieve the task results in excessive concern for oneself.
	Jung	The task for middle age is to make a transition from outer to inner orientation.
		The transition enables middle-aged people to feel secure about their course in life and to balance their four psychological functions: thought, feeling, intuition, and sensation.
	Buhler	The middle years are characterized by expansion and contraction, during which time the person assesses life goals and acknowledges successes and failures.
	Peck	There are four phases of psychological development for middle age: (1) valuing wisdom versus valuing physical powers, (2) socializing versus generalizing in human relationships, (3) cathectic flexibility versus cathectic impoverishment, and (4) mental flexibility versus mental rigidity.
Sociocultural	Havighurst	The developmental task of middle age is to assume a position of social responsibility and guidance of others.

tial to the therapeutic relationship are the middle-aged client's contributions to the identification of goals.

During the contract phase, the nurse and client make decisions about appropriate therapeutic approaches. The general approaches are those used with other adults. Depending on the problem, types of therapy that may be offered are individual, group, and family therapy. Group therapy is particularly useful for middle-aged clients.[13] Butler's use of family therapy that at times includes the grandparents, parents, and children has also proved beneficial. Self-help groups, such as Parents Without Partners, Widow-to-Widow programs, and Alcoholics Anonymous, are also beneficial.

During the working phase, the nurse guides middle-aged clients in an exploration of stressors related to their problem. It is important for the nurse to deal with current realities, rather than early childhood experiences. The goal is to help the client master his problems by confronting them. The nurse assesses the client's potential strength to cope with his problems and helps him develop strategies for constructive resolution. The middle-aged client's fatalistic attitude may reemerge during the working phase. The belief that he is powerless to change events in his life is manifested as resistance to change. Effective work on problems depends on the nurse's understanding that middle-aged clients have a wealth of knowledge and can teach both themselves and others. The skillful nurse teaches clients that they have this capacity and engages in a collaborative relationship instead of patronizing them.

The nurse who becomes angry at the middle-aged client who exhibits helplessness and an inabilty to participate in his care may be manifesting countertransference, which hampers a collaborative relationship. Middle-aged nurses may identify with the middle-aged client and be unable to provide quality care. Young nurses may view the middle-aged client as an authority figure who should be self-sufficient. These perceptions may also indicate countertransference.

Once middle-aged clients make new choices or achieve their consolidated life goals, they are ready for the termi-

nation of the therapeutic relationship. Because of the numerous losses middle-aged clients have experienced, the nurse and client decide on the last meeting several weeks in advance. The usual anxiety, anger, grief, and feelings of rejection of termination may be intensified for middle-aged clients. Depression may replace the more healthy grieving process. A constructive termination with the nurse may contribute to resolving grief from previous losses.

NURSING PROCESS
Assessment

Physical dimension. The most visible physical changes in the middle years, such as graying hair, wrinkling skin, excess fat at the waist, and balding, are influenced by genetic factors. These changes may lead to alterations in body image. People who are anxious about these signs of middle age may try to conceal them. Feelings about getting older and becoming unattractive may be expressed openly or may be disguised in statements referring to someone else, such as "I'm not attractive to my spouse now that I'm getting older." Some people may seek extramarital relationships to prove that they are still attractive to members of the opposite sex.

Of the visible physical changes that affect body image, the most threatening to physical health is obesity. For people who are 30% or more overweight, the probability of dying in middle age increases by 40%.[80] Overeating may be in response to midlife changes or anxiety. Marked obesity may follow major emotional stressors, such as a death in the family, vocational failures, and marital unhappiness. Of course, responses to changes in physical appearance vary with individuals. Clients who derive feelings of worth from their bodies, are likely to be more sensitive to changes in their physical appearance than those who focus on other ways of assessing their value.

Heart disease and stroke, the main causes of death in middle age, are stress-related illnesses and may also be determined by genetic factors. Genetic factors also seem to

Research Highlight

An Analysis of Coping in a Middle-Aged Community Sample

S. Folkman & R.S. Lazarus

PURPOSE

This study was designed to analyze the ways in which community-residing men and women ages 45 to 64 coped with the stressful events of daily life in 1 year and to provide an approach to the assessment of coping.

SAMPLE

The sample was 100 white, primarily Protestant respondents (52 women and 48 men) aged 45 to 64. The participants were selected by telephone from a population previously surveyed.

METHODOLOGY

Information about recently experienced stressful encounters was elicited through monthly interviews and self-report questionnaires completed between interviews. At the end of each interview and questionnaire, the participant indicated on a 68-item checklist the coping thoughts and actions used in the specific encounter. Two methods of coping, problem focused and emotion focused, were analyzed.

FINDINGS

Both problem- and emotion-focused coping were used in 98% of the encounters analyzed. Problem-focused coping was used most often at work and when the person thought something constructive could be done or that additional information was needed. Emotion-focused coping was used in situations related to health and those stressful events the participants viewed as having to be accepted. There was no significant difference between men and women in the methods of coping used, except that men used more problem-focused coping than women.

IMPLICATIONS

Middle-aged adults have the ability to use coping behavior when confronted with problems of daily life. These persons may need to be assisted to increase their use of problem-focused coping with health problems.

Based on data from Journal of Health and Social Behavior **21**:219, 1980.

play a role in predisposing some middle-aged clients to peptic ulcers. These health problems may lead to anxiety over the threat to the client's independence in his job and role in his family. Because cardiovascular disease is the most common cause of death of people in their late 50s, fear of death may be a realistic concern.

Physiological processes of middle age affect all body systems. Changes in these processes influence clients' perceptions of themselves and their ability to function and to relate to others (Table 43-2).

The effect of reproductive changes of middle years on the client's physical functioning needs to be assessed. More information is available about women and their endocrine changes than about men. The onset of the climacteric that includes *menopause* varies; however, ages 40 to 43 is a commonly accepted range for the cessation of menstruation. Women's physiological responses to the climacteric may be characterized by breast pain, hot flashes, and dizzy spells. The emotional and intellectual responses to menopause vary. The stereotypical response portrayed in the literature is often exaggerated. Some women may go from one physician to the next demanding estrogen therapy for treatment of what they consider menopausal symptoms. This response suggests a more serious problem.[53] For many women cessation of menstruation is a happy relief from concern about unwanted pregnancy. Others are depressed.

Osteoporosis is of concern to the middle-aged woman.

This disease results from a decrease in bone mass and calcium loss, begins at about age 40, and becomes more pronounced during and after menopausal changes. It affects 35% to 40% of all women, with the highest incidence among whites and the lowest among blacks. The roundness of the upper back and loss of skeletal height adversely affect body image. Table 43-3 presents risk factors for osteoporosis.

The man's climacteric is referred to as *andropause* because of the decline in the androgen levels during the late 40s and early 50s. Men still produce sperm and are capable of fathering children well into late adulthood.[53] Anxiety and depression may result from a decrease in ability to have an orgasm, which may be viewed as sexual inadequacy or imagined loss of sexual power.

The number of hours of sleep that the middle-aged adult needs varies among individuals; however, the average person requires 6 to 8 hours. As the middle-aged individual approaches his 60s and expends less energy, the need for sleep is approximately 5 to 6 hours a night. More active middle-aged persons may take naps or doze during the day.[73] In a study by Tune[79] sleep charts were kept for an average of 51 days on 509 normal adults ages 20 to 79. As age increased, subjects went to bed earlier and awoke earlier in the morning. Middle-aged participants slept less well than older and younger adults. Complaints of sleeplessness increase with age, but in women there is a sharp increase around the age of 50 that is not found in men. A

TABLE 43-2 Selected physiological changes in the middle-aged adult according to body systems

Body System	Selected Changes
Muscular	Mass, structure, and strength slowly decline as a result of decreased muscle use. Changes in collagen fibers result in thicker and less elastic muscles and cause sagging and drooping of breast, facial, and abdominal muscles.
Skeletal	Bone mass begins to decrease, calcium loss and related bone thinning follows menopausal changes, skeletal changes in the thoracic vertebrae lead to height decrease (more pronounced in women than men), and changes occur in the hip joints.
Integumentary	With adequate nutrition and fluid intake, tissues of the integument remain intact and healthy until age 50 to 55. After this age, wrinkles gradually become noticeable, body water content decreases from 60% to 56%, leading to dry skin; and fat content increases from 14% to 30%, leading to sagging folds, such as under the arms and under the eyes. Too rapid weight reduction causes loose folds that do not readily accommodate the loss of fat. Because of loss of water, the skin is more easily bruised and wounds heal more slowly.
Central nervous	Marked changes usually do not occur until very old age. The high level of intellectual functioning is discussed under assessment of the intellectual dimension. Reflexes begin to slow, and slower response to environmental changes may be observable.
Cardiovascular	Well into middle age, the size of the heart increases to accommodate changes in the arterial system. Functions, rate, and rhythm of the heart are maintained through active work and recreactional activities. As sedentary activities increase, the heart begins to lose its tone, and rhythm and rate changes are noticeable.
Respiratory	The respiratory tissues maintain full vital respiratory capacity (maximal breathing capacity) throughout early middle age, barring cigarette smoking and respiratory disease. By age 55 to 60 there is a gradual decrease in breathing capacity caused by thicker, stiffer, and less elastic lung tissues. Cardiopulmonary diseases may accompany the changes in lung tissue.
Renal	With adequate fluid intake, the normal mechanism of kidney functioning is maintained at full capacity throughout middle age.
Gastrointestinal	Normally, secretions from the gastrointestinal tract are maintained at high levels through early middle age. Decreases in the production of digestive enzymes, acids, and juices may be a factor in the increase in incidence of intestinal disorders, cancer, and gastrointestinal complaints of middle-aged clients.
Metabolic	Onset of diabetes mellitus, hypothyroidism, and adrenal tumors is more common after age 45. Proneness to ulcers and vascular lesions increase because of an increased amount of antiinflammatory hormones. This change in hormones may also affect clients' ability to handle stress.
Special senses	Farsightedness that necessitates correction with glasses or contact lenses develops. Because lenses of eyes gradually become more opaque after age 45, cataract formation becomes a possibility. Blindness may develop as a consequence of diabetes, hypertension, or other cardiovascular conditions. The sense of hearing, smell, taste, and touch are generally maintained at high levels in early middle age. After age 50, noticeable losses in hearing and smell may occur.

controlled trial of the use of estrogens as a hypnotic in postmenopausal women showed that estrogen reduced the number of episodes of sleeplessness.[77]

✳️ *Emotional dimension.* Buhler[9] referred to middle age as the period of the greatest emotional energy because of the various changes to which people have to adapt. Even when the changes do not directly impair functioning, a variety of emotional responses may be identified during assessment.

Clients feel anxiety in response to the changes that signify movement into middle age. This anxiety may motivate them to engage in reassessment of themselves and to work further on accomplishing their life goals. This self-analysis is in response to heightened self-awareness when "life is restructured in terms of time-left-to-live rather than time-since-birth."[58]

Kuhlen[50] proposed that anxiety is a positive source of motivation that may increase and become more generalized in middle age. When people experience the beginning of life contraction, they feel anxious about irreversible physical and social losses. To the extent that people succeed in having rewarding, nonthreatening life experiences, anxiety does not increase appreciably with age. People who capitalize on the benefits of middle age and are not threatened by the visible signs of aging do not feel increased anxiety; those who fear growing old may feel increased anxiety.

Anxiety may be expressed as general malaise or psychophysiological illnesses, such as peptic ulcers, rheumatoid arthritis, and hypertension. When the nurse assesses men between the ages of 40 and 50, she may detect an increase in anxiety over the threat of sudden death from a heart attack. Anxiety over death may be reflected in the

TABLE 43-3 Risk factors for osteoporosis

Factor	Characteristics
Sex	Female
Age	Increases for women after menopause
Race	White
Physical stature	Small frame

client's scanning of the obituary column or writing of a will in response to the death of friends and possibly parents. Ill health and death are threats that give rise to anxiety and influence the middle-aged client's life-style.

Some of the defense mechanisms used in response to such anxiety are denial and rationalization. Use of dissociation, repression, and sublimation may also increase in midlife. Masking common physical changes is coping behavior and may suggest some discomfort about the aging process.

Many experiences of middle-aged clients have the potential for generating anger. At work clients may strive harder as the time for work shortens. They may perceive a young adult as someone who wants to replace them. This real or imagined threat leads to anger as a defense against the anxiety. Clients may also become angry at work when they perceive others trying to hold them back.

When middle-aged clients feel desperate because their needs are not met, they may express anger toward parents and children, whom they perceive as contributing to the lack of need satisfaction. Anger about the role reversal that occurs between middle-aged children and their elderly parents has implications for mental health–psychiatric nursing. The children who perceive themselves as sacrificing their lives for their parents may become frustrated and bitter, and the elderly parents may become the objects of rejection and abuse (see Chapter 36). In the process of striving to become successful clients may have neglected to establish meaningful family relationships; then, in middle age, their lives seem empty.

Middle-aged adults who have neglected or abused their parents may feel guilty. Because of this guilt, adult children may tend to overprotect their parents. Middle-aged clients may also feel guilt when they think they could have done more to achieve their life goals. On the other hand, some people may feel guilt because they surpassed their parents in achieving their career goals. Middle-aged parents may feel guilty about how they raised their children, especially when children do not live up to their expectations.

Most persons approaching middle age feel confident of their ability to make the necessary adjustment. They view it as another milestone in life and may welcome it as a time for further growth. Their positive outlook results from satisfaction with their achievements.

Others respond to midlife changes with despair and depression. Depression is a major threat during the middle years, with increased prevalence of major depression in persons over the age of 45.

Risk factors that increase the likelihood of depression are summarized in Table 43-4.

TABLE 43-4 Risk factors for depression in middle age

Risk Factors	Characteristics
Sex	Female
Age	Declines for women after early 50s; increases for men after late 50s
Social isolation	Absence of intimate, confiding relationships after a change in the nature of the relationship with parents, children, and spouse
Losses	Parental deprivation or loss of a mother before age 14; other losses during midlife, such as a job, career difficulties, marital problems, and physical changes; departure of last child from home; unfulfilled life goals
Family history	History of depression in the family of origin

The losses of middle age need to be assessed as they relate to the client's perceived purpose in life. Lost family ties have traditionally been felt more intensely in midlife by women than by men. The departure of the last child from home may aggravate an already existing middle-aged depression or may precipitate the depression. Working women are less likely to become depressed than housewives, possibly because they are active in another role.

In the past it was believed that hormonal changes associated with menopause played a major role in precipitating depression in middle age. Today many believe that the hormonal changes play no role in the cause of depression in this period. Women who experience severe depression during menopause may be responding to other various losses or may interpret menopausal changes as a loss of femininity. The severe depression that occurs is sometimes referred to as *agitated depression* and is believed to be characterized by a moderate to high level of anxiety, bizarre physical complaints, and paranoid ideation. The essential features of depression in the menopausal years do not differ appreciably from depression in other age groups. Most psychiatrists believe that the clinical features of depression in middle-aged men are no different from those at other times of life.[14] Involutional melancholia, which was once classified as the depression of middle age and may still appear in some texts, was characterized by agitation. This disorder is no longer considered an independent entity. The agitated depression associated with involutional melancholia may still be experienced by middle-aged clients but is not restricted to depression in the middle years.

In addition to the major depressions, an increased incidence of minor depression in middle-aged adults is observed. This occasional mild depression is of short duration and does not require intervention.

The potential for suicide needs to be assessed. Suicide and attempted suicide increase in middle age and are more common among men than women.[15] Suicide is less common between the ages of 40 and 50, after which it increases. Persons who commit suicide are often widowed, separated, or divorced. They may also be socially isolated. Depression and alcoholism in middle age contribute to an increase in the suicide rate. Over 90% of successful suicides are by persons who are depressed, alcoholic, or both.[55]

Intellectual dimension. During middle age, there is decreased efficiency in the functioning of some aspects of the intellectual dimension. However, the peak for other types of intellectual functions occurs at this time.

The special senses are affected in middle age. Most research indicates little change in the ability to taste food up to the age of 60, but taste buds begin to decrease in men at age 50 to 60 and in women at age 40 to 45. Touch sensitivity remains constant up to about the midfifties and then gradually decreases. Individual differences affect the ability to smell, although there seems to be an aging effect on the olfactory sense receptors. Research shows that visual efficiency declines rapidly after 40. Bifocals and trifocals are often needed to correct vision.

The nurse may observe paranoid ideation as a response to failure to achieve life goals. Buhler[19] describes middle-aged clients with this disorder as grandiose failures who have a paranoid lack of insight into their limited abilities or the circumstances that prevent fulfillment of their goals. They become bitter and envious of those who succeed and may blame others for their lack of success.

Short-term memory is believed to decline in middle age. However, the situations in which clients are tested need to be considered when assessing individual memory differences. The middle-aged client's ability to learn is related to the method of presentation. Information heard is generally retained longer than information acquired visually.

Alzheimer's disease is manifested between 45 and 64 years of age. The disease is a dementia with an insidious onset and progressive deterioration. The essential features are loss of memory for recent events and inefficiency in social or occupational functioning. Later, judgment and abstract thinking become impaired, and there may be personality changes. Progressive deterioration results in a vegetative state and death a few years after the onset of symptoms.

Pick's disease, like Alzheimer's disease, is a rare form of premature senile brain degeneration in middle-aged adults. The cerebral cortical degeneration is most significant in the frontal and temporal lobes, which show cellular destruction and gross atrophy. The client has marked personality changes. He may become irritable, belligerent, and morose or euphoric and irresponsible. Early in the illness the client's judgment, emotional control, and reasoning capacities deteriorate. However, gross memory losses and disorientation are not severe early in the disease. Aphasias are common, and deaths occurs in 3 to 10 years. As with Alzheimer's disease, neurologists believe Pick's disease may have hereditary determinants in some cases.[18]

Middle-aged adults who use their intellectual functions have little if any loss of mental ability, whereas those who do not engage in mental activities may experience a decline in intelligence. In middle age people may have a wealth of previous experiences that enhances their present functioning. This experience may be termed *wisdom*.[94]

For some middle-aged adults, vocabulary continues to increase and verbal skills continue to improve. There also may be an improvement in the abilities of the middle-aged

adult to organize and process incoming information and handle larger vocabularies.

Desmond[18] believed that some middle-aged adults are inflexible as a protest against what they view as change for change's sake rather than because they are middle-aged. Generally women are more flexible than men in their capacity for change and growth in middle age.[25]

❊ *Social dimension.* Abuse of alcohol is a major problem in middle age. The nurse will encounter middle-aged clients who have abused alcohol since young adulthood and in some cases since adolescence; these clients may increase consumption of alcohol in middle age in response to changes in their lives. Sometimes clients who have secretly abused alcohol may do so openly when the children leave home. Other clients may lead stable lives before reaching middle age and begin abusing alcohol in their early forties.[70] These clients seem to clearly resort to alcohol abuse in an effort to cope with various midlife changes.

Sometimes, once the children are no longer dependent on parents, one spouse becomes less tolerant of the other's consumption of alcohol or, now aware of the long-standing drinking problem, may seek separation or divorce. The threat of loss of the spouse may motivate the alcoholic partner to seek treatment.

Like alcoholic persons of any age, middle-aged adults may seek treatment because of problems on the job or with physical health. When assessing the health status of the middle-aged alcoholic, the nurse needs to differentiate between depression as a symptom and as a psychiatric illness. Depression as a symptom may result from abrupt abstinence of alcohol and may disappear in days or weeks without a need for antidepressant medication. As a psychiatric illness, depression lasts longer and usually needs to be treated with antidepressant medications and sometimes with ECT.[39]

Role changes in middle age are inevitable and are one of the primary areas to assess. When major role changes are predictable and occur in the normal course of life, they can be anticipated and may lead to limited disruption in clients' sense of themselves. The adjustment to abrupt changes in roles may lead to maladaptive responses. Women are far more eager and have less difficulty than men in changing roles.[22]

Generally the first role change of middle age is the departure of the last child from home. Families may experience the departure of several children, but the departure of the last child is especially significant because the parental responsibility for child rearing ends and the marital relationship becomes the primary one in the family. The extent to which the last child's departure from the home is felt as a negative stressor by the parents is still being debated. Data support the view that most middle-aged women respond positively, seeing it as an opportunity for freedom from child-rearing responsibilities.[30]

With no children at home, the parents may be forced to take stock of their marriage. Thus the nurse assesses the effects of the child's departure on the parents' relationship. The parents' reassessment of their marriage either leads to a strengthening of the relationship or reveals problems. One or both marital partners may become aware of dissatisfaction and seek an extramarital relationship. One may turn to a younger person in actuality or fantasy in a desire to maintain youth. Men are more likely than women to have extramarital affairs with younger partners. Although society greatly disapproves of an older man in an extramarital affair with a younger woman,[28] it is commonly more accepted than a woman having a young partner. However, acceptance of the latter is increasing.

Freidman[28] believed that strong marriages survive the reassessment of middle age and improve as the marital partners spend more time together. Maladaptive marriages tend to survive the midlife crisis because most people in such marriages are so insecure that they do not question the nature of the marital relationship.[28] These people maintain the marriage because they are neurotically dependent on their spouse, fearful of being alone, feel guilty, or are financially dependent on the spouse. However, divorce is a possible outcome of reassessment of the marital relationship in middle age. Partners who divorce after 20 years have usually been incompatible throughout their marriage. Divorce during the postparental years may result when a marriage was maintained for the sake of the children. The external restraints that traditionally bound couples together have been removed for some people. For example, the woman who works outside the home is not financially dependent on the husband and thus may be more likely to divorce if the marriage is not strong. However, divorce in midlife occurs less frequently and unhappy, incompatible marriages continue. The couple may cope by attempting to ignore the difficulties with emotional and physical withdrawal, extramarital relationships, and spending extra time at work.

The death of a spouse is one of the most stressful experiences of middle age. Women especially begin preparing for it in middle age. Women's tendencies to marry older men and the increasing death rate among middle-aged men, especially from cardiovascular disease, increase the potential for widowhood in middle age. Bereavement may lead to the death of widowed persons within 5 years of the spouse's death. Preparation for widowhood may entail anticipatory grief, with the person "rehearsing" with the death of friends and relatives.[78]

Men and women tend to react differently to the loss of a spouse. Men are likely to feel they have lost a part of themselves, while women may feel deserted and abandoned. Men may find it more difficult to express grief than women. However, men tend to recover from the loss more quickly than women and remarry sooner after the death. Women are likely to feel alone once the support of friends and family is no longer available. The majority of widowed persons in their late forties and early fifties remarry because they want companionship, to avoid loneliness, and to have a partner for social activities. Few women in their middle to late fifities remarry.[34]

The nature and the number of social relationships change in middle age. Assessment of these relationships provides data on stressors and social support systems. The changing relationship between the middle-aged adult child and aging parents is significant. Role reversal may lead to some of the stressors discussed earlier (see p. 830). Clients may need to be both parent and child to their own parents while being a parent to children who are older adolescents or young adults. The nurse needs to assess the nature of the relationship between grown children and their parents. If the client's parents are dead, the past relationship needs to be explored.

The decision to institutionalize an aging parent may engender strong feelings of guilt and shame. Caring for the aging parent may remind the client of his own aging and eventual death. The client may be unprepared to deal with this reality, or his experiences with his aging parents may motivate him to come to grips with his own aging and eventual death.

Parents of adolescents may have the additional stress of conflicts with their children. The combination of aging parents, adolescents, and possibly the financial pressures of putting one or more children through college can be a heavy burden for middle-aged parents.

Grandparenthood is a major life event that needs to be explored. Some middle-aged parents eagerly await the day they will become grandparents and may directly or indirectly pressure their children to begin a family. If the children will not accommodate the parent, a conflict may emerge. Transition into the role of grandparent involves a change in the parent-child relationship: for the first time parents share their parental role with an adult child.

The grandchild establishes a bond of common interest between the parent and the grandparent. A comprehensive study by Neugarten and Weinstein[60] indicated that most grandparents derive pleasure and satisfaction from their role. The grandparents in their study had negative experiences when differences arose between the adult child and the parents over child discipline and when grandparents were exploited for baby-sitting services.

Data on the meaning of the role of grandparent can be valuable for the assessment. Neugarten and Weinstein[60] have ascribed five meanings to the role of grandparent:

1. Grandparenthood can be perceived as a source of biological renewal or continuity with the future. In this instance the grandparents view the grandchildren as an extension of themselves, through whom they vicariously experience renewed life.
2. Grandparenthood provides emotional self-fulfillment by giving the grandparents an opportunity to perform the emotional role of grandparent better than they did the role of parent.
3. For a few persons grandparenthood means being a resource person. The grandparents can gain satisfaction by financial or experiential contributions to the grandchild's welfare.
4. A few persons view the grandchild as an extension of the self who will accomplish what neither they nor their children could. Thus the grandchild provides an opportunity for grandparents to aggrandize their ego.
5. Some persons have relatively remote feelings of psychological distance. They imply that they perceive the role as being without meaningful relationships.

In Neugarten and Weinstein's study some of the grandmothers attributed their remoteness to busy work and social schedules. The reasons given seem to have been rationalizations.

The anticipation of and first adjustment to the role of grandmother have not been systematically studied; however, data suggest that the middle-aged woman may consciously and unconsciously relive her own pregnancy and childbirth. She then may develop an anxious overidentification that later interferes with the pleasures of grandparenthood.[7]

Although middle-aged adults are often the givers rather than the receivers of social support, they need to receive social support, too. Social support helps them survive stress by mobilizing the personal resources necessary for coping and serves as a protection against the physical and mental illness that the stress of middle age seems to induce. Social support comes through interaction with family, friends, and acquaintances in informal and formal situations. An assessment of the number and quality of the relationships and the frequency of the interactions provides valuable data on middle-aged clients' support systems.

Because middle-aged adults are often between the older and younger generations in the family, opportunities for them to receive social support may be greatly decreased in this setting. Once the children leave the home, depending on the status of the marital relationship, the spouses may be able to provide mutual social support.

Many middle-aged persons have achieved stability in social competence and have established patterns of socializing that are compatible with their skills and income. This social competence is used to maintain relationships with friends. Friendships are important to middle-aged persons' well-being, and they may serve both as sources of emotional support and as an anchor for integration of the individual with the larger society. However, middle-aged adults may have few friends. Fewer friends in middle age is attributed to a decrease in ego energy rather than a loss of popularity. The relationships with friends that married couples maintain are close and generally develop when children are at home.

Single middle-aged women and men may have been working on friendships since early adulthood. Although some of their friends may be married, most are unmarried. The friendship patterns of the unmarried vary little in middle age. The single woman generally has a strong, stable support system in a group of female friends with whom she has traveled, socialized, and turned to in troubled times. There seems to be no clear pattern of social behavior and friendship patterns for men. The single middle-aged man is likely to have fewer friends than acquaintances. Thus acquaintances may comprise the single man's support system.[42]

The friendship circle diminishes considerably if divorced middle-aged individuals do not remarry. The change in marital status decreases the opportunity for support from friends at a time when the need is great.[42] Relatives may become the divorcee's closest friends and support system. Divorced middle-aged individuals with children at home have limited time for friendships and socializing.

The newly widowed person may at first be flooded with invitations. Later the bereaved person is invited to social functions as an "extra." Gradually this person builds friendships in a small group of other unattached middle-aged individuals.

The nurse may encounter middle-aged adults who avoid meaningful interaction with their peers because of lack of social skills. These clients may not have developed social skills, or during the years of parenting they may have failed to maintain their social relationships with peers. Sometimes clients who are ill at ease in situations with their peers will establish a "pal" relationship with their adolescent children, a relationship that was begun when they attended social activities with their young children. When making an assessment, the nurse may learn that the parent is seeking treatment because the children have broadened their social horizons beyond the parents.

Middle-aged adults are more involved in formal organizations than are young adults. The increased participation in various types of voluntary associations reaches its peak about age 50 and plateaus at the end of middle age.[93]

Middle-aged persons have had sufficient experience in social interaction to determine whom they can or cannot trust. Mistrust of the motives of others may occur at work when they perceive a threat to their position. However, the status they have earned in formal and informal organizations during early middle age also may lead to trust in others.

A changing sense of self results from all of the issues that characterize middle age, such as concerns about physical appearance, aging parents, and work. A number of studies indicate that a positive increase in self-concept usually occurs with advancing age.[41] Neugarten[58] described the self-concept of middle-aged clients in terms of their perception of changes in their careers, families, and status and how they deal with both inner and outer worlds. Women tend to shift their self-image from relationships with others to their own abilities and feelings. Men tend to be more occupationally minded in self-image and have more difficulty as they age.[5] The client who has adjusted well to the changes of middle age will have a positive self-concept. Clients who are insecure and lack self-confidence have a low opinion of themselves.

Middle-aged adults experience a balance between dependence and independence. Healthy dependence may be expressed in any of their life situations. At the same time middle-aged adults have a healthy degree of self-reliance. However, men in this age group have a passive-dependent tendency that increases with age, whereas women become more assertive. As a result of middle-aged adults' development of self, they appreciate the significance of interdependence. For example, parents need their children as vehicles for generativity and spouses rely on each other. Manifestations of an unhealthy imbalance between dependence and independence can be seen in the middle-aged businessman who has cardiac disease yet strives for independence as a defense against dependence.

The psychological implications of retirement are also assessed. The meaning of work to clients affects their adjustment to retirement. For some clients their work gives meaning and structure to their lives. Without preparation for retirement these clients may become physically or mentally ill. Some retiring persons are concerned about finding interests in common with their spouse. Single, divorced, or widowed persons may avoid thinking about retirement if they think it means loss of a position of value in society. Married persons may think of retirement as a joint endeavor. If only the husband is employed, the husband may anticipate retirement with pleasure, whereas the wife may worry about his hanging around the house all day because he may upset her schedule.

✂ *Spiritual dimension.* In middle age people reevaluate their values. The spiritual behavior of middle-aged persons may reflect accumulated wisdom and a value system based on deep philosophical grounds.[45] The middle-aged person may readily accept and understand the spiritual views of others to be legitimate.

Acceptance of the inevitability of one's own death is a significant task that must be completed in middle age. The death of parents increases awareness of vulnerability and death. Awareness of one's mortality also increases as same-age acquaintances become ill and die. The perception of death as a reality leads to taking stock of one's marriage, career, personal relationships, values, and other commitments made earlier in life.

Generally church membership and attendance rise sharply in the 40s and 50s, but both decline after 60. In an effort to cope with some of the changes in midlife, many people turn to religion.

The assessment tool at right contains assessment areas specific to the middle aged adult. It is to be used in conjunction with the assessment tool in Chapter 8.

Analysis

Nursing diagnosis. The following list provides examples of NANDA-accepted nursing diagnoses with causative statements.

1. Disturbance in self-concept related to obesity
2. Sleep pattern disturbance related to menopausal changes
3. Anxiety related to changes in body image
4. Grieving related to departure of children from home
5. Knowledge deficit related to rigidity
6. Impaired social interaction related to divorce
7. Disturbance in self-concept related to lack of job skills
8. Powerlessness related to unfulfilled needs
9. Spiritual distress related to lack of meaningful relationship with God

DSM-III-R diagnoses. The DSM-III-R uses V codes to classify conditions that require treatment or are the focus of attention but are not attributable to a mental disorder. The DSM-III-R does not provide essential features for these conditions. The V codes on p. 834 apply to the middle-aged adult:

HOLISTIC ASSESSMENT TOOL: THE MIDDLE-AGED ADULT

PHYSICAL DIMENSION

What is your reaction to changes in your physical appearance?

What changes have you noted in your sleep pattern?

What are your thoughts about your current weight?

What changes have occurred in your eating habits, for example, the amount of food you eat?

What is your response to menopausal changes? (for women) andropause? (for men)

Since becoming middle aged, how would you rate your sexual experiences on a scale of 1-10, with 10 being high?

What measures are you taking to decrease the risk of osteoporosis?

What changes have you noticed in your vision?

EMOTIONAL DIMENSION

How do you feel about the changes in your life?

How do you express your emotional responses to changes in your life?

What changes have you observed in situations or experiences that you would normally respond to with feelings of anger? guilt? depression?

How do you feel about your responsibility for your aging parents? your children?

INTELLECTUAL DIMENSION

How well do you recall recent events? remote events?

Describe how you have coped with midlife changes.

As you enter middle age, what changes have you noticed in your ability to express yourself? in your vocabulary?

What method of presenting information allows you to best retain it—visually? verbal?

SOCIAL DIMENSION

What do you consider the major role change you have experienced since entering midlife?

Describe your relationship with your spouse now that you are middle aged.

What effect did the last child leaving home have on your marriage? on your life in general?

Describe your adjustment to the death of your spouse. (if a spouse has died)

How is your relationship with your parents different since you entered midlife?

Describe your relationship with your grandchildren. (if a grandparent)

How many friends do you have?

How often do you get together with friends?

Who are the people who constitute your support system?

In what ways have your life goals changed?

What changes have you made in the amount of alcohol you consume?

What preparation are you making for retirement?

SPIRITUAL DIMENSION

In what ways have your beliefs, thoughts, and feelings about death and dying changed since you reached middle age?

What changes have occurred in your church attendance?

What changes have you made in your purpose in life?

1. V61.20 Parent-child problem: Applies to the middle-aged adult who has problem with a child of any age that is not caused by a mental disorder of the parent or child
2. V61.80 Other specified family circumstances: Can be used when the focus of treatment is the middle-aged adult's interpersonal difficulties with a family member other than the client's child or spouse, such as an aged parent or an in-law
3. V62.81 Other interpersonal problem: Can be used to classify a middle-aged adult's problem with someone outside the family, such as a co-worker or a romantic partner, when neither has a mental disorder

Planning

Long-term and short-term goals and outcome criteria appropriate for the for the middle-aged adult are shown in Table 43-5. These are examples of the planning stage of the nursing process.

Implementation

•⦂•⦂• Physical dimension. An adjustment to increased •⦁•⦂• periods of wakefulness and less deep sleep may be achieved as the nurse helps the client understand chang-

ing biological rhythms. Restful sleep provides added energy. The client may know how to relieve insomnia by bedtime rituals, such as a warm bath. Relaxation and exercise may also induce sleep.

The importance of sound nutrition and exercise in maintaining health can be taught. Exercise in middle age helps restore strength to muscles not used regularly. Jogging, swimming, and biking may improve cardiovascular strength and blood circulation. Neugarten[70] uses the term *body monitoring* for activities in which clients engage to keep the body in shape. A good balance of rest and exercise in middle age may contribute to slowing the aging process. Middle-aged clients need to learn to relax and participate in active and passive leisure activities.[16] Today a wide range of methods are used to help clients learn to relax. The nurse can teach some of the age-appropriate methods discussed in Chapter 12.

Intervention in obesity may decrease morbidity and mortality in middle age. Heart disease, hypertension, and diabetes may be prevented if middle-aged clients keep their weight within the limits established for their height and frame.

It is important for the nurse to inform the middle-aged client that the two essential features of a weight maintenance program are controlling caloric intake and expending sufficient energy to burn the calories consumed be-

---

TABLE 43-5 Long-term and short-term goals and outcome criteria related to the middle-aged adult

Goals	Outcome Criteria
NURSING DIAGNOSIS: ALTERATION IN NUTRITION: MORE THAN BODY REQUIREMENT, RELATED TO NORMAL MIDLIFE CHANGES	
Long-term goals	
To prevent obesity	Maintains current ideal body weight
	Consistently consumes nutritional food intake that does not exceed 1,500 calories per day
	Participates in a regular exercise program
To develop adaptive behaviors for coping with normal stressors related to midlife changes	Makes statements that convey understanding and acceptance of the changes
	Initiates at least two leisure activities weekly
	Engages in stress-reduction activities
Short-term goals	
To decrease food intake	Talks about decreased need for excessive food intake
	Eats no junk food
	Eats only at a table in dining room
To participate in an exercise program	Exercises 30 minutes four times a week
To identify midlife changes	Makes statements that indicate knowledge of expected midlife changes
NURSING DIAGNOSIS: INEFFECTIVE INDIVIDUAL COPING RELATED TO ROLE REVERSAL WITH AGING PARENTS	
Long-term goals	
To resolve the conflict related to role responsibility for parents	Fulfills realistic responsibilities for parents
	Makes statements about parents and self as persons in their own right
	Meets parents' and own needs for dependence and independence
To adapt life-style to accommodate responsibility for parents	Arranges for safe living situation for parents
	Sorts out priorities in own needs and those of parents
	Makes statements reflecting knowledge of the need for a change in the relationship
Short-term goal	
To discuss thoughts and feelings about role reversal	Talks about reason for conflict
	Discusses own and parents' need for dependence and independence
	Shares concerns of middle-aged children on care of aging parents

cause of the changes in their eating habits and exercise. The nurse helps the client develop a successful plan for losing and maintaining weight. If the client's program involves major weight loss, he is referred to his physician for a complete physical and a nutritionist for assessment before beginning a diet.

Adhering to a weight control program may be difficult for middle-aged adults. They may now be able to afford fattening foods and may dine in restaurants more often. The client may succeed with his weight maintenance program if he remembers that health and appearance are two of his main goals.

When recommending a caloric intake, a rule of thumb is 15 calories per day per pound. Specific information on diets can be found in many books. The hazards of fad diets, crash dieting, and fasting is discussed.

Regular exercise is an essential aspect of a weight maintenance program. Before the client embarks on a strenuous exercise program, he consults his physician or exercise physiologist. Less rigorous exercises are listed in Table 43-6. Aerobics are beneficial for middle-aged clients. A comprehensive book on aerobics that presents a scientifically sound exercise program and activities for both sexes may be recommended.

Middle-aged clients need to be educated in the relationship between stress and psychological disorders to decrease the potential for developing stress-related illnesses. A general focus for education is the relationship between emotional and physical health. Stress reduction methods and measures used to reduce anxiety (see Chapter 38) are useful. The nurse needs to discuss risk factors that contribute to coronary problems, such as tobacco smoking, diet, intake of alcohol and coffee, and a sedentary lifestyle.

Some menopausal changes may require intervention. The nurse needs to help the client adjust to the declining production of sex hormones. Sometimes an understanding of the biological changes is sufficient to relieve the client's anxiety. Climacteric changes may lead to sexual difficulties that may respond to sex counseling by nurses with specialized preparation (see Chapter 31).

Emotional dimension. Expressing anger rather than internalizing it may prevent physical disorders, such as coronary problems and ulcers. Because today's middle-aged clients may feel guilty about expressing anger and because they may fear loss of control, the nurse can use role playing to provide an opportunity for the client to express anger in a safe situation.

Middle-aged clients who do not successfully grieve for various losses may feel sustained anger and despair that adversely affect functioning. The anger and despair may be manifested as chronic depression. The nurse needs to give these clients an opportunity to successfully complete the grieving process. Anticipatory grieving in preparation for losses is a therapeutic intervention.

Clients may benefit when the nurse conveys her understanding of the intensity of the feelings of bereaved widowed clients and guides them in a healthy expression of the grieving process. Individuals who have lost a spouse through death can be supportive to one another, as described in the Research Highlight on p. 836.

Other losses of middle age need intervention directed toward grief work. Suicide and suicide potential are, of course, problems that require immediate intervention (see Chapter 14). Specific interventions in anxiety, anger, guilt, and despair are discussed in Chapters 11, 12, 13, and 14, respectively.

Intellectual dimension. The nurse capitalizes on the intellectual strengths of middle-aged clients and encourages them, for example, to enroll in refresher courses, continuing education courses, workshops, and courses for college credit. These educational experiences may meet the need for leisure time, a second career, or retirement. Middle-aged clients can also be encouraged to renew past interests in creative activities.

Social dimension. Middle-aged couples may need assistance in adjusting to their postparental marriage. Because of the current attention given to the empty-nest phenomenon and the popular notion of the middle-aged husband's fling with a younger woman, the marital partners may view failure of the marriage in middle age as inevitable. They need to know that their marital relationship in middle age is a new one, one which may be revitalized. Revitalization is based on commitment, communication, and compromise.[20] Commitment entails a willingness to understand each other and to renegotiate the terms of the present marital relationship, instead of focusing on what has been or may have been. Commitment may be based on the survival of the marriage to middle age, which suggests a solid foundation on which to

TABLE 43-6 Nature and examples of activities and calories burned

Nature of Activities	Examples of Activities	Calories Burned per Hour
Sedentary activities	Writing, reading, and watching television	About 100
Light activities	Slow walking, household activities such as dusting, and washing dishes, and average office work	About 150
Moderate activities	Walking at brisk pace, scrubbing, playing golf, bowling, and gardening	About 200
Vigorous activities	Athletic activities usually done away from home such as tennis, walking rapidly, and jogging	300 to 1,000

The Impact of Self-Help Groups on the Mental Health of Widows and Widowers

M.A. Lieberman and L. Videka-Sherman

PURPOSE

The purpose of this study was to examine the impact of self-help groups on the mental health of persons whose spouses had died.

SAMPLE

The sample consisted of 502 bereaved persons who were recruited from mailing lists provided by 71 They Help Each Other Spiritually (THEOS) chapters. Three hundred ninety-four subjects were members of THEOS and 108 were non-members. The sample was opportunistic, and the individuals were self-selected to the self-help group (member of THEOS) and the control group (nonmembers). Ninety-three percent of the study sample were female; 64% of the sample were in their 40s and 50s; and they had been widowed an average of 43 months.

METHODOLOGY

Standard measurement scales used to assess the effects of self-help groups were subscales derived from the Hopkins Symptom Checklist and included depression, anxiety, and somatization; a self-esteem scale, a mastery scale, and a measure of well-being and life satisfaction were also used. In addition, sample members were asked to identify their most pressing widowhood-related problem and to indicate on a nine-point scale the degree of distress that this problem caused. How frequently during the past week the subjects had used alcohol and psychotropic drugs to calm their nerves, create a better mood, induce sleep, or provide energy was assessed. Membership and level of participation in the self-help group was measured by frequency of attendance at meetings and social linkages in the group.

FINDINGS

The findings indicate that members who made social linkages in the group showed higher positive change when compared to members who attended meetings only. Comparisons between self-help participants and members of the control group suggested that the mere passage of time did no account for positive changes. The self-help groups were helpful in alleviating some of the distress experienced by those who had been widowed.

IMPLICATIONS

Self-help groups such as THEOS may decrease the risk associated with prolonged distress related to the loss of a spouse. Such group experiences provide an opportunity for the widowed to meet people and share a common experience.

Based on data from American Journal of Orthopsychiatry **56**(3):435, 1986.

---

build a postparental marital relationship. The nurse guides each partner to recognize the uniqueness of each other and the right of each to grow in flexible roles.

Communication is perhaps the most important component in the new middle-aged marital relationship.[27] The couple may have to learn to risk sharing their feelings and needs. The steps for sharing feelings are (1) to try to get in touch with one's own emotions, (2) to ask the partner when he or she would be receptive to an expression of feelings and needs and then share these to the best of one's abilities, and (3) to learn to listen to all levels of the partner's communication. A simple exercise for beginning to learn to listen is (1) for one spouse to state how he or she feels as clearly as possible and (2) for the other spouse to try to rephrase what was expressed in his or her own words to make sure he or she has understood.

Compromise involves negotiations in which neither person wins (or loses). The partners choose a mutually agreed time and place for discussion of differences. The nurse emphasizes the need to keep the focus of the discussion on the issues at hand. Open communication of thoughts and feelings, listening, and understanding are essential for resolution of conflict.[27]

The middle-aged couple may have problems revitalizing their relationship. Because divorce does not usually come easily to clients who have endured a relationship into midlife, the couple may seek professional guidance. The nurse can suggest preventive counseling. First, she can share with the couple their potential for practicing preventive maintenance in the marriage by using some self-help methods. If the couple's efforts are unsuccessful, the nurse may provide preventive marital counseling or refer them to another professional who specializes in marriage counseling. If the marriage is in serious trouble, counseling prevents divorce in only about 10% to 15% of cases and changes unhappy marriages into happy ones in less than 5% of cases.[20]

If a marriage ends in divorce, each spouse may need assistance to adjust. Even though the marriage was unhappy, the clients need to know that they may respond as they would to a loss and need to complete the grieving process. Clients are encouraged to explore approaches to reorganizing their lives as single middle-aged persons and perhaps as single parents of adolescents. The nurse and other professionals may provide counseling to assist the divorced spouses in their transition to a new life-style.

Clients who become single parents can be referred to Parents Without Partners, the most widely known peer group. Divorced Anonymous is another organization that may be of value. These organizations may help the divorced client to develop a new social life.

The nurse's intervention in middle-aged adult children's responsibility for aging parents begins with relieving their frustration about inadequate information on resources and professional services available for their aged parents. The adult children may benefit from anticipatory guidance in what to expect as the parents age and what they can do to help meet the parents' needs before a crisis develops (see Chapter 44).

Group interventions provide guidance for adults caring for aging parents. When feasible, the adult child and parent can attend community-based educational groups,[48] where adult children and aging parents learn about the aging process and changes from illness. The needs of the parents and the availability of resources may also be presented. This information provides reassurance to the adult children and their parents by allaying anxiety about what to expect. In support groups clients and their parents can confront and discuss their problems from a personal perspective.

Support groups for middle-aged caregiving adults provide an opportunity for them to discuss their concerns in the absence of their parents. The clients can discuss concerns such as the adjustments they are having to make to the role reversal, decisions about living arrangements for aging parents, and strategies for coping with their parents' aging. They can also express anger, guilt, and conflict. Kaplan[48] reports that some group members maintain contact after the group is terminated.

The nurse may recommend an intergenerational family group, which allows all of the children of aging parents to explore feelings and concerns. For example, anger or conflict over who will assist the parents can be expressed. Drawing up a will and making preplanned burial arrangements can be discussed.

Preretirement planning is essential to help prepare clients for retirement. During early middle age, retirement seems remote, and clients may not be interested in a preretirement program. But as they near retirement, clients may indicate an interest in planning for retirement. An important factor that influences preretirement planning is the client's financial status. Will the client's income be sufficient for him to live on? Clients need to include inflation in their assessment of finances. Anticipatory guidance in retirement issues may help potential retirees make a smooth transition into retirement.

Middle-aged clients are less likely than younger workers to lose their jobs. However, when they do, unemployment is often prolonged, and clients may seek mental health services as they adjust to the role of the unemployed job seeker. Employers may perceive a middle-aged job seeker as someone who will become ill or disabled or who will be costly in fringe benefits, such as insurance and pension. Some employers are prejudiced against older job seekers. The experiences of job hunting may lead to mental anguish. After middle-aged clients find work, many

of them may continue to be subjected to displacement through less attractive occupational assignments, lower earnings, and perhaps some damage to their physical and mental well-being.

Interventions for unemployment problems may simply include allowing the client to express his thoughts and feelings about the experiences, or the client may be referred to appropriate community agencies for job counseling. Some special programs are available to prepare middle-aged women for entrance into or return to the work force.

Spiritual dimension. When middle-aged clients enter the health care system, they may need assistance as they reassess their meaning of spirituality and the purpose it can serve in the current transition to midlife. The nurse needs to be aware of this and not impose her own spiritual values. Middle-aged clients' increased focus on religious practices can be reinforced.

Evaluation

Middle-aged clients may participate in the ongoing evaluation of their responses to the nursing intervention. When evaluating the extent to which goals have been achieved, the nurse bases her evaluations on change that is realistic for the client. Middle-aged clients may overemphasize change, want change for the sake of change, and end up with a chaotic life. During evaluation, the nurse emphasizes the continuing potential for growth and fulfillment after therapy is terminated.

BRIEF REVIEW

The middle-aged adult population is currently the fastest growing group in the United States. Although study of this stage of the life cycle is not yet a distinct discipline, nurses and other professionals have begun scientific exploration of the mental health care needs of middle-aged people and interventions to meet these needs.

A person begins transition into the middle years at age 40 and works toward completing the tasks of this stage until age 65 years. Chronological age may not be the best indicator of movement into midlife, because social, positional, physical, and biological cues also indicate the beginning of change.

Havighurst, Erikson, Jung, and Peck have made lasting contributions to theoretical explanation of the experiences of middle age. Havighurst identifies seven tasks related to assuming a position of social responsibility and guidance of others. The task of developing generativity versus stagnation is Erikson's approach to describing the need for middle-aged adults to counsel and direct others. If the client is excessively concerned about himself, he stagnates. Jung and Buhler have similar views that middle-aged people become inner oriented as they engage in a critical assessment of themselves. Peck believes individuals in midlife need to invest their energy in various people and activities to fill the void left by the loss of many significant relationships. His four tasks for middle-aged adults are valuing wisdom versus physical powers, cathectic flexibility versus impoverishment, mental flexibility versus rigidity, and socializing versus sexualizing in human relationships.

Some of the major stressors of middle age result from losses, role changes, and changes in the five dimensions of the person. Physical changes, departure of the last child from the home, renegotiating the marital relationship, and role reversal with aging parents are some of the major events with which the middle-aged adult may have to deal. Obesity is a major health problem. Most middle-aged adults cope effectively with these stressors. If they do not, they may become depressed and abuse alcohol, which may necessitate professional assistance. The middle-aged adult is often able to actively participate in planning his treatment program.

REFERENCES AND SUGGESTED READINGS

1. Aber, R., and Webb, W.B.: Effects of a limited nap on night sleep in older subjects, Psychology and Aging 1(4):300, 1986.
2. Ainlay, S.C., and Smith, D.R.: Aging and religious participation, Journal of Gerontology 39(3):357, 1984.
3. Anorexia nervosa in middle age, Emergency Medicine 14:111, 1982.
4. Atkinson, R.M., and others: Early versus late onset alcoholism in older persons: preliminary findings, Alcoholism: Clinical and Experimental Research 9(6):513, 1985.
5. Back, K.W.: Transition to aging and the self-image, Aging and Human Development 2:4, November 1971.
6. Baruch, G.K., and Barnett, R.: Role quality, multiple role involvement, and psychological well-being in midlife women, Journal of Personality and Social Psychology 51(3):578, 1986.
7. Benedek, T.: Parenthood during the life cycle. In Anthony, E., and Benedek, T., editors: Parenthood: its psychology and psychopathology, Boston, 1970, Little, Brown & Co.
8. Bischof, L.J.: Adult psychology, ed. 2, New York, 1976, Harper & Row, Publishers.
9. Buhler, C.: The general structure of the human life. In Buhler, C., and Massarik, F., editors: The course of human life: a study of goals in the humanistic perspective, New York, 1968, Springer Publishing Co., Inc.
10. Buhler, C.: The course of human life as a psychological problem. In Looft, W.R., editor: Development psychology: a book of readings, New York, 1972, Holt, Rinehart & Winston.
11. Burnside, I.M., Ebersole, P., and Monea, H.: Psychosocial caring throughout the life span, New York, 1979, McGraw-Hill Book Co.
12. Burrows, G.D., and Dennerstein, L.: Depression and suicide in middle age. In Howells, J.D., editor: Modern perspectives in the psychiatry of middle age, New York, 1981, Brunner/Mazel, Inc.
13. Butler, R.N.: Psychiatry and psychology of the middle-aged. In Freedman, A.M., Kaplan, H.I., and Sadock, B.J., editors: Comprehensive textbook of psychiatry IV, ed. 4, Baltimore, 1985, The Williams & Wilkins Co.
14. Chapman, A.H.: Textbook of clinical psychiatry: an interpersonal approach, ed. 2, Philadelphia, 1976, J.B. Lippincott Co.
15. Ciernia, J.R.: Myths about male mid-life crises, Psychological Reports 56:3, 1985.
16. Colarusso, C.A., and Nemiroff, R.A.: Adult development: a new dimension in psychodynamic theory and practice, New York, 1981, Plenum Press.
17. Cooke, D.J.: Social support and stressful life events during mid-life, Maturitas 7(4):303, 1985.
18. Desmond, T.C.: America's unknown middle-agers. In Vedder, C.B., editor: Problems of the middle-aged, Springfield, Ill., 1965, Charles C Thomas, Publisher.
19. Diekelmann, N., and others: The middle years: a special supplement, American Journal of Nursing 75:993, 1975.
20. Donohugh, D.L.: The middle years, Philadelphia, 1981, W.B. Saunders Co.
21. Erikson, E.H.: Childhood and society, ed. 2, New York, 1964, W.W. Norton & Co., Inc.
22. Ecklein, J.L.: Obstacles to understanding the changing role of women in socialist countries, Insurgent Sociologist, 12(1-2):7, 1984.
23. Eden, E.: Factor analysis of a self-concept instrument for older adults, Experimental Aging Research 7(2):159, 1981.
24. Fawell, M.P., and Rosenberg, S.D.: Parent-child relations at middle age. In Getty, C., and Humphreys, W.: Understanding the family: stress and changes in American family life, New York, 1981, Appleton-Century-Crofts.
25. Fiske, M.: Middle age: the prime of life? New York, 1979, Harper & Row, Publishers.
26. Fiske, M., and others: Four stages of life: a comparative study of women and men facing transitions, San Francisco, 1976, Jossey-Bass, Inc., Publishers.
27. Foxall, M.J., and others: Adjustment pattern of chronically ill middle-aged persons and spouse. Western Journal of Nursing Research 7(4):452, 1985.
28. Frieberg, K.L.; Human development: a life span approach, ed. 3, Boston, 1987, Jones & Bartlett, Publishers.
29. Freidman, H.J.: The divorced in middle age. In Howells, J.G., editor: Modern perspectives in the psychiatry of middle age, New York, 1981, Brunner/Mazel, Inc.
30. George, L.K.: Role transitions in later life, Monterey, Calif., 1980, Brooks/Cole Publishing Co.
31. Giele, Z., editor: Women in middle years: current knowledge and direction for research and policy, New York, 1982, John Wiley & Sons, Inc.
32. Goddard, J.: Middle-age crisis: a self-fulfilling prophecy? Nursing RSA Verpleging, 1(9):42, 1986.
33. Golan, N.: Passing through transitions: a guide for practitioners, New York, 1981, The Free Press.
34. Golan, N.: The perilous bride: helping clients through midlife transitions, New York, 1986, Free Press.
35. Gordon, V.C., and others: Growth-support intervention for the treatment of depression in women of middle years, Western Journal of Nursing Research 8(3):263, 1986.
36. Gunter, L.M., and Kolanwsk, A.M.: Promoting healthy lifestyles in mature women, Journal of Gerontological Nursing 12(4):6, 1986.
37. Hamm, J.E., Major, L.F., and Brown, G.L.: Quantitative measurement of depression and anxiety in male alcoholics, American Journal of Psychiatry 46:580, 1979.
38. Harris, R.L., Ellicott, A.M., and Holmes, D.S.: The timing of psychosocial transitions and changes in women's lives: an examination of women aged 45 to 60, Journal of Personality and Social Psychology 51(2):409, 1986.
39. Hayward, M.D., and Hardy, M.A.: Early retirement processes among older men: occupational differences, Research on Aging 7(4):491, 1985.
40. Havighurst, R.J.: Developmental tasks and education, New York, 1972, David McKay Co., Inc.
41. Hess, A.L., and Bradshaw, H.L.: Positiveness of self-concept and ideal self as a function of age, Journal of Genetic Psychology 117:57, 1970.
42. Howells, J.G., editor: Modern perspectives in the psychiatry of middle age, New York, 1981, Brunner/Mazel, Inc.
43. Jacobson, J.M.: A comparison of anxiety levels in midlife women (35-65) who are military spouses and a group of

non-military-affiliated women, Health Care Women International 7(3):241, 1986.

44. Janelli, L.M.: Body image in older adults: a review of the literature, Rehabilitation Nursing 11(4):6, 1986.
45. Jung, C.G.: Modern man in search of a soul, New York, 1933, Harcourt Brace & Co., Inc.
46. Jung, C.G.: Collected works, vol. 17, The development of personality, New York, 1954, Pantheon Books, Inc.
47. Junge, M., and Maya, V.: Women in their forties: a group portrait and implications for psychotherapy, Women and Therapy 4(3):3, 1985.
48. Kaplan, B.H.: An overview of interventions to meet the needs of aging parents and their families. In Ragan, P.K., editor: Aging parents, University Park, Calif., 1979, Ethel Percy Andrus Gerontology Center, University of Southern California.
49. Karp, D.A.: Academics beyond midlife: some observations on changing consciousness in the fifty to sixty year decade, International Journal of Aging and Human Development 22(2):81, 1985-1986.
50. Kuhlen, R.G.: Developmental changes in motivation during adult years. In Birren, J.E., editor: Relation of development and aging, Springfield, Ill., 1964, Charles C Thomas, Publisher.
51. Levinson, D., and others: The seasons of a man's life, New York, 1978, Alfred A. Knopf, Inc.
52. Mancini, J.A., and Blieszner, R.: Return of middle-aged children to the parental home, Medical Aspects of Human Sexuality 19(4):94, 1985.
53. Masserman, J.H.: Psychiatry and health, Port Washington, New York, 1986, Human Science Press.
54. Mattila, V.J.: Paranoid-hallucinatory functional psychoses in later middle age, Psychiatric Fennica, 16:19, 1985.
55. Mirkin, P.M., and Meyer, R.E.: Alcoholism in middle age. In Howells, J.G., editor: Modern perspectives in the psychiatry of middle age, New York, 1981, Brunner/Mazel, Inc.
56. Nahemow, N.: The changing nature of grandparenthood, Medical Aspects of Human Sexuality, 19(4):81, 1985.
57. Neugarten, B.L., editor: Personality in middle and later life: empirical studies, New York, 1964, Atherton Press.
58. Neugarten, B.L.: Adult personality: toward a psychology of the life cycle. In Neugarten, B.L., editor: Middle age and aging, Chicago, 1968, The University of Chicago Press.
59. Neugarten, B.L.: The awareness of middle age. In Neugarten, B.L., editor: Middle age and aging, Chicago, 1968, The University of Chicago Press.
60. Neugarten, B.L., and Weinstein, K.K.: The changing American grandparent. In Neugarten, B.L., editor: Middle age and aging, Chicago, 1968, The University of Chicago Press.
61. Neugarten, B.L., and others: Women's attitudes toward menopause. In Neugarten, B.L., editor: Middle age and aging, Chicago, 1968, The University of Chicago Press.
62. Nolan, J.W.: Work patterns of midlife female nurses, Nursing Research 34(3):150, 1985.
63. Nolan, J.W.: Developmental concerns and the health of midlife women, Nursing Clinics of North American 21(1):151, 1986.
64. Norman, W.H., and Scaramella, T.J.: Mid-life: developmental and clinical issues, New York, 1980, Brunner/Mazel, Inc.
65. Okun, B.F.: Working with adults: individual, family, and career development, Monterey Calif. 1984, Brooks/Cole Publishing Co.
66. Parker, G.: The search for intimacy in mid-life: An exploration of several myths, Australian and New Zealand Journal of Psychiatry 19(4):362, 1985.
67. Peck, R.C.: Psychological development in the second half of life. In Neugarten, B.L., editor: Middle age and aging, Chicago, 1968, The University of Chicago Press.
68. Phifer, J.F., and Murrell, S.A.: Etiologic factors in the onset of depressive symtpoms in older adults, Journal of Abnormal Psychology 95(3):282, 1986.
69. Power, P.W., Hershenson, D.B., and Schlossberg, N.K.: Midlife transition and disability, Rehabilitation Counseling Bulletin. 29:2, 1985.
70. Rosin, A.J., and Glatt, M.M.: Alcohol excess in the elderly, Quarterly Journal of the Study of Alcohol 32:53, 1971.
71. Sands, R.G., and Richardson, V.: Clinical practice with women in their middle years, Social Work 31(1):36, 1986.
72. Schlossberg, N.K.: Counseling adults in transition: linking practice with theory, New York, 1984, Springer Publishing Co.
73. Schuster, C.S., and Ashburn, S.S.: The process of human development: a holistic life-span approach, Boston, 1986, Little, Brown & Co.
74. Shaw, L.B.: Retirement plans of middle-aged married women, Gerontologist 24(2):154, 1984.
75. Stevenson, J.S.: Issues and crises during middlescence, New York, 1977, Appleton-Century-Crofts.
76. Sugiyama, Y.: Sociopsychological changes from the 50's to old age in relation to life satisfaction, Japanese Psychological Review 27(3):317, 1984.
77. Thomson, J., and Oswald, L.: Effect of estrogen on sleep, mood and anxiety of menopausal women, British Medical Journal 2:1317, 1977.
78. Troll, L.E.: Early and middle adulthood: the best is yet to be—maybe, Monterey, Calif., 1975, Brooks/Cole Publishing Co.
79. Tune, G.S.: The influence of age and temperment on the adult human sleep-wakefulness pattern, British Journal of Psychology, 60:431, 1969.
80. Turner, J.S., and Helms, D.B.: Contemporary adulthood, ed. 2, New York, 1982, Holt, Rinehart & Winston.
81. Waring, J.: The middle years: a multidisciplinary view—a summary of the Second Annual Conference on Major Transitions in the Human Life Course, New York, 1978, Academy for Educational Development.

ANNOTATED BIBLIOGRAPHY

Donohugh, D.L.: The middle years: an American College of Physicians book, Philadelphia, 1981, W.B. Saunders Co.

Donohugh presents comprehensive information on all aspects of middle age and includes suggestions for interventions for some of the challenges and obstacles of midlife. The test will be useful to professionals and middle-aged adults.

Golan, N.: The perilous bridge: helping clients through mid-life transitions, New York, 1986, The Free Press.

This text presents theoretical perspectives on late midlife and uses case situations of actual clients to highlight common emotional reactions to the stresses of this period in life. The author includes the range of treatments that were offered to these clients as well as additional interventions she considers effective for assisting middle aged adults through the transitional periods of midlife.

Neugarten, B.L., editor: Middle age and aging, Chicago, 1968, The University of Chicago Press.

This classic text contains a collection of readings describing various aspects of middle age. Some of the articles focus on research related to middle age.

Schlossberg, N.K.: Counseling adults in transition: linking practice with theory, New York, 1984, Springer Publishing Co., Inc.

This resource text presents an overview of the theories of adult development and a framework for intervention that illustrates an integration of knowledge of adult development and counseling skills. The author includes practical techniques for assisting middle aged adults to understand their expeiences and to enhance their ability to successfully cope with the transition.

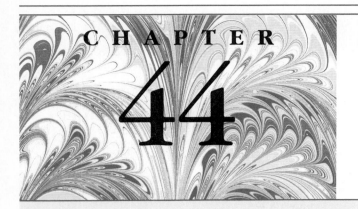

THE AGED ADULT

Cornelia Kelly Beck

After studying this chapter the learner will be able to:

Discuss historical developments related to mental health—psychiatric nursing for the aged adult.

Describe theoretical explanations of the aging process.

Identify important considerations in establishing a therapeutic relationship with aged persons.

Apply the nursing process to the mental health care needs of aged individuals.

Describe specific treatment modalities frequently used for the mental health care needs of aged persons.

At present, the age of 65 years is a socially accepted time for designating a person as aged. However, experiences with the aged have shown that this broad categorization is inappropriate for many since there is no parallel between chronological and psychological aging. Each person ages at a unique rate because of a complex interaction among the physical, emotional, intellectual, social, and spiritual dimensions.

There is a current trend to designate phases within the 65 years and older age span; for example, the young-old are 65 to 75 years; the old-old are 75 to 90 years; and the elite old are older than 90 years. With the recent change in the mandatory retirement age in some industries to 70 years, this age may possibly become the norm for designating someone as aged. However, for the purposes of this chapter, persons who are older than 65 years are considered to be in their later years, and the terms "the aged," "the old," and "the elderly" will be used interchangeably in the discussion of this stage of the life cycle.

Although older people are generally functioning well, there are a significant number of older people who need mental health care to realize their optimal functioning. Approximately 1% of the elderly are in mental hospitals, and an estimated 15% to 25% in the community have significant mental health problems; also, the National Nursing Home Survey[24] found that 30% of nursing home clients had a "diagnosable psychiatric disorder" and 61% had one or more mental impairments or conditions.

Older people are more likely to have multiple chronic disorders, more likely to have encountered a major object loss, and less likely to have supportive people and services available to them than are younger people. Despite these factors that might tend to make their adjustment more tenuous, older people for the most part adapt successfully to their changed circumstances. In fact the majority of older people negotiate the uncertainties of life with success, equanimity, and good humor.[37]

THEORETICAL APPROACHES
Biological

Several alterations in older people's physiology have been explored as explanations for changes in the person's emotional dimension with aging. It is suggested that manic-depressive illness and recurrent depressive disorders in older individuals are primarily caused by the lack of physiological energy and that lithium is effective in treating these disorders because it normalizes the physiological system and prevents the periodic excess and lack of physiological energy.[68] It has also been proposed that the aging of the hypothalamus and the hormonal system leads to a reduced ability to withstand depression-evoking events.[30] A decrease occurs in the synthesis of catecholamines and a compensatory increase occurs in the production of monoamine oxidase (MAO). Increased levels of MAO are especially common in women because of the

🌿 *Historical Overview* 🌿

DATE	EVENT
1900s	Freud advised that psychoanalysis and other forms of psychotherapy were not useful with people over 50 years because of the inelasticity of their mental processes and their ineducability.
1919	Although he agreed with Freud, Abraham was one of the first clinicians to show optimism concerning treatment of the elderly; he found that the weakening of their ego defenses facilitated change in the therapeutic process.
1950	The first nursing textbook on care of the elderly, *Geriatric Nursing,* by Norton[46] was published.
1958	Hanna Segal published the first clinical material describing analytic sessions with an elderly client.
1962	The first gerontological nursing research was published in Britain by Norton and colleagues.
	A small group of geriatric nurses appealed to the American Nurses Association (ANA) for recognition of geriatric nursing as a specialty and held its first national meeting.
1963	Melanie Klein published theoretical formulations on the normal adaptation of the elderly as it affects children and family members.
	Forty percent of the aged mentally ill were in psychiatric institutions, whereas 53% were in nursing homes.
1964	The first American study in gerontological nursing, *The Elderly Ambulatory Patient,* addressed patient health care knowledge, medication errors, food patterns, ambulation, and travel profiles.
	Levin described the impact of loss and change in the therapeutic process with the elderly.
1966	The ANA established the Division on Geriatric Nursing.
1969	The first nursing research was conducted with aged clients in a psychiatric facility.
	Seventy-five percent of the mentally ill aged were in nursing homes, making them the successor to state mental hospitals as the community treatment component of the deinstitutionalization of older mentally ill persons.
1970s	The elderly banded together socially and politically, using "senior power" against being cast as second-class citizens.
1973	Congress established a network of state and area agencies on aging to develop a coordinated system of comprehensive services to meet the needs of older Americans.
	The ANA's division on geriatric nursing published the "Standards for Geriatric Nursing Practice."[2]
1974	The National Institute on Aging was established within the National Institutes of Health to support and conduct biomedical, social, and behavioral research and training related to the aging process.
1977	The term "geropsychiatric nursing" first appeared in the Cumulative Index to Nursing and Allied Health Literature.
1981	At the Third White House Conference on Aging, the American Psychiatric Association and the Committee on Long-Term Care recommended that mental health be an integral part of a comprehensive health and social service delivery system.
	The ANA's division on gerontological nursing prepared a statement that included a definition and philosophy of gerontological nursing practice and presented this statement to the participants in the White House Conference on Aging.
1984	The Middle Atlantic Geropsychiatric Nurses' Association was formed; the group comprises clinical nurse specialists with an interest in the mental health needs of the older adult.
Future	Standards of practice and ANA certification in geropsychiatric nursing will be added to the existing age-specific specialty groups.
	By 1990, 35% of the voting population will be 60 years or above and they will probably strongly support legislation for comprehensive mental health services.
	Economic issues and a growing shortage of long-term care beds will dictate a major rise in the number of aged clients cared for in their own homes.

inverse relationship between levels of estrogen and MAO.[30] The adrenogenic function of the adrenal cortex also decreases progressively with age. The overall effect of these physiological changes is diminished ability to cope with stress.[58]

The data on the association between genetic factors and mental functioning are limited. However, genetic factors have been implicated in the preservation of mental functioning into old age. Chromosome loss has been found to correlate with loss of certain cognitive functions such as memory.[42]

Psychoanalytic

Erikson saw the final stage of life as a time in which individuals evaluate their accomplishments and failures and search for meaning in their lives. He stressed the resolution of integrity versus despair. If older persons can find some meaning in their lives and accept the course that their lives have taken, they can look back on their lives with a sense of integrity. Older persons who evaluate their lives as a waste of time with no meaning may give up hope and end their life journey with a sense of loss, contempt for others, and ultimately despair.

Peck[46] discussed the following three developmental tasks of the older adult:

TASK	EXAMPLE
Body transcendence versus body preoccupation	Establish satisfying relationships and engage in creative activities to transcend self-centeredness and illness
Ego differentiation versus work role preoccupation	Redefine self in terms of roles other than those in the work situation
Ego transcendence versus ego preoccupation	Have one's life extend into the future through children, friendships, and contributions to society

Cognitive

Beck[5] contends that persons' cognitive appraisal of themselves and their situation predominates in establishing equilibrium during the process of adjusting to losses. He proposes that when the cognitive triad (a negative view of the future, environment, and self) is the basis for evaluating a loss, the impact of the cognitive distortions is greater than that of the loss. This cognitive triad is frequently characteristic of older people, and thus their personal cognitive distortions may increase their emotional reactions to loss. For example, they frequently believe that nothing is left in which they can invest their energies. The lack of meaningful roles ascribed to older people by our culture reinforces these cognitive appraisals. However, the degree to which the older person's negative view is cognitive distortion rather than a realistic appraisal is difficult to resolve. In many cases physical disease and isolation worsen the situation and bring about failure in attempts at restitution of the loss, adding feelings of helplessness and hopelessness to the original feelings of sadness over the loss.[60]

Sociocultural

The theory of disengagement developed by Cummings and Henry[15] is one of the earliest and most controversial sociological theories on aging. According to the disengagement theory the individual in middle life realizes his mortality and thus begins to reduce involvement with others and society. At the same time, society is also mutually disengaging itself from the individual. Individuals can use this freedom from restricting ties to society to enjoy old age.

An opposing theory that has been better accepted is the activity theory in which Havighurst[33] proposes that activity promotes well-being and satisfaction in aging. Thus older adults who remain active, engage in social activities, and establish new roles, relationships, hobbies, and interests will age with a sense of satisfaction.

TABLE 44-1 Summary of theories of aging

Theory	Theorist	Dynamics
Biological	Wolpert; Frolkis	The lack of physiological energy results in reduced ability to cope with stress.
Psychoanalytic	Erikson	Acceptance of one's life experiences leads to integrity; viewing one's life as a waste of time results in despair.
	Peck	Achievement of body transcendence, ego differentiation, and ego transcendence leads to successful aging.
Cognitive	Beck	Older persons' negative view of the future, the environment, and themselves increases their negative emotional reactions to loss.
Sociocultural		
Disengagement	Cummings and Henry	The individual voluntarily reduces involvement with society as society disengages itself from the individual.
Activity	Havighurst	The individual who remains active ages with a sense of satisfaction.
Continuity	Neugarten	Individuals maintain a consistent level of activity as they age.
Interactionist	Spence	Individuals move from one role to another depending on their characteristics and circumstances.

The continuity theory proposed by Neugarten[45] suggests that individuals' personalities do not change as they age and that their behavior becomes more predictable. They maintain continuity in their habits, commitments, preferences, and particularly the way they adapt to social situations. Thus their pattern of aging can be predicted from knowledge of these factors.

The interactionist theory proposed by Spence[58] views age-related changes as resulting from the interaction of the individual characteristics of the person, circumstances in society, and the history of social interaction patterns of the person. Roles that the individual fulfills during a lifetime are the focus of the interactionist theory. People try to plan and balance their roles, move from one role to another, and assume a complex pattern of roles. However, with aging, their major roles end and they take on new roles of their own choosing.

Table 44-1 summarizes theories of aging.

RELATING TO THE CLIENT

Most older clients have had limited or no previous contact with mental health professionals and are unsure what to expect. They have also formed their attitudes during a time when seeking help for mental health problems was not accepted by society. Therefore they may be fearful and suspicious in their initial contacts, and it may take repeated contacts and careful explanations by the nurse to allay their fear.

Essential to developing a trusting relationship with an aged client are the nurse's beliefs about and attitude toward her own aging and toward this age group. There are six hurdles or stereotypes that can affect the establishment of a therapeutic relationship with an aged client.[32] The first is the "can't teach an old dog new tricks" syndrome. If nurses view the older person as incapable of change, they will not be motivated to invest energy in facilitating change. In addition, nurses may unwittingly convey infantilizing, pitying attitudes. The second hurdle is entitled "My God, I'm mortal too." If nurses are having difficulty accepting their own aging process, including the issues of illness, loss, and mortality, the wrinkled skin and gray hair of the older person will activate their own fears and uncertainties about aging.

The next hurdle involves the "why bother?" or the "senility is natural" attitude. If nurses view the aged person as a composite of multiple deficits accumulated through aging, they will have difficulty recognizing the client's inner resources. If they forget that the client has a history of successful accomplishments and self-responsibility and treat him as if he has always been old, they may see him as incapable of handling certain kinds of information or responsibilities. These attitudes may result in a fourth hurdle of "ministering to" and unnecessarily "doing for" aged persons rather than helping them use the resources they have to maintain control over their own lives.

The last two hurdles involve the role confusion that often occurs in interactions with aged persons: the "I'm the child" attitude and the "client is a child" attitude.

With the first attitude, the nurse may assume the role of a child rather than that of an adult and thus may respond to an elderly client as though to a parent. With the "client is a child" attitude, the nurse may treat the elderly person as a child. This has been termed "infantilization" of the elderly.

It is helpful to share personal and mutual interests in order to bridge the generation gap and facilitate the human bond. Nurses who are much younger than the client may have some difficulty in understanding the experiences of their older clients. Their understanding and empathy with older persons may be enhanced by imagining what it may be like to be in the older person's situation. Nurses' understanding of the aging person's situation may also be increased by their life experiences with other older persons such as parents or grandparents and by a sound knowledge base of the process of aging.

Developing a trusting relationship with an aged person begins with calling the client by his title and last name. This is a sign of respect that boosts self-esteem. Seemingly endearing terms such as "Grandpa" or "Grams" may convey a hidden message about the person's value and contribute to loss of self-esteem. As the relationship develops, the nurse can ask clients the name they prefer.

The nurse needs to sit in a chair in full view of the client. It is important to convey acceptance that the interaction may need to be paced slower and that the nurse has time for the slower interaction process. As indicated in the Research Highlight on p. 844, communication is maximized when it can be paced by the elderly client.

After an initial level of trust has been established, the working phase of the relationship begins. Society has frequently forced the elderly into a dependent role, and they in turn have often adopted society's negative stereotypes toward them. Thus fostering the client's sense of interdependence and self-responsibility is frequently difficult. Negative emotional reactions to life changes often affect the way a client participates in the assessment and planning process. To encourage participation, the nurse can have elderly persons relate meaningful life events, feelings about these incidents, and feelings about anticipation of events such as the birth of a great-grandchild or a long-awaited trip. Clients also may tell about fears associated with the aging process—fear of loneliness or becoming unwanted, fear of becoming a burden on others, or fear of death. Elderly clients may also describe feelings about the physical changes that accompany aging. The nurse needs to recognize that these fears may be based on reality and to use clients' assets to help them in meeting their needs.

Aged persons need to have control over the basic decisions affecting their lives rather than to have the values and decisions of others imposed on them. For example, they can participate in decisions about relocation rather than having their children decide for them that their home is no longer an appropriate place for them to live. Given the opportunity to make such decisions, aged persons also need to know that others will accept their decisions. Just as clients are given the chance to take part in planning their care, they need the opportunity to choose alternatives as the plan is implemented. The opportunity

Research Highlight

Response Time and Health Care Learning of Elderly Patients

K.K. Kim

PURPOSE

The purpose of this study was to determine if elderly clients perform better in health care learning when provided slower or self-paced response conditions. Learning performance was defined as the scores on a knowledge test following nutrition instruction. Response time was the number of seconds to recall or recognize nutrition information during the nurition posttest.

SAMPLE

The study was conducted at a midwestern hospital serving adult patients with chronic diseases. A total of 105 clients were randomly assigned to one of three response groups: fast paced, slow paced, and self-paced. Ages of the sample clients ranged from 60 to 92 years with a mean of 73 years. There were 70 men and 35 women; on the average, the clients had 9.4 years of education.

METHODOLOGY

A nutrition knowledge pretest was given. Immediately following the pretest, nutrition instruction on 10 calcium-rich foods was completed. Approximately 24 hours after the nutrition instruction, the posttest of nutrition knowledge was administered to patients under the three different conditions: fast-paced responses, slow-paced responses, and self-paced re-

sponses. At the end of the posttest, clients were asked their opinions about the amount of time available in answering questions during the posttest. Immediately after the posttest, the Hearing Handicap Scale was administered. Demographic data were collected at the end of each interview.

FINDINGS

Learning performances under the fast- and slow-paced conditions did not differ. Learning performances under the self-paced condition were superior to the two experimenter-paced conditions. There was a significant positive relationship between the experimental conditions and clients opinions about the available response times. The clients in the self-paced group were more likely to say that they had enough time in answering questions. Likewise, more clients in the slow-paced group said that they had enough time when compared with the fast-paced group.

IMPLICATIONS

The findings of this study document that a self-paced response condition is advantageous for elderly clients. In questioning elderly clients, the nurse needs to give a person as much time as needed to respond. If an elderly person is not given time to respond to a question, the performance may be poor even though the response is known.

Based on data from Research in Nursing and Health 9:3, 1986.

to change approaches displays sensitivity between the nurse and the aged person.

The client's psychological mindedness and introspectiveness are important when planning one-to-one therapy with the elderly. Clients with a lifelong disregard and aversion to "talking" about psychological processes are often threatened in a one-to-one encounter. However, many elderly have the capacity to deal with ideas with little emotional bias and respond readily to suggestions and interpretations of the nurse therapist.[6]

Long-standing defenses may be rigidly adhered to and prohibit change. In contrast, often there is a weakening of defenses with age that can facilitate psychotherapy and make the elderly less rigid than many younger clients. Often clients realize this may be the last chance to change and are willing to work on issues they could not face at an earlier time.[13]

Transference is a major therapeutic problem in working with the elderly because of the usual age difference between the client and the nurse. An example of transference is the client who attributes characteristics possessed by a son or daughter to the nurse or treats the nurse as a

son or daughter. Negative transference is usually attributed to the elderly's unresolved conflicts toward their own children. These hostile and envious feelings are transferred to the nurse. Positive transference occurs when the elderly client attributes his feelings of love and attachment for his own children to the nurse. In countertransference, traits are ascribed to the client that are related to the nurse's feelings or experiences with older persons. Although a trend has developed to accept transference as a tool in treating the older client, problems may occur when they result in an overattachment between the older client and the nurse.

Termination of the therapeutic relationship with the older client is approached with the recognition that because elderly persons have frequently lost many of their social contacts, the nurse can become a major component of the older person's social support system. A truly meaningful relationship may be crucial in an older person's life; thus nurses need to be particularly concerned about providing alternate support persons for the aging client. If the elderly person has developed other social supports, the process of termination with the nurse will be less difficult.

NURSING PROCESS
Assessment

✦ ***Physical dimension.*** A summary of the physical changes in aging is presented in Table 44-2.

The older adult may have characteristic alterations in sleep patterns that are noted in the data collection process. The first alteration relates to the latency period of sleep, that is, the time it takes a person to fall asleep. A latency period of about 10 minutes is typical until 60 years of age. At 70 to 79 years the latency period reaches a mean of 23 minutes.[28] The latency period may also be lengthened if the older person is afraid to fall asleep for fear he will never awaken.

Since the older person's physiological tolerance for sleep deprivation is lower than that of the younger person, insomnia is also important to note. The periods of wakefulness during the night are frequent and longer. Awakenings are often caused by nocturnal micturition and may also be caused by fear, anxiety, and depression about the realities of decline and inevitable death.[35] Frequently these occurrences interrupt rapid eye movement (REM) sleep. Adequate REM sleep is particularly important in maintaining the integrity of the older person's central nervous system. The amount of stage 4 non-REM sleep is reduced by about 50% in the elderly person. Mental agility declines as stage 4 sleep declines, and the person finds it more difficult to learn psychomotor skills. Also, older people who go to bed very early in the evening may awaken early in the morning and complain of insomnia because they are unable to return to sleep.[27]

The older person's pattern of napping, as well as the reason for napping, is noted. Daytime naps seem to increase with age. This may indicate changes in sleep patterns, or it may be the result of boredom from lack of stimulation. Naps following fatigue or exhaustion are useful in providing relaxation. Daytime naps may compensate for loss of impaired sleep at night; however, this compensation does not always occur, and the person who naps during the day may still suffer from the effects of impaired sleep at night. Frequent daytime napping because of an unstimulating environment can lead to difficulties in sleeping at night. Aged persons who do not nap during the day may take several rests while sitting in a chair.

Because daytime naps are associated with particular sleep patterns, the time of day during which the older person naps is also important. REM sleep predominates during morning naps and is a continuation of the sleep from the prior evening. The client awakens feeling refreshed because it is a light stage of sleep. In addition, because REM sleep has the purpose of organizing recent memory data, morning naps enable the client to think more lucidly. Afternoon naps, on the other hand, predominate in stage 4 sleep, which is the deepest of all the sleep levels. On awakening the client is likely to feel groggy and exhausted. The more stage 4 sleep in the afternoon, the longer the latency, or falling-asleep, stage will be that evening.[28]

Because of the many changes in observable features with aging and the value that American society places on a youthful appearance, the elderly may experience problems with their body image. For example, the characteristics of the aging skin, the thinning of hair, or the loss of teeth may alter the individual's body image and result in the lowering of self-esteem.

Some physical manifestations of depression are particularly noteworthy in older persons. In some depressed older persons nocturia is unaccompanied by daytime urinary frequency. Thus, if the explanation of nocturia is inadequate, depression needs to be considered as a possible cause. The psychomotor agitation sometimes present in depression tends to disappear in the older depressed person, except when the depression is severe.[52] This is probably due to the weakened affectivity that accompanies aging. Because physical problems at this time are normal and acceptable, the aged tend to use physical complaints to express their depression and these are seen as the predominant feature of depression in aged persons.

However, many of the symptoms of depression in older people are wrongly considered a part of normal aging, and therefore depressive states in the elderly are often not diagnosed by mental health care providers. For example, an older person with the classical depressive picture of perpetual fatigue, and gastrointestinal symptoms of anorexia, epigastric distress, and constipation can easily be viewed as experiencing the normal processes of aging rather than being a depressed person.

✻ ***Emotional dimension.*** Researchers generally agree that physical decline and the need to conserve energy may result in the older person's manifestation of emotions being subtler than it was at an earlier stage in the life cycle. Also, the era in which older people grew up promoted stoicism, and they were not encouraged to show their feelings. For these reasons, the overt clues for assessing the older person's emotional dimension may be fewer and sensitivity is needed to detect subtler clues. However, in older persons with organic brain changes, display of some emotions may be more pronounced because of a decreased ability to control emotional expression.

Anxiety is common in old age and is frequently caused by the multiple losses experienced by the aged person, particularly the loss of self-esteem and adaptive capacity. Severe anxiety is not as common in elderly persons because of the many strategies they have developed to handle stress during their long lives. The common manifestations of anxiety in the aged person are similar to those in other age groups. However, because of changes in the larynx with normal aging, voice changes, which are signs of anxiety, are not as easy to detect in the older person as they are in the younger person. Drastic changes in the semantic content of conversation may also signal mounting anxiety.

Anxiety may be especially difficult to detect in frail, debilitated older persons who are confined to bed and have little energy to expend. They may manifest their anxiety by turning their heads away, watching television, closing their eyes, or looking out the door or window in an effort to avoid eye contact.

TABLE 44-2 Physical assessment findings in the elderly

Characteristics	Findings
Cardiovascular changes	
Cardiac output	Heart loses elasticity; therefore decreased heart contractility in response to increased demands
Arterial circulation	Decreased vessel compliance with increased peripheral resistance to blood flow resulting from general or localized arteriosclerosis
Venous circulation	Does not exhibit change with aging in the absence of disease
Blood pressure	Significant increase in the systolic, slight increase in the diastolic, increase in peripheral resistance and pulse pressure
Heart	Dislocation of the apex because of kyphoscoliosis; therefore diagnostic significance of location is lost
	Increased premature beats, rarely clinically important
Murmurs	Diastolic murmurs in over half the aged; the most common heard at the base of the heart because of sclerotic changes on the aortic valves
Peripheral pulses	Easily palpated because of increased arterial wall narrowing and loss of connective tissue; feeling of tortuous and rigid vessels
	Possiblity that pedal pulses may be weaker as a result of arteriosclerotic changes; colder lower extremities, especially at night; possiblity of cold feet and hands with mottled color
Heart rate	No changes with age at normal rest
Respiratory changes	
Pulmonary blood flow and diffusion	Decreased blood flow to the pulmonary circulation; decreased diffusion
Anatomic structure	Increased anterior-posterior diameter
Respiratory accessory muscles	Degeneration and decreased strength; increased rigidity of chest wall
	Muscle atrophy of pharynx and larynx
Internal pulmonic structure	Decreased pulmonary elasticity creates senile emphysema
	Shorter breaths taken with decreased maximum breathing capacity, vital capacity, residual volume, and function capacity
	Airway resistance increases; less ventilation at the bases of the lung and more at the apex
Integumentary changes	
Texture	Skin loses elasticity; wrinkles, folding, sagging, dryness
Color	Spotty pigmentation in areas exposed to sun; face paler, even in the absence of anemia
Temperature	Extremities cooler; decreased perspiration
Fat distribution	Less on extremities; more on trunk
Hair color	Dull gray, white, yellow, or yellow-green
Hair distribution	Thins on scalp, axilla, pubic area, upper and lower extremities; decreased facial hair in men; women may develop chin and upper lip hair
Nails	Decreased growth rate
Genitourinary and reproductive changes	
Renal blood flow	Because of decreased cardiac output, reduced filtration rate and renal efficiency; possibility of subsequent loss of protein from kidneys
Micturition	In men possiblity of increased frequency as a result of prostatic enlargement
	In women decreased perineal muscle tone; therefore urgency and stress incontinence
	Increased nocturia for both men and women
	Possibility that polyuria may be diabetes related
	Decreased volume of urine may relate to decrease in intake but evaluation needed
Incontinence	Increased occurrence with age, specifically in those with dementia
Male reproduction	
Testosterone production	Decreases; phases of intercourse slower, lengthened refractory time
Frequency of intercourse	No changes in libido and sexual satisfaction; decreased frequency to one or two times weekly
Testes	Decreased size; decreased sperm count; diminished viscosity of seminal fluid
Female reproduction	
Estrogen	Decreased production with menopause
Breasts	Diminished breast tissue
Uterus	Decreased size; mucous secretions cease; possibility that uterine prolapse may occur as a result of muscle weakness
Vagina	Epithelial lining atrophies; narrow and shortened canal
Vaginal secretions	Become more alkaline as glycogen content increases and acidity declines

From Ebersole P. and Hess, P., Toward healthy aging: human needs and the nursing process, ed. 2; Data from Malasanos, L., and others: 1985. Health assessment, 3rd ed., The C.V. Mosby Co., St. Louis; Blake, D.: 1979. Physiology and Aging Seminar for Nurses, Napa, Calif., May; and Wardell, S., editors, 1979. Acute interventions: nursing process throughout the life span, Reston Publishing Co., Reston, Va.

TABLE 44-2 Physical assessment findings in the elderly—cont'd

Characteristics	Findings
Gastrointestinal changes	
Mastication	Impaired because of partial or total loss of teeth, malocclusive bite, and ill-fitting dentures
Swallowing and carbohydrate digestion	Swallowing more difficult as salivary secretions diminish
	Reduced ptyalin production; therefore impaired starch digestion
Esophagus	Decreased esophageal peristalsis
	Increased incidence of hiatus hernia with accompanying gaseous distention
Digestive enzymes	Decreased production of hydrochloric acid, pepsin, and pancreatic enzymes
Fat absorption	Delayed, affecting the rate of fat-soluble vitamins A, D, E, and K absorption
Intestinal peristalsis	Reduced gastrointestinal motility
	Constipation because of decreased motility and roughage
Musculoskeletal changes	
Muscle strength and function	Decrease with loss of muscle mass; bony prominences normal in aged, since muscle mass decreased
Bone structure	Normal demineralization, more porous
	Shortening of the trunk as a result of intervertebral space narrowing
Joints	Become less mobile; tightening and fixation occur
	Activity may maintain function longer
	Normal posture changes; some kyphosis
	Range of motion limited
Anatomic size and height	Total decrease in size as loss of body protein and body water occur in proportion to decrease in basal metabolic rate
	Increased body fat; diminished in arms and leg, increased in trunk
	Decreased height from 2.5 to 10 cm from young adulthood
Nervous system changes	
Response to stimuli	All voluntary or automatic reflexes slower
	Decreased ability to respond to multiple stimuli
Sleep patterns	Stage IV sleep reduced in comparison to younger adulthood; increased frequency of spontaneous awakening
	Stay in bed longer but get less sleep; insomnia a problem
Reflexes	Deep tendon reflexes responsive in the healthy aged
Ambulation	Kinesthetic sense less efficient; may demonstrate an extrapyramidal Parkinson-like gait
Voice	Decreased range, duration, and intensity of voice; may become higher pitched and monotonous
Sensory changes	
Vision	
Peripheral vision	Decreases
Lens accommodation	Decreases, requires corrective lenses
Ciliary body	Atrophy in accommodation of lens focus
Iris	Development of arcus senilis
Choroid	Atrophy around disk
Lens	May develop opacity, cataract formation; more light necessary to see
Color	Fades or disappears
Macula	Degenerates
Conjunctiva	Thins and looks yellow
Tearing	Decreases; increased irritation and infection
Pupil	May be different in size
Cornea	Presence of arcus senilis
Retina	Observable vascular changes
Stimuli threshold	Increased threshold for light touch and pain
	Ischemic paresthesias common in the extremities
Hearing	Less perceptible high-frequency tones; hence greatly impaired language understanding; promotes confusion and seems to create increased rigidity in thought processes
Gustatory	Decreased acuity as taste buds atrophy; may increase the amount of seasoning on food

Older people have a tendency to reminisce about previous events in their lives. Although this process can serve a reorganizing function, as discussed later in this chapter, it can also result in reality-based or imagined guilt feelings. Because most older people grew up in an environment that promoted a strict conscience, they may have strict rules for themselves. When they do not live up to these unrelenting standards, they may feel bad, worthless, and guilty.

Older persons may tend to hide their feelings about themselves and the way they are treated. This often means that their anger is repressed and is manifested by depression. They may be unable to accept that they even feel anger because they have learned to suppress it well. Aphasia, brain damage, or various other physical, emotional, and social reasons may also impede the expression of anger. Often older persons talk about their feelings of anger only indirectly. For example, they may complain about food, staff, relatives, or various world events.

On the other hand, some people may be more apt to express anger in their later years than at other stages in their lives. These people may become less inhibited with age, or their defenses may not be as effective in helping them control their anger. Aggressive reactions by dis-turbed older persons often arise out of a need to gain attention, a need to feel in control, or violations of lifelong dietary preferences and privacy needs.[4] The catastrophic responses that result from these precipitating factors interfere with proper care, cause distress to the individual and other persons, may induce serious emotional problems, and often aggravate existing physical disorders.

The nurse needs to assess both the older client's multiple losses and their ways of coping with these losses. If older people have something to look forward to during the remainder of their life or in their afterlife, they have a strong resource in coping with the losses of aging. The investment of emotional energy in new objects is a way of relieving this loss. However, this investment is often more difficult for the older client because of their fatigue and reluctance to enter into new enterprises. If the older client is not able to cope with the losses of aging, depression will probably occur. There is an increase in the length and frequency of depressive episodes resulting from multiple losses.

Other precipitants of depression include organic mental disorders, and cerebral arteriosclerosis . As the individuals become aware of their progressive loss of intellectual faculties, depression ensues.

TABLE 44-3 Distinguishing depression, delirium and dementia*

Features	Depression	Delirium	Dementia
Confusion	Client may complain of problems with remembering; concern with these problems; impairment probably mild	Client is likely to deny problems exist, selective impairment, major disruption in daily living	Confusion is noticed by others, staff, family; major memory disturbance
Hallucinations and delusions	Absent (usually)	Vivid hallucinations and well-developed delusional systems	Sometimes paranoid accusations present, illusions, personality changes possible
Onset	Can be abrupt or gradual; look for a precipitant: life changes, losses, change in health	Abrupt and rapid	Slow and insidious
Progress	Not progressive	Symptoms become severe in a few days	Gradual or step-wise progression
Fluctuations	Client may feel worse in the morning	Large fluctuations even hour to hour	Some change in severity possible, but not large (clients with multiinfarct dementia exhibit greater fluctuations in mental status and behavior than clients with Alzheimer's disease)
Duration	From 2 weeks to 6 months; may last years	A few days or weeks	Months or years
Mental status exam	Usually no errors, or no more than one	Connotative errors likely	Two or more errors (number or errors correlates to severity of disease)
Neurological	Normal aging pattern; performance on tests requiring speed	Selective impairment especially attention	Global deficit that becomes worse as the disease progresses

Modified from Goss, A., and King, K.: Based on data from Zarit, S., Orr, N., and Zarit, J.: The hidden victims of alzheimers's disease: families under stress, New York, 1985, New York University Press.

In fact, depression as an early feature of dementia has been observed so frequently that depression was believed at one time to actually progress to dementia. However, when the organic mental syndrome becomes severe, the loss of psychological capacity, including mood reactivity, is so great that the individual's ability to react with depression is significantly diminished or absent. Therefore the symptoms of depression are modified and overshadowed by the forgetfulness, poor judgment, and confusion of organic mental disorders.

Because the verbal response patterns and overt behaviors of depressed persons and persons with organic mental disorders are similar, the depressed older person may be misdiagnosed as cognitively impaired. However, a number of signs and symptoms distinguish between depression, delirium, and dementia (Table 44-3).

Related to the problem of depression is suicide, which is the leading cause of death of the elderly. Although the elderly make up about 11% of the population, they account for roughly 25% of reported suicides. In 80% of older persons' suicide attempts, depression is present; 12% of elderly persons who attempt suicide will try again within 2 years, usually in a setting identical to that of the first attempt.[44]

Older persons choose suicide so that they die while they are still physically and mentally able to make decisions; this is especially true if they are facing a debilitating terminal illness and are alone. They may attempt suicide as a way of controlling or beating death and may not see death as an end to the person. They may consider suicide as a way to rejoin deceased loved ones and frequently choose the anniversary date of an important loss for the suicide attempt. Even when they have been taught that suicide is wrong, their guilt feelings may be ovecome by a strong belief that they have a right to choose when and how to die.

Older people are more likely to succeed in their suicide attempts because they generally choose more dangerous methods. Thus the elderly person who states a wish to die is considered at high risk. This is especially true if plans include a violent method and a suicide note is left.

Although elderly persons' active suicide attempts are more violent, they are not nearly as common as the indirect self-destruction called benign suicide or subintentional suicide. This self-destructive behavior is frequently seen in the older person who finds it impossible to deal with widowhood and dies shortly after the spouse's death. It also occurs frequently among the aged who reside in nursing homes. Examples of subtle self-destructive behavior are refusing to eat, refusing medication, and not taking care of one's physical needs. These behaviors often are not viewed as suicide attempts by those caring for the elderly, and the intent behind such suicidal behavior often is not considered. Thus if clients refuse medications, their behavior may be interpreted as being stubborn, cantankerous, or confused; their not taking care of their own physical needs could be viewed as forgetfulness or carelessness. However, any behavior that is potentially harmful to the individual needs to be explored for self-destructive intent.

✳ *Intellectual dimension.* Sensory alterations common with aging can have an effect on aged persons' perceptions of their world. For example, the decline in peripheral vision in the elderly may result in their viewing others as intruding on their own personal space without warning. Data on a person's orientation and memory indicate the reliability of subsequent information. Having data on the person's cognitive abilities or level of understanding assists the nurse in asking questions and giving information to the client at an appropriate level of understanding. Because the older person is frequently distracted by irrelevant stimuli, questions need to contain only one thought and be clear and concise. Older persons' increased response time requires that questions be paced according to their speed in answering the questions. For the confused older client whose attention span is short, the nurse provides a period of rest between data collection sessions.

Sensory deprivation is a common problem among the elderly, particularly those who are institutionalized. Body changes, such as hearing loss, that alter the reception or perception of sensations; a decrease in life space, such as with a loss of mobility; or a decrease in the amount or variety of environmental stimuli may all result in sensory deprivation. Thus stimulation in older persons' environments is particularly important as their life space decreases. The sources of stimulation to each of the five senses, interpersonal contacts, and the meaningfulness of the stimuli to clients are important areas for assessment.

If the older person's activities are limited to a particular community, building, or room, sensory deprivation is more likely. For example, the older person who is transferred from his home to a high-rise apartment building may stay primarily in his apartment where he may experience inadequate sensory stimulation. Such sensory deprivation is believed to accelerate the normal degenerative changes that accompany aging by enhancing the loss of functional cells in the central nervous system. In general, it has been found that isolation leads to sensory deprivation, loss of mental function, and personality disintegration in the elderly.[4] Signs that the individual is receiving too much stimulation, such as confusion or lack of response, are also important to note.

Although memory for past events usually remains intact in the older person, memory for recent events is frequently impaired. The preservation in memory of past events may be the result of the greater importance of these events or the frequent mental rehearsal of them by the older person.

Older persons' degree of defensiveness about their aging needs to be assessed as an indicator of their adaptation. Patterns of denial may frequently interfere with their acceptance of aging and their recognition of physical limitations. An example is elderly people who are secretive about their age, overuse hair dyes and cosmetics to appear young, exaggerate their physical prowess, and ignore physical impairments. This denial impedes healthy adaptation to the reality of aging. The older person who refuses to plan ahead may be failing to face the decline of aging and may awaken one day with the realization that "I am old."

An intense, almost morbid preoccupation with health, called *hypochondriacal preoccupation*, may be present. Frequently this preoccupation is concerned with the gastrointestinal and cardiovascular systems. These complaints may have a bizarre quality and may be the beginning of somatic delusions. This preoccupation with one's body may provide the elderly with an acceptable "sick role" and allow them to deny their loss of independence, success, and prestige.

If a client who is rehabilitating well from a stroke or other physical illness begins to decline, depression needs to be considered. The hypochondriacal complaints characteristic of depression need to be distinguished from a necessary and normal preoccupation with the body. Taking an active interest in personal preventive health care, in conserving one's body stamina, or in the symptoms of a chronic disease may be adaptive and necessary preoccupations with the body, particularly in old age.

The older client who is confused may engage in *wandering*, which is a tendency to move about either in a seemingly aimless or disoriented fashion or in pursuit of an indefinable or unobtainable goal. The client who wanders is particularly troublesome to families and institutions who have a moral and legal obligation for the client's safety.

Wandering most often is an avoidance behavior in response to stress. In comparison to clients who do not wander, those who are wanderers move about more, spend more time screaming or calling out, spend less time in social behavior, and are more disoriented.

In assessing wandering behavior, the following questions need to be considered:

1. What is the person's pattern of wandering?
2. Is it overtly goal-directed or searching behavior, combined with calling out or looking for an unobtainable person or goal, for example, a dead spouse?
3. Is it overtly goal-directed or searching behavior directed toward an obtainable but lost object, for example, dentures?
4. Is it apparently non-goal-directed behavior with multiple goals and aimless or poor attention span?
5. Is it the result of a lifelong pattern of coping with stress, as in walking or running away from stress?
6. Is it related to previous work roles, such as mail carrier?
7. Is the individual searching for security in the face of fear or anxiety?
8. What is the individual's usual wandering route?
9. What is the timing of the wandering; is it seasonal or at a particular time of day?
10. What is the individual's usual affect and behavior during incidents of wandering?[19,38]

Expressive functions may also be affected by aging or by the disease processes that frequently accompany aging. The older person with dementia often experiences language disturbances that begin with a general decline in vocabulary and range of expression and lead to repetitious and concrete speech. Although the language disturbances are similar to the aphasias caused by focal lesions, some qualitative differences are evident. The errors and delays in naming, which are the most-documented speech abnormalities in dementia, may result partly from a failure to adequately recognize objects. Therefore asking the person with aphasia to name easily recognized objects will not improve his errors and delays. However, the person with dementia may show improvement in naming objects with rehearsal.

Incoherent or repetitious speech, sometimes called *sounding*, can also result from nonorganic causes. It often occurs when meaningful communication has been interrupted and is frequently seen as meaningless babble. However, sounding can serve several purposes for older people, including (1) reaffirming their presence, (2) testing how people respond to their needs, (3) discharging pent-up tension, (4) providing self-stimulation, and (5) establishing their personal space or territorial boundaries.[22]

❀ ***Social dimension.*** One of the developmental tasks of older persons is adjusting to changes in their relationship to significant others, including spouses, children, grandchildren, and friends. Because of the illness or death of significant others or changes in older person's mobility, the number of people who are significant to them frequently declines. This often results in an increase in significance being given to people who remain. For example, children's returning home for special occasions may become extremely important to the aged parent.

The older person's relationship with his spouse and the level of satisfaction with this relationship are important assessment areas. Generally the pattern of satisfaction or dissatisfaction with marital relationships continues into old age. Frequently older people believe that since their children have grown, their lives are calmer, they are more free to do as they please, and they are drawn closer together by mutual leisure interests. However, many potential marital stressors may emerge, including retirement, financial concerns, disagreements about moving, and health problems. As in any other life stage, these stressors may serve to draw the couple closer together or separate them.

Role reversal may occur in the marriages of older persons. Older men who have been actively involved with the world may become more introverted and submissive. Women who have been passive earlier in life may become more domineering and aggressive. The degree to which role reversal occurs depends on the individual characteristics of the couple and their past patterns of decision making. It may range from the woman simply sharing more in decision making to her assuming the role of family authority and primary decision maker.

The prevailing attitude of society is to glamorize youth and disparage old age. This frequently results in low self-esteem that can lead to depression. Low self-esteem is usually not expressed in the elaborate delusions about unworthiness characteristic of younger people but rather in more subtle expressions such as "I'm useless now" or "You don't need to waste your time on me."

Some depressed older persons believe that they are of no value; they think of themselves as ugly, lonely, hopeless, and undeserving. They are unable to see the invalidity of their thoughts; they do not understand that these beliefs do not represent who they really are.

The older person's level of social interaction and social support needs to be assessed. This includes the loss of relationships and goals because of the deaths of friends and family; migration of the person, family members, and friends; and retirement. The Research Highlight below shows that there may be a relationship between the older person's social support and his well-being.

Relationships with family members make up the nucleus of the social life of most older people and tend to be more important than relationships with their friends. Therefore the degree of satisfaction that older people have in their relationships with their children is assessed. The elderly often have some definite expectations of their children, such as believing that they should visit or write often. Aged parents also need to shift perspectives toward their children and view them as adults rather than as children.

Retirement is a significant developmental event. Most retired persons are able to adapt over time. However, the meaning that work has held for the older person, how the older person views his retirement, whether retirement was mandatory or voluntary, how prepared the person is, and how the spouse reacts to retirement are important areas of data collection. If work played a central and sig-

nificant role in the person's life, the loss of work may be felt severely; these intense feelings of loss may hinder the person from beginning to find substitutes for the work. In these cases the aged individual is likely to become depressed. What appears to be a problem with retirement may actually be a reaction to aging, or vice versa, and this also is considered in the assessment.

Some older people may view retirement as a privilege, welcome the relief from a rigid schedule, and look forward to some leisure years. Others may view retirement as a threat and vigorously oppose it, especially if their self-worth is based primarily on worker identity. If retirement is compulsory, older people may think that they are being discriminated against because of their age or that their personal dignity has been affronted. Thus they may enter retirement resentful toward society and brooding over the injustice done to them. Persons who are able to make their own decisions about retirement are generally happier in their retired years. Voluntary retirees have significantly greater emotional satisfaction, feelings of usefulness, emotional stability, self-confidence, positive attitudes, and positive striving. Some wives of retirees look forward to their husband's retirement, and others have grave reservations about it. Unemployed wives may find that having their husbands around all day interferes with their daily routines and necessitates major adjust-

---

Research Highlight

The Relationship of Social Support to Health in Elderly People

S.J. Laschinger

PURPOSE

This study investigated the relationship between the quality of social support and the elderly person's level of health. It was hypothesized that elderly persons with a high quality of social support also experience a high level of functional health and psychological well-being. Functional health was defined as a person's ability to perform activities of daily living. Psychological well-being was defined as how people feel about themselves.

SAMPLE

Twenty-five subjects were randomly selected from 400 participants in a central urban program for elderly people in the province of Quebec. The sample included 11 women and 14 men. Their ages ranged from 60 to 84 years, with a mean age of 74 years. Seven subjects were older than 80 years and 18 were younger. One was divorced, two were married, ten were widowed, and twelve were single.

METHODOLOGY

All subjects were interviewed by the investigator and asked to identify all persons who were "important" to them.

Nurses in the program collected the functional health data and the psychological well-being data from the subjects. The functional health measure was a 15-item set of observer ratings of competence in activities of daily living.

FINDINGS

The hypothesized relationship beetween the quality of social support and the older person's level of health was not demonstrated in this study. However, there was a relationship between social support and psychological well-being in males, but not in females. Also for subjects above 80 years a relationship between functional health and psychological well-being was found, but this was not the case for subjects below 80 years of age. All subjects perceived a better quality of social support from professionals as compared to nonprofessionals.

IMPLICATIONS

The quality of older persons' social support needs to be a part of the nurse's assessment. The role of the nurse in providing social support to the elderly is important.

Based on data from Western Journal of Nursing Research 6:3, 1984.

ments. If the wife is still employed when the husband retires, stress may also be encountered.

The older person's participation in leisure activities is assessed. Persons who become more active after retirement usually experience greater life satisfaction than those whose participation in activities decreases or remains unchanged.

Although financial needs may decrease after retirement, financial matters are a very realistic concern of old age and account for a large portion of the problems in adjusting to retirement. Economic problems often necessitate adjustments in older persons' life-styles; for example, they may be unable to join or maintain membership in various organizations, to give gifts to family or friends, or to retain their home. Most older people who have had an adequate income are able to adjust their life-styles and find adequate financial resources. However, the onset of health problems frequently creates a financial crisis.

Housing is an important element in the life of the older person and can have a decisive impact on the well-being and life-style of older persons. Because most older people prefer to live in their own homes, the loss of this meaningful possession can be a major stressor; living with children or other relatives can lead to another set of stressors.

Many older people move to the Sunbelt after retirement. The function of such relocations in achieving life satisfaction is inconclusive. Some of these "transplanted" people experience serious loneliness for the family and close friends they have left behind and find it difficult to cope with an unfamiliar environment and to adapt to one-season weather. For others a new environment is beneficial and leads to renewed vitality and a greater interest in life.

Maintaining a sense of trust in himself and the world is a substantial challenge for the person facing the multiple losses of aging and living in an environment in which he is fearful of physical harm. Older people who do manifest a sense of trust have usually been able to achieve the developmental tasks discussed earlier in this chapter. Those who have not developed a sense of trust and who are under stress are likely to exhibit symptoms of mistrust ranging from suspiciousness to paranoia.

The loss of sensory acuity, especially auditory loss, has been associated with suspiciousness. Failing memories may also lead to suspiciousness in aged persons who choose to project their problems onto others rather than accept a decrease in memory. Major environmental changes such as moving to a nursing home may precipitate suspiciousness, especially since the change involves stress. Social isolation has also been found to be highly correlated with the development of paranoia.

Older adults may make vague complaints about external forces, such as landlords, nurses, or relatives, controlling their lives. These may be generalized feelings of desertion or of being abused by the younger generation, the government, or negative outside forces. This suspiciousness may be a lifelong style that becomes exaggerated as a result of the situational changes accompanying aging. Individuals who have consistently used the defense mechanism of projection may be predisposed to heightened suspiciousness in their later years when multiple losses occur.

Because of cultural biases and discrimination against the aged, the older person's paranoid ideation is examined. His ideation may be accurate; for example, the bank officer may indeed be reluctant to give the older person a loan, the store clerk may avoid answering his questions, or someone may be planning to steal his Social Security check. The suspiciousness of the older person may not always be unrealistic.

While there are true paranoid disorders that occur for the first time in old age, most of the paranoid symptoms seen in the elderly reflect social isolation and misinterpretations of environmental events rather than delusions. When multiple losses challenge people's sense of control over the world, they may search for some explanation for the losses. If they are unable to find such an explanation, they may attempt to reduce the ambiguity of the unknown by resorting to mystical or primitive interpretations of their world. This is especially true in individuals whose character predisposes them toward suspiciousness.

Aged persons' level of independence, their ideas about dependence-independence, and their reactions to the loss of independence are all important areas of assessment. Unless there is a specific illness, most individuals between 65 and 75 years continue with normal activities and by 85 years are usually showing the effects of age. Most individuals older than 85 years need assistance in carrying out normal activities. Thus individuals as they age usually need to give up some of thier independence; adjusting to dependence then becomes a major developmental task of old age. The independence that older people have is related not only to their health, but also to such specific factors as income, mobility, housing, and life-style.

Older people usually view dependence negatively. The desire to remain independent in one's later years can be adaptive or maladaptive depending on the reason for and the degree of this desire. In a society that places a high value on independence, making decisions and doing things for oneself give older persons a sense of pride and can be a major source of self-esteem. They may also want to remain independent so as not to be a burden on others, since this not only inconveniences others but also may lower the esteem given older people.

In addition, fear and mistrust may be motives for remaining independent. The older person may mistrust people's reasons for wanting to help him and fear that he may be used or manipulated. Older people may also want to maintain their independence because it serves to preserve a vulnerable self-concept; that is, individuals can remain isolated from others and keep from becoming dependent. This isolation helps them avoid any negative reactions from others. These last two motives are maladaptive because they can lead to withdrawal and isolation. Therefore the motives that the aged person has for maintaining independence are important in the assessment.

The majority of older men and women with intact relationships continue to enjoy themselves sexually and consider sensual pleasure a rewarding part of being an older person. The time necessary to reach adequate levels of excitement before orgasm is increased and the period of orgasm decreases, but the overall pattern of sexual activity a couple has achieved remains intact.

Older people often distinguish between intercouse and intimacy. Some research suggests that the nonintercourse aspects of love peak in the later years, since more and more persons are likely to have experienced the full range of human loving, which allows them to share empathic affection. However, the expression of sexuality may be hampered by lack of privacy, unavailability of partners, or negative caregiver attitudes.[38]

In the assessment, nurses are concerned with the status of past as well as present loving relationships and the degree to which the client was or is satisfied with these relationships. Even if a person is no longer sexually active, asking questions regarding sexuality shows recognition of the individual's past and present. The nurse inquires as to the older person's current sexual outlets, the importance of sexual activity in his life, and any physical, emotional, or mental problem regarding sex.

Most older people highly value independence. Thus when they lose their independence, they may despise themselves and their situation and are extremely unhappy; many say they would prefer to die rather than become dependent. Older people often depend on their children; this usually puts a great strain on their relationship, causing an authority crisis of perhaps greater proportion than that seen in childhood. This situation may also lead to abuse of the older person by the family, (see Chapter 36).

Some older people may enjoy dependence, particularly those for whom it has been a lifelong pattern. They may use helplessness to attract and hold the love of family, friends, or caregivers. Dependence may be culturally influenced; for example, elderly southern women were socialized to depend on their husbands. An older person may have a need for dependence that originated early in life but lays dormant until many of the resources are lost; these losses affect the individual's sense of mastery and activate feelings of helplessness.

In evaluating an older person's level of dependence, it is important for nurses to differentiate actual disability from excess disability. *Excess disability* is the loss of function that is associated with emotional perceptions of the client or nurse. An example of excess disability is the mentally impaired client who because of staff shortage and scheduling is dressed by an aide in the morning. The elderly person may actually be capable of dressing himself with assistance. However, this skill may be lost because it is more efficient to have someone dress him. Family members caring for impaired elders may also contribute to such artificially created dependence.[38]

✿ ***Spiritual dimension.*** The final stage in the life cycle often provides time to think about spiritual matters. Issues such as mortality and immortality, love relationships, and transcendence take on new meanings as death approaches and are important areas of assessment for the nurse.

Religion has been found to correlate with feelings of happiness, usefulness, and personal adjustment in older people, especially in men and those older than 70 years.[7] When the older persons of today were being reared, religion and church- or temple-related activities were emphasized and church activities were often the main social events. Most studies indicate that older people who have grown up with these values continue these activities if possible. Those who have not been active church or temple members during their young and middle adult years often reestablish these ties as they become older. Membership in a church or synagogue is often retained longer than membership in any other voluntary organization. Religious activities may decrease only when the older person becomes ill or cannot find transportation. When religious activities outside the home decrease, those within the home, such as listening to religious services on the radio or television, may increase. Because of the importance of religion to many older clients, it is a component of the nurse's assessment.

The finiteness of life takes on added significance in later years; at this time older persons may reclarify the significance of death and achieve their last developmental task, the acceptance of death. Their readiness for death and their specific fears about dying are important factors in the assessment of the spiritual dimension. Having put their affairs in order and having achieved their major goals, many older persons are ready for death while continuing to live their lives to the fullest. For many of these people establishing a legacy or passing something on to the next generation is important. Clients who are discussing the meaning of life may become despairing and find no meaning. They may think that God is punishing them for their sins and turn away from God as their depression increases. A few older people feel cheated by life and robbed of opportunities to fulfill their hopes. These people do not accept death and may approach it with a sense of despair.

Many older people do not fear death, and older people with strong religious beliefs are generally less anxious about death that those who are not religious. Those who are anxious usually have fears about the process of dying rather than about death itself. They fear losing control as death approaches, being unable to obtain help when they need it, and being abandoned.

The holistic assessment tool below contains assessment information specific to the aged adult. It is to be used in conjunction with the assessment tool in Chapter 8.

Measurement tools. Table 44-4 lists measurement tools that are useful in assessing the older adult.

Analysis

Nursing diagnosis. The following list provides examples of NANDA-accepted diagnoses with causative statements.
1. Disturbed self-concept related to the aging process,
2. Potential for self-harm related to loss of spouse,
3. Social isolation related to relocation to nursing home
4. Powerlessness related to recent retirement

HOLISTIC ASSESSMENT TOOL: THE AGED ADULT

PHYSICAL DIMENSION
Genetic History

At what age did members of your family die?
Is there any history of Alzheimer's disease or multi-infarct dementia in your family?

Activities of Daily Living
Diet and Elimination
Describe any problems you have with incontinence.

Exercise and Activity
Describe physical limitations you have that prohibit adequate exercise.

Sleep and Rest
Describe any fears you have that keep you from falling asleep at night or keep you awake during the night.
Do you take naps and at what time of the day?
What is your consumption of tobacco, alcohol, and drugs?

General Appearance
Body Image

In what ways has the aging process altered your body image?

Sexuality

Describe any vaginal pain or irritation.
Describe any difficulty you have with sexual functioning.

EMOTIONAL DIMENSION

How have you responded to your own aging?
What losses have occurred as an older adult? What have these losses meant to you? In what ways have you coped with the losses of aging?
Describe your feelings about your aging and your present circumstances.
Does anything about your physical health concern you?
In what ways are you satisfied with your accomplishments?
Describe any major regrets you have about your life.

INTELLECTUAL DIMENSION

What changes have occurred in your vision, hearing, taste, smell, and feeling? In what ways have you compensated for these sensory changes?
Describe any difficulty you have with your memory. What strategies have you used to help with your memory?
In what ways have you been able to adapt to the changes taking place in your world?

SOCIAL DIMENSION
Self-Concept

In what ways has your self-concept been altered by the aging process?

Interpersonal Relations

In what ways has your relationship with your spouse and children changed during your older adulthood.
What kinds of social interactions do you engage in? Describe your satisfaction with your level of social interaction.

Environmental Factors

Are you retired? If so, was it a mandatory or voluntary retirement? Was retirement forced because of illness?
Describe any preretirement preparation.
Describe any difficulty in adjusting to retirement.

Trust-Mistrust

Do you feel safe going out during the day or night?
Describe your satisfaction with your level of control of your life.

Dependence-Independence

In what areas have you been required to become more dependent because of the aging process? How have you adjusted to this change in dependence?

SPIRITUAL DIMENSION

How has your philosophy of life changed during your later years?
What meaning does your life have?
Describe your sense of purpose and usefulness.
What do you fear about your own dying?
Describe how you have achieved the major goals in your life.

TABLE 44-4 Measurement tools

Instrument	Description
Home Assessment Checklist[64]	A 50-item questionnaire that evaluates environmental and safety conditions of the older person's general household, kitchen, bathroom, and bedroom
Older Americans' Resources and Services Instrument (OARS)[28]	A multidimensional functional assessment tool that covers social resources, economic resources, mental health, physical health, and activities of daily living
Short Portable Mental Status Questionnaire (SPMSQ)[47]	A 10-item questionnaire that assesses the presence and degree of cognitive deficit in regard to orientation, long- and short-term memory, and information necessary for activities of daily living

Planning

Table 44-5 provides long-term goals, short-term goals, and outcome criteria for diagnoses related to the aged adult. These serve as examples of the planning stage of the nursing process.

Implementation

✦ Physical dimension. Older persons' rest and sleep can be promoted by helping them become aware of their biorhythms and plan their activities and rest to be in synchrony with their body functions. They also need information about the normal characteristic changes in the sleep patterns of older people.

Plans need to be made for a balance between activity and rest during the day. Since it takes older people three times as long to get to sleep later in the evening if they take afternoon naps, it is helpful to schedule social and recreational activities in the afternoon and to allow ample time for a nap before lunch. Scheduling purposeful activities in the afternoon also helps prevent boredom and provides exercise conducive to evening sleep. Short rest periods intermittently during the day, such as sleeping, reading, watching television, or listening to the radio, help increase the efficiency of activities that follow. Rest periods of about 20 minutes in a reclining position are particularly helpful after the noon and evening meals. Before the person rests, the nurse or client loosens clothing around the neck, wrist, ankle, and pelvic girdle to allow for proper circulation. Clients need to be encouraged to nap in their beds because when they nap in a chair, the neck is often hyperflexed or hyperextended. This may cause compression of the arteries in the neck; changes in cerebral blood flow and decreased vascular resistance may then lead to mental confusion or hypotension.

If older persons are institutionalized, arrangements are made to follow their usual bedtime rituals, including allowing time to perform these rituals before retiring. Since older clients are sometimes fearful of other people entering their room or home during the night, their safety and the safety of their personal belongings are ensured. A call or telephone system that is answered promptly may provide the sense of security needed for resting. Foods rich in protein and milk products before bedtime help promote sleep and provide alternatives to sleep medications.

By their acceptance and positive regard for older persons, nurses can assist in promoting a positive body image. Encouraging older persons to take pride in their appearance is also important and may include discussing hairstyles or the use of cosmetics to cover blemishes. In an institutional setting nurses can assist in preventing any unsightly appearance that may be caused from stained dentures, soiled clothing, and unkempt hair, fingernails, and beards. Older people sometimes fail to maintain their appearance because their hands are crippled with arthritis or they lack awareness, energy, or incentive; the strategic placement of mirrors can help to improve their awareness.

If changes in body image have produced negative self-evaluations, older people need reassurance and positive reinforcements for the aspects of themselves that transcend physical appearance.

TABLE 44-5 Long-term and short-term goals and outcome criteria related to the aged adult

Goals	Outcome Criteria
NURSING DIAGNOSIS: FEELINGS OF POWERLESSNESS RELATED TO ADMISSION TO A NURSING HOME	
Long-term goals	
To develop a feeling of hope about existence	Makes future-oriented statements
To maintain control over existence	Is assertive in asking for his needs to be met
Short-term goals	
To exercise self-determination	States that his actions have an influence on the outcome of events or experiences
	Assumes responsibility for as much self-care as possible
To make decisions about important aspects of daily living	States preferences about activities such as bedtime and frequency and timing of baths
NURSING DIAGNOSIS: SOCIAL ISOLATION RELATED TO THE RECENT LOSS OF SPOUSE	
Long-term goals	
To develop needed or desired intimate relationships and roles	Describes present relationships and roles that are meaningful
	Expresses feelings of belonging and being needed
Short-term goals	
To complete grief work for coping with loss of sources of intimacy	Decreases frequency of feelings of sadness over loss
To decrease frequency of feelings of loneliness	Prepares for contacts with people for high-risk periods such as evenings, meals, holidays, and anniversaries
	Seeks out surrogates for human intimacy such as pets
	Removes barriers to desired social contacts

Emotional dimension. It is often effective to combine several techniques when dealing with anxiety in elderly clients. Attentive listening, touch, or mild exercise can help to alleviate anxiety. Anxiety can also be treated by using deep muscle relaxation followed by systematic desensitization. Then positive reinforcement can be used to condition alternate or competing responses. A combination of self-efficacy training, modeling, operant shaping of alternate responses, and supportive counseling is especially effective if feelings of helplessness underlie the elderly person's anxiety.[18]

Older people often need encouragement to express their anger. Letting them know that their anger is sensed and accepted is important. Because they frequently hold in a lot of angry feelings, when they are given a chance to express them, their outbursts may be strong. They need to be encouraged to explore the causes for their feelings and to receive direction in getting back to the initial cause or loss. Nurses' acceptance, encouragement, and caring may help clients feel better about themselves and thus respond less angrily toward others. Older persons' indirect expression of anger in defiant or sarcastic behavior may have kept loved ones away. Thus, after being able to expose their anger, they may need some assistance in reestablishing relationships with loved ones. Constructive physical activities may also provide for some release of anger. Examples of such activities are hammering, digging in a garden, painting, and squeezing clay.

Loneliness is one of the most frequent causes of depression in the elderly (see Chapters 14 and 19).

Older persons often do not understand the relationship between their physical complaints and their depression. It is helpful to first establish rapport by listening to clients' complaints fully and intently; then assistance can be given in helping them to be as comfortable as possible. This conveys understanding and hope. The nurse explains that some of the physical symptoms may be a manifestation of depression and that in dealing with the depression some of the physical symptoms may be relieved.

Since repetitious talking about symptoms does not help the client, behavior modification may be useful. For example, expressions of feelings and interest in activities, people, and living can be reinforced with positive responses. Preoccupation with self and physical symptoms is given no response or only minimal matter-of-fact attention. "How are you?" is not asked as an opening remark because it may encourage statements about physical complaints. Instead, conversation can be directed to the person's emotional state, to important past experiences, or to involvement with present interests.

Preoccupations or actual problems with defecation, particularly constipation, frequently accompany depression in the older person. However, because of their habit-forming effect, laxatives and enemas need to be used only when necessary. When an enema is used, its meaning to the depressed older person needs to be considered, since it can be viewed as an invasion, a well-deserved punishment, or a means of control. Natural laxatives, such as raw or bulk food, are a preferable substitute. Fluid intake and exercise are also encouraged.

Cognitive psychotherapy is a helpful therapy for depression with older persons. Cognitive restructuring is a way for them to cope with situations that cannot be changed in reality but can be changed in the way they are perceived.

The nurse refrains from being overly optimistic in dealing with depression in older people. The depressed older person with a severe physical illness may not be helped substantially by psychotherapy. The physical illness causes a decrease in vitality already reduced by aging and depression.

Intellectual dimension. Promoting sensory stimulation is one way in which the nurse can assist in preventing sensory deprivation. In elderly people the intensity of the stimuli often needs to be increased if an increase is not contraindicated. For example, sound may need to be louder, and foods may need to be more highly seasoned. The family or friends of the elderly are encouraged to promote sensory stimulation by extending elderly persons' life space, for example, by taking them to restaurants, on walks, to sports events, or to shopping centers. Frequently family or friends who are willing to do these things are fearful that they may not know how to cope with the client's physical problems, such as being too unsteady to feed oneself or being unable to walk without assistance. Therefore the nurse assists them in anticipating difficulties and preparing to either avoid or deal with them.

The nurse makes every effort to prevent sensory overload before it occurs. Since older people often take longer to comprehend and to react, questions need to be phrased so that only one thought is being asked and sufficient time is given to formulate a response. Irrelevant stimuli are also eliminated. For example, directions or instructions to the elderly need to be brief and concise.

The older person generally takes a longer time to process stimuli accurately. The nurse needs to watch and listen for verbal and nonverbal cues, such as fear or doubt, because they may indicate perceptual confusion. If the older person's perception seems inaccurate, the nurse can help him to reconstruct the event, to look at all aspects of it, and to determine what actually occurred.

Orientation to time, place, and person helps to improve the older person's memory. Memory reminders, such as brief notes or instruction cards, need to be concise and well organized; they can help the individual cope with excessive stimuli and function more independently. Giving the older person a choice of responses or offering alternative solutions when asking questions is also helpful, since recognizing information is usually easier then recalling information.

Memory skills training can also be used for older adults with memory difficulty such as forgetting names. Generally this training consists of *mnemonic techniques* such as visual imagery associations or categorization. For example, the older person learns a series of logical steps for reconstructing a person's name on presentation of the face, as follows:

1. Identify a prominent facial feature (such as a large nose).

TABLE 44-6 Strategies for teaching aged adults

Instructional Variable	Strategies
Rate of presentation of information	Present new information at a fairly slow rate
	Let adult learner proceed at his own rate whenever feasible
	Provide adult learner with ample time to respond to questions
	Present a limited amount of material in any single presentation to prevent swamping effects
Organization of information	Present new information in a highly organized fashion
	Use section headings, handouts, summaries, etc., so that adult learner can get a "handle" on material
	If memory processes are taxed in a learning project, encourage adult learner to use retrieval plans
	Avoid introduction of irrelevant information in order to prevent confusion
	If visual displays are used, employ simple stimulus configurations
Mode of presenting information	Use auditory mode of presentation when presenting discrete bits of information to be used immediately
	Use visual mode when presenting textual materials to capitalize on opportunity for review during reading
	Utilize models to facilitate strategy development
Covert strategies	Encourage adult learner to generate his own mediators
	Supply adult learner with mediators when necessary
	With concrete material, imagery mediators are superior to verbal mediators and interacting images better than conjunctive images
	Whenever feasible, train adult learner in use of mnemonic devices
	Encourage adult learner to generate covert monitoring verbalizations and provide training when necessary
Meaningfulness of material	Present information which is meaningful to adult learner
	Assess cognitive structure of adult learner to ensure that material is introduced at appropriate level
	Use examples, illustrations, etc., which are concrete
Degree of learning	Provide ample opportunity for adult learner to over-learn material before moving on to new material
	Remove time constraints from instructional and evaluation process
Introduction of new material	As initial step in learning, identify and eliminate inappropriate responses which may "compete" with appropriate response
	Organize instructional units so that potentially interfering materials are spaced far away from each other
	Stress differences between concepts before similarities
	Make instructional sequence parallel hierarchy of knowledge in any given area
	Instructional procedures should be premised on knowledge of conditions required for a type of learning based on task analysis
	Introduce a variety of techniques for solving problems
Transfer effects	Take advantage of experience the adult learner possesses
	Relate new information to what adult learner already knows
	Develop learning sets which maximize opportunity for positive transfer effects
Feedback effects	Provide verbal feedback concerning correctness of responses after each component of task is completed
	Do not assume that initially poor performance on a novel, complex task is indicative of low aptitude
Climate	Establish a supportive climate
	Engage adult learner in information-oriented, collaborative evaluation
	Encourage adult learner to take educated guesses

Adapted from Burnside, I.M.: One-to-one relationship therapy. In Burnside, I.M.: Nursing and the aged, ed. 2, New York, 1981, McGraw-Hill Book Co., pp. 77-78; based on data from Okun, M.A.: Adult Education **27**(3):1977.

2. Derive a concrete, high-imagery transformation of the person's name ("Beck" becomes "Beak").
3. Form an interacting visual image associating the prominent facial feature with the name transformation.[69]

Combining relaxation with memory skills training enhances the ability of elderly persons to benefit from memory training programs.[70]

A series of games called Eldergames has also been used to work with the memory problems of older clients experiencing cognitive decline. They concentrate, for example, on evoking earlier memories when short-term memory, but not long-term memory, has begun to erode.[50]

In teaching-learning situations with the elderly, the nurse needs to assure older persons that they will be given ample time and that their efforts will be accepted without ridicule. A task that seems overwhelming to the older person can be divided into smaller, more manageable parts, thus providing increased opportunities for success. Other suggestions for teaching older adults are presented in Table 44-6.

Cognitive functioning in the elderly may also be stimulated by physical exercise and music and may be improved by adequate sleep. Elderly people who participated in exercise therapy for a 12-week period were found to have a significant improvement in cognitive functioning. Music therapy has also been found to improve the older person's memory and cognitive functioning.[9] Since lack of sleep interferes with cognitive functioning, any of the activities discussed earlier for promoting sleep are also helpful in improving cognitive functioning.

The most common approach to the management of wandering behavior is the use of medications, door locks, gerichairs, and other restraining mechanisms. However, these actions may, in fact, produce or exacerbate wandering behavior. Restraints may increase hostility, as well as decrease security, orientation, and stimulation.

Interventions for wandering need to be tailored to the mood of the wanderer. The placid wanderer who may be bored or repeating a real or imagined activity needs to be approached casually and perhaps channeled into a less disturbing behavior. Agitated wanderers, who may be releasing frustration and tension through motor activity, need to be listened to, kept at a fair distance, and provided outlets for their aggression. "Happy wanderers," who may be exploring, need to be left alone but watched or taken on "guided tours." In general, wandering decreases if a regular regimen of exercise, walking, or getting outside is established.[37]

Social dimension. Self-esteem is promoted by reinforcing positive achievements in both present and past experiences. One approach is asking the client to make a list of his attributes and then to assess them as positive, negative, or neutral. Another technique is to use a prepared self-concept scale on which the client is asked to characterize his usual functioning with regard to a set of bipolar adjectives. The nurse then interjects traits the client may not have included, as well as helps the client formulate goals for self-improvement from the negative

qualities that he perceives. Usually, the number of positive traits suggested by clients outweighs the number of negative traits. This in itself is helpful in that it suggests to clients that they are not totally negative or deficient.[37]

The elderly tend to overattribute their negative physical symptoms to aging. Therefore another approach to improving self-esteem is redirecting the negative attributes that the elderly associate with aging to environmental factors instead. For example, when the client attributes his tiredness to "being old," he can be reminded that he was awakened at 5:30 AM. Explanations for feelings and behavior are thus refocused on situational factors that are amenable to change. This type of intervention can improve self-esteem in the elderly by changing negative, defeatist attitudes into hopeful, problem-solving approaches.[50]

The recognition by the elderly and by society of the continuing need for social interactions can be promoted through the mass media, pamphlets, posters, and discussion groups. On an individual basis, the nurse can use skillful interviewing to help the elderly person become aware of social interaction needs, validate them as real and important, and accept the need as normal. Clients can then be assisted in identifying realistic and acceptable solutions and, if possible, in making their own choices from among the alternatives. The nurse may need to introduce older persons to neighbors or others in the community, help them form new relationships by identifying common interests and experiences, help them revive old relationships, or involve them in group activities. The choices that the older person makes to meet social interaction needs are supported; the nurse can also assist in evaluating the effectiveness of the choice.

In addition, the nurse may form small discussion groups with elderly clients to provide opportunities for social interaction, to teach social skills, or to offer a continuing support system for members. The use of alcoholic beverages during social events has also helped increase the socialization of elderly persons. Friendly visitor services and telephone reassurance programs are examples of community-based services that have been successful in providing social support to the elderly.

Elderly widowed persons' needs for assistance vary depending on their ability to adjust to the changes from the loss of a spouse. When the older person needs support from others who understand or assistance in becoming involved in old or new activities, the nurse can help by providing the client with information about organized support groups for widowed persons.

Preretirement counseling is a way to prevent some of the problems that elderly persons frequently encounter during retirement. A postretirement program is also needed to help retirees review their past accomplishments, cope with the realities of retirement, adjust to the new role, and identify ways they can continue to make valuable contributions to society. For example, some firms offer retired workers part-time employment in a special workshop; volunteer groups may provide workshops and craft centers for the elderly; and elderly business people may be organized to provide advisory services to businesses or organizations. Also several programs for retired persons have been sponsored by the U.S. government. The Retired Senior Volunteer Program (RSVP) helps the aged meet the expenses incurred doing volunteer work; in the Foster Grandparent Program elderly people are paid a small fee for providing emotional support to children in institutional settings. A sense of comradeship and community is fostered by such participation, which also diminishes feelings of hopelessness and social rejection.

Although nurses cannot usually directly affect the income of the elderly, they can be advocates for them in supporting governmental and other efforts that will help ensure an adequate income in retirement. Nurses can also assist elderly clients in obtaining needed information on such topics as budgeting, tax benefits, insurance, wills, estates, investments, and reduced rates offered to senior citizens.

The nurse may be able to counsel older people regarding their decision to move or with their selection of appropriate housing. An evaluation of their present residence and a thorough investigation of other possible residences need to be done before the client makes the decision to relocate. If a decision is made to relocate, a trial move may be suggested. In the older person with brain dysfunction, any relocation, even within the same facility, is disruptive. Therefore the nurse provides a thorough orientation to the new environment.

If there is paranoid behavior related to isolation, as in the client who has recently moved, the nurse intervenes in the process that created the individual's social isolation. Restoring a pattern of social communication is essential; relocating the older individual may be necessary. Because the individual's paranoia may cause people to stay away from him and thus exacerbate the condition, "shuttle diplomacy" may be necessary.[23] This involves contacting individuals living in close proximity to the client who are aware of the client's condition and may have been targets of the client's accusations. The client's conditions can be explained to these people, and they can be informed that the client is being treated and that the prognosis is good. This prevents further social isolation of the client. Planned visits to the client by members of an outreach team are also helpful in the client's resocialization.

Giving the older person control and participation in decision making may help to prevent suspicion. Knowledge of the nature of the problem by the family and staff can help them deal with the client's accusations and reduce the hostility directed toward the client. Older persons may also benefit from help in organizing their possessions or from techniques that will help their memory, such as those described earlier.

Interventions for helping the older person maintain as much independence for as long as possible involve social policy issues, such as providing adequate supplementary income for the elderly, and expanding community services that allow older people to stay in their homes, such as homemaker services, visiting nurses, Meals on Wheels, and adequate public transportation. Nurses can be advocates for the elderly in securing the provision of such services.

Negative reactions to dependence can be reduced by respecting older people's desire for independence and by giving them as many choices as possible. For example, individuals in an institutional setting can be allowed to choose meals from a menu, recreational activities, or the timing of their baths.

Excess disability or dependence is discouraged by not hurrying or assisting a client who is capable of self-care. This approach also discourages helplessness that fosters further dependence. Examples include eliminating a wheelchair when a client can walk or establishing a bladder-retraining program rather than using catheterization.[41]

✄ ***Spiritual dimension.*** Intervening in the older person's spiritual dimension frequently involves collaboration with clergy. Recognition is given to the support that religious institutions offer to the elderly. Nurses can also become involved in encouraging churches to develop meaningful services and opportunities for the aged. They may provide opportunities for the older and younger generations to interact and for older people to interact with each other through programs such as Adopt-a-Grandparent, the sharing of resources, or crisis assistance.

The use of visualization and meditation can be fostered by the nurse to increase the meaning of existence for the client. Connecting a present need with a past memory image can help to partially ease the present need. For example, aged persons recently relocated to a nursing home may long for the familiar environment of their home. Directing them to visualize their past familiar environment in as much detail as possible will help reconstruct these perceptions and may ease the present need for the familiar and provide a sense of comfort. Nurses may also teach the elderly to meditate and encourage them to keep a dream diary, practice yoga, recite poetry, or play a musical instrument. These are all mechanisms of release and renewal that may add meaning to their existence.

Another mode of self-transcendence for the older person is the mentor relationship. This mode is infrequently used but can add meaning and purpose to older people's lives, and others may benefit from their wisdom and special abilities. The nurse can encourage the aged person to act as an adviser or guide in furthering the development of younger persons. For example, an aged person with business experience assists a younger person in business endeavors.

The nurse can facilitate the meeting of older people's needs for transcendence by encouraging them to share their experiences through some type of legacy, such as sharing their memories in an oral or written form, teaching skills to others, giving away monetary assets or objects of significance, or donating body organs. Establishing a legacy may become a major concern before a person's death. Legacies can serve as a way of extending one's meaning to others through handing down something from the past. Sharing experiences allows older persons to see how their lives have had an impact and prepares them to leave the world with a sense of meaning. It can also give a feeling that one's life will continue, will be tied with survivors, and will provide younger generations with an important sense of continuity.[22]

Often older people have particular objects that they

identify as their most cherished possessions. These objects usually represent important memories and are often an expression of the person's transcendence of themselves. For example, one woman who had raised many cats during her lifetime had also collected figurines of cats that she kept near her bed in her nursing home room. These objects represented important memories and were obviously her most cherished possession. She guarded them with great care and needed to make decisions concerning when and to whom these objects were dispersed. Insensitive distribution of these objects by staff or family members conveys a negative message to the older person, such as "Your death is imminent." When older people approach death, they may want to distribute their important possessions or plan for this distribution as a way of expressing their transcendence; nurses can provide assistance and support to the client in this process as well as help family members graciously accept these gifts.

To assist older people to establish legacies the nurses may ask older people what has been the most meaningful contribution in their lives, what impact their generation has had on the world, or what they would like to leave to the younger generation. After the person's interests are elicited, a method needs to be established for recording the legacy, identifying the recipients, and distributing the legacy as planned. The older person also needs feedback on how the legacy is received.[22]

If older persons are unable to gain a sense of satisfaction by recalling their individual accomplishments, another approach is to tap into their past. Questions about the accomplishments of their generation may be asked. Mentioning important historical events, eliciting their reactions to these events, and asking questions such as "What happened during your lifetime that changed the world?" are activities that may give the person a feeling of collective accomplishment.

Other people, particularly if they are angry or denying their mortality, may not be concerned with establishing a legacy and need not be pushed to do so. These persons need assurance of God's love or that of a supreme being and need help to find a sense of hope. The assistance of clergy may be needed.

Evaluation

The adequacy of nursing interventions is evaluated by the extent to which they build on the older client's available strengths and do not promote excess disability. Care is appropriate if the unique characteristics and needs of the elderly are taken into consideration. The effectiveness of nursing interventions is related to the extent to which needed changes are incorporated into the older person's long-established life patterns and values. Finally, the issue of efficiency in caring for the elderly needs to address the requirement of increased time in implementing many nursing care activities with this age group.

By this stage in their lives, older people often have the self-awareness to make an important assessment of changes in their sense of well-being. Therefore their reports can be an important aspect of the evaluation process.

SPECIFIC TREATMENT MODALITIES

Each of the treatment modalities discussed in Part 3 of this text can be used with the aged client. Reality orientation, validation therapy, remotivation therapy, resocialization, reminiscent therapy, and pet therapy will be discussed in this chapter because these are used most often with older persons.

Reality Orientation

One of the first psychological therapies used with institutionalized elderly, reality orientation (RO) is a behavioral therapeutic approach that attempts to increase an individual's awareness of time, place, and person. Two basic approaches are used in RO: 24-hour RO and classroom RO. Twenty-four–hour RO involves everyone who comes in contact with confused elderly clients by presenting them with basic information about time, place, and person. For example, when bringing supper to the elderly client, the nurse might say, "Hello, Mr. Darrell. I am Ms. Kelly. It is 6 o'clock in the evening. Here are some meat loaf and black-eyed peas for your supper." This is a team approach in which every contact with the person helps reorient him. It is often an early phase of rehabilitation used in conjunction with more traditional techniques such as activity therapy, physical and occupational therapy, and remotivation. As a supplement to 24-hour RO, many institutions provide RO classes. These may be scheduled on a daily to a weekly basis. Classes are divided into basic and advanced courses. The therapist can work best with only three or four moderately to severely confused clients, but six or eight are usually involved in the advanced class for those who are less confused.

RO was designed for use with mildly to severely confused persons regardless of the source of their confusion. It can also be used to help maintain orientation and prevent confusion. The effectiveness of RO may depend on the degree, duration, type, and cause of the confusion.

Since the goal of RO is to reduce confusion, its effectiveness as a treatment is evaluated by progress in the individual's ability to accurately state time, place, and date. Changes in other behavioral indicators of confusion also need to be monitored.

Validation Therapy

It is possible that disoriented behavior is not meaningless and that continually correcting a client's disoriented responses (language or behavioral) systematically neglects the meaning inherent in the confused behavior.[74] Such neglect not only is perceived by the client, but also effectively increases his anxiety and isolation. For example, cooperative nursing home residents who believe that they are still at home may become upset when an RO program is aimed at giving up this belief. If an individual is happier in a confused state than in an oriented one, the wisdom of using RO with this person needs to be addressed.

This concern about RO led to the development of validation therapy[24] for use with the confused client. This therapy involves searching for the meaning and emotion in the client's words and validating these with the client. For example, if a nursing home client tells the nurse that she has to leave because she has to see her mother (who has been dead for many years), the nurse would respond as follows:

Client: I have to go. I have to see my mother.
Nurse: What does she look like? You must have loved her very much. Do you still miss her?

This dialogue leads to a warm discussion of the client's relationship with her mother. If the same client had been forced to face the reality that her mother is dead, the client would likely have become resistant and uncooperative.

Remotivation Therapy

An offshoot of the reality orientation concept is remotivation therapy. In remotivation the focus is on the individual's self-concept and self-perception through reminiscences of the individual's past life, which are shared with a group. The individual is thus strengthened in two ways: (1) by encouragement to describe the self concretely as a person with roles and specific social functions and (2) by encouragement to speak accurately about past and present experiences.[10]

Resocialization

In studies designed to explore the relative effectiveness of reality orientation and *resocialization*, it has generally been found that resocialization is more effective.[10,20,53] Each study reported increased responsiveness, increased socialization with staff and with each other, increased participation in self-care, and less hostile, disruptive behavior. Some techniques reported to facilitate socialization and group interaction among cognitively impaired persons include the following:

1. Create unity and a sense of group through touching and joining hands to both initiate and terminate a session.
2. Plan group time so that it is least likely to be changed or disrupted by other activities.
3. Minimize outside distractions by holding the group session in a convenient but quiet room. Establish the norm with other staff that clients are not to be disturbed during group time.
4. Structure the group session as follows:
   a. Announce a topic that is familiar.
   b. Stimulate memories and reminiscing through use of associated foods, objects, and pictures.
   c. Incorporate activities that are likely to both evoke relevant memories and encourage active participation of all members (for example, cutting cake, stirring lemonade, singing a familiar theme-related song).
5. Do not separate friends, and do sit next to a member who seems particularly anxious or confused.
6. Be careful to design activities to meet the needs of the group members; activities that evolve from the needs of the leader or staff are likely to be too abstract or complicated.

Reminiscent Therapy

Reminiscent therapy involves recalling or reminiscing about the past for the purpose of assigning new meanings to past experiences. Whether it is used as an individual or a group process, *reminiscent therapy* is a journey through or a summation of one's life in which the client integrates experiences into their self-concept by mentally reliving them. Repressed and painful material is reviewed, and some of the sting is taken out of the past by altering the perception of the past. Early memories may be reconstructed in such a way that they serve the individual's needs, fears, and interests. Or reminiscence may be adaptive in reducing the dissonance between older people's expectations of themselves from the past and their present situation and behavior.

As in other group work with the aged, the number of group members needs to be kept at about eight or nine. Persons who have been isolated and who have not had much opportunity for exploring and resolving long-held conflicts are at psychological risk in a reminiscent group; feelings of guilt and remorse, which frequently emerge during the life review process, may develop into obsessive rumination and even suicidal panic.[12,19] Older individuals who are confused or suffering from brain damage can also participate in reminiscent therapy; however, caution is needed to prevent the heightened anxiety called catastrophic reaction that occurs when they cannot answer or perform.

Reminiscing groups can be conducted by professionals from a variety of disciplines, including nurses, art therapists, occupational therapists, music therapists, and social workers. Successful completion of the life review process is more likely to occur if the person is able to experience the process in a cohesive, supportive group in which trust and security are available. Since the group is a supportive rather than a therapy group, skills in listening and communication are adequate preparation for leading such a group.

The life review is a crucial process in the aged person's adaptation and, if successfully completed, assists in the following:[16]

1. Personality reintegration
2. Feelings of serenity
3. Acceptance of life as meaningfully resolved
4. Greater understanding of life's ambiguities
5. Transfer of culture and value to others
6. Examination of intrapsychic conflicts
7. Reconciliation of family relationships
8. Richer sharing of present experiences
9. Acceptance of death

Unstructured reminiscing groups may be spontaneously stimulated by a special occasion at which people begin remembering the past. More structured groups may be short term (about 10 weeks) or may go on indefinitely with a periodic evaluation of the group's goals.

Pet Therapy

The use of pets in therapy with the elderly has been shown to have many beneficial effects. In some institutional settings pets, including dogs, cats, birds, and rabbits, have been given permanent residence. In other situations, animals are brought in on a daily or weekly basis. Since animals show affection without restraint, they are often helpful in bringing about positive changes in the client's physical and mental status. All clients, especially those who have poor eyesight or are hard of hearing, can benefit from the increased tactile stimulation that pets provide. Pet therapy is not a replacement for human contact but is an additional alternative that is especially useful for reaching the frail or withdrawn older client.[37]

BRIEF REVIEW

As the number of aged persons has grown, increased attention has been focused on their mental health care. Nursing has had a primary role in providing care to this age group, and the geropsychiatric nurse has a prominent role in caring for their mental health needs.

Although a variety of theoretical approaches have been proposed for explaining the changes in the aged, this remains a fertile field for new understandings. Erikson describes the major developmental task of this age group as ego integrity vesus despair. Peck describes their tasks as (1) ego differentiation versus work role preoccupation, (2) body transcendence versus body preoccupation, and (3) ego transcendence versus ego preoccupation.

The nurse's attitude toward the aged is an important consideration in establishing a therapeutic relationship with an elderly client. Older people, because of their many years of experience, are often uniquely qualified to participate in planning their care.

The nurse is frequently involved in designing interventions to both prevent and treat the loneliness, depression, and paranoid behavior common to this age group. The issues of retirement, relocation, dependence, and death are also frequently paramount concerns for elderly persons. The behavioral manifestations and dynamics of these conditions have some distinctive features in this age group that are important to consider when assessing the older person and when deciding which aspects of intervention are most crucial.

A number of specific individual and group treatment modalities have been used successfully with the older adult client. These include reality orientation, validation therapy, remotivation therapy, resocialization, reminiscent therapy, and pet therapy.

REFERENCES AND SUGGESTED READINGS

1. Abel, B.J., and Hayslip, B.: Locus of control and retirement preparation, Journal of Gerontology 42(2): 1987.
2. American Nurses' Association: Standards of gerontological practice, Kansas City, 1976, The Association.
3. American Nurses' Association, Division on Gerontological Nursing: Gerontological nursing: the positive difference in health care for older adults, Kansas City, 1980, The Association.
4. Aronson, M.K.: Bennett, R., and Gurland, B.J., editors: The acting-out elderly, New York, 1983, Haworth Press.
5. Beck, A.T.: The development of depression: a cognitive model. In Friedman, R.J., and Katz, M.M., editors: The psychology of depression: contemporary theory and research, Silver Spring, Md., 1974, V.H. Winston & Sons.
6. Bibrine, G.L.G.: Old age: its liabilities and its assests. A psychobiologic discourse. In Lowenstein, R, editor: Psychoanalysis: a general psychology, International Universities Press, New York, 1980.
7. Blazer, D., and Palmore, E.: Religion and aging in a longitudinal panel, Gerontologist **16**:82, 1976.
8. Bornstein, R.: Cognitive and psycho-social development in the older adult. In Schuster, C.S., and Ashburn, S.S., editors: The process of human development, Boston, 1980, Little, Brown & Co.
9. Burnside, I.M.: Nursing and the aged, ed. 2, New York, 1981, McGraw-Hill Book Co.
10. Burnside, I.M.: Working with the elderly: group processes and techniques, ed. 2, Monterey, California, 1987, Wadsworth Health Sciences.
11. Busse, E.W., and Glazer, D.G.: Handbook of geriatric psychiatry, New York, 1980, Van Nostrand Reinhold Co.
12. Butler, R.N., and Lewis, M.I.: Aging and mental health, ed. 3, St. Louis, 1982, The C.V. Mosby Co.
13. Clunn, P.: Psychiatric–mental health nursing, New York, 1985, Medical Examination Publishing Co., Inc.
14. Cole, J.O., and Barrett, J.E., editors: Psychopathology in the aged, New York, 1980, Raven Press.
15. Cummings, E., and Henry, W.E.: Growing old, New York, 1961, Basic Books, Inc., Publishers
16. Davis, A.J., and Kalkman, M.E.: New dimensions in mental health—psychiatric nursing ed. 5, New York, 1980, McGraw-Hill Book Co.
17. Davis, J.H., and others: The human/companion animal bond: how nurses can use this therapeutic resource, Nursing and Health Care, **5**(9): 1984.
18. Davison, G.C., and Neale, J.M.: Abnormal psychology: an experimental clinical approach, New York, 1982, John Wiley & Sons, Inc.
19. Dawson, P. and Reid, D.W. Behavioral dimensions of patients at risk for wandering, the Gerontologist **27**(1), 1987.
20. Donahue, E.: Reality orientation: a review of the literature. In Burnside, I., editor: Working with the elderly, Monterey, Calif., 1984, Wadsworth Publishing Co.
21. Dye, C.A.: Assessment and intervention in geropsychiatric nursing, Orlando, Fl, 1985, Grune & Stratton, Inc.
21a. Duke University Center for the Study of Older Americans: Duke University Medical Center, Durham, N.C., 1975, Duke University Press.
22. Duke University Center for the Study of Aging and Human Development: Duke University Medical Center. Durham, N.C., 1975.
23. Ebersole, R., and Hess, R.: Toward healthy aging: human needs and nursing response, St. Louis, 1985, The C.V. Mosby Co.
24. Eisdorfer, C.: Conceptual models of aging: the challenge of a new frontier, American Psychologist **38**:197, 1983.
25. Eisdorfer, C. and Cohen, D. Mental health care of the aging: a multidisciplinary curriculum for professional training, New York, 1982, Springer Publishing Co., Inc.
26. Erikson, E.H.: Childhood and society, ed. 2, New York, 1964, W.W. Norton & Co., Inc.
27. Feil, N. Validation: The Feil method., Cleveland, Ohio, 1982, Edward Feil Productions.
28. Feinberg, I.: Functional implications of changes in sleep py-

siology with age. In Terry, R.D., and Gershon, S., editors: Neurobiology of aging, New York 1976, Raven Press.

29. Forbes, E.J., and Fitzsimmons, V.M.: The older adult: a process for wellness, St. Louis, 1981, The C.V. Mosby Co.

30. Frolkis, V.V.: Physiological aspects of aging. In von Hahn, H.P., editor: Practical geriatrics, Basel, Switzerland, 1975, S. Karger AG.

31. Grauer, H.: Depression in the aged: theoretical concepts, Journal of the American Geriatrics Society 25:447, 1977.

32. Hagebak, J.E., and Hagebak, B.R.: Serving the mental health needs of the elderly: the case for removing barriers and improving service integration, Community Mental Health Journal 16:4, 1980.

33. Havighurst, R.J.: Successful aging. In Williams, R.H., Tibbits, C., and Donahue, W., editors: Processes of aging, vol. 1, New York, 1963, Atherton Press.

34. Horton, A.M., editor: Mental health interventions for the aged, New York, 1982, Praeger Publishers.

35. Kales, J.D.: Aging and sleep. In Goldman, R., and Rockstein, K., editors: The physiology and pathology of human aging, New York, 1977, Academic Press, Inc.

36. Kaluger, G., and Kaluger, M.F.: Human development: the span of life, ed. 3, St. Louis, 1984, The C.V. Mosby Co.

37. Kermis, M.D.: Mental health in late life, Boston, 1986, Jones & Bartlett Publishers, Inc.

38. Kermis, M.D.: The psychology of human aging: theory, research and practices, Newton, Mass., 1984, Allyn & Bacon, Inc.

39. Lazarus, L.W., editor: Clinical approaches to psychotherapy with the elderly, Washington, D.C., 1985, American Psychiatric Press, Inc.

40. Lewinsohn, P.M., and Teri, L.: Clinical geropsychology: new directions in assessment and treatment, New York, 1983, Pergamon Press.

41. Lewis, C.: Facilitating a better reality: a treatment approach for the confused and disoriented. In Horton, A.M., editor: Mental health interventions for the aged, New York, 1982, Praeger, Publishers.

42. Matsuyama, S.S., and Jarvik, L.F.: Genetics and mental functioning in senescence. In Birren, J.E., and Sloane, R.B., editors: Handbook of mental health and aging, Englewood Cliffs, N.J., 1980, Prentice-Hall, Inc.

43. McCracken, A., Emotional impact of possession loss, Journal of Gerontological Nursing, 42(2):1987.

44. Murray, R., Huelskoetter, M., and O'Driscoll, D.: The nursing process in later maturity, Englewood Cliffs, N.J., 1980, Prentice-Hall, Inc.

45. Neugarten, B.L.: Personality in middle and late life, New York, 1964, Atherton Press.

46. Norton, K.: Geriatric nursing, St. Louis, 1950, The C.V. Mosby Co.

47. Peck, R.: Psychological developments in the second half of life. In Neugarten, B., editor: Middle age and aging, Chicago, 1968, The University of Chicago Press.

48. Pfeiffer, E.: A short portable mental status questionnaire for the assessment of organic brain deficit in elderly patients, American Geriatric Society 23:433, 1975.

49. Pierce, P.M.: Intelligence and learning in the aged, Journal of Gerontological Nursing 6:267, 1980.

50. Rodin, J., and Langer, E.: Aging labels: the decline of control and the fall of self-esteem, Journal of Social Issues, 36(2):12, 1980.

51. Rovner, S.: Alzheimer's disease: games and reality, Washington Post, p. 16, May 7, 1986.

52. Roybal, E.R.: Federal involvement in mental health care for the aged, American Psychologist, 39: 163, 1984.

53. Schuster, C.S., and Ashburn, S.S., editors: The process of human development, Boston, 1980, Little, Brown & Co.

54. Schwab, M., Radar, J., and Doan, J.: Relieving the anxiety and fear in dementia, Journal of Gerontological Nursing, 11:8, 1985.

55. Schwartz, D., Henley, B., and Zeitz, L.: The elderly ambulatory patient: nursing and psychosocial needs, New York, 1964, Macmillan Publishing Co., Inc.

56. Scogin, F., Storandt, M. and Lott, L.: Memory skills training, memory complaints, and depression in elderly adults, Journal of Gerontology 40(5):562, 1985.

57. Smyer, M.A., and Gatz, M., editors: Mental health and aging: programs and evaluations, Beverly Hills, Calif., 1983, Sage Publications.

58. Spence, D.L.: The meaning of engagement, International Journal of Aging and Human Development 6: 193, 1975.

59. Stanley, B., editor: Geriatric psychiatry: clinical, ethical and legal issues, Washington, D.C., 1985, American Psychiatric Press.

60. Stenback, A.: Depression and suicidal behavior in old age. In Birren, J.E., and Sloane, R.B., editors: Handbook of mental health and aging, Englewood Cliffs, N.J., 1980, Prentice-Hall, Inc.

61. Stephens, L.P.: Reality orientation, Washington, D.C., 1969, American Psychiatric Association and Community Psychiatry Service.

62. Storandt, M.: Counseling and therapy with older adults, Boston, 1983, Little, Brown & Co.

63. Thomas, H.: Personality and adjustment to aging. In Birren, J.E., and Sloane, R.B., editors: Handbook of mental health and aging, Englewood Cliffs, N.J., 1980, Prentice-Hall, Inc.

64. Thomasma, D.C.: Freedom, dependency and the care of the very old, Journal of the American Geriatrics Society 32: 906, 1984.

65. Tideiksaar, R.: Home assessment checklist, Ritter department of geriatrics and adult development, The Mount Sinai Medical Center, New York, 1983.

66. Wells, T.: Aging and health promotion, Germantown, Md., 1982, Aspen Systems Corp.

67. Wolanin, M.O., and Phillips, L.R.: Confusion: prevention and care, St. Louis, 1981, The C.V. Mosby Co.

68. Wolpert, E.A.: Manic-depressive illness as an actual neurosis. In Anthony, E.J., and Benedek, T., editors: Depression and human existence, Boston, 1975, Little, Brown & Co.

69. Woodruff, D.S., and Birren, J.E., editors: Aging: scientific perspective and social issues, Monterey, Calif., 1983, Brooks/Cole Publishing Co.

70. Yesavage, J.A.: Imagery pretraining and memory training in the elderly, Gerontology 29:271, 1983.

71. Yesavage, J.A.: Relaxation and memory training in thirty nine elderly patients, American Journal of Psychiatry 141: 770, 1984.

72. Zarit, S., Orr, N., and Zarit, J.: The hidden victims of Alzheimer's disease: families under stress, New York, 1985, New York University Press.

73. Zimmer, J.G., Watson, N., and Treat A.: Behavioral problems among patients in SNF's, American Journal of Public Health 74:1118, 1984.

74. Zung, W.: A self-rating depression scale, Archives of General Psychiatry 12:63, 1965.

75. Zung, W.: Depression in the normal aged, Psychosomatics 8:286, 1967.

Burbank, P.M.: Psychosocial theories of aging: a critical evaluation, Advances in Nursing Science **9**:73, 1986.

This article presents a summary and evaluation of the three major psychosocial theories of aging: activity theory, disengagement theory, and continuity theory. Some important problems are identified with each of the theories.

Burnside, I.M., editor: Working with the elderly: group process and techniques, North Scituate, Mass, 1987, Duxbury Press.

This textbook begins with a brief history of group work with the elderly and gives an overview of a variety of types and levels of the group process. Theoretical concepts are adapted for group work with the elderly, and many practical suggestions are given. The book concludes with a discussion of curriculum changes needed to prepare professionals for group work with the elderly.

Kermis, M.D.: Mental health in late life: the adaptive process, Boston, 1986, Jones and Bartlett Publishers, Inc.

This text presents a comprehensive and practical approach to mental health care of the elderly. The etiology, symptoms, and treatment of pychiatric disorders of the elderly are addressed as well as mental health policy and its social and behavioral consequences.

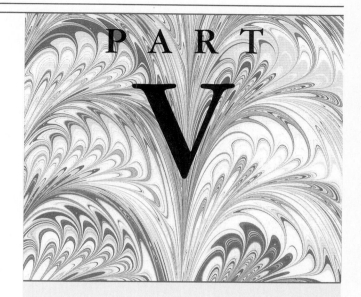

PART V

Issues and Trends

The practice of mental health–psychiatric nursing, while having its foundation in the one-to-one therapeutic relationship, occurs within the context of a social structure in which legal, ethical, and professional issues exert a significant influence on the care provided. Informed deliberation on these issues is a dynamic, ongoing process essential to the accountable, caring practice of mental health–psychiatric nursing.

The nurse is continually faced with situations in which value judgments are made, thus necessitating the clarification, reaffirmation, or reexamination of values. Chapter 45 reviews major ethical orientations and discusses ethical issues in mental health–psychiatric nursing over the life cycle.

The laws that relate to mental health–psychiatric nursing generally reflect the major ethical principles accepted by society. In Chapter 46 an overview of the legal system is presented as a background for understanding the federal and state laws of concern to mental health–psychiatric nursing practice. Malpractice, assault and battery, false imprisonment, confidentiality, commitment, and consent are explicated, and the nurse's role in influencing changes in the law is reviewed. Content on patient classification systems is presented.

As the body of knowledge that provides a basis for the professional practice of mental health–psychiatric nursing is expanded through research, the quality of client care is enhanced. In Chapter 47, the development of research in mental health–psychiatric nursing is reviewed and major research studies are highlighted. The measurement of behavior is discussed and particular measurement, ethical, and legal considerations in mental health–psychiatric nursing research are examined.

Society has a right to expect a reasonable degree of excellence in the provision of mental health–psychiatric nursing care. Chapter 48 reviews the approaches that have been developed for ensuring a standard of care. Pro-tocols, peer review, and auditing are discussed as mechanisms for implementing the ANA's Standards of Nursing Care in Psychiatric–Mental Health Nursing. Professional development, credentialing, and third-party payments are examined within the context of mental health–psychiatric nursing practice.

Finally, psychiatric consultation liaison nursing is discussed in Chapter 49. Types of consultation-liaison are explained, and the qualifications for the role of psychiatric consultation liaison nurses are reviewed. A conceptual model that describes the processes of consultation and liaison and an integration of the two processes is presented. Practice issues related to psychiatric consultation liaison nursing are addressed.

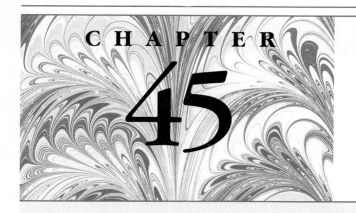

ETHICAL ISSUES

Elsie L. Bandman   Bertram Bandman

After studying this chapter the learner will be able to:

Discuss the origin and development of moral issues in the treatment of the mentally ill.

Examine ethical issues in mental health–psychiatric nursing from a historical perspective.

Analyze each of the ethical views presented in relation to client problems encountered in mental health–psychiatric nursing.

Identify the major ethical issues in mental health–psychiatric nursing of the infant, the child, the adolescent, and the adult.

Analyze the ethical principles relevant to individual, group, and family therapy.

Apply logical principles to the examination of ethically justifiable norms in mental health–psychiatric nursing

The values placed on the care of the mentally disabled are a measure of the ethical sensitivity of a society. The worth placed on the mentally ill as human beings by religious, educational, social, and health care institutions of society determines whether they are to be treated as persons in need of help, punished as objects possessed, or simply rejected and ignored.

Current psychiatric nursing emphasizes the role of the nurse as a therapeutic agent. Such involvement and responsibility inevitably raise moral questions and conflicts. Psychiatric nurses are faced with choices regarding continuation of medication or electroconvulsive therapy when the client refuses. Conversely some clients demand medications or treatment regarded as unnecessary by nurses. Nurses are confronted by involuntarily admitted clients who refuse recommended individual, group, or family therapy. Such situations raise dilemmas regarding the client's right to respect, to receive, and to refuse treatment versus the client's best interests.

The moral issues that affect mental health–psychiatric nursing often overlap and conflict. This makes ethics seem complicated and multifaceted, appearing now like a science, now like an art, sometimes like a religion, and at other times like a game or a business. Whatever ethical orientations the nurse chooses as the "right" ones and no

matter how hard the struggle to avoid imposition of the nurse's values on clients, the selection of therapeutic interventions among alternatives is value laden. The selection of one intervention rather than another supports or opposes a particular moral framework oriented by an emphasis on rights, justice, duty, goals, love, power, or self-interest. Thus the nurse is inescapably a moral agent in relation to clients, her own good, and the good of society.

VALUE CLARIFICATION

Ethics attempts to justify what is good and to distinguish good and evil. To act ethically persons need to identify their notions of right and wrong. Value clarification is a process for making a person's preferences and priorities explicit. It begins with a choice of a value from among alternatives, then moves to a prizing of that value, and finally to a decision to act on that value.[16] In the first stage, one sifts through one's preferences and ranks them; in the second stage, one reflects on which of the chosen values are worthwhile; and in the third stage, one maps a strategy of action to achieve the values one has chosen and prized on reflection (Figure 45-1).

A drawback of value clarification is that the expression of an individual's preferences does not imply that these

✿ *Historical Overview* ✿

DATE	EVENT
500 BC	Greeks and Romans subjected mentally ill persons to cruel and inhumane treatment. A few societies treated mentally ill persons as prophets who possessed insight and vision.
500 AD	For Europeans, treatments such as hydrotherapy, music, gymnastics, rocking, and massage were available mainly for the rich with acute disorders. Chronically ill patients were thought to be incurable.
1200s	Care of the sick was considered a religious duty.
1200s-1500s	There was a vigorous rebirth of interest in human personality, values, and affairs. Books on depression, mother-child relationships, and the mentally retarded were published.
1500s	At the time of the Reformation and the Inquisition mentally ill persons were persecuted as witches and allies of the devil.
1600s	Moral treatment of mentally ill persons included respect, individualized care, privacy, confidentiality, and forms of occupational therapy, drama, and psychotherapy based on commitment to a rational, scientific approach and rejection of supernatural causation.
1700s-1800s	Benjamin Rush introduced moral treatment and scientific investigation of mentally disabled individuals in the United States in 1783. Dorothea Dix reformed the brutal care and neglect of mentally ill persons and created or expanded hospital facilities in America, Canada, and Europe.
1884	The American Psychiatric Association advocated humanization of treatment of mentally ill individuals through specialized care for alcoholic, acute, and chronic patients; family care; and legislative reform.
1908	The National Committeee for Mental Health was organized to make issues of mental health and care of mentally ill persons a matter of national concern.
1980s	The role of the psychiatric nurse as client advocate is developed.
Future	The mental health–psychiatric nurse will become increasingly more involved in ethical issues afffecting clients.

preferences are justifiable or that these preferences should be preferred. No matter how much a person reflects on his choice of values, the prizing of a value raises serious question as to whether the prized value is morally justifiable to other persons and groups. Value clarification, while providing a preliminary and intial stage in value deliberation, calls for further development in the process of justification. This further development involves the study of ethical prinicples.

ETHICAL ORIENTATIONS

Ethics arises whenever good or harm results. Almost anything one does in interpersonal relations may cause good or harm. The most difficult aspect of ethics concerns how one defines good or harm. Good for whom, oneself or others? Is Aunt Mary's divorce good for her, her alcoholic husband, her six children, her community? What is the good? Several major ethical issues will be presented in the following discussion along with several major moral positions. These positions attempt to provide reasoned answers but no definitive conclusions to major ethical issues in mental health–psychiatric nursing.

Paternalism Versus Libertarianism

A major ethical issue that affects the treatment of psychiatric clients concerns paternalism versus libertarianism. Paternalism holds that the state (or, literally, "one's father") knows best and that each individual is subordinate and duty bound to comply with the authority figure, be it a parent, physician, nurse, or state, who is said to know best. The antithesis of paternalism is libertarianism, which holds that the individual is sovereign and may choose without intereference as long as the individual does not harm others. For example, a 24-year-old psychiatric client is seriously disturbed and suspicious but is no danger to others. She can improve if given drug X, which has a side effect of dystonia, but she values her appearance more than improving her mental condition. If the client

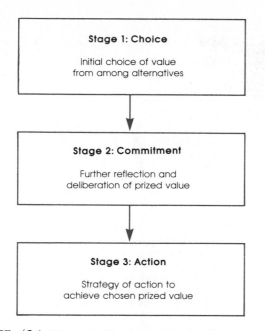

FIGURE 45-1 Value clarification process. (Adapted from Steele, S.M., and Harmon, V.M.: Values clarification in nursing, New York, 1979, Appleton-Century-Crofts.)

prefers not to take drug X, but the nurse knows that this drug will restore the client's rationality through reduction of paranoid thoughts, the nurse is justified in giving the client the drug on rational paternalist grounds. On libertarian grounds, however, the client has the right to decide whether to take drug X.

Egoism Versus Altruism

A second moral issue that affects mental health–psychiatric nursing is that of egoism versus altruism. Egoism holds that one does and also should think and act in one's own interest exclusively.

A difficulty with egoism is that people generally live together and need one another. Therefore they need to control one another's behavior by avoiding harm and giving help. For every person to act without considering others is inappropriate in contexts involving the sensitivities and welfare of others, such as not heeding traffic lights.

Some difficulties with egoism and paternalism lead to another moral-based view, sometimes identified as altruism, or love-based ethics. Most notable in this regard is the ethics of Christianity, which holds that one ought to love God and to love one's neighbor as oneself. Love-based ethics also means teaching disturbed clients the importance of developing love, care, affection, and consideration for the needs of others.

One difficulty with a love-based view of ethics is that "love" is ambiguous. It may refer to child-parent relationships, romantic or sexual relationships, or an ideal, such as "brotherhood" or "sisterhood" between people. Second, love sometimes discriminates unfairly, singling out

some to be loved while rejecting or ignoring others. A third, related difficulty of a love-based ethics is that it is difficult for any person to show or give love to more than a small number of persons on a continuing basis. Despite these difficulties, love is an antidote to selfishness.

Majority Rule Versus Principles

Mill, chief advocate of the greatest happiness, or majority rule (also known as utilitarianism) held that "actions are right in proportion as they tend to promote happiness, wrong as they tend to produce the reverse of happiness."[8]

A major proponent of principled morality, Kant believed that an act is good if everyone ought, in similar circumstances, to do the same act without exception. This is known as the *universalizability principle*. In practice, the universalizability principle means no one may commit suicide, and everyone must keep every promise made.

A close philosophical cousin to Mill's utilitarianism is the *doctrine of double effect*. This doctrine holds that a lesser good or even an evil is morally permissible if done to achieve a greater good, provided that certain conditions are fulfilled. One condition is that the evil side effect is not intended directly. Warning the police that one's psychiatric client intends to commit murder is a lesser wrong if it prevents the greater wrong, murder, from occurring. Critics of double effect, however, say that the wrong done has nothing to do with the good aimed at. In different terms, the end does not justify the means.

Acts of utilitarianism and double effect are sometimes viewed as being unprincipled expediency and a mockery of morality. Defenders of utilitarianism and double effect counter that ethics, being practical, is by definition contaminated by the conditions in the real world. For example, if a drug stabilizes a seriously disturbed person but has side effects, administering the drug is justified on double effect grounds by the good it does for the client.

A strength of Kantian ethics is that it reminds persons of ideals and principles that ought to govern human conduct. Telling the truth, for example, is a vital obligation nurses need to fulfill in treating psychiatric clients. Correspondingly, a strength of utilitarian ethics is that it often minimizes disaster and harm and maximizes benefits to the majority, such as giving a beneficial behavior-controlling drug to a client. A difficulty of utilitarian ethics, however, is that appeal to the majority may overlook minorities, such as mentally afflicted persons, who also need help. The needs of mentally afflicted persons may require tax revenues that the majority opposes. In psychiatric nursing practice scarce personnel, facilities, or resources may be used to rationalize custodial or inadequate treatment of clients who need help.

Omissions Versus Commissions

A fourth moral issue is whether omissions are equivalent to commissions. In psychiatric nursing terms, the question is whether failing to treat a client is morally equivalent to mistreating the client.

TABLE 45-1 Models of ethics

Model	Characteristics	Leading Figures	Advantages	Drawbacks
Paternalism	"Father knows best"; emphasis on single authority figure as sole decision maker; in nursing and health care, "captain of the ship" doctrine	Plato Hobbes Lord Patrick Devlin	One authority figure; unity; line and staff authority; appropriate if one person knows better than others what to do, for example, some physicians and psychiatrists	Denies pluralism, variety, democracy, shared decision making, and distribution of rights, responsibilities, and powers; inappropriate if person in charge is less competent than subordinate co-workers
Libertarianism	Premium placed on individual liberty; unjustified interference is morally impermissible; taxation is used solely to minimize "force and fraud;" other forms of taxation for social and economic causes constitute "forced labor"	J.S. Mill R. Nozick R. Sade M. Friedman	Liberty is a cherished value and is related to individual initiative, achievement of merit (sometimes identified as meritocracy), and individual independence, principle of informed consent respects individual liberty	Undue attention to good aspects of individual liberty and not enough regard paid to social and communal responsibilities such as public education, hospitals, and sanitation
Utilitarianism	Greatest happiness for greatest number, emphasis on consequences of acts aimed at maximizing pleasure and minimizing pain; provides basis for calculation of cost/benefit/risk ratio	J.S. Mill J. Bentham	Pleasure and desire for happiness come easily to people; one can appeal to people to seek happiness; concerned with acts and consequences, leading to prudence and care to achieve one's desired results (for example, avoidance of sexually transmitted diseases); also based on cost/benefit/risk ratio; considers majority interests	Ignores minorities; fails to give attention to nonnegotiable values such as justice, truth telling, doing good for its own sake, and avoiding evil for the same reason, if necessary (for example, not torturing or killing just because these may pay off)

The philosophical justification for rating omissions with commissions comes from existentialism, which holds that one exists by taking responsibillity for all decisions in all aspects of one's life in which one has a conscious, reflective process at work. For example, a person who recognizes the plight of a psychiatric client is responsible for acting as if the client's situation depends on that person's ability to correct the client's plight. To fail to correct an evil is to show "bad faith" and is as bad as doing an evil. Watching another person abused without intervening is as bad as being the abuser. To attempt to evade decisions is to make decisions.

A strength of existentialism is its emphasis on honest and responsible human relationships. A difficulty of existentialism is the practical impossibility of being responsible for all the world's difficulties

Absolute Rights Versus Prima Facie Rights

A fifth moral issue concerns the view that rights are absolute versus the view that rights can be overridden, since they are rights on the surface or face, that is, *prima facie rights*.

There are three conditions that attend any right. To have a right is to be free to exercise it or not as one chooses. Second, to have rights implies that other relevant persons have corresponding duties to comply with the terms and provisions of one's rights. Third, to have rights means that one's rights are consistent with rationally defensible principles of justice. Rights thus imply freedom, duties or responsibilties, and justice. In the absolute view of rights the contention is that individual rights to property or to refuse treatment can never be overridden by any other moral considerations. In contrast, treating rights

TABLE 45-1 Models of ethics—cont'd

Model	Characteristics	Leading Figures	Advantages	Drawbacks
Kantian ethics	Emphasis on moral character, good will, intentions, obligations, not inclination, interests, or desires; emphasis on principled action no matter what the personal consequences; acts are moral only if universal, result of free will, rational, impartial, and exceptionless	I. Kant J. Rawls	Values such as promising, helping the needy, truth telling, and being just are uncompromising (for example, slavery is absolutely wrong and is never made right by consequences); torture, murder, lying, and injustice are always wrong	Fails to consider aspirations, interests, drives, motivations, consequences, and contexts that call for adaptation of principles; inflexible
Existentialism	Conscious human beings have a free will and are therefore responsible for their acts; Human acts include commissions and omissions (This issue arises if one considers whether not doing is morally equivalent to doing; for example, is failure to treat tantamount to murder?); according to theory, one is as responsible for not acting as for acting; according to Descartes, a forerunner of existentialism, one is responsible for what one is conscious about; to know, for example, that a client needs help and to do nothing is as serious as harming that client (that is, passive euthanasia = active euthanasia)	S. Kierkegaard J.P. Sartre	Increases responsibility for omissions, negligence, unconcern (for example, Kitty Genovese murdered in a New York apartment with 37 neighbors looking on and doing nothing; the 37 onlookers are regarded as being as evil as the murderer)	To identify omissions with commissions places undue burden of responsiblity on people's shoulders; we cannot, as a practical matter, be held responsible for all the starvation and suffering in the world
Absolute rights versus prima facie rights	Absolute rights stress exceptionless rights and their application to all contexts; prima facie rights refer to rights that are assumed until further notice, and these may be overridden if more morally compelling interests arise	J. Feinberg J. Rawls R. Dworkin R.B. Brandt	Absolute rights: the people of a society know that some values in the form of rights have priority over all other values; prima facie rights: flexible, practical	Absolute rights too stringent; prima facie rights treated as interests that may be overridden by more powerful interests; rights are not steadfast or assured values

as prima facie means that rights may be overridden by stronger conflicting rights or by other values. For example, a psychiatric client's right to the freedom of the nursing unit may be overridden by seclusion or restraints if the client physically abuses others.

A strength of the prima facie view is that an individual's absolute right may be overridden in favor of the rights of others or the person's own best interests. In the prima facie view the rights of a larger number of persons morally outweigh the rights of a small number when the rights of the two groups conflict. Another strength of the prima facie view is its practical advantage in coping with conflicts of rights and in suggesting a scale of priorities among rights, to avoid arbitrariness, for example. A difficulty, however, is that prima facie rights may be treated as weaker than rights need to be; rights are then too easily

overturned by every pressure that comes along. Rights without built-in constraints against their erosion are not worth the respect accorded them as rights. On the other hand, rights written in stone, without possibility of change, are too brittle to withstand the ardors of practical moral life. The ideal is to have rights that are well entrenched, sturdy, and well respected, but open to reasoned modifications. At any rate the differences between these two views of rights are a matter of degree. Both views hold that rights are important to moral discourse.

Human rights are generally regarded as the union of self-determination and subsistence rights, or the right to be helped when one is in need. Compromises and arguments frequently concern the limits and extent of such rights. One issue is that some subsistence rights impose intolerable burdens on those expected to provide for such rights. For example, giving all psychiatric clients optimal psychiatric care, including prolonged psychoanalysis, is regarded by opponents of subsistence rights as too expensive. In relation to other urgent social goals, such as education or care of elderly persons, this means of reducing mental illness consumes an inordinate amount of available resources.

A summary of the models of ethics, their characteristics, leading figures, advantages, and drawbacks is presented in Table 45-1.

A Trilogy of Clients' Moral Rights

Despite the controversies over the meaning, limits, and significance of rights, three important moral rights of psychiatric clients emerge: (1) the right to respect, (2) the right to receive treatment, and (3) the right to refuse treatment. Each of these rights has an impact on nurse-client relations and issues of care.

The right to respect includes the right to dignity and regard for a psychiatric client as a potentially rational person and as an "end," not as a means or instrument of someone else's will. The right to respect also implies the right to privacy, confidentiality, and informed consent.

The right to receive treatment includes the client's right to know the diagnosis, the treatment that is proposed, the anticipated procedures and processes, and the expected results.

The third right in this trilogy of health care rights is the client's right to terminate or refuse a proposed treatment at any time. If after a true and adequate explanation, including a statement of consequences, the client believes that the proposed treatment is either too risky or burdensome or painful to bear or if the competent client simply wishes to discontinue treatment, he has the right to do so.

Macklin[9] cites three reasons clients give for refusing treatment: (1) the client perceives inhumane conditions; (2) drugs or treatments (for example, electroconvulsive therapy) have undesirable side effects; and (3) the client's consenting organ, the mind, is affected. A ground for overriding a psychiatric client's right to refuse treatment is that such a client's rational powers and autonomy would be increased as a result of treatment. In Macklin's view, only for the third reason may a client's right to refuse be overridden.

There are several views on whether to override a mental client's right to refuse treatment. Table 45-2 summarizes the views that are held by a libertarian, a paternalist, a utililtarian, and a rational paternalist.

Competence and the Rights of Psychiatric Clients

The judgment that a person is competent gives reason to trust that the person will avoid doing harm. This judgment is a basis for awarding or denying a person's right to decide. The concept of competence is ambiguous. The scenes presented in Table 45-3 help clarify the concept.[4]

These scenes and moral-philosophical positions show that each position has strengths and weaknesses and that no position seems appropriate for all cases. Libertarian val-

TABLE 45-2 Ethical positions toward a psychiatric client's right to refuse treatment

Position	Attitude
Libertarian	The client may refuse any treatment if the client does not harm others.
Paternalist	The mental health–psychiatric nurse (acting on behalf of the state) may override a client's rights for the good of the client.
Utilitarian	The mental health–psychiatric nurse (acting on behalf of the state) may override the client's rights if doing so serves the greatest happiness of the greatest number.
Rational paternalist	The client's right may be overridden if the client would later retrospectively regard such an action as being in his rational interest, in contributing to the client's autonomy as a person.

ues are what psychiatric clients' rights are largely about. But to restore their rationality, paternalism or rational paternalism may be appropriate. In other cases, utilitarian values of caring for the greatest good of the greatest number are called for.

ETHICAL ISSUES THROUGHOUT THE LIFE CYCLE
Infancy and Childhood

The mental health–psychiatric nurse who counsels prospective parents needs to consider several moral issues. Couples with a family history of mental illness fear the genetic transmission of schizophrenia or major affective disorders. The nurse needs to inform these couples that the nature versus nurture controversy is still unresolved. Currently only a few genetic defects out of a vast number of possibilities can be identified. The nurse counselor can clearly recommend genetic screening as useful in identifying such diseases as Tay-Sachs and hemophilia. The nurse can also recommend amniocentesis during pregnancy as a test for Down's syndrome with the choice of aborting the pregnancy. However, only as the scientific evidence regarding questions of genetic vulnerability to mental illness develops can the nurse provide definitive answers to questions of the inheritance of mental illness. Until then, nurses need to clearly identify their moral positions regarding sterilization, contraceptives, or abortion for a mentally disabled person. The mentally ill or defective person is greatly in need of information, education, counseling, and concrete help in carrying out procedures for avoiding an unwanted pregnancy. If pregnant, the client is in need of prenatal care, delivery support, and help for planning the disposition of herself in relation to the baby. Again, the nurse uses the nursing process and the moral principles of striving to do good and to do no harm in helping these vulnerable individuals.

Other examples of ethical problems threatening the

TABLE 45-3 Five scenes showing how "competence" gives a reason for overriding a psychiatric client's right to receive or refuse treatment

Scene	Conflict	Conclusion
Dr. Doe: "I cannot prescribe drug X for you because it will do you physical harm." Mr. Roe: "But you are mistaken. It will not cause me physical harm."	Dr. Doe and Mr. Roe disagree factually about drug X.	Mr. Roe is factually incompetent (the layperson is presumed wrong when disagreeing with a physician).
Dr. Doe: "I cannot prescribe drug X to you because it will cause you physical harm." Mr. Roe: "That's just what I want. I want to harm myself."	Dr. Doe and Mr. Roe disagree whether drug X, which harms Mr. Roe, is good.	Mr. Roe is incompetent (it is presumed that Mr. Roe's values in wanting to harm himself are irrational).
Dr. Doe: "I cannot prescribe drug X to you because it is likely to do you physical harm." Mr. Roe: "I don't care if it causes me physical harm. I'll get a lot of pleasure first, so much pleasure, in fact, that it is well worth running the risk of physical harm. If I must pay a price for my pleasure, I am willing to do so."[4]	Dr. Doe and Mr. Roe disagree that drug X, which harms Mr. Roe, causes enough pleasure to justify drug X despite its harm.	Mr. Roe is competent (moral stalemate between Dr. Doe and Mr. Roe).
Dr. Doe: "You need a blood transfusion to stay alive." Mr. Roe: "A blood transfusion is against my religious principles as a Jehovah's Witness. I'd rather die first."	Dr. Doe and Mr. Roe disagree that a blood transfusion will serve Mr. Roe's ultimate good.	Mr. Roe is competent (moral, religious conflict of values between Dr. Doe and Mr. Roe).
Dr. Doe: "I cannot release you because of your continuing insistence that you are the historical Napoleon and the savior of France." Mr. Roe: "I refuse to stay in your institution precisely because I am the historical Napoleon, and I am urgently needed in the immediate liberation of France."	Dr. Doe and Mr. Roe disagree on Mr. Roe's identity, Mr. Roe believing himself to be the historical Napoleon.	Mr. Roe is incompetent (no stalemate since there is a factual basis for going against Mr. Roe's claim).

mental health of the family are the birth of a baby with Down's syndrome or serious deformities. The use of high-level technology can save the lives of many infants, and the decision to treat or not to treat and let nature take its course is not always considered to be an option for the parents. Parents need time to evaluate the facts and the advice in order to arrive at their own decision. The decision is not the surgeon's or the pediatrician's. It is an ethical decision with which the couple lives all of their lives; therefore, they need to give serious consideration to the rights of the infant and to their own capacities and resources.

Moral questions arise about the extent to which a family is obligated to subordinate its energies, goals, and resources to the care and well-being of the abnormal, dysfunctional child. Value choices are between the sanctity of life and the rights of the parents and siblings to a full life without the lifelong expense and anguish of the handicapped child. In all cases any contemplated treatment needs to be carefully explained in nontechnical language so that the parents understand exactly what the prognosis, risks, and alternatives are, especially when there will be lifelong impairment and dependence. The nurse with awareness of the ethical orientations previously discussed can assist the parents with their choice by clearly articulating the moral presuppositions of available choices.

Adolescence

Increasingly, adolescents seek health care such as counseling, contraceptives, or abortion on a confidential basis without parental knowledge. The age of 18 is now recognized as the age of majority in all states, but adolescents who are minors may be provided health care without parental consent in the following situations: in emergencies when necessary to protect life; for contraceptive services; for abortion services (in litigation in some states); for parental abuse or neglect; for treatment of venereal disease; for detection of pregnancy; when married, divorced, or self-supporting and living away from parents; and when age 16 or older and requesting admission to a psychiatric hospital for treatment.[18] Persons who fall into these categories have not only the right to respect and the right to receive treatment, but also the right to refuse treatment. This means that adolescents' rights to self-determination give them authority that requires the nurse to give them a full explanation of the risks and benefits of the proposed treatment, the diagnosis, prognosis, and the alternatives as the basis for fully informed consent. However, there are limits to the rights of even emancipated adolescents, including the right to be sterilized, to donate an organ, and to receive electroconvulsive therapy. Parental consent, a court order, or both are required in these procedures. When parents disagree over health services provided or refuse lifesaving treatment for their dependent adolescent, a court order is usually sought by the health care facility.

The adolescent's right to psychiatric treatment has not received the same degree of support from the courts, from family, and from public opinion as has the adolescent's right to medical care for physical illness. Parents may deny an adolescent's right to psychiatric treatment on grounds of shame, guilt, or threat to their status as "good parents." Where public community mental health facilities are available, the adolescent's right to treatment and to moral self-determination is respected. In recent years no psychiatrist, physician, or surgeon has been found liable by the courts for the proper treatment of minors of 15 and older without parental consent.[7] Most states now permit minors to consent to medical treatment without specifying psychotherapy. Seemingly, this immunity from parental interference includes standard forms of psychotherapy given by recognized professionals. However, the right of the adolescent to receive nontraditional or bizarre forms of treatment, such as those emphasizing sexual expression, presents moral dilemmas to even those parents most supportive of adolescent's rights to self-determination. The parents' right to care for their children in ways they consider beneficial may in this case conflict with the adolescent's right to receive treatment. This dilemma is sometimes resolved by parental appeal to the adolescent on grounds of love-based or goal-based ethics, since resorting to power-based ethics usually results in the termination of the relationship between parent and child. The ultimate parental appeal is to their overriding concern for the adolescent's best interests. A lawsuit by the parents charging that the nontraditional treatment contributes to the delinquency of a minor may be the last resort, which may irreparably damage the parent-child relationship.

The adolescent's right to refuse treatment is fraught with complications by the adolescent's struggle toward individual standards, values, ethics, and beliefs. If these are radically different from those of the parents, the parents may require psychiatric care for what they consider abnormal behavior. The adolescent's right to refuse psychiatric treatment on grounds of parental objection to long hair, sexual activity, use of marijuana, and failure to attend church, for example, is morally justifiable on grounds of the adolescent's right to his own standards, values, ethics, and beliefs. The parents can impose limits such as curfews, allowances, and use of the family car to curb behavior, but forcing an adolescent to participate in treatment is difficult and antitherapeutic. Such force violates the individual's right to self-determination.

It is diffiicult to support the adolescent's unqualified right to refuse treatment when confronted with an adolescent's serious suicidal or homicidal tendencies. Yet, as the commitment of "normally" rebellious minor adolescents to mental hospitals by parents demonstrates, parents do not always have the best interests of the child at heart. The adolescent so treated has the right to refuse treatment and to receive available help and protection in exercising due process rights. The same rigorous standards for commitment that apply to adults—danger to self and others—apply to adolescents. There is, however, a difference in degree between an adolescent's rights and an adult's rights. An adolescent's autonomy rights cannot be as extensive as those of an adult because of the general dependence, inexperience, underdeveloped capacities, and needs of an adolescent.

Genuine dilemmas exist, in instances where adolescents leave home and family to join religious groups that control all aspects of the young person's life. In such groups, the adolescent is severely conditioned and programmed into a state of total allegiance and obedience to the community and is regarded as part of the communal property. Desperate parents have abducted adolescents from such groups and placed them in psychiatric care involuntarily. Some adolescents in this situation have refused psychiatric intervention and returned to the religious community. Others were relieved at the actions of their parents in their best interests and participated in therapy. The moral dilemma is whether the adolescent is able to make a rational decision to refuse treatment or is responding in terms of the behavior control strategies used by the religious group.

In most cases involving adolescents, the dilemma is between the adolescent's right of self-determination and parental duty to respect the young life by preserving it in whatever ways are possible and necessary. Clearly the facts and risks of the situation need to be carefully evaluated by parents, mental health–psychiatric nurses, and others involved in providing care as a basis for a decision. In this way a decision is the result of careful assessment and deliberation justified on the moral principles deemed most appropriate to save the young life. Appeal to love-based, duty-based, or goal-based ethical orientations may also be included in the basis for decision by parents, nurses, and other health professionals who respond to the adolescent's rights to respect, to receive treatment, and to refuse treatment.

Adulthood

For various reasons, not all adults are able to achieve developmental tasks of independence and ego-enhancing interdependence in the process of living. Persons with psychiatric problems sometimes behave and dress in ways that are unconventional, odd, distasteful, disgusting, and unacceptable to the public. A fundamental ethical issue for the community becomes the extent to which it tolerates deviant behavior. One example is whether harmless old "bag ladies" carrying their belongings in shopping bags, dressed in layers of long-worn, shabby clothing, and sometimes smelling of urine should be allowed to roam the subways and train stations of cities at will. One view is that such persons are to be regarded as mentally ill and placed in public institutions, or as vagrants and placed in prison, or as mandatory residents and placed in community facilities. Vagrants, beggars, alcoholics, and delusional and hallucinating persons in the streets are examples of individuals whose behavior poses a problem mainly to themselves. This issue concerns individual liberties versus the social offense given to the general public. One libertarian argument is that, since the offensive behavior falls short of actually harming anyone else, interference is unjustified. The counterargument by legal paternalists is that these persons set a negative example by demeaning themselves and disrespecting others. To allow them to continue is to sanction their behavior and set a bad example to the community.

Ethical dilemmas arise concerning the right to end one's life because of the conflict between the value that all life is sacred and the value of self-determination and freedom. The moral principle of autonomy is pitted against the rights of individuals in families and in society to preserve life. One view holds that all suicidal clients be locked up "for their own good" until their ideas change in favor of living. This may take years or may never occur. One concern is with the hospitalized client who, despite therapy and drugs, makes repeated attempts to end his life. The paternalistic person, who believes that all life is sacred, cares for the mentally ill and prevents all suicide on the assumption that these persons are unable to care and to think for themselves. The counterargument is that the chronically ill, institutionalized client discharged into an indifferent community suffers isolation, loneliness, and alienation. These conditions may be enough to mobilize the person's wish to end life. In this view an individual has a fundamental right to control his life. The dilemma, nevertheless, persists concerning the individual's right to end life when the impaired organ is the organ of judgment. This argument for autonomy is supported in the case of clients who decide to end their lives at lucid intervals. The dilemma of valuing the freedom of an individual versus interference in peoples' lives by protecting them against their own wishes is virtually unsolvable. Critics of paternalism view the increasing use of behavior control techniques of all kinds as threatening freedom of choice over one's own body.

The principle of fully informed consent, contained in the *Code for Nurses* and other codes, is a necessary condition for all forms of therapy. It is especially signifcant in the individual relationship of nurse to client if the seeds of trust are to be planted and grow into a therapeutic alliance, in which nurse and client work together toward agreed-upon therapeutic goals. An ethically justifiable relationship is based on clearly stated presumptions of the client's autonomy to enter into treatment, collaborate in the direction of the treatment, seek consultation freely, and terminate at will, after analysis of the reasons for ending therapy. Clients have these rights and the expectation that they will be supported by the nurse. The client with clearly expressed problems has the right to expect that therapy will be directed toward modification of these problems, rather than toward satisfaction of the nurse's needs. It is expected that in a therapeutic relationship the nurse will respect the client in every way possible, including the client's nondestructive values, even if different from social norms. Respect for clients means that they are respected as ends and not as means to the nurse's ego aggrandizement or sexual satisfaction. Respect for persons includes the client's right to privacy and confidentiality.

No client will be discussed, compared, or mentioned in any way to another client, family member, health professional, or agency without the client's knowledge and consent.

All persons seeking psychiatric help need to be asked basic questions of value, such as whether the client, family, or group want to change behavior; to what extent; and for what purpose. In some therapeutic relationships the client's values are in harmony with those of the nurse and with societal norms of behavior. But the nurse's values may be opposed to those of clients in other cases.

The central ethical issue in family therapy may be the need to establish a balance between the needs and rights of an individual in relation to the rights of other individuals in the family and society. Rights of the individual are sometimes in conflict with the rights of other family members. For example, if a father continues incestuous sexual relations while in family therapy, the nurse is faced with deciding whether to refuse to continue therapy on the grounds of the father's use of the child as a means to satisfy his sexual drives, and reporting the practice to the police or continuing therapy toward ending incest. The nurse may use this moral issue as the focus of family therapy with the objective of helping the family to clarify the rights and duties of parents and children in relation to each other. Another issue is whether the nurse has the right or duty to remain morally neutral while the family works through its moral principles and choices, as in the case of drug-abusing parents adversely influencing their child.

Another ethical issue concerns the role of the nurse in family therapy in relation to the family's values. The nurse may perceive her role as that of a referee who takes a neutral ethical stance, helping the family develop its own ethical norms, or, in contrast, she may communicate her ethical views to the family in problematic situations. Moral problems arise concerning whether it is possible for the nurse to deny her own values in evaluating behavior.

Whatever ethical orientation nurses choose as most expressive of their values and no matter how hard nurses try not to impose their values on families, the very process of selecting interventions is value laden. Selected interventions are for or against a particular framework of right-based, justice-based, duty-based, goal-based, or love-based ethics. For example, if a nurse asks family members deadlocked in a conflict of rights what they think about a situation in terms of greatest individual need and the least advantaged person in the family, the nurse is using a justice-based framework. If, on the other hand, the nurse asks the same family what would make the most people happy in this situaton, the nurse is intervening from a goal-based orientation. If, in contrast, the nurse asks what would be right for everyone with no exception, the nurse is intervening on the basis of a duty-based orientation.

The nurse cannot remain neutral when values oppose a common morality as in cases of violence or incest. Yet nurses may not express their ethical orientations in all situations. It may be unnecessary when the family has well-formulated moral principles in accordance with a common morality for guiding conduct. In most cases, however, nurses can help families explore their moral choices on the basis of mutual respect and enhancement of personhood. Such principles as autonomy, beneficence, and justice are continually refined through dialogue and applied to strengthening human relationships that are socially wholesome and individually fulfilling.

ETHICAL APPROACHES TO RESOLUTION OF VALUE CONFLICTS

Ethical principles apply to nursing practice and health care throughout the life span. A wide range of choices is available in most situations of health and illness. Moreover, one cannot decide in matters of health and illness, since to do nothing is in fact to decide in favor of the status quo, or the situation as it is. The availability of options has important implications for the client since every choice carries different degrees of intrusiveness. Generally clients expect to maintain control and to make decisions based on their values and goals, an application of the principle of self-determination. On the other hand, the nurse is knowledgeable and possesses expertise by virtue of her education and experience. Serving the client's well-being by facilitating the improvement of health is the justification for the existence of nursing and for all other health care disciplines. The justification of nursing is to look after the well-being of clients by applying the principles of beneficence (to do good, justice as fairness, and equal consideration) and nonmaleficence (to prevent harm). The union of these principles with autonomy is essential to shared decision making. Shared decision making provides consideration of the family's goals, values, and well-being. The principle of equity (treating like cases alike) is also considered in shared decision making. Application of this principle suggests that nursing resources are fairly distributed and that nurses treat all clients with equal respect as individuals.

Conflict between principles is at times unavoidable. In psychiatric nursing practice, an acutely psychotic, violent, and assaultive client needs to be restrained to prevent harm to self or others. This is an example of the use of the principle of well-being, namely, to do good and prevent harm, to override the principle of the client's self-determination. Clearly, the safety of the client and others overrides the client's need to physically express his rage and frustration against self or others. The principle of equity (treating like cases alike) is applied to the client by the use of restraints and explanations exactly as it would be applied to similarly violent and assaultive clients.

The goal of shared decision making in psychiatric care facilitates clients' control and responsibility for decisions relating to their lives and health. Suggested steps in ethical decision making are to (1) define the problem through nursing assessment; (2) clarify the client's problem in relation to life-style, values, goals, resources, and relationships; (3) assess the client's level of competence, communication, and understanding as the basis of consent or refusal; (4) separate ethical issues from administrative, medical, or legal considerations; (5) identify major ethical issues in relation to desires and competing or conflicting options; (6) justify the moral choice through use of ethical principles; (7) evaluate the moral choice and justifica-

tion in relation to professional codes, the law, and the institutional mission; (8) implement the moral decision based on fully informed, freely given rational choice; and (9) appeal an irrational or coerced decision not supportive of the client's well-being through legitimate channels of authority.

The ethical principles and guidelines discussed are illustrated in the following example.

Case Example

Betty, a beautiful 19-year-old college student with schizophrenia, is urged to take medication X, known to benefit clients with similar symptoms by making their behavior less irrational. Possible side effects include uncontrollable muscular and facial movements that do not always respond to treatment. Betty refuses to take X.

The question in the preceding case is whether paternalism, libertarianism, or utilitarianism applies. The nurse can choose from several moral orientations. For example, a nurse, Ms. N., may be a libertarian. Ms. N. supports Betty's right to refuse. Another health team member with a utilitarian orientation may challenge Ms. N. in a moral dialogue by asking, "Have you considered what effects her refusal will have on her as well as on other people? Betty may never function in a responsible position without drug X." Or a paternalist-oriented nurse may ask Ms. N., "Are you thinking of Betty's long-term good? Betty's chances of a hospital discharge and return to college will be helped by taking drug X and hindered by not taking it."

By referring to the suggested steps in decision making, Betty's problem can be summarized as follows:

1. The problem is Betty's refusal to take drug X because of its side effects.
2. Possible side effects affecting her appearance can interfere with her single life-style, intimate relationships, and hopes for a successful career and marriage.
3. The client is competent enough to understand the options.
4. Administrative and legal considerations emphasize her well-being.
5. The major ethical issues are the client's moral right to refuse treatment versus the paternalistic position of forcing drug administration in support of her best interests.
6. The client's right to free choice can be justified by the principle of liberty rights to her own body. The paternalistic position of requiring the drug can be supported by principles of beneficence (do good), nonmaleficence (do no harm), equal consideration, and utility (the greatest good for the greatest number).
7. Nursing and medical professional codes of ethics support principles of doing good and avoiding harm. The client may be seriously harmed by failure to take the drug for control of her symptoms.
8. The nurse as client advocate implements the decision by educating the client about the significant aspects of this drug in relation to her life-style, her career and marriage goals, and the control of side

effects by the selective use of additional drugs and drug moratoriums. As a result of the nurses's relationship and educational activities, Betty agrees to take the drug for control of her symptoms with monitoring and systematic follow-up.

There are two difficulties with ethical decision-making views. The first is that ethical values are part of the very process of identifying and selecting data and considering who should decide. A second difficulty of ethical decision making is that after the nurse considers the alternatives, she is still left having to make a justifiable moral decision as to what is the best thing to do. There is no verification that shows that libertarianism, paternalism, utilitarianism, or any other position has the conclusively justifiably right answer.

Each moral or ethical view sets out its catalog of virtues or priorities. The mental health–psychiatric nurse, knowing alternative value-based views not as closed systems but as overlapping, dynamic value priorities in flux, has to decide in particular cases. The decisions are all value laden, and each part of the process is also value laden. Some moral decisions seem right, others wrong. Approximately a dozen viable ethical views merit consideration without providing the absolutely right answer for all time. Yet some ethical principles provide a relatively stable residue of hard-core moral strength, shared by neighboring moral views. Some behaviors and conditions are justifiably regarded as bad, such as slavery, segregation, abuse, torture, rape, and murder; by implication, their opposites, such as freedom, desegregation, kindness, and consideration, are regarded as good.

However, the nurse can apply logical principles of evaluation to supplement ethical decision making in mental health–psychiatric nursing. She observes logical *do's* and *dont's*, such as not having more in the conclusion than there is in the premises or not concluding with more than the evidence warrants. To know what is unwarranted may sometimes be just as valuable as knowing what is warranted.

Ethical alternatives need to be considered in a nondogmatic way. A useful rule of thumb is to begin with the libertarian presumption of respect for the personhood of the client and seriously consider the client's word, but to override the client if compelling reasons justify doing so. Knowing the strengths of paternalism and utilitarianism helps when the libertarian view is too frail to help the psychiatric client. For example, restoring a depressed suicidal client to rationality and autonomy may justify coercing the client to take medications he refuses.

One moral philosophical move is to regard the ethical principles that apparently collide and categorize some of these as goals or "ends" principles and others as instrumental, intermediary, or "means" principles. One then works toward harmonizing ethical ends and means. For example, self-determination or autonomy may be regarded as an aim of mental health–psychiatric nursing. The means for achieving a client's autonomy or liberty may then be seen to consist of temporarily controlling a client's behavior. But such control is only a means toward achieving the goal of the client's self-determination.

Another moral philosophical move is to convert apparently conflicting ends statements into convergent, harmonious ends and means as an identifiable goal, such as a client's autonomy (a Platonic-Kantian value), and then note its compatibility with other end state values, such as self-realization and happiness (Aristotelian and utilitarian ethical values). An example is having to decide between two equally deserving persons when demands outrun resources. One case is to decide who receives very expensive medical care between two beloved children, both of whom need care. One needs long-term psychiatric care; the other has leukemia that sometimes responds to treatment. One can toss a coin or throw one's hands up in the air. There is no ethical solution, only tragedy.

At times, deciding between two equally deserving persons is also the moral dilemma of the mental health–psychiatric nurse. To fail to recognize tragedy and stalemates is to ignore the predicaments of the human estate, which is that everything in this world is not so tidy and clear as some persons would like to have it. However, one can still work to improve the human relations that can be improved. This is what the ethics of mental health–psychiatric nursing is largely about.

BRIEF REVIEW

A brief historical review of psychiatric clients from Greek antiquity to the present shows a largely contemptuous attitude on the part of most people toward mentally disturbed and retarded persons. Neglect and cruelty characterize the early history of the treatment of the mentally ill. Character attributions based on ignorance chronicle the long, arduous history of gradual reform from superstition to early psychiatry. Trained intelligence based on verifiable assessments of human nature, along with extended sensitivity, has refined older, less efficient forms of treatment.

Ethical issues in the treatment of mental health–psychiatric clients include paternalism versus libertarianism, egoism versus altruism, majority rule or goal-based ethics versus fixed principles, omissions versus commissions, absolute versus prima facie rights, and negative versus positive rights. These moral "-isms" also present ways of looking at issues. No final answers can be expected regarding an absolute standard of right and wrong that applies to mental health–psychiatric nursing. However, some fairly well-entrenched values and principles, such as respect for rights and the golden rule morality implied by utilitarianism, have good reasons behind them.

A trilogy of client rights—the right to respect, the right to treatment, and the right to refuse treatment—has a major role in moral values. But dilemmas easily arise in dealing with the rights of mentally disturbed persons. A case in point is the psychiatric client's right to refuse the kind of treatment that the client needs to become more rational. Further dilemmas surrounding the right to respect, to receive treatment, and to refuse treatment arise in individual, group, and family therapy. The emphasis is on a rights-based view, one that shows respect for clients as ends rather than as means.

REFERENCES AND SUGGESTED READINGS

1. Annas, F.L., Glants, L.H., and Katz, B.F.: The rights of doctors, nurses, and allied health professionals, New York, 1981, Avon Books.
2. Bloch, D.A.: The family of the psychiatric patient. In Arieti, S., editor: American handbook of psychiatry, vol. 1, ed. 2, New York, 1974, Basic Books, Inc., Publishers.
3. Davidhizar, R.: Beliefs and values of the client with chronic mental illness regarding treatment, Issues in Mental Health Nursing 6(3-4)261, 1984.
4. Feinberg, J.: Social philosophy, Englewood Cliffs, N.J., 1973, Prentice-Hall, Inc.
5. Flanagan, L.: Psychiatry: a question of ethics, Nursing Times, 82(35):39, 1986.
6. Hobbes, T.: The leviathan, Oxford, England, 1861, Blackwell Press.
7. Holder, A.R.: Legal issues in pediatrics and adolescent medicine, New York, 1977, John Wiley & Sons, Inc.
8. Kant, I.: Fundamental principles of the metaphysics of morals, Indianapolis, 1948, Bobbs-Merrill. (Originally published in 1785).
9. Macklin, R.: Man, mind, and morality: the ethics of behavior control, Englewood Cliffs, N.J., 1982, Prentice-Hall, Inc.
10. Mill, J.S.: Utilitarianism, liberty and representative government, London, 1910, J.M. Dent & Sons, Ltd. (Originally published in 1859).
11. Mill, J.S.: Utilitarianism, Indianapolis, 1957, Bobbs-Merrill. (Originally published in 1861).
12. Peplau, H.E.: Some reflections on earlier days in psychiatric nursing, Journal of Psychosocial Nursing and Mental Health Services 20(8):17, 1982.
13. Plato: The republic, Indianapolis, 1974, Hackett Publishing Co., Inc. (Translated by G.M.A. Grube).
14. Sandelowski, M.: The politics of parenthood. . . competing maternal-fetal, parent-child, and individual-family claims, Maternal Child Nursing, 11(4)235, 1986.
15. Sharfstein, S.S., and Beigel, A., editors: The new economics and psychiatric care, Washington, D.C., 1985, American Psychiatric Press.
16. Steele, S.M., and Harmon, V.M.: Values clarification in nursing, New York, 1979, Appleton-Century-Crofts.
17. Trotter, C.M.F.: I never promised you a rose garden but I must remember to tell you about the thorns. . . the ethics involved in psychotherapy, Journal of Psychosocial Nursing and Mental Health Services 23(4)6, 1985.
18. Wieczorek, R.R., and Natapoff, J.N.: A conceptual approach to the nursing of children, Philadelphia, 1981, J.B. Lippincott Co.

ANNOTATED BIBLIOGRAPHY

Bandman, E.L., and Bandman, B.: Nursing ethics in the life span, Norwalk, Conn., 1985, Appleton-Century-Crofts.

This book addresses the moral issues and problems of everyday nursing practice throughout the life span of clients. Models of nurse-patient-physician relationships are described as well as approaches to making ethically justifiable decisions based on nursing strategies, guidelines, and canons of critical reasoning.

Dyer, A.: Ethics and Psychiatry, Washington, D.C., 1987, American Psychiatric Press.

This book examines the current issues affecting health professionals in psychiatric care. Issues addressed include confidentiality, informed consent, and autonomy. Psychiatry's contribution to ethics is also discussed.

CHAPTER 46

LEGAL ISSUES

Virginia Trotter Betts   Gloria Birkholz

After studying this chapter the learner will be able to:

Identify sources of mental health law.

Describe common potential civil liability interactions.

Explain the role of a nurse witness in client consent and legal proceedings.

Identify how guaranteed rights may be applied to mental health settings.

Describe the civil and procedural rights of clients with mental health problems.

Distinguish between voluntary and involuntary commitment of adults and minors.

Identify issues in the commitment of mentally ill criminal clients.

Identify the main issues in client consent to and refusal of treatment.

Describe ways in which a nurse can influence legislation.

Laws reflect social norms. Laws may differ between governmental branches as well as from state to state. The legislative process is often slow and reflects compromises between varying beliefs and attitudes. Although the law may not always seem just, there exists a legal behavior that society enforces through sanctions such as money awards, fines, or imprisonment. It is important to know the current law that affects psychiatric nursing practice; if mental health–psychiatric nurses know the law, use it effectively, and help change it as necessary, the mental health client can receive respectful care and the nurse will be recognized as a knowledgeable professional.

OVERVIEW OF THE LEGAL SYSTEM

When analyzing the legal trends throughout the United States on matters of mental health, it is necessary to know the relevant Supreme Court decisions and federal statutes. In addition, the particular state mental health code and significant court interpretations on both the state court and the federal appeals court level need to be determined. State statutes can then be compared to national precendents.

Civil suits. A law generated by the branches of government may be enforced by initiating a lawsuit. A *civil suit* results from a dispute between persons and is resolved by a variety of remedies, most often by monetary settlement. An example of a civil suit might be a client suing a hospital director for not following state mental health laws. The most common civil actions brought against nurses working in mental health settings include malpractice, assault and battery, false imprisonment, and breach of confidentiality.

Malpractice. Malpractice is a civil action that may be brought against a professional when breach of the professional standard of care causes injury to the client. The nurse's professional standard of care is to do what a reasonably prudent nurse would do for the client. To assess and keep up to date on what a reasonably prudent nurse would do, the nurse:

1. Practices within national standards of practice
2. Follows the policies and procedures of an agency
3. Reads and discusses current articles and texts written for mental health–psychiatric nursing
4. Attends professional continuing education courses

Historical Overview

DATE	EVENT
1700s-1800s	The mentally ill lost many of their rights with institutionalization: the right to vote, to make wills or contracts, and to keep their professional licenses.
Early 1900s	The state legislature created an alternative to state involuntary commitment proceedings by providing care and permitting voluntary hospital admissions.
1951	Almost every state permitted the mentally ill to avoid involuntary commitment by volunteering themselves for confinement.
Late 1960s	The rights of the mentally ill experienced renewed attention as a spin-off of the civil rights movement.
1970s	There was legal recognition that confinement in a mental hospital involves a massive curtailment of liberty; the courts and lawmakers began to examine the questions of who can be institutionalized and how this institutionalization is to be accomplished.
1980s	Because of deinstitutionalization, society is being pressured to better absorb the mentally ill into communities, jobs, housing, and education.
Future	The rights of the mentally ill will probably be expanded, making it extremely difficult to institutionalize a client.

If the nurse does not do what the prudent nurse would have done in a similar situation and the act or failure to act injures the client, the client may recover money damages by suit. Typically the injury of the client must be actual physical harm, such as attempted or actual suicide. However, some courts are beginning to recognize severe emotional distress without physical injury.

In 1980 a Connecticut hospital was successfully sued for $3.6 million for the malpractice of its nurses. Ms. Pisel had been placed in a seclusion room as her orientation deteriorated. No one checked her for 4 hours, after which time she was found semicomatose, having wedged her head between the mattress and rail of a metal bed. In this case there were multiple violations of the nursing standards of care, including failure to properly monitor a secluded client and failure to notify the physician of a change in the client's condition. A nurse also revealed that a few days after the injury the nursing director told the staff to rewrite the nursing notes, which they did, raising a professional issue beyond malpractice (*Pisel v. Stamford Hospital,* 1980).

The most common malpractice cases against psychiatric nurses are those dealing with inadequate observation or judgment. Such a case is exemplified by failing to prevent a suicide by not synthesizing data which indicate that the client needs closer supervision or not initiating precautions to ensure the client's safety. A client who has threatened suicide cannot be left with open windows or free access to materials that can cause injury. The client needs to be closely observed.

Assault and battery. The legal definition of *assault* is a threat of touching without client consent. *Battery* is the actual unconsented touch. An assault and battery suit can be brought both as a civil suit by a person and as a criminal suit by the state. A person can sue civilly for assault and battery without an injury. In the health care setting, any treatment of a client who has not been declared legally incompetent is a battery if the treatment is given without his consent, unless an emergency situation exists.

If the client is incompetent, the guardian must give consent before treatment. Threatening to give a medication when the client refuses is assault. Giving any medication the client refuses is battery.

False imprisonment. False imprisonment is the wrongful confinement of a client in such a way that he has no escape or exit. A potential situation of false imprisonment arises when the client is locked on a ward or placed in seclusion or restraint or when a voluntarily hospitalized client wishes to leave but is not released. To avoid suits for false imprisonment, a hospital needs to have a policy defining when a client may be confined. Confinement is permitted when the client is dangerous to himself or others. Documentation of the events justifying such restraint is critical. Continued observation and adherence to policy on releasing the client are also important. It has been argued, but is not widely accepted, that medication beyond therapeutic need is also a form of false imprisonment (*Amicus brief,* 1977). Excessive use of medication is similar to imprisonment because in addition to restricting the client's thought process, it also restricts his movement.

Breach of confidentiality. Under the American Nurses' Association's (ANA's) *Code of Ethics*[2] and certain state laws, the nurse has the responsibility to keep information about a client confidential. This means that information received from clients or their records should be released only by an appropriate release of information protocol.

In law there is a concept called *privileged communication.* Privileged communication means that, even in court proceedings, selected persons do not have to reveal a client's communication to them. When called to court to tell what the client said about any feelings, thoughts, or actions, the nurse needs an attorney's assistance to know how the concept of privileged communication applies in the court or proceedings of hearing. By legislative enactment state by state, the privilege may apply only to certain professionals (for example, lawyers, clergy, psychologists) and may not apply to nurses. In fact, privileged communication statutes that include the nurse exist in only a few states. In the other states the nurse is required to reveal client communication if requested to do so during a court proceeding. Thus a legal and ethical dilemma arises if the nurse is called as a witness in a variety of legal proceedings. In any court proceeding the nurse is sworn to tell the truth. If the nurse lies, she commits perjury; if the nurse in a state without privilege refuses to speak, her behavior may be considered criminal contempt of court.

The clinical purpose of privileged communication statutes is to encourage clients to communicate honestly with the practitioner treating them. Making communication with a professional a privileged communication encourages truthful sharing of information. Legally whether the nurse is called as a witness for or against the client determines the status of the communication. In court the general rule is that the client may at any time permit the professional to release information. It is the client's privilege not the professional's. Therefore, if the client asks the professional to testify, the professional must truthfully give all information, including any communication of the client. However, if the nurse is a witness against the client, the nurse must keep the information confidential if the privileged communication statute exists for nurses.

The issue of confidentiality may arise in a commitment hearing. If the nurse is asked by the client or the client's attorney to testify, the nurse has no choice. However, if the nurse is asked by the state to testify in order to commit the client, the nurse should refuse to speak about client communications if state law recognizes communication to the nurse as privileged.

In a malpractice suit, privileged communication is not an issue. When a client is suing a nurse for the care given, the client has already put the issue of nursing care before the court and therefore waived his privilege of confidentiality. Thus the nurse is free to reveal all communications with the client.

The nurse may also be asked to appear at court as an expert witness on the standard of care for nursing. As an expert witness, the nurse's testimony is based on experience and education as a nurse, so there is no problem with client confidentiality. Before giving a deposition or appearing in court, the nurse examines the records of the case and is asked to give an opinion as to the appropriateness of the nursing care.

A new legal trend also requires professionals to disclose confidential information outside court proceedings. Some states have now imposed a duty on professionals to disclose confidential information when a known potential victim is at serious risk of harm. This duty, called the duty to warn, was first recognized in the case of *Tarasoff v. Board of Regents of the University of California* (1976). In this case the client confided to his psychotherapist that he intended to kill Tatiana Tarasoff when she returned from her summer vacation. The psychotherapist did not warn Tatiana or her parents of the threat. When the client did kill Tatiana, her parents won a lawsuit based on the therapist's failure to warn.

The law has not gone so far as to say a therapist must warn of every threat. A therapist must warn only about those threats that pose a serious danger and only if a victim has been identified specifically by the client or when the therapist is able to identify the victim. This duty has been imposed by courts on psychiatrists and psychotherapists, and it seems likely that nurses engaged in psychotherapy would also be required to warn potential victims.

The argument against further expansion of this duty to warn victims is that the effectiveness of therapy will be reduced if therapists must breach their clients' confidences to warn potential victims. If a client's trust is diminished, the client may cease to admit anger, and successful treatment may be impossible. The duty to warn has placed mental health workers in a double bind. If they break a client's confidence, they may be sued for breach of confidentiality. If they fail to break the confidence and a potential victim is injured, the mental health professional may be sued for negligence in a failure to warn.

CURRENT LAW

This section focuses on specific federal and state laws that influence mental health care today. The U.S. Constitution and selected federal laws are examined with current application to mental health. Discussion of state law focuses particularly on civil rights, commitment proceedings, and consent issues.

Federal Law

Several constitutional amendments have significant application to mental health law (Table 46-1).

The First Amendment to the Constitution states that "Congress shall make no law respecting an establishment of religion, or prohibiting the free exercise thereof; or abridging the freedom of speech." Freedom of speech as guaranteed by the First Amendment has been interpreted in one court to include a person's mental processes and the communication of ideas (*Kaimowitz v. Department of Mental Health,* 1973). This means that persons have the right to have their own thoughts, even if the thoughts are bizarre or out of the norm. This interpretation is not accepted by most states. Similarly it has been argued that because medication interferes with free generation of thoughts, the First Amendment also protects against the altering effects of medication. Again, this interpretation has not been adopted nationally because these cases did not reach the Supreme Court.

TABLE 46-1 Amendments to the U.S. Constitution as related to mental health care

Amendment	Possible Interpretations
First: Freedom of speech	Right to generate abnormal thought
	Right to express abnormal thought
First: Freedom of religion	Right to practice religion
	Right to refuse treatment if it conflicts with religious beliefs
Fifth: Federal right to due process of law	Procedural rights
Eighth: Freedom from cruel and unusual punishment	Freedom from treatment used as punishment
	Freedom from poor institutional conditions
	Freedom from excessive medication
Fourteenth: State right to due process of law and equal protection	Procedural rights
	Privacy
	Equal treatment

Freedom of religion has been held to mean the right to practice one's religion even when institutionalized. This includes the right to refuse medication or treatment on the grounds that it conflicts with religious beliefs (*Winters v. Miller,* 1971). Although a client does have a right to practice a religion, the courts have not recognized an absolute right to refuse treatment on religious grounds. The constitutional amendments can be argued to guarantee rights, but under certain conditions these rights may be overridden by the courts.

The Eighth Amendment to the Constitution says that "Excessive bail shall not be required, nor excessive fines imposed, nor cruel and unusual punishment inflicted." It is still unclear in the law whether freedom from cruel and unusual punishment applies only to criminals or can be applied to noncriminal hospitalized mentally ill clients as well. It does apply to the mentally ill when treatments such as medications, restraints, seclusion, aversive stimuli, electroconvulsive therapy, and psychosurgery are used as punishment rather than therapy. Other violations of the Eighth Amendment have been considered to be institutional conditions such as unsanitary living conditions, inadequate exercise or nutrition, and insufficient staffing (*Lessard v. Schmidt,* 1974). It has also been argued that an excess of medication and forced medication are cruel and unusual punishment (*Lessard v. Schmidt,* 1974).

The Fifth Amendment to the Constitution, "No person . . . shall be compelled in any criminal case to be a witness against himself, nor be deprived of life, liberty or property, without due process of law," and the Fourteenth Amendment, Section 1, "Nor shall any State deprive any person of life, liberty, or property, without due process of law; nor deny to any person within its jurisdiction the equal protection of the laws," require that citizens be guaranteed due process of law. Due process means that certain procedural safeguards, such as the right to notice, counsel, a hearing, access to documents, client's own professional examination, client's presence at the hearing, and client's cross-examination of witnesses, must take place before the state can place persons in hospitals against their will. The Fifth Amendment applies due process to the federal government, and the Fourteenth Amendment applies this principle to all states. Because the Supreme Court has recognized that involuntary commitment to a mental hospital involves a grave deprivation of liberty, any law that commits a person to a mental hospital must meet due process requirements (*Humphrey v. Cady,* 1972). State statutes, state courts, and lower federal courts have been active in defining due process procedures. These procedures will be further discussed under "Civil Commitment."

Besides creating a fundamental right to be free from incarceration and requiring due process before commitment, the Fifth and Fourteenth Amendments guarantee a fundamental right to privacy. Privacy has thus far been used by courts to protect family and body privacy. The most familiar privacy case is *Roe v. Wade* (1973), the Supreme Court case granting a woman the right to a first-trimester abortion. The right to privacy may also apply to a mental health client's right to refuse treatment. The concept of privacy is still being defined by the courts and is an area in which new mental health precedent may be set.

Equal protection under the law, which is also mandated by the Fourteenth Amendment, means that neither the federal or state government can treat one group of people differently from another unless there is a rational reason to do so. If the government has an appropriate reason for unequal treatment, the government can proceed differently. For example, if a mentally ill criminal is committed to a mental hospital under the guarantee of equal protection, the criminal should have the same procedural safeguards and the same rights as those required for a noncriminal client committed to a mental institution. However, this is not true because the state has a rational reason (to protect the community from the criminal) for treating the criminal and noncriminal unequally.

Civil Rights

Constitutional rights apply to every U.S. citizen. They apply to nonpatients as well as clients in all settings: inpatient, outpatient, and community. However, these rights are very broad and somewhat difficult to apply to daily situations.

Besides the rights that courts find in the U.S. and state constitutions, other sources of clients' rights exist. In 1980 Congress passed the Mental Health Systems Act (MHSA), creating a bill of rights for mentally ill clients (see list below). Because the rights found in the MHSA are only a recommendation from Congress to the states, they are now law. However, this act does suggest rights that reflect federal lawmakers' agreement on what rights states should adopt. Table 46-2 illustrates how states have complied with the Mental Health Systems Act. The rights that a state adopts as actual rights in its health code have the force of law for that state's residents. Following are the rights most frequently listed in state statutes for residential clients:[37]

1. Right to completeness and confidentiality of records
2. Right to access to records
3. Right to access to personal belongings
4. Right to freedom from restraints and isolation
5. Right to treatment, including individual medical plan, least restrictive alternatives, and periodic review of examinations.
6. Right to daily exercise
7. Right to access to visitors
8. Right to use of writing materials and uncensored mail
9. Right to use of telephone
10. Right to access to courts and attorneys
11. Right to employment compensation
12. Right to be informed of rights

The Mental Patient's Bill of Rights should be checked against what is in the state's mental health code, federal and state statutes, federal and state constitutions, and hospital or ward policies.

All rights, whether constitutional or statutory, are merely on paper unless they are made known to the client and the client has some way to secure them. Nurses need to be aware of the client's rights. The nurse acts as the client's advocate by informing the client of his legal rights and then supporting his decision on how or if a right is pursued. Some state statutes provide a residential grievance procedure for clients who believe their rights are not being granted, but other states have no grievance procedure. In the latter case, clients may secure their rights through lawsuits. A violation of a right guaranteed by the U.S. Constitution may be brought before federal or state court, and clients may sue an individual state or federal government official if that official violated their clear constitutional right by ignoring the law or acting maliciously (*Wood v. Strickland,* 1975).

Rights may also be withdrawn under certain circumstances. If state law is unclear on when such rights can be curtailed, there needs to be a written agency policy that defines the criteria for denial of rights. For example, although there may be a right to freedom from physical isolation, a client who has attacked another client may be placed in isolation. When the right to freedom is denied, documentation in the client record should state the events. Then the agency policy should be followed. For example, the policy might state, "Isolation must take place within 15 minutes of an incident; there must be a written order; the order is valid for a maximum of 3 hours; the client shall have access to toilet facilities every hour and exercise every 3 hours." Nursing notes should indicate that an assessment of client's behavior plus the implementation of the agency procedures did take place.[44]

TABLE 46-2 State compliance with Mental Health Systems Act

Right of Client	Level of Compliance*		
	Y	N	P
Right to treatment and least restriction of liberty	19	3	29
Right to individual treatment plan	6	7	38
Planning of participation	8	38	5
Explanation of treatment	4	32	15
Right to refuse treatment	16	11	24
Right to refuse participation in experimentation	11	28	12
Freedom from restraint or seclusion	31	11	9
Right to humane treatment environment	19	8	24
Right to confidentiality of records	46	2	3
Right to access to records	35	12	4
Right of private conversation	12	22	17
Right to telephone use, mail, and visitors	38	3	10
Right to information regarding rights	8	12	31
Right to assert grievances	9	31	11
Right to referral on discharge	13	29	9

Adapted from Lyon, M., Levine, M., and Zusman, J.: Mental Disability Law Reporter **6:**184, 1982.
*Y, Substantial compliance, N, state law contradicts MHSA subsection or has no corresponding provision; P, partial compliance or substantial variation.

State Law

Commitment. The commitment of a client to a mental institution is the exercise of a strong power of the state. The state is able to commit a person under its police power to protect others from harm or under its *parens patriae* power to protect or help the person. A person may be committed to a mental hospital through the civil court or the criminal court system. The civil court system requires that the person meet the criteria set up in the state mental health code. The criminal system requires that the person is being prosecuted for a crime but is either incompetent to stand trial or is not guilty of the crime because of insanity. Civil commitment may be initiated by the client, a physician, the police, a state attorney, a family member, or others listed in the state statute. There are two types of civil commitments: voluntary and involuntary.

Civil commitment. Voluntary entry into the hospital is by consent of the client or someone acting for the client. Almost every state permits voluntary admission[6] although public hospital bed space is increasingly limited.

When admission is voluntary, there is a statutory right to be released if and when the client no longer wishes to remain. The time it takes to release the client should only be the reasonable time it takes to go through normal hospital exit procedures, unless the client meets the state requirements for involuntary commitment.

Voluntary clients are likewise considered competent unless otherwise adjudicated and therefore have the right to refuse treatment, including psychotropic medications unless they are dangerous to themselves or others, as in a violent episode on the treatment unit (*Rennie v. Klein,* 1981). This right to refuse medications is one important difference in the care of voluntary clients from that of clients of involuntary status. Thus it is important for nurses to be able to clearly identify the admission status of clients in their care.

State codes have two types of involuntary commitment: *emergency* and *indefinite* involuntary. The indefinite involuntary commitment usually has subdivisions of *initial* and *extended* commitments.

When a person's conduct poses an immediate danger of serious harm to himself or others, the client may be held temporarily for his safety or the safety of others through the emergency involuntary commitment statutes in most states. Unfortunately, it may be a police officer who first encounters the client, and detection may be at a jail until transfer to a health facility is possible. State statutes differ on this point; some permit several days' detention in a jail, whereas others require immediate transfer. In a health facility an examination is done to determine that an emergency does indeed exist. The person required to perform the admitting examination varies from state to state and can be the psychiatrist, physician, or in some states, the psychiatric nurse.

Statutes should specify when the examination must be done and how long emergency detention can last. The suggested statute on civil commitment of the American Bar Association (ABA) recommends no longer than 72 hours for an emergency.[43] Because no hearing is required, emergency treatment can be started although no review or diagnosis takes place. It is in everyone's interest to have the shortest time period for emergency holds and a hearing as quickly as possible.

If the initial screening does not validate the existence of an emergency, the client must be released. The client must also be released when the emergency ceases or at the expiration of the state statutory emergency detention time if there has been no petition for involuntary commitment.

Due process. The exact procedures for involuntary commitment that meet due process are not created by the U.S. Congress but by each state's legislature in its mental health code. The mental health code defines what a mental disorder is, the conditions that must be met to commit someone involuntarily, the procedure for the hearing, the length of an initial and extended commitment, and the rights of the institutionalized client. If the state legislature does not create a constitutionally acceptable code, the courts will. In 1975 the U.S. Supreme Court in *O'Connor v. Donaldson* said that the presence of mental illness alone was not enough to justify involuntary institutionalization. In this case, Mr. Donaldson was 50 years old when his father successfully had the state of Florida commit him for delusional ideation. Mr. Donaldson was diagnosed as paranoid schizophrenic, but he had never committed a dangerous act. He was institutionalized for 15 years despite his repeated requests for release. For those 15 years he received little treatment and at times his environment consisted of being in a room with 60 other clients. The Supreme Court decided that "a state cannot constitutionally confine without more [sic] a non-dangerous individual who is capable of surviving safely in freedom by himself or with the help of willing and responsible family members or friends" (*O'Connor v. Donaldson,* 1975, p. 578). "Without more" means the client must at least receive more than milieu therapy. The court, however, did not enumerate what treatment would be enough to justify confinement of a nondangerous person. Future court cases will be necessary to define the minimal treatment.

It is clear that a state may commit a person for mental illness plus dangerousness. By 1979, 46 states adopted the criteria of mental illness and danger to self or others as the grounds for involuntary commitment. About 30 states also declared that nondangerous mentally ill persons can be committed if they are "gravely disabled" or "in need of care or treatment." Gravely disabled or in need of care or treatment typically means that because of a mental condition the client is unable to care for his basic needs of nutrition, clothing, shelter, safety, and medical care.[46] An example of a gravely disabled client is one who does not eat because of disorientation.

Because almost every state permits indefinite involuntary commitment on the grounds of danger to self or others, it is important to know what this means. Danger to self may include the range of behavior from attempted suicide to not meeting basic needs. Danger to others may include behavior ranging from threats of violence to actual attacks. In all these situations the exact statutory language is important. When specific language is present, the client's actual conduct must reflect the statutory language. For example, if the state commitment statute requires substantial threat of imminent harm and the statement "I feel so bad I would like to die" is the client's only action, it may not be sufficient evidence to commit the client. However, if his statement were accompanied by the act of holding a loaded gun to the temple, the conduct then becomes more statute specific.

Using dangerousness as the criterion for state commitment has been criticized. Research shows that no one, including psychiatrists and judges, can accurately predict who will be dangerous.[12] Research also supports the fact that mentally ill clients are no more apt to be dangerous than people in the general population.[12] Thus to place mentally ill persons in hospitals when they have committed no dangerous act is to place them there merely for their mental illness.

The ABA recommends in its model act that the following be the criteria for involuntary commitment:[43]
1. Severe mental disorder
2. Likelihood of inflicting serious physical harm on self or others as manifested by an overt act
3. Incompetency to make own treatment decisions
4. Treatability (including availability of treatment resources as well as improvements in condition)

The model act does not recommend involuntary commitment of the gravely disabled but suggests a legal incompetency hearing and appointment of a guardian.

In any civil commitment proceeding, the state will

STATE COMMITMENT PROCEDURAL RIGHTS

1. Right to remain silent—client does not have to say anything that can be used to determine if commitment criteria are met, for example, talking about acts of violence during examination or hearing. Not in majority of states.
2. Right to notice*—client must be given information about time, date, place of hearing, witnesses who will speak for commitment, and what they will speak about.
3. Right to counsel*—client has a right to an attorney who will represent the client's interest, including private talks with his attorney, uncensored communication, and absolute right to call. In a few states, counsel has the right to be present at mental examination.
4. Right to hearing*—client has a right to a meeting with a judge, including presentation of evidence and witnesses on client's behalf before nonemergency detention can continue. May be held at hospital.

5. Right to jury—client has a right to a jury hearing if long-term commitment is being sought (long term means 90 days or more). No U.S. constitutional right in civil commitment hearings and not a right in majority of states.
6. Right to review documents*—the chart, Kardex, medication sheets, as well as the psychiatrist's examination report must be made available to client's counsel.
7. Right to own professional examiner*—client can choose psychiatrist to do an independent examination and testify in the hearing.
8. Right to be present at hearing*—client can hear full testimony about his mental illness and dangerousness unless the judge finds client disruptive in the proceedings. It can be argued that the client who is excessively medicated is not present.
9. Right to cross-examine witnesses*—client or attorney can ask questions of any witnesses, including health professionals.

*Most frequently listed in state statutes.

---

have to prove by clear and convincing evidence (a higher standard of proof than in most civil litigation) that the client meets the state's criteria for commitment (*Addington v. Texas,* 1979). What constitutes clear and convincing evidence depends on the facts of the case. An example of clear and convincing evidence of dangerousness is found in *In the Matter of N.B.* (1980). The client in this case was hostile and aggressive to the hospital staff and tried to choke another client. He was determined by the court to be dangerous and an appropriate candidate for involuntary commitment.

Besides meeting the state criteria or definition for commitment, the process of nonemergency involuntary civil commitment of an adult must also be procedurally fair in order to meet the constitutional right of due process of law before freedom can be taken away. This means that certain procedures have been recognized as giving the client a fair chance at presenting his version of the situation so the client will not be incarcerated unfairly or incorrectly. The typical procedural rights for short- or long-term commitment are found in the box above. The commitment hearing is conducted with all rights that the state constitution recognizes, after which the judge either finds clear and convincing evidence for commitment or insufficient evidence, in which case the client is not hospitalized.

The ABA recommends that the initial involuntary commitment be no more than 90 days. If during that 90 days the client exhibits new threats or acts of harm, another 90-day commitment is sought.[43] Most states, however, permit initial commitments of 6 months to 1 year.

Commitment of minors. Commitment of minors differs from commitment of adults because minors, who in most states are persons under 18 years of age, are considered legally incompetent to perform adult activities. Therefore

parents make decisions for them, traditionally deciding when their children need to receive counseling or medication and if they need to be placed in a mental hospital. The unique situation with minors is that their parents voluntarily commit them, although in fact the child may strongly protest. The question is whether this situation is actually voluntary or involuntary commitment. If in fact it is a type of involuntary commitment, the minor needs to be allowed some constitutional procedural safeguards because his liberty is being taken away.

Cases dealing with children represent a clash between two legal concepts: the right of the family to be free from state intrusion and the *parens patriae* responsibility of the state to protect citizens with a disability, in this case, minors. In the past most states did not intervene when parents voluntarily committed their children to mental institutions.[13]

However, over time, states have changed their statutes to include more procedural safeguards before institutionalization of children.[14] Typically these rights include a right to counsel for the child and a right to a hearing.

The issue of whether states could permit voluntary commitment of minors to mental institutions without substantially increased procedural safeguards was finally decided by the U.S. Supreme Court in 1979. The case, *Parham v. J.L.* (1979), challenged the Georgia statute permitting voluntary commitment without an adversarial hearing. The Supreme Court held that, although the child has a right to be free of unnecessary body restraint and not to be labeled erroneously, parents could place their children in institutions without a hearing. The court said that the child's rights are adequately safeguarded by a physician's examination and review of the child's history. The physician is considered by the court to be a neutral fact finder who determines if a child meets the state's statutory requirements for commitment. If in the physician's judgment the child does not, the parent may not admit the child to the hospital. Instead of a formal hearing, the physician's examination can act to counteract potential parental abuse. Although this is the current law, state statutes that do require a hearing are valid, since a state can always have more stringent safeguards than the U.S. Constitution requires; however, it may not have fewer safeguards. In the Supreme Court decision in the *Parham* case, three justices dissented, saying that children need even more procedural safeguards than adults because they are confined longer, are more vulnerable, and bear an emotional scar for life if erroneously labeled. The *Parham* decision has been criticized in both the legal and the psychiatric fields, and it is possible that as a result of this dissent more procedural safeguards for minors will be recognized by the Supreme Court in the future.

Criminal commitment. Persons may also be placed in mental institutions through criminal proceedings. When citizens are accused of a crime, they may plead that they should not be held guilty because they were insane. Criminal law defines insanity somewhat differently than the health care professions, which are concerned with descriptive symptoms and prognosis, not merely a time-specific state of mind. Currently, state courts recognize three different definitions of criminal insanity[7]:

1. The M'Naghten Rule—at the time of committing the act the person under defect of reason did not know the nature and quality of the act or did not know it was wrong.
2. The Irresistible Impulse Test—at the time of the act the person was of such mental condition that even if he knew the act to be wrong, his actions were beyond control.
3. The American Law Institute, Model Penal Code Section 4.01 (1)—at the time of the conduct, as a result of mental disease or defect, the person lacked substantial capacity either to appreciate the wrongfulness of his conduct or to conform his conduct to the requirements of law.

Whichever definition that a state utilizes for an insanity defense, if the accused is found by a jury to meet the criteria, then the accused is found not guilty of the crime. The client is then committed to a mental hospital for evaluation and treatment. Continued treatment requires that the hearing process continue to find the client "committable." When no longer in treatment, the client is free.

This commitment process may not be appropriate for criminal clients. There is continuing controversy over ways to approach the criminal treatment problem, including sentences of "guilty but insane" and giving criminals a time sentence in a mental institution if mental illness is present.[25] These findings allow treatment for the mental illness if resources are available while still holding the client responsible and punishable for the crime. When criminals are found mentally ill, they have a right to be treated for their illness. However, if they are already in jail, they may not be transferred to a mental institution just because a psychiatrist now finds them mentally ill. They have a right to counsel and a hearing before a

change in their commitment from a jail to a mental hospital (*Vitek v. Jones,* 1980).

The criminal system also funnels clients into mental institutions because of questions of competence to stand trial. *Competence to stand trial* refers to the mental condition necessary for a criminal defendant so that he may (1) confer with an attorney about his defense, (2) understand the nature of charges against him, and (3) understand courtroom procedure. If a criminal defendant cannot meet these criteria, the client is placed without a commitment hearing in a mental hospital for evaluation or treatment. Periods of observation and treatment can be long, and if competence is never regained, the client has in fact received a life sentence. To remedy this potential problem, the Supreme Court held in *Jackson v. Indiana* that a 27-year-old client who did not have competence to stand trial for a theft of $9 worth of property could not be "held more than a reasonable time necessary to determine whether there is substantial probability that he will attain capacity in the foreseeable future" (*Jackson v. Indiana,* 1972, p. 728). If regaining competence is not foreseeable, a civil commitment proceeding may be initiated if state criteria are met; otherwise, the client goes free.

Minors who are charged with crimes but who are also mentally ill typically have their criminal charges dropped or are placed on probation if they spend a specified amount of time in a mental institution or receive outpatient treatment. The facility acceptable to the court will depend on the minor's illness, the crime, and the resources of the facility.

Right to treatment and least restrictive alternative. There are two emerging concepts that affect the commitment process: the right to treatment and the least restrictive alternative principle.

The theory behind a right to treatment comes from the concept of due process in that a state should not institutionalize a person unless it can treat the person. If a person is gravely disabled and there is no treatment, perhaps it would be more appropriate to appoint a guardian than to institutionalize a person without treatment. A right to treatment was first articulated in a criminal case (*Rouse v. Cameron*) in 1966, when Mr. Rouse applied for release from a mental hospital on the grounds that he had received no treatment. He had avoided a criminal charge of carrying a dangerous weapon when he was found to be insane and then spent 4 years involuntarily committed to a mental hospital without treatment; however, the maximum sentence for carrying a dangerous weapon was 1 year. Interpreting the Washington, D.C. statute that said mental patients are entitled to treatment, the judge in this case ruled that a criminal had a right to treatment if he was insane or a right to be released if he was no longer insane.

By 1979, following the dicta in *Wyatt v. Stickney* (1974), 27 states had some form of right to treatment through statutory or case law.[37] Some states have explicit rules about what treatment entails, including a treatment plan with objectives, activities, and evaluation criteria. Others are not specific, stating only that there is a right to treatment.

It is unclear legally whether a right to treatment is an obligation to treat or merely a right to be released from a hospital when treatment is not available. But if a state does have a right-to-treatment law, a person who cannot be treated may not be committed to a hospital.

The *least restrictive alternative (LRA) principle* means that the least restrictive treatment and placement possible should be ordered for a client. The principle can be applied to any mentally disabled client, from mentally ill clients to clients with Down's syndrome. The LRA principle ensures that when a state has the right to intervene, the state will do so with minimal intrusion into the client's life. The LRA principle has been applied to the commitment process by some federal courts and by at least 10 states.[41] The following are some examples of the application of the LRA principle:

1. Placing a client in the care facility closest to his home rather than in a state hospital far from his home
2. Placing a client who can maintain daily employment in a weekend and night care facility rather than a 24-hour hospital
3. Providing home care services instead of full-time hospitalization to a gravely disabled client

Unfortunately one of the difficult problems with the LRA principle is the limited availability of needed outpatient facilities and services.

The LRA principle has sometimes been applied to conditions within the institution after commitment.[49] This means that other medications are to be tried before psychotropic drugs, psychotherapy before medication, and closer observations before seclusion (*Wyatt v. Stickney,* 1974; *Rennie v. Klein,* 1981).

Consent to treatment. In legal terminology *consent* has three elements, all of which must be present for validity: capacity, voluntariness, and information.[56]

Capacity means the ability to understand or comprehend, although total comprehension is not necessary. There are certain classes of people the law says do not have capacity: minors (usually persons under 18 years of age), persons declared incompetent by the court, and criminals who have successfully proved incompetency. Individuals may have varying degrees of capacity. For instance, a mentally disabled client may have the capacity to know that he does not want electroconvulsive therapy but may be unable to understand a complex contract or manage financial matters.

For persons who are recognized as lacking capacity under the law, a guardian may be appointed to give consent. Parents of a minor are automatically the guardians. In the case of an adult, a court proceeding must first take place to determine if the adult is competent. Competency hearings usually take place when a client refuses hospitalization or treatment, when parental rights over children are at issue, or when the validity of a will is in question. Unfortunately there is no single national definition of legal incompetency; it is the legal conclusion that, because of an impairment, the person is no longer able to make responsible decisions for himself, his dependents, or his property.

If a court determines incompetency, a guardian is appointed for that adult. Typically the court appoints a family member as the guardian. If no family member is available, a friend, a staff member, or other interested person can be appointed. The guardian the court appoints may have power of consent for the person, the power to use his property as necessary, or power over both the person and his property. Most courts have held that the guardian must represent the judgment the client would make, not what the guardian believes is best for the client.[36] For example, a mentally ill client is declared incompetent and the guardian is asked to consent to electroconvulsive therapy. Although the guardian may believe strongly that the client would benefit from the treatment, the guardian's beliefs should not be controlling. If the client had previously said that electroconvulsive therapy was not personally desirable, or if the client had experienced electroconvulsive therapy and indicated that it would be unacceptable in the future, the guardian should present these views.

Besides capacity, the valid consent must be *voluntary,* not forced, threatened, or given under fraud or distress. Some abuses in this area have arisen in forced or uninformed experimental projects (for example, treatment for syphilis with placebos) or in requiring the client to be part of an experiment in order to gain admittance to a particular unit or residential center (for instance, admittance only if consent is given for a hepatitis study).

Several gray areas may constitute duress for clients. The client who is a voluntary client but who is threatened with discharge or involuntary commitment if he does not consent to medications, treatment, or continued hospitalization may be a victim of coercion. It has also been suggested that because of the inherent inequality of the physician-client relationship, it is impossible for the client to escape coercion totally (*Kaimowitz v. Department of Mental Health,* 1973).

The third part of valid consent is that it must be *informed;* that is, the person must have sufficient information to make a choice about the treatment (*Cobbs v. Grant,* 1972). Typically the following information must be given a client about the treatment, experiment, or surgery (*Salgo v. Leland Stanford Jr. University Board of Trustees,* 1957):

1. Procedure to be performed
2. Purposes of the procedure
3. Expected result
4. Risks involved
5. Medical alternatives

How much information needs to be given to the client is determined by what other professionals would do in similar circumstances. Legally most states require that the practitioner tell the client what other practitioners would tell him, although some courts hold that at a minimum the client needs to be told of any risk of death, permanent injury, or delayed recuperation (*Cobbs v. Grant,* 1972). The medical alternatives include only those recognized by medicine as alternatives. It does not include information on nontraditional treatments, such as those of Indian medicine men. It is also necessary to inform the client of the probable results of refusing the treatment or medication

(*Young v. Group Health Cooperative of Puget Sound,* 1976).

The person who is to perform the procedure is legally responsible for explaining the procedure. Informed consent is the result of one or more conversations between client and physician and is usually evidenced by a written document between the parties. An oral consent is as valid as a written consent but more difficult to prove.

Typically, the more intrusive the procedure, the more likely it is that a written consent will be obtained because the written document can be used as proof that consent was given. A written consent, however, does not always mean the consent is valid. If any of the three elements of consent is missing, the consent is not valid. A lack of valid informed consent in the health care context makes health professionals vulnerable to suits for battery (see earlier discussion). In such a lawsuit, if the treatment and its results have had a serious negative consequence on the client, the court will likely examine the prior presence of each element of informed consent.

It is advisable for the nurse to be present during the physician's explanation of the procedure so information can be used in the client's care and teaching. The nurse may also witness the client's signature to the consent. When nurses act as consent witnesses, they are acknowledging that the client was the one who signed the form. The remainder of the nurse's role as a consent witness is unclear in the courts. The nurse may be responsible for observing indications of disorientation or noting that the information was understood. If the client is very disoriented or indicates misunderstanding, the nurse does not have the client sign the form but notes the disorientation and tells the physician. The major factor at issue in consent in the mental health context is the capacity of the client to be truly informed. Therefore documentation and assessment by the nurse as to capacity and knowledge are significant.

In certain circumstances treatment may be given even though consent was not obtained or a full explanation was not given to the client. Treatment may be begun if there is an emergency and the client is unable to consent. An emergency is defined differently under each state's law but usually refers to the possible loss of life, an extremity or an eye, or other potentially serious, irreversible physical harm. The client may be unable to consent to treatment because he is semiconscious as a result of medication overdose. An emergency may also exist if a client is about to injure another person. In an emergency, an attempt to obtain consent from a relative, court, or hospital administrator may be required by state statute. However, if serious consequences may result from such a delay, treatment may be begun without consent.

Consent of minors. In the matter of consent of minors for treatment, the ABA recommends that children be given some independent right to consent to specific forms of treatment.[45]:

> Children over 14 years old can consent for themselves to psychotherapy, whereas children under 14 years must have parental consent.
> Parental consent is required for all minors' medication,

but a child over the age of 14 years has an independent right to refuse medication. The refusal by the child may be overturned by a court.

Right to refuse treatment. Another side of the issue of informed consent is the right to refuse treatment or to withhold consent. It is usually true that every person has a right to accept or refuse medication or other medical treatment for any reason whatsoever, even whim. There is, however, a tension between the client's right to his body and what the physician or society may decide is best for that person.

The mentally ill client's right to refuse medical treatment is not absolute. Clients can usually refuse treatment because it is against their religious beliefs. This was established for mental clients in *Winters v. Miller* in 1971. Ms. Winters was a 59-year-old client with no dependents who had been involuntarily placed in a New York hospital. Although a practicing Christian Scientist, she was continually medicated despite her objections on religious grounds. She had never been declared by a court to be mentally incompetent. A federal district court found that if a person is competent, the person may refuse treatment. Many states have now included in their statutes a right to refuse treatment because of religious beliefs[36].

Even when refusal is not on religious grounds, a right to refuse treatment is still generally recognized. However, unique problems arise with mental health clients. First, competent clients always have the right to refuse treatment. The problem is determining if a mentally ill client is in fact competent. Most states, in statutes or through courts, hold that until there is a separate hearing to determine legal incompetency, the client who acts incompetently has all the rights of a competent person, including refusing treatment. Once a person is legally incompetent, the guardian has the power of consent. A guardian does not rely on his own beliefs but should decide as the client would if the client were competent using the client's previous decisions and religious beliefs, the complications of the treatment, and the prognosis in determining whether to consent to or refuse treatment (*Superintendent of Belchertown State School v. Saikewicz,* 1977; *In the Matter of Guardianship of Richard Roe III,* 1981).

In 1979 the voluntary and involuntary clients at the Massachusetts state mental health facilities asked for a definition of when clients could be forcibly medicated. The federal appeals court said that medication could be forced only after legal determination of incompetency, unless there was an emergency. However, the court said that even before a declaration of incompetency, an emergency could be defined as including not only physical harm but also mental deterioration. Because state laws are clear in stating that an emergency treatment can begin without the client's consent, this broad interpretation of emergency situations has far-reaching consequences (*Mills v. Rogers,* 1982). To protect the client's rights, the court did say that in an emergency, psychotropic medications can be forced on the client only after other alternatives had been ruled out. In other words, forced medication in a psychiatric emergency is subject to the LRA principle.

Some states have granted the right to refuse treatment

that is based not on a client's competency but on whether the client has a voluntary or an involuntary admission. Such states conclude that voluntary clients have a right to refuse treatment but involuntary clients do not.[42] The Mental Health Systems Act of 1980 (Section 9501) recommends that all states adopt a right to refuse treatment for voluntary clients but does not mention this same right for involuntary clients. The issue of whether a competent involuntarily committed client can refuse medication when there is no emergency was introduced in the case of *Rennie v. Klein* (1981). Mr. Rennie, 38 years old, was involuntarily committed to a New Jersey psychiatric hospital in 1976. He had a previous history of suicidal, homicidal, and delusional episodes and 11 previous hospitalizations. He was not declared incompetent. When Mr. Rennie refused medication, the lower federal court found that involuntarily committed clients have a partial right to refuse treatment. But because the state also has a right to protect other hospitalized clients, there may be some instances in which medication can be forced on involuntarily committed competent clients. To protect the involuntary client's right to refuse treatment, the appeals court said that state regulations which provide review of medication refusal by a treatment team must meet the constitutional due process requirement. The rights of involuntarily committed clients to refuse medication remain less clearly defined and are open to further litigation.

NURSES' INFLUENCE ON CHANGES IN THE LAW

Nurses need to be sure their viewpoints are being heard and can do so by influencing changes in the law. Expert witnesses, especially on the nursing standard of care, will change the case law of the future by increasingly demanding a national standard of nursing practice utilizing ANA generic and psychiatric–mental health standards.

When state and federal legislators introduce bills, they collect input from their constituents. Nurses need to have input into the legislation before it is passed because it may determine everyone's rights and obligations.

The first step in ensuring that legislation reflects nurses' input is to elect a person to the state legislature who has the views the nursing profession supports. A nurse can do this by knowing candidates' opinions, working in the campaign of a sympathetic candidate, and voting. There is an American Nurses' Association Political Action Committee (ANA-PAC) with state branches. ANA-PAC and its state political action committees are organized to support candidates who are proponents of health care resources and alternative providers.

After electing a candidate who listens to nurses, the next step is to know what bills are being presented to the state or federal legislature. To affect the bill and have it reflect nursing's viewpoint, nurses need to lobby. This can be done individually or through a group, especially the state nurses' association. Individually, nurses can attend committee hearings on the bill and at times testify. Nurses can also express their viewpoints to representatives or senators by telephone, telegram, or letter. A nurse who has helped with a legislator's campaign or is a voter in the legislator's district may get a better reception. A viewpoint needs to be objective and based on factual data that are presented to validate a position.

Although it is not easy to affect legislation, it is possible. In one state a nurse who attended a state subcommittee meeting on the mental health code was able to influence the bill so that it reflected a nursing concern. The proposed bill stated that institutionalized clients were required to have a complete physical examination every 2 years. The nurse knew this was too infrequent and reported this to the committee, which voted in the nurse's suggestion that a physical examination be done every 6 months.

Belonging to professional associations and lobbying through them are truly useful. Each state nurses' association has a legislative committee and a lobbyist who are aware of current state legislation affecting nursing and who know how to influence that legislation. Often state associations have workshops during legislative sessions to teach nurses about the legislative process. They are worthwhile and enable a nurse to watch a representative in action, become familiar with the process, and begin lobbying. Special interest groups in the area of mental health, such as the state mental health associations and the ANA Council on Psychiatric Mental Health Nursing, also are aware of current mental health legislation, both federal and state.

BRIEF REVIEW

Legally, the mental health client has many rights and the nurse has concurrent obligations. Laws that influence mental health care are made by state legislatures, the Congress, and state and federal courts. To know the law for the state in which the nurse practices, it is necessary to know both state and federal statutes as well as recent cases decided by the state courts, the federal circuit courts and courts of appeals, and the Supreme Court.

The nurse is vulnerable to a malpractice suit when the nursing standard of care is breached and a client is injured. The nurse may also be sued for assault and battery, false imprisonment, or breach of confidentiality. The nurse may reveal client communication if the client consents, if the client brings a malpractice action against the nurse, or if there is a duty to warn a known potential victim of a client's threat of serious harm. The nurse must reveal client confidences in a court proceeding unless a state's privileged communication statute applies to her.

The U.S. Constitution and state laws have given the mentally ill client many rights. Constitutional amendments have been interpreted in courts as permitting mental health clients to be free from punishment, to be given due process of law, and to have the right to have or refuse treatment. Civil rights for mentally ill clients have been suggested by Congress for states to adopt, and many states have in fact adopted guaranteed rights.

Mentally ill clients may be institutionalized either by their own consent or through the power of the state. A client may not be involuntarily committed by the state merely for being mentally ill, but most states permit commitment when a client is dangerous to himself or others or is gravely disabled. Proving that the client meets the state criteria for commitment involves numerous procedural safeguards concerning the hearing, counsel, and length of commitment. If clear and convincing evidence of the client's dangerousness or grave disability is presented and due process is followed, the state may involuntarily commit the client. A right to treatment and the LRA principle are two emerging trends influencing the commitment process. Minor children may also be committed to mental hospitals, but the law typically does not guarantee them the full due process rights guaranteed to adults. Criminal clients enter mental hospitals if they are found not guilty by reason of insanity or are found incompetent to stand trial.

In dealing with the mental health system the client has the right to consent to treatment if the client has the mental capacity, has voluntarily given consent, and is informed. The client who is competent has a right to refuse treatment, but the courts have still not fully decided if involuntarily committed clients can refuse treatment. If a client is not competent, a legal guardian may consent to what the client would permit if the client had the capacity to consent.

Mental health law will change with new statutes and court decisions. The nurse needs to be aware of the most recent legislation to know the client's rights and the nurse's obligations. The nurse may also influence the law by testifying about the nursing standard of care as an expert witness and by active participation in the political process.

REFERENCES AND SUGGESTED READINGS

1. *Addington v. Texas,* 441 U.S. 418 (1979).
2. American Nurses' Association: Code of ethics, Kansas City, 1976, The Association.
3. Amicus brief in *Okin v. Rogers,* Mental Disability Law Reporter **2**:43, 1977.
4. Andrade, P., and Andrade, J.: Malpractice of psychiatric nurse, Proof of Facts 2d **26**:363, 1981.
5. Beck, J.C.: The potentially violent patient and the Tarasoff decision in psychiatric practice, Washington, D.C., 1987, American Psychiatric Press.
6. Brakel, S.J., and Rock, R.S., editors: The mentally disabled and the law, Chicago, 1971, The University of Chicago Press.
7. Brooks, A.D.: Law, psychiatry, and the mental health system, Boston, 1974, Little, Brown & Co.
8. *Cobbs v. Grant,* 8 Cal. 3d 229, 104 Cal. Rptr. 505, 502 P. 2d 1 (1972).
9. Cole, R.: A patient's right to refuse antipsychotic drugs, Law, Medicine and Health Care 9(4):19, 1981.
10. Cooke, G., editor: The role of the forensic psychologist, Springfield, Ill., 1980, Charles C Thomas, Publisher.
11. Creighton, H.: Law every nurse should know, ed. 4, Philadelphia, 1981, W.B. Saunders Co.
12. Diamond, B.L.: The psychiatric prediction of dangerousness, University of Pennsylvania Law Review **123**:439, 1974.
13. Ellis, J.: Volunteering children: parental commitment of minors to mental insitutions, California Law Review **62**:840, 1974.
14. Ellis, J.: Commitment proceedings for mentally ill and mentally retarded children. In Schetky, D.H., and Benedek, E.P.,

editors: Child psychiatry and the law, New York, 1980, Brunner/Mazel, Inc.
15. Greenlaw, J.: On concealing mistakes, Nursing Law and Ethics 1(8):5, 1980.
16. Hickman, F.J., and Abrams, R.: The preparation and trial of a civil commitment case, Mental Disability Law Reporter **5**:201, 1981.
17. *Humphrey v. Cady,* 405 U.S. 504 (1972).
18. *In the Matter of Guardianship of Richard Roe III,* 421 N.E. 2d 40 (Mass. 1981).
19. *In the matter of N.B.,* 620 P.2d 1228 (Mont. Sup. Ct. 1980).
20. *Jackson v. Indiana* 406 U.S. 715 (1972).
21. *Kaimowitz v. Department of Mental Health,* 2 Prison L. Rptr. 433 (Cir. Ct. Mich. 1973).
22. Kjervik, D.K.: The psychiatric nurse's duty to warn potential victims of homicidal psychotherapy outpatients, Law, Medicine and Health Care 9(6):11, 1981.
23. Klein, J.I., MacBeth, J.E., and Onek, J.N.: Legal issues in the private practice of psychiatry, Washington, D.C., 1984, American Psychiatric Press.
24. Laben, J.K., and McLean, C.P.: Legal issues and guidelines for nurses who care for the mentally ill, Thorofare, N.J., 1984, Slack, Inc., Publishers.
25. Legal issues in state mental health care: proposals for change—civil commitment, Mental Disability Law Reporter **2**:75, 1977.
26. *Lessard v. Schmidt,* 349 F. Suppl. 1078 (E.D. Wis. 1972), remanded 414 U.S. 473 (1974), on remand 379 F. Suppl. 1379 (1974), remanded 421 U.S. 957 (1975).
27. Matthews, D.B.: The right to refuse psychiatric medication, Medicolegal News 9(2):4, 1980.
28. Mental Health Systems Act, PL 96-398. U.S. Congress, 96th Congress, 1980.
29. *Mills v. Rogers,* 102 S. Ct. 2442:(1982).
30. National Mental Health Act, PL 79-487, U.S. Congress, 79th Congress, 1946.
31. *O'Connor v. Donaldson,* 442 U.S. 584 (1979).
32. *Parham v. J.L.,* 442 U.S. 584 (1979).
33. Pavalon, E.I.: Human rights and health care law, New York, 1980, American Journal of Nursing Co.
34. *Pisel v. Stamford Hospital,* 180 Conn. 314, 430 A2d 1 (1980).
35. *Rennie v. Klein,* 476 F. Suppl. 1294 (D.N.J. 1979), modified and remanded 653 F.2d 836 (3rd Cir. 1981), cert. denied 49 U.S.I.W. 3911 (U.S. 1981).
36. Right to refuse treatment under state statutes, Mental Disability Law Reporter **3**:350, 1979.
37. Rights of disabled persons in residential facilities, Mental Disability Law Reporter **3**:350, 1979.
38. *Roe v. Wade,* 410 U.S. 113 (1973).
39. *Rouse v. Cameron* 373 F (D.C. Circuit) 2451 1966.
40. *Salgo v. Leland Stanford, Jr., University Board of Trustees,* 154 Cal 2 560, 317 p. 170 (1st District, 1957).
41. State laws governing civil commitment, Mental Disability Law Reporter **3**:206, 1979.
42. A.A. Law, Psychiatry and morality essays and analysis, Washington D.C., 1984, American Psychiatric Press.
43. Suggested statute on civil commitment, Mental Disability Law Reporter **2**:127, 1977.
44. Suggested statute on mental health standards and human rights, Mental Disability Law Reporter **2**:305, 1977.
45. Suggested statute on mental health treatment for minors, Mental Disability Law Reporter **2**:473, 1978.
46. *Superintendent of Belchertown State School v. Saikewicz,* 370 N.E.2d 417 (Mass. 1977).

47. *Tarasoff v. Board of Regents of the University of California,* 131 Cal Reptr 14, 551 P 2d 334 (1976).

48. Tiano, L.V.: *Parham v. J.R.:* Voluntary commitment of minors to mental istitutions, American Journal of Law and Medicine **6:**125, 1980.

49. Turnbull, H.R., editor: The least restrictive alternative: principles and practices, Washington, D.C., 1981, American Association on Mental Deficiency, Inc.

50. *Vitek v. Jones,* 445 U.S. 480 (1980).

51. *Winters v. Miller,* 446 F.2d 65 (2nd Cir. 1971), cert. denied, 404 U.S. 985 (1971).

52. *Wood v. Strickland,* 420 U.S. 308 (1975).

53. *Wyatt v. Stickney,* now *Wyatt v. Aderholt,* 325 F. Suppl. 781 (M.D. Ala. 1971), 344 F. Suppl. 373 (M.D. Ala. 1972), 344 F. Suppl. 387 (M.D. Ala. 1972), aff'd 503 F.2d 1305 (5th Cir. 1974).

54. *Young v. Group Health Cooperative of Puget Sound,* 535 F. Suppl. 776 (D. Ark. 1976).

ANNOTATED BIBLIOGRAPHY

American Bar Association: Mental Disability Law Reporter, Washington, D.C.

This bimonthly magazine focuses on the disabled, including the mentally ill. It presents current cases and laws that affect this population. Although it is written mainly for lawyers, it is the most comprehensive summary of current law on the disabled.

Ennis, B.J., and Emergy, R.D.: The rights of mental patients, New York, 1978, Avon Books.

This is an American Civil Liberties Union handbook for mental patients. It presents current law in lay terms on involuntary hospitalization, civil and criminal commitment, and rights in or out of the hospital. It also has fact sections on the problem of defining mental illness and an appendix on drug descriptions, side effects, and dosages.

Simon, R.I.: Clinical Psychiatry and the Law, Washington D.C., 1986, American Psychiatric Press, Inc.

An up-to-date case review and instructive commentary on legal concerns in the psychiatric practice.

Turnbull, H.R., editor: The least restrictive alternative: principles and practices, Washington, D.C., 1981, American Association on Mental Deficiency, Inc.

This is a guide to understanding the meaning of the legal term "least restrictive alternative." Its descriptions of various alternatives are useful for client referrals.

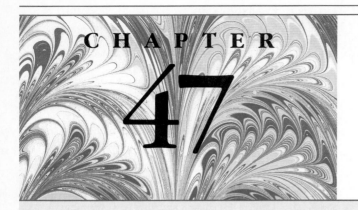

CHAPTER 47

RESEARCH

Lynne Brooks   Marilyn M. Bunt
Mary Patricia Ryan

After studying this chapter the learner will be able to:

Discuss the history of mental health–psychiatric nursing research.

Explain research approaches in mental health–psychiatric nursing.

Discuss concerns of measuring human behavior.

Identify major sources of instruments to measure behaviors associated with the five dimensions of the person.

Discuss important legal and ethical considerations.

Research provides nurses with information needed for making clinical decisions. Generally nurses' clinical decisions are intuitive. Practice was historically by trial and error; what seemed to work well was passed on by word of mouth. As nurses organized, more information was gathered, giving nurses more of a scientific base for their intervention. The participation of nurses in academic research in the past 30 years has given credibility to professional nursing practice. Scientific research is necessary to generate, support, or refute knowledge.[22]

The interpersonal nature of psychiatric nursing lends itself to a combination of subjective and objective data. However, designing research studies of human behavior is difficult. Variables used are often abstract and hard to define precisely. Measurements of human behavior are mostly indirect. Smoyak[51] reports that mental health–psychiatric nurses have trouble applying research findings to practice. Therefore, research from other disciplines involving human responses is often used as a guide in nursing interventions.

Research, integral to nursing, is included in the American Nurses' Association's (ANA) Standard of Psychiatric–Mental Health Nursing[3] (see the box on p. 894). Mental health–psychiatric nurses need to be familiar with the structure, process, and outcome criteria outlined in Standard XI.

The increasing number of clinical studies in mental health–psychiatric nursing is documented in a monograph by the Western Interstate Commission for Higher Education,[60] which summarized the number and topics of studies from 1954 through 1980. The majority of studies in the professional and graduate student literature concern nurses themselves. However, there is increasing investigation of clinical issues.

APPROACHES TO RESEARCH

One basic distinction among research approaches is that between experimental and nonexperimental research. In *experimental research*, the investigator deliberately manipulates some condition or phenomenon to assess the effects of the manipulation on some other condition or phenomenon. In *nonexperimental research* the investigation centers on the description of existing conditions or phenomena.

Another distinction concerns the type of data to be evaluated. Quantitative data are those which are represented numerically and may be handled through some statistical technique. Qualitative data may be verbally descriptive of some phenomenon but may be difficult or impossible to convert into a logical numerical framework.

A detailed discussion of the various research approaches, including conditions under which each is most appropriately applicable, may be found in Campbell and Stanley[12], Kerlinger[33], Fox[26], Polit and Hungler[40], and Seaman and Verhonick.[47] However, several research ap-

Historical Overview

DATE	EVENT
1915	Tucker conducted one of the earliest surveys in mental health–psychiatric nursing service that demonstrated the conditions under which mental health–psychiatric nurses functioned.
1928	Taylor did a study on educational qualifications of mental health–psychiatric nurses.
1946	The training grants provided by the National Mental Health Act of 1946 had a significant impact on psychiatric nursing research.[14]
1949	The establishment of the National Institute of Mental Health and psychiatric nursing as a clinical specialty provided funds for psychiatric nursing education and enabled psychiatric nurses to develop research expertise.
1950s	Early studies on nursing care of neuropsychiatric patients exceeded research in all other clinical fields in volume and quality.[48] Nurses participated in and co-authored broad studies of psychiatric care with other professionals.
1956	At the First Midwest Conference on Psychiatric Nursing, Marian Kalkman emphasized the pressing need for nursing research in state hospitals.
1960s	After the community mental health movement, psychiatric nursing research began to deal with the nurse-client relationship.
1983	Monograph reported that the number of studies on psychiatric nursing care increased from 28 between 1954 and 1959 to 825 from 1975 to 1980 (Table 47-1).
Future	With increasing emphasis on short-term hospitalization and prevention of illness, nurses will conduct research on healthy people.

TABLE 47-1 Mental health–psychiatric nursing topics of master's theses in nursing and selected literature

Concept Name	Number of Studies from 1954 to 1980	Concept Name	Number of Studies from 1954 to 1980
Nursing activity		Locus of control	11
Teaching individual	22	Compliance	19
Teaching group	20	Substance abuse	18
Therapy, individual	44	Obesity	9
Therapy, group	47	Life events	34
Behavior modification	12	Social and emotional need	16
Inpatient (hospital, nursing home)	91	Death and dying (suicide)	16
Outpatient (clinic)	54	Loss and grief	6
Child (0-12)	70	Empathy	9
Adolescent (13-19)	41	Stress	20
Adult (20-60)	29	Coping and adjustment	18
Elderly (61+)	57	Instrument development	9
Family (marital and parenting)	49	Instrument use	7
Nonpsychiatric diagnosis	66	Studies of nurses and others	267
Psychiatric diagnosis	133	Nursing management functions	23
Depression	16	Nursing care delivery	37
Anxiety	31	Health care delivery	3
		Self-esteem	28

Modified from Western Interstate Commission for Higher Education: A sourcebook: research in psychiatric mental health nursing, Boulder, Colo., 1983, Western Interstate Commission for Higher Education, p. 3.

ANA PSYCHIATRIC MENTAL HEALTH
STANDARD XI: RESEARCH

The nurse contributes to nursing and the mental health field through innovations in theory and practice and participation in research.

RATIONALE

Each professional has responsibility for the continuing development and refinement of knowledge in the mental health field through research and experimentation with new and creative approaches to practice.

STRUCTURE CRITERIA

1. Formal opportunities exist for nurses to conduct and/or participate in research at appropriate educational levels.
2. Mechanisms ensure protection of human rights.

PROCESS CRITERIA

The nurse:

1. Approaches nursing practice with an inquiring and open mind.
2. Uses research findings in practice.
3. Develops, implements, and evaluates research studies as appropriate to level of education.
4. Uses responsible standards of research in investigative endeavors.
5. Ensures that a mechanism for the protection of human subjects exists.
6. Obtains expert consultation and/or supervision as required.

OUTCOME CRITERION

The nurse has published contributions to theory, practice, and research.

---

proaches deemed particularly relevant for mental health–psychiatric nursing will be briefly discussed, with examples of their use.

Qualitative Comparative Analysis

A fairly recently described method or approach to research is that of *qualitative comparative analysis,* or grounded theory, described by Glaser and Strauss.[30] This approach is important for theory development, especially in an area in which theoretical bases for explaining phenomena are lacking. Using the qualitative comparative analysis approach, the researcher enters the situation without having formulated specific hypotheses or questions, armed only with the general area of interest. Observations are made in great detail and with great breadth. The researcher then leaves the situation and attempts to discover, from the qualitative data gathered, the variables that are present in the situation. Gradually as variables and relationships are identified through a series of entries into the situation followed by organization and conceptualization of the data accumulated, the researcher constructs the theory by using a combination of inductive and deductive reasoning. The theory is grounded in the phenomena in question through this process. The theory then needs to be tested in some new situation, with the researcher using a more formal research approach to validate its construction.

The method of qualitative comparative analysis was used by Wilson[59] in generating explanatory propositions concerning the process of limiting intrusion. Wilson's research setting was an experimental treatment community for individuals suffering from schizophrenia. This research approach may be of potentially great significance for mental health–psychiatric nursing, in which theory development is a major goal.

Case Study

The *case study* is a descriptive survey that focuses on one or a limited number of units. The unit of study may consist of an individual, a group, or an institution. The method involves an attempt to discover, in depth, multiple attributes of the unit. Typically the case study involves a longitudinal approach, with intense study of changes that occur over time. Data may not be subject to statistical interpretation but may require qualitative analyses.

Case studies may be conducted to aid in understanding phenomena or may involve an attempt to fully understand a problematic situation in which intervention is needed. The study may provide a baseline from which to proceed. The researcher is able to employ a dynamic process, moving in the most appropriate direction as information unfolds and interpretations are made. Many researchers in mental health–psychiatric nursing have used the case study method. Two classical examples are Freud and Piaget. Freud, in his study of Dora,[28] used the case study method in his intense analysis of the events involving an 18-year-old woman who came to him with severe attacks of coughing. Freud was able to qualitatively analyze current and remembered events in Dora's life, including two significant dreams, to understand the young women's hysterically based cough.

Piaget clearly used the case study in his detailed observations of his three children in their early months of life in *Play, Dreams and Imitations in Childhood.*[38] Again, the in-depth longitudinal approach allowed Piaget to come to a full understanding of the development of imitation and other phenomena in his infant children.

Causal Comparative Research

Causal comparative research is an extension of correlational research in that the researcher attempts not only to discover relationships among variables of interest but also to identify the possible cause after the effects have already occurred. With this approach, as with other descriptive approaches, the research cannot manipulate or directly control the variables. The investigator selects two or more groups that are known to differ on some phenomenon of interest and works retrospectively form the effect in attempting to discover variables that might be related to or explain the observed differrences.

For example, a researcher who is interested in depression in the elderly may wish to identify factors that are related to and possibly causative of depression in this group of individuals. She may begin by selecting a sample of elderly persons who either were clinically diagnosed as depressed or scored in the depressed range of scores on an instrument designed to identify depressed persons, such as the Depression Inventory.[6,7] She may then select a second sample of elderly persons who are identified either clinically or by the instrument to be within the normal range. Thus the subjects fall into the appropriate groups on the basis of their diagnoses or scores. The researcher then gathers data on a variety of factors that she has determined to be related to or presumably causative of depression.

The researcher needs to recognize that causal comparative research is descriptive; that is, any factors which are identified must not be interpreted as causative of the condition being investigated. Because the variables are uncontrolled and the subjects are not randomly selected or assigned to groups, any relationships identified are descriptive and may be interpreted only as possible causes. Further study and a more rigorous approach is needed to establish a true causal relationship.

MEASUREMENT OF BEHAVIOR

Research in mental health–psychiatric nursing often involves the measure of behavior. These measurements can be indirect or direct. Direct measurements are mostly physiological, such as laboratory tests and blood pressure, pulse, and respiration measurement. Accurate measurement of abstract psychological characteristics such as anxiety, dependency, and hope are more technical and therefore difficult to achieve when compared to measuring physical characteristics such as body temperature and blood pressure. Tools or instruments, such as questionnaires, are used most often in mental health–psychiatric nursing research. These instruments may be constructed by investigators or borrowed from journals or books. A number of authors have prepared collections of instruments for the mental health–psychiatric nursing researcher.[13,15,37,41,43]

The researcher tries to identify instruments that measure the variables of the study as accurately and precisely as possible, which generally is not an easy task.

Many difficulties with instrumentation have been addressed by nurse researchers; an entire issue of *Nursing Research* (September-October 1981) was devoted to this problem. Reliability and validity of instruments especially are areas of concern in the study of human behavior. *Reliability* refers to the consistency or repeatability of measurement of the same behavior under similar conditions. It is difficult to establish reliability in behavioral research, in part, because repeated measurements may affect the characteristics the researcher wishes to measure. Fluctuation in the individual, poorly standardized instruction, and errors resulting from measurement subjectivity are examples of influences that lower the reliability of psychological measurements. The nurse can improve reliability by (1) writing clear items for the measuring instrument, (2) adding more items of equal kind and quality, and (3) writing clear and standard instructions.[33]

More doubt is expressed by professionals concerning the validity rather than reliability of psychological measurement. *Validity* refers to the extent to which an instrument is purported to measure. A precondition for validity is reliability. An instrument cannot be valid if it is unreliable. There is often congruence between objects being measured such as physical qualities and relatively simple characteristics of persons and the measurement instrument; however, less is evident in the measurement of complex behavior. The nurse can attempt to validate the measurement instrument by (1) content validation—judging the representativeness of the content of the measuring instrument, (2) criterion validation—a comparison of the scale scores with external variables, criteria, believed or known to measure the characteristic of the person under study, and (3) construct validation—validating the theory that explains the differences in the behavior measured.[33]

Dingeman and others[17] conducted a study to determine the reliability and factor structure of the Nurses' Observation Scale for Inpatient Evaluation (NOSIE) using a group of 247 short-stay psychiatric clients. Items were grouped into six or seven factors: social competence, social interest, personal neatness, irritability, manifest psychosis, retardation, and depression. The clients were rated on each item of the NOSIE by two psychiatric nurses independently. The results were very similar among American, English, and Dutch patients (except for the social competence and personal neatness subscales in the Dutch). Therefore the instrument's reliability and validity were supported.

The competence of clients to complete the instrument as expected is also a concern. Medication and particular symptoms, such as psychosis, may affect clients' ability to respond validly. Any differences in the measurement setting may affect the results for a particular client. Thus the researcher needs to be thoroughly familiar with the instrument to be used.

SOURCES OF RESEARCHABLE QUESTIONS

Researchable questions or problems in mental health–psychiatric nursing may stem from a variety of sources, including theory, the literature, and nurses' own experience. The practitioner in mental health–psychiatric nursing needs to collaborate with the nurse researcher to develop questions and problems for study directly relevant to clinical practice. Questions arise in daily practice that, when placed in an appropriate framework and properly developed, can be researched. Questions about the clinical area are frequently initiated this way. A study may be suggested by a specific problem or a more general need. In either case research questions may involve the client, nurse, client-nurse interactions, setting, interventions, or anything of curiosity.

Cohen's study[16] exemplifies research of a client problem. He noted the high anxiety levels in clients about to undergo ECT and used specific emotional support as an intervention. Stricklin's study[53] demonstrates research on

TABLE 47-2 The highest fifteen priorities of mental health–psychiatric nurses

Rank	Item
1	After identifying factors that contribute to repeated hospital admissions, determine and evaluate interventions that reduce readmission among VA clients with chronic problems.
2	Explore the factors that relate to continuity of care after hospitalization, with emphasis on the nurse's role.
3	After developing criteria to assess clients compliance, explore those interventions that enhance the client's response to the health maintenance program.
4	After examining contributing factors to staff burnout, determine various ways to deal with this phenomenon in the VA system.
5	Identify factors that influence and increase psychiatric symptomatology in hospitalized VA patients.
6	Identify assessment criteria to predict potentially suicidal clients and preventive nursing interventions for self-destructive behavior.
7	Evaluate the effectiveness of various approaches to care planning on client care and nursing staff satisfaction.
8	Develop reliable and valid criteria to assess client's readiness to learn, and evaluate the effects of teaching clients.
9	Explore and evaluate supportive measures to enhance the care of terminally ill clients and their families (for example, hospice, Brompton's solution, and family counseling).
10	Explore the effects of treatment approaches such as milieu therapy, chemotherapy, and specific nursing interventions for clients with psychiatric problems..
11	After exploring the role of the VA in providing health maintenance and prevention programs, identify and evaluate effective methods for accomplishing this.
12	Determine effective approaches to motivate staff to provide quality care for veterans.
13	Define quality nursing care and develop valid and reliable criteria to measure it.
14	Identify factors that contribute to successful implementation of primary nursing in VA health care settings.
15	Explore nursing comfort measures to help clients manage and tolerate pain.

Adapted from Ventura, M.R., and Waligora-Serafin, B.: Study priorities identified by nurses in mental health settings, International Journal of Nursing Studies **18**:41, 1981.

the nurse. She looked at interobserver reliability in documenting the assessment record of the mentally ill client. Many questions about the interaction between the client and nurse can be posed. An example is an investigation of the effect of the nurse's leadership style on client behavior in group therapy. Questions about setting may include a comparison of the effects of rape victim counseling in the hospital emergency room with counseling in the victim's home. Many studies have been done to evaluate interventions. A 1973 study by Anderson[4] evaluated the use of videotape feedback as a psychotherapeutic nursing approach with long-term psychiatric clients. A number of questions have come from researcher curiosity: What are the characteristics of elderly persons who choose to attend a program on human sexuality? Are there differences among various cultural groups in coping styles? What changes occur in relationships with significant others in younger compared with older bereaved individuals in the first year after the death?

To establish priorities in mental health–psychiatric research, a study was conducted using the Delphi Technique. Opinions of 367 Veteran Administration (VA) nurses were gathered to identify areas in which nurses needed to conduct research.[56] As seen in Table 47-2, a top priority was to identify factors that contributed to re-

TABLE 47-3 Ideas for research from ANA standards

Nursing Intervention	Client Outcome
Psychotherapeutic	Regains or improves previous coping ability
Health teaching	Prevents further disability
	Demonstrates acquisition of knowledge
Activities of daily living	Attains level of ability in self-care in acute and rehabilitation phases
Somatic therapies	Incorporates knowledge of somatic and drug therapies into self-care activities
Therapeutic environment	Is oriented to schedule and rules for milieu
	Knows reasons for and condition of release from restraint or seclusion
	Demonstrates awareness of environmental effects on health
Psychotherapy (individual, group, or family)	Articulates elements of therapeutic contract
	Demonstrates responsibility for therapeutic work
	Shows movement toward goals of therapy

From Western Interstate Commission for Higher Education: A sourcebook: research in psychiatric nursing, Boulder, Colo., 1983, Western Interstate Commission for Higher Education.

peated admissions and effective assessment and interventions. Client teaching, care planning, and methods to assist staff with motivation were also seen as high priorities.

The ANA standards of nursing practice provide ideas for research that focuses on testing relationships between nursing interventions and client outcomes (Table 47-3).

Research questions may also arise from the literature. Studies published in *Nursing Research* and other journals often conclude with suggestions for related research. Juxtaposition of several studies may create an idea for another. Descriptions of particular interventions, an instrument, or methods may serve as a stimulus for a project. Often a study may be replicated with another sample, another setting, or some variation that can increase knowledge about the problem being investigated.

Theory may serve as a source of researchable problems. According to Stevens,[52] theory serves a descriptive or explanatory function, whereas research is intended to test the description or explanation.

Researchable questions may develop as the nurse interacts with professionals from related disciplines. The nurse researcher may wish to compare aspects of her practice with those of others. For example, how do nursing interventions compare with interventions used by social workers or clinical psychologists? Because nursing is a practice discipline, theories of many other disciplines have served to stimulate ideas for nursing research in the past and are likely to continue to do so in the future. Theories on stress, families, change, and adaptation are only a few that are relevant to mental health–psychiatric nursing. Behavioral theories are particularly significant.

ETHICAL AND LEGAL CONSIDERATIONS

ANA's Human Rights Guidelines for Nurses in Clinical and Other Research[2] provide a framework for involving clients in investigation. It identifies human rights—the right to freedom from intrinsic risk or injury and the right of privacy and dignity. Informed consent means that a person knowingly, voluntarily, intelligently, and in a clear and manifest way gives consent to participate in experimental procedures.[18]

Several principles in ANA's Code for Nurses[1] emphasize the nurse's obligation to safeguard confidential information about a client obtained from any source. The researcher explicitly ensures confidentiality by the consent form given to each prospective subject asked to participate in research.

FUTURE RESEARCH

The question of what lies ahead for nursing was the subject of an issue of *The American Nurse.*[1] The future of nursing is seen to be focused on prevention, the aging populations, and distributive care. Research emphasis will move from basic to applied areas of excesses, such as smoking and obesity.

Sills[48] proposed that mental health–psychiatric nursing research focus on determination of boundaries of health,

which subsume the boundaries of nursing care. Sills also recommended research on healthy individuals and quality of life rather than existing illness. Fleming[25] also urged that research be done in areas of preventive health, nursing care, and conditions likely to persist in the future.

In the 1984 and 1985 forum to discuss issues in psychiatric nursing the Council of Directors of Graduate Programs identified the need for research studies to examine the relationship between clinical research and public policy decisions. The council also stated that research needs to examine the concept of reversibility in organic disorders and that research must demonstrate what nurses offer as clinicians. Research also needs to examine the effects of rapid societal changes.

The uses of psychotherapy and family therapy are instances of the nurse's expanded role that need to be explored. Interpersonal systems theories and crisis and rhythm theory are presented in the expanded role.[23]

Smoyak[51] wrote that research on interactions between therapists and clients is needed. Generally, she identified a need for research that documents which interventions work and when they work with families. Specifically she gave direction to an area of study by investigating the contract between therapist and client. Smoyak raises the question, "Is the contract one that the therapist wants or the client wants?"

Classifying psychiatric patients will also require research. The problems of identifying behaviors and the less defined procedural emphasis makes classification difficult, largely because of the interpersonal nature of mental health–psychiatric nursing. Confidence in a given system depends on being certain of its validity and reliability. Some systems sufficiently classify clients according to nursing care needs, whereas other systems have not been adequate. Psychiatric client classification systems need to incorporate identifiable behaviors and have less emphasis on procedural aspects. Studies like Schroder and others'[47] need to be done to determine the validity and reliability of a client classification system on psychiatry.

The future direction of research in this field is toward health and wellness, incorporating a more holistic approach to client care.

BRIEF REVIEW

Research is important for mental health–psychiatric nurses to add to their knowledge base, improve practice, and move toward professionalization of the discipline. The focus of research in nursing has moved from the study of educational programs and functions and characteristics of nurses to clinical issues in client care, influenced throughout by current issues and needs and major professional nursing organizations.

Recent studies focus on one or more of the five dimensions of the person. Methodological approaches relevant to mental health–psychiatric nurse researchers are descriptive-nonexperimental and experimental methods. Research questions may be generated from within nursing practice or related areas. Sources of researchable questions include theory, published or unpublished literature, and the nurse's own practice.

Measurement of behavior is problematic because of the individual's complexity. An important prerequisite to reliable and valid research is the selection of instruments that appropriately measure the variables in question. Traditional standardized tests and other instruments can be found in compendiums on nursing or psychological variables and published and unpublished studies. Uniformity in administration is essential for valid research.

Future research in mental health–psychiatric nursing is likely to be applied as opposed to basic, focusing on healthy individuals, preventive health issues, and problems that are likely to persist. Also, theory testing and classification systems will be investigated.

REFERENCES AND SUGGESTED READINGS

1. American Nurses' Association: Code for nurses with interpretive statements, Kansas City, 1976, American Nurses' Association.
2. American Nurses' Association: Human rights guidelines for nurses in clinical and other research, Kansas City, 1975, The Association.
3. American Nurses' Association: Standards of psychiatric and mental health nursing practice, Kansas City, 1982, The Association.
4. Anderson, C.: Use of videotape feedback as a psychotherapeutic nursing approach with long-term psychiatric patients: a pilot study, Nursing Research 22:507, 1973.
5. Baker, B., and Lynn, M.: Psychiatric nursing consultation: the use of an inservice model to assist nurses in the grief process, Journal of Psychiatric Nursing and Mental Health Services 17(7):43, 1979.
6. Beck, A.T.: Depression, Philedelphia, 1967, University of Pennsylvania Press.
7. Beck, A.T., and others: An inventory for measuring depression; Archives of General Psychiatry 4:561, 1961.
8. Brandt, P., and Weinert, C.: The PRQ: a social support measure, Nursing Research 30:277, 1981.
9. Brooking, J.: Psychiatric nursing research, City?, Year?, John Wiley & Sons, Inc.
10. Brower, H., and Tanner, L.: A study of older adults attending a program on human sexuality: a pilot study, Nursing Research 28:36, 1979.
11. Brown, E.: Newer dimensions of patient care. II. Improving staff motivation and competence in the general hospital, New York, 1962, Russell Sage Foundation.
12. Campbell, D., and Stanley, J.: Experimental and quasi-experimental designs for research, Skokie, Ill., 1963, Rand McNally & Co.
13. Cattell, J., and Warburton, F.: Objective personality and motivation tests, Chicago, 1967, University of Illinois Press.
14. Chamberlain, J.: The role of the federal government in development of psychiatric nursing, Journal of Psychosocial Nursing and Mental Health Services 21(4):11, 1983.
15. Churn, K., Cobb, S., and French, J., Jr.: Measures for psychological assessment, Ann Arbor, Mich., 1975, Survey Research Center.
16. Cohen, R.: The effect of specific emotional support on anxiety levels prior to electroconvulsive therapy, Nursing Research 19:169, 1970.
17. Dingemans, P.M., and others: A cross-cultural study of the reliability and factorial dimensions of the nurses' observation scale for inpatient evaluation (NOSIE), Journal of Clinical Psychology 40(1):169, 1984.
18. Downey, M.: A bill to regulate Defense Department experimental procedures in human subjects (HR 13457), U.S. Senate, 94th Congress, second session, April 29, 1976. In Arniger, B., Sr.: Ethics in nursing research, Nursing Research 26:334, 1977.
19. Downs, F.S.: A sourcebook of nursing research, Philadelphia, 1984, F.A. Davis Co.
20. Downs, F.: The relationship of findings of clinical research and development of criteria: a researcher's perspective, Nursing Research 29:94, 1980.
21. Dracup, K., and Meleis, A.: Compliance: an interactionist approach, Nursing Research 31:31, 1982.
22. Fawcett, J.: A declaration of nursing independence: the relationship of theory and research to practice, Journal of Nursing Administration 10(6):36, 1980.
23. Fitzpatrick, J.J., and others: Nursing models and their psychiatric mental health applications, Bowie, Md., 1982, Robert J. Brady Co.
24. Flaskerud, J.: Perceptions of problematic behavior by Appalachians, mental health professionals, and lay non-Appalachians, Nursing Research 29:140, 1980.
25. Fleming, J.: The future of nursing research. In Downs, F., and Fleming, J., editors: Issues in nursing research, New York, 1979, Appleton-Century-Crofts.
26. Fox, D.: Fundamentals of research in nursing, ed. 4, New York, 1982, Appleton-Century-Crofts.
27. Fox, D., and Leeser, I.: Readings on the research process in nursing, New York, 1981, Appleton-Century-Crofts.
28. Freud, S.: Dora: an analysis of a case of hysteria, New York, 1963, Thomas Y. Crowell Co., Publishers.
29. Friedeman, J.: Development of a sexual knowledge inventory for elderly persons, Nursing Research 28:372, 1979.
30. Glaser, B., and Strauss, A.: The discovery of grounded theory: strategies for qualatative research, Chicago, 1967, Aldine Publishing Co.
31. Gortner, S.: Nursing research: out of the past and into the future, Nursing Research 29:204, 1980.
32. Haller, K., Reynolds, M., and Horsley, J.: Developing research based innovation protocols: process, criteria, and issues, Research in Nursing and Health 2:45, 1979.
33. Kerlinger, F.: Foundations of behavioral research, New York, 1964, Holt, Rinehart & Winston
34. Krampitz, S., and Pavlovich, N., editors: Readings for nursing research, St. Louis, 1981, The C.V. Mosby Co.
35. Marram, G.: Barriers to research in psychiatric–mental health nursing: implications for preparing the nurse researcher, Journal of Psychiatric and Mental Health Services 14(4):7, 1976.
36. Miller, T.: Life events scaling: clinical methodological issues, Nursing Research 30:316, 1981.
37. Pfeiffer, J., and Heslin, R.: Instrumentation in human relations training, Iowa City, 1973, University Associates.
38. Piaget, J.: Play, dreams, and imitation in childhood, New York, 1962, W.W. Norton & Co., Inc. (Translated by C. Gattegno and F.M. Hodgson.)
39. Pincus, H.A., and Pardes, H.: Clinical research careers in psychiatry, Washington, D.C., 1986, American Psychiatric Press.
40. Polit, D., and Hungler, B.: Nursing research: principles and methods, ed. 2, Philadelphia, 1982, J.B. Lippincott Co.
41. Robinson, J., and Shaver, P.: Measures of social psychological attitudes, Ann Arbor, Mich., 1973, Institute for Social Relations, University of Michigan.
42. Rose, L.E.: Ethical considerations of patient involvement in clinical psychiatric research, Canadian Mental Health 34(2):8, 1986.

43. Rugh, J., and Schwitzgebel, R.: Instrumentation for behavioral assessment. In Ciminero, A., Calhoun, K., and Adams, H., editors: Handbook of behavioral assessment, New York, 1977, John Wiley & Sons, Inc.

44. Schanding, D., and others: A small study of how the staff of an inpatient psychiatric unit spends its time, Perspectives in Psychiatric Care 10(2):91, 1982.

45. Schmidt, S.: Withdrawal behavior of schizophrenics: application of Roy's model, Journal of Psychosocial Nursing and Mental Health Services 19(11):26, 1981.

46. Schroder, P.J., and others: Testing validity and reliability in a psychiatric patient classification system, Nursing Management 17(1):49, 1986.

47. Seaman, C., and Verhonick, P.: Research methods, ed. 2, New York, 1982, Appleton-Century-Crofts.

48. Sills, G.: Research in the field of psychiatric nursing, 1952-1977, Nursing Research 26:201, 1977.

49. Simmons, L., and Henderson, V.: Nursing research: a survey and assessment, New York, 1964, Appleton-Century-Crofts.

50. Slavinsky, A., and Krauss, J.: Two approaches to the management of long-term psychiatric outpatients in the community, Nursing Research 31:285, 1982.

51. Smoyak, S.: Clinical practice: institute or based on research, Journal of Psychosocial Nursing and Mental Health Services 29(4):9, 1982.

52. Stevens, B.: Nursing theory: analysis, application, evaluation, Boston, 1979, Little, Brown & Co.

53. Stricklin, M.L.: The mental health patient assessment record: interobserver reliability, Nursing Research 28:11, 1979.

54. Topf, M., and Dambacher, B.: Predominant source of interpersonal influence in relationships between psychiatric patients and nursing staff, Research in Nursing and Health 2(1):35, 1979.

55. Ventura, M., Hinshaw, A., and Atwood, J.: Instrumentation: the next step, Nursing Research 30:257, 1981.

56. Ventura, M.R., and Waligora-Serafin, B.: Study priorities identified by nurses in mental health settings, International Journal of Nursing Studies 18:41, 1981.

57. Western Interstate Commission for Higher Education: A sourcebook: research in psychiatric mental health nursing, Boulder, Colo., 1983, Western Interstate Commission for Higher Education.

58. Williams, M., and others: Nursing activities and acute confusional states, Nursing Research 28:25, 1979.

59. Wilson, H.: Limiting intrusion: social control of outsiders in a healing community, an illustration of qualitative comparative analysis, Nursing Research 26:103, 1977.

60. Wilson, H.: Deinstitutionalized residential care for the mentally disordered: The Soteria House approach, New York, 1982, Grune & Stratton, Inc.

61. Wilson, H.S., and Hutchinson, S.A.: Applying nursing research, Reading, Mass., 1986, Addison-Wesley Publishing Co., Inc.

62. Youssef, F.A.: Adherence to therapy in psychiatric patients: an empirical investigation, International Journal of Nursing Studies 21(1):51, 1984.

ANNOTATED BIBLIOGRAPHY

American Nurses' Association Commission on Nursing Research: Human rights guideline for nurses in clinical and other research, Kansas City, 1975, The Association.

This gives detailed consideration to the protection of human rights and free informed consent. Also stated is the expectation that protocols will document procedures to be followed in obtaining consent.

Chaska, N., editor: The nursing profession: a time to speak, New York, 1983, McGraw-Hill Book Co.

This excellent compendium of important nursing issues devotes a section to research.

Fox, D.: Fundamentals of research in nursing, ed. 4, New York, 1982, Appleton-Century-Crofts.

This book presents specific steps for planning and implementing nursing research projects using any of a wide variety of methodologies.

Polit, D., and Hungler, B.: Nursing research: principles and methods, ed. 2, Philadelphia, 1982, J.B. Lippincott Co.

This comprehensive text provides a background for selecting, defining, and placing a nursing research problem appropriately into theoretical context and developing the problem into a proposal from which a study can be implemented and a report written.

U.S. Department of Health and Human Services: Psychiatric–mental health nursing: proceedings of two conferences on future directions, Washington, D.C., 1986, U.S. Government Printing Office.

These proceedings document current perspectives on specific systems that affect psychiatric–mental health nursing. Strategies for implementing goals to improve education, practice, research, and policy are developed.

Western Interstate Commission for Higher Education: A sourcebook: research in psychiatric mental health nursing, Boulder, Colo., 1983, Western Interstate Commission for Higher Education.

This monograph discusses issues in psychiatric–mental health nursing. A summary of topics of master theses and literature and a listing of studies in psychiatric–mental health nursing are presented.

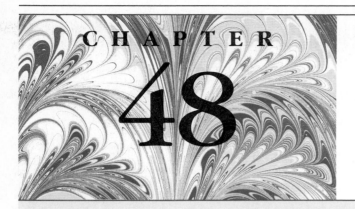

CHAPTER 48

QUALITY ASSURANCE

Elizabeth B. Brophy   Diane M. Hedler

After studying this chapter the learner will be able to:

Define the concept of quality assurance.

Critique the American Nurses' Association standards of care in mental health–psychiatric nursing.

Give examples of protocols for nurses.

Integrate the key components of a quality assurance program.

Analyze modes of professional development in terms of their effects on client care.

Differentiate among licensure, certification, and accreditation.

Understand the concept of third-party payments.

Show how the quality assurance concept can be applied to various nursing models.

Quality assurance is the process by which the maintenance of excellence in the provision of health care is ensured. The term quality encompasses such descriptions of care as acceptability, affordability, effectiveness, and comprehensiveness. *Assurance* refers to a process that includes the identification of values and standards, specification of criteria, measurement of observable aspects of care, and remedial action if indicated. In this chapter quality assurance is defined more specifically as a process by which (1) appropriate criteria related to client care are identified and (2) mechanisms are developed to ensure the measurements and achievement of specified criteria.

Quality assurance is an important aspect of mental health–psychiatric nursing for several reasons. First, federal funds, particularly those provided through Medicare, Medicaid, and maternal and child health programs, are available only after evidence is provided that predetermined standards of care have been met. Similar procedures have also been assumed by state agencies. Other external forces requiring formal assessment programs are accrediting groups such as the Joint Commission on Accreditation of Hospitals (JCAH).

Second, quality assurance programs help nurses monitor their own practices in a systematic way. Mental health–psychiatric nurses want to ensure that the quality of their care contributes to the optimal mental health of

the person, the family, and the community. By developing and implementing procedures that demonstrate the quality of care rendered and by designing programs to lessen the deviations from the established criteria, nurses can maintain the standards and ideals they have developed.

Finally, quality assurance is important to the public's confidence in health care professionals. The increased involvement of insurance companies and other private and public organizations in the evaluation of health care systems suggests that the general public's confidence in the quality of services delivered by health professionals has eroded. Thus quality assurance programs are one way in which professional nurses regulate their profession in order to maintain a high level of nursing practice and at the same time retain the confidence of the public.

KEY COMPONENTS IN QUALITY ASSURANCE

Quality assurance programs involve several key components. *Standards of care* in mental health–psychiatric nursing practice, *criteria* specific to practice, and *protocols* for nursing interventions provide the basis for developing *audits* or review of care procedures on the institutional, departmental, or unit basis. Reviews may also be conducted within an individual or *peer-review* format. The *levels of practice* manifested by the therapeutic skills

Historical Overview

DATE	EVENT
1858	Florence Nightingale documented her attempts to raise the standards of health care in the Crimean War.
1912	E.A. Codman introduced the first system of medical audit.
1913	American College of Surgeons introduced accreditation for medical education and performance.
1923	Goldmark Report recommended closing substandard nursing schools, instituting 48-hour workweek, and encouraging staff nurses rather than student nurses to assume responsibility in hospitals.
1948	Brown Report, funded by Carnegie Foundation, recommended national accreditation for nursing schools and affiliation of hospital schools with universities.
1955	*Hospital Progress* made reference to evaluation by means of nurses' notes. American Nurses' Foundation was formed to conduct, sponsor, and stimulate research.
1956	Commission on Professional and Hospital Activities, Inc. was formed.
1957	Thayer Hospital, Waterville, Maine, developed the nursing audit plan.
1960	Sr. M. Deeken developed a guide for the nursing service audit.
1965	American Nurses' Association (ANA) wrote its position paper on entry into practice. National League for Nursing (NLN) provided a self-evaluation guide to assess nurses' functions and skills.
1967	Yura and Walsh defined evaluation as one of the four functions of the nursing process. D. Slater developed a rating scale with six dimensions of nursing behavior.
	Amendments were made to Medicare and Medicaid legislation.
	Utilization review committees were created.
1970	Wandelt and Agar developed the Quality Patient Care Scale (Qual-PaCS), based on observation and rating.
	JCAH shifted focus from provision of minimal to optimal care by means of retrospective medical care audits.
1971	ANA Commission on Economic and General Welfare and Congress for Nursing Practice recommended work on peer review, joint practice, and audits.
1972	Carter and others developed the nursing process criteria.
	Phaneuf published *The Nursing Audit: Profile for Excellence.* Amendments to the Social Security Act created the PSROs in an effort to overcome the deficiencies of the utilization review committees; this shifted the responsibility for assessing care from hospitals to local groups of physicians.
	American Hospital Association's Patient Bill of Rights, Social Security amendments (PL92-603), and patient evaluation procedure (PEP) for health professionals were introduced.
1973-1974	ANA published generic and division standards based on the nursing process.
1974	Medicus/Nursing Care Systems recommended development of process and outcome criteria and use of retrospective and concurrent monitoring.
	JCAH developed discharge outcome criteria and critical management elements for disease-oriented diagnostic categories.
1975	Federal government reviewed regulations regarding institutional review requirements consistent with Professional Standards Review Organizations (PSRO) system.
1976	ANA formed interdivisional Council on Certification.
	ANA set forth model for implementing standards of care and published the *Quality Assurance Workbook.*
	A section on the quality of professional services was added to JCAH *Accreditation Manual for Hospitals.*
1979	The credentialing study was reported in Madison, Wisconsin.
	Revision of mental health–psychiatric standards of practice was initiated.
	JCAH accreditation manual for hospitals was totally revised, with problem-focused approach to quality assurance activities.
1982	Revised standards of psychiatric–mental health nursing practice were published.
1983	Passage of H.R. 1900 (PL98-21), the Social Security Amendment of 1983, established prospective payment system based on 467 diagnostic-related group (DRG) categories for pretreatment diagnosis billing.
1984	Psychiatric, rehabilitation, and substance abuse hospitals or units were exempted from DRGs.
Future	The development of patient classification systems and nursing diagnoses for psychiatric clients will contribute to the effective utilization of mental health–psychiatric nurses and more precise interventions.

of nurses may also be addressed during the review process.

Professional development activities, as part of a quality assurance program, may be part of the continuing education program within the hospital or agency being reviewed or in other institutions, such as colleges, in which programs are made available by qualified nurse educators. Another form of professional development is graduate education in nursing. Nurses may enroll in master's or doctoral programs for advanced level preparation in clinical practice, research, education, administration, or a combination of these. Professional development is an important factor in the maintenance and upgrading of care.

Allied concepts (for example, credentialing) are also considered. *Credentials* provide evidence of credibility and competence. Three types of credentials are commonly considered within the context of the quality assurance process. *Licensure* involves the legal right of nurses to provide nursing services for remuneration. *Certification* is a nongovernmental recognition of the achievement of predetermined standards in a specialized area of nursing.

The quality assurance process will vary, depending on the practice model being implemented. Mental health–psychiatric nurses function in institutional and noninstitutional settings and focus on a variety of age groups and categories of illness in any given setting. Quality assurance programs are planned to explore the particular aspects of care that are pertinent to a specific setting.

Many nurses today believe that improvement in access to, and quality of care is linked to securing *third-party reimbursement* for their services.[17] To secure such allocation of funds for nursing services, professional nursing care will need to be differentiated from that rendered by allied professionals. Finally, participation in professional activities is one mark of the professional individual and is inextricably linked with quality assurance.

Quality assurance programs elicit evidence of effectiveness, efficiency, and accountability. Data of this nature may be used to request funding, report costs, plot future courses of action, gain community support, provide immediate feedback to nurses, and improve the quality of institutional or agency care of the client.

Overall, the major ramifications of quality assurance activities are an increased awareness and upgrading of the degree of excellence required in mental health–psychiatric care in any given institution and the provision of feedback to individual nurses who are directly involved in providing this care. For truly professional nurses this systematic kind of evaluative response, both positive and negative, is desirable.

Standards of Care

In mental health–psychiatric nursing standards of care are drawn from the available knowledge about human behavior, the norms of the groups who care for the mentally ill, and the values that have been identified by those who call themselves mental health–psychiatric nurses. Examples of such norms and values include the right of clients to be safeguarded in whatever settings they may be placed while receiving care, to experience a sense of personal acceptance, and to be provided with therapeutic modes of intervention. Standards of care derived from such bases provide guidelines for professional behaviors through which the desired quality of care can be achieved. The ANA *Standards of Psychiatric and Mental Health Nursing Practice*[8] constitute just such a firm and carefully developed basis for nursing interventions.

For a number of reasons the implementation of the ANA standards in everyday practice is a difficult task. First, the complexity of each client—his situation, personal dynamics, and responses—cannot be underestimated and needs to be considered in specific ways. At the same time the role functions and expectations of the nurse may vary according to the setting. For example, the clinic nurse may assume primary responsibility for individual therapy. Consequently, standards of care that are generally comprehensive in nature need to be applied in a manner that is consistent with the characteristics of each client and each setting.

Second, nurses are frequently involved in dependent functions (such as implementing physicians' orders) and independent functions (such as the ongoing assessment of nursing care) at the same time. The psychiatrist and the nurse basically share responsibility for planning the client's treatment. Realistically, however, not all physicians accept this position. Therefore nurses strive to implement standards of care based on the nursing profession's expectations regarding their capabilities. These standards may or may not be accepted by health professionals with whom nurses work. To add to the complexity of the situation each nurse brings a unique knowledge and skill base to the nursing role. When procedures are designed to assess whether the accepted standards of care have been implemented, it becomes a difficult task to identify which aspects of client outcome are directly attributable to nursing intervention. When psychiatrists and nurses collaborate in therapy four factors regarding standards of care are in operation: the ANA standards representing the expectations of the nursing profession, the nurse's personal belief and value systems, the American Medical Association (AMA) standards representing the expectations of the medical profession, and the psychiatrist's personal belief and value systems.

Nurses owe primary loyalty to the client rather than to the institution, the profession, or the physician. However, institutional regulations often impinge on aspects of care and modes of therapeutic intervention. Various sources of conflict are possible. Nurses functioning as client advocates may find themselves in contention with the institution, the physician, or both. The physician and the nurse together may not agree with the institutional position. For example, a psychiatrist and a nurse may believe that a female client can benefit from visits by her 15-year-old son who is her only child. However, the institution has a strict rule that does not allow minors to visit in the psychiatric unit. Obviously, important factors have been introduced, including the nurses's relationship and responsibility to the employer as well as to the client. Consequently, when involved in client care nurses are not able to use the ANA standards of care or any other set of standards in isolation but need to generalize the intent and characteristics of the standards while incorporating their own abilities and the possibilities of the setting in which they function.

Several sources of standards of nursing care have been identified; however, the question "Who really sets standards of nursing care?" may legitimately be asked. In many cases specific nursing standards and nursing protocols have been developed in response to the requirements set by JCAH when hospital accreditation is the major goal. Nurses, particularly those functioning in middle-management roles, tend to seek guidelines from professional nursing organizations. Consequently, publications such as the ANA's *Standards of Psychiatric and Mental Health Nursing Practice*[8] significantly influence professional nurses in their standard-setting activities. Concepts and ideals presented in ANA and NLN publications are reviewed by nurses in clinical practice and evaluated within the context of clinical realities. In addition, input is available and often mandated by government agencies. state boards of nurse examiners, state nursing organizations, and state health departments. The result is a unique combination of ideas flowing from experience, situational realities, professional ideals, and individual personalities.

Some commonalities in the standards of nursing care may be identified from hospital to hospital and from agency to agency. At the same time, idiosyncratic features may also be found and are often related to the availability of technological facilities or to cultural viewpoints in a particular state or region. This is a desirable situation because the various institutions in which nurses practice are indeed different, and the standards of nursing care need to be appropriate and relevant to the setting.

The manner in which standards for mental health–psychiatric nursing practice are developed often involves a task force or other committees and presentations of preliminary statements of standards to the members of the organization for criticism and revision. Nurses who are most influential in the development of standards are probably those who have achieved a significant level of expertise in a particular functional area, who have completed graduate education, and who have been recognized by their peers as being outstanding in some professional nursing role.

Criteria

Criteria are specific, predetermined rules or principles developed by health care professionals for a given setting and against which the health care practices implemented in that setting are compared. Three types of criteria are generally used: structure, process, and outcome criteria.

Structure criteria indicate the aims and purposes of the institution, agency, or program and can be designed for the institution or agency, the client, or the nurse. In structure criteria, statements may be made about the philosophy and objectives of the institution or agency, the physical facilities, the administrative organization, fiscal management, government and accreditation regulations and standards, and the policies and procedures of the institution or agency. Examples of structure criteria in mental health–psychiatric nursing practices are (1) the expectation that staff nurses have completed a course in group therapy and (2) the requirement that each client in the mental health unit have a primary and associate nurse assigned to provide care. Accreditation manuals provide additional structure criteria. Accreditation agencies require that administrators organize and record the specific processes that provide the means by which structure criteria are used during a quality assurance review.

When structure criteria are used it is necessary to verify that adequate resources are available to provide necessary services. In other words, nurses need adequate knowledge, equipment, support personnel, and facilities for the provision of quality care.

Process criteria are used in the evaluation of actions and the sequence of behaviors and events during the provision of client care. During a concurrent audit the activities of professional and nonprofessional personnel during the assessment and management phases of client care are evaluated. Examples of a process review as it may occur in mental health–psychiatric nursing include (1) documentation of the therapeutic one-to-one relationship and progress notes related to clients' movement toward identified goals, (2) evidence that clients for whom medication has been ordered receive instruction about the medication, and (3) data to indicate whether or not the nursing care plan was developed, with input from the client and the primary nurse within 72 hours of admission.

The use of process criteria is an opportunity to identify problems that occur while caring for clients and to take immediate measures that can change or improve the final outcome of care. These criteria also enable the nursing department to evaluate the extent to which nursing care activities are completed, the implementation of policy and procedures, and the activities of the team coordinator of each component of care.

Outcome criteria are developed to evaluate the end result of the care and services provided to the client. A discernible change occurs in the health status of the client after medical and nursing care has been implemented. Only when outcome factors are compared to pertinent criteria can the nurse know that the goals and objectives of care have been reasonably achieved.[2] Examples of outcome criteria are the client's orientation to time, place, and person and his responsibility for activities of daily living when discharged from the hospital.

One difficulty with the use of outcome criteria is the fact that only the outcomes or effects of intervention are reviewed. If the outcomes are evaluated as not reaching the level stated in the predetermined criteria, it is difficult to determine whether some aspects of the nursing process were poorly implemented or client motivation and cooperation were lacking. For example, a withdrawn client may be discharged without having responded verbally except with close family members. If the client's communication patterns were apparently unchanged, it would be helpful to analyze the steps of the nursing process as they were implemented during treatment and the client characteristics and behaviors observed by the caregivers. In such a situation a process audit becomes desirable.

Once the desired criteria are chosen, quality assurance administrators may need to consider whether the audit is to be discipline specific. For example, nurses may choose to audit only a particular aspect of care within their clinical specialty. Auditors may choose to evaluate nursing interventions to promote sleep in depressed clients whose sleep patterns are disturbed.

Protocols

A protocol is "an instrument that guides a practitioner in the collection of data and recommends specific action based on that data."[11] Protocols are used primarily by nurses in primary care facilities and in rural areas. Usually a protocol is a written statement of signs and symptoms, with a list of necessary or desirable laboratory or other diagnostic procedures, and of specific indications of therapeutic interventions that may be followed by the care provider when the person functioning in this role is not a physician. Another type of protocol is composed of guidelines to be used in chronic illnesses when a health care provider is overseeing the progression of the disease in the client. Interventions may be limited with the expectation that during acute phases, referrals to physicians will be made.

In hospital quality assurance programs protocols may be defined as statements of behaviors identified as discrete steps used by nurses in the clinical role. These activities are employed by nurses in the attainment of long- and short-term goals. By stating nursing behaviors precisely and in sequence, nurses become more aware of procedures and are able to identify specific stages in client care that have been accomplished well or poorly.

In mental health–psychiatric nursing, particularly in community mental health nursing, protocols involving the use of medications may become more commonly used than at present. Certain factors influence the acceptability of protocols such as the number and availability of qualified psychiatrists, the difficulty in assessing and evaluating symptoms, the frequency with which specified conditions are encountered, and the expected severity of the client's responses.

Protocols for mental health–psychiatric nurses are usually developed by a multidisciplinary committee composed of professional health providers who function within that setting. Members of the committee are most often physicians because they are recognized as health team leaders and have the right to prescribe medications. It is acceptable for such a committee to review published protocols for adaptation and use in a given setting.

Such committees may also develop protocols after a careful review of the literature that is focused on biochemistry, manifestations of psychiatric disorders, and appropriate treatment modalities. Pathological conditions that may be seen need to be identified and diagnostic tests specified. For example, a client may come into a community mental health clinic complaining of being depressed

and unable to cope with life's demands. The protocol includes such biological assessments as a complete physical examination, urinalysis, SMA-18, chest x-ray study, and perhaps the rapid dexamethasone suppression test or the thyrotropin stimulation test. Psychological tests may include the Minnesota Multiphasic Personality Inventory, the Beck Depression Scale, and the standardized National Institute of Mental Health Diagnostic Interview. Finally, guidelines related to intervention need to be stated as clearly and concisely as possible.

While protocols are being developed arrangements are made for emergency referrals to appropriate consultants or, at a later time, to the psychiatrist responsible for the unit or agency. Nurses using protocols also need to seek a periodic review of client records to validate the effectiveness of the treatment modalities employed.

The most critical problem with protocols is the legal constraints placed on nursing practice. The nurse practice acts in many states limit the definition of nursing functions. Only physicians are licensed to sign prescriptions for medications and x-ray and laboratory studies. In using protocols nurses seek to perform the functions that lie within their area of expertise, thus making certain procedures available to clients when a physician is not present and furnishing the physician with necessary data about complex conditions that require medical review, diagnosis, and treatment.

The use of the standardized procedures found in protocols may also be viewed as limiting nursing interventions because approaches need to be highly individualized. The degree of restriction in what the nurse is allowed to do may be related to the number and availability of physicians and primary care nurses in a given state, region, or community.

Protocols may be written in such a way as to reduce the legal vulnerability of the health care provider or the agency. For instance, the possibility exists that the required number of diagnostic procedures may be excessive. The freedom to order basic diagnostic tests as recommended in the protocol, without being forced to order unnecessary tests, is critical if nurses are to be able to use protocols effectively.

In summary, protocols may be used in several ways: (1) to direct nursing interventions, (2) to intervene in client care when physicians are not available, and (3) to serve as specific statements of nursing behaviors that can be incorporated into quality assurance activities.

Patient Classification Systems

To the professional nurse today, patient classification systems and nursing diagnoses are important and related constructs. Both, if carefully developed and used, can help to identify the knowledge base and the nursing behaviors that are specific to mental health–psychiatric nurses.

The term *patient classification system* refers to the "identification and classification of patients into care groups or categories, and to the quantification of these categories as a measure of the nursing effort required."[15] Classification systems may be used to estimate staffing patterns for nurses by describing what nurses do. A major problem in the care of mentally ill clients is the difficulty in establishing broad categories and/or methods of quantification—for example, when the focus of care is on an adolescent who is "acting out."

In an attempt to use the nursing diagnoses developed by NANDA in the care of mentally ill clients, many mental health–psychiatric nurses have tended toward the DSM-III-R classification system because it includes behavioral terms and is used by allied health professionals, such as psychiatrists and psychologists. However, in 1984, because of a lack of relevant psychiatric nursing diagnoses, a task force was set up by the Executive Committee of the ANA Division of Psychiatric and Mental Health Nursing Practice to identify and classify nursing diagnoses that can be used by mental health–psychiatric nurses. To date the task force has developed a classification system for nursing diagnoses organized according to three response classes: individual, interpersonal/family, and community/environment. They have concentrated their initial work in developing 12 response patterns within the individual response class.[21]

Patient classification systems and nursing diagnoses may foster effective use of nurses and precise intervention by nurses; however, it is important to remember that quality care is not guaranteed as a result of efficiency.[15]

Audits

Auditing in nursing is the verification that the nursing care given to clients is appropriate and in accord with the predetermined standards of nursing care in a particular clinical area. The JCAH, an organization that has had a great impact on quality assurance activities in health care agencies, has expanded the term audit to mean nursing care review and evaluation. This expanded term implies not only that many indicators of the quality of care need to be examined but also that the audit process needs to be continued as the framework for assessment of nursing care. Therefore, the terms audit and nursing care review will be used interchangeably in this chapter.

JCAH standards for nursing care require that professionally qualified nurses direct nursing care, that an organizational working plan and written procedures related to nursing care be maintained, that evidence of safe therapeutic care be presented, and that ongoing plans to update nurses' knowledge and skills be developed. In addition to JCAH, federal and state governments have mandated quality assurance activities on client care involved in federal- or state-funded health care programs.

Publications such as the *Statement on Psychiatric and Mental Health Nursing Practice*[3] and *A Plan for Implementation of the Standards of Nursing Practice*[1] provide guidelines for client care and nurses' actions. The ANA Congress of Nursing Practice also publishes a *Quality Assurance Update* to address current issues in the quality assurance process. In responding to the requirements of accrediting groups and in seeking to achieve the level of expertise recommended by nursing organizations, administrators of hospitals and agencies may choose to develop

standards and review procedures specific to their own setting or to adapt standardized review plans that are commercially available.

Audit programs developed by individual hospitals or agencies have the advantage of being specific to the setting and therefore probably have a high degree of validity. However, such institution-developed plans may suffer from some unclear, untested, and unreliable statements. On the other hand, carefully developed standardized audit programs or instruments contain clear, tested statements with indexes of reliability and validity.

One such standardized review program is Medicus, which was developed jointly by the Rush-Presbyterian–St. Luke's Medical Center in Chicago, the Baptist Medical Center in Birmingham, and the Medicus Systems Corporation. The Medicus Nursing Quality Assurance Monitoring System may be used in a mental health–psychiatric nursing unit.[26]

Six major objectives and 32 sub-objectives are used in the Medicus Nursing Monitoring System. The major objectives include the following[13]:

1. Formulation of a nursing care plan
2. Attention to the client's physical needs
3. Attention to the client's emotional, mental, and social needs
4. Evaluation of nursing care objectives
5. Attention to unit procedures for the protection of all clients
6. Collaboration in the delivery of nursing care by administrators and managerial personnel

This monitoring system is implemented by applying client-specific and unit-specific criteria related to the nursing process at the various levels of care.

Other instruments that may be used as a part of an ongoing audit process are also available. The Slater Nursing Competencies Rating Scale includes 84 items related to observable or measurable nursing behaviors that represent the critical elements of the nursing process. The following items, focused on actions directed toward meeting the psychosocial needs of individual clients, are taken from the Slater Scale[33]:

1. Gives full attention to the client
2. Is a receptive listener
3. Approaches the client in a kind, gentle, and friendly manner
4. Responds in a therapeutic manner to the client's behavior
5. Recognizes anxiety in the client and takes appropriate action

As implied in its title this scale requires a nurse observer and allows for ratings on a continuum from "best nurse" to "poorest nurse."[33] The Quality Patient Care Scale (Qual-PaCS) is a 68-item instrument derived from the Slater Scale. The Slater Scale is focused on the nurse's performance and involves observation of nursing interventions, whereas Qual-PaCS is focused on the client as the recipient of care. Both scales permit comparison of the quality of care received from different care-providing groups by various client groups in a variety of settings. The greatest challenge to persons using such standardized programs or instruments is to adjust them to the specific needs and characteristics of the setting.

Auditing, then, is a mechanism used to assess and verify the quality of client care. By referring to JCAH, PSRO, ANA, and government requirements for health care agencies, nurses can develop or adapt quality assurance activities that are specific to their area of practice and can become part of the client care review and evaluation process.

There are three types of audit: concurrent, retrospective, and prospective. These types of audits are discussed within the context of nursing care, although the concept may be applied in terms of the care provided by any group of health professionals, such as physicians and pharmacologists.

A *concurrent audit* is a method of evaluating ongoing activities (see Table 48-1). In mental health–psychiatric nursing, concurrent auditing involves an assessment, at the time of review, of one particular aspect of care provided to clients in treatment. For example, in a psychiatric unit the evaluators may want to ascertain whether side rails are up on the beds of confused elderly clients. During a concurrent audit, client charts, care plans, staff and client interviews, and observations of nursing care are components of the review. This type of audit allows corrective action to be taken immediately, thereby quickly improving the quality of care being rendered in the area. Immediate feedback also provides the nurse with a growth experience and an opportunity to develop greater capabilities in the clinical role.

In a *retrospective audit* the nursing process as it was applied during treatment is evaluated after services have been rendered (see Table 48-1). In this type of audit direct observation of nursing care is impossible; the completed medical record, nursing care plans, nurses' charts, interviews with staff members and former clients, staff conferences, and questionnaires are used to arrive at a realistic picture of past events. This kind of audit is the means by which corrective actions may be developed for clients who will require treatment in the future. One potentially serious problem in this kind of audit is that people are often forgetful. The length of time since treatment and the impact of the experience on the client or nurse influence the degree of retention of some of the facts that are essential for the evaluation. This emphasizes the importance of accurate recording to the auditing process.

A *prospective audit* resembles a descriptive study. Criteria are set, and a review of a defined number of clients with a specific diagnosis is made. For example, the care given to the next 20 clients diagnosed as being depressed may be studied. After a prospective review it is possible to develop criteria based on the observation of the care provided to the selected client sample.

Nurses may also be involved in a *multidisciplinary audit*. In this approach a particular client problem or diagnosis is selected. A multidisciplinary group establishes specific criteria appropriate to this problem or diagnosis. In the multidisciplinary audit process the performance of the various health professionals, such as the psychiatrist, psychologist, psychiatric nurse, and psychiatric social worker, who work to meet the criteria is reviewed. Reviewers may elect to audit the specific assessment procedures employed by the members of the team in working with suicidal clients. In multidisciplinary audits the total treatment may also be assessed with the goal of increasing the overall quality of care provided by the health team. In such a review nurses need to be sure that nursing standards are addressed and that they do not find themselves auditing only medical care and dependent nursing functions.

Operation of a Quality Assurance Program

In large institutions it is common for quality assurance committees for nursing to oversee all nursing review activities. The nursing quality assurance committee usually sets standards of care and may suggest specific criteria to be used in evaluation procedures. This group generally organizes the mechanical details of the program, setting up audit deadlines and frequently arranging for analysis of data.

When the audit or review takes place it is important to isolate the factors that negatively affect the quality of client care. Such factors can be identified from external and internal unit or area sources.[19] External source input is that from outside the unit or area: government reports of care in similar situations, client complaints, suggestions from other units, professional literature, and agency or department lists of nursing goals and objectives. Internal data sources include the unit's medical records, incident reports, surveys of clients and staff members, research and evaluation by staff members, previous audit results, and staff members' suggestions.

Once the problem or topic is identified, the type of criteria is chosen by the unit quality assurance committee members, unit administrator, and unit staff nurses. Decisions on the number and type of clients to be surveyed are then made. Criteria include statements of what is measured (for example, assessment of emotional needs), what source of data is used (for example, client interviews, medical records, and nursing care plans), and at what

TABLE 48-1 Types of audits: Differentiating factors

Factors	Concurrent	Retrospective	Prospective
Time of care	Ongoing	Past	Future
Data	Observation Records Interviews	Records Interviews	Predetermined criteria and plan of care
Significant consideration	Provides immediate feedback	Danger of forgotten or nonrecorded data	Focused on a specific diagnostic group

level the criteria need to be met (for example, 100% or 85%). Any exceptions to the criteria are stated (for example, disoriented clients will not be interviewed).

The topic, rationale, and criteria are then submitted to the quality assurance committee for review and evaluation before the study can be undertaken. Final approval for the study occurs on the unit level but only after the recommendations of the nursing quality assurance committee have been taken into account.

When the study plan is ready for implementation, data may be collected by the nursing quality assurance committee, unit staff members, or a person designated by the committee. After the data are obtained it is advisable for the unit staff nurses and supervisors to review the study process and make comments. The data are then analyzed either by institutional personnel or by computer. Computers are being used with increasing frequency because of the volume and complexity of the data collected and the time required for analysis.

When the data analysis is complete the unit staff nurses are informed of the results of the audit. Problems and probable causes are identified, criteria are reviewed with the nursing staff, corrective actions are recommended, and an appropriate follow-up plan is formulated. An audit summary report is then submitted to the quality assurance committee of the institution or agency.

Peer Review

Peer review is a process by which the quality of nursing care rendered by an individual nurse is evaluated by other psychiatric nurses actively involved in clinical nursing practice. The ANA[6] has identified peer review as a vital component of a quality assurance program, and it is now required for eligibility for third-party reimbursement by Civilian Health and Medical Program of Uniformed Services (CHAMPUS). Evaluation of individual nurse performance in quality assurance programs is different from the general evaluation of performance often initiated by employers. The goal of quality assurance programs is not only to review an employee's performance in terms of reward systems but also to improve overall client care.

Standards of care now constitute the foundation of the evaluation inherent in quality assurance programs, protocols provide step-by-step guidelines for nursing interventions, audits verify the appropriateness and outcomes of client care, and peer review allows the contributions of individual nurses to be appraised.

At present a staff nurse's performance is frequently assessed by means of self-evaluation, peer evaluation, and supervisor evaluation. Peer review procedures promote individual accountability and are often the primary way of recognizing clinical expertise. Peer review procedures also document nursing care and establish the degree of consistency between practice and predetermined standards. Obviously, observation of specific role behaviors is the best basis for evaluation. Many peer review programs have been fashioned after a behavioral model that is consistent with the concept of levels of practice.

Record keeping as a nursing responsibility has become a function that needs to be carefully incorporated into any peer review process. The use of DRGs in the care of hospitalized Medicare clients has influenced the nursing role. Because the allocation of federal funds is based on the utilization of hospital resources required by clients with similar health needs, the documentation of effective interventions has become essential for reimbursement. Nurses have always been expected to provide adequate charting of nursing care. Currently, however, nurses are asked to document nursing interventions and the specific effects of such procedures. They are expected to review the charting of client services rendered in ancillary departments and to note the completeness of medical reports and diagnoses.

A number of variables regarding the nursing role are included in a peer review. The provision of client care includes the nursing processes of assessment, analysis, planning, implementation, and evaluation, as well as collaboration with other health professionals. Professional development may include such behaviors as self-direction, maintenance of consistently high standards of care, and attendance at workshops and other educationally oriented activities. Client teaching may be categorized as part of the provision of nursing care or as a separate nursing function. Leadership and management skills may be considered another facet of the role, including such activities as delegation of responsibility, planning and implementation of in-service programs, and, in some cases, consultation. Research has long been recognized as a function of the nursing role, but it is only now being considered in peer review and performance appraisal activities.

Levels of Practice

The concept of levels of practice may be defined as a ranking or a degree of performance supported by a particular knowledge base and the development of required skills. Operationally, specific nursing behaviors that reflect comparable levels of practice are identified.

Client care may be evaluated by means of accepted standards of care, recognizing that all staff nurses are capable of specific basic role functions. However, the quality of care can be enhanced if attention is systematically given to the "fit" that exists between the client's specific needs and the nurse's level of expertise. The inclusion of the levels of practice concept in a quality assurance program provides a more precise description of the unit being evaluated and the level of care being rendered.

In mental health–psychiatric settings it is necessary to identify the beginning levels of theoretical knowledge and clinical practice that may be legitimately expected. The activities in this clinical area differ from those in other clinical specialties and need to be clearly defined in behavioral terms. Levels of practice need to be related to reasonable skill development; for example, the new baccalaureate graduate can be expected to participate in group therapy but not to assume full responsibility for a weekly therapy group of clients. Specific examples of criteria related to levels of practice are represented in Table 48-2.

TABLE 48-2 Criteria related to levels of practice in mental health–psychiatric nursing

Function	Level of Practice	Criteria
Communication	I	Uses communication skills of listening and problem-solving goals in the stages of the nurse-client relationship
		Participates in regular supervision of own nursing interventions
	II	Uses communication skills of confrontation and reflection to intervene in the expression of feelings and provide for attainment of therapeutic goals
		Participates in regular supervision of own nursing interventions
	III	Uses a therapeutic framework (for example, psychoanalytic, interpersonal, gestalt); interventions reflect appropriate communication responses and insight into nursing therapy
		Participates in regular supervision of own nursing interventions
	IV	Uses appropriate communication responses in the implementation of interventions; nursing therapy reflects a theoretical framework and definition of therapy issues and goals
		Participates in regular supervision of own nursing interventions
Education	I	Identifies need for personal and professional growth; attends all required unit and hospital in-service programs
		Attends formal education programs or earns a minimum of 8 to 12 continuing education units each year
	II	Initiates topics for in-service programs
		Identifies in-service needs for self and unit to continuing education committee member and unit nursing managers
	III	Conducts a minimum of one in-service program each year
		Provides orientation session for new graduate nurses
	IV	Plans, implements, and evaluates a continuing education or client education program
		Plans, implements, and evaluates an educational program relating to a mental health issue on or off the unit at least once a year

Levels of practice are based on the institutional philosophy and objectives, the nursing department's philosophy and objectives, and ANA standards of nursing practice. In addition, the ANA standards for mental health—psychiatric nursing are used when mental health–psychiatric nurses are involved.

Initially, a levels of practice committee is organized. This committee is composed of representatives of the different groups of nurses, such as administrators, clinical specialists, and staff nurses. After nursing criteria are complete and approved by the overall department, the mental health–psychiatric nursing group develops specific additional criteria.

When specific nursing behaviors are identified and correlated with levels of practice, staff nurses are provided with a system in which (1) increased knowledge and skills can be efficiently used and (2) continued professional development can be recognized. Until the concept of levels of practice was used, staff nurses who sought promotion within the system were usually forced to leave the clinical role and seek the next level of status and salary benefits in an administrative or educational role within the hospital. Nurses who remained at the bedside may have received salary increments based on length of service, but the staff nurse role remained static, placing the new graduate and veteran nurse on the same level within the organizational structure. A recognition of levels of practice therefore provides a way to acknowledge the experienced nurse as well as to differentiate skills among nurses with similar preparation and experience.

The need for precision in the utilization of nursing resources and for documentation of appropriate nursing care has been reemphasized with the advent of DRGs and similar cost-containment measures. Medicare funding for client care is dependent on the achievement of specific client goals, accurately reflected in written records that are clearly understood by the hospital community and the various funding agencies. With time such groups as the major insurance companies may not only review the skill level of the professional nurse who provided a particular aspect of client care, but even require that specific nursing functions be rendered only by those who can provide evidence of advanced practice or skill development.

Integration of Key Components in Quality Assurance

When standards of care, protocols, audit procedures, peer review, and levels of practice are discussed, it is important to be able to translate the theoretical ideas into practical behaviors that are observable and are either directly or indirectly related to client care. Behavioral interpretations of three standards of care are presented in Table 48-3. These standards are among the ANA standards for mental health-psychiatric nursing.[8]

It is also important to recognize that evaluation, when considered as a part of a broader audit procedure, involves all professional nurses who function in a particular area of an agency or institution. Although the data for quality assurance programs are obtained from individuals, final reports are made in terms of the group within the

TABLE 48-3 Application of three ANA standards of mental-health–psychiatric nursing practice to three quality assurance components

Protocol	Audit	Peer Review

STANDARD V-A—PSYCHOTHERAPEUTIC INTERVENTIONS: THE NURSE USES PSYCHOTHERAPEUTIC INTERVENTIONS TO ASSIST CLIENTS IN REGAINING OR IMPROVING THEIR PREVIOUS COPING ABILITIES AND TO PREVENT FURTHER DISABILITY

Protocol	Audit	Peer Review
Involvement of primary nurse in one-to-one therapeutic care	Review nursing care plan and progress notes to assess nursing interventions with alternate behavior patterns, limit setting, and interpersonal relationships Informally discuss progress and direction of therapy Interview client about nurse's attention to client's time and needs Interview other health professionals who are collaborating in client care about apparent changes in client problems identified in nursing care plan	Interview unit nurses about primary nurse's attention to client conferences, awareness of client problems, and so on Report progress of therapy, with expectation of peer feedback; provide evidence of appropriate consultation Provide written process recordings, audiotapes, and videotapes of individual sessions
Clarification of communication as part of coordination of client care, with professional personnel such as physicians, other nurses, and administrators and with nonprofessional personnel such as aides and nursing assistants	Ascertain effectiveness of communication among health professionals at unit staff conferences Review written progress notes Monitor end-of-shift report about understanding and implementation of care plan Interview nonprofessional personnel about their knowledge of care plan and awareness of pertinent intervention in a given situation based on information received from the primary nurse	Observe input provided by primary nurse at the multidisciplinary conferences Evaluate, over an extended period, the effectiveness of the end-of-shift report Review written progress notes Expect peers to substitute for primary nurse, using her care plans

STANDARD VIII—CONTINUING EDUCATION: THE NURSE ASSUMES RESPONSIBILITY FOR CONTINUING EDUCATION AND PROFESSIONAL DEVELOPMENT AND CONTRIBUTES TO THE PROFESSIONAL GROWTH OF OTHERS

Protocol	Audit	Peer Review
Determine quality of informal educational methods of professional development for individual nurse by means of discussions with peers and supervisors, consultations with other professional personnel, and use of institutional information resources on unit	Interview nurse Interview supervisory personnel Review number and types of professional books and periodicals checked out of library by nursing staff Note verbal or nonverbal indications of new awareness of therapeutic concepts, theories, or strategies	Evaluate informal discussions Note introduction of new ideas or concepts in unit meetings or reporting sessions Note any tendency to share new insights or strategies that can improve client care in unit
Determine extent of organized informational experience planned to improve knowledge and skills in areas of clinical expertise that have not been well developed in nurse	Review all continuing education activities at least annually Review budget in terms of amount of money made available for continuing education on a given unit Provide evidence of attendance at meetings, courses, and the like Confer with nurses involved in continuing education program to determine if they disseminate information obtained at workshops, courses, and the like Interview nurses on regular basis to review learning needs and achievements	Document whether or not new knowledge has been incorporated in provision of client care Invite persons to present in-service program based on workshops attended Interview peers in terms of improvement of care provided
Determine if any contributions were made to client care in units in which student nurses are placed	Observe staff nurses' responses when student nurses are functioning in area Interview clients about collaboration between staff nurses and student nurses in therapeutic matters Use interview or questionnaire to determine staff nurses' perceptions regarding student nurses on unit	Interview peers about perceptions of individual staff nurses regarding presence of student nurses on unit Interview student nurses in terms of their acceptance and learning experiences in psychiatric area

Continued.

TABLE 48-3 Application of three ANA standards of mental-health–psychiatric nursing practice to three quality assurance components—cont'd

Protocol	Audit	Peer Review

STANDARD XI—RESEARCH: THE NURSE CONTRIBUTES TO NURSING IN THE MENTAL HEALTH FIELD THROUGH INNOVATIONS IN THEORY AND PRACTICE AND PARTICIPATION IN RESEARCH

Protocol	Audit	Peer Review
Encourage an awareness of need for and appreciation of nursing research	Interview nurses about attempts to incorporate research findings in nursing practice and willingness to participate in research projects Review unit research activities on an annual basis Review budget in terms of funds requested or allocated for research purposes	Determine if staff members incorporate research factors in case presentations Interview staff nurses regarding their attitudes toward nursing research by identifying degree of support and assistance provided for individual research projects planned and implemented by individual nurses

From The American Nurses' Association: Standards of psychiatric and mental health nursing practice, Kansas City, Mo., 1982, The Association.

unit or the institution being reviewed. If the findings indicate a need for change this is considered in terms of the group or unit and not of the individual.

It is critical to coordinate standards of care, protocols, audit procedures, and peer review in such a way as to complete the quality assurance activities with a sense of having accomplished something of value. The result of these activities is improved client care. However, to attain the level of nursing care desired it is important to critique nursing interventions in a constructive manner to avoid alienating or dampening the enthusiasm of those involved. (For example, criticisms can be made by describing a specific behavior instead of assuming that one knows the nurse's rationale for her actions.) If while making an emphatic statement the nurse has the habit of shaking her finger at the person with whom she is speaking, this can be pointed out as an observed behavior. The pointing out of a specific behavior by the person providing feedback may allow the criticism to be accepted and acted on.

PROFESSIONAL DEVELOPMENT

The JCAH has established standards requiring staff development in health care institutions. This mandate is based on the assumption that such programs provide a method by which corrective responses may be made to negative findings in personnel and outcome audits. The objective of this attempt to meet identified needs or deficits and to encourage active participation in specialized roles and functions is improved client care.

The ANA[4] has taken the stand that professional nurses have the serious responsibility to become involved in a continuous learning process that builds on previously acquired knowledge and skill development. The various evaluation procedures involved in a quality assurance program provide a constructive way to improve one's skills and the quality of care rendered. Professional development and quality assurance programs are closely allied, and the relationship benefits the facility, clients, and nurses.

The term professionalism implies certain levels of competence in nursing practice and educational accomplishments that reflect breadth of knowledge, skills, and personal maturity. Nurses most commonly become involved in continuing education programs or in some form of graduate education.

Continuing Education

Continuing education includes short-term planned programs of courses under the direction of staff educators or academicians. Learning experiences are designed to enhance previously acquired knowledge and skills. Situational needs in each hospital or agency influence the content in continuing education programs. When planning inservice programs staff directors may refer to several ANA publications, such as the *Standards for Nursing Services*[2] and the *Standards for Continuing Education in Nursing.*[4]

If continuing education programs are to be successful it is important that nurse administrators approve of and facilitate their implementation. To do this, nurse administrators need to be in a position of authority, with the ability to channel the necessary funds and personnel required for well-conceptualized and well-organized programs.

Interinstitutional collaboration is one way in which the cost of continuing education may be contained. Audiovisual hardware, library materials, and personnel of one health agency may be involved in programs in another institution on an exchange basis.

College or university-based programs, sometimes called degree-completion or educational mobility programs, are also a form of continuing education. This enterprise is characterized by an effort on the part of nurse educators to differentiate between content considered essential to a generic baccalaureate nursing program and content that may be lacking for registered nurses working for a bachelor's degree in nursing. One solution is to require nurses to complete challenge examinations. This approach seems reasonable if the evaluators have a clear conception of what content is essential.

Graduate Education

Graduate education includes organized programs of study under the direction of professional educators in a college or university. The primary function of graduate education is to prepare nurse specialists with the additional knowledge and skills necessary to exercise independent judgment. The graduate of the basic baccalaureate program is considered a generalist; the graduate of the clinical master's program is considered a specialist. In other words, the professional nurse, the generalist, is expected to understand the basic principles of multiple clinical areas, such as medical-surgical and psychiatric nursing. On the master's level the nurse has the opportunity to study a specific clinical area in depth, combining specialized experiences and knowledge and thereby becoming a specialist in that area.

Nursing programs that terminate with a clinical master's degree usually focus on mastery of a common core of knowledge, expertise in a specialty area of nursing, and a research orientation designed to foster inquiry in the specialized area of study. In graduate mental health–psychiatric nursing programs, emphasis is usually placed on assessment, awareness of the most frequently encountered emotional problems and pathological conditions, appropriate nursing interventions, modes of evaluation, and research related to this clinical area. Nursing skills usually include practice in individual therapy as well as group and marital or family therapy. Students are given the opportunity to function in a variety of settings and are encouraged to practice collaboratively with other health professionals in the care of mentally ill clients. Graduates are also expected to have a critical understanding of issues relevant to mental health–psychiatric nursing and the promotion of mental health.

The doctorate is a critical degree for the advancement of the nursing profession. Members of any discipline who are prepared at this level are expected to preserve, expand, and transmit the knowledge that is critical to the discipline. Nurses prepared at this level are needed to teach in graduate programs, to function in clinical roles and administrative positions, and to conduct research in every aspect of nursing. Each year more doctoral programs in nursing are made available. As a result, the degrees of Doctor of Nursing Science (D.N.Sc.), Doctor of Nursing Education (D.N.Ed.), Doctor of Philosophy in Nursing (Ph.D.), Doctor of Public Health (D.Ph.), and others are awarded in much larger numbers than were awarded in the past.

In summary, professional development, whether through continuing education or graduate education, is important in order to retain the concept of quality assurance and quality nursing care. Nurses returning to the clinical area with a master's or doctoral degree contribute not only specialized knowledge but also broadened perspectives on their own capabilities and on the health care delivery system itself.

Use of structure, process, and outcome criteria for review of educational programs as well as for clinical practice helps identify and maintain the levels of excellence that are essential if the quality of care is to be assured.

CREDENTIALS

A *credential* attests to the institution's or person's qualifications to function in a particular area of expertise. To acquire a credential an institution or individual is identified by a recognized authority as having attained a predetermined set of standards at a given point in time. The purposes of credentials are to ensure quality care of clients and to protect the public. These purposes are inherent in any quality assurance program, and the possession of appropriate credentials constitutes a part of the audit process.

Any discussion of credentials is incomplete without reference to *The Study of Credentialing in Nursing*[5]; this study was conducted in Milwaukee in 1978 and 1979. The report identified four fundamental features of the process of acquiring credentials: quality, identity, protection, and control. These features will be referred to in the following comments. Within the context of nursing, critical credentials include licensure, certification, and accreditation of the educational programs involved in the preparation of professional nurses and clinical nurse specialists.

Licensure

Licensure is the process by which the legal right to practice nursing is accorded a person in a given state. It is the oldest, most familiar mechanism used in the United States to regulate the quality of services rendered. In most states, once a license is issued the person is required only to pay the annual fee and seek renewal of the license in question. Therefore licensure is used to identify the practitioner. In addition, it protects the recipient of care insofar as practices that do not reach minimal standards leave the practitioner open to legal action; thus limited control is possible.

Programs involving licensure of nurses are developed within the state legislature. Various states define the scope of practice differently and allow varying degrees of diagnosis and intervention by registered nurses. Furthermore, as the nursing profession has expanded, the states have granted the same licensure to graduates of diploma, associate degree, and baccalaureate degree programs.

In the 1978 ANA statement of resolutions, the profession identified two categories of nursing practice: the professional and the technical. Similar resolutions were upheld at the 1986 ANA Convention. The underlying premise is that the minimal preparation for entry into professional nursing needs to be the baccalaureate degree. In 1982 the NLN agreed with this premise, reaffirming it at the 1983 NLN National Convention[28] and again in 1986.[27]

Under the present system a board of nurse examiners or a similar group is part of the state structure involving the licensing of nurses. This allows for some degree of input or power by nurses within the implementation of the state law. Currently, in some states, consideration is being given to a type of institutional licensure. This approach places the power to grant or withhold licenses in the hands of hospital and agency administrators.

On the one hand advocates of institutional licensure

imply that state nursing licensure boards are self-serving. They suggest that institutional licensure will cut costs and promote efficiency by: (1) providing opportunities for evaluation of individual on-site performance, (2) allowing for innovative continuing education programs in hospitals, and (3) facilitating career mobility. On the other hand nurses focus on individual accountability for the quality of nursing care provided. If institutional administrators were to develop job descriptions for all health workers, nurses would probably no longer determine the scope of their own practice, job mobility might be hindered, formal nursing educational programs could be considered inappropriate, and nurses could be hired because of a salary category rather than on the basis of level of expertise.[16] Several basic questions deserve to be posed. Would institutional licensure improve the quality of health care? Would institutional licensure influence the current standards of nursing practice in a positive or negative way? Would the cost of an institutional licensing program be passed on to the consumer of health care, that is, the client?

Certification

Certification is the process by which a nongovernmental agency provides a reliable endorsement that a person has met certain predetermined standards in a specialized area of nursing. Certification procedures in nursing have been developed in order to protect the consumer and to recognize clinical expertise. This type of credentialing is voluntary, and nurses who elect to forego this process are not sanctioned. Professional organizations are primarily involved in certification procedures, although states and institutions have initiated programs seeking a legal endorsement of competency, particularly in areas of clinical specialization.

Specialty organizations, for example, the Association of Operating Room Nurses, provide specialized certification for members of their group. Mental health–psychiatric nurses are among those who have chosen to use the ANA certification program. Two levels of certification are available for mental health–psychiatric nurses. Registered nurses may apply for certification as mental health–psychiatric nurses after having practiced direct client care for at least 4 hours weekly, with 2 years of mental health–psychiatric nursing experience within the last 4 years and having had access to supervision. Certification as a clinical specialist may be obtained in adult or child and adolescent care. Requirements include a master's or higher degree in nursing with a specialty in mental health–psychiatric nursing, access to supervision, and experience in clinical practice in at least two different treatment modalities. Applicants on both levels must complete a comprehensive written examination.

In 1987 the ANA reported that 8,214 mental health–psychiatric nurses had been certified at the generalist level, 2,756 at the clinical specialist level in adult psychiatric nursing, and 317 at the clinical specialist level in child psychiatric nursing.[1]

The major problem in any consideration of certification is the lack of a standardized system that can be recognized by the profession and by the public. A major advantage to an acknowledged professional system of certification is the recognition of competency as a necessary basis for treatment and third-party payments.

PARTICIPATION IN PROFESSIONAL ACTIVITIES

Acquiring professional credentials involves evaluation of both individuals and institutions. By belonging to professional organizations either as an individual or as a member of a group, the professional nurse contributes to the maintenance of quality care. Following is a list of nursing organizations to which the mental health–psychiatric nurse may belong.

American Association of Colleges of Nursing
American Nurses' Association
   Cabinet on Nursing Education
   Cabinet on Nursing Practice
   Cabinet on Nursing Research
   Cabinet on Human Rights
   Council on Psychiatric–Mental Health Nursing
American Academy of Nursing
American Hospital Association
   Assembly of Hospital Schools of Nursing
   Staff Specialists in Nursing Education
International Council on Nursing
National League for Nursing
   Council of Baccalaureate and Higher Degree Programs
   Council of Home Health Agencies and Community Health Services
Nurses' Coalition for Action in Politics
Sigma Theta Tau (nursing honor society)

Mental health–psychiatric nurses frequently also belong to such nonnursing professional groups which include the following:

American Association of Suicidology
American Orthopsychiatric Association
American Personnel and Guidance Association
American Psychological Association
American Red Cross
American Society of Allied Health Professions
Association for Specialists in Group Work
Health Standards and Quality Bureau (formerly Bureau of Quality Assurance)
International Academy of Professional Counseling and Psychotherapy
National Alliance for Mental Illness
Women and Health Care

Although these lists are not exhaustive it is apparent that many nursing groups emphasize a particular clinical area or minority interest. This diversification of interest may reflect fragmentation among professional nurses; this is a critical aspect of professional development and quality assurance in nursing that needs attention.

Ineffective communication among the various interest groups tends to foster parochialism in professional nurses. *Networking* is a system of sharing information that creates links among people. This system focuses on reciprocal relationships. For example, a mental health–psychiatric nurse, working as a team member in an alcohol abuse program, contacts a nurse educator, requests and receives help in locating a research instrument, and at the same time agrees to share insights with students regarding the care of alcoholic clients. Networking helps develop resources that enable participants to satisfy their professional needs and to expand their professional interests. It allows for collaborative planning and the development of effective techniques for identifying, storing, retrieving, and linking resources.

THIRD-PARTY PAYMENT

A third-party payment is a reimbursement for services provided to a client by a person or group who is neither the provider nor the receiver of the services, for example, payment by an insurance company. For years nurses have sought a change in reimbursement policies related to health care services. Nurses believe that they can provide health maintenance programs and community-based care, especially in long-term illnesses, that would reduce the need for hospitalization and the overall cost of health care. Much of this is impossible at the present time because reimbursement policies, for the most part, are focused on the delivery of medical care. This approach emphasizes pathology and reinforces the practice of hospitalization.[17]

Although the concept of third-party payment to nurses has not been implemented widely, one event that may prove to be significant to a general acceptance of third-party reimbursement is the approval in 1982 of CHAMPUS, a provision in the Defense Appropriations Act. CHAMPUS is a federally supported medical program designed specifically for active and retired military personnel and their spouses and children. Certified psychiatric nurses and nurse practitioners are eligible for direct reimbursement for their services under CHAMPUS.

State insurance laws need to be considered in any discussion of third-party payments. Many health care providers and consumers recognize that the law in each state defines the limits of nursing practice, but not everyone realizes that the state insurance laws allow or disallow reimbursement to specific health professionals for health care services. In many states registered nurses may not be reimbursed by third parties because of restrictions in the insurance laws. For example, in August 1984 a bill providing third-party reimbursement for nursing services was vetoed by Governor Mario Cuomo of New York. In his veto message Governor Cuomo recognized this approach as a cost-efficient alternative for health care but found the bill "unacceptable" because it would lead to "fragmentation of payment."[9]

At the present time mental health–psychiatric nurses in Michigan, Washington, New Jersey, and West Virginia may be reimbursed for health care services but with varying stipulations in each state. Consequently, professional nurses seeking third-party reimbursement need to examine not only the definition of nursing in each state but also the insurance laws of the state. In practice many mental health–psychiatric nurses elect to function as therapists in community clinics or outpatient departments where third-party payments for services rendered are made to the agency. In this way mental health–psychiatric nurses function in the therapeutic role but are not paid directly for these activities.

It is obvious then that changes are indicated. Jennings[17] pointed out, however, that whereas technological advances in the health care industry have occurred rapidly, practices related to the economics of health care have tended to lag. Professional nurses need to work to be recognized by physicians and by the public as essential health care providers. It may happen that policy makers on the state and national levels will not make third-party payment a reality for professional nurses until evidence is available showing that quality health care rendered by nurses is cost-effective.

PRACTICE MODELS

Practice models may be defined as various patterns in the delivery of nursing services by which health care is made available to diverse groups of people in different settings. The most obvious distinction in practice models can be made when comparing nursing practice in institutional and noninstitutional settings. In the institutional setting the administrators delegate the responsibility for client care to the health professionals they employ. In noninstitutional situations the individual health professional is held directly responsible for the care rendered. It is especially important that nurses functioning in noninstitutional facilities implement review procedures on a regular basis because they assume a degree of responsibility that is more widely shared in a hospital setting.

Within the psychiatric hospital or the psychiatric unit of a general hospital, the staff nurse is usually responsible for a specific number of clients. The nurse is expected to confer with the psychiatrist, be sure the client receives the medications ordered, and assess the client in terms of nursing interventions that may include individual or group therapy. There is a certain sense of security in this practice site because the client is safeguarded during the entire period of hospitalization.

Joint practice represents another institutional practice model. Shortly after The National Joint Practice Commission was established in 1971, a study was funded by the Kellogg Foundation that allowed professional personnel in four American hospitals to work together to explore nurse-physician relationships. The five elements that were found to be essential in joint practice were (1) a joint practice committee, (2) primary nursing, (3) individual clinical decision making by nurses, (4) an integrated client record, and (5) a joint client care record review. The final evaluation of the project indicated that the quality of care was improved with joint practice.

The clinical nurse specialist role in either the hospital or the agency setting involves direct care responsibilities. In addition, the clinical specialist serves as a consultant for staff nurses and other nursing personnel, organizes and presents in-service educational programs, and identifies research findings that may be pertinent to clinical interventions. Whether the clinical specialist functions in a staff or line position depends on the organizational structure of the agency or institution and on the conditions of employment stipulated at the time that the clinical nurse specialist agrees to function as a member of the clinical staff.

In the outpatient department of a hospital or in a community mental health center, the nurse is assigned a caseload and arranges appointments for individual, group, marital, or family therapy. In this setting the nurse has a greater degree of autonomy than in the hospital units because clients are exposed to multiple stimuli outside the therapeutic milieu. Frequent intra-agency conferences involving health professionals within the agency provide opportunity for consultation.

The mental health–psychiatric nurse who functions in the school, industrial plant, or military agency is also a member of an institutional group. Although the nurse in the school or the factory may work alone or as one of a small group of nurses, the nursing activities that constitute the role are usually clearly described and may be limited.

The clinical nurse specialist who functions in a noninstitutional setting is involved with clients in a way that is considerably different from that observed in hospital settings. The nurse who chooses to function in private practice is the most obvious example. A mental health–psychiatric nurse in private practice functions on a fee-for-service basis not unlike that used by the private-duty nurses of the 1950s. The major difference, however, is that the private-duty nurse assumes responsibility only for the implementation of the physician's orders. In contrast, the nurse practitioner in private practice is responsible for data collection, problem identification, and intervention. This professional collaborates with a medical doctor or a group of health professionals or assumes sole responsibility for the care rendered.

In a 1985 issue of *Pacesetter,*[7] the newsletter of the Council on Psychiatric and Mental Health Nursing, the following guidelines for mental health–psychiatric nurses involved in private practice were provided. Clinical nurse specialists in psychiatric and mental health nursing should:

1. Identify themselves to clients as members of the nursing profession and display or have credentials (R.N. license, diploma, certification certificate) to show if requested
2. Are certified, eligible for, or in the process of becoming certified by ANA or a state nurses' association or both
3. Use factual information in advertisements regarding their qualifications and competence
4. Carry malpractice and premises liability insurance
5. Manage financial arrangements as follows
   a. Request a fee that is clear and understandable to the client
   b. Complete insurance forms to facilitate reimbursement to the client or provider
   c. Should the client be unable to pay a requested fee, negotiate a lower fee or refer to an appropriate source
   d. Should the client's financial circumstances worsen

during the course of treatment, making payment of the agreed-upon fee impossible, continue treatment until referral to another setting can be accomplished
   e. Should efforts to collect the fee fail, may employ a collection agency, small claims court or other legal action after informing the client
6. Outline clearly with clients the conditions of service such as frequency and duration of appointments, fee for missed or canceled sessions, and confidentiality
7. Conform to the ANA *Standards of Psychiatric and Mental Health Nursing Practice*
8. Respect clients' rights to confidentiality; maintain and safeguard appropriate records; when such data are to be shared (with other professionals on referral, with courts or lawyers in case of lawsuits), inform the client in advance; when such data are used for professional publications, reframe data to prevent recognition of the client
9. Do not engage in social, sexual, or business contacts with the client or those close to the client; may engage in professional contacts with the client or those close to the client
10. Are available to the client outside regular business hours in emergencies; when unavailable for such reasons as illness and vacations, provide a qualified substitute who will respond to emergency calls
11. Recognize limits of statutory accountability in relation to client needs and use referrals to other professionals for necessary services, such as medications or hospitalization; collaborate with these professionals when appropriate and authorized by the client
12. Report unethical behavior by another nurse to the appropriate body within the professional organization
13. Respect institutional policies when granted staff privileges to continue professional services to hospitalized clients
14. May elect to sell her practice to a professionally qualified successor

Finally, mental health–psychiatric nurses are also active as nursing consultants in medical-surgical settings, hospices, convalescent homes, and other agencies and programs. This practice model is more fully developed in Chapter 49.

BRIEF REVIEW

Quality assurance programs are now a formal part of hospital and agency care. Standards of nursing care developed with the professional organization are the bases on which quality assurance activities in nursing are built. Probably the most difficult aspect of quality assurance is the process of developing realistic criteria and designing monitoring procedures within the context of constantly changing conditions.

The concepts of levels of practice and the use of protocols provide an opportunity for mental health–psychiatric nurses to expand the implementation of the nursing role based on the development of clinical competencies in the clinical setting. Peer review processes and professional development through continuing education or the completion of advanced degrees are methods by which professional nurses enhance their knowledge base and the ability to provide the kind of nursing care that is expected of a professional member of the health care delivery team. Credentials serve as a protection for the consumer by providing identification of individual nurses' qualifications in particular clinical areas.

It is important to note that systematic evaluation of nursing care is a priority for professional nurses, not only in terms of their responsibility to the public but also in terms of their commitment to themselves and to the profession.

REFERENCES AND SUGGESTED READINGS

1. American Nurses' Association: Certification catalog, Kansas City, Mo., 1988, The Association.
1a. American Nurses' Association: A plan for implementation of the standards of nursing practice, Kansas City, Mo., 1975, The Association.
2. American Nurses' Association: Quality assurance workbook, Kansas City, Mo., 1976a, The Association.
3. American Nurses' Association: Statement on psychiatric and mental health nursing practice, Kansas City, Mo., 1976b, The Association.
4. American Nurses' Association: Standards for continuing education in nursing, vol. 1, Kansas City, Mo., 1979a, The Association.
5. American Nurses' Association: The study of credentialing in nursing: a new approach, Kansas City, Mo., 1979b, The Association.
6. American Nurses' Association: Pacesetter, Kansas City, Mo., 1981, The Association.
7. American Nurses' Association: Guidelines for private practice, Pacesetter 12:3, Spring 1985.
8. American Nurses' Association: Standards of psychiatric and mental health nursing practice, Kansas City, Mo., 1982, The Association.
9. American Nurses' Association: Legislature passes reimbursement bill, Governor vetoes it, The American Nurse 16(9):19, 1984.
10. Bulechek, G.M., and Maas, M.L.: In McCloskey, J.C., and Grace, H.K., editors: Current issues in nursing, ed. 2, Palo Alto, Calif., 1985, Blackwell Scientific Publications.
11. Bullough, B.: The law and expanding nursing role, New York, 1980, Appleton-Century-Crofts, Inc.
12. Caterinicchio, R.P., editor: DRG's, what they are and how to survive them, Thorofare, N.J., 1984, Slack, Inc.
13. Coordinators Manual: nursing quality monitoring methodology, May 1983, Medicus Systems Corp.
14. Evans, C.L.S., and Lewis, S.K.: Nursing administration of psychiatric–mental health care, Rockville, MD, 1985, Aspen Systems Corp.
15. Giovannetti, P.: Understanding patient classification systems, Journal of Nursing Administration 9(2):4, 1979.
16. Grippando, G.M.: Nursing perspectives and issues, Albany, N.Y., 1977, Delmar Publishers.
17. Jennings, C.P.: Nursing's case for third party reimbursement, American Journal of Nursing 79:111, 1979.
18. Joel, L.A.: DRG's and Rim's: implications for nursing, Nursing Outlook 32:42, 1984.
19. Joint Commission on Accreditation of Hospitals: The quality assurance guide: a resource for quality assurance, Chicago, 1980, The Commission.
20. Kurose, K., and others: A standard care plan for alcoholism, American Journal of Nursing 81:1001, 1981.
21. Loomis, M.E., and others: Development of a classification system for psychiatric–mental health nursing: Individual response class, Archives of Psychiatric Nursing 1(1):16, 1987.
22. Maas, M.L.: Nursing diagnosis in a professional model of nursing: Keystone for effective nursing administration, Journal of Nursing Administration 16(12):39, 1986.
23. Mailbusch, R.M.: Evolution of quality assurance for nursing in hospitals. In Schroeder, P.S., and Mailbusch, R.M., editors: Nursing quality assurance, Milwaukee, Wis., 1984, Aspen Systems Corp., pp. 3-28.
24. Martin, J.M., and Finneran, M.R.: Standards of practice as a basis for peer review, Perspectives in Psychiatric Care 18:242, 1980.
25. Meisenheimer, C.G., editor: Quality assurance, Rockville, Md., 1985, Aspen Systems Corp.
26. Miller, M.C., and Knapp, R.G.: Evaluating quality of care, Germantown, Md., 1979, Aspen Systems Corp.
27. National League for Nursing: Interpretive statement on NLN position in support of two levels of nursing practice, Publication No. 11-2158, New York, 1986, National League for Nursing.
28. News: NLN reaffirms its BSN stance despite "technological nursing" rift, American Journal of Nursing 83:985, 994, 1983.
29. Reed, L.S., Meyers, E.S., and Scheidemandel, P.L.: Health insurance and psychiatric care: update and appraisal, Washington, D.C., 1984, American Psychiatric Press, Inc.
30. Schroeder, P.S., and Mailbusch, R.M., editors: Nursing quality assurance, Milwaukee, Wis., 1984, Aspen Systems Corp.
31. Smith, M.H., editor: Graduate education in nursing: issues and future directions, Atlanta, 1981, Southern Regional Education Board.
32. United States Government: The federal register, January 3, 1984.
33. Wandelt, M., and Stewart, D.: The Slater Nursing Competencies Rating Scale, New York, 1975, Appleton-Century-Crofts, Inc.

ANNOTATED BIBLIOGRAPHY

Albiez-Gibbons, A.: Mental health acuity system: the measure of nursing practice, Journal of Psychosocial Nursing and Mental Health Services 24:7:16, 1986.

This article presents the development of an acuity system in a mental health–psychiatric setting that reflects the variable intensity of client care on each shift. By nursing staff developing standards of care for clients in behavioral crises, the quality of care is addressed without increasing documentation during crisis periods. The use of a mental health acuity system in projecting staffing needs is also discussed.

Kaplan, K.O., Hopkings, J.M., and Longabaugh, R.: Quality assurance guide for psychiatric and substance abuse facilities, Chicago, 1981, Joint Commission on Accreditation of Hospitals.

This book provides a comprehensive, problem-focused approach to quality assurance from the point of view of the Joint Commission. It includes goals and objectives, identification and resolution of problems, priority setting, sample programs, critiques of quality assurance plans, and examples of assessment methods.

CHAPTER 49

PSYCHIATRIC CONSULTATION LIAISON NURSING

Joyce S. Levy   Anita Lewis

After studying this chapter the learner will be able to:

Define psychiatric consultation and liaison nursing.

Identify the historical facts that have influenced the development of psychiatric consultation liaison nursing.

Identify the steps in the psychiatric consultation liaison process.

Identify the overall goals of psychiatric consultation liaison nursing.

Describe models of practice within psychiatric consultation liaison nursing.

Identify techniques and strategies for effective consultee-consultant alliance building.

Identify the sources of power, benefits, and challenges of consultation liaison work.

Describe the educational preparation, professional experience, and clinical supervision of the psychiatric consultation liaison nurse.

Identify future avenues for license and creativity in the practice of psychiatric consultation liaison nursing.

Mental health consultation is "the provision of clinical expertise regarding the delivery of psychological care in response to a request from a health care provider."[20] *Liaison* is "the facilitation of the relationship that exists between the patient, the illness, the consultees and the hospital/ward milieu."[20]

The goals of liaison practice are consistent with the goals of consultation; a dynamic, complementary relationship exists between consultation and liaison work. Consultation is the rendering of an expert opinion. Liaison activates, expands, and brings to life that expert opinion. Consultation practice precedes liaison practice. Slowly they become mutually dependent. The following example illustrates this relationship. A consultation was requested to determine why a client was refusing to complete a course of intravenous antibiotic treatment. He gave no reason for his refusal. The assessment by the psychiatric consultation liaison nurse revealed that the major reason for the client's refusal was not related to his feelings or any misunderstanding regarding the treatment but rather

his loss of confidence in his primary nurse. The consultation developed into a need for liaison practice.

A *consultation alliance* is a relationship between the consultant and the consultee characterized by an understanding that clinical dilemmas will and can be approached together. A *liaison alliance* is a relationship between the consultant and the consultee that signifies some clinical dilemmas can be understood and resolved by reflecting on the interactions among care providers and clients. In the previous example a liaison alliance is essential before the client's loss of confidence in his primary nurse can be addressed.

The essence of consultation is personal and professional respect. Consultants are "invited in." Regardless of the type of consultation being provided, the consultee is ultimately responsible for the client. A second invitation to consult is rarely issued when the consultee feels devalued. If the consultant behaves or is viewed as a supervisor, an arrogant expert, or a judge, the effectiveness of clinical practice will be impaired. Consultation liaison nurse, con-

Historical Overview

DATE	EVENT
1902	First inpatient psychiatric unit in a general hospital, was established at Albany hospital in New York.
1920	Models of psychosomatic medicine emerged.
1934	Rockefeller Foundation provided funds for five psychiatric liaison departments in general hospitals.
1940s	Psychiatric nursing consultation was provided in general hospitals.
1950s	Mental health consultation and psychiatric units in general hospitals were further expanded.
1960	Nursing departments in many general hospitals recognized the need for the role of consultation liaison nurses.
1960s	Discussions of the concept of nursing consultation appeared in the literature.
1970s	Gerald Caplan[4] published research and development data relating to mental health consultation. Formal graduate education programs in consultation liaison nursing were developed at University of Maryland and at Yale University.
1974	*Liaison Nursing: A Psychological Approach to Patient Care,* was the first textbook on psychiatric consultation liaison nursing.
1982	*Psychiatric Liaison Nursing: The Theory and Clinical Practice,* by Anita Lewis and Joyce Levy, was published. It established a theoretical base for practice.
Future	The increased emphasis on the biological basis of mental illness will create a need for more mental health–psychiatric nurses to function as consultation liaison nurses.

sultants, and liaison nurse will be used interchangeably in the chapter. The types of consultation discussed in this chapter are client centered and consultee centered. Listed below are types of mental health consultation[4]:
1. Client-centered
2. Consultee-centered
3. Program-centered administrative
4. Consultee-centered administrative

CHARACTERISTICS OF THE PSYCHIATRIC CONSULTATION LIAISON NURSE
Qualifications

The psychiatric consultation liaison nurse is a registered nurse with a master's degree, clinical experience in general nursing, advanced clinical skills in psychiatric nursing, and administrative or supervisory experience. The psychiatric consultation liaison nurse should be clinically competent, proficient in assessing complicated nursing care situations, and insightful and knowledgeable about transference and countertransference issues.

The hallmarks of psychiatric consultation liaison nursing are objectivity, flexibility, personal and professional maturity, and the ability to take reasonable risks and to tolerate the intolerable. Expert skills in the art of listening

for process, themes, and agendas are required. Problems presented for consultation are frequently quite complex and filled with hidden agendas. Identifying the essence of the problems, expanding consultation to include liaison principles, and formulating and implementing interventions form the core of practice. The ability to practice autonomously is essential.

Roles

The major focuses of the role of the liaison nurse are enhancement of the delivery of psychological nursing care and the effective management of care. She also serves as a catalyst in facilitating effective negotiations with staff and clients and is responsible for promoting a professionally supportive, nonevaluative, collaborative relationship with the consultee. The liaison nurse practices predominantly in the general hospital, although the role has been and is adaptable to community settings.

Development and implementation of the role are a continuous process. This process is altered, tested, and influenced by the liaison nurse, the health care system, and external forces. When she enters a health care system to provide psychiatric consultation liaison nursing, the nurse carefully assesses the hospital or organization. Appraisal of reporting relationships, formal and informal power, job descriptions, previous history of the system, and identification of subsystems are important aspects of implementation of the role within the system. Maintaining high visibility, availibility, flexibility, and credibility in response to requests is essential, while continuing to carefully attempt to achieve clinical goals. The pressure to gain acceptance may tempt the newly hired liaison nurse to use inappropriate situations to implement her role. For example, a consultee may be warm, friendly, and welcoming to the liaison nurse and attempt to involve her in a struggle with the administration.

The role can be implemented by involvement in the established structure of the nursing department, through inservice and orientation programs, committee participation, support to staff, and support to clients with cardiac or respiratory arrests, dying clients and their families, and victims of violence.

The clinical responsibilities of liaison nurses are based on the goals of practice. Clear goals are the foundation of practice and continue to serve as guidelines as the role develops. The goals are:

1. To teach the concepts of effective psychological care and its implementation
2. To support nursing staff in providing psychological nursing care
3. To aid in maintaining alliances, respect and esteem with the consultee
4. To encourage acceptance and tolerance of insolvable care issues

The goals may be implemented by formal or informal teaching, direct or indirect client intervention, client care conferences, support groups for consultees, multidisciplinary conferences, and role modeling.

CONCEPTUAL MODEL

Although consultation and liaison practice become a portion of every encounter with a client or a consultee, for purposes of clarity they are discussed separately.

The Consultation Process

The consultation process involves four steps, listed below. These steps are carefully thought through and expanded in the context of building an alliance with the consultee[20]:

1. Invitation
2. Evaluation of appropriateness
3. Problem identification
4. Direct or indirect care

The first step, the invitation to consult, is accompanied by assessment of several issues. First is identification of the consultee. Who is requesting consultation—nurse, doctor, social worker, family member, client? Next, the psychiatric consultation liaison nurse reviews prior experience with the consultee making the request. It is also important to consider when consultation is sought in the course of hospitalization and illness and to identify whether there is any significance to the "timing" of the request. For example, has the client been admitted the day of the request, and has this somehow created sufficient anxiety among the consultees to warrant immediate consultation? Has the client been in the hospital for weeks, being managed by the consultee and now consultation is indicated? What has changed to warrant this request?

The second step involves evaluation of the appropriateness of the consultation request. All requests for consultation are, at the very least, opportunities to illustrate and clarify the role of the liaison nurse and explore issues relative to the psychological care of clients. Each consultation request is a potential opportunity to role model, teach, or learn more about the consultee, the unit, and the system. Some common consultation requests are shown in the box below. Every request is a potential springboard for enhancing consultation alliances, since each request is a call for help.

Problem identification is the third step of the consultation process. Clarifying the nature of the request and the focus of the problem are important if the consultation provided is to be useful and the goals of practice achieved.

Consultation requests are both overt and covert. The former usually reflects a legitimate difficulty (for example, client noncompliance with medical treatment). The latter typically reflects the consultee's wish for or fear of the client or an emotional reaction to the situation that may be unacceptable. Often the covert question reflects unconscious reactions. In the noncompliant client, the covert level of the request may be "this client is infuriating—tell us that we've tried long enough, and can be angry and can abandon him." Noting the descriptive language used in expressing the problem is helpful.

The problem necessitating consultation is initially defined by the consultee. Just as the client may accurately or inaccurately identify his problems, so may the consultee. Perhaps the language is misleading. Perhaps the con-

---

COMMON CONSULTATION REQUESTS

A consultation is frequently requested for the client who:

Is depressed
Is manipulative
Is frequently asking for pain medication
Wants staff to do everything for him
Is refusing treatment
Is threatening to leave AMA
Is a drug abuser or addict
Has a psychiatric history
Has a terminal illness
Refuses surgery
Needs support
Is verbally abusive
Is physically abusive
Is seductive

ELEMENTS OF DIAGNOSING THE TOTAL CONSULTATION

1. Consultation request
2. Consultee
3. Doctor
4. Unit
5. Family
6. Medical illness
7. Chart
8. Client (direct consultation model)

From Lewis, A., and Levy, J.: Psychiatric liaison nursing: the theory and clinical practice, Reston, Va., 1982, Reston Publishing Co.

sultee's diagnosis of the problem is incorrect. While maintaining a client care focus, the liaison nurse endeavors to "diagnose the total consultation." This process involves comprehensively assessing aspects of the consultation that are beyond the consultant-client interaction (see the box above).[20] Reviewing issues pertinent to the client's family, the doctor, the ward, and the medical illness and reviewing the client's chart, aid the consultant in clarifying the consultation problem before determining the intervention. Consultees may have unrealistic or unconscious expectations of the liaison nurse and her ability to solve the problem that becomes apparent as the total consultation is diagnosed.

The final step of the consultation process involves a decision about a direct or indirect model of care. This determination is primarily based on the nature (seriousness, intensity, impact) and the focus (client, consultee, family, other) of the consultation request. In the direct model of consultation, the client and family are interviewed by the liaison nurse, who then provides psychological intervention. With the indirect model of consultation, a consultee-centered/case-centered conference is held and intervention is planned. Follow-up, reassessment, and evaluation are ongoing and essential to both models. These activities are best shared by consultant and consultee as their alliance strengthens. Documentation in the client's record is the consultee's responsibility with the indirect model. The liaison nurse is responsible for documentation with the direct model.

The following guidelines may aid in determination of a direct or an indirect model approach.

Direct care is indicated when:

1. The nature of the problem presented remains unclear or complex
2. The consultant's role is new or not well understood; clinical involvement may enhance system entry
3. The required intervention is complex and beyond the level of the consultee's expertise
4. Consultee anxiety is high and inhibits problem resolution
5. Consultee resistance is rigidly fixed
6. The same or similar problem(s) have been previously presented by the same consultee, at which time an indirect model was unsuccessful
7. Alliances will be enhanced
8. The "problem" is of special interest to the consultant and a direct model will not hamper alliances

Indirect care is indicated when:

1. The problem is clear and easily formulated
2. The consultee has formulated an appropriate intervention plan and is merely asking for support and validation from the consultant
3. Consultee anxiety is sufficiently low and her clinical skill is sophisticated enough to implement the required intervention
4. The consultee is appropriately motivated to carry out the intervention
5. Resistence to carrying out the intervention is low and chances are high that the plan can be successfully implemented
6. The problem can be resolved fairly easily by the consultee, who has become too dependent on the consultant
7. The problem is not client focused, but rather consultee focused
8. A direct model will weaken alliances and may be interpreted as a lack of confidence in the consultee on the part of the consultant

The Liaison Process

Liaison is a method by which to detect, prevent, and manage psychiatric problems and to resolve difficulties between clients and consultees. Liaison symbolizes the clinical partnership between the consultant and consultee. Liaison also denotes an abstract process that may be regarded as manipulative, interpretive, or intrusive by the consultee.

The liaison process comprises the following elements. Each element emerges from the one that proceeds it. All of the elements are of equal importance for understanding liaison work and enacting the process.

Education and socialization

During nurses' education, they are socialized into three basic positions that they can assume in the process of providing client care: "can do," "should do," and "can't do." As the nurses begin their professional practice, they often believe they "can do" everything for clients. With additional experience, they feel they "should do" everything for clients. Frequently nurses experience frustration and discouragement in their efforts to intervene with clients, based on the first two positions. This experience results in nurses thinking they "can't do" anything for clients.

A triangle serves as a useful, concrete image for depicting these three positions, because they can be superimposed on the three points of each triangle (Figure 49-1). The lines between the points represent the roads every nurse can travel in her psychological and behavioral approach and her reaction to each clinical encounter. These encounters can be with clients, their families, peers, other members of the health care team, and the liaison nurse.

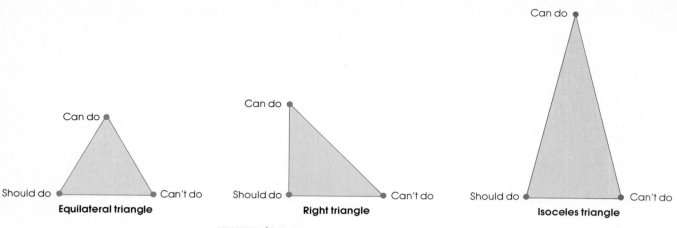

FIGURE 49-1 Education-socialization triangle.

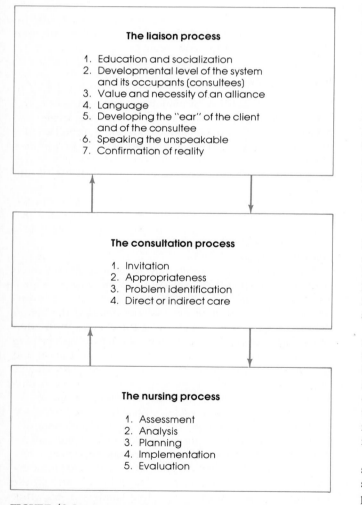

FIGURE 49-2 Interdependence of three clinical processes.

The size and shape of the triangle change with each clinical encounter. The shape can be an equilateral, a right, or an isosceles triangle, as in Figure 49-1. Women's issues, the gestalt of the ward, the quality of leadership, performance expectation, client/family responses, the illness and its course, and identification and transference issues are significant factors that blend to influence the shape of the triangle. The quality of care delivered and the satisfaction of the nurse are reflected in the triangle.

The lines between the points are the paths the consultee travels in her efforts to provide care. These paths contain all the memories, emotions, and specific clinical care approaches tried and their results. Not all three paths are traveled in each situation. The lines between the points and the three basic positions reflect the length of the paths the consultee traveled and the amount of time taken to get from one point to the next. The liaison nurse notes where the consultee started and where she is now in terms of the education and socialization triangle.

When the inexperienced consultee encounters her first help-rejecting client, she discovers that sympathy, time, energy, alternative teaching methods, or threats of future illness are ineffective. She then may feel responsible, believing that she "should" be able to intervene. Through increased experience with help-rejecting clients, the consultee may feel defeated at the onset—"can't do."

Psychiatric consultation liaison nurses travel the same triangle as the consultee—what can be done, what should be done, what can't be done. Liaison nurses attempt to intervene in client or consultee behaviors and emotional responses that interfere with care delivery and health recovery. It is impossible to intervene in all the ramifications of insufficient staffing, inadequate nursing management, or in the behavior of a client who is invested only in a life of drug abuse.

With additional clinical experience, consultee and liaison nurse learn to set priorities and become increasingly skillful in delineating realistic client care outcomes. Appreciating the triangle's existence and the position of each individual aids in understanding the total consultation.

Developmental level of the system and the consultee(s) within the system

The developmental level of the system refers to the quality of nursing care practice, leadership, relationships among health care providers, and the psychological sophistication characteristic of the delivery of care within a health care system. As some consultees remain and others move on, as leaders develop, a dynamic, ever-changing system is created. The developmental stage of each consultee is reflected in her position on the education-socialization triangle, her relationships with other health care providers, and the quality of care she provides. For example, when the consultee adheres to the "can do" position, believing she can always meet the client's needs, a therapeutic intervention may be difficult.

Case Example

Mrs. Rose, a 59-year-old woman, was hospitalized on a general surgical unit in a small community hospital, having had a radical mastectomy for breast cancer 3 days earlier. She was attempting to conceal her grief by constantly requesting "little things" of her nurse, and the nurse attempted to meet her requests. Although these unending requests enabled her to have frequent contact with her nurse, they also prevented the client and nurse from discussing Mrs. Rose's psychological reaction to her mastectomy.

With education and continued professional experience, nurses increase their knowledge and sophistication about the meaning of a client's behavior. There are nurses who tend to hold on to the "should do" position, sometimes demonstrated in the belief that all clients should be as independent as possible and that the nurse should consistently encourage their independence. For example, for Mrs. Thomas, a 42-year-old woman who was recovering from a subarachnoid hemorrhage, dependency meant renewed closeness with her estranged husband. This was evidenced by his attentiveness, including feeding her. Although she was able to feed herself, she experienced this as very supportive. Attempting to tamper with this dependency would have proved nontherapeutic. There are situations in which independence is not the most desirable goal for the client.

The value and necessity of an alliance

The potential power of consultation and liaison alliances is reflected in the honest valuing of the consultee's work, views, and expertise. It is important to tactfully recognize gaps in knowledge and not question the consultee unnecessarily. The consultant communicates to the consultee her belief that the request was appropriate, that she tried in some way to deal with the problem, and that anxiety and fear can influence problem-solving skills.

Anxiety and fear can influence the consultee's approach to the psychiatric consultation liaison nurse in other ways, as shown in the Case Example below.

Case Example

A highly competent staff nurse with years of clinical experience angrily approached the liaison nurse. The staff nurse demanded that the liaison nurse help her stop a 51-year-old business executive, who had had gallbladder surgery 5 days earlier, from "regressing." " He's refusing to do anything for himself. He's on the light constantly and always pointing out my inefficiencies," she said. The consultee's affect was hostile and demanding. It was apparent that she had not approached the client about her concerns. This behavior was uncharacteristic of her. The consultee was affectively doing to the consultant what the client was doing to her. In addition to solving the stated problem, it would be appropriate for the liaison nurse to diagnose the total consultation with special attention to the covert dilemma—the esteem needs of the consultee.

Language

The language used by the consultee to describe the problem in nursing care is significant. The quality, intensity, potential symbolic meaning, and concurrent affect expressed in the language are noted by the liaison nurse to enhance information previously gathered in diagnosing the total consultation. It is important to ask the consultee whether the client describes the problem in the same way as the consultee. A consultee may label a client "manipulative and seductive," whereas the client describes himself as "angry and frightened." For example, Mr. Micheal, a 46-year-old married father of four, two days after a femoropopliteal bypass graft, is described by the nurse as "doing well but very withdrawn for no apparent reason." However, Mr. Michael describes himself as not doing well because he is still in the intensive care unit, his family has not visited, and he is experiencing mild confusion with poor memory and is trying to conceal it.

Developing the "ear" of the client and the "ear" of the consultee

This element of the liaison process involves perfecting the clinical skill of hearing and conceptualizing issues from the perspective of the client as well as the consultee. This results in the development of a "larger" ear. If the client is described as "appropriately depressed," questions the consultant may raise are: How are his behavior and responses to illness being heard and felt? and By whose standards are the client's psychological responses being judged? Understanding the affects coloring the experience, the possible perceptions and feelings of all involved, and the quality of their communication are inherent in developing the larger ear. This understanding is primarily for the benefit of the liaison nurse. Depending on the intensity of the problem and the strength of the alliance, such understanding may or may not be shared directly with consultees or clients.

The liaison nurse remains sensitive to everyone's opinion. By gathering views, the consultant illustrates that although consensus may not be possible, an intervention that takes each view into consideration may be developed. This is the value of developing the larger clinical ear.

Speaking the unspeakable

There are times when offering an interpretation—putting into words what others are unaware of and therefore unable to say—can be useful. The value of speaking the unspeakable is often illustrated in the clarification of transference and identification issues for a consultee who may be suffering in the course of her attempts to care for a client.

Case Example

Mr. Fine, a 28-year-old law student diagnosed with acute renal failure necessitating dialysis, was described as tearful, compliant, and withdrawn. The nursing staff knew he was depressed, but could not move beyond their own sadness and identification. The liaison nurse intervened by speaking the unspeakable, which involved addressing the consultee's fear, vulnerability, and helplessness.

Assessing alliances is crucial when speaking the unspeakable. Will speaking out help or hinder? Will interpretation open the door for additional understanding and intervention? Caution is necessary. If the consultee is feeling vulnerable or suspicious or has experienced a narcissistic injury, an interpretation may merely serve to pointlessly add unwelcome insight to injury.

Confirmation of reality

This final element of the liaison process involves describing and examining a situation as it actually is. This perspective is especially useful in labeling intolerable situations, some of which must endured. It involves verbalizing what others are painfully aware of but too frightened or inhibited to say. There are situations in which confirming reality provides clarity and an atmosphere conducive to problem solving.

Case Example

When a 31-year-old client with AIDS began to throw his urine and feces at the nurses, prompt intervention was in order. The liaison nurse stated that in reality the client needed his health care team more than they needed him, and that nurses do not have to tolerate such behavior. This resulted in an increased willingness to understand what may have motivated the client's actions. Empathic limits were developed.

When in the midst of a chaotic, provoking clinical situation, it is not uncommon for a sense of reality to become elusive. Confirming reality can dramatically reduce the tension experienced by consultees when in a difficult clinical situation. It can lead not only to problem resolution but also to the enhancement of alliances.

Assessment of Consultations

A five-dimensional approach for assessing consultations serves as an additional tool in psychiatric consultation liaison practice. The significance of each dimension varies with the problem, the client, and the consultee.

Physical dimension. The liaison nurse assesses the physiological impact of the illness. All physical illness is a psychological event; it is rarely possible to experience an illness exclusively in the body or the mind. Data are compiled concerning biological causes of the illness, natural history, treatment, symptomatology, present and projected degree of debilitation, absense or presence of pain, and prognosis. The typical experience of a partic-

ular illness and whether or not this is an unusual or typical presentation are key in formulating useful interventions. How have normal body processes been affected by the illness? Is the illness visible, and has this influenced body image? Visible signs and symptoms of illness are not a prerequisite for an alteration or distortion of body image. When a young woman with long-standing diabetes was asked to described how she felt about her body, she tearfully responded, "That's easy—I feel terrible; my body is dirty and marked."

The client's physical status, health history, and usual health care practices before becoming ill are noteworthy. The possibility of an underlying organic cause for the psychological presentation of a physical illness is considered. For example, pancreatic cancer can often be first expressed as a clinical depression. In addition, medications, treatments, and metabolic imbalances can alter cognitive status and influence physical presentation. It is imperative to note that the relationship between the physical and psychological causes and presentations of illness are fluid.

Emotional dimension. The client's psychological and emotional responses to illness and hospitalization are best evaluated in the context of his premorbid status. Significant psychological history, personality style, defensive structure, mode of adaptation, affect, mood, and present level of psychological functioning are relevant. Four psychological behaviors are necessary to work through an illness. These include "egocentricity, constriction of interests, emotional dependency, and hypochondriasis."[20] These behaviors are expected stages in the client's response to illness. They also may not occur or may vary in intensity, and they are individualized. The client who is having difficulty sharing his nurse with other clients may be described as egocentric. The client intensely focused on his intravenous line is demonstrating constriction of interests. The client who is unable to make even the smallest decision on his own is exhibiting emotional dependency. Hypochondriasis is evident in the client who becomes focused on minor body aches and pains and is unable to give them up. The client may move from one stage to another as well as return to a previously experienced stage.

The experience of giving and receiving care is filled with emotional reactions, mutual expectations and assumptions, identifications, and transference responses among clients and health care providers. Deciphering these complex issues is crucial. The psychological developmental levels of client and consultee are also significant. Illness often holds special meaning for the client and consultee. Depending on the nature of the illness, its symptomatology, its treatment course, the nursing care required, the part of the body affected, and previous knowledge or experience, meanings of illness may vary. Eight categories have been identified that elucidate the subjective, psychological meanings of illness: "a challenge, an enemy, a punishment, a weakness, a relief, a strategy, irreparable loss or damage, a value."[23]

The degree of emotional conflict the client experiences in relation to illness may be a result of the meaning it signifies and or the degree of life disruption it precipitates.

These facets of the emotional dimension may be difficult to assess directly.

✳ ***Intellectual dimension.*** This dimension includes a mental status examination of the client. Knowledge of the neurological and metabolic ramifications of the illness, potential side effects of medication and treatments, and signs and symptoms of pseudodementia, dementia, and delerium are noted.

The liaison nurse evaluates whether a formal mental status examination would be appropriate, based on the overall psychological presentation of the client, degree of physical illness and discomfort, and the nature of the problem. The client's educational history, intellectual capacity memory and ability to apply knowledge are factors to assess.

It is also useful to identify the consultee's level of comprehension of the "problem" as well as her ability to understand and carry out a psychologically based nursing care intervention.

✤ ***Social dimension.*** This dimension can be especially powerful in influencing the outcome of a consultation. When social norms and family dynamics and values brought to the care situation by client and consultee are at odds, their conflict precipitates the consultation. These situations often become intense.

Clinical dilemmas symptomatic of conflicts in the social dimension, often presented as interpersonal problems among clients and consultees or between consultees, represent complex challenges to effective intervention.

Important areas for consideration include the milieu of the ward; leadership or management style; the degree, nature, and sources of professional esteem and cohesion among consultees; and relationships among care providers. Environmental factors also necessitate review—for example, the social significance of the hospital and its location to the client; the consultee; the community; whether the client is in a private room, a semiprivate room, or a ward; and whether room change occurs and why. The degree of life disruption that illness and hospitalization creates for the client and for his family is significant. Culture and ethnicity also mold the relationship between client and consultee. They may also color the client's and the consultee's beliefs concerning the liaison nurse and the utilization of consultation.

✤ ***Spiritual dimension*** Assessment of religious and philosophical beliefs concerning general life values, ethical standards, views of illness, death, hope, and our purpose, provide the liaison nurse with an even richer understanding of the client, the consultee, and their responses of each other. Recognizing the importance of the values and teachings of individual religions in the life of client and consultee is central. For example, the refusal to have an abortion or to receive blood products is not only a reflection of a religious viewpoint, but also a potential area of conflict between client and consultee. Clients, consultees, and liaison nurses may find that their values are in conflict when faced with defining comfort measures for the terminally ill client. Clients who have strong, supportive religious beliefs may be better equipped to face the stresses of a long and complex illness.

PRACTICE ISSUES

The complex practice issues of identification, transference, countertransference, and resistance are the most difficult to assess, understand, and intervene. Assessment requires an understanding of these issues, which can influence the consultee, the client, and the liaison nurse.[8] It is often these very issues that serve as strong roadblocks to the liaison nurse's effective implementation of her recommendations.

After careful assessment of the clinical situation it may become apparent that the interaction between the client and the caregiver is interfering with the care of the client.

Case Example

Mr. Josh, a 32-year-old lawyer with an 8-year history of drug abuse, was demanding, disruptive, and had threatened to sign out against medical advice. Mr. Josh had been admitted with an infected leg. A multidisciplinary case conference was organized to address his nursing needs and to formulate a management plan. The primary nurse described Mr. Josh's behavior as obnoxious and divulged without embarrassment the hostile techniques she used to maintain control. She further revealed how she used these techniques with her children. What effect did Mr. Josh's behavior have on the nurse and on his care? It is possible that he raised conflictual issues that had not been resolved for the nurse.

Nurses in nonpsychiatric settings are less aware of the need for self-understanding in the delivery of psychological care. Often psychological care problems encountered in the medical-surgical settings are a result of this lack of awareness.

The inner distress of the consultee can be transformed into a problem that is labeled as the client's problem. The responsibility of the liaison nurse is to include the possibilities of the impact of the nurse-client relationship in her formulation of the clinical situation. The client may be too dependent or the nurse too intolerant of dependence.

The experience of illness and hospitalization and the psychological regression that occurs are the precipitants for identification, transference, and countertransference. The power of the client's psychological regression is often overlooked. The most common issues involved in these psychological processes are aggression, loss, grief, separation, sexuality, intimacy, dependency, control, autonomy, and integrity. When possible it is clinically helpful to determine, for example, whether the consultee's urgency in medicating a client is an expression of the client's need or the nurse's. Which one is depressed, withdrawn, angry or hostile? The challenge is to intervene effectively without more complete knowledge regarding transference or countertransference issues involved in a particular situation. There may be neither time nor permission for this understanding. The relationship between the liaison nurse and the consultee does not include license to explore these issues. In the previous Case Example, it might have been helpful to simply acknowledge the intense feelings between Mr. Josh and his nurse by stating to his nurse that Mr. Josh appeared to be making her suffer. Such comments feel supportive without being intrusive.

Identification, a conscious process, raises issues usually

CLUES TO TRANSFERENCE AND COUNTERTRANSFERENCE

Listed below are behavioral and emotional clues of transference or countertransference.

Increased or decreased interest in the client
Depression
Affectionate feelings
Inability to set limits
Arguing with the client
Desire to impress the client
Sadistic, hostile feelings
Disapproving and angry feelings
Special need to be reassuring
Provoking acting-out behavior
Thinking or dreaming about the client
Desire to assist client in special ways
Strong desire to provide care for client
Deriving unusual satisfaction or gratification from the care of the client.

---

recognized and more easily understood than transference or countertransference. Identification may occur around similar life situations between client and consultee (age, sex, type of illness, appearance, or occupation). Identification issues can also evoke the unconscious process of transference or countertransference and complicate the understanding of the consultee-client relationship. There are behavioral clues to transference and countertransference (see the box above). A staff nurse may overidentify with a client who is also a nurse, the same age, and suffering from a dreaded disease such as cancer of the reproductive system. On an unconscious level the client may evoke in the nurse previous feelings such as rivalry, rage, or depression. These powerful feelings can cloud the path to intervention. At these times postponing action while observing and listening is advisable.

Transference and countertransference can be positive or negative and can benefit or interfere with the client-nurse relationship.

Transference includes unconscious feelings and expectations related to relationships and events in the past. An important aspect of understanding clients who are physically ill is speculating on possible unconscious motives that may be influencing their present adaptation. Why is the client overcompliant? What does it mean when a young man cannot bear to be separated from his wife before surgery? Why does an elderly woman become hostile when her CAT scan is postponed? Is it simply fear, is there a reawakening of feelings from the past, or could this just be an expression of her compulsiveness?

Clients may revive unresolved conflicts in the health care provider.[40] These conflicts may interfere with meeting the care needs of the client. *Countertransference* can lead to defensive maneuvers that either destroy the alliance with the client, as with Mr. Josh in the preceding

Case Example, or lead to positive maneuvers that may help the client overcome isolation and suffering.

Case Example

Ms. Patrick, in contrast to the other nurses, approached an elderly woman client in a warm, caring, solicitous manner that was out of proportion to the client's nursing care needs. Ms. Patrick was constantly doing things for the client. The extra attention clearly helped. The client had demonstrated increasingly demanding behavior after her CAT scan was rescheduled. It is important for the liaison nurse to recognize that Ms. Patrick's behavior may be a positive countertransference response that has led to a positive adaptation for the client.

The consultant refrains from articulating the consultee's countertransference when diagnosing the total consultation. The nurse is responsible for her own behavior. However, if the nurse's personal struggles or conflicts interfere with safe care, if there is potential for harm to the client, or if the nurse asks for help, tactful intervention including a recommendation for psychotherapy may be indicated.

As concentrated attention is given to both positive and negative ramifications of transference and countertransference, the impact on the consultee and the client becomes more obvious. The more a consultee seeks direct personal satisfaction from caring for the client, the more likely that emotionally charged issues will be avoided or acted out by either party instead of being felt or verbalized in a helpful manner. It is also possible that client care can be used by the nurse as a defense against what is evoked by the client. What does it mean for the client who, after expressing fear and sadness about pending renal transplant surgery, is provided prompt attention to his physical needs and then is left to rest—along with his worries? If the nurse's wish is to have her sense of competence and self-worth mirrored by the client's appreciation and recovery, it may be intolerable for her to bear the client's affect. She may provide him with competent care in one dimension while abandoning him in another.

Liaison nurses are not immune to the issues of identification, transference, and countertransference. The role as consultant does allow some distancing from the clinical situation. However, psychiatric education and clinical supervision assist the consultant in remaining vigilant to these issues in clinical situations and in professional interactions. What does it mean when the staff nurse compliments the nurse consultant by saying, "We knew you would figure something out," or I'm so glad to see you. We don't know what to do—we've tried everything." Does the consultee magically want the consultant to fix it? Does the consultant wish to be viewed as superior?

When a clinical case is presented for consultation a parallel process may occur among the consultee, client, and liaison nurse. *Parallel process* refers to the reenactment of the relationship between client and consultee within the relationship between consultee and consultant. For example, the client may express hopelessness to his nurse (consultee). The consultee may then in turn describe the client's clinical situation as hopeless to the consultant. The liaison nurse needs to be attuned to feelings of helplessness, depression, anger, or hopelessness in herself and recognize the presence of parallel process. It is possible that the consultee is unwittingly communicating and reenacting the client's feelings to the consultant. After a careful assessment and analysis, if a consultation remains unclear, the diagnosis might be parallel process.

Case Example

The psychiatric consultation liaison nurse was asked to see Mr. Thomas, a 41-year-old married father of three, who was in the intensive care unit (ICU) after suffering a massive myocardial infarction. Mr. Thomas was very accepting of his care, the experience of being in the ICU, and his diagnosis. The ICU nurses described him as a "real nice guy" without any problems, but they thought he would need some support when he left their unit. Since it was stressful in the ICU with many admissions and transfers, the liaison nurse intervened directly. The liaison nurse had the same impression of Mr. Thomas as the consultee but began to wonder why the consultation was requested. More importantly, she found herself visiting the client more often than his psychological discomfort warranted. When Mr. Thomas casually mentioned his hope for the television he had requested 2 days earlier, the liaison nurse, quite out of character, bypassed the usual procedure for obtaining TV sets and personally issued his second request. The next day, when Mr. Thomas still had not received his TV, the liaison nurse tracked down the TV hostess and insisted that Mr. Thomas get his set immediately.

It was likely that the client's passivity was the reason for the consultation and that the active role of the liaison nurse mirrored the active role the ICU nurses assumed in requesting consultation. Perhaps Mr. Thomas evoked identification issues, transference, or countertransference.

An ongoing challenge for the liaison nurse is determining how to deal with these practice issues. Acknowledgement of personal conflicts with a consultee may best be addressed by a general statement such as, "It seems that this client is really getting to you." It is important to recognize that sometimes conflicts with clients are based on inexperience rather than on unconscious wishes or fantasies. The inexperienced nurse who becomes too involved with the depressed client may want to be therapeutic and may not be experiencing countertransference. As the liaison nurse continues to observe and study behavior and relationships, more questions arise about the relationships between consultee, client, and the liaison nurse.

Resistance is another issue that influences the practice of psychiatric consultation liaison nursing. *Resistance* is an overt or covert force that is opposing in nature. Resistance may emanate from conscious and unconscious feelings and may often not be understood. It is not simply rejection. As the liaison nurse continues the task of establishing and developing an alliance and becoming more credible in the system, resistance takes on a variety of shapes and forms. Some examples of resistance as demonstrated by the consultee are:

Reluctance or refusal to carry out interventions
Asking for help but failing to allocate time to discuss the problem

Not communicating major changes in a client's condition
Consistently stating that there are no psychological care problems

The risk for the liaison nurse rests with personalizing the resistance, becoming hurt, angry, or withdrawn. The liaison nurse listens to what the consultees are saying, recognizes verbal as well as nonverbal communications, hears the urgency in their requests, and their discomfort, fear, or terror. These observations are combined with the consultant's own feelings as a mirror to the parallel process that may be occurring. The goals of psychiatric consultation liaison nursing always guide intervention. However, if the observation or recognition of resistance is not included, diagnosing the total consultation may never be achieved. The liaison nurse needs to be cautious and not view all questioning of psychiatric nursing as resistance. There may be realistic reasons for this questioning; perhaps the consultee feels that the client's unstable medical condition would make an intervention impossible or inadvisable.

The liaison nurse can be more effective when she considers all of the possibilities regarding resistance rather than limiting herself to one interpretation. A skilled liaison nurse considers that resistance may be present but recognizes that it is not the only opposing force to successful interventions. Clinical supervision by an experienced psychiatric consultation liaison nurse, when possible, is helpful in identifying resistance and it's effect on practice. For example, a liaison nurse who was new to her role was troubled by the consultees' lack of interest in intervening directly with their clients. The consultees insisted that the consultant see every client. Her supervisor suggested that perhaps the consultees felt inadequate, were overworked, or were demonstrating some resistance by requesting that the liaison nurse do what they were clinically capable of doing. Their resistance might have been a wish that the psychiatric consultation liaison nurse should "work" and not just talk to them. Perhaps the consultation alliance was not strong enough. The goals of psychiatric consultation liaison nursing practice are not attainable without understanding resistance.

Other practice issues that warrant attention are the benefits and hazards associated with practicing psychiatric consultation liaison nursing in one system over time. Benefits occur when the liaison nurse remains in a system enduring resistance while maintaining alliances. These benefits include the following:

1. The system is likely to reward the demonstrated competence of the consultant with power.
2. Explanation of roles and goals decreases.
3. The quality of consultation increases.
4. Increased competence of the consultee results in a trend away from crisis intervention toward preventative management.
5. An increase in the quantity of consultations.

Hazards that may result when the liaison nurse remains in a system are as follows:

1. Increased clinical competence and acceptance can lead to entitlement, elitism, false safety, and boredom.

2. Consultees may want to continue to ascribe magical attributes to the liaison nurse. The consultant may no longer try to dispel the myth. The following is an example of the hazard of deemphasizing this mystical conception. Dr. Adam requested Ms. Gottlieb, the liaison nurse, to assess Mr. Harvey's depression after his myocardial infarction. He told the head nurse that no one was as efficient or thoughtful as Ms. Gottlieb. The hazard for Ms. Gottlieb is feeling flattered, complimented, honored, or superior rather than assessing the meaning of this statement in terms of the total consultation.

3. Sharing secrets and becoming more involved with the group that was initially taboo is more tempting. This is the time to identify new and productive professional paths and to avoid the pitfalls of staying in the system. The consultation-liaison process is illustrated through application to a clinical Case Example.

Case Example

Consultation Request

"I need your help with Mr. Slaten. He's screaming, being impossible, and refusing care!"

Assessing the Consultation Request

Who: Request for consultation is initiated by the client's primary nurse, Ms. Brown.

What: The request is for help in dealing with Mr. Slaten, a 53-year-old, divorced father of one 19-year-old daughter. The client has a 15-year history of diabetes mellitus. Two years ago he had a mild, right-sided cerebrovascular accident, is legally blind, has chronic congestive heart failure, and presently suffers from a severely infected left leg. Approximately 6 months before admission, he developed a chronic deep-vein thrombosis of the left leg. After delaying hospitalization and trying to "follow doctor's orders at home," Mr. Slaten felt he no longer had a choice but to be admitted to the hospital. Severe vascular insufficiency to his lower left leg and foot was diagnosed. A below-the-knee amputation is recommended. Despite intense pain, Mr. Slaten is refusing the procedure.

When: Consultation is requested on day 6 of hospitalization.

How: The request is expressed by telephone to the consultant. Ms. Brown is talking rapidly. She sounds frightened, upset, and asks if the consultant can be available today.

Why: Mr. Slaten's behavior and psychological response to his illness, hospitalization, and prescribed treatment is interfering with the delivery of comprehensive care. The consultee is clearly worried, frustrated, and distraught about Mr. Slaten's physical and emotional status.

Consultation Questions

Overt consultation question: "Why is Mr. Slaten, who is familiar with this hospital and staff, being so disruptive and refusing care? Please evaluate his behavior and possible depression."

Covert consultation question: a strong, implied wish on the part of the consultee that the consultant "get Mr. Slaten to stop being crazy and sign the surgical permit—how can he treat us like this?"

Analysis: Problem identification. The type of consultation being requested is client-centered.

The consultee: The liaison nurse has worked with the consultee before. Ms. Brown has been a registered nurse for 2 years and is frequently in charge of the ward on the night shift. Ms. Brown is bright, insightful, highly motivated, encourages client participation in care planning and delivery, individualizes care plans, and sets realistic care goals. Ms. Brown is convinced that the consultant will know what to do. Of note is that Ms. Brown has a tendency to respond personally to clinical nursing failures.

The doctor: Dr. Martin has been caring for Mr. Slaten for many years. He is clearly quite angry with Mr. Slaten and tells the liaison nurse that Mr. Slaten "should have come in sooner, does as he pleases, and is merely taking up our time. If he doesn't want the amputation, he doesn't have to have it." It is apparent from the ensuing discussion that Dr. Martin has put in an enormous effort with Mr. Slaten. Dr. Martin is worried and upset with him and convinced that the client's decision to refuse surgery is not in his best interest. The liaison nurse has never worked with Dr. Martin, who has a reputation for rarely seeking psychiatric consultation, preferring to manage things himself. Dr. Martin is friendly and polite, but obviously skeptical of what may be accomplished.

The unit: The unit is a busy, 35-bed medical-surgery unit. It is well staffed, and primary nursing is practiced. The head nurse has been in her position for many years and is supportive of staff, but only occasionally calls the consultant. However, the head nurse does support and encourage her staff in their requests for consultation.

The family: Mr. Slaten has one child, Amy. She had been living with him, but recently moved in with her fiance and is very involved in planning her wedding. There has been no contact with Mrs. Slaten for many years. Amy visits her father daily, sometimes accompanied by her fiance. Reportedly the client is in better spirits when his daughter is present. There is no other family. Mr. Slaten was working and living independently until he developed the thrombosis. This, coupled with his chronic illnesses, forced him to retire from a 20-year career as an art critic. Mr. Slaten gave up his apartment and moved to a low-cost housing development.

The medical illness: Mr. Slaten is an insulin-dependent diabetic. His present medical regimen includes neutral protamine Hagedorn (NPH)-insulin, methyldopa (Aldomet), furosemide (Lasix), a low-salt, 1200-calorie diet and mild fluid restriction warranted by congestive heart failure. Mr. Slaten suffers from bilateral vascular insufficiency and peripheral neuropathy. His left leg is the most seriously effected with many deep, infected skin lesions and probably osteomyelitis. The leg is quite swollen, extremely painful, and is not responding to routine wound care (intravenous Keflex and elevation). Meperidine (Demerol) and hydroxyzine pamoate (Vistaril) are not successful in controlling pain and the client is refusing to try other analgesic, stating that they make him feel "sick" and "cloud" his head. Dressing changes are painful and Mr. Slaten sobs and swears if and when he allows them to be done. He is on strict bed rest and is sleeping poorly with minimal appetite, constipation, low-grade fevers, and headaches. He has never been as ill as he is now.

The chart: Mr. Slaten's chart reflects a long association with the hospital. He has always complied with prescribed medical regimens. He has been hospitalized over the years for pneumonia, pulmonary edema, a foot ulcer, and most recently the CVA. Mr. Slaten was well known and loved by the staff and was previously described as "quiet, cooperative, appreciative, and a fighter." Notes in the present chart suggest that the client's present behavior is uncharacteristic of him, ("hostile, demanding, uncooperative, and verbally abusive to staff"). The chart is now filled with notations concerning the progressively deteriorating status of Mr. Slaten's leg and his equally deteriorating emotional state. At times he refuses to bathe and eat and is further described as "depressed, irritable, and mildly confused." The chart indicates that Mr. Slaten is in metabolic balance, and his neurological evaluation is normal.

Determination of Model of Care

Direct consultation: Ms. Brown's efforts to solve the problem herself by client education, support, and empathic limit setting have failed. Ms. Brown feels she has failed because she is unable to change Mr. Slaten's behavior. Ms. Brown's anxiety is quite high. The problem is very complex. Identification and or transference issues may be involved (consultee is similar in age to client's daughter). Direct service may provide an opportunity to intervene regarding Mr. Slaten, and also to further assess, understand, and perhaps intervene with Ms. Brown's concerns. Also, Dr. Martin is resistant and doubtful regarding the usefulness of psychiatric consultation. Direct service would potentially clarify and illustrate the clinical skills and work of the psychiatric consultation liaison nurse. Additional factors include the busy pace of the unit and Mr. Slaten's limited social supports.

In further diagnosing the total consultation, each dimension necessitates careful assessment, either by direct examination or indirectly by observation and listening. The liaison nurse endeavors to answer questions formulated for each dimension.

Dimensions

Physical: What would have been Mr. Slaten's overall psychological state if he were a healthy 53-year-old man? Was his behavior a direct result of persistent, unremitting physical deterioration? Is this a typical presentation? With recognition of the effects of diabetes on the body, consideration would be given to factors such as sexual potency, energy level, and neuropathy. What is it like to experience the worst complications of diabetes? How did Mr. Slaten deal with his loss of visual acuity? What is the illness experience with a severely infected leg? Is there much pain?

Emotional: If Mr. Slaten was described as a fighter, what happened to that spirit? What is the experience of viewing oneself as a competent fighter and now as hopeless, incompetent, and useless? What does it mean when a formerly passive, self-contained gentleman is shouting obscenities at doctors and nurses? What has been the general psychological meaning of illness for Mr. Slaten? Has this meaning changed? If Mr. Slaten no longer views illness as a challenge, is he struggling with whether or not he can continue to fight? What meaning does this conflict and this illness hold for Ms. Brown and Dr. Martin? Do the visible signs of deterioration have a special impact on Mr. Slaten? Is his behavior an example of externalization as a defense against anxiety, emotional dependence, and/or ambivalence regarding the recommended amputation?

Intellectual: Is it possible that Mr. Slaten has experienced mental status changes? How does he perform on a mental status examination? Is he experiencing organic changes that are resulting in alterations in behavior? Has his short-term memory loss been induced by depression? Has his previous pride in his intellectual abilities contributed to his response to illness?

Social: Will Mr. Slaten be able to maintain his present living situation? What is the impact of his daughter's recent separation from him and her future marriage? Would it be helpful for Mr. Slaten to explore these issues with Ms. Brown? To what degree has progressive illness isolated Mr. Slaten?

Spiritual: What part has hope and faith served in Mr. Slaten's being a "fighter"? Does he want to die now? What was involved in his earlier trusting belief in God? Does he now feel betrayed? Does he believe that he has now been given more than he can bear?

Practice issues

The issues raised for Dr. Martin and Ms. Brown were different. These issues were influenced by the course of Mr. Slaten's illness and these two consultees' previous personal and care giving experiences. Was Dr. Martin experiencing sympathy, depression, and sadness? Was Ms. Brown feeling manipulated and angry?

What unconscious issues were raised for each by Mr. Slaten's affect and behavior? How was Mr. Slaten's psychological conflict experienced by Dr. Martin and Ms. Brown? Why does Ms. Brown tend to personalize care failures? Does Mr. Slaten hold some special sigificance for Ms. Brown, and what did her upset and concern mean to him? How are these issues experienced by the psychiatric consultation liaison nurse?

Nursing diagnoses

The following list provides NANDA-approved nursing diagnoses with causative statements to be considered in this case:

1. Ineffective coping related to complex medical illness
2. Potential for self-harm related to abandonment and depression
3. Potential for dysfunctional grieving related to an alteration in support system
4. Extreme powerlessness related to progressive illness
5. Noncompliance with nursing and medical care measures related to ineffective coping
6. Disturbance in self-concept related to alterations in body image
7. Unresolved grief related to retirement, major life changes, separation from daughter
8. Severe social isolation and lack of diversional activity related to the ramifications of medical illness

Liaison Elements

In further assessing the consultation and determining intervention, the liaison nurse endeavors to answer the following: Does Ms. Brown believe that she "should" or "can," with consultation, provide Mr. Slaten with successful interventions herself? Does Dr. Martin believe that he "should" intervene, but know that he "can't"? How did the previous relationship between Ms. Brown and the consultant influence this case? How can the developing alliance with the head nurse and Dr. Martin be addressed? Did Mr. Slaten's language communicate criticism, despair or, helplessness? Was it heard as manipulation or devaluation? Did Mr. Slaten hear things differently? Was the unspeakable issue the wish for the client to leave or to die?

Intervention

Following are interventions planned for Mr. Slaten.

1. Direct assessment of Mr. Slaten and ongoing grief work by the liaison nurse
2. Consultation with a psychiatrist for psychotropic and pain medication and evaluation of competency and suicidality
3. Social service consultation with daughter and fiance for evaluation of needs
4. Team meeting—liaison focus, includes the head nurse. Mr. Slaten's intrapsychic conflict is explained, clarified; his affect is described and a care plan is developed
5. Care plan
   a. Therapeutic limit setting
      (1) Meals and snacks are provided as usual. If Mr. Slaten refuses these, he is not offered special foods.
      (2) Verbal abuse is to be ignored, but when Mr. Slaten becomes physically abusive, he is to be restrained.
      (3) Struggles over bathing and dressing changes are to be avoided: offer several different times for care and assistance while making Mr. Slaten responsible for refusing care.
   b. The consultees are encouraged to recognize the real stresses in Mr. Slaten's life and that his behavior is a mirror of his internal conflict. (Ms. Brown and Dr. Martin are not responsible for Mr. Slaten's responses, reactions, or care choices.)
   c. Consistent visibility and availability of the liaison nurse needs to occur.
   d. Regular team meetings need to occur.

BRIEF REVIEW

Psychiatric consultation liaison nursing incorporates theoretical concepts from nursing, psychiatry, crisis intervention, systems theory, and adult learning theory. Clinical practice is based on a blending of consultation and liaison theory, and focuses on the enhancement and effective management of psychologically based nursing care. A framework for assessment is also used that includes the five dimensions. Historically, psychiatric consultation liaison nursing emerged as a subspecialty of psychiatric nursing and developed in response to increased recognition of the mind-body relationship in physical illness and recovery, and additional clinical responsibilities of nursing staff, coupled with technological advances in medicine.

Mental health consultation is "the provision of clinical expertise regarding the delivery of psychological care in response to a request from a health care provider."[20] Liaison is "the facilitation of the relationship that exists between the patient, the illness, the consultees and the hospital/ward milieu."[20] The goals of psychiatric consultation liaison practice are (1) to teach the concepts and implementation of effective psychological care, (2) to support nursing staff in providing psychological care, (3) to aid in maintaining alliances, respect, and esteem with the consultee, and (4) to encourage acceptance and tolerance of insolvable care issues. Consultation and liaison alliances are developed as the work progresses and are powerful elements. The liaison nurse remains available, visible, objective, nonevaluative, and collaborative with consultees. Consultation and liaison alliances are strengthened as the psychiatric consultation liaison nurse implements the steps of the consultation process—assessment of the invitation to consult, evaluation of the appropriateness of the request, problem identification, and the determination and implementation of a direct or indirect intervention. The total consultation is diagnosed in order to further understand the needs of the client and the consultee.

Consultation practice is complementary to liaison practice. The elements of the liaison process are (1) education and socialization, (2) developmental level of the system and the consultee(s), (3) value and necessity of an alliance, (4) language, (5) developing the "ear" of the client and the "ear" of the consultee, (6) speaking the unspeakable, and (7) confirmation of reality. Liaison symbolizes the clinical partnership between the consultant and consultee.

Practice issues that affect the consultation liaison process are identification, transference or countertransference issues, parallel processing, or resistance involved in the consultation liaison relationship.

Psychiatric consultation liaison nursing practice can become quite powerful in the creation of a respectful, competent, clinical partnership with consultees. It is as detrimental to the achievement of clinical goals for the liaison nurse to accept an idealized or overly intimate status with client or consultee as it is for her to personalize resistance and rejection. Using the skills and knowledge of a nurse, a psychiatric clinician, and a consultant, the numerous pieces of the consultation liaison process are identified and implemented to enhance client care.

REFERENCES AND SUGGESTED READINGS

1. Barbiasz, L., and others: Establishing the psychiatric liaison nurse role: collaboration with the nurse administrator, Journal of Nursing Administration 14:8, 1982.
2. Barry, P.: Psychosocial nursing assessment and intervention, Philadelphia, 1984, J.B. Lippincott Co.
3. Blake, P.: The clinical specialist as nurse consultant, Journal of Nursing Administration 7:10, 1977.
4. Caplan, G.: The theory and practice of mental health consultation, New York, 1970, Basic Books, Inc, Publishers.
5. Davitz, L.L., and Davitz, J.R.: Nurses' responses to patients' suffering, New York, 1980, Springer Publishing Co., Inc.
6. Fife, B., and Lemler, S.: The psychiatric nurse specialist: a valuable asset in the general hospital, Journal of Nursing Administration 13:14, 1983.
7. Goldstein, S.: The psychiatric clinical specialist in the general hospital, Journal of Nursing Administration 9:3, 1979.
8. Groves, J.: Taking care of the hateful patient, New England Journal of Medicine 298(16):883, 1978.
9. Hamric, A., and Spross, J.: The clinical nurse specialist in theory and practice, New York, 1983, Grune & Stratton, Inc.
10. Hedlund, N.L.: Mental health nursing consultation in the general hospital, Patient Counseling and Health Education 1:85, 1978.
11. Hendler, N., Wise, T., and Lucas, M.J.: The expanded role of the psychiatric liaison nurse, Psychiatric Quarterly 51:135, 1979.
12. Holstein, S., and Schwab, J.: A coordinated consultation program for nurses and psychiatrists, Journal of the American Medical Association 194:5, 1965.
13. Howard, J.S.: Liaison nursing, Journal of Psychiatric Nursing and Mental Health Services 16:35, 1978.
14. Jackson, H.: The psychiatric nurse as a mental health consultant in a general hospital, Nursing Clinics of North America 4:327, 1969.
15. Kahana, R., and Bibring, G.: Personality types in medical management. In Zinberg, N.E., editor: Psychiatry and medical practice in a general hospital, New York, 1964, International Universities Press, Inc.
16. Kohnke, M.F.: The case for consultation in nursing designs for professional practice, New York, 1977, John Wiley & Sons, Inc.
17. Kucharski, A., and Groves, J.: The so-called "inappropriate" psychiatric consultation request in a medical or surgical ward, International Journal of Psychiatry in Medicine 7:209, 1976-1977.
18. Kuntz, S., Stehle, J., and Marshall, R.: The psychiatric clinical specialist: the progression of a speciality, Perspectives in Psychiatric Care 18:2, 1980.
19. Langman-Dorwart, N.: A model for mental health consultation to the general hospital, Journal of Psychiatric Nursing and Mental Health Services 17(3):29, 1979.
20. Lewis, A., and Levy, J.: Psychiatric liaison nursing: the theory and clinical practice, Reston, Va., 1982, Reston Publishing Co.
21. Lipowski, Z.J.: Consultation liaison psychiatry: an overview, American Journal of Psychiatry 131:623, 1974.
22. Lipowski, Z.J.: Liaison psychiatry, liaison nursing, and behavioral medicine, Comprehensive Psychiatry 22:6, 1981.
23. Lipanski, Z.J.: Physical illness, the individual and the coping process, International Journal of Psychiatry in Medicine 1(2):98, 1970.
24. McKegney, F.P., and Beckhardt, R.: Evaluative research in consultation liaison psychiatry—review of the literature 1970-1981, General Hospital Psychiatry 4:197, 1982.

25. Meyer, E., and Mendelson, M.: Psychiatric consultations with patients on medical and surgical wards: patterns and processes, Psychiatry **24**:199, 1961.
26. Moos, R.H.: Coping with physical illness, New York, 1977, Plenum Medical Book Co.
27. Nelson, J., and Schilke, D.: The evolution of psychiatric liaison nursing, Perspectives in Psychiatric Care **14**(9)61, 1976.
28. Pasanau, R.O.: Consultation-liaison psychiatry, New York, 1975, Grune & Stratton, Inc.
29. Pati, B.: Nursing consultation: a collaborative process, Journal of Nursing Administration **10**(11):33, 1980.
30. Peteet, J.: A closer look at the concept of support, General Hospital Psychiatry **4**(1):19, 1982.
31. Rankin, E., editor: Psychiatric/mental health nursing, Nursing Clinics of North America, **21**:3, 1986.
32. Robinson, L.: Liaison nursing: psychological approach to patient care, Philadelphia, 1974, F.A. Davis.
33. Robinson, L.: Psychiatric liaison nursing 1962-1982: a review and update of the literature, General Hospital Psychiatry **4**:139, 1982.
34. Samter, J., Scherer, M., and Shulman, D.: Interface of psychiatric clinical specialists in a community hospital setting, Journal of Psychiatric Nursing and Mental Health Services **19**(1):20, 1981.
35. Schwab, J.J.: The psychiatric consultation, Journal of Continuing Education in Psychiatry **40**(2):17, 1979.
36. Simmons, M.K.: Psychiatric consultation and liaison. In Critchey, D., and Mourin, J., editors: The clinical specialist in psychiatric mental health nursing, New York, 1985. John Wiley & Sons, Inc.
37. Simons, R.C., and Pardes, H., editors: Understanding human behavior in health and disease, Baltimore, 1977, Williams & Wilkins.
38. Stein, H.: The psychodynamics of medical practice: unconscious factors in patient care, Berkeley, Calif., 1985, University of California Press.
39. Stickney, S., Moir, G., and Gardner, E.: Psychiatric nurse consultation: who calls and why, Journal of Psychiatric Nursing and Mental Health Services **19**(10):22, 1981.
40. Strain, J., and Grossman, S.: Psychological care of the medically ill, New York, 1975, Appleton-Century-Crofts.
41. Termini, M., and Ciechoski, M.: The consultation process, Issues in Mental Health Nursing **3**:1, 77, 1981.

ANNOTATED BIBLIOGRAPHY

Barry, P.: Psychosocial nursing assessment intervention, Philadelphia, 1984, J.P. Lippincott Co.

General psychiatric concepts are used to develop a psychosocial assessment and intervention model for nonpsychiatric settings. The emphasis is on the functioning of nonpsychiatric clients who are having psychological responses to physical illness. The first part of the book presents a theoretical base including the implications of psychosocial issues and stress in physical illness, organic brain syndromes, use of defense mechanisms, and major personality styles. The second part includes nursing interventions with the emotionally complex client, psychosocial aspects of specific physical conditions, and the coping challenge of chronic illness. This book is a helpful guide for the psychiatric consultation liaison nurse.

Hackett, T., and Cassem, N.: Massachusetts General Hospital handbook of general hospital psychiatry, St. Louis, 1978, C.V. Mosby Co.

A handbook for professionals involved in the care of medical and surgical clients. This book contains helpful and practical information about the psychological care of the physically ill. Chapters on drug addiction, the pain patient, confusion, delirium, dementia, and coping with illness and depression are of special interest. The chapter on the role of nurse clinicians in liaison psychiatry describes the evolution and scope of the role at Massachussetts General Hospital.

Lewis, A., and Levy, J.: Psychiatric liaison nursing: the theory and clinical practice, Reston, Va., 1982, Reston Publishing Co.

A comprehensive textbook that provides a theoretical model based on a holistic approach to clinical practice. Geared primarily for graduate students in psychiatric nursing and practicing clinicians, the text traces the evolution of nursing consultation, the consultation process, and the experience of illness and hospitalization. Rich with examples from the authors' extensive clinical experience this text is practical as well as theoretical. This book, which was the American Journal of Nursing Book of the Year in 1982, is an essential addition to the psychiatric consultation liaison nurse's library.

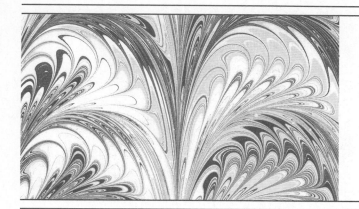

APPENDIX A
DSM-III-R Classification: Axes I-V Categories and Codes

All official DSM-III-R codes are included in ICD-9-CM. Codes followed by an asterisk (*) are used for more than one DSM-III-R diagnosis or subtype in order to maintain compatibility with ICD-9-CM.

A long dash following a diagnostic term indicates the need for a fifth digit subtype or other qualifying term.

The term *specify* following the name of some diagnostic categories indicates qualifying terms that clinicians may wish to add in parentheses after the name of the disorder.

NOS = Not Otherwise Specified

The current severity of a disorder may be specified after the diagnosis as:

Mild ⎤
Moderate ⎬ Currently meets diagnostic criteria
Severe ⎦

In partial remission (or residual state)
In complete remission

Disruptive Behavior Disorders

314.01	Attention-deficit hyperactivity disorder
	Conduct disorder
312.20	group type
312.00	solitary aggressive type
312.90	undifferentiated type
313.81	Oppositional defiant disorder

Anxiety Disorders of Childhood or Adolescence

309.21	Separation anxiety disorder
313.21	Avoidant disorder of childhood or adolescence
313.00	Overanxious disorder

Eating Disorders

307.10	Anorexia nervosa
307.51	Bulimia nervosa
307.52	Pica
307.53	Rumination disorder of infancy
307.50	Eating disorder NOS

Gender Identity Disorders

302.60	Gender identity disorder of childhood
302.50	Transsexualism
	Specify sexual history: asexual, homosexual, heterosexual, unspecified

DISORDERS USUALLY FIRST EVIDENT IN INFANCY, CHILDHOOD, OR ADOLESCENCE

Developmental Disorders
Note: These are coded on Axis II

Mental Retardation

317.00	Mild mental retardation
318.00	Moderate mental retardation
318.10	Severe mental retardation
318.20	Profound mental retardation
319.00	Unspecified mental retardation

Pervasive Developmental Disorders

299.00	Autistic disorder
	Specify if childhood onset
299.80	Pervasive developmental disorder NOS

Specific Developmental Disorders

	Academic skills disorders
315.10	Developmental arithmetic disorder
315.80	Developmental expressive writing disorder
315.00	Developmental reading disorder
	Language and speech disorders
315.39	Developmental articulation disorder
315.31*	Developmental expressive language disorder
315.31*	Developmental receptive language disorder
	Motor skills disorder
315.40	Developmental coordination disorder
315.90*	Specific developmental disorder NOS

Other Developmental Disorders

315.90*	Developmental disorder NOS

302.85*	Gender identity disorder of adolescence or adulthood, nontranssexual type
	Specify sexual history: asexual, homosexual, heterosexual, unspecified
302.85*	Gender identity disorder NOS

Tic Disorders

307.23   Tourette's disorder
307.22   Chronic motor or vocal tic disorder
307.21   Transient tic disorder
          Specify: single episode or recurrent
307.20   Tic disorder NOS

Elimination Disorders

307.70   Functional encopresis
          Specify: primary or secondary type
307.60   Functional enuresis
          Specify: primary or secondary type
          Specify: nocturnal only, diurnal only, nocturnal and diurnal

Speech Disorders Not Elsewhere Classified

307.00*   Cluttering
307.00*   Stuttering

Other Disorders of Infancy, Childhood, or Adolescence

313.23   Elective mutism
313.82   Identity disorder
313.89   Reactive attachment disorder of infancy or early childhood
307.30   Stereotype/habit disorder
314.00   Undifferentiated attention deficit disorder

ORGANIC MENTAL DISORDERS

Dementias Arising in the Senium and Presenium

          Primary degenerative dementia of the Alzheimer type, senile onset
290.30   with delirium
290.20   with delusions
290.21   with depression
290.00*   uncomplicated
          (Note: code 331.00 Alzheimer's disease on Axis III)

Code in fifth digit:
1 = with delirium, 2 = with delusions, 3 = with depression, 0* = uncomplicated

290.1x   Primary degenerative dementia of the Alzheimer type presenile onset, _____
          (Note: code 331.00 Alzheimer's disease on Axis III)
290.4x   Multi-infarct dementia, _____
290.00*   Senile dementia NOS
          Specify etiology on Axis III if known
290.10*   Presenile dementia NOS
          Specify etiology on Axis III if known (e.g., Pick's disease, Jakob-Creutzfeldt disease)

Psychoactive Substance-Induced Organic Mental Disorders

          Alcohol
303.00   intoxication
291.40   idiosyncratic intoxication
291.80   Uncomplicated alcohol withdrawal
291.00   withdrawal delirium
291.30   hallucinosis
291.10   amnestic disorder
291.20   Dementia associated with alcoholism
          Amphetamine or similarly acting sympathomimetic
305.70*   intoxication
292.00*   withdrawal
292.81*   delirium
292.11*   delusional disorder

          Caffeine
305.90*   intoxication
          Cannabis
305.20*   intoxication
292.11*   delusional disorder
          Cocaine
305.60*   intoxication
292.00*   withdrawal
292.81*   dilirium
292.11*   delusional disorder
          Hallucinogen
305.30*   hallucinosis
292.11*   delusional disorder
292.84*   mood disorder
292.89*   Posthallucinogen perception disorder
          Inhalant
305.90*   intoxication
          Nicotine
292.00*   withdrawal
          Opioid
305.50*   intoxication
292.00*   withdrawal
          Phencyclidine (PCP) or similarly acting arylcyclohexylamine
305.90*   intoxication
292.81*   delirium
292.11*   delusional disorder
292.84*   mood disorder
292.90*   organic mental disorder NOS
          Sedative, hypnotic, or anxiolytic
305.40*   intoxication
292.00*   Uncomplicated sedative, hypnotic, or anxiolytic withdrawal
292.00*   withdrawal delirium
292.83*   amnestic disorder
          Other or unspecified psychoactive susbstance
305.90*   intoxication
292.00*   withdrawal
292.81*   delirium
292.82*   dementia
292.83*   amnestic disorder
292.11*   delusional disorder
292.12   hallucinosis
292.84*   mood disorder
292.89*   anxiety disorder
292.89*   personality disorder
292.90*   organic mental disorder NOS

Organic Mental Disorders Associated with Axis III Physical Disorders or Conditions, or Whose Etiology is Unknown

293.00   Delirium
294.10   Dementia
294.00   Amnestic disorder
293.81   Organic delusional disorder
293.82   Organic hallucinosis
293.83   Organic mood disorder
          Specify: manic, depressed, mixed
294.80*   Organic anxiety disorder
310.10   Organic personality disorder
          Specify if explosive type
294.80*   Organic mental disorder NOS

PSYCHOACTIVE SUBSTANCE USE DISORDERS

          Alcohol
303.90   dependence
305.00   abuse

Amphetamine or similarly acting sympathomimetic
304.40   dependence
305.70*   abuse
Cannabis
304.30   dependence
305.20*   abuse
Cocaine
304.20   dependence
305.60*   abuse
Hallucinogen
304.50*   dependence
305.30*   abuse
Inhalant
304.60   dependence
305.90*   abuse
Nicotine
305.10   dependence
Opioid
304.00   dependence
305.50*   abuse
Phencyclidine (PCP) or similarly acting arylcyclohex-
    ylamine
304.50*   dependence
305.90*   abuse
Sedative, hypnotic, or anxiolytic
304.10   dependence
305.40*   abuse
304.90*   Polysubstance dependence
304.90*   Psychoactive substance dependence NOS
305.90*   Psychoactive substance abuse NOS

SCHIZOPHRENIA

Code in fifth digit:
1 = subchronic, 2 = chronic, 3 = subchronic with acute exacerbation, 4 = chronic with acute exacerbation, 5 = in remission, 0 = unspecified.

Schizophrenia
295.2x   catatonic, _____
295.1x   disorganized, _____
295.3x   paranoid, _____
    Specify if stable type
295.9x   undifferentiated, _____
295.6x   residual, _____
    Specify if late onset

DELUSIONAL (PARANOID) DISORDER

297.10   Delusional (Paranoid) disorder
    Specify erotomanic, grandiose, jealous, persecutory, somatic, unspecified;

PSYCHOTIC DISORDERS NOT ELSEWHERE CLASSIFIED

298.80   Brief reactive psychosis
295.40   Schizophreniform disorder
    Specify: without good prognostic features or with good prognostic features
295.70   Schizoaffective disorder
    Specify: bipolar type or depressive type
297.30   Induced psychotic disorder
298.90   Psychotic disorder NOS (Atypical psychosis)

MOOD DISORDERS

Code current state of Major Depression and Bipolar Disorder in fifth digit:
1 = mild, 2 = moderate, 3 = severe, without psychotic features, 4 = with psychotic features (*specify* mood-congruent or mood incongruent), 5 = in partial remission, 6 = in full remission, 0 = unspecified

For major depressive episodes, *Specify* if chronic and *specify* if melancholic type.

For Bipolar Disorder, Bipolar Disorder NOS, Recurrent Major Depression, and Depressive Disorder NOS, *specify* if seasonal pattern.

Bipolar Disorders

Bipolar disorder
296.6x   mixed, _____
296.4x   manic, _____
296.5x   depressed, _____
301.13   Cyclothymia
296.70   Bipolar disorder NOS

Depressive Disorders

Major Depression
296.2x   single episode, _____
296.3x   recurrent, _____
300.40   Dysthymia (or Depressive neurosis)
    Specify: primary or secondary type
    Specify: early or late onset
311.00   Depressive disorder NOS

ANXIETY DISORDERS (or Anxiety and Phobic Neuroses)

Panic disorder
300.21   with agoraphobia
    Specify current severity of agoraphobic avoidance
    Specify current severity of panic attacks
300.01   without agoraphobia
    Specify current severity of panic attacks
300.22   Agoraphobia without history of panic disorder
    Specify with or without limited symptom attacks
300.23   Social phobia
    Specify if generalized type
300.29   Simple phobia
300.30   Obsessive compulsive disorder (or Obsessive compulsive neurosis)
309.89   Post-traumatic stress disorder
    Specify if delayed onset
300.02   Generalized anxiety disorder
300.00   Anxiety disorder NOS

SOMATOFORM DISORDERS

300.70*   Body dysmorphic disorder
300.11   Conversion disorder (or Hysterical neurosis, conversion type)
    Specify: single episode or recurrent
300.70*   Hypochondriasis (or Hypochondriacal neurosis)
300.81   Somatization disorder
307.80   Somatoform pain disorder
300.70*   Undifferentiated somatoform disorder
300.70*   Somatoform disorder NOS

DISSOCIATIVE DISORDERS (or Hysterical Neuroses, Dissociative Type)

300.14   Multiple personality disorder
300.13   Psychogenic fugue
300.12   Psychogenic amnesia
300.60   Depersonalization disorder (or Depersonalization neurosis)
300.15   Dissociative disorder NOS

SEXUAL DISORDERS

Paraphilias

302.40   Exhibitionism
302.81   Fetishism
302.89   Frotteurism
302.20   Pedophilia
          Specify: same sex, opposite sex, same and opposite
          sex
          Specify if limited to incest
          Specify: exclusive type or nonexclusive type
302.83   Sexual masochism
302.84   Sexual sadism
302.30   Transvestic fetishism
302.82   Voyeurism
302.90*   Paraphilia NOS

Sexual Dysfunctions

Specify: psychogenic only, or psychogenic and biogenic
(Note: If biogenic only, code on Axis III)
Specify: lifelong or acquired
Specify: generalized or situational

          Sexual desire disorders
302.71   Hypoactive sexual desire disorder
302.79   Sexual aversion disorder
          Sexual arousal disorders
302.72*   Female sexual arousal disorder
302.72*   Male erectile disorder
          Orgasm disorders
302.73   Inhibited female orgasm
302.74   Inhibited male orgasm
302.75   Premature ejaculation
          Sexual pain disorders
302.76   Dyspareunia
306.51   Vaginismus
302.70   Sexual dysfunction NOS

Other Sexual Disorders

302.90*   Sexual disorder NOS

SLEEP DISORDERS

Dyssomnias

          Insomnia disorder
307.42*   related to another mental disorder (nonorganic)
780.50*   related to known organic factor
307.42*   Primary insomnia
          Hypersomnia disorder
307.44   related to another mental disorder (nonorganic)
780.50*   related to a known organic factor
780.54   Primary hypersomnia
307.45   Sleep-wake schedule disorder
          Specify: advanced or delayed phase type, disorga-
          nized type, frequently changing type
          Other dyssomnias
307.40*   Dyssomnia NOS

Parasomnias

307.47   Dream anxiety disorder (Nightmare disorder)
307.46*   Sleep terror disorder
307.46*   Sleepwalking disorder
307.40*   Parasomnia NOS

FACTITIOUS DISORDERS

          Factitious disorder
301.51   with physical symptoms
300.16   with psychological symptoms
300.19   Factitious disorder NOS

IMPULSE CONTROL DISORDERS NOT ELSEWHERE CLASSIFIED

312.34   Intermittent explosive disorder
312.32   Kleptomania
312.31   Pathological gambling
312.33   Pyromania
312.39*   Trichotillomania
312.39*   Impulse control disorder NOS

ADJUSTMENT DISORDER

          Adjustment disorder
309.24   with anxious mood
309.00   with depressed mood
309.30   with disturbance of conduct
309.40   with mixed disturbance of emotions and conduct
309.28   with mixed emotional features
309.82   with physical complaints
309.83   with withdrawal
309.23   with work (or academic) inhibition
309.90   Adjustment disorder NOS

PSYCHOLOGICAL FACTORS AFFECTING PHYSICAL CONDITION

316.00   Psychological factors affecting physical condition
          Specify physical condition on Axis III

Personality Disorders
Note: These are coded on Axis II

Cluster A

301.00   Paranoid
301.20   Schizoid
301.22   Schizotypal

Cluster B

301.70   Antisocial
301.83   Borderline
301.50   Histrionic
301.81   Narcissistic

Cluster C

301.82   Avoidant
301.60   Dependent
301.40   Obsessive compulsive
301.84   Passive aggressive
301.90   Personality disorder NOS

V CODES FOR CONDITIONS NOT ATTRIBUTABLE TO A MENTAL DISORDER THAT ARE A FOCUS OF ATTENTION OR TREATMENT

V62.30   Academic problem
V71.01   Adult antisocial behavior

V40.00   Borderline intellectual functioning (Note: This
          is coded on Axis II)

V71.02   Childhood or adolescent antisocial behavior
V65.20   Malingering

V61.10	Marital problem
V15.81	Noncompliance with medical treatment
V62.20	Occupational problem
V61.20	Parent-child problem
V62.81	Other interpersonal problem
V61.80	Other specified family circumstances
V62.89	Phase of life problem or other life circumstance problem
V62.82	Uncomplicated bereavement

ADDITIONAL CODES

300.90	Unspecified mental disorder (nonpsychotic)
V71.09*	No diagnosis or condition on Axis I
799.90*	Diagnosis or condition deferred on Axis I

V71.09*	No diagnosis or condition on Axis II
799.90*	Diagnosis or condition deferred on Axis II

MULTIAXIAL SYSTEM

Axis I	Clinical Syndromes
	V Codes
Axis II	Developmental Disorders
	Personality Disorders
Axis III	Physical Disorders and Conditions
Axis IV	Severity of Psychosocial Stressors
Axis V	Global Assessment of Functioning

SEVERITY OF PSYCHOSOCIAL STRESSORS SCALE: ADULTS

CODE	TERM	EXAMPLES OF STRESSORS	
		Acute Events	**Enduring Circumstances**
1	None	No acute events that may be relevant to the disorder	No enduring circumstances that may be relevant to the disorder
2	Mild	Broke up with boyfriend or girlfriend; started or graduated from school; child left home	Family arguments; job dissatisfaction; residence in high-crime neighborhood
3	Moderate	Marriage; marital separation; loss of job; retirement; miscarriage	Marital discord; serious financial problems; trouble with boss; being a single parent
4	Severe	Divorce; birth of first child	Unemployment; poverty
5	Extreme	Death of spouse; serious physical illness diagnosed; victim of rape	Serious chronic illness in self or child; ongoing physical or sexual abuse
6	Catastrophic	Death of child; suicide of spouse; devastating natural disaster	Capitivity as hostage; concentration camp experience
0	Inadequate information, or no change in condition		

SEVERITY OF PSYCHOSOCIAL STRESSORS SCALE: CHILDREN AND ADOLESCENTS

CODE	TERM	EXAMPLES OF STRESSORS	
		Acute Events	**Enduring Circumstances**
1	None	No acute events that may be relevant to the disorder	No enduring circumstances that may be relevant to the disorder
2	Mild	Broke up with boyfriend or girlfriend; change of school	Overcrowded living quarters; family arguments
3	Moderate	Expelled from school; birth of sibling	Chronic disabling illness in parent; chronic parental discord
4	Severe	Divorce of parents; unwanted pregnancy; arrest	Harsh or rejecting parents; chronic life-threatening illness in parent; multiple foster home placements
5	Extreme	Sexual or physical abuse; death of a parent	Recurrent sexual or physical abuse
6	Catastrophic	Death of both parents	Chronic life-threatening illness
0	Inadequate information, or no change in condition		

GLOBAL ASSESSMENT OF FUNCTIONING SCALE (GAF Scale)

Consider psychological, social, and occupational functioning on a hypothetical continuum of mental health-illness. Do not include impairment in functioning due to physical (or environmental) limitations.

Note: use intermediate codes when appropriate, e.g., 45, 68, 72.

Code

90
|
81   **Absent or minimal symptoms** (e.g., mild anxiety before an exam), **good functioning in all areas, interested and involved in a wide range of activities, socially effective, generally satisfied with life, no more than everyday problems or concerns** (e.g., an occasional argument with family members).

80
|
71   **If symptoms are present, they are transient and expectable reactions to psychosocial stressors** (e.g., difficulty concentrating after family argument); **no more than slight impairment in social, occupational, or school functioning** (e.g., temporarily falling behind in school work).

70
|
61   **Some mild symptoms** (e.g., depressed mood and mild insomnia) **OR some difficulty in social, occupational, or school functioning** (e.g., occasional truancy, or theft within the household), **but generally functioning pretty well, has some meaningful interpersonal relationships**

60
51   **Moderate symptoms** (e.g., flat affect and circumstantial speech, occasional panic attacks) **OR moderate difficulty in social, occupational, or school functioning** (e.g., few friends, conflicts with co-workers).

50
41   **Serious symptoms** (e.g., suicidal ideation, severe obsessional rituals, frequent shoplifting) **OR any serious impairment in social, occupational, or school functioning** (e.g., no friends, unable to keep a job)

40
|
31   **Some impairment in reality testing or communication** (e.g., speech is at times illogical, obscure or irrelevant) **OR major impairment in several areas, such as work or school, family relations, judgment, thinking, or mood** (e.g., depressed man avoids friends, neglects family, and is unable to work; child frequently beats up younger children, is defiant at home, and is failing at school).

30
|
21   **Behavior is considerably influenced by delusions or hallucinations OR serious impairment in communication or judgment** (e.g., sometimes incoherent, acts grossly inappropriately, suicidal preoccupation) **OR inability to function in almost all areas** (e.g., stays in bed all day; no job, home, or friends)

20
|
11   **Some danger of hurting self or others** (e.g., suicide attempts without clear expectation of death, frequently violent, manic excitement) **OR occasionally fails to maintain minimal personal hygiene** (e.g., smears feces) **OR gross impairment in communication** (e.g., largely incoherent or mute).

10
1   **Persistent danger of severely hurting self or others** (e.g., recurrent violence) **OR persistent inability to maintain minimal personal hygiene OR serious suicidal act with clear expectation of death.**

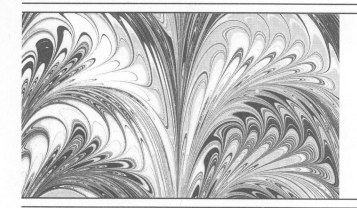

APPENDIX B

ANA Standards of Psychiatric and Mental Heath Nursing Practice

Standard I–Theory

The nurse applies appropriate theory that is scientifically sound as a basis for decisions regarding nursing practice.

Standard II–Data Collection

The nurse continuously collects data that are comprehensive, accurate, and systematic.

Standard III–Diagnosis

The nurse utilizes nursing diagnoses and standard classification of mental disorders to express conclusions supported by recorded assessment data and current scientific premises.

Standard IV–Planning

The nurse develops a nursing care plan with specific goals and interventions delineating nursing actions unique to each client's needs.

Standard V–Intervention

The nurse intervenes as guided by the nursing care plan to implement nursing actions that promote, maintain, or restore physical and mental health, prevent illness, and effect rehabilitation.

Standard V-A–Psychotherapeutic Interventions

The nurse (generalist) uses psychotherapeutic interventions to assist clients to regain or improve their previous coping abilities and to prevent further disability.

Standard V-B–Heath Teaching

The nurse assists clients, families, and groups to achieve satisfying and productive patterns of living through health teaching.

Standard V-C–Self-care Activities

The nurse uses the activities of daily living in a goal-directed way to foster adequate self-care and physical and mental well-being of clients.

Standard V-D–Somatic Therapies

The nurse uses knowledge of somatic therapies and applies related clinical skills in working with clients.

Standard V-E–Therapeutic Environment

The nurse provides, structures, and maintains a therapeutic environment in collaboration with the client and other health care providers.

Standard V-F–Psychotherapy

The nurse (specialist) utilizes advanced clinical expertise in individual, group, and family psychotherapy, child psychotherapy, and other treatment modalities to function as a psychotherapist and recognizes professional accountability for nursing practice.

Standard VI–Evaluation

The nurse evaluates client responses to nursing actions in order to revise the data base, nursing diagnoses, and nursing care plan.

Standard VII–Peer Review

The nurse participates in peer review and other means of evaluation to assure quality of nursing care provided for clients.

Standard VIII–Continuing Education

The nurse assumes responsibility for continuing education and professional development and contributes to the professional growth of others.

Standard IX–Interdisciplinary Collaboration

The nurse collaborates with interdisciplinary teams in assessing, planning, implementing, and evaluating programs and other mental health activities.

Standard X–Utilization of Community Health Systems

The nurse (specialist) participates with other members of the community in assessing, planning, implementing, and evaluating mental health services and community systems that include the promotion of the broad continuum of primary, secondary, and tertiary prevention of mental illness.

Standard XI–Research

The nurse contributes to nursing and the mental health field through innovations in theory and practice and participation in research.

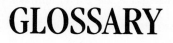

GLOSSARY

abreaction Process whereby repressed material is brought back to consciousness and reexperienced affectively.

absolute rights Veto powers that moral agents have against majorities or rulers.

abstract thinking Stage in the development of cognitive thought processes. Thoughts are characterized by adaptability, flexibility, and the use of abstractions and generalizations.

accommodation Process of change that enables the individual to manage situations that were previously beyond his abilities.

acquaintance rape A rape committed by a man known to the victim.

acrophobia Fear of high places.

acting out Indirect expression of feelings through behavior, usually nonverbal, that attracts the attention of others.

active listening Alert hearing, with an attitude of wanting to hear what the client has to say.

active-passive Concept that characterizes persons as either actively involved in shaping events or passively reacting to events.

actualized religions Religions that stress trust in one's own nature and encourage self-direction and growth.

activity theory Theory in which Havighurst proposes that activity promotes well-being and satisfaction in aging.

acute or functional grief The process of acknowledging and expressing feelings associated with loss.

acute pain A subjective sensation of hurt, caused by a harmful stimulus, that warns of current or impending damage to tissue.

adaptation Striving to find equilibrium between oneself and one's environment.

adaptive dependence Behavior in which a person is dependent when the external and internal environments preclude autonomous functioning.

adaptive independence Behavior that occurs when the individual is able to act according to his own judgment.

adaptive maneuvering Manipulative responses of newborns.

addiction Physical dependence on a substance.

adjunctive groups Groups with specific activities and focuses, such as socialization, perceptual stimulation, sensory stimulation, and orientation to reality.

administrative consultee–centered consultation Expert advice to caregivers in conflict.

administrative program–centered consultation Expert advice regarding a program or a policy of an organization.

Adult ego state Part of the self that computes and solves problems, using information received from the Parent and Child ego states.

affect Outward manifestation of a person's feelings and emotions.

affection Feeling or emotion expressed toward another; a loving attachment; fondness.

affiliation Closeness or connection with another (as achieved by affiliative behavior).

agape Greek for the highest form of love.

agapeism Practice of love-based ethics.

aggression Forceful, self-assertive action or attitude that is expressed physically, verbally, or symbolically. It may arise from innate drives or occur as a defensive mechanism and is manifested by either constructive or destructive acts directed toward oneself or against others.

aggressive maneuvering Type of destructive manipulative behavior that is characterized by multiple demands, threats, requests for special consideration, and playing members of the health care team against each other.

aggressive-radical therapy Therapy that proposes that clients should be radicalized through the therapeutic process. Making all values explicit results in the client's viewing the solution of emotional conflict and the raising of political consciousness as one and the same.

agnosia Total or partial loss of the ability to recognize familiar objects or persons through sensory stimuli as a result of organic brain damage.

agoraphobia Anxiety disorder characterized by a fear of being in an open, crowded, or public place, where escape may be difficult or help not available in case of sudden incapacitation.

agraphia Impairment in intellectual functioning characterized by the loss of the ability to write.

aim Characteristic of an instinct directed toward removing a body need.

akathisia Side effect of antipsychotic medication that is manifested by a feeling of restlessness and frequently accompanied by complaint of a twitching or crawling sensation in the muscles.

akinesia Impaired motor function.

Al-Anon Self-help group in which family members of alcoholics are taught how to understand and give healthy support to the drinker.

alarm reaction (AR) Initial response to stress characterized by a generalized expression of the body's defense system; first stage of the general adaptation syndrome.

Alateen Self-help group for teenage members of families in which they are taught how to understand and give healthy support to the drinker.

Alcoholics Anonymous (AA) Organization of recovering alcoholics whose purpose is to help alcoholics stop drinking and maintain sobriety through group support, shared experiences, and faith in a power greater than themselves.

alcoholism Condition in which a person's drinking behavior constitutes a social and health problem, characterized by psychosocial and biochemical causes, physiological effects, including brain damage, and public and personal consequences.

Alexander technique Alternative therapy founded by Frederick Alexander that focuses on the body musculature, posture, and breathing process. The goal of treatment is reintegration of the body through reeducation.

alexia Impairment in intellectual functioning characterized by the inability to comprehend written words.

all-channel pattern of communication Messages may originate at any point and all members may interact.

altruism Love-based ethics that involve loving and doing for others what one does for oneself.

ambivalence Simultaneous conflicting feelings or attitudes toward a person or object.

amnesia Loss of memory of a specific time or event or a loss of all past memories.

anaclitic depression Syndrome occurring in infants usually after sudden separation from the mothering person and characterized by severe impairments in the infant's physical, emotional, intellectual, and social development.

analysis Categorization of data, identification of gaps in data, and determination of patterns from pieces of data. Used to interpret and give meaning to collected data.

andropause Change of life in men when a reordering of their life takes place, for example, career change and divorce.

anger Strong feeling of annoyance or displeasure.

anhedonia Inability to feel pleasure or happiness for experiences that are ordinarily pleasurable.

anilingus Oral stimulation of the anal area.

anima Female archetype in the male.

animus Masculine archetype in the female.

anorexia General loss of appetite resulting from physical and psychosocial causes, contributing to a state of malnutrition and related mental health problems.

anorexia nervosa Extreme form of anorexia, usually seen in adolescent girls, characterized by distorted body image and prolonged inability to eat, with marked weight loss, amenorrhea, and other symptoms resulting from emotional conflict. Creates life-threatening condition and retarded growth.

anticholinergic Pertains to the blockade of acetylcholine receptors resulting in inhibition of transmission of parasympathetic nerve impulses.

anticipatory adaptation Act of adapting in advance of a potentially distressing situation, such as when a person tries to relax before calling to receive the results of a laboratory test.

anticipatory grief Feelings experienced in anticipation of a loss that has not yet occurred.

anticipatory guidance Helping persons anticipate vivid details of an expected challenge and consider the accompanying unpleasant emotions and fantasies.

antisocial behavior Lack of socialization with behavior patterns that bring a person repeatedly into conflict with society.

antisocial personality disorder Disorder characterized by repetitive failure to abide by social and legal norms and to accept responsibility for own behavior.

anxiety State of feeling of apprehension, uneasiness, agitation, uncertainty, and fear resulting from anticipation of a threat or danger, usually of intrapsychic origin, whose source is generally unknown or unrecognized.

anxiety disorders Emotional illness characterized by the feeling of fear and by symptoms associated with the autonomic nervous system, such as palpitations, tachycardia, dizziness, and tremor.

anxiety hierarchy Hierarchial relationships among anxiety-producing stimuli.

anxiolytic An antianxiety medication.

aphasia Abnormal neurological condition in which language function is defective or absent because of an injury to certain areas of the cerebral cortex.

approach-approach conflict Conflict resulting from the simultaneous presence of two or more incompatible impulses, desires, or goals, each of which is desirable.

approach-avoidance conflict Conflict resulting from the presence of a single goal or desire that is both desirable and undesirable.

apraxia Impairment in the ability to engage in purposeful activities, even though muscle strength and coordination are present.

arbitrary inference Type of cognitive distortion in which a negative conclusion is drawn from insufficient evidence.

archetypes Symbols that are derived from the collective experiences of the race.

Arica therapy Alternative therapy founded by Oscar Ichazo that focuses on consciousness and provides tools to systematize and describe the human psyche. The goal of therapy is to increase the powers of the mind.

art therapy Type of therapy that focuses on expressing oneself and portraying one's feelings by use of various forms of artwork.

asceticism Defense mechanism commonly used in adolescence that involves repudiation of all instinctual impulses.

assault Threat of touching without the client's consent.

assertiveness Behavior that is directed toward claiming one's rights without denying the rights of others.

assertiveness training Alternative therapy that focuses on the development of behaviors for self-expression of feelings, attitudes, wishes, opinions, and rights.

assessment First phase of the nursing process, which involves the collection of data about the health status of the client.

assimilation Process by which the child develops the ability to handle new situations and problems with his existing mechanisms.

assurance Process that includes the identification of values and standards, specification of criteria, measurement of observable aspects of care, and remedial action if indicated.

asterixis Hand-flapping tremor often accompanying metabolic disorders.

atman Innermost spirit and highest controlling power of a person.

atypical somatoform disorder Physical symptoms and complaints that appear to be a preoccupation with some imagined defect in physical appearance or ability.

audit Review and evaluation of nursing care procedures.

authenticity Quality of being trustworthy and genuine; emotional and behavioral openness in a relationship.

authoritarian personality Constellation of traits indicative of one who advocates obedience and strict adherence to rules.

autism Preoccupation with the self and with inner experiences.

autistic thought Ideation that has a private meaning to the individual.

autoerotic Sensual, self-gratifying.

autogenic therapy Alternative therapy founded by Wolfgang Luthe that focuses on the brain-directed processes. The goal of treatment is establishing functional harmony by using natural forces in the brain.

automatic thoughts Type of habitual shorthand conclusion about a situation that is not subjected to critical evaluation.

aversion therapy Application of the behavioral model of psychiatric care. A painful stimulus is given to create an aversion to another stimulus, which leads to a behavior that the individual wishes to change.

avoidance responding Performing a behavior before a conditioned stimulus appears.

avoidance-avoidance conflict Conflict resulting fror the confrontation of two or more alternative goals or desires that are equally aversive and undesirable.

avoidant personality disorder Condition characterized by hypersensitivity to rejection, a need for uncritical acceptance, and low self-esteem.

awareness context of death What each individual involved with a dying client knows of the client's defined status or condition and the client's recognition of others' awareness.

balancing factors Events that contribute to the production and outcome of a crisis.

basic anxiety Profound insecurity and vague apprehensiveness.

battered wife Any woman who is beaten by her mate, regardless of the legality of the marital relationship.

battery Touching the client without his consent.

battle fatigue Physically and psychologically disabling condition caused from participation in a war.

behavior Any observable, recordable, and measurable act, movement, or response of an individual.

behavior modification Type of therapy that attempts to modify observable, maladaptive patterns of behavior by the substitution of a new response or set of responses to a given stimulus.

behavioral treatment Modality of treatment that helps the individual modify behavior by changing learned behavior responses.

benign suicide Indirect self-destructive behavior; also called subintentional suicide.

benzodiazepines Group of chemically related antianxiety drugs.

bibliotherapy Type of group therapy in which articles, books, poems, and newspapers are read in the group to help stimulate thinking about events in the real world and secondarily to foster relating to each other.

bioenergetic therapy Alternative therapy founded by Alexander Lowen that focuses on the body musculature and breathing process. The goal of treatment is to release the body armor and permit the flow of energy.

biofeedback Process providing a person with visual or auditory information about the autonomic physiological functions of his body, as blood pressure, muscle tension, and brain wave activity, usually through the use of instrumentation.

biorhythms Any cyclic biological event or phenomenon, such as the sleep cycle, the menstrual cycle, or the respiratory cycle.

bipolar affective disorder Subgroup of the affective disorders that is characterized by the occurrence of at least one episode of manic behavior, with or without a history of episodes of depression.

bisexuality Ability to achieve orgasm with a partner of either sex.

blocked communication Incongruent verbal and nonverbal messages; also, discrepancies and inconsistencies in messages.

blocking Spontaneous loss of thought.

blunting Decreased intensity of emotional expression from that which one would normally expect.

body image Person's subjective concept of his physical appearance.

body language Transmission of a message by body position or movement.

body monitoring Activities in which individuals engage to keep the body in shape.

borderline personality disorder Condition characterized by instability in many areas, with no single feature present. Some characteristics are unstable interpersonal relationships, impulsive behavior, and wide mood swings.

boundary Index of family health in which the generations are clearly marked and issues are dealt with by the appropriate generation; the limit set between the family and the larger society.

bruxism Grinding of the teeth.

bulimia nervosa Form of anorexia nervosa in which the victim alternates periods of anorexia and fasting with periods of gorging and then purging with induced vomiting. Victims may rapidly consume up to 50,000 calories of food in a few hours and then induce vomiting, sometimes repeating the behavior as often as three or four times in one day.

butyrophenones Group of chemically related antipsychotic drugs.

cachectic State of malnutrition resulting from excessive dieting.

caffeinism Condition of nervous stimulation resulting from excessive use of caffeine-containing beverages or drugs. Characterized by typical drug withdrawal symptoms when caffeine intake is restricted or removed.

capacity Ability to understand or comprehend. Total comprehension is not necessary.

catastrophic reaction Heightened anxiety that occurs in confused persons when they are not able to answer or perform.

cao gio Folk practice that consists of applying oil to the back and chest of a child with cotton swabs, massaging the skin until warm, and then rubbing it with the edge of a copper coin until marks appear.

case study Descriptive survey that focuses on one or a limited number of units; a unit may be an individual, a group, or an institution.

catatonic State of psychologically induced immobilization, at times interrupted by episodes of extreme agitation.

catatonic excitement State of extreme agitation that occurs when a person is unable to maintain catatonic immobility.

catatonic stupor Apparently unresponsive state that is related to a fear of loss of impulse control.

catharsis Release that occurs when the client is encouraged to talk about things that bother him. Thoughts and feelings are brought out in the open and discussed.

causal comparative research Extension of correlational research in which in addition to discovering relationships among variables of interest, the researcher also identifies the possible cause after the effects have already occurred.

causal connecting statements Process by which the nurse helps the client relate the cause and effect between two events that are the outcome of the client's specific feelings, behavior, or responses.

certification Process by which a nongovernmental agency provides a reliable endorsement that a person has met predetermined standards in a specialized area of nursing.

chain pattern of communication Messages are initiated at one point and are passed from one receiver to the next until the message reaches the end of the chain.

chakras In Hindu belief, centers of swirling pranaic energy that act as centers of consciousness.

ch'i In Chinese philosophy, fundamental life energy that flows in orderly ways through the body along meridians.

child abuse or neglect Physical or mental injury, sexual abuse, negligent treatment, or maltreatment of a child under eighteen years of age.

Child ego state Part of self that includes feelings, wishes, and memories; part of this ego state is the natural use of feelings as they arise, and part is learned behavior as one responds to others by adapting to their wishes or by rebelling.

child psychiatry Subspecialty area of psychiatry that focuses on the study and treatment of emotionally disturbed children.

chlorpromizine equivalent Approximation of the quantity of drug necessary to equal 100 mg of chlorpromazine's antipsychotic efficacy.

chromosome Any of the threadlike structures in the nucleus of a cell that function in the transmission of genetic information.

chronic care Modality of care, usually clinic based, requiring monitoring of a chronic, long-standing clinical health problem.

chronic mental distress Set of behaviors representing a role created by society as a result of observations of individuals exhibiting behaviors troublesome to society and labeled mentally deviant.

chronic pain Subjective sensation of hurt, with or without pathological findings and of longer duration.

chronicity The continuation of a health disruption until it has a possibly permanent impact on the overall identify and life style of the client.

chronopsychophysiology Science that studies the physiological cyclic processes in the body.

Chua K'a System of muscle tension release that emphasizes clarification and cleansing of both mind and emotions.

circadian rhythm Pattern based on a 24-hour cycle, especially the repetition of certain physiological phenomena, such as sleeping and eating.

circumstantial speech Type of speech in which there is the inclusion of many unnecessary and trivial details before the person reaches his goal.

civil suit Dispute between two persons that is resolved by a variety of remedies, most often monetary.

clang associations Combining of words that rhyme.

clarification Intervention technique designed to guide the client to focus on and recognize gaps and inconsistencies in his statements.

claustrophobia Fear of closed places.

client-centered consultation Expert advice regarding care of person needing service.

climacteric Menopausal period in women; sometimes used to refer to the corresponding period in men.

clinical psychologist Psychologist who specializes in the selection, administration, and interpretation of psychological tests.

closed awareness context of death Attempts are made to prevent the client from knowing of his possible death.

closed groups Groups in which all members are admitted at the same time and vacancies occurring in membership are not filled.

coaching Method of engaging spouses in dialogue about alternative actions while leaving the choice to clients.

coalitions Family members uniting with one parent against the other.

cognition Process of logical thought.

cognitive Referring to the mental process of comprehension, judgment, memory, and reasoning, as contrasted with emotional and volitional processes.

cognitive appraisal Process that probably takes place in the cerebral cortex and intervenes between the environmental stimulus and the reaction.

cognitive restoration Intervention technique designed to restore cognitive functioning.

cognitive restructuring Change of attitudes, values, or beliefs that limit the person's self-expression as a result of insight or behavioral achievement.

cognitive structuring The therapist reviews with the client the changes that have occurred in a client's thinking in order to give the client a sense of change and a sense of playing an active role in producing the change.

cohabitate To live together in a sexual relationship when not legally married.

coitus Sexual intercourse with a partner of the opposite sex.

collective bargaining Use of collective action in negotiating client care and economic issues with one's employer, including wages, hours, and work conditions.

collective unconscious Inherited, racial foundation of the personality structure.

collusion Active process by which each mate unconsciously chooses a partner based on his unmet infantile needs with the expectation that the partner chosen will meet the need.

communication Totality of human behavior, including both how people behave and how they exchange meanings about their behavior.

companion animals Animals that serve as substitutes for people.

compensation Defense mechanism by which the individual attempts to make up for real or fancied deficiencies.

competence to stand trial Mental condition necessary for a criminal defendant so that he may confer with an attorney about his defense, understand the nature of charges against him and understand courtroom procedure.

complementary transactions Transactions that can go on indefinitely as the persons keep relating from the same ego states.

compulsion Insistent, repetitive, intrusive, and unwanted urge to perform an act that is contrary to one's usual wishes or standards.

compulsive personality disorder Disorder characterized by limited ability to express tender emotion, the need for perfection, and irrational adherence to order; rules and rituals interfere with functioning.

concreteness Difficulty with abstract thinking manifested by the literal interpretation of messages.

concrete thinking Stage in the development of the cognitive thought processes in which thoughts are logical and coherent. The individual is able to sort, classify, order, and organize facts, but is incapable of generalizing or dealing in abstractions.

concurrent audit Method of evaluating ongoing activities.

confabulation Fabrication of experiences or situations, often recounted in a detailed and plausible way to fill in and cover up gaps in memory.

confession Act of seeking expiation through another from guilt for an actual or imagined transgression.

confidentiality Disclosure of certain information only to another specifically authorized person.

confinement deprivation Disorder that occurs when individuals are separated from familiar surroundings or denied contact with familiar persons or objects, as when one is confined to a single hospital room or one-room apartment.

conflict Opposition between two drives that are experienced simultaneously in response to the same situation.

confrontation Communication that invites another to examine some aspects of his behavior that exhibit a discrepancy between what he says and what he does.

congruent communication Communication pattern in which the sender is communicating the same message on both verbal and nonverbal levels.

conjoint family therapy Therapy in which a single nuclear family is seen and the issues and problems raised by the family are addressed by the therapist.

conscience Prohibiting aspect of the ego that relates to that which is morally wrong.

conscious Experiences within awareness at the moment.

consensually validated symbols Symbols that are accepted by enough people that they have an agreed upon meaning.

consensus Device individuals use to establish unanimous social meaning.

consent Voluntary agreement by the person who has the capacity to do so, given the appropriate information.

consort abuse Battering of an emancipated minor or female 18 years of age or older, involving an intentional act or acts of physical violence that occur during the course of an intimate, interpersonal relationship with a spouse or male partner.

constructive manipulation Using one's strengths and abilities in interpersonal situations to promote successful relationships.

consultation alliance Relationship between the consultant and the consultee characterized by an understanding that clinical dilemmas will and can be approached together.

consultee-centered consultation Expert advice to the consultee to clarify the details of the client's situation to increase the consultee's cognitive understanding and awareness of her feelings involved in caring for the client.

continuity theory Theory about aging which suggests that people's personalities do not change as they age and that their behavior becomes more predictable.

contract Agreement within the one-to-one relationship involving setting goals and a plan of action for carrying out the goals to achieve behavior change.

conversion disorder Somatoform disorder characterized by a loss of, or alteration in, physical functioning that is an expression of psychological conflict.

coping Active process of using personal, social, and environmental resources to manage stress.

coping mechanisms Balancing factors that affect individuals' ability to restore equilibrium following a stressful event.

corrective emotional experience Process by which the client gives up old patterns of behavior and learns and relearns new patterns through reexperiencing early unresolved feelings and needs.

counterconditioning Process used by the behavioral therapist in which a learned response is replaced with an alternative response that is less disruptive for the person.

countertransference Conscious or unconscious emotional response of a psychotherapist to a client.

couples therapy Therapy in which couples, married or unmarried and living together, are seen in therapy.

credential Global term referring to a recognition that a person or institution has attained a predetermined set of standards at a given point in time. In this text, licensure, certification, and accreditation are discussed as types of credentials.

crisis Event experienced when a person faces an obstacle to important life goals that is, for a time, insurmountable through the use of usual problem-solving methods.

crisis intervention Active entering into the life situation of an individual, family, or group experiencing a crisis to decrease the impact of the crisis event and to assist the client or clients to mobilize personal resources and regain equilibrium.

crisis-prone person Individual who has no available support system, or, if social supports are available, is unable to use them in his efforts to cope with everyday stress.

crisis resolution Development of effective adaptive and coping devices to resolve a crisis.

criteria Specific rules or principles against which health care practice may be compared. In this text, structure, process, and outcome criteria are discussed.

cue Stimulus that determines the nature of the person's response.

cultural group Class of people who share some common characteristics but do not necessarily share a culture.

culturally relativistic perspective Understanding the behavior of transcultural clients within the context of their culture.

cultural relativity Fitting within the context of a particular culture.

culture Learned patterns of values, beliefs, customs, and behaviors that are shared by a group of interacting individuals.

cunnilingus Oral stimulation of the female genitals.

curandero Type of folk healer used by Hispanics.

dance therapy Type of therapy that involves expression of feelings through the rhythmic body movements of dance.

daydreams Future states during which the child withdraws from the real world to a world of fantasy and wish fulfillment.

death instincts Instincts aimed at destruction

defense mechanism Unconscious intrapsychic reaction that offers protection to the self from a stressful situation. Also called "ego defense."

defensive radical therapy Therapeutic process viewed as a survival tactic; the therapist begins at the client's present state and uses encouragement of the client with self-defeating behaviors.

deinstitutionalization At the individual client level, the transfer to a community setting of a client who has been hospitalized for an extended period of time, generally many years; at the mental health care system level, a shift in the focus of mental health care from the large, long-term institution to the community-based care, accomplished by discharging long-term clients and avoiding unnecessary admissions.

deja vu Sensation that what one is experiencing has been experienced before.

delayed or dysfunctional grief Syndrome that results when there is failure to experience or express grief at the time of loss.

delirium Acute organic mental disorder characterized by confusion, disorientation, restlessness, clouding of the consciousness, incoherence, fear, anxiety, excitement, and often illusions, hallucinations, and delusions.

delirium tremens Mental diagnostical term that has been replaced with the diagnosis "alcohol withdrawal delirium."

delusion Fixed false belief contrary to evidence. It may be persecutory, grandiose, nihilistic, or somatic in nature.

delusion of grandeur False belief that one has great money, power, and prestige. It is frequently manifested in the belief that the individual is a famous person.

delusion of persecution False belief that one has been singled out for harassment.

delusion of poverty False belief that one is impoverished.

dementia Chronic organic mental disorder characterized by personality disintegration, confusion, disorientation, stupor, deterioration of intellectual capacity and function, and impairment of control of memory, judgment, and impulses.

denial Defense mechanism used to resolve emotional conflict and allay anxiety by disavowing thoughts, feelings, wishes, needs, or external reality factors that are consciously intolerable.

density Concentration of people in a given location.

dependent personality disorder Mental disorder characterized by an inability to function independently and lack of self-confidence.

depersonalization disorder Emotional disorder characterized by a feeling of self-estrangement in which a dream-like atmosphere pervades.

depression Mood disturbance characterized by feelings of sadness, despair, and discouragement resulting from some loss or disappointment.

depression position Normal stage of development during which the child learns to modify ambivalence and sustain loss of the "good mother."

dereistic thought Type of mental activity in which fantasy is not tempered by the laws of logic, experience, and reality.

destructive manipulation Using or "playing" others for one's own purposes.

detoxification Process of withdrawal from alcohol in a controlled environment.

detriangle Process by which one avoids participating in a triangular interpersonal situation.

developmental crisis Stress that occurs when a person is unable to complete the tasks of a psychosocial stage of development and is thus unable to move on to the next stage.

developmental lines Concept developed by Anna Freud that considers the child's chronological age and expectations for ego maturation at each stage of development.

deviant behavior Everyday transactions that exceed the usual accepted behavior and involve failure to comply with a social norm.

dietician Health professional who is concerned with the nutritional needs of the client.

differentiation Degree to which the emotional and intellectual systems of a person are integrated. High differentiation results in goal-directed, mature behavior. Also called *individuation.*

direct practice roles Roles in which the nurse meets the mental health needs of the community through various treatment modalities.

discounts Actions that devalue by not recognizing a person, a problem or a problem's importance and solvability, or the person's ability to solve the problem.

disengagement Term describing the rigid, fixed boundaries that can exist between subsystems in a family. These rigid boundaries lead to distance and discourage communication.

disjunctive Relationship in contextual therapy characterized by distancing.

disorientation Inability to correctly identify the self in relation to time, place, or person.

disparaging maneuvering Type of destructive manipulative behavior exemplified by reprimands and self-pity.

displacement Shift of an emotion from the person or object toward which it was originally directed to another, usually neutral or less dangerous, person or object.

dissociation System of processes for minimizing or avoiding anxiety by which parts of the individual's experience called "not me" are kept out of consciousness.

dissociative disorders Conditions characterized by a sudden, temporary alteration in the integrative functions of consciousness, identity, or motor behavior.

distancing Movement away from another.

distracting maneuvering Type of destructive manipulative behavior exemplified by changes of subject, flattery, expressions of helplessness, tearfulness, dawdling, and last-minute stalling.

disturbed communication Communication that is not clear and is impeded by various factors.

diurnal mood variation Changes in mood that are related to the time of day.

doctrine of double effect Doctrine that a lesser good or an evil is morally permissible if done to achieve a greater good, provided that certain conditions are fulfilled.

dominance Fact or state of controlling or prevailing over others.

double approach-avoidance conflict Conflict resulting from the presence of two goals, both of which are desirable and undesirable.

double bind Two conflicting messages from someone who is crucial to one's survival. One message is usually verbal, one nonverbal. See also *incongruent communication.*

dream analysis Primary method of gaining access to uncensored material from the unconscious.

drive Stimulus that has sufficient strength to impel the person into activity.

dysarthria Impaired, difficult speech, usually a result of organic disorders of the nervous system or speech organs.

dysfunctional thought record Record on which a client is instructed to record his thoughts whenever a strong emotion is experienced; this record is explored by the therapist and the client to examine the evidence that supports or refutes the automatic thoughts and to explore alternative interpretations.

dysfunctional stereotype Stereotyping in which the dysfunctional aspects of a culture are emphasized.

dyskinesia Impairment of the ability to execute voluntary movements.

dysmnesia Impairment in the ability to retain and recall information.

dyspareunia Pain during sexual intercourse.

dystonia Side effect of antipsychotic medication that is characterized by muscle spasms, particularly of the head, neck, and tongue.

echolalia Repeating exactly what is heard.

echopraxia Imitation of the body position of another.

eclectic approach Use of a combination of theories from more than one framework.

ecology Study of organisms in their home; the study of people as they influence and are influenced by one another and their environment.

ectomorph Person whose physique is characterized by slenderness and fragility. See also *endomorph; mesomorph.*

egalitarian group leadership Groups led by coleaders of equal status; a collegial relationship.

ego Executive of the personality that maintains harmony among the id, the superego, and the external world.

ego boundaries Individual's perception of the boundary between himself and the external environment.

ego dystonic Elements of a person's behavior, thoughts, impulses, drives, and attitudes at variance with the standards of the ego and inconsistent with the total personality. Also called "ego alien."

ego state Consistent pattern of feelings accompanied by a related set of consistent behavior patterns.

ego syntonic Aspects of a person's behavior, thoughts, and attitudes viewed as acceptable and consistent with the total personality.

egoism Ethical position that one does and should think and act in one's interest exclusively.

elderly abuse Any willful or negligent act that results from negligence, malnutrition, physical assault or battery, or physical or psychological injury inflicted against an elderly person by other than accidental means.

electroconvulsive therapy (ECT) Electric shock delivered to the brain through electrodes placed on the temple(s) to artificially produce a grand mal seizure.

emancipated minor Person under the age of 18 who is totally self-supporting.

embarrassment State of feeling self-conscious or ill at ease.

emic Defining of normal and abnormal behavior by members within a cultural group.

emotional abuse Use of implicit or explicit threats, verbal assault, or acts of degradation that are injurious or damaging to an individual's sense of self-worth.

emotional cutoff Breaking away from an emotional attachment to family to differentiate oneself.

emotional object constancy Ability to hold a mental symbolic picture of the loved object when the object is absent.

emotional neglect Lack of maintaining an interpersonal atmosphere conducive for psychosocial growth and development of a sense of personal worth and well-being.

emotional system Emotional chain reactions that occur among family members and tie the emotional functioning of one family member integrally to that of another.

emotionally disturbed child Child whose personality development is arrested or interfered with so that he shows impairment in reasonable and accurate perceptions of the world, impulse control, learning, and social relations with others.

empathy Ability to recognize and, to some extent, share the emotions and states of mind of another and to understand the meaning and significance of that person's behavior.

encopresis Fecal incontinence.

encounter group Group that focuses more on emotional experiencing; especially valued are emotional honesty, self-exposure, confrontation, and obtaining an intense positive emotional experience.

encounter therapy Alternative therapy developed by William Schultz that focuses on the client's blocks to better function. The goal of the treatment is to assist the client in making the most satisfying use of personal capabilities.

enculturation Process by which culture is transmitted from one generation to the next.

endomorph Person whose body build is characterized by a soft, round physique with a large trunk and thighs, tapering extremities, an accumulation of fat throughout the body. See also *ectomorph; mesomorph.*

enmeshment Excessive tightness at the expense of individual independence; occurs in families in which sharing is intense and engulfing.

entitlement Underlying assumption of people which holds that the world owes them something.

enuresis Incontinence or involuntary urination; particularly problematic for children. Also called "bed-wetting."

environmental modification Intervention that focuses on making changes in the client's environment that decreases stress and the potential for another crisis.

equilibrium Balance among the parts of a system.

Erhard seminar training (est) Alternative therapy developed by Werner Erhard that focuses on four basic principles: belief, experience, reality, and self. The goal of the treatment is a transformation in the participants' nature of experiencing.

erogenous zones Areas of the body (mouth, anus, and genitals) in which tension becomes concentrated and can be relieved by manipulation of the region.

eros Lust or sexual drive; a type of physical love.

ethic Standard of valued behavior or beliefs adhered to by an individual or group; a goal to which one aspires.

ethical dilemma Issue for which moral claims conflict with one another: (1) a difficult problem that seems to have no satisfactory solution or (2) a choice between equally unsatisfactory alternatives.

ethnocentricity Attitude that one's own cultural group is superior.

ethnocentric perspective One's judgment of the behaviors of persons of a different culture by the standards of one's own culture.

etic Defining of normal and abnormal behavior by persons outside a cultural group.

evaluation Category of the nursing process in which a determination is made and recorded regarding the extent to which the established goals of care have been met.

excess disability The loss of function that is associated with the perceptions of the client or nurse but is not a true disability.

exhibitionism Achievement of sexual pleasure by exposing one's sexual organs to another, usually a stranger.

existential School of philosophical thought that focuses on the importance of experience in the present and the belief that people find meaning in life through their experiences.

experimental research Research in which the investigator deliberately manipulates some condition or phenomenon to assess the effects of intervention on some other condition or phenomenon.

expiatory behavior Repentant, atoning, or some kind of reparative behavior resulting from a guilty conscious.

exploitative character Term used by Fromm to describe a person who takes what he wants by exploiting or using everyone, enhancing his stance of interpersonal power in the process.

expressive aphasia Inability to express ideas in words.

expressive functions Observable behaviors from which mental activity is inferred, including speaking, writing, drawing, physical gestures, facial expressions, and movements.

expressive groups Groups that focus on feelings. In groups for the elderly, these are contrasted with the more concrete and structured groups commonly used, such as remotivation, reminiscence, and life review groups.

external locus of control Belief that an outcome is determined by fate, chance, or powerful others and is thus beyond personal control.

extinction Decrease in the occurrence of a behavior when the behavior is not reinforced.

extrapyramidal effects Side effects of an antipsychotic medication that resemble the symptoms of parkinsonism, including tremor, drooling, and altered gait.

extrasensory perception (ESP) Awareness or knowledge acquired without using the physical senses.

factitious disorders Symptoms of illness that are caused by the deliberate effort of the person, usually to gain attention. Attempts to gain attention by this means are often repeated even when the individual is aware of the hazards involved.

false personification Security operation that involves stereotyping, such as labeling or prejudging others.

false transactions Transactions in which communication is stopped or crossed up by one individual relating from a different ego state than the other person expected.

family myths Series of fairly well-integrated beliefs shared by all family members concerning each other and their mutual position in the family life.

family projection process Primary mechanism by which the multigenerational transmission process operates; the family members attribute their thoughts and impulses to other family members.

family therapy Therapy modality that focuses treatment on the process between family members that supports and perpetuates symptoms; a way of conceptualizing human relationship problems that focuses on the context in which an emotional problem is generated.

fan pattern of communication Messages originate at one source and are directed downward to several receivers who do not interact with each other.

fear Emotion that results from tension and pessimism arising from the danger of actual physical harm to one's existence.

feedback Response to the sender of a message.

Feldenkrais therapy Alternative therapy founded by Moshe Feldenkrais that has as its central focus awareness and the movements of the body. The goal of the therapy is for the client to establish a good self-image through correction of the movements of the body.

fellatio Oral stimulation of the male genitals.

female sexual dysfunction Medical term for psychosomatic and pathological conditions that interfere with normal female sexual activity.

feminist therapy Alternative therapy that is both a philosophical approach to the conduct of therapy and a specific type of therapy, that is, consciousness raising (CR). The focus of both types is the presence of sexism and sex role stereotyping in society. The goal of therapy is consciousness raising.

fetishist Person who obtains sexual pleasure from an inanimate object, such as a shoe or leather garment.

first-order change Change within a system that itself remains unchanged.

fixation Arrest at a particular stage of psychosexual development, such as anal fixation.

fixed feature space Internal and external design of a building and its relationship to other buildings and environmental factors.

flat affect Affect of a client who does not communicate feelings in verbal or nonverbal responses to events.

flexibility Ability to adapt or to respond to changing conditions; the state of mind that permits consideration of new ideas and information.

flight of ideas Alteration in thought processes resulting in a sudden rapid shift from one idea to another before the preceding one has been concluded with some relatedness of the train of thought.

flight to health Resistance process occurring when the client chooses to abruptly terminate therapy, seeing himself as "cured," rather than experiencing a reactivation of painful feelings.

flight to illness Client's effort to demonstrate to the therapist that the client is too ill to terminate therapy and continued support is needed.

flooding Form of desensitization that uses real or imaginary situations to evoke strong feelings of anxiety.

focused activity Technique that serves the purpose of actively focusing the client toward his adaptive coping abilities and away from maladaptive ones.

folk illnesses Illnesses that are attributed to nonscientific causes; two major categories are naturalistic and personalistic illnesses.

foreplay Sexual pleasuring preceding orgasm.

formative evaluation Judgments made about the effectiveness of nursing interventions as they are implemented.

free association Spontaneous verbalization of thoughts and emotions entering the consciousness during psychoanalysis.

free-floating anxiety Type of neurotic anxiety that is characterized by general apprehensiveness and pessimism.

Freudian character Term used by Fromm to describe a miserly person who holds on to what he has.

frigidity Inability of the female to achieve orgasm.

frustration Feeling resulting from an interference with one's ability to attain a desired goal, satisfaction, or security.

function of communication That which communication accomplishes for the person or persons involved (as distinguishable from the structure of communication).

functional analysis Discovery of the sequence of events involved in producing and maintaining undesirable behavior.

functional disorder Mental or emotional impairment that is believed to be psychosocial in origin.

fusion Tendency of two people experiencing an intense emotional attraction to unite.

fusion-exclusion Compensatory mechanism by which two people can stay in close contact with each other and avoid fusion-generated anxiety either by excluding a third person from their relationship or by focusing their energies on a third person.

galactosemia Genetic condition in which one is unable to metabolize galactose.

Gamblers Anonymous Self-help group that helps gamblers and uses a modified version of the Alcoholics Anonymous program as its approach.

game Series of learned unconscious maneuvers that lead to a well-defined payoff; an ulterior transaction that leaves the players with bad feelings.

gender identity Inner sense of maleness or femaleness that identifies the person as being male or female.

gender role Image a person presents to others and to himself that declares him to be male or female.

general adaptation syndrome (GAS) Process by which the body's nonspecific responses to stress or noxious agents evolve through stages of adaptation.

general anxiety disorder Anxiety state characterized by persistent anxiety of at least a month's duration, excluding symptoms associated with a phobic, panic, or obsessive-compulsive disorder.

general female sexual dysfunction Condition in which the female feels no sexual pleasure from sexual stimulation and is unable to have erotic feelings and responses.

generic approach A treatment approach to crisis based on the premise that certain identifiable patterns of behavior are characteristic of each type of crisis and that psychological tasks specific to the type of crisis are required if the crisis is to be successfully resolved.

genetic insight Deepest level of self-understanding.

genetics Branch of biology dealing with the phenomena of heredity and the laws governing it.

genogram Multigenerational diagram of a family.

genuineness Quality characterized by openness, honesty, and sincerity. The nurse possesses genuineness when she is self-congruent and authentic and relates to the client without a defensive facade.

geropsychiatric nursing Mental health–psychiatric nursing care of the older adult.

gestalt Whole picture.

gestalt therapy Alternative therapy founded by Frederick Perls that focuses on the barriers that block awareness. The goal is authentic growth in the here and now.

globus hystericus Feeling of a lump in the throat that interferes with swallowing.

grandiosity Overappraisal of one's worth and ability.

grandstanding Form of manipulation of others to satisfy one's needs.

gravely disabled Because of a mental condition, the client is unable to care for his basic needs of nutrition, clothing, shelter, safety, and medical care.

grief Emotional response that follows loss or separation.

group content Work of a group; specific tasks and problems; goals to be accomplished.

group dynamics All that takes place within a group from the time of its inception until termination.

group norms Acceptable group behaviors. These will vary from one group to another. In one group it is acceptable to be open with feelings, but this is not acceptable in another group that is primarily concerned with accomplishing a concrete task.

group process Interaction continually taking place between members of a group.

group therapy Modality of therapy in which common problems are confronted in a group setting by individuals experiencing similar difficulties.

guilt Remorseful awareness of having done something wrong.

guilty fear Emotional response that occurs when a person is in the process of doing something that is immoral, disapproved of, or illegal. The fear is of getting what is deserved.

habeas corpus Right retained by all psychiatric clients that provides for the release of an individual who claims he is being deprived of his liberty and detained illegally. The hearing for this determination takes place in a court of law in which the client's sanity is at issue.

habit Link or association between a stimulus and a response.

half life Time it takes for half of a medication to be eliminated, destroyed or decayed in the body.

hallucinations Sensory perception that does not result from an external stimulus. It can occur from any of the senses and is classified auditory, gustatory, olfactory, tactile, or visual.

hatha yoga Step-by-step system of physical training that involves use of the entire body and stretching exercises and holding postures.

helplessness Belief that no one can do anything to aid one; an inability to make autonomous decisions.

hepatic encephalopathy Brain damage caused by liver disease and consequent ammonia intoxication and by deficiency of thiamin and other nutrients. Usually seen as a consequence of alcoholism and its attendant malnutrition.

heterogeneous groups Groups composed of members of both sexes, with a variety of ages, backgrounds, behaviors, and needs.

histrionic personality disorder Mental disorder characterized by dramatic and exaggerated behavior that draws attention to oneself.

holism Philosophy in which all entities are viewed more in terms of relationships and processes than as separate parts that can be adequately analyzed in isolation.

homeostasis Maintenance of a normal steady state in the body.

homogeneous groups Groups composed of members of the same sex and similar ages, backgrounds, behaviors, and needs.

homosexuality Sexual preference for someone of the same sex.

homunculism Notion that children are miniature adults.

hope Mental state characterized by the desire to gain end or accomplish a goal combined with some expectation that what is desired is attainable.

hopelessness Belief that no help can be obtained.

hospice System of family-centered care provided outside the hospital designed to assist the dying client to maintain a satisfactory life-style through the terminal phases of dying.

hostile aggressiveness Pattern of behavior ranging from threatening physical violence to voicing challenging, demeaning, and criticizing remarks.

hostility Feeling of anger and resentment characterized by destructive behavior.

hot flash Common symptom of menopause in which the body becomes warm with an excessive period of perspiration followed by chillness; may involve only the face and neck or may extend over the entire body.

human ecology Study of people in their multiple environments.

human potential movement Social transition of values from a child-centered focus to an adult-centered focus on development potential.

humanism Philosophy in which people, as well as their interests, developments, fulfillment, and creativity, are made central and dominant.

hydrotherapy Various forms of therapy entailing the use of water to bring about a therapeutic and tranquilizing effect.

hyperkinesis Unusual or excessive activity in children with resulting behavioral problems and learning difficulties. Theories of the cause vary and include allergies and sensitivities to food additives.

hypertensive crisis Syndrome characterized by rapidly changing neurologic abnormalities. Occurs after eating certain foods containing a high concentration of tyramine in reaction to the injestion of MAO inhibitors.

hypervigilance Increased state of watchfulness.

hypnosis An altered state of consciousness whereby distraction is minimized and concentration is heightened to reduce pain.

hypnotic A trance like state.

hypochondriacal pain Pain described by persons who have a constant preoccupation with their bodies, fear disease or body dysfunction, and experience pain.

hypochondriacal preoccupation An intense, almost morbid, preoccupation with health.

hypochondriasis Somatoform disorder characterized by an exaggerated concern for one's health, an unrealistic interpretation of signs or sensations as abnormal, and preoccupation with the fear of having a serious disease.

hypomania Clincial syndrome that is similar to, but less severe than, that described by the term *mania* or "manic episode."

hypothesis A level of interpretation based on theoretical formulations that can be validated but are tentative and can be changed as new data is collected.

hysteria Disorder in which symptoms of physical illness appear without any underlying organic pathological condition. Also known as conversion reaction.

hysterical pain A type of conversion disorder brought on by a specific, highly charged emotional event related to earlier unconscious emotional conflicts.

id Basic system of the personality structure that consists of all psychological processes that are present at birth.

ideas of reference Obsessive delusion that the statements or activities of others refer to oneself, usually taken to be deprecatory.

identification Unconscious defense mechanism by which a person patterns his personality on that of another person, assuming the person's qualities, characteristics, and actions.

identity Organizing principle of the personality system that accounts for the unity, continuity, uniqueness, and consistency of the personality. It is the awareness of the process of "being oneself" that is derived from self-observation and judgment and is the synthesis of all self-representations into an organized whole.

identity confusion Lack of clarity and consistency in one's perception of the self, resulting in a high degree of anxiety.

idiosyncratic behavior Variation from the dominant cultural pattern encountered in one person.

illusions False interpretation of an external, usually visual or auditory, sensory stimulus.

imagery Formation of mental concepts, figures, and ideas.

immediate memory Type of memory that involves the fixation of information that is selected for retention during the registration process.

immobility deprivation Inability to respond to physical stimulation resulting from decreased physical activity, such as that caused by traction, casts, or paralysis.

impetus Strength or force of an instinct.

implementation Phase of the nursing process in which nursing actions are carried out that assist the client to maximize his health capabilities and provide for client participation in health promotion, maintenance, and restoration.

implosive therapy Form of desensitization therapy in which there is repeated exposure to a highly feared object.

impotence Inability by the male to obtain or maintain an erection of sufficient strength to allow performance of the act of intercourse.

incest Sexual activity performed "on a child by a member of the child's family group," not limited to sexual intercourse but including any action performed to sexually stimulate the child or use of the child to stimulate other persons.

incompetency Legal status that must be proved in a special court hearing. As a result of the hearing the person can be deprived of many of his civil rights. Incompetency can be reversed only in another court hearing that declares the person competent.

incongruent communication Communication pattern in which the sender is communicating a different message on the verbal and nonverbal levels and the listener does not know to which level he should respond. See also *double bind.*

indirect practice roles Roles in which the nurse participates in care by providing clinical expertise and knowledge to other health care providers who use that knowledge to meet the mental health needs of the community.

individual approach A treatment approach to crisis that emphasizes assessment of the intrapsychic and interpersonal processes of the person in crisis by a mental health professional.

individual family therapy Therapy in which each family member has a single therapist and the family may meet together occasionally with one or two of the therapists to see how the members are relating to one another and work out specific issues that have been defined by individual members.

individualization Caring for each client as an individual and unique being with a singular outlook on the world and life situations.

individuation Gradual development of psychological autonomy—a self that is separated from the mother; sense of separate identity but simultaneously a deep attachment to the family. Also called *differentiation;* interrelated with *separation.*

indoklon therapy Treatment with indoklon, a colorless, volatile liquid given with oxygen inhalation to induce convulsions, used for emotional disturbances.

informal space Personal distances maintained in interpersonal encounters.

informed consent Disclosure of a certain amount of information to the client about the proposed treatment and the attainment of the client's consent, which must be competent, understanding, and voluntary.

infradian rhythms Encompassing cycles that are longer than 24 hours, such as the menstrual cycle.

injunctions Convert script messages given from the Child ego state of the father and mother.

insight Self-understanding; extent of one's understanding of the origin, nature, and mechanisms of behavior.

instincts Inborn psychological representation of a need.

insulin coma therapy (insulin shock therapy) Insulin given in progressive amounts to a fasting client to produce hypoglycemia and coma for the treatment of psychiatric disorders.

integration Stage, as described in Moreno's theory of emotional release, that the individual feels restored with self and others following the release of anger; also, the tendency for all aspects of a culture to function as an interrelated whole.

intellectualization Defense mechanism in which reasoning is used as a means of blocking a confrontation with an unconscious conflict and the emotional stress associated with it.

intentionality General goal of self-mastery in psychotherapy; seen as self-actualization by Maslow and congruence by Rogers.

interactional synchrony Nonverbal body positioning and adjustments very young children make to adult verbalizations that enhance learning the relationships of verbalizations and gestures.

interactionist theory Theory about aging that views age-related changes as resulting from the interaction between the individual characteristics of the person, the circumstances in society, and the history of social interaction patterns of the person.

internal locus of control Belief that an outcome is a consequence of the individual's actions and is thus under his personal control.

interpersonal communication Communication between two or more persons, characterized by expressive action, the conscious or unconscious perception of that action by another or others, and the perception that the expressive action was perceived by others.

interpersonal perceptions Concept of norms, social responsibility, and justice growing from role taking and understanding of the meaning of situations to other people.

interpretation Assigning an underlying cause or meaning to a behavior.

intervention Any act by the nurse that implements the nursing care plan or any specific objective of the plan.

intimacy Capacity to commit; reciprocal involvement with others personally, sexually, occupationally, and socially.

intimate zone The area within 18 inches of the body; the space in which physical activity occurs.

introjection Intense type of identification in which the person incorporates qualities or values of another person or group into his own ego structure.

introspection Act of examining one's own thoughts and emotions by concentrating on the inner self.

isolation Defense mechanism in which an unacceptable idea, impulse, or act is separated from its original memory source, thereby removing the emotional charge associated with the original memory.

Johari's window A two-way matrix that provides an analysis of the known and unknown aspects of self as they relate to self-awareness and awareness of others.

kinesic behaviors Nonverbal cues of communication that function to achieve and maintain bonds or attachments between people.

kinesiology Scientific study of muscular activity and of the anatomy, physiology, and mechanics of the movement of body parts.

Korsakoff's syndrome Form of amnesia often seen in chronic alcoholism, characterized by a loss of short-term memory and an inability to learn new skills.

kwashiorkor Form of protein malnutrition, seen in weaned infants, characterized by physical and mental growth intervention and fluid-electrolyte imbalances.

lability Frequent or unpredictable mood changes.

language Collection of signs or symbols of which two or more communicators or interpreters understand the significance.

language acquisition device (LAD) Innate, schematic central nervous system neuromotor structure that is species specific and matures as the child develops, providing the mechanisms for speech.

latency Stage of development occurring between the ages of 6 and 12 years in which the major task is the achievement of a sense of competence.

learned helplessness Behavioral state and personality trait of a person who believes that he is ineffectual, his responses are futile, and he has lost control over the reinforcers in his environment.

learning disorder Condition affecting children and characterized by difficulties in reading, writing, and numerical calculation.

leftover guilt Type of guilt resulting from early conditioning and shaped by patterns of thinking, feeling, reacting, and behavior within the family.

lesbian Woman whose sexual preference is for another woman.

lethality Estimation of the probability that a person who is threatening suicide will succeed based on the method described, the specificity of the plan, and the availability of the means.

levels of practice Identified nursing behaviors related to degrees of knowledge and skill development.

leverage Therapeutic influence developed by the helping person as a result of the helping person's efforts on the client's behalf.

liaison The facilitation of the relationship that exists between the patient, the illness, the consultees, and the hospital/ward milieu.

liaison alliance A relationship between the consultant and the consultee that signifies some clinical dilemmas can be understood and resolved by reflecting on the interactions among care providers and clients.

libertarianism Ethical orientation that the person is sovereign and may choose without interference as long as he does not harm others.

libido See *psychic energy.*

licensure Process by which the legal right to practice nursing is accorded a person in a given state and based on evidence of minimal standards of competence.

life change units Term assigned to the kinds of social changes an individual experiences and the amount of stress that the changes cause.

life instincts Instincts directed toward survival and propagation of the species.

life review Reminiscence usually occurring in old age as a consequence of the realization of the inevitability of death.

limit setting Act of making a person aware of his rights and responsibilities while communicating the expectation that he will respect the rules; also, the application of appropriate sanctions if the person does not obey the rules.

locus of control Person's perception of the power he has over events that affect his life.

logotherapy Approach to psychotherapy based on the existential model and developed by Viktor Frankl. The focus is on the search for meaning in present experiences.

long-term memory Type of memory that is also referred to as learning and involves a person'a ability to store information.

loneliness The absence of expected relationships.

loose associations A communication pattern characterized by lack of clarity or connection between one thought and the next.

love Strong affection for another arising out of personal relations.

lunacy Archaic term referring to the belief that the moon affects behavior, especially psychopathological behavior.

machismo Hispanic concept of the man, which includes their culturally desirable traits of courage and fearlessness and the dysfunctional behaviors of heavy drinking, seduction of women, and domineering and abusive spouse behaviors.

magical thinking Belief that merely thinking about an event in the external world can cause it to occur; result of regression to an early phase of development.

magnification Cognitive distortion in which the effects of one's behavior are magnified.

maladaptive behavior Behavior that does not adjust to the environment or situation and interferes with mental health.

maladaptive independence Behavior that interferes with an individual's ability to attain a high level of health.

male sexual dysfunction Medical term for psychosomatic and pathological conditions that interfere with normal male sexual activity.

malingering Willful and deliberate feigning of the symptoms of a disease or injury to gain some consciously desired end.

mal ojo The practice of casting the "evil eye."

mandala Universal religious symbol spontaneously drawn by most children.

mania Condition characterized by a mood that is elevated, expansive, or irritable.

manipulation Process of influencing another to meet one's own needs and desires, regardless of the needs and desires of another; a technique of some alternative therapies that involves physically working on the body with the hands or elbows for the purpose of correcting malfunctioning muscles.

manipulative religions Religions that emphasize the inability of individuals to trust their own nature and encourage helplessness.

mantra Unique secret sound that is selected specifically for each participant by the therapist in transcendental meditation.

mapping Process of handing down a set of patterns from one generation to another.

marasmus Form of protein and calorie malnutrition in infants and young children, often associated with maternal and other deprivation with life-threatening physical and mental consequences.

marathon group Form of group originated by George Bach that meets for an extended time, for example, several days in a row or a whole weekend. The intensity of the group and its extended time frame are believed helpful in the breaking down of defenses built to protect one from knowing and understanding one's inner self.

marketing character Term used by Fromm to describe a person who takes in whatever the authority of others provides.

marriage contract (couple contract) Situation in which two people join in a committed relationship, each with a separate understanding of expectations within the relationship.

Maslow's hierarchy of needs Pyramid of human needs (physiological, safety, security, love and belonging, self-esteem, and self-actualization) theorized by Abraham Maslow.

masochism Pleasure derived from physical or psychological pain inflicted either by oneself or by others.

masochist One who gains feeling of satisfaction by allowing another to inflict pain.

massage Technique of some alternative therapies that involves rubbing or kneading of the body, usually with the hands, to stimulate circulation.

masturbation Production of orgasm by self-manipulation of the genitals.

matter-of-factness Avoidance of emotional responses and reassurance; treatment of requests, pleas, or manipulative maneuvers with casualness.

material abuse The theft or misuse of an individual's property or money.

matiasma The beliefs and practices surrounding the healing practice of the "evil eye."

maturational crisis Transitional or developmental periods within a person's life when his psychological equilibrium is upset.

mechanical restraints Any of several means of restricting a client's freedom of movement. Includes camisoles, wrist and ankle restraints, sheet restraints, and sheet packs.

meditation Technique of tension reduction in which the person closes his eyes, relaxes the major muscle groups, and repeats a cue word silently to himself each time he exhales.

megavitamin therapy Treatment that includes giving the psychiatric client large doses of special vitamins and minerals.

melancholy Feeling of deep sadness or depression.

menopause Termination of menstruation, usually between the ages of 48 and 50.

mental health consultation The provision of clinical expertise regarding the delivery of psychological care in response to a request from a health care provider.

mental health–psychiatric nurse A nurse who specializes in the care of clients with mental health problems.

mental health–psychiatric nursing Interpersonal process that strives to promote and maintain behavior that contributes to integrated functioning. It employs the theories of human behavior as its science and purposeful use of self as its art. It is directed toward both preventing and treating mental disorders and promoting optimal mental health for society, the community, and the individuals who live within it.

mentor One who guides; a teacher.

mesomorph Person whose physique is characterized by a predominance of muscle, bone, and connective tissue. See also *ectomorph; endomorph.*

metacommunication Communication that refers to how a given message is to be understood.

midlife transition Bridge between early adulthood and middle adulthood that lasts from 40 to 45 years of age.

milieu Environment or setting.

milieu therapy Use of the total environment of a setting for treatment purposes.

minimization Cognitive distortion in which the effects of one's behavior are minimized.

mnemonic techniques Techniques for improving memory such as visual imagery associations or categorization.

modal operators Term within neurolinguistic programming that refers to grammatical structures which imply contingencies, possibilities, and necessities.

momentary adaptation Ability to be effective at the moment a distressing situation actually occurs.

monoamine oxidase (MAO) inhibitors Group of chemically related antidepressant medications.

moral anxiety Type of anxiety that is experienced in response to fear of the ego.

morbid grief reaction Delayed or distorted reaction to the loss of a significant person.

Morita therapy Alternative therapy founded by Shoma Morita that has as its focus the neurotic symptoms of the client. The goal of the therapy is character building, which enables the client to live responsibly and constructively even if the symptoms persist.

morphogenic families Families characterized by flexible rules and communication that are appropriate to the developmental level of family members.

mourning All psychological processes set in motion within the individual by a loss. The process of mourning is resolved only when the lost object is internalized, bonds of attachment are loosened, and new object relationships are established.

multidisciplinary audit An audit done by a group of health care professionals.

multigenerational transmission process Emotional process by which unresolved family problems are carried from one generation to another.

multi-infarct dementia Condition in which a succession of strokes has destroyed enough brain tissue to cause dementia.

multiple family therapy Therapy in which four or five families meet weekly to confront and deal with problems or issues they have in common.

multiple impact therapy Therapy in which families come together for intensive work, usually over a 3-day weekend or week-long encounter.

multiple personality disorder Condition characterized by the existence of two or more complete personality systems that are usually very different from one another.

Munchausen's syndrome Term applied to persons who repeatedly come to acute care settings with convincing but false symptoms of illness or injury, and with falsified documents to support evidence of the disease.

muteness Disorder characterized by a complete loss of speech.

mutual collaboration Concept that emphasizes the nurse and client working together to identify client problems and plan desired outcomes.

mutual pretense context of death The client and others know that he is dying but pretend otherwise.

myoclonus Spasm of a muscle or a group of muscles.

narcissism Abnormal interest in oneself, especially in one's own body and sexual characteristics; self-love.

narcissistic personality disorder Condition characterized by an exaggerated sense of self-importance.

narcotherapy Intravenous administration of barbiturates or stimulants to produce a physiological effect conducive to therapeutic change.

Narcotics Anonymous Organization similar to Alcoholics Anonymous for drug-dependent individuals.

National Alliance for the Mentally Ill (NAMI) National organization for family members of psychotic persons.

naturalistic illnesses Illnesses caused by impersonal factors, that is, entities without regard for the persons.

nature versus nurture controversy Long-standing debate as to a child's personality potential, with "nature" proponents emphasizing instincts, genetics, and biological factors and "nurture" proponents emphasizing environment and socialization.

neglect Condition that occurs when a caregiver is unable to or fails to provide minimal emotional and physical care to a person entrusted to his care.

neologisms Words that are invented by the person and understood only by him.

networking Informal communication system by means of which resources and information are pooled or shared.

network therapy Therapy conducted in people's homes in which all persons interested or invested in a problem or crisis that a particular person or persons in a family are experiencing take part.

neuroleptic Medication that produces an altered state of consciousness, characterized by quiescence, reduced motor activity, and reduced anxiety.

neurotic anxiety Type of anxiety that arises when perception of danger is from the instincts of the id.

Neurotics Anonymous Self-help group for persons with emotional problems that uses the format of the Alcoholics Anonymous program.

neurotic behavior Behavioral dysfunction that is characterized by anxiety but in which reality is not distorted.

neurotransmitter Chemical compounds serving as transmitters of neuromuscular impulses. A number of these substances have nutrient precursors and hence may be affected by diet.

night terrors Nightmares after which the child has difficulty reorienting to reality.

nightmare Frightening dream accompanied by feelings of helplessness and suffocation.

nihilistic delusion False belief that the self, part of the self, or another object has ceased to exist.

nirvanic state State in which mental processes cease.

nodal events Occurrences that may cause anxiety, such as birth, death, divorce, marriage, or a child leaving home.

noncompliance Failure of the individual to carry out the self-care activities prescribed in a health care plan.

nonexperimental research Research in which the investigator centers on description of existing conditions or phenomena.

nonpossessive warmth Nurse's warm acceptance of the client's experience as being part of that person with no conditions on acceptance.

nonverbal communication Messages that do not involve the spoken or written word and are conveyed by behavior.

normal grief reaction Syndrome manifested by bereaved people that consists of somatic distress, preoccupation with the image of the deceased, guilt, hostile reactions, and generally increased anxiety.

norms Ideal cultural patterns that represent what most members of the society believe persons ought to do in a particular situation.

nuclear family emotional system How a single generation deals with their level of differentiation.

nuclear problem Underlying reason for an individual's reaction to a precipitating event.

numinous Spiritually elevating.

nursing audit Type of clinical evaluation of nursing care that may focus on a nursing activity (process audit) or on the behavior of a client in response to the nursing care that has been provided (outcome audit).

nursing diagnosis Statement of a health problem or a potential problem in the client's health status that a nurse is licensed and competent to treat. A number of nursing diagnoses have been identified and accepted by the National Group on the Classification of Nursing Diagnosis (Fifth National Conference).

nursing process Process that serves as an organizing framework for the practice of nursing. It encompasses all of the steps taken by the nurse in caring for a client: assessment, analysis, planning, implementation, and evaluation. The rationale for each step is founded in theory.

obesity Condition in which the individual weighs at least 20% more than his ideal weight.

object Means by which the aim of an instinct is achieved.

object permanence Capacity to perceive that things exist even when not seen.

object relations Emotional bonds between one person and another, as contrasted with interest in and love for the self; usually described in terms of capacity for loving and reacting appropriately to others.

obsession Intrusive, repetitive thought, image, or impulse that the person finds distressing and unwanted because of its repulsive or inane nature. Content may be of aggressive, sexual, blasphemous, or obscene quality.

obsessive-compulsive Characterized by or relating to the tendency to perform repetitive acts or rituals, usually as a means releasing tension or relieving anxiety.

occupational therapist Health professional who assists the clint in activities of daily living, the development of work tolerance, the development of muscle strength and skills, and resocialization.

oculogyric crisis Side effect of antipsychotic medication that is characterized by the uncontrollable rolling upward of the eyes.

one-to-one relationship Mutually defined, collaborative goal-directed client-therapist relationship for purpose of psychotherapy.

open awareness context of death The client and others know that he is dying and relate to each other openly.

open groups Groups that admit new members whenever vacancies occur in membership.

operant behavior Behavior whose strength is controlled by the stimulus events that precede and follow it.

operant conditioning Process by which the results of a person's behavior determine whether the behavior is more or less likely to occur in the future.

operationalization of behavior Stating the client's complaints or problems in specific, observable behavioral terms.

organic brain syndrome (OBS) Any psychological or behavioral abnormality associated with transient or permanent brain dysfunction caused by a disturbance of the physiological functioning of brain tissue.

organic mental disorders Psychological or behavioral abnormalities associated with brain dysfunction caused by a disturbance of the physiological functioning of brain tissue with a known etiology.

orgasm Sexual climax, a sense of strong involuntary contractions of the muscles of the genitals experienced as exceedingly pleasurable, set off by sexual excitement.

orgasmic dysfunction Inability of the female to achieve orgasm in sexual activity.

orientation Ability to correctly relate the self to time, place, and person.

orientation phase Phase of the therapeutic relationship in which the nature and purpose of the relationship is explained.

orthostatic hypotension Drop in blood pressure related to change in position. A common side effect of psychotropic medications.

outcome criteria Criteria developed to evaluate the end result of the care and services provided to the client.

overgeneralization Cognitive distortion in which that which is true for one event is assumed to be true for all others.

overloading Talking too much and too fast; a common way for the elderly to handle anxiety.

overreaction Term applied to responses that are appropriate to a situation but go beyond what one would normally expect from the situation.

pain prone person Person who expresses pain predominantly in response to loss, anger, hostility, rejection, and guilt.

panic Attack of extreme anxiety that involves the disorganization of the personality. Distorted perceptions, loss of rational thought, and an inability to communicate and function are evident.

panic disorder Anxiety state characterized by recurrent panic (anxiety) attacks that occur at times unpredictably, although certain situations may become associated with a panic attack.

panic state Type of neurotic anxiety that is accompanied by acute and extreme anxiety, intense physiological arousal, and disorganization of personality and functional abilities.

paradoxical interventions Approach to treatment of dysfunctional communication that addresses difficulties in problem formulation and resolution.

parallel process Reenactment of the relationship between client and consultee within the relationship between consultee and consultant.

paranoid delusion False belief that one is being persecuted.

paranoid disorders Mental disorders with persistent delusions or persecution or jealousy.

paranoid ideation Exaggerated belief or suspicion, not of a delusional nature, that one is being harrassed, persecuted, or treated unfairly.

paranoid personality disorder Mental disorder characterized by extreme suspiciousness and mistrust of others, a fear of losing independence, and a desire to be dominant.

parapsychology Study of experiential phenomena that occur outside of the usual limits of sensory awareness, including extrasensory perception and precognition.

parataxic distortion Use of a parataxic mode of thinking by an adult.

parataxic mode of experience Type of thinking in which the person thinks there is a causal relationship between events that occur at the same time but are not logically related.

parens patriae Power of the state to commit a person to protect others from harm.

Parent ego state Part of self with messages (tapes) that sound like one's parents; the tapes contain advice and value messages with many "oughts" and "don'ts."

Parents Anonymous Self-help group for abusive parents.

Parents Without Partners (PWP) Self-help group for single parents, whether widowed, separated, or divorced.

passive Behavior that subordinates the individual's own rights to the demands of others.

passive-aggressive personality disorder Disorder characterized by an indirect resistance to social and occupational demands, procrastination, and inefficient functioning.

paternalism Ethical orientation that the state knows best and that each person is subordinate and duty bound to comply with the authority figure who is said to know best.

pathological or morbid grief Excessive grief response resulting in health problems

patient classification system Identification and classification of clients into care groups or categories and the quantification of these categories as a measure of the nursing effort required.

patterned operations Patterns of behavior that are observable and manifested either verbally or nonverbally.

pedophile Person whose sexual preference is for a child.

peer review Process by which the quality of nursing care rendered by one nurse is evaluated by other nurses actively involved in clinical nursing practice.

perception Process by which a person interprets stimuli.

perceptual deprivation Inability to recognize stimuli from the environment often because of medications that alter the level of consciousness, cerebral dysfunction, or thought disorders.

performationism Theory that all human life has some form and function and that the embryo is a tiny, fully formed adult that has to grow in size and stature only.

perseveration Involuntary and pathological persistence of an idea or response.

persona Social mask that a person wears in social situations.

personalistic illness Illness resulting from punishment or aggression, directed specifically toward the individual.

personal set Sensory apparatus, beliefs, and patterned operations that the nurse brings to the relationship with a client.

personal unconscious The aspect of the mind that consists of experiences that were once conscious but that have been transformed by repression, suppression, or other mechanisms.

personal zone Similar to a protective zone, the boundaries of which expand and contract according to contextual characteristics; from 18 inches to approximately 4 feet.

personalistic illnesses Illnesses that result from punishment or aggression that are specifically directed toward a person.

personification Image that individuals have of themselves and others.

pet therapy Use of pets to bring about positive changes in the client's physical and mental status.

phenomenological groups Groups that focus on the experiencing of persons: getting to know and understand them as "real people."

phenomenology Study of phenomena.

phenothiazines Group of chemically related antipsychotic medications.

phenylketonuria (PKU) Genetic disease caused by lack of the cell enzyme that controls metabolism of the essential amino acid phenylalanine. Accumulated abnormal metabolites cause severe mental retardation in unscreened and untreated infants. Therapy is nutritional: low phenylalanine diet with special formula and foods.

philosophy Search for understanding about the basic truths and principles of the universe, life, and morals by logical reasoning.

phobic reaction Persistent fear of some object or situation that presents no actual danger to the person or in which the danger is magnified out of proportion to its actual seriousness.

Photophobia Intolerance or fear of light.

photosensitivity Excessive response to sunlight.

physical abuse Intentional injury, harmful deed, or destructive act inflicted by a parent, guardian, mature child, or caregiver on another person with whom an interpersonal or advocacy relationship is shared.

physical dependence Characteristic of drug addiction that is present when withdrawal of the drug results in physiological disruptions.

physical neglect Volitional deprivation of essential care necessary to sustain life, growth, and development.

physiological conversions Physiological changes that accompany anxiety and serve no constructive purpose. However, they can form the basis for pathological changes in function that may progress to structural changes and irreversible organic changes.

placebo Any medical or nursing measure that is effective because of its implicit or explicit therapeutic intent rather than its specific chemical or physical properties.

planning Act of determining what can be done to assist the client in restoring, maintaining, or promoting health. This phase involves judging priorities, establishing goals, developing objectives, and identifying strategies for implementation.

pleasure-pain Concept that characterizes persons as drawn to events that are positively reinforcing versus repelled from those that are negatively reinforcing.

pleasure principle Seeking immediate gratification of needs in order to experience pleasure and avoid pain.

point behaviors Refers to how body parts move within space and how they orient themselves in some direction

positive regard State of conveying attitudes of warmth, caring, liking, interest, and respect to another.

positive reinforcement Reward for a response.

positive thinking Coping strategy that serves as a defense against environmental obstacles and encourages a pursuit of happiness.

possession trance Belief that the body has been taken over in its function by a spiritual entity.

postcrisis period Period characterized by a return to the steady state, with the person resuming his precrisis level of functioning or perhaps a higher or lower state of functioning, depending on the effectiveness of the crisis resolution.

posttraumatic stress disorder Anxiety state precipitated by a traumatic event that involves reexperiencing the traumatic event.

posturing Voluntary assumption of inappropriate or bizarre posture.

poverty of speech State in which one's vocabulary is increasingly diminished.

practical nurse Nurse who works under the supervision of a registered nurse.

pragmatic Belief that ideas are valuable only in terms of their consequences.

prana Life energy that unites the physical body into a whole and organizes the life processes.

precognition Having foreknowledge of events.

preconscious Perceptions and memories that are outside awareness but are immediately available to consciousness when the need arises.

precrisis period Period during which the person maintains his equilibrium through the use of his usual coping mechanisms.

precursor therapy Type of treatment relating chemical compounds tht are influenced by diet to neurological clinical conditions.

predisposing factors Conditioning factors that influence both the type and amount of resources that the individual can elicit to cope with stress. They may be biological, psychological, and sociocultural in nature.

preformationism Dominant theory before the seventeenth century that viewed all human life with the same form and function (for example, children are small adults).

preinteraction phase First phase of the nurse/client relationship whereby the nurse becomes aware of her thoughts and feelings about the interaction.

premature ejaculation Lack of voluntary control over the reflex of ejaculation by the male before the female has achieved orgasm in the act of sexual intercourse.

premonition Sense of an impending event without prior knowledge of it.

premorbid personality Characteristics of one's personality occurring before the development of disease.

preparatory grief Preparation of oneself for separation and impending losses; occurs in stage IV of the process of dying.

prepubescent period Period of development before puberty; period of accelerated growth proceeding gonadal maturity.

pressured speech Type of speech in which the person may talk without being interrupted and may be difficult to interrupt.

preventive psychiatry Use of theoretical knowledge and skills to plan and implement programs designed to achieve primary, secondary, and tertiary prevention.

prima facie rights Rights on the surface or face that may be overridden by stronger conflicting rights or by other values.

primal scream therapy Alternative therapy developed by Arthur Janov that focuses on the repressed pain of infancy or childhood. The goal of the therapy is for the client to surrender his neurotic defenses and become real.

primary anxiety First stage of anxiety related to the developmental process and that evolves out of the birth process.

primary care Phase of health care that is considered to be the initial entry into the health care system, usually community-based care.

primary drives Drives that are innate and in close contact with physiological processes.

primary gain Decrease in anxiety resulting from the individual's efforts to cope with stress.

primary process thought Primitive thought processes that are normally kept unconsciously by use of the coping mechanism of repression; impulsive infantile ideation that involves the use of an image of an object to relieve tension.

primitive anxiety Fearlike state induced by the anxiousness of the mothering one.

privileged communication Legal term that applies only in court-related proceedings and means that the right to reveal information belongs to the person who spoke and the listener cannot disclose the information unless the speaker gives permission. It exists between a client and health professional only if a law specifically establishes it.

process criteria Criteria used in the evaluation of actions, sequence of behaviors, and events during the provision of client care.

process of communication Manner in which something is said or done, as in asking a direct question; content of communication; literal meaning of words and symbols.

procrastination Putting off doing something until some future time.

professional development Enhancement of the theoretical knowledge and level of skill in the nurse in order to remain effective in the nursing role.

projection Attributing one's own thoughts or impulses to another person. Through this process the individual can attribute his own intolerable wishes, emotional feelings, or motivations to another person.

projective character Term used by Fromm to describe a person who is unable to use his powers and to realize the potentiality inherent in him.

prospective audit Audit that reviews a defined number of clients with a specific set of criteria.

protocol Guideline or statement of behaviors identified as discrete steps to be taken by nurses in the clinical role.

prototaxic mode of experience Type of primitive experience characterized by sensations, feelings, and fragmented images of short duration and which are not logically connected.

proxemics Study of the interaction of spatial features of an environment.

pseudodementia Delirium that masquerades as dementia.

pseudodenial Client's denial of his illness to another person or failure to tell another person about his illness to protect that person.

pseudohomosexuality Occurring during adolescence when there is a preference for members of the same sex and inordinate amounts of time are spent with members of the same sex.

pseudohostility Term used to describe families that quarrel excessively to cover up their real need and affection for each other.

pseudomutuality An extreme family defense against individualization.

pseudoparkinsonism Having Parkinson's disease-like symptoms which include tremors and muscle rigidity.

pseudoplacidity Characteristic of individuals who use a limited range of human emotions because of their rigidity and excessive control of their emotions.

pseudoposition Compensatory mechanism in which spouses assume "pretend" polarized positions with one another.

pseudoself That part of the self that fluctuates with the emotionality of the moment.

psychiatric nursing See *mental health–psychiatric nursing*

psychiatric social workers Social workers who deal with the social and psychological problems of clients.

psychiatric technician Technician who assists the nurse in performing client care activities.

psychiatrist Physician who specializes in the treatment of mental disorders.

psychic energy (libido) Body energy used for psychological tasks such as thinking, perceiving, and remembering.

psychoanalysis Branch of psychiatry founded by Sigmund Freud devoted to the study of the psychology of human development and behavior; a system of psychotherapy based on the concept of a dynamic unconscious and the use of techniques such as free association, dream interpretation, and analysis of defense mechanisms.

psychoanalytic treatment Process of therapy in which the irrational belief systems from the unconscious realm are eradicated through gaining of insights and correcting the system so that normal functioning can be assumed by the individual.

psychodrama Therapeutic use of dramatic techniques developed by Moreno, enabling group members to act out and receive feedback about stressful life experiences.

psychodynamics Explanation of the forces that motivate behavior; emphasizes the influence of past experiences on present behavior and the influence of mental forces on development and behavior.

psychodynamic insight Behavioral change resulting from uncovering the roots of origin of one's behavior.

psychogenic Originating within the mind.

psychogenic amnesia Condition characterized by either a partial or total inability to recall the past.

psychogenic fugue Condition characterized by amnesia and physical flight from an intolerable situation.

psychogenic pain Pain in the absence of adequate physiological explanations when psychological explanations may clarify the cause.

psychogenic pain disorder Somatoform disorder characterized by the complaint of pain in the absence of physical findings and evidence of an etiological role for psychological factors.

psychological dependence Characteristic of drug addiction that is manifested in a craving for the abused substance and a fear that it will not be available in the future.

psychological testing Diagnostic tool used by the psychologist to aid in assessment of the client; includes administration of a battery of cognitive and projective tests.

psychology Study of the mind.

psychomotor retardation Slowing of motor activity related to a state of severe depression.

psychosexual development Series of developmental phases throughout the life cycle that promotes growth of the individual in the areas of psychological and sexual development.

psychosomatic Relating to, characterized by, or resulting from the interaction of the mind, or psyche, and the body; the expression of emotional conflict through physical symptoms.

psychosurgery Surgical interruption of selected neural pathways that involve the transmission of emotional impulses in the brain.

psychosynthesis Alternative therapy developed by Robert Assagioli that focuses on three levels of the unconscious: lower, middle, and higher conscious, or superconscious. The goal of the treatment is the recreation or integration of the personality.

psychotherapy Any of a great number of related methods of treating mental or emotional disorders by psychological techniques rather than by physical means.

psychotic behavior Severely dysfunctional behavior characterized by a panic level of anxiety, personality disintegration, and regression behavior. The person experiences a reduced level of awareness and has great difficulty functioning adequately.

psychotic disorders Category of health problems distinguished by the following characteristics: severe mood disorder, regressive behavior, personality disintegration, reduced level of awareness, great difficulty in functioning adequately, and gross impairment in reality testing.

puberty Developmental period during which the secondary sexual characteristics begin to appear and sexual reproduction capability is present.

pubescence Stage of maturation in which the individual becomes physiologically capable of reproduction.

public space Space that extends outward from approximately 12 feet, with the individual in the center.

qualitative comparative analysis Research approach used to generate theory from a combination of inductive and deductive reasoning; also referred to as "grounded theory."

quality assurance Process by which (1) appropriate criteria related to client care are identified and (2) mechanisms to ensure the measurement and achievement of specified criteria are developed.

radical therapy Alternative therapy that is really more an attitude about the therapeutic process than a specific type of treatment. The focus is on the social and political value systems of the therapist, client, and society. The goal is for the client to be better able to cope with society and to become active politically for change.

rage Violent, intense, and short-lived anger.

rape Legally defined as the forcible perpetration of the act of sexual intercourse on the body of a woman not one's wife. A more contemporary definition would include acts of oral and anal sodomy and allow for its occurrence within marriage as well.

rapport Sense of mutality and understanding; harmony, accord, confidence, and respect underlying a relationship between two persons; an essential bond between a therapist and a client in psychotherapy.

rational responses Alternative interpretations that support or refute automatic thoughts.

rational-emotive therapy (RET) Alternative therapy founded by Albert Ellis that focuses on the client's irrational belief systems. Through an ABC approach the client is assisted to acquire effective self-analysis skills that he continues to use after treatment termination.

rationalization Defense mechanism in which the individual attempts to justify or make consciously tolerable, by plausible means, feelings, behavior, and motives that otherwise would be intolerable.

reaction formation Defense mechanism in which a person avoids anxiety through overt behavior and attitudes that are opposite of his repressed impulses and drives and that serve to conceal those unacceptable feelings.

reality anxiety Type of anxiety that is equated with fear and is based on the perception of danger in the external world.

reality principle Postponement of immediate gratification of needs until a more appropriate object for satisfaction of needs is available.

reality testing Process of evaluating one's environment so as to differentiate between external reality and one's inner imaginative world.

reality therapy Alternative therapy founded by William Glasser that focuses on the three *r's:* responsibility, reality, and right and wrong. The goal of the therapy is to assist the client in fulfilling basic needs for love and self-worth.

rebirthing Alternative therapy developed by Leonard Orr that focuses on the breath and breathing apparatus. The goal of treatment is the health of the birth-damaged breathing apparatus so the person is able to use the breath as a supportive and creative part of daily life.

recent memory Type of memory that involves retention of information for an hour or so to 1 to 2 days.

reception deprivation Inability to receive stimuli properly because of damage in tissue receptors, resulting in partial or total loss of sensation.

receptive aphasia Inability to recognize or manipulate words as symbols of ideas.

receptive character Term used by Fromm to describe a person who takes in whatever the authority of others provide.

receptive functions Functions that involve one's ability to acquire, process, classify, and integrate information.

reciprocal inhibition Response inhibitory to anxiety that occurs in the present of the anxiety-evoking stimuli, thus weakening the connection between the stimuli and the anxiety response.

Recovery Self-help group that provides support for persons discharged from inpatient psychiatric hospitals.

referential index deletions Term in neurolinguistic programming that refers to the omission of the specific person being discussed.

reflecting Communication technique in which the nurse picks up the feeling tone of the client's message and repeats it back to the client. Reflection encourages the client to continue with clarifying comments.

reframing Finding alternative ways for viewing behavior.

regression Return to an earlier, more primitive form of behavior.

reinforcement Any event, contingent on the response fo the organism, that alters the future likelihood of that response.

rejunctive Relationship in contextual therapy characterized by moves toward trustworthy relatedness.

relaxation therapy Type of therapy that focuses on learning and practicing relaxation techniques in a group using such modalities as deep breathing exercises, muscle relaxation, fantasies of being in one's favorite place, fantasizing with music, and guided imagery.

religiosity Excessive concern with spiritual and religious matters.

reminiscent therapy Therapy that aims at integrating the client's life experiences into their self-concept by mentally reliving them.

remotivation group Type of group that uses a give-step format developed for regressed or withdrawn persons.

repetition compulsion Concept central to the psychoanalytical explanation of play, which states that when a child is exposed to experiences unable to be understood he will set up the experience in play and reexperience the situation again and again until the overload is reduced.

repression Involuntary exclusion of a painful or conflictual thought, impulse, or memory from awareness. It is the primary ego defense, and other mechanisms tend to reinforce it.

repressive-inspirational approach Approach used in some groups that discourages the breaking down of defense mechanisms. Members are encouraged to focus on positive feelings and group strengths. This approach is commonly used in groups of chronically mentally ill clients.

resentment Indignation or ill will resulting from a real or imagined offense.

resistance Attempt of the client to remain unaware of anxiety-producing aspects within himself. Ambivalent attitudes toward self-exploration in which the client both appreciates and avoids anxiety-producing experiences are a normal part of the therapeutic process.

resocialization Use of the techniques to facilitate socialization and group interaction, usually among cognitively impaired persons.

restating Reflecting back that which has been said, using the client's choice of words.

retarded ejaculation Condition in which the male fails to complete an orgasm with the act of ejaculating semen.

retrospective audit Audit that evaluates services after they have been rendered.

rigidity Inability to acquire new responses to changing conditions. The state of mind that rejects information and remains unyielding and opinionated.

ring pattern of communication Messages that are initiated at one point and are passed from one receive to another with the last receiver reporting to the sender.

risk factors Situations in the environment that are potentially hazardous to the child's mental health.

role ambiguity Form of role stress that occurs when one or more roles are not clearly articulated in terms of behavior or levels of expected performance.

role behaviors Behaviors used repeatedly by individuals; specific behaviors recognized as part of one's usual way of relating.

role change Occurs in situations in which status is retained but role expectations remain the same.

role conflict Role stress that occurs when a person is required to enact roles that are in conflict with his value system or to play two or more roles that conflict with one another.

role incompetence Role stress that results from a person's inability to fulgill role obligations.

role incongruence Role stress that occurs when an individual undergoes role transitions requiring a significant modification in attitudes and values.

role induction interview. Therapeutic technique that provides information to the client in advance of ways the client is expected to behave.

role overload Type of role stress that occurs when excessive demands are made of a person in a particular role and insufficient time is available to fulfill obligations.

role overqualification Type of role stress that occurs when a role position does not require full use of a person's resources.

role playing Psychotherapeutic technique in which a person acts out a real or simulated situation as a means of understanding intrapsychic conflicts.

role reversal Act of assuming the role of another person in order to appreciate how the person feels, perceives, and behaves in relation to himself and the other.

role stress Situation that occurs when the demands for a person's position in the social structure are difficult, conflicting, or impossible.

roles Patterns of behavior expected of persons.

rolfing, or structural integration therapy Therapy developed by Ida Rolf that focuses on the body posture and musculature. The goal of therapy is to realign the body posture with the earth's gravity.

romanticism Social and esthetic movement in art, literature, and music characterized by a revolt against society and social institutions.

rumination Persistent thinking about and discussion of a particular subject.

sadist Individual who gains a feeling of power by inflicting pain on others.

sadomasochism Pleasure derived from pain and suffering inflicted on self by self or others and the inflicting of physical or psychological pain or suffering on others.

samadhi State of total enlightment in which the body, mind, and spirit function as a harmonious whole.

Santero A type of folk healer used by Hispanics.

scapegoat Person who bears the blame for others.

schema Innate knowledge structure that allows the child to organize in his mind ways to behave in his environment.

schizoid personality disorder Disorder characterized by aloofness, lack of warmth, indifference to the feelings of others, and a serious defect in interpersonal relationships.

schizophrenia Manifestation of anxiety of psychotic proportions, primarily characterized by inability to trust other people and disordered thought processes, resulting in disrupted interpersonal relationships.

schizotypal personality disorder Emotional illness characterized by unusual speech, behavior, and thought content. There are also problems in interpersonal relationships.

school phobia Child's state of anxiety related to separating him from his parents by his attending school. It is a form of separation anxiety; the child is not afraid of school per se.

script Transactional analysis term that refers to a person's life plan that was adopted during childhood.

seclusion Form of physical restraint in which the individual is placed in a single room, which may be locked, to decrease stimuli and allow the agitated client to gain control of his behavior.

secondary drives Drives that evolve during the process of growth and incite and direct behavior.

secondary gain Indirect benefits, usually obtained through an illness or disability.

secondary intervention Early diagnosis and prompt and effective treatment to reduce the duration of a significant number of psychiatric disorders that occur.

secondary process thought Conscious thought processes that are under the control of the ego and are characterized by logic.

second-order change Change that changes the system itself.

security operations Term related to the interpersonal model of psychiatric care that refers to mental mechanisms which are developed to deal with anxiety-provoking experiences.

sedative Substance that has a calming effect.

selective abstraction Type of cognitive distortion in which focus on one aspect of an event negates all other aspects.

selective inattention Security operation occurring when the person avoids anxiety by not attending to what is said or what is happening.

self-actualization Tendency toward maximal realization and fulfillment of one's human potential.

self-care model Framework for nursing care directed toward self-care by the client to the greatest degree posible. The model requires an assessment of the client's capability for self-care and need for care.

self-concept Composite of ideas, feelings, and attitudes that a person has about his own identity, worth, capabilities, and limitations. Such factors as the values and opinions of others, especially in the formative years of early childhood, play an important part in the development of self-concept.

self-destructive behavior Any behavior, direct, or indirect, that if uninterrupted, will ultimately lead to the death of the individual.

self-disclosure Revelation that occurs when a person reveals information about his self, ideas, values, feelings, and attitudes.

self-esteem Judgment or evaluation of one's worth in relationship to one's ideal self and to the performance of others.

self-help groups Therapeutic groups without health professional leadership. Some have been started jointly by health professionals and lay persons, but group members take on the leadership responsibility.

self-ideal Perception of how one should behave based on certain personal standards. The standard may be either a carefully constructed image of the kind of person one would like to be or merely a number of aspirations, goals, or values that one would like to achieve.

self-imposed guilt Restictive type of guilt that the individual is aware of and from which he is unable to free himself.

self-management approach Treatment approach in which the client assumes responsibility for his behavior, for changing his environment, and for planning his future.

self-other Concept aht characterizes persons believing that sources of power are within the self as opposed to those who believe the source of power is in others.

self-responsibility One of the concepts of holism by which individuals assume responsibility for their own health.

self-system Significant aspect of personality that develops in response to anxiety.

semifixed feature space Objects in the environment that have some degree of mobility, for example, furniture.

sensate focus technique Therapeutic program for the treatment of erectile dysfunction.

sensitivity training group Group developed for the purpose of increasing self-awareness, increasing understanding of group process, or increasing awareness of the effects of one's behavior in groups.

sensory deprivation involuntary loss of physical awareness caused by detachment from external sensory stimuli; often results in psychological disorders such as panic, mental confusion, depression, and hallucinations.

sensory overload Bombardment by multiple sensory stimuli as in an intensive care unit.

sensory-based language Nonverbal behavior.

separation At the end of infancy, psychological disengagement from the mother, who is now perceived as distinct and apart from oneself; interrelated with *individuation.*

separation anxiety Anxiety that becomes manifest at separation from a significant person, especially and beginning with the mother. This is normal behavior toward the end of the first year.

set Predisposition to behave in a certain way.

sexual abuse Engagement of dependent children or developmentally immature individuals in forms of exploitive or physically intimate sexual activity.

sexual dysfunction Psychosomatic disorder experienced as a difficulty for individuals to have/or enjoy sexual encounters.

sexual hormones Chemical substances (estrogen, testosterone, progesterone) produced in the body that produce specific regulatory effects on the activity of certain organs of the reproductive system.

sexual intercourse Heterosexual intercourse involving penetration of the vagina by the penis.

sexuality Totality of sensations, attitudes, thoughts, feelings, and actions related to one's maleness or femaleness.

sexual masochism Sexual pleasure and gratification derived by experiencing physical or mental pain and humiliation.

sexual mores Fixed, morally binding customs (about sexual activities) or a particular group.

sexual sadism Sexual pleasure and erotic gratification obtained from inflicting physical or psychological pain on another person.

sexual tasks Specific skills learned in various phases of development in the life cycle continuum to allow an adult to function normally in the sexual realm.

sexual therapist Professional with specialized knowledge, skill, and competence in assisting individuals who experience sexual difficulties.

sexual therapy Modality of counseling that aids in the resolution of pathological conditions so that a healthy sexuality can be maintained to allow life and relationships to be enjoyed.

shadow Archetype that represents the unacceptable aspects and components of behavior.

shame Painful emotion caused by a strong sense of guilt, embarrassment, or disgrace.

sibling position Birth order of the person in relation to his siblings.

Silva mind control Alternative therapy founded by José Silva that focuses on the client's consciousness. The goal of treatment is to increase the powers of the mind, including being able to project the mind into inanimate objects, animate objects, animals, and, finally, humans for the purpose of diagnosing and possible healing the pathological condition they identify.

simple deletions Term in neurolinguistic programming that refers to the omission of detailed information.

simple phobia Irrational fear of a specific object or situation, such as fear of snakes or elevators. The fear seldom persists beyond adolescence.

situational crisis Crisis that occurs when a specific external event upsets an individual's psychological equilibirum.

situational loneliness Loneliness precipitated by a specific life event.

situational supports Persons who are available in the environment and who can be depended on to help the individual solve problems.

skills training Teaching of specific verbal and nonverbal behaviors and the practicing of these by the client.

sleep apnea Absence of spontaneous respirations occurring during sleep.

sleep deprivation Inability to receive adequate rest resulting in fatigue, heaviness of eyelids, tremors, apathy, and visual distortions.

social anxiety Discomfort in the presence of others.

social character Set of characteristics common to most people in a cultural group or society.

social ideal Society's conception of the ideal behavior pattern.

social interaction Action mutually affecting two or more persons.

social interaction pattern Milieu treatment pattern wherein the physician, client, and staff are viewed as team members, all of whom have information valuable to the client's care.

social learning theory Theory that explains the development of aggressive behavior as part of the socialization process.

social phobia Irrational fear of being observed or scrutinized, such as fear of speaking or performing in public.

social radical therapy Intent to bring about change by merging into the larger radical political movement.

social relationship Continuing pattern of social interaction.

social roles Patterns of attitudes, values, goals, and behaviors that are expected of individuals by virtue of their position.

social skills training Type of training that focuses on assisting the person to function more effectively in everyday social interaction.

social space Area about 4 to 12 feet from the person; in this zone no touching is possible.

social support systems Members of one's social environment who are perceived by the individual as "significant others" and who provide some degree of emotional support, task-oriented help, feedback and evaluation, social relatedness and integration, and access to new information.

socialization Basic process by which the human organism becomes a person, acquires norms and values, and becomes a functioning member of society.

societal regression How society deals with the anxiety generated by dwindling food and material sources and increasing threats of atomic annihilation.

sociogram Diagram or picture portraying people relating to each other. Usually people are indicated by circles. Lines drawn between circles represent people relating to each other.

solid self That part of the self that is thought out and not influenced by attempts at emotional negotiation.

somatic Pertaining to the body.

somatic delusion False belief that all or a part of the body is impaired in some way.

somatic therapies Specific medical intervention techniques to treat an emotional disorder.

somatization disorder Somatoform disorder characterized by repeated and multiple physical complaints of several years' duration for which no physical cause can be identified, although medical attention has been sought.

somatoform disorders Group of disorders characterized by recurrent and mutliple physical symptoms for which there are no demonstrable organic findings or identifiable physiological bases.

somnambulism Dissociative manifestation of sleepwalking.

somniloquy Dissociative manifestations of talking while sleeping.

sounding Incoherent or repetitious speech resulting from nonorganic causes.

source Body needs related to instincts.

specificity Component of psychotherapy that facilitates the clear, explicit expression of thoughts and feelings.

spiritualism Any philosophy, doctrine, or belief emphasizing the spiritual rather than the material.

spirituality Core of an individual's existence, integrating and transcending the physical, emotional, intellectual, and social dimensions.

spontaneity An energy force that propels an individual toward a creative state of being.

stage of exhaustion (SE) Third stage of the general adaptation syndrome that results from prolonged experiences with stress.

stage of resistance (SR) Second stage of the general adaptation syndrome characterized by resistance to change in body organs that leads to homeostasis and survival.

standards of care Comprehensive statements indicating the level of nursing care expected of the practitioner.

status Position in society.

status epilepticus Medical emergency characterized by continual attacks of convulsive seizures occurring without intervals of consciousness.

statutory rape Legal term for the act of sexual intercourse with a female under the age of consent determined by state law.

stereotype Opinion held by a group that is represented by a lack of critical judgment.

stigma Attribute that is deeply discrediting.

stimulus hierarchy List of arousing aspects of a phobic object in increasing order of the level of fear produced.

stranger anxiety Anxiety at the appearance of unfamiliar persons, normal and expected at 6 to 9 months of age. This is a sign of development of the awareness of the existence of a special, loved person.

stress Body's arousal response to any demand, change, or perceived threat.

stress inoculation Procedure useful in helping clients control anxiety by substituting positive coping statements for statements that bring about anxiety.

stress management Methods of controlling factors that require a response of change within the person by identifying the stressors, eliminating engative stressors, and developing effective coping mechanisms to constructively couteract the response.

stressors Stimuli that the individual perceives as harmful or threatening and produce a state of tension.

strokes Transactional analysis term that refers to unit of recognition that one person can give another or that a person can give to himself.

structural analysis Segregation and analysis of ego states.

structural modification Technique of structured family therapy in which the therapist changes the structure of the boundaries between generations.

structure criteria Criteria that indicate the aims and pruposes of the institution, agency, or program.

subculture Group of individuals within a society who share values, beliefs, and behaviors that differ from those of the dominant society.

sublimation Unconscious process of substituting socially more acceptable activity patterns that partially satisfy a need for an activity that would give rise to anxiety.

submission Type of kinetic reciprocal activity in which one person resigns themselves to another.

subsequent anxiety Second stage of anxiety that is experienced with maturation of the ego and superego.

substance abuse Use of any mind-altering agent to such an extent that it interferes with the individual's functioning.

substance dependence Physiological dependence on drugs characterized by the development of tolerance for drugs or withdrawal symptoms when drugs are not taken.

succorance Act of client seeking help following loss of parent or friend by asking the nurse to take the part of a significant other.

succession The state of every system being in a constant state of change.

suicide Self-inflicted death.

suicide attempt Any action deliberately undertaken by the individual that, if carried to completion, will result in his death.

suicide gesture Suicide attempt that is planned to be discovered in an attempt to influence the behavior of others.

suicide threat Direct, indirect, verbal, or nonverbal warning that the individual plans to attempt suicide.

summative evaluation Judgments about the effectiveness of nursing care when it is terminated.

superego Aspect of the personality concerned with prohibitions of parental figures.

supervision Process by which a nurse of lesser experience is assisted by a nurse clinician of greater experience to develop self-awareness and therapeutic skills.

supportive psychotherapy Therapy designed to assist the client to modify interpersonal relationships, change perceptions and cognitions, and reward behavior contingencies.

suppression Process that is the conscious analogy of repression. It is the intentional exclusion of material from consciousness.

surface structure Term within neurolinguistic programming that refers to the meaning expressed in the sentence as spoken, which is usually not well formed or complete.

suspicion awareness context of death When client becomes suspicious, usually because of personal physical clues, that information about his condition is being withheld.

symbiosis Mutually reinforcing relationship between two persons who are dependent on each other.

Synanon Residential center that uses a therapeutic community approach to provide rehabilitation for drug abusers.

syntaxic mode of experience Type of thinking that is logically interrelated with experience and involves the use of consensually validated symbols.

synthesia Perceptual distortion tht involves the tasting of color.

system Set of parts meshing with each other within a boundary.

systematic desensitization Technique of behavior therapy that involves the pairing of deep muscle relaxation with imagined scenes depicting situations that cause the client to feel anxious. The assumption is that if the person is taught relaxation rather than anxiety while imagining such scenes, the real-life situation that the scene depicted will cause much less anxiety.

system recomposition Technique of structured family therapy in which the therapist intentionally changes the composition of roles so that all members have an opportunity to interact within their designated role.

symptom focusing Technique of structured family therapy in which the therapist takes control of the symptom by prescribing that the client intensify the symptom.

tabula rasa Description of the receptive "blank stare" condition of the child's mind at birth.

tangential speech Loss of goal direction in communication; failure to address the original point of discussion.

tardive dyskinesia Serious side effect of antipsychotic medication characterized by the buccolinguomasticatory triad of head, jaw, and facial movements, athetoid and choreiform movement of the extremities, and tonic contractions of the back and neck muscles.

telegraphic speech Type of language disturbance commonly experienced by persons with OBS and characterized by irrelevant replies to questions.

telepathy Communication of thought from one person to another by means other than the physical senses.

temper tantrums Unpredictable, violent outbreaks of anger during which the person is out of control, screaming, kicking, and striking at others.

termination phase Conclusion of the nurse-client relationship in which both participants evaluate outcomes achieved and project future changes.

thanatology Study of dying and death.

theme interference Type of transference reaction often identified during consultation.

theme interference reduction Method of consultation that reduces the potential displacing of conflict on future clients.

themes Underlying issues or problems experienced by the client that emerge repeatedly during the course of the nurse-client relationship.

therapeutic alliance Joining of the client's rational adult ego with the therapist in a collaborative effort to study the client's conflicts.

Therapeutic communication Communication in which there is an intent of one or more of the participants to bring about a change in the communication pattern of the system.

therapeutic community Use of a treatment setting as a community with the immediate aim of full participation of all clients and the eventual goal of preparing clients for life outside the treatment setting.

therapeutic impasse Roadblock in the progress of the nurse-client relationship that arises for a variety of reasons and may take different forms.

therapeutic milieu General setting where treatment occurs, regardless of the philosophy of treatment.

therapeutic nurse-client relationship Mutual learning experience and a corrective emotional experience for the client in which the nurse uses herself and specified clinical techniques in working with the client to bring about behavioral change.

Therapeutic reminiscing Sharing events about the past in a way that makes one feel good about the past.

therapeutic touch Specialized kind of touching in which there is an intent to heal.

therapist Person in charge of directing the change of another person who skews communication in such a way that the client is exposed to situations and message exchanges that eventually bring about more gratifying social relations.

theraplay Form of treatment that uses active physical contact and control of the child.

third-party payment Reimbursement for nursing services provided by a person or group, neither of which is the provider or recipient of the services.

thought retardation Disturbance of thought characterized by extremely slow thought formation.

thought stopping Type of behavior modification that helps the client to limit negative thoughts about himself.

tolerance Characteristic of drug addiction that refers to the progressive need for more of the abused substance to achieve the desired effect.

tort Civil wrong for which the injured party is entitled to compensation.

total institution Institution that provides complete facilities for personnel who choose to use them.

trance Generally interpreted as soul absence of some kind and frequently linked to hallucinations or visions.

transaction Stimulus from an ego state of one person and the corresponding response from the ego state of another person.

transactional analysis (TA) Therapeutic modality based on the communications model of psychiatric care and developed by Eric Berne. Therapy takes place through the identification and interpretation of communication units (transactions) leading to understanding of interpersonal games that underlie behavioral disturbances. The goal is to develop the ability to communicate directly without using games.

transcendent Pertaining to the ability to go beyond one's ordinary everyday limits and to experience more than one's usual existence.

transcendental meditation (TM) Alternative therapy, introduced into the United States by Maharishi Mahesh Yogi, that focuses on consciousness. Through meditating, the client is assisted to achieve a state of enlightenment and reach his full human potential.

transcutaneous electrical nerve stimulators Use of an electrical current at or near the pain site to control pain.

transference Unconscious mechanism by which feelings and attitudes originally associated with important people and events in one's early life are attributed to others in current interpersonal relationships.

transformation rules Reordering of words into sentences to convey meaning in the process of learning language.

transient loneliness Loneliness that lasts only a few minutes or hours and is relieved by the client.

transitional crisis Crisis period related to the movement from one stage of development to another.

transsexual Person who is genetically an anatomical male or female but expresses, with strong conviction, that he or she has the mind fo the opposite sex, lives as a member of the opposite sex either part or full time, and seeks to change his or her original sex legally, through hormonal and surgical sex assignment.

transvestite Person who cross-dresses, or puts on the garments of the opposite sex, by choice.

triadic childbearing Parental constellation in which the father and mother are equally significant to the child's personality, maturation and development.

triangle Emotional process that deflects the conflict in a dyad by focusing on a third person, issue, or thing.

tricyclics Group of chemically related antidepressant medications.

tyramine Amino acid; restricted in diet for persons on monoamine oxidase (MAO) inhibitor drugs used as antidepressants because of the nutrient-drug interaction, which may bring on a hypertensive crisis.

ulterior transactions Transactions that are bilevel. The first level is usually of relevant statement; the second level is usually nonverbal and has hidden psychological meaning.

ultradian rhythms Pattern based on a cycle of less than 24 hours such as stomach contractions and brain wave rhythms.

unconscious Level of awareness that characterizes memories, thoughts, and feelings that have undergone repression.

underlying assumption Set of rules one holds about oneself, others, and the world; these rules are regarded as unquestionably true.

undifferientiated family ego mass Emotional fusion in families in which all members are similar in emotional expression.

undoing Defense mechanism in which something unaccpetable and already done is symbolically acted out in reverse, usually repetitiously, in the hope of relieving anxiety.

universal qualifiers Term within neurolinguistic programming that refers to general impressions of limitations; all, common, every, only, and never are examples of universal qualifiers.

universalizability principle Principle that an act is good if everyone should, in similar circumstances, do the same act without exception.

unspecified verbs Term within neurolinguistic programming that refers to verbs that are more or less specific to observable actions.

vaginismus Condition in the female in which normal genitalia are present, but the vaginal muscle tightly close when penal penetration is attempted.

validation Agreement of the nurse with certain elements of the client's communication.

validation therapy Therapy that involves searching for the meaning and emotion in the client's words and validating these with the client.

value clarification Method whereby a person can discover his own values by assessing, exploring, and determining what his personal values are and what they hold in personal decision making.

values Concepts that a person holds worthy in his personal life. They are formed as a result of one's experiences with family, friends, culture, education, work, and relaxation.

vector Direction of forces related to change in behavior.

venting Technique that allows the client to freely express his thoughts and feelings about a crisis situation.

verbal communication Written and spoken messages exchanged in the form of words as the elements of language.

violation of rights Form of elderly abuse that occurs when an individual is forced from his home or coerced nto a nursing home unnecessarily.

violence Acting out of destructive aggression by assaulting people or objects in the environment.

visualization Intervention aimed at guiding the client in a relaxed state to visualize positive experiences and promote more effective use of one's imagination.

voluntary consent Consent that is not forced threatened, or given under fraud or distress.

voyeurism Achievement of sexual pleasure by observing the nudity or sexual activity of others.

wandering Tendency to move about either in a seemingly aimless or disoriented fashion or in pursuit of an indefinable or unobtainable goal.

we-group Group that provides the chronically mentally ill client with safe opportunities to socialize with others who are familiar with the problem of chronic mental illness.

Wernicke's syndrome Syndrome associated with thiamine and sometimes niacine deficiency that consists of memory loss, confabulation, progressive dementia, ataxia, clouding of consciousness, and maybe coma. The disorder mainly affects alcoholics.

wheel pattern of communication Messages originate at a central position; interaction may occur between the message sender and any one of the receivers as well as between the receivers positioned next to each other.

wholistic counseling Alternative therapy developed by William Woodson that focuses on the whole person—mind, body, and spirit—and health. The goal of therapy is growth of the total person.

wisdom The ability to make the best choices from the alternatives that are available.

withdrawal Attempt to avoid interaction with others and thus avoid relatedness; also, the occurrence of specific physical symptoms when substance intake is reduced or discontinued.

withdrawal syndrome Occurrence of specific symptoms when a person who is physically addicted to a chemical substance discontinues its use.

word salad Communication pattern characterized by a jumble of disconnected words.

work of worrying Coping strategy by which inner preparation through worrying increases the level of tolerance for subsequent threats.

working phase Phase of the nurse-client relationship in which dysfunctional patterns of behavior are identified and new ways of coping with stress are explored and tested.

working through Process by which repressed feelings are released and reintegrated into the personality.

worry Concern at the present time about a future situation or event.

yang Polarized aspect of *ch'i* that is active or positive energy.

yin Polarized aspect of *ch'i* that is passive or negative energy.

yoga (hatha) Alternative therapy of ancient lineage that focuses on the body's musculature, posture, breathing mechanism, and consciousness. The goal of this ancient practice is attainment of physical and mental well-being through mastery of the body, achieved by exercising, holding postures and proper breathing, and "one-pointedness" meditation.

Zen Alternative therapy that differs from yoga only in the meditation techniques. In Zen the goal is to achieve mindfulness. The meditator aims for full awareness of any and all thoughts of the mind. All are given equal value.

zoophile Person whose sexual preference is for an animal.

INDEX

Page numbers in *italics* indicate boxes and illustrations.
Page numbers followed by *t* indicate tables.